THE NERVOUS SYSTEM

Volume 1

Basic Neurosciences

EDITORIAL ADVISORY BOARD: VOLUME 1

THE NERVOUS SYSTEM

A Three-Volume Work Commemorating the 25th Anniversary of the National Institute of Neurological and Communicative Disorders and Stroke

Editor-in-Chief:
Donald B. Tower, M.D., Ph.D.

VOLUME 1

THE BASIC NEUROSCIENCES

Volume Editor:

Roscoe O. Brady, M.D.
Chief, Developmental and Metabolic Neurology Branch
National Institute of Neurological and Communicative
Disorders and Stroke

RAVEN PRESS, PUBLISHERS ▪ NEW YORK

1975
Raven Press, 1140 Avenue of the Americas, New York City, New York 10036

Made in the United States of America

International Standard Book Number 0–89004–075–3
Library of Congress Catalog Card Number 75–33499

Contents

Contributors

Bernard W. Agranoff, M.D.
Professor, Department of Biological Chemistry
University of Michigan
Ann Arbor, Michigan 48104

Richard R. Almon, Ph.D.
Research Assistant Professor, Department of
  Biology
University of California, San Diego
La Jolla, California 92037

Ellsworth C. Alvord, Jr., M.D.
Professor of Pathology
University of Washington
School of Medicine
Seattle, Washington 98195

Clifford G. Andrew, M.D., Ph.D.
Intern, Department of Medicine
Duke University
School of Medicine
Durham, North Carolina 27710

Stanley H. Appel, M.D.
Department of Medicine, Division of Neu-
  rology
Duke University Medical Center
Box M2900
Durham, North Carolina 27710

Julius Axelrod, M.D.
Chief, Section on Pharmacology
Laboratory of Clinical Science
National Institute of Mental Health
National Institutes of Health
Building 10, Room 2D47
Bethesda, Maryland 20014

Pearce Bailey, M.D., Ph.D.
4513 Q Street NW
Washington, D.C. 20007

Samuel H. Barondes, M.D.
Professor, Department of Psychiatry
University of California, San Diego
School of Medicine
Box 109
La Jolla, California 92037

Soll Berl, M.D.
Research Professor, Department of Neurology
Mount Sinai School of Medicine
Fifth Avenue and 100th Street
New York, New York 10029

Floyd E. Bloom, M.D.
Laboratory of Neuropharmacology
Division of Special Mental Health Research
St. Elizabeth's Hospital
WAW Building
Washington, D.C. 20032

Samuel Bogoch, M.D., Ph.D.
Dreyfus Medical Foundation
2 Broadway
New York, New York 10004

Milton W. Brightman, M.D.
Head, Section on Neurocytology
Laboratory of Neuropathology and Neuro-
  anatomical Sciences
National Institute of Neurological and Com-
  municative Disorders and Stroke
National Institutes of Health
Building 36, Room 3B24
Bethesda, Maryland 20014

Richard P. Bunge, M.D.
Department of Anatomy
Washington University
School of Medicine
St. Louis, Missouri 63110

R. E. Burke, M.D.
Acting Chief, Laboratory of Neural Control
National Institute of Neurological and Com-
  municative Disorders and Stroke
National Institutes of Health
Building 36, Room 5A29
Bethesda, Maryland 20014

David A. Butterfield, Ph.D.
Assistant Professor, Department of Chemistry
University of Kentucky
Lexington, Kentucky 40506

W. Maxwell Cowan, M.D., Ph.D.
Chairman, Department of Anatomy and Neurobiology
Washington University
School of Medicine
660 South Euclid Avenue
St. Louis, Missouri 63110

John Dowling, Ph.D.
Professor of Biology
Harvard University
The Biological Laboratories
16 Divinity Avenue
Cambridge, Massachusetts 02138

Bernard Droz, M.D., Ph.D., D.Sc.
Professor of Physiology at l'Universite Pierre et Marie Curie
Paris, France
and
Conseiller Scientifique au Commissariat a l'Energie Atomique
Centre d'Etudes Nucleaires de Saclay
B.P. 2, 91190 Gif-sur-Yvette, France

Edward V. Evarts, M.D.
Chief, Laboratory of Neurophysiology
National Institute of Mental Health
National Institutes of Health
Building 36, Room 2D13
Bethesda, Maryland 20014

Joseph D. Fenstermacher, Ph.D.
Head, Membrane Transport Section
Division of Cancer Treatment
National Cancer Institute
National Institutes of Health
Building 37, Room 5C23
Bethesda, Maryland 20014

Jordi Folch-Pi, M.D.
Director, Biological Research Laboratory
McLean Hospital
Belmont, Massachusetts 02178

Thomas V. Getchell, Ph.D.
Associate Professor, Department of Physiology
Yale University
School of Medicine
New Haven, Connecticut 06510

Norton B. Gilula, Ph.D.
Assistant Professor
The Rockefeller University
66th Street and York Avenue
New York, New York 10021

Avram Goldstein, M.D.
Director, Addiction Research Foundation
and

Professor of Pharmacology
Stanford University
710 Welch Road
Palo Alto, California 94304

Murray Goldstein, D.O., M.P.H.
Director, Extramural Affairs
National Institute of Neurological and Communicative Disorders and Stroke
National Institutes of Health
Bethesda, Maryland 20014

Bernice Grafstein, Ph.D.
Department of Physiology
Cornell University Medical College
1300 York Avenue
New York, New York 10021

Harry Grundfest, Ph.D.
Department of Neurology
Columbia University
College of Physicians and Surgeons
630 West 168th Street
New York, New York 10032

James W. Gurd, Ph.D.
Department of Zoology
University of Toronto
Scarborough College
West Hill, Ontario, Canada

Gordon Guroff, M.D.
Chief, Section on Intermediary Metabolism
Laboratory of Biomedical Sciences
National Institute of Child Health and Human Development
National Institutes of Health
Building 6, Room 310
Bethesda, Maryland 20014

Frederick H. Harvey, M.D.
Fellow in Neuropathology
University of Washington
School of Medicine
Seattle, Washington 98195

Alfred Heller, M.D., Ph.D.
Professor and Chairman, Department of Pharmacological and Physiological Sciences
The University of Chicago
947 East 58th Street
Chicago, Illinois 60637

Sarka Hruby
Research Associate, Department of Pathology
University of Washington
School of Medicine
Seattle, Washington 98195

Masao Ito, M.D., Ph.D.
Department of Physiology
Faculty of Medicine

University of Tokyo
Hongo, Bunkyo-ku
Tokyo, Japan

Eric R. Kandel, M.D.
Professor of Physiology and Psychiatry
Director, Division of Neurobiology and
  Behavior
Columbia University
College of Physicians and Surgeons
630 West 168th Street
New York, New York 10032

Arthur Karlin, Ph.D.
Department of Neurology
Columbia University
College of Physicians and Surgeons
630 West 168th Street
New York, New York 10032

Robert Katzman, M.D.
The Saul R. Korey Department of Neurology
Albert Einstein College of Medicine
1300 Morris Park Avenue
Bronx, New York 10461

John S. Kauer, Ph.D.
Postdoctoral Fellow, Department of Phys-
  iology
Yale University
School of Medicine
New Haven, Connecticut 06510

Seymour S. Kety, M.D.
Department of Psychiatry
Massachusetts General Hospital
Fruit Street
Boston, Massachusetts 02114

Richard D. Keynes, D.Sc., F.R.S.
Professor of Physiology
Physiological Laboratory
University of Cambridge
Downing Street
Cambridge CB23EG, England

Marian W. Kies, Ph.D.
Chief, Section on Myelin Chemistry
Laboratory of Cerebral Metabolism
National Institute of Mental Health
National Institutes of Health
Building 36, Room 1A27
Bethesda, Maryland 20014

Igor Klatzo, M.D.
Chief, Laboratory of Neuropathology and
  Neuroanatomical Sciences
National Institute of Neurological and Com-
  municative Disorders and Stroke
National Institutes of Health
Building 36, Room 4D02
Bethesda, Maryland 20014

George B. Koelle, M.D., Ph.D.
Professor and Chairman, Pharmacology De-
  partment
University of Pennsylvania
School of Medicine
Philadelphia, Pennsylvania 19174

Abel Lajtha, Ph.D.
Director, New York State Research Institute
  for Neurochemistry and Drug Addiction
Ward's Island
New York, New York 10035

Rodolfo R. Llinás, M.D., Ph.D.
Division of Neurobiology
University of Iowa
Oakdale, Iowa 52319

Werner R. Loewenstein, Ph.D.
Professor and Chairman, Department of Physi-
  ology and Biophysics
University of Miami
Box 875
Biscayne Annex
Miami, Florida 33152

Oliver H. Lowry, M.D., Ph.D.
Professor of Pharmacology
Washington University School of Medicine
660 South Euclid Avenue
St. Louis, Missouri 63110

Anders Lundberg, M.D.
Professor, Department of Physiology
University of Gotenborg
Faculty of Medicine, Universitet
I. Gotenberg, Vosaparken, S-411–24, Sweden

Edward F. MacNichol, Jr., Ph.D.
Assistant Director, Research Services
Marine Biological Laboratories
Woods Hole, Massachusetts 02543

Henry R. Mahler, Ph.D.
Research Professor, Department of Chemistry
and
Center for Neural Sciences
Indiana University
Bloomington, Indiana 47401

Richard L. Masland, M.D.
Department of Neurology
Columbia University
College of Physicians and Surgeons
630 West 168th Street
New York, New York 10032

Dale E. McFarlin, M.D.
Chief, Neuroimmunology Branch
National Institute of Neurological and Com-
  municative Disorders and Stroke
National Institutes of Health
Building 36, Room 5D12
Bethesda, Maryland 20014

Henry McIlwain, D.Sc., Ph.D.
Professor of Biochemistry
British Postgraduate Medical Federation
Institute of London
De Crespigny Park, Denmark Hill
London SE5 8AF, England

Guy M. McKhann, M.D.
Chairman, Division of Neurology
The Johns Hopkins University
School of Medicine
Baltimore, Maryland 21205

James O. McNamara, M.D.
Assistant Professor, Division of Neurology
Duke University
School of Medicine
Durham, North Carolina 27710

Blake W. Moore, Ph.D.
Professor of Biochemistry in Psychiatry
Department of Psychiatry
Washington University
School of Medicine
600 South Euclid Avenue
St. Louis, Missouri 63110

Bryce L. Munger, M.D.
Professor and Chairman, Department of Anat-
omy
The Milton S. Hershey Medical Center
The Pennsylvania State University
500 University Drive
Hershey, Pennsylvania 17033

Toshio Narahashi, Ph.D.
Professor and Vice-Chairman, Department of
Physiology and Pharmacology
Duke University Medical Center
Durham, North Carolina 27710

William T. Norton, Ph.D.
Professor of Neurology and Neurosciences
The Saul R. Korey Department of Neurology
Albert Einstein College of Medicine
1300 Morris Park Avenue
Bronx, New York 10461

Sidney Ochs, Ph.D.
Department of Physiology
Indiana University Medical Center
1100 West Michigan Street
Indianapolis, Indiana 46202

William Oldendorf, M.D.
Brentwood Hospital
Veterans Administration
Wilshire and Sawtelle Boulevards
Los Angeles, California 90073

Michael B. A. Oldstone, M.D.
Department of Experimental Pathology
Scripps Clinic and Research Foundation
476 Prospect Street
La Jolla, California 92037

Sanford L. Palay, M.D.
Department of Anatomy
Harvard Medical School
25 Shattuck Street
Boston, Massachusetts 02115

George D. Pappas, M.D.
Department of Neurosciences
and
Department of Anatomy
Albert Einstein College of Medicine
The Rose F. Kennedy Center for Research in
Mental Retardation and Human Develop-
ment
1410 Pelham Parkway South
Bronx, New York 10461

Lee Peachey, Ph.D.
Professor, Department of Biology
University of Pennsylvania
Philadelphia, Pennsylvania 19174

John P. Perkins, Ph.D.
Department of Pharmacology
University of Colorado
School of Medicine
Denver, Colorado 80220

Rosemarie Petersen
Research Technologist, Department of Pa-
thology
University of Washington
School of Medicine
Seattle, Washington 98195

Shirley E. Poduslo, Ph.D.
Neurochemistry Laboratory
The Johns Hopkins University
School of Medicine
1721 East Madison Street
Baltimore, Maryland 21205

Dominick P. Purpura, M.D.
Professor and Chairman, Department of
Anatomy
and
Director, The Rose F. Kennedy Center for
Research in Mental Retardation and Human
Development
Albert Einstein College of Medicine
1410 Pelham Parkway South
Bronx, New York 10461

Richard Quarles, Ph.D.
Research Chemist
Developmental and Metabolic Neurology
Branch
National Institute of Neurological and Com-
municative Disorders and Stroke
National Institutes of Health
Bethesda, Maryland 20014

Thomas S. Reese, M.D.
Chief, Section of Functional Neuroanatomy
Laboratory of Neuropathology and Neuro-
anatomical Sciences
National Institute of Neurological and Com-
municative Disorders and Stroke
National Institutes of Health
Bethesda, Maryland 20014

Eugene Roberts, Ph.D.
Director, Division of Neurosciences
City of Hope National Medical Center
1500 East Duarte Road
Duarte, California 91010

J. David Robertson, M.D., Ph.D.
Chairman, Department of Anatomy
Duke University Medical Center
Box 3011
Durham, North Carolina 27710

Allen D. Roses, M.D.
Assistant Professor, Division of Neurology
Duke University
School of Medicine
Durham, North Carolina 27710

Charles H. Sawyer, Ph.D.
Professor, Department of Anatomy
University of California, Los Angeles
School of Medicine
Los Angeles, California 90024

Cheng-Mei Shaw, M.D.
Professor of Pathology
University of Washington
School of Medicine
Seattle, Washington 98195

Gordon M. Shepherd, M.D., Ph.D.
Department of Physiology
Yale University
School of Medicine
333 Cedar Street
New Haven, Connecticut 06510

Richard L. Sidman, M.D.
Department of Neuropathology
Harvard Medical School
25 Shattuck Street
Boston, Massachusetts 02115

Peter B. Smith, Ph.D.
Postdoctoral Fellow, Division of Neurology
Duke University

School of Medicine
Durham, North Carolina 27710

Solomon H. Snyder, M.D.
Professor of Pharmacology and Psychiatry
Department of Pharmacology and Experi-
mental Therapeutics
The Johns Hopkins University
School of Medicine
725 North Wolfe Street
Baltimore, Maryland 21205

Kunihiko Suzuki, M.D.
Professor of Neurology and Neuroscience
The Rose F. Kennedy Center for Research in
Mental Retardation and Human Develop-
ment
Albert Einstein College of Medicine
1410 Pelham Parkway South
Bronx, New York 10461

Ichiji Tasaki, M.D.
Chief, Laboratory of Neurobiology
National Institute of Mental Health
National Institutes of Health
Building 36, Room 1D02
Bethesda, Maryland 20014

Donald B. Tower, M.D., Ph.D.
Director, National Institute of Neurological
and Communicative Disorders and Stroke
National Institutes of Health
Bethesda, Maryland 20014

Silvio S. Varon, M.D.
Professor, Department of Biology
University of California, San Diego
La Jolla, California 92037

Yng-Jiin Wang, M.S.
Brain Research Group
Chemical Laboratory
Indiana University
Bloomington, Indiana 47401

Norman Weiner, M.D.
Professor and Chairman, Department of
Pharmacology
University of Colorado Medical Center
4200 East Ninth Avenue
Denver, Colorado 80220

The Nervous System, Donald B. Tower, Editor-in-Chief. *Vol. 1: The Basic Neurosciences.* Raven Press, New York, 1975.

Introduction

Donald B. Tower

Shortly after assuming the position of Director of NINCDS in June 1974, I realized that the Institute would mark its 25th Anniversary in one year's time. Public Law 692 (81st Congress) creating the National Institute of Neurological Diseases and Blindness was signed into law on August 15, 1950. In staff meetings we discussed how best to take cognizance of this event. These three volumes represent our choice of the most appropriate, tangible way to celebrate the Institute's silver anniversary. By coincidence the oldest neurological society in the world, the American Neurological Association, celebrated the centennial of its founding in June 1875, so that 1975 is indeed a banner year for American neurology.

For 22 of the 25 years of the Institute's existence I have had the privilege of being a staff member and a part of its development. At the invitation of Pearce Bailey and Milton Shy, I joined the clinical division of NINDB as head of the Section of Clinical Neurochemistry in July of 1953. Like many of the original clinical staff I came from the Montreal Neurological Institute. In fact at one time there were more MNI alumni at the NIH in Bethesda than anywhere else outside Montreal. Today few may appreciate the contribution that the Montreal Neurological Institute has made to the American neurological scene, particularly in neurosurgery and the neurosciences. The MNI was opened in 1934, funded by Rockefeller Foundation money, and it began turning out a modest but significant number of clinicians and researchers trained under the guidance of Wilder Penfield, William Cone, Colin Russell, and their colleagues. A fair proportion of the American neurological community today had part of their training there and/or at Queen Square in London. Certainly the MNI provided the nucleus for the NINDB intramural program at its inception, and together with the neurology units of the Veterans Administration it helped to bridge the academic training gap until the NINDB training programs could join in.

In those early days, the NIH was a more intimate community than it is now. At Top Cottage, which stood on the site of the present Building 31 office building, the laboratory chiefs from all institutes met weekly for luncheon discussions of ongoing research. I was not then a lab chief but was invited to talk to them about our work on the neurochemistry of epileptogenic cerebral cortex. One has a certain nostalgia for the time when most of the NIH research talent could sit together at informal luncheon seminars. In a similar vein, Pearce Bailey would call together at his home in the Spring Valley area of Washington all the NINDB scientists to go over the grants which the National Advisory Neurological Diseases and Blindness Council would review and to seek our advice for his testimony before the Congressional appropriations committees. Pearce Bailey enjoyed this latter task perhaps more than any other of his responsibilities and he was a master at it. Today with thousands of grants and several hundred on-campus scientists it is difficult to realize how small and intimate our NINDB group was in those days.

There are other piquant recollections from the early years. When Mait Baldwin operated on his first case of focal epilepsy in the new NINDB surgical suite on the 10th floor of the Clinical Center, the surgical team was new, and the procedure, carried out in classic Penfield fashion, took a good deal longer than expected. When 5 P.M. came, with the patient's head still open, the O.R. supervisor told her staff to go home because she could not authorize overtime. Baldwin prevailed on her to leave one hustle nurse and an orderly so that he could complete the operation. Like other growing pains of the newly opened NIH Clinical Center, it took a high level conference downtown to resolve the issues raised by this incident.

Shortly after I arrived Milton Shy showed me in our area of the Clinical Center an empty room which, he said, was to be a soundproof room, the nucleus of the NINDB intramural communicative disorders program. He was never able to initiate that program; in fact it took another 21 years before I had the satisfaction of recruiting Jorgen Fex and of seeing the intramural Laboratory of Neuro-otolaryngology opened in 1974. We had other constraints in the early 1950s. Domestic meeting travel money was restricted, so that we had great difficulty in getting to national meetings. At one point in 1954 the Bureau of the Budget suspended NIH intramural funds because they thought the daily cost to house a Clinical Center patient was too high. We did not get paid for a month, until Congressional pressures came to our rescue. For the historian very little is really new.

I was more fortunate than most of my intramural colleagues in being able to participate in the extramural phases of the NINDB programs. I can remember meeting with Betsy Hartman and a few colleagues to review the early groups of special fellowship applications, the inception of a program which contributed much to the development of special talents among clinical teachers and investigators in the American neurological community. It was also my privilege to serve for 8 years (1954 to 1962) on the Neurology Study Section of the NIH Division of Research Grants. Tom O'Brien, the executive secretary, wanted a neurochemist, and I seemed to be the only one foolish enough to rush in where others were reluctant to tread. As all study section members know, it was a most rewarding experience. Finally, the late Heinrich Waelsch joined me on the study section, and I was able to retire after what must have been one of the longer tours of study section duty. On one occasion I remember the concern that Paul Bucy, Bob Galambos, and I expressed that all of Molly Brazier's salary was to come from grant funds and none from her institution (at that time, Harvard University). How ironic that seems in today's climate.

For a year in 1967 to 1968, at Dick Masland's request, I substituted for Murray Goldstein as Acting Associate Director of NINDB for Extramural Programs, while Murray spent a year in neurology at the Mayo Clinic. Except for my study section experience I knew essentially nothing about the operation and nature of the extramural research grants and training programs. Dedicated staff—Malcolm Ray, Betsy Hartman, Mathilde Solowey, Elsa Keiles, and many others—helped me to learn and kept me from erring too often. The high points of the extramural year are the meetings of the advisory council, when allocations of the Institute grant funds are recommended. As short a time ago as 1968, we were able to fund virtually all the grants recommended for approval by the study sections. But that was nearly the end of the expansionist era; as yearly appropriations began to level off, numbers of applications still increased, and costs per grant began to climb.

Most of my years at NIH have been in the Institute's intramural program. What started as a modest two-room clinical neurochemistry section on the 4-north corridor of the Clinical Center progressed to an 8-room unit in the 10-D wing and eventually to a 21-room laboratory in the 3-D wing. A Laboratory of Neurochemistry had been on paper even before 1950, but only two sections were ever activated during the NINDB-NIMH combined basic intramural program—one on lipid chemistry headed by Roscoe Brady (assigned to NINDB) and one on physical chemistry headed by Alex Rich (assigned to NIMH). When the joint basic program was split between the two institutes in 1960, Wayne Albers (from the Laboratory of Neuroanatomical Sciences), Roscoe Brady, Beni Horvath (a muscle chemist in my section), and I proposed to Milton Shy that we form within the NINDB a four-section Laboratory of Neurochemistry. This idea was generally concurred in, and the present laboratory came into being. It and its various predecessors have graduated a small but distinguished group, among whom are many of today's leaders in the field. Moreover, Brady's program prospered so that it has become a separate laboratory, the Developmental and Metabolic Neurology Branch, in 1971.

Perhaps these fragmentary reminiscences may convey something of the high regard I have for this Institute, its staff and supporters, and its programs. Few people, relatively speaking, live through a major period of history, yet those of us who have participated in these last 25 years have had just such an experience. Clinical neurology and neurosurgery and the clinical disciplines in the disorders of human communication (otorhinolaryngology, audiology, speech pathology, and the like) have begun to flourish after years, even decades, of neglect and undermanning. The infusion of academicians — teachers and clinical investigators — catalyzed by the NINDB training programs represent, in my opinion, a very major contribution. Most importantly it was paralleled by the truly remarkable growth of neuroscience and communicative science research. To our admittedly partisan eyes, this has been the most significant biomedical event of the last several decades. And again the NINDB and later the NINDS provided most of the stimulus directly or indirectly.

Consider for a moment the contrast between 1975 and 1950. My examples come from areas of my interests and experiences, but they will suggest many others. At the time the NINDB was founded our knowledge of the Krebs cycle of intermediary metabolism was newly established. The importance of vitamin B_6 to CNS function was still to be demonstrated. Gamma-aminobutyric acid (GABA), serotonin, and dopamine were still to be discovered. And we knew nothing of reserpine and the subsequent host of psychomimetic drugs. The concept of the mechanism of neuromuscular transmission had just changed from an electrical to a chemical one, and the mechanisms of action of cholinesterase and the anticholinesterase agents were just in the process of elucidation. The electric eel and the squid were among the earliest of "exotic" species to prove especially valuable to the neuroscientist. Effective procedures for measuring human cerebral blood flow and metabolism were still awaited, and the dynamic, bidirectional transport nature of the blood-brain barrier was not yet suspected. Central inhibition was not understood; axoplasmic flow was known, but its bidirectional transport characteristics were still unknown. The voltage clamp technique and studies of the details of axonal conduction were in their infancy, and a decade would elapse before sodium-potassium-activated ATP-ase and the enzymatic basis for ion transport would be discovered.

Isotopic tracers were few and not widely used. The liquid scintillation counter and isotopic scintiscanning were still to be developed. The mainstays of modern biochemical analysis, thin-layer chromatography and gas-liquid chromatography, were unknown. The preparative ultracentrifuge was just coming off the drawing boards, so that subcellular fractionation, lysosomes, synaptosomes, and membrane and receptor isolations were far in the future. There were no fluorescence techniques for tracing anatomical pathways, identifying antigen-antibody reactions, or conducting microanalytical quantifications. Computer technology as we know it today was hardly imagined. And that novelty the electron microscope had not yet proved applicable to the examination of neural tissues.

We knew something about the macromolecular arrangement of the myelin sheath — one of the first biological membranes subjected to study by physical techniques such as X-ray crystallography. But we did not yet understand the intricacies of its structure or the role of oligodendroglia or Schwann cells in its genesis and maintenance. The details of the biosynthesis of neural lipids — fatty acids, phospholipids, and sphingolipids — were still obscure. Even the basic structures of glycolipids, mucopolysaccharides, and glycoproteins remained to be elucidated. Knowledge of protein synthesis and turnover and the role of ribosomes in neural cells was still to come. Similarly the nature of RNA, DNA, and the genetic code, and their importance to cellular development and function, were years away. Such key processes as glycogen synthesis and mobilization to provide energy as glucose were not understood, and the key role of the cyclic nucleotides in these processes was not even suspected. To suggest in 1950 that we could isolate acetylcholine receptors by means of a Taiwanese snake venom toxin, alpha-bungarotoxin, and that we could make antibodies to the receptor for analytical studies and to provide a model for human myasthenia gravis would have seemed highly improbable.

We were beginning to learn about the simple peptide nature of the posterior pituitary hormones, but we had only rudimentary appreciation of the role of the hypothalamus in pituitary hormone control. The hypothalamic releasing factors would not be discovered for another decade. We knew about inborn errors of metabolism, but we did not know about enzyme deletions or attenuations, so that the biochemical lesions responsible for phenylketonuria (PKU), galactosemia, and the like were still to be demonstrated. The dietary management of PKU had to await the isolation or synthesis of the amino acids required for the synthetic phenylalanine-free diet. Diagnostic tests for PKU screening would also come later. Neuroviruses like rabies and polio were known, but the polio vaccines were still experimental and would require the development of tissue culture for commercial production to become feasible. The rubella virus had not yet been isolated, and a vaccine would not be developed for another 15 years. The recognition of the role of slow and latent viruses in dementias was nearly 20 years away.

In 1950 there were only three really effective anticonvulsant drugs, in comparison to 15 now. There was no effective therapy for Parkinson's disease; only neostigmine was available for myasthenia gravis; antibiotics were just beginning to make inroads into the bacterial infection of the nervous system, with some of them creating new problems because of their ototoxicity; and the steroids for edema, immunosuppression, etc., were still to come.

For all these advances and a great many more we must credit the biomedical research and research training effort spearheaded by the NIH and contemporary federal and private sector organizations in the post-World War II era. For the neurosciences and the communicative sciences the NINDB provided the major resources through its research grant, training grant, and special training programs. Some of the highlights of the development and progress of these programs are recounted in the following chapters contributed by my predecessors as directors of NINDB and NINDS, Pearce Bailey, Richard L. Masland, and Theodore F. MacNichol, Jr. The rest of the story is covered in large measure by the 160 chapters that follow in these three silver anniversary volumes. To the many contributors who joined in, despite short deadlines, we are most grateful. There are gaps and omissions that we acknowledge with regret, but I think that, on balance, what is written here about the highlights of the basic and clinical neurosciences and the communicative sciences provides a sufficiently full accounting of the 25 years of our endeavors.

A very great many people have contributed to those endeavors. The Institute has been the catalytic instrument, vitalized by a dedicated cadre of professional and administrative employees. But the scientific community, the academic community, the practitioners, the voluntary organizations and the patient community, the Congress, the rest of the NIH, and, yes, even the bureaucrats of DHEW have all played significant roles. These volumes are significant milestones for the accomplishments of which all can be proud. But they are just milestones. Much remains to be accomplished to solve the problems of stroke, paraplegia, deafness, multiple sclerosis, muscular dystrophy, epilepsy, parkinsonism, cerebral palsy, the vast group of genetic disorders, the many viral and immunological disorders, and so many more. Not only is the NINCDS concerned with leading causes of death in the United States like stroke and CNS trauma, but it is also concerned with the major problems of morbidity confronting our country. The numbers — over 40 million patients — are enormous; the costs to society — many times the 20 billions of dollars for care alone — are staggering. What we have learned about the nervous system, as recorded here, is truly impressive and significant. But it is very sobering to realize how much still remains to be learned.

I hope that at the next appropriate anniversary celebrated by the NINCDS, the director at that time can cite the foregoing unsolved problems and point proudly to their solutions as a result of Institute-supported research. I expect the next decade to be the decade of the nervous system, when our knowledge can truly advance by quantum leaps. But the pace of research must be sustained — and that will require dedicated teachers to inspire and proselytize medical and science students to make the nervous system their career; it will require resources for training, resources for basic research, and resources for clinical applications and delivery to the practicing physician and the patient; and surely it will require even greater research efforts by the neuroscience community. For, as so aptly put by John Donne, the greater the island of knowledge, the longer the shoreline of the unknown.

The Nervous System, Donald B. Tower, Editor-in-Chief. *Vol. 1: The Basic Neurosciences*. Raven Press, New York, 1975.

National Institute of Neurological Diseases and Blindness: Origins, Founding, and Early Years (1950 to 1959)

Pearce Bailey

Government organizations and support of biomedical research and development did not reach conspicuous dimensions until the 1940s and 1950s. The development and production of atomic energy under government sponsorship gave rise to a growing belief that analogous efforts in biomedical research could lead to a conquest of many diseases.

The discovery and development of antibiotics coupled with greater refinements of surgical techniques added to a greater public awareness of public health problems and to a greater optimism of their eventual control through research. Between 1937 and 1950 the death rate in the United States declined 15%. From 1937 to 1952 federal funds for biomedical research increased 10-fold. An increasing portion of these federal outlays was flowing to the National Institutes of Health (NIH), the principal research arm of the Public Health Service (PHS).

The mounting control of some acute infectious diseases following World War II led to a switch of public concern from acute conditions to more chronic ones of obscure metabolic origins. The disease targets, to be highlighted then as now, were cancer, heart disease, and mental health.

Even before the close of World War II, large private endowments for the promotion of medical research and medical programs were dwindling to a trickle in the light of increased taxes and fear of inflation. These individual endowments were superseded by the creation of large foundations aimed at broad health and social goals; but most important from the standpoint of neurology was the postbellum growth of voluntary health agencies dedicated to the conquest of categorical diseases. These voluntary groups were made up mostly of patients already afflicted or threatened or of members of their families and their friends. They devised ingenious methods of fund raising through door-to-door subscriptions, public relations, displays, and competitions on radio and television. They enjoyed tax exemption.

Soon the notion developed that another effective way to raise research funds in large amounts was for citizen groups to plead before the Congress to establish and appropriate funds to federal research institutes at the NIH for the scientific investigation of disease problems with which they were concerned. In 1946 only one voluntary group of consequence was concerned with a neurological disease: The National Foundation for Infantile Paralysis, the goals of which were far too circumscribed to constitute a platform for an across-the-board approach to neurological research. There was yet no way at a layman's level to group all organic diseases of the nervous system together and demonstrate their significance as a public health and socio-economic problem.

Moreover there was a lack of unanimity, even among neurologists, as to how neurological medicine should be classified and defined. Was it a branch of internal medicine as originally intended or was it a part of a neuropsychiatric hegemony as treated in the United States government medical organizations? Or should it be an autonomous discipline? There were no clear answers to the question at that time.

Two things were abundantly clear by 1946, however: (1) a definite trend to increase funding by the federal government of biomedical research programs, particularly those projects having a disease orientation; and (2) academic neurology, regardless of its place in the medical hierarchy, must acquire a greater degree of fiscal autonomy if it were to compete successfully for the federal dollar. Government medical and scientific thinking in 1946 considered neurological research as an appendage of psychiatry, and the various areas of investigation were grouped together under the hybrid term "neuropsychiatry." The first modern notion of neuropsychiatry probably took root in the doctrine of organic psychiatry championed by Meynert and others during the late nineteenth century.

In this country extensive use of the term neuropsychiatry first came into being as a military expedient during World War I. The Division of Neurology and Psychiatry, independent of internal medicine, was established in the Army Surgeon General's Office in 1917, organized and directed by a neurologist.[1] The physicians of the newly created division were mostly psychiatrists, but the neurologists were described as being more aggressive and better qualified as men of the world. Members of the American Neurological Association had a significant representation in this program.[2]

Most of the psychiatrists were recruited from state hospital systems and had secured their education through the routine performance of their duties. They were essentially hospital administrators with wide experience in management of the psychoses but little in treating the psychoneuroses. Their training in organic diseases of the nervous system was almost nil. The neurologists were trained in organic nervous diseases but had had office experience in psychoneuroses, and they lacked hospital experience in management of the psychoses.

Because of their divergent backgrounds of experience it was considered expedient to pool neurologists and psychiatrists into a single operating unit by giving supplementary training to both groups in the areas where their experience was defective. Thus military neurology and psychiatry were united under the all-inclusive label of neuropsychiatry. The war neuroses turned out to be the number one medical problem in the army.

The impact of the newly created military neuropsychiatry division soon extended into civilian teaching and practice. Despite sporadic resistance it had the strong backing of J. Ramsey Hunt[3] in neurology and Adolph Meyer[4] in psychiatry. The use of the term neuropsychiatry reached a peak during the 1930s, after which it

began to decline only to be reactivated by mobilization in World War II.

During World War II, unlike World War I, the divisions of neuropsychiatry of all the medical departments of the armed services were headed by psychiatrists as were most of the administrative posts. As in the first world war, the war neuroses were again considered the number one medical problem, but this time the psychiatrists were the ones who were the more aggressive and more men of the world. The neurologists usually played a secondary role as consultants to neuropsychiatric services.

Toward the close of the war, all government medical departments of the armed services and Veterans Administration had divisions of neuropsychiatry headed by psychiatrists. Departments of neuropsychiatry or psychiatry were becoming mandatory for accreditation in the nation's medical schools. The term neuropsychiatry had obviously become almost synonomous with psychiatry, as attested to by the decline of candidates being certified then in both neurology and psychiatry by the American Board.

Hence in 1946 neurological medicine and research was not sufficiently organized or defined at a professional or fiscal level to justify a national institute in Bethesda. Should neurologists therefore merely stand by, tread water, and watch while other programs in biomedical science were spiraling? Not necessarily. The renovated medical program of the Veterans Administration provided a promising vehicle for the advancement of academic neurology until the day when a greater degree of organization would allow for a more direct, concerted attack through the establishment of a national institute.

When I was separated from my neurological duties at the Philadelphia Naval Hospital in 1946, I was offered the opportunity to take charge of the neurology program in the division of neuropsychiatry of the Department of Medicine and Surgery of the Veterans Administration (VA), replacing Howard D. Fabing who had temporarily occupied the post on a short-term detail from the army and who wished to return to private practice in Cincinnati.

Here was an opportunity and the only one at the time for the new Chief of VA Neurology to aid academic neurology and help plan for its future. The VA appointment was approved by the Council of the American Neurological Association.

A complete renovation of medical departments of the old Veterans Bureau began around 1945 under the direction of two veteran generals of the European Theatre of Operations, General Omar N. Bradley, the new VA administrator, and General Paul R. Hawley, a physician and the new chief medical director. The new leadership was further inspired and supplemented by the appointment of a civilian, Paul B. Magnuson, the dynamic professor of orthopedic surgery at Northwestern University, as head of the VA education and research service.

Under the VA medical program, grant applications related to neurology were first reviewed by a subcommittee on neurology and then by a committee on neuropsychiatry. There was no direct line between the heads of the VA professional services with the research grant applicants or with the National Research Council (NRC). The central mission of the VA medical program was directed toward better care and facilities of veteran patients, not research. The director of the neurology section, however, was able to keep abreast with the trend of these research grants by attending committee meetings of the NRC as a guest.

When I accepted the position of chief of neurology in the central office, I was already imbued by ancestry and training with a fervor to contribute to the advancement of academic neurology through increasing facilities for training and research. To attain these objectives, the best opportunity appeared at the time to be in the *Dean's Committee Plan* of the VA medical program. This was one of several new programs and was instituted to bring VA medicine in close association with academic medicine. I was permitted to join the teaching staff at the Georgetown School of Medicine and to have limited consultations with private patients in order not to lose the human touch.

In 1946 the VA neurology section was under the neuropsychiatric division, headed by Daniel Blain, a psychiatrist. The relationship with the head of the division was good; budgetary allotments to neurology were generous even though it was regarded as a minor appendage of neuropsychiatry.

The first act of the chief of neurology was to procure a medical advisory committee selected by the council of the American Neurological Association (ANA). The ANA committee was of inestimable help in shaping the nascent VA neurological program and guiding it along lines conducive to furthering the development of academic neurology and to establishing better care for veteran patients.

Planning a program such as this necessarily entailed considerable travel to medical centers and scientific institutions throughout the country in order to take the national pulse with respect to the development of neurology. Wherever possible interviews were held with deans, department heads of internal medicine and psychiatry, and neurologists on the teaching staffs. The purpose was to explore ways in which neighboring VA facilities could be supplemented to be of use to their training and research programs in neurology.

In addition, a questionnaire survey was conducted under VA auspices to test the number and availability, and above all the interest, of qualified neurologists in neurological teaching, practice, or research. The questionnaire was mailed to physicians certified either in neurology alone or in both neurology and psychiatry prior to July 1947 by the American Board of Psychiatry and Neurology. The results of the survey were encouraging from the standpoint of interest in neurological medicine, but they showed that there were many inadequate facilities.[5]

The VA neurological training program breathed new life into residency training throughout the country, and within 2 years 34.6% of the 170 neurological residents in the country were in VA hospitals. Many of the VA programs provided university hospitals with additional beds and facilities and a way to add to their professional staffs. On completion of residency training, those residents who were ill-adapted to full-time academic careers or loath to enter private practice could still remain on VA staffs. Many did.

In 1946 the patient centers of neurologically disabled veterans from both world wars were large — approximately 20% to 30% of the patient population in general medical and surgical hospitals and 10% in psychiatric hospitals. Moreover, there were special categories of neurological patients from World War II who required special rehabilitation programs—50,000 epileptics, 20,000 craniocerebral injuries, 600 post-traumatic head injuries, 3,000 serious spinal cord injuries (paraplegics and quadriplegics). The special centers for paraplegics (except the largest one at the VA Hines Hospital in Chicago under L. J. Pollock) were not of direct concern to the neurology section. They required a multidisciplinary administration from the chief medical director's office in which R. Glen Spurling, consultant in neurosurgery, and Howard A. Rusk, consultant in physical medicine and rehabilitation, played leading roles.

As previously mentioned, the support of individual research projects was not an outstanding feature of the early VA program, since its central mission was directed to the improvement of medical care. However, the Neurology Section did organize, with the help of civilian consultants, several intramural pilot and demonstration projects directed to the improvement of medical care of veterans. All these programs contained research components, but they were too general and diffuse or too goal-seeking to be classified as research projects. They were viewed and passed on by an intramural VA committee and were organized as national treatment and research centers.

In 1947 the VA Neuropsychiatric Division changed its name to the Psychiatry and Neurology Service, thus giving to the neurology program greater exposure and enhancing its prestige. The VA Chief of the Neurology Section also became assistant chief of the Psychiatry and Neurology Service,* which added weight to his administrative position and maneuverability.

A variety of factors too numerous to enumerate here contributed to the expansion of VA medical research in little over a decade. It seems probable that it could not have happened were it not for the *Dean's Committee Plan* and the principle of locating VA hospitals and clinics near or on medical school campuses— determinations which originated in the early

---

* Recently (1972) the neurology service in the VA Central Office for the first time became a separate service under the directorship of Warren V. Huber.

Hawley-Magnuson era and welded VA medicine closely to academic medicine.

During the late 1940s several neurologists were bemoaning the state of academic neurology, stressing its decline in prestige and authority, and its lack of power to determine its own destiny. Some of these opinions were articulated as presidential addresses before the American Neurological Association. The most comprehensive survey report on this subject was given by Lewis J. Pollock[6] and his ANA committee on public relations before an executive session of the ANA in 1949 under the presidency of Stanley Cobb.

The American Academy of Neurology (AAN) was founded the year before by A. B. Baker and a cohort of young "Turks." Its main purposes were to: (1) provide an opportunity for younger men, down to the residency level, to participate in the scientific and administrative programs of a national neurological society; (2) set up active year-round committees for the advancement of neurology; and (3) provide low-cost professional courses for its members at annual meetings. It also struck for a greater autonomy of neurology as a medical discipline.

During the late 1940s there were rumblings that neurological research could never attain its rightful place in the sun until a separate institute for these conditions was established at the NIH. Harvey Cushing was the first to petition for the establishment of a federally supported national institute for the investigation of combat injuries to the nervous system incurred during World War I; but lacking public knowledge and support this effort soon evanesced. It was not until the late 1940s and early 1950s that voluntary health agencies devoted to the research and care of neurological diseases gained sufficient substance and momentum to impress legislators. These voluntary agencies were composed mostly of neurological patients and their families and friends, who for the first time saw an opportunity to press for aid for their afflictions which for centuries had been synonomous with social embarrassment, shame, and despair. Among the earlier of these groups was the National Multiple Sclerosis Society (1946), United Cerebral Palsy (1951), Muscular Dystrophy Association of America (1950), Myasthenia Gravis Foundation, and National

Epilepsy League (1950). Many more were eventually to be added.

Several members of the ANA testified before Congress on behalf of these voluntary groups. Among them, for multiple sclerosis, were H. Houston Merritt, Tracy Putnam, and Hans Reese; and for epilepsy, William G. Lennox.

Unlike the American Heart Association and the National Cancer Society, the new neurological voluntaries did not push for a single institute dedicated to the whole spectrum of neurological disabilities, but they confined their efforts to a particular disease in which their membership was involved. Accordingly, at least four bills were introduced in Congress for four neurological conditions as well as one more for blindness.

The administrative feasibility of establishing multiple institutes was soon challenged. During late 1949 Senator Tobey (New Hampshire) with the assistance of Senator O'Mahoney (Wyoming) offered a substitute bill for the National Multiple Sclerosis Act which Senator Tobey had introduced previously. The new bill proposed the organization of a national institute for neurological diseases within the framework of the PHS. The new bill would cover all neurological disorders and blindness, eye research being considered sufficiently close to the nervous system to justify its inclusion. The new bill was acceptable to the neurological and blindness voluntaries and to the Surgeon General (Leonard Scheele), and resulted in the legislative authorization of a neurology and blindness institute in Bethesda.

The National Institute of Neurological Diseases and Blindness (NINDB), later changed to the National Institute of Neurological Diseases and Stroke (NINDS), and still later to the National Institute of Neurological and Communicative Disorders and Stroke (NINCDS), was authorized in August 1950 by Public Law 692 (81st Congress). Consequently the NINDB became one of the National Institutes of Health of the Public Health Service, which at that time were under the jurisdiction of the Federal Security Agency. The Department of Health, Education, and Welfare (HEW) with a secretary of cabinet rank was not created until 1953, whereupon PHS and the NIH were absorbed into the swelling domain of HEW.

When NINDB was authorized, it was granted essentially the same organizational pattern as other institutes then in existence at NIH:* microbiology (the original PHS research authority), cancer (1937), heart (1948), mental health (1949), arthritis and metabolic diseases (1950), and dental research. Another important research facility was the Division of Research Grants, which as we shall see later processed and (through nonfederal committees called study sections or training committees) reviewed the scientific merit of all grant applications and passed their recommendations to the various national advisory councils.

As previously mentioned, eye research was an integral component of the NINDB program. Because of this, it soon appeared practical to include disorders of all the special senses, especially hearing, in the purview of NINDB. Then NINDB became an institute of neurological and sensory diseases. While this was true in practice, it was not adopted as an official title. However, in 1975, as noted earlier, the Institute's name was again changed to give more visibility to the communicative disorders dealt with by the Institute. The component of sensory disease research and training averaged about 20% of the Institute's activities. Ophthalmologists were never completely happy about being under the aegis of neurology; in the course of time, as they broadened their research interests and capabilities, sufficient strength was mobilized from citizen's groups to establish in 1968 a separate National Institute for Eye Research at NIH.

The provisions of Public Law 692 empowered the Institute through the Surgeon General to conduct intramural research and training on the Bethesda campus in neurological diseases and blindness, and to support such research and

---

* The names of many of the original institutes have been changed; the original microbiological institute is now the National Institute of Allergy and Infectious Diseases; arthritis and metabolic diseases is now the National Institute of Arthritis, Metabolism, and Digestive Diseases; the heart institute is now the National Heart and Lung Institute. New institutes have appeared: the National Institute of General Medical Sciences; the National Institute of Eye Research, separated from the Neurology Institute; the National Institute of Child Health and Human Development; and the National Institute of Aging.

training at universities and other institutions related to the causes, prevention, diagnosis, and treatment of these disorders. Like the other national institutes, the NINDB had a national advisory council of 12 persons who were non-federal appointees with statuary authority (six professionals and six public-spirited citizens) usually appointed for 4 years by the Surgeon General of the PHS. There were also *ex officio* members representing the Department of Defense and the VA. The Council made the final recommendations concerning approval and disapproval of research and training applications, but their activities related more to the guidance and determination of Institute policy.

The bulk of the review on the scientific merit of grant applications was under the jurisdiction of the Division of Research Grants (DRG), part of the NIH Director's Office, which was not aligned with any particular institute. DRG was the first to receive grant applications, process them, and then assign them for scientific review by appropriate study sections or training committees. The study sections are nonfederal groups of experts who rotate in specialized fields of basic and clinical disciplines. The members of study sections are selected by the DRG, not by the Institute directors. If existing study sections did not possess sufficient scientific expertise for the evaluation of a given application, DRG could appoint a special ad hoc review committee.

After an application was reviewed by a study section and assigned a priority, it was then passed on to the Council for final NIH determination and recommendations to the Surgeon General. Rarely was an approved application rejected by the Council.

While the original mandate of NINDB was broad and flexible, no money whatsoever had been appropriated by the Congress for the new Institute and hence no full-time director could be appointed. Therefore the Institute's routine affairs during 1950 were administered by the National Institute of Mental Health (NIMH). True, a National Advisory Council for NINDB was appointed and two of its members were neurologists: Henry W. Woltman and H. Houston Merritt. The cost of the NINDB Council meetings and the funding requirements for reimbursements to DRG for the review of grants and maintenance, housekeeping, utilities,

rent, etc. were assumed as part of the operating expenses of NIH under the purview of the NIH director.

The first NINDB Advisory Council did review a number of grant applications submitted by the study section of the DRG. This was an interesting academic exercise but, in a sense, an exercise in futility. The NINDB Council could and did approve many of these applications, but without any budget the Institute could not fund any of them. Some eventually were funded by other institutes. The NINDB during 1950 was definitely a standby program and so remained until the summer of 1951 when it obtained its first annual budget of $1.25 million.

This first NINDB budget, however, was misleading. It was not independent, being part of the general operating expenses of the NIH, administered by the Office of the Director of NIH. Most of the budget was not for new programming or the support of new research projects. It consisted mostly of comparative transfers of old but still active research projects of a neurological and sensory disease nature and the funds to support them from other institutes, particularly from NIMH.

What there was of new money in the 1951 NINDB budget nevertheless did allow for the appointment of the first Institute director, Pearce Bailey, early in the fall, and provided him with a secretary and an administrative officer. A few months later the Institute was fortunate in procuring the services of an imaginative science administrator, Frederick L. Stone, on temporary loan from DRG. Accordingly, during 1951 and 1952 NINDB emerged from its original standby phase to an active planning phase.

Prior to the appointment of an NINDB director, the NIH director had decided, largely owing to influence exerted from NIMH, to combine the basic science programs of NIMH and NINDB into a single unit under Associate Director (NIMH-NINDB) Seymour S. Kety.

Under this pattern of program organization, part or all of the NIMH basic science branches were transferred to NINDB. Those transferred to NINDB together with their eventual heads were biophysics (Kenneth Cole), neurophysiology (Karl Frank, I. Tasaki), experimental neuropathology (Jan Cammermeyer), neuroanatomical sciences (William F. Windle).

During 1950 and 1951 NIMH underwrote the cost of this program including the associate director's salary. The associate director for basic research was therefore wearing two hats, being responsible to two separate institutes. Such an arrangement can be disadvantageous especially if one of the institutes (NIMH) is bigger and richer than the other (NINDB); but here the arrangement had a positive aspect. It afforded an opportunity to initiate at least part of the NINDB intramural program.

By the time the NINDB director arrived in Bethesda there was no money to launch any new programs; no laboratory or clinical space had been allocated to the new institute. To requests for space, the proverbial response was: "If you have no money, what would you do with the space?" But the combined NIMH-NINDB basic science program was gaining momentum, thus adding some prestige to NINDB. It was fortunate too that the associate director of the combined program, Seymour Kety, was a mature and creative scientist of rare ability and bounding with imagination and energy.

Kety remained in charge of the combined program until 1956. He was succeeded by Robert L. Livingston. The combined (NIMH-NINDB) endeavor continued until the 1960s, when it was split into two separate programs — one in mental health, the other in neurology and blindness.

In 1952 the Institute's annual budget was increased from $1,252,233 to $1,992,300, but again the bulk of the increase still consisted of comparative transfers of already active research projects from other institutes and from the DRG and for allocations for reimbursements to the NIH for central housekeeping services. There was little new money for the support of new research projects or training grants or for the activation of intramural programs in clinical investigations. No clinical or laboratory space had been allocated to NINDB in the new clinical center (scheduled for completion in 1953). The Institute's basic research programs were still almost entirely supported by NIMH. The survival of NINDB appeared questionable to many.

The lean years of 1951 and 1952, however, did allow time for hard and serious planning.

NINDB had many vulnerabilities which were crying for reorganization and reform. On the political front, the Institute was signally vulnerable because: (1) the voluntary health agencies testifying before the Congress did not present a united front; and (2) the NINDB budget had not been organized as a line item in the President's budget, like cancer, heart, and mental health.

The voluntary health agencies backing the Institute during these early austerity years made a splintered and disjointed presentation to the members of the Congressional appropriations committee. So involved were they in their own programs, they were prone to testify on behalf of the diseases to which they were dedicated and not on behalf of the whole range of neurological disabilities and their serious public health consequences. Sometimes they appeared competitive, making their testimony confusing to the committee members of the Congress who at best were only dimly aware of the potential scope of neurological and sensory disease research.

To alleviate this situation, the NINDB director, in his capacity then as President of the American Academy of Neurology, appointed an AAN liaison committee to meet with the heads of the interested voluntary agencies. The purpose of the meeting was to form a national committee of professional and lay groups for promulgating a concerted program in neurological research.

The meeting took place July 25, 1952 in Bethesda. The liaison committee members representing the AAN were A. B. Baker, Sidney Carter, F. M. Forster, R. W. Graves, A. S. Rose, T. J. von Storch, and Hans H. Reese, then President of the American Neurological Association, who represented the ANA. Representing the voluntary health agencies were their respective directors or their delegates who were dedicated to epilepsy, multiple sclerosis, muscular dystrophy, and cerebral palsy. Also represented was the National Society for Crippled Children and Adults (Chicago). In this manner the National Committee for Research in Neurological Disorders (NCRND) was born. A. B. Baker was elected Chairman of the new national committee and continued in this post until 1970, when he was succeeded by Paul C. Bucy.

The NCRND immediately appointed several standing committees to promote a more cohesive approach to the problems of neurological research. The committee most relevant to the growth of NINDB was the Committee on Public Education, chaired by Mrs. Ruth McCormick Tankersly, former publisher of the *Washington Times Herald,* and president of the then National Epilepsy League. She lived near Washington and was well known in political circles. The purpose of her committee was to enlighten the people and the Congress, especially the subcommittees on appropriations, on the significance of neurological research. Early important committee members in these frontier days were the late Cornelius H. Traeger (then Medical Director) and Sylvia Lawry (then Secretary, now Executive Director) of the National Multiple Sclerosis Society. The national committee still flourishes today but with a greatly enlarged membership.

After the NCRND was placed in operation and its impact felt, it was not long before (with the help of John E. Fogarty, Chairman of the House Subcommittee on Appropriations) NINDB was broken out as a line item in the federal budget and given its own identifiable appropriation. At last the iron ring of fiscal repression had been broken, and for the first time the Institute had relevant recognition.

Accordingly, NINDB in 1953 procured an increase in its annual appropriations from $1.97+ million to $4.50 million. Now the Institute was able to pay its full share of the intramural basic research grants, to have new money to fund new research grant applications; and for the first time, the appropriation contained funds for training grants in neurology and ophthalmology in the amount of $504,000. At approximately the same time, the DRG had organized a separate Neurology Study Section for the scientific evaluation of NINDB research grant applications. By the end of the year, the momentum of the Institute's growth had automatically made available clinical and laboratory space in the new clinical center for the eventual pursuit of a clinical investigations program.[7]

A plan for organizing graduate training programs, both clinical and basic, in neurological and sensory disorders was carefully planned before funds became available for funding them. They related both to clinical and basic training.

At the time, training programs were not popular proposals either within the NIH or the PHS. The top leaders were more careful then than now about antagonizing organized medicine or the medical schools. A possible accusation of socialized medicine was the *bête noire* to be avoided. The NINDB training proposal had an unusual twist, however, for it was designed solely to train teachers and investigators to add persons of experience and talent to the existing research pool for the probable event that more research funds would become available. It was understood that some of the training recipients would stray away from their academic pursuits to enter private practice, but this was not considered too amoral for at that time at least 15 states did not have a single qualified neurologist. Studies to date have consistently shown that the vast majority of NINDB trainees continue to pursue academic careers, many now holding important chairs in leading medical schools, hospitals, and other institutions.

The review and approval of graduate training applications followed channels essentially similar to those of research grant applications, passing from committee to council. The graduate training applications were reviewed first by special training committees in neurology, ophthalmology, and later in otolaryngology—all under the aegis of DRG. Individual stipends for research trainees or fellowships were usually reviewed by a special ad hoc committee appointed by the council.

In 1956 a program in special clinical traineeships was activated by the late Gordon Seger to give to physicians who had completed a residency additional training in their own disciplines of neurology, ophthalmology, or otolaryngology and in such allied fields as internal medicine, pediatrics, and neuropathology—fields in which such supplementary training seemed needed for teaching and research in clinical neurology.

Still remaining to be inaugurated at NINDB in 1953 was a program of intramural clinical investigations. The basic investigations were already under way in the joint NIMH-NINDB set-up. To the director the clinical program should be an important segment of the Institute's program for it would add a human touch to the grants and laboratory programs and keep the administrative activities in intimate touch with the life scene in neurological medicine. At the beginning this project seemed no more than a wish-fulfilling dream owing to financial insufficiency and lack of clinical space. However, with the increase in the 1953 appropriation, the completion of the Clinical Center, and finally the allocation of space from NIMH to NINDB in 1953, the dream became a reality.

On May 1 of the same year, G. Milton Shy and Maitland Baldwin took up their duties as directors of the NINDB intramural branches of medical and surgical neurology, respectively. Associated with the bedside examination and research program, certain clinical laboratories at the Clinical Center were soon established in neurochemistry (Donald B. Tower), neuropathology (Igor Klatzo), neurophysiology and EEG (Cosimo Ajmone-Marsan), applied pharmacology (Richard L. Irwin), and neuroradiology (Giovanni Di Chiro).

The Institute's clinical investigations program did not have residents in a strict sense, but it soon gained approval for training by the American Board and therefore employed young men as clinical associates. Several of these are already well known in neurological circles and are ANA members. Among them are: W. King Engel (now in charge of the medical neurology clinical investigations at the Institute), Kenneth R. Magee, Lewis P. Rowland, and Elsworth C. Alvord, Jr. (ANA associate member).

NINDB was not successful in immediately recruiting a director of the intramural eye research unit owing to the dearth of ophthalmologists at that time who were dedicated primarily to full-time positions in ophthalmic research. It was not until 1954 that Ludwig von Sallmann could be persuaded to leave New York for Bethesda. A better choice could not have been made. The structure of the Institute's clinical eye research program was essentially the same as that of neurology. A devoted advisor in the early promulgation of a sound intramural program in eye research was the late Jonas S. Friedenwald of Johns Hopkins (a member of the NINDB Council, 1954 to 1956).

Patients entering all institutes at the Clinical Center are called study patients and are admitted only by physician referral and only if considered suitable for inclusion in an ongoing research project. On discharge they are returned to the care of the referring physician.

Transportation to the Clinical Center and back home is borne by the patient except in certain emergencies. There is no charge for treatment or diagnostic procedures. All such procedures must have approval by a medical board appointed by the director of the Clinical Center.

The clinical staff at NINDB during its first decade of activity was greatly aided by the presence of several distinguished visiting scientists. The visiting scientist program permitted mature and independent investigators from elsewhere to spend varying times not exceeding 6 consecutive months on the Bethesda campus to participate and collaborate in the Institute's programs. There were many of these, but two come most vividly to mind: the late J. Godwin Greenfield of Queen Square, who beginning in February 1955 spent three 6-month periods at the Institute where he also finished his textbook in neuropathology, and E. Arnold Carmichael, a superb teacher.

Another aspect of the NINDB planning which the Institute started to develop at the beginning was a collaborative field investigations program. The NINDB thinking embraced the concept that many neurological diseases and problems could be most effectively attacked by a concerted approach often at multidisciplinary, multi-institutional levels wherein the Institute would function as a coordinating center and a central laboratory for the compilation and evaluation of data. Both the extramural and intramural programs (when indicated) were involved.

At the time there seemed to be good reasons for such an approach. Neurological research then, as practiced by clinical neurologists, appeared to be isolated from workers in allied medical fields and in the basic sciences. The study of many neurological diseases, if confined to one institution, did not contain sufficient patients for the production of valid statistical results. Scientific epidemiological studies in neurology requiring information from many sources both here and abroad had not yet begun. Research in the neurological diseases of infancy and childhood was a relatively neglected field.

Finally, there were many unsolved problems, such as the optimum structure of neurological education, which needed clarification. These, it was thought, could be aided by organizing problem-oriented symposia attended by leading authorities of institutions and disciplines. Thus NINDB was to become a sponsor for forums to air problem-oriented points of view in the general field of academic neurology and medicine. Many (too many to enumerate) such symposia were held throughout the history of NINDB, usually organized in cooperation with other institutions or societies. A rather intellectually sophisticated one was the National Conference on Education in the Neurological Sciences held in White Sulphur Springs in 1966, under the sponsorship of the AAN and the ANA, and supported by NINDB.[8]

The first collaborative field investigation, inaugurated in 1952, related to the uncovering of the precipitating causes of retrolental fibroplasia, a disease that was then only about a decade old but already the most common cause of blindness in infants. The project involved collaboration with eight hospitals and the National Society for the Prevention of Blindness. In a short time the offending agent was identified as the administration and duration of oxygen given to prematures in incubators. The completion of the project took about a year and did much to give early recognition to NINDB research.

Within its history NINDB has initiated many collaborative field investigations, most of them fruitful; there are too many to name here. Many related to epidemiological problems, such as the geographic distribution of multiple sclerosis (Kurland et al.), the genetic basis of one form of amyotrophic lateral sclerosis in Guam, the problems of kuru in New Guinea, and that of slow virus diseases (Gajdusek).

From 1951 onward the Institute's director was struck by published observations on the high mortality and morbidity of infants, especially during the perinatal period of human development. He therefore conceived the notion of promulgating a far-reaching, long-term pathological investigation of nervous disorders arising from nervous system injuries sustained during the perinatal period. Such a prospective study covered many disciplines and needed the collaboration of numerous institutions, involving the study of thousands of patients and their offspring. During the early 1950s neurological examinations of the newborn were imprecise or lacking; often a neurological

diagnosis was not made until the child was 3 to 5 years old. Obstetrical records in hospitals were usually incomplete; then there was a customary lack of liaison between the obstetrician and pediatrician, and between the pediatrician, internist, and neurologist.

In brief, the slate had to be wiped clean, so a proposal was prepared for the formulation of new uniform protocols and for structuring a vast prospective study involving 15 medical schools and calling for the examination of 50,000 women and their offspring for at least 10 years. The Institute, serving as a central laboratory, would pool, process, and integrate the data.

Because of the many difficulties involved, plans for the perinatal project evolved slowly. By 1952 the director obtained sufficient funds to explore further the organization of the project. After many more years of planning, pretesting, and many meetings with expert committees, the first patient was admitted to the main phase of the study in 1958. Fortunately, during 1958 the Institute procured the appointment of R. L. Masland as assistant director; his primary duties then were to take charge of the perinatal study. A monograph by Niswander and Gordon[9] on the subject was published in 1972.

A more subtle motive behind the perinatal project was to bring into bold relief the relative neglect of research into neurological diseases of early childhood, as well as the lack of interdisciplinary cooperation in this field of research. Among other things, more clinical neurologists with training in pediatrics and more pediatricians with training in neurology were needed. These needs were highlighted in symposia and conferences, which undoubtedly contributed to the significant growth of training programs in child neurology during the 1960s. In this endeavor Sidney Carter and others greatly contributed to the cause.

By 1956 the basic organizational frame of NINDB was already carved and formed. The three-pronged attack (extramural, intramural, collaborative and field) comprising research projects, field investigations, graduate training programs, traineeships, and fellowships was well off the ground. The annual appropriations had reached about $10 million. From 1956 through 1959, when the first NINDB director resigned to join another neurological research mission, all Institute programs had proliferated extensively, the annual appropriation reaching almost $30 million; approximately 25% of this amount was allocated to research and training related to research of diseases of vision.

Much of whatever progress the NINDB has made in the past was due largely to the unstinted services given by physicians and scientists serving on its various advisory boards, study sections, training committees, and its board of scientific counselors (this group appointed by NIH evaluated, guided, and advised the intramural programs in clinical and basic research). The highest echelon in the advisory hierarchy was the National Advisory Council which was the only one given statutory authority by the Congress. Selected by HEW and PHS, its membership comprised medical leaders, medical school deans, educators, and public-spirited citizens, basic scientists, and distinguished physicians in neurology, ophthalmology, and otolaryngology. At least two neurologists were always found on the Council; all were members of the ANA, and many were or were to become president of the association. The ones who served one or more terms were H. Houston Merritt (1950 to 1953, 1954 to 1958, 1960 to 1964); H. W. Woltman (1950 to 1954); Roland P. Mackay (1953 to 1957); Raymond D. Adams and Clark H. Millikan (1961 to 1965); A. B. Baker (1962 to 1966); John Stirling Meyer (1964 to 1968); A. L. Sahs (1967 to 1970); Augustus S. Rose (1969 to 1972).

With a few notable individual exceptions, neurosurgeons as a group were reluctant, despite many overtures, to participate in NINDB affairs until 1960 for fear of federal dominance of their own program; hence they had no official group representation on the Council until 1961. In 1958, however, the late Winchell McK. Craig of the Mayo Clinic was appointed as a neurosurgical consultant to the Council for matters relating to neurosurgical projects.

It was not until 1960, according to Guy L. Odom, "that the neurosurgeons realized that federal support was essential."[10] During the same year neurosurgical representation on the National Advisory Council was officially requested. In 1961 Paul C. Bucy, who had already served on the neurology study section, was appointed to the Council. Successive neurosurgical appointments followed: A. Earl Walker (1965 to 1969); Bronson S. Ray (1971 to 1973).

Once neurosurgical participation was committed, it added new vigor to the Institute's planning and programming. The neurosurgeons scored heavily in adding to the Institute's research potential and to their own graduate training program. They also entered the political arena. Bucy in 1972 became chairman of the National Committee for Research in Neurological Disorders, succeeding A. B. Baker.

During the latter part of 1959 Richard L. Masland became the Institute's director and deftly guided its course until 1968, when Edward F. MacNichol, Jr. took over the helm. Under Masland there were changes in program emphasis. Several partial research gap areas were filled, particularly in virology, immunology, and genetics; and additional space at Bethesda was acquired, even a new building for the basic research program. A program for career investigators was developed and expanded. The annual appropriations, as in other institutes at NIH, spiraled to approximately $116 million.

During the Masland era there was considerable proliferation of the training grants program, reaching 62 neurological programs in 30 states, 23 neurosurgical programs in 14 states, and 11 programs in child neurology and nine in neuroradiology in six states. The development of training programs and the motivations involved have been graphically depicted by Severinghaus.[11] More projects, both extramural and intramural, were funded by contract rather than the usual form of processing. Contract grants were unknown at NINDB until 1960, but the original program architecture and the central mission of NINDB remained essentially intact.

In 1968 eye research was broken out of NINDB and transformed into a separate National Institute of Eye Research. The budgetary slack at NINDB created by this movement was soon more than compensated for by increased research and training activities in neurosurgery and in otolaryngology and otology. During the same year the name NINDB was changed to National Institute of Neurological Diseases and Stroke. The change in name was resisted by the NINDB directorate but took place anyway owing to outside influence.

Recently emerging, innovative concepts on medical education and on health care delivery systems aimed at meeting the needs of our changing times may well modify the original facade of the national neurology institute. Since 1970 the NINDS training programs have been brought to a virtual standstill. The surge and dramatization of knowledge in the basic sciences may overshadow the popular appeal of disease-oriented research in many categories.

While these emerging trends are struggling to attain more concrete form, one thing seems certain for the remainder of this century: the government organization and funding of biomedical research and development will continue. Who else can afford it?

REFERENCES

1. Bailey, P., Sr., Williams, F. E., and Kamora, P. O. (1929): *Medical Department of the United States Army in the World War. Vol. 10: Neuropsychiatry.* War Department.
2. Weisenberg, T. H. (1924): *Military History of the American Neurological Association, Semicentennial Anniversary Volume, American Neurological Association (1875–1924).* Boyd Printing Company.
3. Hunt, J. R. (1934): The domain of neuropsychiatry and the training of the neuropsychiatrist. *Arch. Neurol. Psychiatry,* 31:1078.
4. Meyer, A. (1922): Inter-relations of the domain of neuropsychiatry. *Arch. Neurol. Psychiatry,* 8:11.
5. Bailey, P. (1949): The present outlook of neurology in the United States. *J. Assoc. Med. Coll.,* 24:214.
6. Pollock, L. J. (1949): Report of the committee on public relations. *Trans. Am. Neurol. Assoc.,* 74:16–47.
7. Bailey, P. (1953): America's first national neurologic institute. *Neurology (Minneap.),* 3:321.
8. Conference on Education in the Neurological Sciences, White Sulphur Springs, West Virginia, November 13–16, 1966. *Arch. Neurol.,* 17:449, 1967.
9. Niswander, K. R., Gordon, M., et al. (1972): *The Women and Their Pregnancies.* Saunders, Philadelphia.
10. Odom, G. L. (1972): Neurological surgery in our changing time. *J. Neurosurg.,* 37:255.
11. Severinghaus, A. E. (1971): *Neurology: A Medical Discipline Takes Stock.* DHEW Publication No. (NIH) 72–175.

The Nervous System, Donald B. Tower, Editor-in-Chief. *Vol. 1: The Basic Neurosciences*. Raven Press, New York, 1975.

National Institute of Neurological Diseases and Blindness: Development and Growth (1960 to 1968)

Richard L. Masland

The period of 1960 to 1968 represented a period of fantastically rapid growth during which the annual budget of the Institute increased from $41.5 million to $128.6 million. The results were a transitional period during which many new programs were developed and many methods of fostering, supporting, and evaluating the research effort were explored.

Throughout this period there was a continuous effort to achieve a meaningful participation of the NINDB Advisory Council in the ongoing extramural and collaborative programs, including both grant and contract. The work of the Council was greatly facilitated by the use of Council subcommittees for training and research, as well as special task forces of Council members and consultants to study and advise on special program areas. The greatest strength of the program was the unusual ability and dedication of both lay and professional members of the Council.

This report traces the evolution of certain program areas that were of particular importance either by reason of scientific potential, national interest, or neglect, and which for such reason acquired special program emphasis. It is important, however, that the broad base of the program from its inception and throughout this period was generated by the individual and nongovernmental scientists, and supported on a competitive basis within the regular grants program of the Institute.

Ironically, the intramural program of the Institute might be looked on in a similar light. The broad program areas of this facet of the Institute's activities were determined by the disciplines and research interests of the scientists selected as laboratory and branch chiefs. The nature of the research evolved without external manipulation.

A great impetus for this program occurred when the basic research segment of the intramural program, previously shared with that of the National Institute of Mental Health (NIMH), became independent, and Dr. Milton Shy was appointed Associate or Scientific Director of the intramural program. The following laboratories and branches were established at that time:

Medical Neurology Branch (chief: Dr. G. Milton Shy)

Surgical Neurology Branch (chief: Dr. Maitland Baldwin)

Ophthalmology Branch (chief: Dr. Ludwig von Sallmann)

Electroencephalography and Clinical Neurophysiology Branch (chief: Dr. Cosimo Ajmone-Marsan)

Laboratory of Biophysics (chief: Dr. Kenneth Cole)

Laboratory of Neurophysiology (chief: Dr. Wade Marshall; this continued as a joint laboratory of NINDB and NIMH)

Laboratory of Neuroanatomical Sciences (chief: Dr. William Windle)

Laboratory of Neurochemistry (chief: Dr. Donald Tower)

The intramural program also received additional strengthening when, on the recommendation of the Boisfeullet Jones Committee, the decision was made and funds appropriated for the construction of additional laboratory space for the Institute's direct operation. The justification for this important program expansion stemmed from two sources. Historically, the NINDB was established after most of the space within the Clinical Center had been assigned to other institutes. The new building was to rectify this inequity. Equally important, at the time of this decision NINDB was undergoing an impressive expansion of its collaborative and field activities. A major part of the justification for the new building (building 36) was to provide office and laboratory space for these programs on the Bethesda campus. Unfortunately, even before the building was finally occupied in 1968, the expansion of these and other programs had made this goal unattainable, and large segments of the collaborative and field program continued to be housed off-campus.

Initially, from 1950 to 1956, Dr. Seymour S. Kety held the post of director of basic research, administering a joint laboratory research program for NIMH and NINDB. Dr. Shy was appointed NINDB clinical director in 1953, reporting to the director of the NINDB. In 1956 Kety was succeeded by Dr. Robert B. Livingston; and in 1960, when the joint NIMH-NINDB basic program was dissolved, Dr. Shy assumed additional duties as scientific director of the NINDB in charge of the entire intramural program. After his departure, Dr. Karl Frank served briefly in that capacity (1965 to 1968) and was succeeded by Dr. Henry G. Wagner in 1968. During this time Dr. Baldwin served as clinical director for the intramural program.

During the 1960s additional laboratories were established: Laboratory of Molecular Biology (chief: Dr. Ernst Freese), Laboratory of Perinatal Physiology (Dr. William Windle), and Laboratory of Neural Control (chief: Dr. Karl Frank); and the Collaborative and Field Research (C&FR) division was formalized to include the collaborative perinatal project (under Dr. Heinz Berendes); head injury and epilepsy programs (under Drs. William Caveness and J. Kiffin Penry, respectively); and the slow and latent virus studies (under Drs. Carleton Gajdusek and Clarence J. Gibbs, Jr.). During this period (to 1968) the C&FR activities were directed by Dr. William Caveness.

Almost from the beginning, one of the major program areas of the NINDB had been the search for the causes and prevention of cerebral palsy, mental retardation, and related neurological and sensory disabilities (now being spoken of as the developmental disabilities). Drs. Pearce Bailey, William Windle, and Henry Imus, in consultation with a number of non-governmental scientists (including Stewart Clifford, Nicholson Eastman, and George Anderson) had developed a broad and imaginative program for this objective.

The focal point for clinical investigations was in neuropathology. George Anderson had spent a lifetime studying the neuropathological findings in infants and adults suffering from cerebral palsy. His efforts had been frustrated by the inadequacy of clinical data regarding the patients coming to autopsy. It was agreed that neuropathological investigation was at a dead end unless a study could be made of a series of patients for whom adequate clinical data were available. From this developed the concept of a collaborative study in which a large number of pregnant women would be carefully studied, extensive data recorded, and the events of pregnancy and labor carefully followed. Detailed information would thus be available in those instances where there was a defective outcome, and where the patients came to post-mortem examination.

The concept of the collaborative investigation drew support from the dramatic effectiveness of the cooperative project for the study of retrolental fibroplasia. Stewart Clifford, Nicholson Eastman, and Henry Imus moved progressively to launch this program. They blitzed the country on a tour of major medical centers, and by the time I became director almost all of the 13 centers which ultimately participated in the project had been signed up.

Each of these centers had agreed to study a given number of pregnancies in accordance with a standardized protocol to be worked out within the collaborating institutions and the central office in Bethesda. In addition, in accordance with a basic NIH philosophy that investigators should be free to follow imaginative and creative leads as they developed, each institution was also authorized to carry out "ancillary" studies which involved a variety of clinical and laboratory investigations relative to the problem of perinatal pathology. This concept provided an additional incentive to participating institutions through which to invest the interest and participation of creative and imaginative scientists. In addition, it was protection against a sterile pedestrian undertaking and gave the project the character of a broad "program project" in which a diversity of approaches would be encouraged.

The collaborative project was an "epidemiological" approach—the basic philosophy being to observe but not to experiment. It was recognized that within a clinical population of pregnant women there were sharp limits, and no experimentation or manipulation was involved. It was to extend this area of the program that Drs. Bailey and Windle developed the primate colony in Puerto Rico. Within the free-ranging colony on Cayo Santiago, it was proposed to have observations of pregnancy in the wild. This study would be paralleled by laboratory investigations carried out in the small temporary buildings constructed on the grounds of the quarantine station in San Juan.

From the outset this program came under bitter attack on scientific and philosophical grounds. At that time, goal-directed research had not received the popular support it currently enjoys. There was bitter opposition from prestigious members of the scientific community who resented the channeling of large amounts of money into a government-sponsored project. Certain members of the human embryology and development study section, which had been attempting to develop a program in this area, were especially resentful that the usual individual review of specific grants was being bypassed, and that government funds were allocated to research, details of which, in their view, had not been adequately spelled out. There was also bitter criticism of the project itself on the thesis that it was a "fishing expedition" without a defined hypothesis.

Because of the sizable sums of money involved in obtaining the base data for neuropathological study, its objectives had been markedly broadened in recognition of the fact that the number of patients available for pathological study would be very limited and that there was other important information that could be obtained from the follow-up of the surviving individuals. No protocol had been developed which provided an adequate study design for this undertaking. To this end Drs. Jacob Yerushalmy and Carroll Palmer, each an experienced man in epidemiological studies, were recruited to assist in the development of a set of objectives and a study design.

Owing to this still further broadening of the concept of the study, Dr. Yerushalmy was concerned that even with the large number of pregnancies to be studied the number of defective offspring might be so small as to provide limited opportunity for statistical analysis. To correct this defect he developed the concept of the "extensive" (later referred to as "ex-pensive") phase of the study. It was felt that by having a more limited perinatal protocol—in fact a revised set of standard obstetrical forms—and inducing collaborating institutions within the cities where the project was in progress to use these protocols, at least good obstetrical data would be available at very limited expense on a much larger population. At some subsequent date a review of the defective individuals within the community could provide a much larger number of handicapped offspring for investigation, but without the large sums to be expended within the directly collaborating institutions. A good deal of initial planning went into this facet of the study, but it was never implemented for lack of funds and leadership. However, possibly as a result of these deliberations, Dr. Yerushalmy himself recognized a similar potential within the Kaiser Permanente foundation program. Within this group it was possible to obtain standardized obstetrical data, as well as follow-up on a large proportion of the defective offspring.

The NINDB study design and objectives thus worked out were reviewed by the collaborating institutions and approved, and the study was launched as a pilot phase from 1959. The revised protocol was also reviewed by the members of the Human Embryology and Development Study Section at a workshop held at the Arden House in 1958. The stated objectives of the study envisioned the investigation of known causes of "unfavorable outcome," and also the "search for the presently unknown" causes. The major criticism of the project related to the question of whether there was, in fact, a hypothesis being tested within the study.

As the project evolved there was also continuing pressure for a critical scientific review of the ancillary studies. The justification for this question was strengthened as the project developed, since there had not been a sharp restriction on the allocation of funds within each collaborating institution between the funds spent for the standard protocol and those allocated to ancillary studies. Because the project was slow in development, very large proportions of the budget had become allocated to the ancillary projects. It thus became necessary to sharpen the distinction between these two components of the grant. Ultimately, the ancillary studies were separated from the core activities

and reviewed as independent projects. (In the
further evolution of this program, there was
continuing emphasis on adherence to the set
protocol that had been developed by the entire
group, and to this end the later years of the
program were supported as contracts rather
than as regular research grants.)

An interesting example of "spinoff" from the
ancillary studies was the work of Dr. Robert
Guthrie in the development of the screening
tests for phenylketonuria (PKU). This was
probably the first demonstration of the feasibility of broad screening during the neonatal
period for an inborn error of metabolism. Subsequently, laws were passed in a number of
states making such screening mandatory. There
was considerable resentment on the part of
some pediatricians who felt that this was a rare
disease and that such legislation required the
allocation of disproportionate resources of
funds and manpower. It has always seemed to
me that a major shortcoming of this program
was its limited scope—that having established
the logistics for obtaining a neonatal specimen,
one then had the obligation to scan as broadly
as possible, even though the other inborn
errors of metabolism which might be recognized
were even less prevalent and less treatable than
was PKU. A series of workshops were held at
NINDB, the purpose of which was to bring
together scientists interested in screening for
genetic defects with instrument manufacturers
from industry, in the hopes that industrial know-
how might be brought to bear on the development of a multiscreening "instrument."

The laboratory at Puerto Rico, although
originally thought of as having some interaction
with the clinical investigations, evolved along
a completely independent but highly productive
course. Under able supervision the free-ranging
colony on Cayo Santiago continued to multiply
and became a laboratory for the study of social
anthropology in the more or less normal environment. In addition, when the colony became
crowded, a certain number of animals were
made available for special virological studies, it
having been demonstrated that the animals in
this isolated environment had had little exposure
to contagious diseases.

In the San Juan laboratory Dr. Windle demonstrated that animals could well be raised in
captivity in this environment. In collaboration

with Drs. Jeffrey Dawes in England and
Calderia Garcia from Argentina, a series of
highly imaginative and sophisticated studies
were carried out, including demonstration of
the mechanism of action of kernicterus and
asphyxia in combination, and of some of the
remedial procedures. There were, however,
never enough pregnant animals for the many
studies that were being attempted, and it became evident that the productivity of this laboratory could be markedly enhanced by enlarging
the resources.

It should be noted that the work of this laboratory was of particular interest to Congressman
John Fogarty. It is fair to say that all of the activities of the Department of Health, Education,
and Welfare (HEW) were of particular interest
to Mr. Fogarty. In the hearing room of the congressional office building were photographs of
many of the installations of HEW. In my initial
testimony to Mr. Fogarty, I was astounded at
his intimate knowledge of the program. He
made it a practice to visit the Bethesda installation and a number of the off-site laboratory
stations as well. He made annual visits to
Puerto Rico to review the work of the perinatal
laboratories. In the spring of 1964, Mr. Eckart
Wipf (NINDB executive officer) and I went
with Mr. Fogarty to Puerto Rico to look over
the program. We met with Dr. Windle, and it
was evident that there was a need for expansion. Space was available at the quarantine
station, and Dr. Marvin S. Cashion, in charge
of that installation, agreed that a major extension of the perinatal laboratory at the quarantine
station could be accomplished without detri-
ment to the other activities at the quarantine
station. Mr. Fogarty was impressed with the
desirable nature of this location. Plans were
drawn up, and it was agreed that an additional
temporary building would be constructed on
the quarantine station.

However, before this program could be implemented it had to be reviewed and approved by
NIH. The following autumn, in preparation for
the congressional hearings, Dr. James Shannon
(director of NIH) and I again went to Puerto
Rico to review the facilities. During the interim
there had been very important developments in
that environment. Specifically, the Common-
wealth had established the new Centro Medico
at the site of the hospital at Rio Piedras. A

decision had been made to move the medical school to that site. Thus the opportunity existed to establish a research laboratory within the orbit of the university and within which there could be created meaningful cooperation with the community of scientists which hopefully would be developed in that expanding environment. The Atomic Energy Commission had already constructed a research laboratory at the Centro Medico. It was indicated that space could be made available to NINDB for a primate laboratory. The decision was made that rather than expanding the laboratory at the quarantine station, where it would continue to develop in relative scientific isolation, it would be preferable both from the point of view of the laboratory and of the University of Puerto Rico to establish a new center at the Centro Medico. Unfortunately, this concept was not discussed with Mr. Fogarty prior to the congressional hearings. When, at these hearings, Mr. Fogarty inquired about the status of the laboratory in San Juan, I reported on this plan for a new laboratory. Mr. Fogarty's response was, "Masland, you have been brainwashed."

The sensitive history of this laboratory is a saga of bureaucratic frustration. The funds were appropriated by Congress the following year. In spite of the most intensive efforts by Mr. Wipf, it required several more years before title could be obtained to property at the Centro Medico. There were further delays while a decision was made regarding the contractor for the plan. It was logical that this construction be carried out by a Puerto Rican contractor, but those responsible for construction in the government selected a New York-based agency for this work. It was at approximately this point that there was an expressed need for a similar laboratory space for the Institute of Child Health and Human Development, and a decision was made that the laboratory should be operated as a joint venture, and that it should be enlarged in order to provide adequate resources for both institutes. It was necessary to return to the Congress for the additional funds required for this expanded laboratory. This was accomplished, and planning went forward for this additional development to build a very impressive laboratory center at the Centro Medico. However, as a result of subsequent budgetary cutbacks, this laboratory has never been built.

In retrospect, there is much to be said for temporary buildings.

An example of what can be done on a shoestring is a program developed by Drs. D. Carleton Gajdusek and Clarence J. Gibbs, Jr. at the Department of Interior's Patuxent Wildlife Research Center in Laurel, Maryland. Like so many important developments, this program started by chance. Carleton Gajdusek had been sent by the Ford Foundation to the Near East to investigate an epidemic of poliomyelitis and to work in immunology at the Eliza Hall Institute in Australia. On his way home he learned of an epidemic of a peculiar neurological disease in Australian New Guinea, and with characteristic curiosity took off to investigate directly. He saw enough kuru in the jungles of New Guinea to become completely fascinated. He remained with these Stone Age people for a year during which time he worked out the full epidemiology of kuru and attempted to determine its etiology. On his return to the United States, arrangements were made through Dr. Joseph Smadel, associate director of NIH, for Dr. Bailey to provide the resources for Gajdusek within NINDB for the investigation of this strange neurological disorder.

Dr. Gajdusek established a field station in New Guinea and continued his epidemiological investigations, the general consensus being that this degenerative disease must be the expression of an unusual gene. Gajdusek carried on extensive epidemiological investigations but was not fully convinced of the genetic hypothesis, and we agreed that a program should be established to search for an infectious etiology.

It was about this time that reports came from Iceland that an infectious agent had been isolated from sheep suffering from scrapie—a disease which heretofore had been considered an inherited disorder. After conversations with Dr. Hilary Kaprowski, Dr. Gajdusek arranged to visit the laboratories in England and Iceland, and he returned with several specimens of infected material in his pocket and the conviction that scrapie was indeed a virological disease. The initial laboratory studies were carried out in building 9 on the Bethesda campus.

It was immediately recognized, however, that for inoculation studies of kuru we would have to use primates, and there would be a long incubation period during which animals would have to be protected from intercurrent infection. I discussed with Dr. Smadel the thesis that this could best be accomplished on an island in the Puerto Rico area similar to Cayo Santiago where the animals could be kept carefully isolated, and where breeding could be carried out in a favorable environment. Dr. Smadel was opposed to this thesis, pointing out that supervision would be difficult in that remote environment and that isolation was probably more effectively accomplished in a more accessible laboratory under more direct supervision. He could also have pointed out the problems of staffing in a remote laboratory. As an alternative, arrangements were made to build a small temporary building on the grounds of the Patuxent Wildlife Research Center, Laurel, Maryland. In addition, there was laboratory space available within their newly completed research laboratory there which had not been completely filled.

Shortly after the laboratory had been occupied there was quite a furor generated by the Department of Agriculture whose laboratories were adjacent in the Beltsville area. This group, responsible for the health of agricultural animals in the United States, were less than enthusiastic when they discovered that Dr. Gajdusek had introduced the scrapie-infected material into the United States. They were somewhat mollified by Dr. Gibbs' assurances regarding the care with which the studies were being carried forward. They demonstrated a complete change of attitude when Dr. Gajdusek, wandering around the hills of Kentucky, demonstrated that there were many infected animals already in the United States that were being quietly buried, without comment, in the hinterland. Scrapie thus became a problem of equal priority for our own agricultural welfare.

However, the project was not yet home free. Difficulties now arose at the other end. Although Dr. Gajdusek had had excellent cooperation in New Guinea from the health officers charged with the welfare of the New Guinea natives, officials in Australia were not entirely happy to have Dr. Gajdusek running free among the New Guinea natives. Although his relations with them were excellent, the official relations within this protectorate were of a sensitive nature, and it was felt that his

activities should be under official restraints. In addition there were scientists in Australia who felt that it was their responsibility to solve this difficult medical problem and that they were being impeded by outside interference. At any rate, a genetic hypothesis had been well established for which Australian scientists were claiming priority. At one time there was an official recommendation in Australia that Dr. Gajdusek not be permitted to return to the trust territory. Fortunately, better judgment prevailed; arrangements were made for collaboration within the research station in New Guinea and new work was permitted to proceed.

There has been too little recognition of the fantastic logistical problems involved in obtaining fresh specimens in the New Guinea jungles and having them shipped in liquid nitrogen for inoculation into various animals in the laboratories at Patuxent. Some of these specimens at Patuxent arrived within 72 hr of the death of the patient. The feat was made possible through Carleton Gajdusek's dynamic personality, his creative imagination, and the boundless energy with which he attacked the problem. However, it was also the result of a team effort, since the responsibilities for maintenance of the laboratories at Patuxent fell on the capable shoulders of Clarence Gibbs, and the logistical support was ably provided by the NINDB executive officer Mr. Eckart Wipf and his staff. It was the latter who had to wrestle with some of the more sticky administrative details. For example, how does one justify an expenditure of $15 for a pig—especially when the pig is to be used for purchasing a wife for the head bearer? I would like to feel that I made some contribution to this program in staving off the skeptics at NIH who were not convinced that this was the best way to find the virus.

In fact, many of us within NINDB were convinced that neurovirology was an important and overlooked field, and a number of steps were taken to foster research in this area. Drs. Gajdusek and Gibbs sponsored an important conference on slow viruses. Around 1963 word filtered from the Soviet Union that viruses had been isolated from patients with multiple sclerosis, and that a monkey in Sukhumi had developed the picture of amyotrophic lateral sclerosis after being inoculated with human material. An exchange mission was sent to the Soviet Union to investigate these claims, and pathological material was brought back for study in this country. It has not been possible to substantiate these claims.

Research on infectious agents also formed an important aspect of the collaborative perinatal project. Discovery of the role of the rubella virus in congenital malformations highlighted interest in the possible role of other agents, and it was determined that blood specimens should be obtained from all the pregnant women in the study and made available for prospective and retrospective studies. Dr. John Sever was recruited to carry forward these investigations, and within a short time his laboratory had developed an unusual potential for mass screening of sera and for the development of antigens.

At the same time that Dr. Sever was processing material from the collaborative project, he had also been attempting to isolate the rubella virus from soldiers afflicted with German measles at various camps throughout the country. It was through this combination of facts that Dr. Sever and I became involved in a confrontation with other virologists relative to the "discovery" of the rubella virus. Several years previously, a British scientist had discovered that the presence of one virus could be demonstrated by its ability to block infection of a tissue culture by a second virus. Dr. Paul Parkman at Walter Reed laboratories then used this technique to demonstrate that materials obtained from soldiers suffering from "recruit fever" (rubella) contained an infective agent, and he reported these findings. Dr. Sever recognized the probability that this was the rubella virus, further modified the technique, and using the resources available to him conducted a very rapid series of studies on material from his previous investigations of rubella in military personnel. Dr. Sever and his staff were the first to infect volunteers with tissue-culture-grown rubella virus and to produce clinical rubella in the volunteers. The first I knew of Dr. Sever's discovery was when he came to me in great distress saying that a newspaper reporter, while visiting a laboratory elsewhere in the United States, had learned of Dr. Sever's discovery and that he intended to publish this finding in the press.

Dr. Sever did not wish to be in the embarrassing position of appearing to report his scientific findings through this media and came to me for advice as to how this should best be handled. After consultation with several other scientists we came to the conclusion that these data should be reported to the members of the collaborative project with whom Dr. Sever had been working in other areas. We arranged such a meeting to be attended by representatives of the press in addition to the scientists, and invited a number of others to attend. I was completely unprepared for the hostile reception I received. It turned out that Dr. Tom Weller and Dr. Franklin Neva from the Harvard School of Public Health had independently isolated the rubella virus. They had not made this result broadly known but were proposing a joint publication in order that they could share the credit with the Walter Reed investigators. They were completely unbelieving that Dr. Sever could have accomplished in such short time the actual studies that he had. In spite of this, the die was cast since word had leaked to the press, and it was necessary for us to proceed with our report. However, Dr. Sever's paper, which he had submitted to the *Journal of the American Medical Association,* was held up for publication until after the reports of Weller and Parkman had been published.

Dr. Sever's work with the rubella virus put him in the ideal position to carry forward these studies during the great epidemic which struck the collaborative project at approximately that time. Working closely with scientists at The Johns Hopkins University and using serum available from the collaborative project, it was possible to obtain (hopefully for the last time) extensive epidemiological data regarding the impact of the rubella virus during pregnancy.

Viewed in perspective it is safe to say that during the 1960s the Institute was directly or indirectly involved in three of the most exciting developments in neurovirology of this era— discovery of the role of an infectious agent in scrapie, kuru, and Jakob-Creutzfeldt disease; final isolation of the rubella virus and development of a vaccine for the prevention of prenatal rubella; and discovery of the role of measles virus in the production of subacute sclerosing panencephalitis (SSPE). Whether the long-term effort launched at that time for a similar (viral) solution to the problems of multiple sclerosis, amyotrophic lateral sclerosis, and parkinsonism may have a similar payoff remains for the future to disclose.

The development of studies on parkinsonism has been another area of exciting development in neurology. Concern for parkinsonism was high on the priorities of NINDB—if for no other reason than that it represented one of the major neurological causes of disability. In addition, evolving research made it clear that advances were to be looked for in this field. Specifically, as early as 1962 in my congressional testimony I reported on the "unique chemical characteristics which render the basal ganglia unusually susceptible to certain toxic agents" and reported that "the recent discovery that certain of the tranquilizing agents are capable of producing parkinsonism is a development of tremendous importance. One substance called dopamine has now been demonstrated to exist in unusually high concentrations within certain of the basal ganglia. Differences of the urinary excretion patterns in various types of parkinsonism have been demonstrated. An accurate knowledge of biochemical abnormalities offers promising hope for a more effective chemical control of this great affliction." Working with the Parkinson's Disease Foundation, the Institute supported a series of workshops and conferences having to do with the role of the basal ganglia, as well as of chemical mediators in neural function.

The discovery by Dr. Leonard Kurland of a focus on Guam of parkinsonism-dementia associated with Alzheimer's-like cell changes in the neurons provided another fascinating clue to parkinsonism—a clue which still remains to be unraveled. The association of this disorder with the unusual form of amyotrophic lateral sclerosis also seen in that Guamanian environment led to epidemiological studies which demonstrated that the Alzheimer's cell changes are present in unusual frequency throughout the Chamorro population of Guam. In the early stages of these investigations, major emphasis was on a possible role of the cycad nut, a common source of nourishment in this environment. To exploit the research possibilities presented by this focus, a small NINDB-supported research facility was established on Guam and continues to be maintained.

However, it was not until the development of the program for the neurological research centers that the Institute was able to provide powerful impetus for a national Parkinson's disease research program. The research center program was the natural evolution of a series of efforts spurred by congressional pressures to develop a more systematic approach to a national program for the control of neurological diseases. The initial efforts of the Institute were engendered primarily through the support of individual research projects, and the direction and emphasis of the program were determined by the interest of the scientific community at large. Early exceptions to this were specific collaborative projects directed toward the solution of specific disease problems or questions. The first of these most successfully carried through under Dr. Bailey's directorship was that which settled the questions of the role of oxygen in retrolental fibroplasia. The collaborative perinatal project was a broad and far more ambitious undertaking of this sort. That program was shortly followed by cooperative studies for evaluating anticoagulant therapy and stroke, and the surgical treatment of intracranial aneurysm. This form of approach was particularly exploited in the efforts which the Institute made to encourage a more aggressive program for the evaluation of medical and surgical therapies. A small "collaborative study of the role of ACTH in myasthenia gravis" seemed to demonstrate that this therapy is of no value. Later, there was a cooperative study developed for the evaluation of ACTH in multiple sclerosis, a study which unfortunately had inconclusive results. Evaluation of therapy in multiple sclerosis has been and will always be an extremely difficult undertaking because of the unpredictable course of the illness. The long-term commitment required makes it difficult to retain the interest of the large group of collaborators needed for a sufficiently long period of time.

The development of the research center concept, with authorization for the development of centers for clinical investigation, offered a new opportunity for the development of broad problem-oriented programs. By 1963, 15 research centers and program projects had been established; by 1964 the number had jumped to 21. These centers were particularly effective in providing a focus on the major objectives of the Institute such as cerebrovascular disorders, epilepsy, and muscle disease. The Congress, however, increasingly questioned whether the Institutes were sufficiently monitoring the national research effort, and there was a demand for assurances that the program was actually directed toward the national interest. As mentioned, a variety of techniques were used to provide program review for the Institute staff and to be presented to the Congress. In several instances individual investigators were recruited to conduct a program review, such as that on epilepsy carried out by Dr. Preston Robb and on head injury by Dr. Alex Taylor. Some committees of the Council were also designated for certain program areas. Prior to establishment of the National Eye Institute, the NINDB Council subcommittee conducted a broad review on blindness. A similar subcommittee carried out an unusually broad and valuable review of the field of speech and hearing. Included in their recommendations was establishment of an intramural program in this field—a recommendation which was not finally completed until 1974, well after I had left the Institute.

One of the most effective of the Council subcommittees was that on cerebrovascular disease. Because of overlapping program interests, this was developed as a joint subcommittee with the National Heart Institute and was carried forward with Dr. Murray Goldstein (associate director for NINDB extramural programs) as the executive secretary of the committee. The results of this committee's efforts were most impressive and included periodic conferences on cerebral vascular disease, establishment of research centers, development of a cerebrovascular information center, and a number of cooperative projects for the evaluation of therapy. Included also was a series of projects on the classification of cerebrovascular disease, a development that has done much to provide standardization of nomenclature in this important field.

In spite of these several efforts, however, two key issues remained unresolved. Senator Hill and others were firmly convinced that the exchange of scientific information was inadequate —that there were scientific advances lying unrecognized, which if disseminated through the scientific community and to the practitioners could have a major impact on scientific advances and national health. The second concern was that the Institutes were not accurately monitoring their programs and scientific advances to be certain that federal funds were being used to the fullest advantage. Desirable though these objectives seemed, there was no immediate prospect that the staff of the Institute would ever be of sufficient size to carry out this type of review, and serious doubt that should such a staff be recruited specifically for this job they would be of the scientific caliber and wisdom to provide this type of scientific leadership. In an effort to resolve this dilemma, we developed the concept of the scientific information center. This concept envisaged the establishment and support of a research center staffed by scientists of unquestioned ability and stature within a given field. Affiliated with such a research center would be the establishment of a scientific information center within which data and reports in this area of science would be collated to be reviewed by the appropriate scientist. The results of these reviews would be disseminated to the scientific community through publications and research seminars, and then anything regarding the progress of science would be made available to NINDB to provide program direction at the national level. This concept was reviewed and approved by the Senate, and in 1963 Dr. James Shannon (director of NIH) and I met with Dr. H. Houston Merritt and his associates to consider the establishment of such a center at the Neurological Institute in New York where there was a group of scientists partly supported by the Parkinson's Disease Foundation who were mounting a multidisciplinary attack on this problem. Columbia had an unusually powerful medical library and staff, and it appeared an ideal center for an information program in clinical neurology. Subsequent to this other centers were established: human communication at The Johns Hopkins University; brain sciences at the University of California, Los Angeles; and, proposed but not implemented, vision at Harvard University. As the program evolved there was considerable modification of the original concept, with a greater emphasis on broad review and dissemination of bibliographic and abstract material, and less emphasis on program review within a scientific community.

At the same time these extramural activities were evolving, Dr. Edgar Bering and his staff in program analysis undertook the task of evaluating the thrust of the individual grants being supported within the intramural and extramural programs in terms of their program objectives in relation to national need. These projections were used to provide and highlight areas not being adequately attended (such as the neurological disorders of aging) and to mobilize support and interest in a more aggressive approach to neglected areas. It was partly on the basis of such deliberations that Dr. William Caveness was recruited to provide greater emphasis to the national program for head injury, and shortly afterward Dr. J. Kiffin Penry was appointed to provide greater emphasis and coordination of the attack on convulsive disorders. Through conferences, publications, collaborative projects, and the establishment of research centers, these neglected areas have moved ahead with dramatic swiftness throughout the ensuing years.

It is instructive to recount the vicissitudes of efforts to establish a national epilepsy program. In 1965, as a result of a meeting with the secretary of DHEW Anthony J. Celebrezze, the Secretary's Committee on Epilepsy was established to focus national attention on the problems and needs in the various areas of the epilepsies in the conquest of this disorder. The following year this group was redesignated the Public Health Service Advisory Committee on the Epilepsies under the Surgeon General, PHS, with two subcommittees: the Research and Research Training Subcommittee to assist the NINDB in evaluating ongoing programs and recommending new efforts; and the Service and Service Training Subcommittee to advise the Bureau of State Services (Neurological and Sensory Disease Service Branch) concerning services and manpower needs. The latter was abolished in 1970, and the Committee was renamed the Secretary's Advisory Committee on the Epilepsies, with authority delegated to the Assistant Secretary for Health and Scientific Affairs. Finally the Research and Research Training Subcommittee of the PHS Advisory

Committee was restructured and established in 1971 as the Epilepsy Advisory Committee at NIH. Under Dr. Penry's guidance the latter committee has functioned effectively since then, with three subcommittees: on basic research, epidemiology, and anticonvulsant drugs (with liaison with the Food and Drug Administration and the pharmaceutical industry).

At various points during the 1960s attention was directed toward the problem of instrument development. Events of science and medicine have repeatedly demonstrated the tremendous advance that follows the development of a new instrument or technological advance. During the early 1960s industry became aware of the increasing importance of the health industry, and we were frequently approached by representatives from industry inquiring about methods whereby their expertise could be brought to bear on medicine. Requests for funds specifically for this purpose were included on several occasions in the congressional testimony. However, because of the very large amounts of money that would be required at that time to achieve a significant involvement from a major industry and because of the logistical difficulties, these plans were never implemented on a large scale. During extensive discussions that were held with scientists and representatives from industry, it became evident that the most effective approach would require representatives from interested industry to work closely with laboratory scientists in order to obtain a really meaningful knowledge of the type of problem involved. In several instances research centers were established in which this concept could be implemented.

An area where instrumentation had a particularly appealing application was in the development of prosthetic devices. I had approached Dr. Wendell Krieg (author and illustrator of *Functional Neuroanatomy*) regarding the possibilities of developing some training films to be used in connection with a planned basic course in the neurosciences. It was our concept that these films might be part of a carefully worked out basic science program. Dr. Krieg was particularly interested in using photographed models with animation for the teaching of neuroembryology. In the course of these discussions Dr. Krieg brought up another of his areas of interest – the possibility of replacing defective human sense organs (eyes, ears) with artificial prostheses. There already had been some preliminary experiments indicating that the cerebral cortex could be stimulated artificially, and Dr. Krieg felt that if a large research center were established and devoted to this purpose some prostheses could be developed. However, throughout the scientific community there was much greater interest in a simpler approach—the development of visual aids and mechanically activated prosthetic devices for those with physical impairments. We held a series of discussions with personnel from the prosthetics laboratory at MIT, and a program for the development of prosthetic devices was in fact funded by the DHEW Office of Vocational Rehabilitation.

During his term as associate director for intramural activities, Dr. Karl Frank was involved in some of these negotiations with industry and became increasingly aware of the potential for the utilization of contracts in this general area. In parallel with broad programs for the development of the artificial heart and artificial kidney, it was recognized that there was an equal need for the artificial eye, artificial ear, and booster devices for implementation of thought processes in paralyzed individuals. At one of the scientific meetings Dr. Frank demonstrated the activation of effector devices through an electromyographic pick-up. Although technically very difficult, the required basic steps were obvious. There was need for a clear understanding of the basic mechanisms of nervous action, with precise appreciation of the role of each segment of the nervous system so that this role could be duplicated by instrumentation—by a mechanical or an electronic device. Finally the means would have to be developed whereby one could interface with the human nervous system, providing for recordings from it or stimulation of it over long periods of time. In regard to these three aspects of prosthesis development, the Institute's whole program in basic neurophysiology in reality addressed itself to the first issue. In fact, with respect to the justification for fundamental science, one would need no further objective to justify manifold the national effort in basic science at this time. The second requirement—duplication of such instrumentation—was probably the least difficult step (although when one recognized that the retina probably

represented an instrument containing 100 million computers, its duplication might not be so simple). However, the neglected area, and in many respects the key problem, was that of obtaining an effective input into the nervous system. The new laboratory of neural control under Dr. Frank was established (in 1968) to address itself to these challenging problems. I suppose instrument development and such research as that cited above represented a fringe area in the broad spectrum ranging from laboratory science to the delivery of health services to the sick. The respective boundaries have been an area of continued uncertainty.

Especially within the training program of NINDB there was continued criticism of that part of the program which provided funds for training in the clinical sciences. At the time the Institute was established in 1950, there were only a handful of clinical neurologists. It was recognized by Dr. Bailey and the Advisory Council that it would be most difficult to mount a program of clinical investigation unless there were adequate clinicians in the field of neurology and unless those being trained had a solid scientific background. The training program was established and developed on this basis, i.e., the training of academicians. The major initial emphasis was adult neurology. During the early 1960s a child neurology program was added, and programs in ophthalmology and human communication paralleled these developments. It should be noted that the program in child neurology created a group of neurologically trained specialists to address themselves to a field that had been largely overlooked at least from this approach. The experience of the NINDB training program as a whole was periodically reviewed, and it was repeatedly demonstrated that a very large proportion of the trainees, in spite of their clinical training, remained in research and academic posts. Whereas during the 1950s there were very few universities with significant departments of neurology, by the end of the 1960s there were hardly any universities without such departments. The Severinghaus report published in 1971 noted that in 1947 there were only 32 residency positions in neurology but the number had since grown to over 700. In 1955 there were only 15 independent departments of neurology in comparison to 61 associated with departments of medicine, psychiatry, or neuro-surgery. By 1970 the respective totals were 49 independent departments and 36 associated with other departments.

The NIH was under continuing pressure to become involved in the delivery of health services, since it was clearly recognized that the expertise developed by the institutes and their contacts with the university community could have a powerful impact on this problem. In 1962, under pressure from Senator Hill, the Congress appropriated $4 million to the NINDB for the delivery of health services and the implementation of scientific knowledge. The NINDB was prepared to administer this program. However, the decision was made that it was more properly the responsibility of the DHEW Bureau of State Services, with an experimental program to be established in the Bureau of State Services for training and research on the delivery of health services in the neurological and sensory disorders. This program was gradually merged into the broad program of the Bureau of State Services, and ultimately lost its identity with the merger of the Bureau of State Services into other branches of the DHEW. Thus, in spite of a very broad mandate spelled out in the initial legislation, the NINDB confined its program to the conduct and support of research. The implementation of this policy decision also involved a continuing pressure for elimination of the clinical research training programs which in fact died several times before their most recent apparent demise within the last few years.

A view of NINDB during the 1960s would not be complete without reference to the Institute's efforts to promote a world-wide program in neurology and the neurosciences. The post-war years were ones of enthusiasm for international cooperation. Within the devastated European countries where able and outstanding scientists trained and prepared for scientific research, they were entirely lacking in material resources and technical assistance. Many of these scientists felt entirely isolated; there was a great need for personal communication with exchange of scientific knowledge and training of personnel, and there was a desire and willingness for international collaboration. To further this effort, Dr. Bailey assisted in establishment of the World Federation of Neurology (WFN) under the presidency of Dr. Ludo van Bogaert. The NINDB made a grant to assist in the establishment of "problem commissions" which could bring scientists together to consider the world's needs in neurological research and to provide a forum for exchange of scientific information. One of the most effective of these problem commissions was that of which Dr. Leonard Kurland served as chairman for a number of years and which developed a world-wide program in epidemiology, especially of multiple sclerosis. Following Dr. Bailey's retirement as director of NINDB, he served as representative to the WFN in further developing an international program. There was particular interest in epidemiological investigations of cerebrovascular disease. Dr. A. B. Baker developed a protocol for evaluating pathological material, and from this evolved a number of collaborative undertakings in this area.

It was soon recognized at that time that certain types of research could be justifiably supported by the United States only if American scientists were directly involved. As a result, the concept of the "paired grant" developed. This involved collaboration between United States scientists and a scientific group in a foreign country. In many instances such grants were used to exploit the availability of unusual material or expertise in a foreign country. Collaboration of the investigator in the United States assured appropriate use of resources, guaranteed that the problem was one of interest to this country, and made possible a training center both in this country and abroad within which the scientific competence of each group could be enhanced. A number of paired grants of this sort were developed. This concept formed the basis of the subsequently evolving projects under the "PL-480" program.

During and following the war the United States had sold large quantities of material and food to countries on the fringes of the Iron Curtain. Such countries did not have dollars for repayment but paid in local currency retained in the country for expenditure by the United States under Public Law 480 (83rd Congress). It was determined by the Congress that some of these funds were to be made available for medical research. To assure that these funds would in fact be utilized in the interest of the United States, it was decided that a philosophy similar to that developed for paired grants would be utilized in the exploitation of these funds. I was sent to Poland in 1961 as chairman of a task force to undertake the development of the first of these programs involving our Institute. Through previous contacts we had obtained a list of Polish scientists in the neurological sciences who were well recognized in the United States. It was interesting that many of these men had been brought to the United States immediately after the war by the Rockefeller Foundation, had completed scientific training in this country, and then returned to establish laboratories in Poland. Naturally these men were known and respected by their mentors in the United States. We arrived in Poland to find the members of the Polish Ministry of Health rather suspicious of our intent. However, a meeting was arranged with members of the Ministry, members of our task force, and selected scientists within the Polish scientific community in whom we had expressed a particular interest. We sat on opposite sides of a long table something in the fashion of a small United Nations conference. I led off with a brief introduction indicating the purpose of our mission and stating our conviction that health knew no national boundaries and that it was our desire to find means for the support of outstanding scientists in Poland. I explained the paired grant concept and suggested that each of the scientists present might give us a brief summary of his research interests as an introduction. The concept was well received, and the remainder of that session was taken up with discussions by the Polish scientists. At the conclusion of this session it was decided that each member of the visiting team would undertake a visit to a group of Polish scientists in accordance with their areas of scientific interest and expertise. From these visits research programs would be devised which then might be brought back to the United States for review by American scientists who might be interested in collaborative research. This mission was much facilitated by the participation of Dr. Igor Klatzo whose knowledge of the Polish language and of Polish

scientists was of inestimable value. A number of collaborative projects were developed, those in neuropathology and muscle disease having been particularly productive.

In September 1965 I undertook a similar venture in Yugoslavia. A number of scientists from Belgrade had worked at the Brain Research Institute at UCLA. Some collaboration especially involving exchange of personnel was already in progress. Under the International Brain Research Organization (IBRO), in collaboration with UNESCO, a plan had been created for establishment of an international research laboratory on the Adriatic coast at Kotor. This proposal had received very enthusiastic support from the Yugoslav administration, and during the course of our visit we had an interview with Mr. Avdo Humo, vice-president of the Republic and commissioner for research. He expressed great enthusiasm for this project, pointing out that they recognized the need for the stimulus which their scientific community would receive from visits by foreign scientists and from collaboration with scientists from both East and West. They looked on the Kotor project as an ideal focus for East-West cooperation. Finally, he hoped that scientists from other countries who visited Yugoslavia would develop an affection and appreciation for their country.

With Dr. Mary Brazier and others we visited the proposed site at Kotor. It consisted of an abandoned chalet, "the palace of the Adriatic Guards," located on a beautiful point projecting into Kotor Bay. Nearby was a small biological research station. Meeting with selected representatives of the University of Belgrade, we then spent several days refining a draft proposal for establishment of a laboratory for marine neurobiology to be developed at Kotor under sponsorship of the University of Belgrade and cooperating with a new laboratory to be built in Belgrade as well as the Brain Research Institute at UCLA. During this visit we also consulted with scientists in Zagreb and Ljubljana. With Dr. Brazier a project was developed at the research laboratory in Zagreb originally established by the Rockefeller Foundation. A project of Dr. Milan R. Dimitrijevic, developed in Ljubljana, was subsequently funded by other federal agencies.

In retrospect the United States has benefited in several ways from these foreign individual research grant, paired grant, and PL-480 programs. The informal "diplomacy" achieved by these programs created in many countries — such as Italy, Sweden, Poland, and Yugoslavia — a truly significant measure of postwar good will. In several countries these programs provided the needed interim support until local resources could be mustered to support their biomedical research. Subsequent research contributions by these foreign scientists have benefited American medicine as well as their own. Moreover, specific projects have generated new knowledge often from unique foreign resources and often at a fraction of the domestic United States cost, with very practical benefits to the American public. An example was the use of the PL-480 mechanism by Dr. Roscoe

Brady in the NINDB intramural program to provide the essential radiolabeled substrates for demonstrating the enzymatic defect in the various sphingolipid storage diseases and for development of appropriate diagnostic and screening tests. In this case, the talents at Israel's Weizmann Institute of Dr. David Shapiro, the world's leading authority on organic chemical synthesis of sphingolipids, were enlisted to provide the needed chemicals through a PL-480 agreement. The results in improved clinical management of this group of genetically determined disorders, including Gaucher's, Niemann-Pick, Tay-Sachs and Fabry's disease, have provided dramatic testimony to the value of such programs — one of many, both domestic and international, that forwarded the research and training missions of the NINDB during the 1960s.

The Nervous System, Donald B. Tower, Editor-in-Chief. *Vol. 1: The Basic Neurosciences*. Raven Press, New York, 1975.

National Institute of Neurological Diseases and Stroke (1968–1973)

Edward F. MacNichol, Jr.

By the fall of 1968 a number of events had occurred which demanded a detailed re-examination of the goals, policies, and organization of the National Institute of Neurological Disease and Stroke (NINDS). The National Eye Institute (NEI) had just been created so that it became necessary for NINDS personnel to operate NEI as a separate entity until a permanent director and other key personnel could be recruited and adequate funds appropriated to permit transfer of programs to an independent institute. Approximately 25% of the NINDS budget was identified as activities directly related to research on eye disease, vision, and blindness.

The long period of NIH prosperity had come to an end. Budgets for all the institutes were no longer increasing annually, and cutbacks in funding had begun and were to continue throughout the entire period, while inflation and decreased personnel ceilings would continue to take their toll of NIH programs. We at NINDS often felt that we were sustaining more than our fair share of the cutbacks. During the years when bountiful support caused rapid program expansion the Institute grew so rapidly that its organizational framework had difficulty in keeping up with the increases in programs and responsibilities. Furthermore, as is inevitable in any situation involving rapid growth, some programs were less successful than others and needed to be dropped in favor of more promising new ones. However, federal personnel policies make such reprogramming of internal operations very slow, if not impossible, to accomplish.

There was evident an urgent need for program reorganization, particularly in the collaborative and field research (C&FR) area. In particular, the Collaborative Perinatal Study, by far the largest single program of NINDS, was moving from its data-gathering phase into intensive data analysis. This demanded not only changes in organization but personnel with skills other than those needed for patient examination and record keeping. There was also an evident need to expand some activities in the C&FR program (such as epilepsy, communicative disorders, and stroke), to redirect the program in head injury research, and to transfer some strictly in-house laboratory operations such as virus studies to the intramural program so that standards for review, promotions, supervision, and budgeting would be the same for all NINDS laboratories.

In addition, the question had arisen whether the Laboratory of Perinatal Physiology (LPP), an intramural program, should continue as a semiautonomous operation in Puerto Rico or whether it should be returned to Bethesda where its scientists could interact more directly with their colleagues. The relevance to the mission of NINDS of the most interesting and productive behavioral studies, being carried out by groups unrelated to NINDS on the free-ranging monkeys of the LPP, had also been seriously questioned by the Board of Scientific Counsellors. Finally, it was painfully evident that not only was no work on communicative disorders being done in C&FR, but there was none in the intramural program either. Yet research on communicative disorders is one of the major fields of NINDS responsibility.

The history of NINDS during the period 1968 to 1973 from an administrative point of view consists largely of attempts with varying success to cope with these key problems facing it at the outset, as well as with others, such as the need for an effective equal employment opportunity (EEO) program, and the move of the Slow Virus Laboratory from the Patuxent Wild Life Reservation—needs which became evident during the period. In spite of the attention that was needed for these major administrative problems and in spite of reductions in both funds and positions, it was also possible to initiate a few modest programs. Among these were the implementation of a program to develop neural prostheses and the funding of two major extramural centers for research in multiple sclerosis, three stroke acute care research units, and six studies for planning acute spinal cord injury research centers. In addition, a collaborative study of cerebral death was undertaken, a Stroke Commission was convened to advise on the future course of stroke research, and a National Commission on Multiple Sclerosis was chartered by Congress but funded and housed by NINDS.

By the end of the 1968 to 1973 period, planning for an intramural communicative disorders laboratory had been completed, permission secured to establish it, and search for a laboratory chief initiated. In the C&FR program, sections on stroke, communicative disorders, and bioengineering were established and the epilepsy program was expanded. Although the advisability of establishing one or more large centers for research on, training in, and treatment of epilepsy had been agreed on, and several conferences were held to decide how this was to be done, lack of funds precluded implementation of the program at that time.

In addition to the need for reorganizing individual program areas it became more and more evident that the entire structure of the Institute should be reorganized on the basis of diseases and the scientific research areas relating to them rather than on the basis of administrative support mechanisms. The Institute appeared most of the time to function as three separate institutes: intramural research, collaborative and field research, and extramural grants. Each of these was headed by an associate director who rarely had contact with the others except at executive staff meetings. Below the associate director there seemed to be little contact between individuals in the different divisions responsible for the same program areas. Furthermore, it was frequently the case that in a given program area no single person had complete information on the total activities of the Institute in that area. During the congressional hearings which established the National Commission on Multiple Sclerosis, Congressman Rogers severely criticized the Institute for having no one person who served

as a focus of activity for this disease. The deputy director of NIH had long been urging the Institute to reorganize along programmatic lines. Unfortunately no consensus on a reorganization plan was achieved during the period in question.

The Perinatal Research Branch (PRB) had the responsibility for coordination, data collection, and data analysis for the large collaborative perinatal study which had involved as many as 15 separate contractors. Until 1968 it was attached to the Director's Office instead of being part of C&FR where it obviously belonged under the then existing structure of the Institute. Neither it nor C&FR were subject to the rigorous technical merit reviews that were mandatory for the other scientific programs of the Institute. No firm plans had yet been made for a coordinated data analysis or the preparation of a comprehensive guide to the study data (the basic document). Furthermore, PRB and the Office of Biometry, also attached to the Director's Office, were not interdigitated in such a way as to make such efforts possible. Accordingly, the Perinatal Research Committee, which had heretofore confined itself to reviews of the activities of the outside contractors, was asked to review in detail the operation of the PRB itself. The upshot of this review was the assignment of responsibility for operation of the PRB to the Perinatal Research Committee until a reorganized PRB containing elements of the Office of Biometry and the Office of Biometry itself could be incorporated into a reorganized C&FR. In due course the first volume of the Basic Document appeared, and preliminary analyses revealed some important findings, among which were the observations that a moderate weight gain by a pregnant woman did not increase the probability of toxemia and correlated significantly with the health of the offspring, and the observation that babies with low birth weight or who were premature were far more likely to be mentally retarded and to have other defects than babies who were born heavier or later. The effects of such other factors as maternal age, number of previous pregnancies, smoking, socioeconomic status, and ethnic group were also investigated. In addition, a group at Tufts and Boston University used the perinatal research data for extensive correlative studies on the effects of drugs and medicines on the outcome of pregnancy.

The Virus Laboratory of the PRB continued its studies of maternal rubella and broadened its investigation to include cytomegalovirus, herpes, and other common infectious agents by developing improved immunological and serological techniques to screen the vast number of serum samples collected during the study. It also studied the rare children's disease subacute sclerosing panencephalitis (SSPE) and showed that the etiologic agent was almost certainly a defective measles virus. A serious problem had been the processing of the large number of pathological specimens resulting from the study. This was finally solved by discontinuing attempts to do the pathology in-house and contracting outside for this work.

The change in emphasis in the Collaborative Perinatal Study from data collection to data analysis had serious consequences for many of the PRB personnel. Numerous file and coding clerks were no longer needed, and some of the physicians, nurses, and other personnel used in conducting and monitoring patient examination and follow-up studies also became superfluous. Consequently we undertook a program of retraining and of identifying other positions inside and outside NINDS to which the surplus personnel could be transferred with the least possible traumatic effects. These employees had worked long, diligently, and loyally for NINDS, which now had an obligation to make every effort to place them in other suitable positions.

By 1968 C&FR had become a loosely knit collection of projects involving in-house investigations and external contracts. We adopted the policy of administering all research contracts through C&FR, even though some, such as the neural prosthesis program, might have project officers and scientific direction from the intramural program, and of transferring all laboratory operations to the intramural program unless there were special reasons for keeping them elsewhere. For example, the PRB virus laboratory was to remain in C&FR until its large responsibility to the collaborative perinatal program was ended. Furthermore, all laboratory operations wherever located now came under

regular review by the Board of Scientific Counsellors, and a uniform system for review of the promotion of laboratory scientists was adopted. All C&FR activities were consolidated into five branches: The Perinatal Research Branch, Applied Neurologic Research Branch, Epidemiology Branch, Office of Biometry, and Infectious Disease Branch. Sections on communicative disorders and biomedical engineering were added subsequently. The slow virus studies were transferred to the intramural program and became the Laboratory of Central Nervous System Studies. The pathology section of PRB was abolished and its image-processing activities were transferred to the National Cancer Institute.

A number of major changes in the intramural program were accomplished. Probably the most important of these was the transfer of the Laboratory of Perinatal Physiology (LPP) from Puerto Rico to Bethesda. The principal reason for its original location in Puerto Rico was the need for pregnant rhesus monkeys, which at the time had not been successfully raised in cage colonies. When the latter was accomplished there was no need for the free-ranging monkeys in the program. Furthermore, dated pregnancies could be secured only from the cage colonies. It was evident also that the young LPP scientists in Puerto Rico were suffering from the lack of contact with scientists in closely related disciplines. On the other hand, the laboratory was doing very valuable work on fetal anoxia and the effects of anesthetics and other perinatal factors on fetal development. This research was highly productive and justified both continuation of the laboratory and freeing it from extraneous responsibilities. The behavioral studies on free-ranging monkeys to which the laboratory devoted a major effort, appeared to be valuable and interesting but only peripherally related to the mission of NINDS. Furthermore, the animals were of great potential value in the studies of primate reproduction, circulation, aging, immunology, and many other fields more closely related to the missions of other institutes. It would have been short-sighted to have abolished this very valuable scientific resource merely because of its dubious relevance to the mission of NINDS. The primate holdings were therefore transferred to a contract-supported operation by the University of Puerto Rico and as soon as the transfer had been satisfactorily completed, operating funds and supervisory responsibility were transferred to the Division of Research Resources for operation as a general primate facility.

Another major change in the intramural program was the creation of the Developmental and Metabolic Neurology Branch by the merger of the Section of Lipid Chemistry of the Laboratory of Neurochemistry with the Developmental Neurology Section of the Surgical Neurology Branch. This came about largely because of the brilliant work done in the Laboratory of Neurochemistry on the identification of the enzyme deficiencies causing a number of inherited lipid storage diseases such as Tay-Sachs, Fabry's, Niemann-Pick, and Gaucher's diseases. It became evident that the time was ripe to start applying this knowledge clinically to prevent or alleviate the deleterious effects of the genetic lesions underlying this group of diseases.

In addition, a Laboratory of Experimental Neurology was established to study the development of experimental epilepsy in primates, and a Section on Neuronal Interaction was created in the Laboratory of Neurophysiology to house the personal research programs of the NINDS Director and the Associate Director, IR.

The most severe problems facing the NINDS extramural program during the entire period was the impossible task of maintaining the previous levels of research grant and training programs in the face of very considerable decrease in the buying power of the funds apportioned for research and the mandatory attrition of NIH training grants. The number of approved research grant applications increased at an accelerating rate presumably owing to decreases in funds available for support of research in areas of mutual interest by the Department of Defense, Atomic Energy Commission, National Aeronautics and Space Agency, National Science Foundation, and even the National Institute of Mental Health, which appeared to have curtailed much of its support both for research in neuroscience and mental retardation. The quality of the new applications was as good as ever, since the usual approximately 50% passed study-section technical merit review, but a much smaller fraction of approved grants could be funded, dropping below 10% at several National Advisory Neurological Diseases and Stroke (NANDS) council meetings.

In spite of the temptation to fund only what might be considered areas of special need, the NANDS Council wisely refused to guess that some categories of research were likely to pay off more than others, and continued to recommend funding in all categories, with continued reliance on technical excellence as the primary criterion for support. The Council continued to give special attention to young investigators with brilliant but untried ideas and to a few projects in important areas in which little scientific progress was being made. The main reliance for the development of special program areas continued to be on "programming" efforts by the extramural program staff. This consisted of identifying persons and organizations having strong capabilities in the desired program area and encouraging them to prepare grant applications of outstanding merit. Thus the methods that had previously been used so successfully to establish an extramural stroke research centers program was used to establish programs in research on acute care for spinal cord injury and for stroke, and for the establishment of comprehensive multiple sclerosis research centers.

The decreasing support and eventual cutoff of training programs reversed an important trend which had had far-reaching and beneficial results in the improvement of medical care, particularly in the so-called minor specialties. As Dr. Pearce Bailey so eloquently pointed out, prior to the advent of governmentally funded training programs the state of knowledge in neurology, otolaryngology, and ophthalmology was static. Although diagnosis in neurology was highly refined, improvements in treatment occurred rarely. The training programs created an atmosphere of scientific curiosity and permitted clinical specialists to obtain training in the basic sciences relevant to their research needs. The programs also provided financial support for the time faculty members spent in teaching clinical research which they could not otherwise afford to do. Also, the programs accelerated the development of important subspecialties such as neuroradiology, neuropathology, and child neurology. In addition, by providing deans with seed money the training programs encouraged them to establish departments of neurology, neurosurgery, and otolaryngology instead of reserving all available funds for general medicine and other major specialties. The reduction in training funds was felt first at the newer medical schools in which training programs had just been established. These could no longer compete for renewals with older programs of established excellence, so the programs terminated, and students and faculty members drifted back from part-time teaching and research to fulltime practice. Unless training programs are revived rapidly the rate of progress in the medical research specialties necessary to furtherance of the NINDS mission may soon be what it was 25 years ago.

The impact of the demise of the training programs on the basic sciences was thought to be less severe than on the clinical sciences since graduate students could be supported as assistants on research grants (albeit at severalfold higher indirect costs). However, comprehensive multidisciplinary training such as neurobiology or animal behavior, as taught in a number of institutions, has proved to be outstandingly successful in broadening the base of skills and concepts of young investigators, fitting them for more effective and more imaginative kinds of research. This training is very expensive because of the variety of faculty skills and of expensive equipment and materials they require, as well as the limited number of students who can be trained if each is to get careful individual attention. Hence it would be nearly impossible to fund them without government support.

The government-wide requirements for equal employment opportunity (EEO) programs to ensure equal pay for equal work, the hiring of minority group individuals and women to positions in which their skills and abilities could be fully utilized and the training of able and intelligent people for more meaningful and remunerative jobs all generated a great deal of activity within NINDS and the other NIH institutes. At first there was insufficient understanding of the problem and goals of EEO or of how one went about preparing an affirmative action plan. However, thanks to a dedicated group of NINDS employees of diverse backgrounds and levels in the institute hierarchy,

aided by specialists provided by the Office of the Director, NIH, and a firm of employee relations specialists under contract to NINDS, things soon began to move. Two retreats lasting several days each were held off-campus while selected individuals representing majority and minority groups, aided by our consultants, argued, talked, cajoled, and confronted each other. Armed with a better understanding of the situation a committee under the deputy director was able to prepare an excellent affirmative action plan, and steps were begun to implement it at all levels.

Unfortunately, our specified commitment to EEO came at a time when the budgeted positions in NINDS were being progressively reduced as a part of attempts to decrease overall federal employment. Thus the opportunity to implement EEO through new hirings was drastically curtailed. We were not permitted even to reprogram the positions vacated by the closing of the Puerto Rico operation. They were simply taken away and additional cuts were imposed. Furthermore, by executive order all government agencies were required to reduce their overall grade point averages, effectively stalling promotions. This made a mockery of attempts to implement upward mobility. In spite of these obstacles, NINDS made a healthy start in implementing EEO.

Perhaps the most spectacular research supported during 1968 to 1973 by NINDS (in this case largely intramural) was identification of the enzyme defects in a number of lipid storage diseases having serious effects on the development of the nervous system. Tay-Sachs, Fabry's, Niemann-Pick, and Gaucher's diseases are typical. Tests of both heterozygous carriers and of the unborn fetus were developed, permitting immediate control by prevention or termination of pregnancy, and giving the hope of future control by supplying substitutes for the missing or defective enzymes.

The studies of slow-acting neurotropic viruses largely by intramural scientists led to many important increases in our knowledge. The identification of the cause of Jakob-Creutzfeldt disease as such a virus showed that such human viruses must be more prevalent than the very isolated example of kuru previously identified by NINDS scientists as of infectious origin. The partial characterization of this group of transmissible agents showed them to be un-usually resistant to heat and chemical agents and to have an affinity for membranes, and led to the determination of the size of the infectious unit and to the establishment of their inability to provoke an immune response. That this has been done in a relatively short time, in spite of the fact that the only assay has been the de-velopment of the clinical disease one or more years after inoculation, has been possible only because of very effective planning and experi-mental design. Identification of the cause of subacute sclerosing panencephalitis (SSPE) as an incomplete measles (or closely related) virus was a remarkable piece of scientific detection, involving the recovery of whole virus in a mixed tissue culture. The development of an animal brain tumor model in dogs by using the Rous sarcoma virus deserves mention.

The studies of neurohormones and synaptic and neuromuscular transmitters, new knowledge about the mechanisms of synaptic transmission, identification of a large variety of transmitters, delineation of the ultrastructure of synaptic junctions, and chemical identification of receptor sites have been important additions to our under-standing of nervous system function. Develop-ment of an effective treatment for parkinsonism showed how such knowledge could be applied to the treatment of a severely incapacitating disease and provided strong impetus for the support of further studies in this area. The development of effective therapies for my-asthenia gravis and hypokalemic periodic paralysis was a major achievement and, along with the development of an effective treatment for parkinsonism, has given hope for the de-velopment of effective therapies for other in-capacitating diseases of the nervous and mus-cular system.

The development of an effective organization within NINDS in collaboration with outside institutions for research on epilepsy has been an outstanding accomplishment. A "pipeline" for animal and clinical testing of promising anticonvulsant drugs was established and used for the evaluation of several compounds. An excellent series of collaborative monographs to facilitate research in various aspects of epilepsy has been published. Very sensitive assays for established and new anticonvulsant drugs were developed. These have permitted rational evaluation of the effects of therapy on the basis of blood levels of the therapeutic agents rather than on the basis of the dosage the patient has allegedly been taking. Methods of telemetering and recording electroencepha-lographic activity in free-ranging patients to determine the frequency and severity of petit mal seizures were developed, and progress has been made in planning for the development of one or more comprehensive epilepsy research programs. None could be implemented during the period in question owing to lack of funds. Much progress was made by NINDS-supported scientists in the study of simple animal nervous systems with individually identifiable neurons. These investigators have shown that even very simple systems are capable of varied and com-plex behavior, even of primitive learning. It appears likely that the laws of interaction de-veloped from such studies will form the basis for analysis of more complex systems such as the primate CNS.

The development of improved neuroradio-logical and isotope scanning techniques by NINDS intramural scientists and grantees and by industry and others has been spectacular. High-resolution cerebral and spinal cord angio-graphy made possible the identification of very small vascular lesions. Isotope scanners and cameras using technetium and positron emitters have made it possible to identify tumors and infarcted areas of too-small radiological con-trast to be identified by conventional radio-graphy. The development of scanning X-ray densitometers such as the computerized axial tomography scanners (e.g., the EMI scanner) has made it possible to visualize such lesions and the cerebrospinal fluid system without isotopes or air or contrast media.

The Nervous System, Donald B. Tower, Editor-in-Chief. *Vol. 1: The Basic Neurosciences*. Raven Press, New York, 1975.

NINCDS Manpower Recruitment and Training Programs (1950 to 1975)

Murray Goldstein

BACKGROUND

The Problem

In 1950 research and clinical manpower in the neurological and communicative disorder areas were taxed to the extreme. Clinical neurologists were a rarity; academic neurologists in research and teaching were limited to a few national centers. Clinical neurosurgeons shouldered the responsibility for providing most neurological diagnostic and therapeutic services; neurosurgical teaching and research were essentially the "free time" activities of busy practitioners associated with major centers. Otolaryngology was primarily a clinical, private practice discipline; as in neurosurgery, teaching and research were the "free time" activities of busy practitioners associated with major centers. Basic neuroscientists were principally concerned with gross neuroanatomy, electrophysiology, and light microscopy; each research area suffered from acute shortages of trained personnel. The areas of cell biology, molecular biology, human genetics, and biochemistry were in their "modern infancy" and thought hardly relevant yet to the problems of the nervous system, hearing, or speech.

Thus the NINDB identified as its initial training priorities: (1) the recruitment and training of a cadre of teacher-clinicians and teacher-investigators to provide the personnel necessary for the development of academic departments; (2) the recruitment and training of basic scientists prepared to apply evolving technology to the problems of the nervous system and the special senses; and (3) the training of a core of neurological clinicians to begin to provide needed diagnostic and therapeutic clinical services.

Legislative and Executive Authorities, 1950 to 1973

On August 15, 1950, P.L. 692 (81st Congress) created the National Institute of Neurological Diseases and Blindness (NINDB). In addition to responsibilities for research, the law specified: "The Surgeon General is authorized to provide training and instruction and establish and maintain traineeships and fellowships, in such Institute and elsewhere, in matters relating to the diagnosis, prevention, and treatment of such disease or diseases with such stipends and allowances (including travel and subsistence expenses) for trainees and fellows as he may deem necessary and, in addition, provide for such training, instruction, and traineeships and for such fellowships through grants to public and other nonprofit institutions."

The Senate report accompanying H.R. 7035, the Fiscal Year 1962 Appropriation Act, which was subsequently passed into law, authorized for the NINDS "a program of professional and technical assistance. . . . These activities, in the view of the committee would include . . . support of professional training and health educational activities. . . ." The amount of $4.2 million was appropriated and apportioned to NINDB for professional and technical assistance activities. However, these programs were not activated within the NINDB, but rather initiated as the Neurological and Sensory Disease Service Program in the Public Health Service (PHS), Bureau of State Services (BSS), later transferred as the Neurological and Sensory Disease Control Program to the Regional Medical Programs Service of the Health Services and Mental Health Administration, now operationally terminated.

On November 5, 1962 the surgeon general wrote by memorandum to the director of NIH, on the "Support of Residency Training in Neurology, Ophthalmology and Otolaryngology: This memorandum will summarize my decisions following the several recent discussions among NIH, BSS, and OSG. Basic residency training in the subject fields will be operated as a single program with the NINDB having primary responsibility for the present fiscal year. NINDB will have the future responsibility of making adequate arrangements so that BSS can program to meet its needs, the objective being to correct deficits for personnel in community service and practice as well as in research and teaching to the maximum extent possible. . . . It is understood and agreed that both NIH and BSS can operate separate post-residency training programs designed to meet their respective needs. . . ."

P.L. 89–199, authorized on September 23, 1965, provided NINDB with a supplemental appropriation of $2.850 million for additional research and training activities in cerebrovascular disease. In addition to funds for research and for the training of teacher-investigators and research personnel in the stroke area, funds were allotted to the NINDB to be used for the training of clinical specialists in the cerebrovascular diseases and for providing physicians with the latest information about stroke diagnosis, treatment, and prevention.

On August 16, 1968, P.L. 90–489 (90th Congress) created the National Eye Institute, assigning to that institute responsibility for training in ophthalmology and the visual sciences and changing the name of the NINDB to the National Institute of Neurological Diseases; this name was subsequently changed to the National Institute of Neurological Diseases and Stroke (NINDS) on October 24, 1968.

Through legislation and executive decision, the NINDS had been assigned the responsibility for program activities aimed at providing adequate numbers and quality of professional and scientific personnel to meet the research, teaching, and clinical needs in the areas of the neurological and communicative disorders. The strategy for program implementation was derived from these authorities and the opportunities available.

Initial Program Activity

The Institute received its first appropriation during fiscal year 1952, an appropriation of approximately $1.5 million of which $79,167 was utilized for training purposes. During fiscal year 1952 the special traineeship and research fellowship programs were initiated with the awarding of a total of 26 stipends, 11 special traineeships, and 15 research fellowships. During fiscal year 1953 the Institute initiated its graduate training grant program by the administration of six graduate training grants awarded with National Heart Institute funds to facilitate the training of teacher-investigators in rehabilitation medicine. The research career and career development programs were initiated during fiscal year 1965 with the awarding of 14 research career awards and 74 research career development awards. By fiscal year 1970 the Institute's training programs had developed to include an active program involving 219 graduate training grants, 68 research career development awards, 12 research career awards, 226 special traineeships, and 89 postdoctoral fellowships.

Training Program Objective

The overall objective of the training programs of the NINDS has been the recruitment and training of skilled professional and scientific personnel to develop and apply the knowledge needed for prevention and cure of the neurological and communicative disorders. (Prior to fiscal year 1970, this responsibility also included the visual disorders.) Each training area effort had to be considered individually and specific program subobjectives and methods developed to meet those specific training needs. This was accomplished by establishing advisory and peer review committees in the three major areas of Institute responsibility: basic sciences, neurological disorders, and communicative disorders.

The following disciplinary and program areas were identified by the Institute as those requiring special consideration for training support from the NINDS:

1. *Clinical neurological sciences*
   Medical neurology
   Child neurology
   Neurological surgery
   Neuroradiology
   Cerebrovascular disease
2. *Clinical communicative sciences*
   Otolaryngology
   Communicative disorders (audiology; speech pathology; multidisciplinary)

3. *Neurological and sensory basic sciences* (e.g., neuroanatomy; developmental neurology, neurophysiology; neurochemistry; neuropharmacology; neurobiology; sensory physiology; biophysics; neurovirology; neuroimmunology)
4. *Neuropathology and otopathology*
5. *Ophthalmology and visual sciences — prior to fiscal year 1970*

NINDS TRAINING PROGRAMS, 1950 TO 1973

The training programs of the NINDS utilized three major approaches for promoting the development of personnel of the quality and number required to accomplish its assigned mission. These approaches included the development and support of superior training environments, the stipend support of trainees during periods of specialized scientific and professional training, and the establishment of trained personnel in academic careers of teaching and research.

Development and Support of Superior Training Environments

In each of the preclinical and clinical science areas of NINDS responsibility, first priority was given by the Institute to the development of superior teaching environments as a base for the recruitment and training of all trainees participating in the training program, regardless of career objectives or source of stipend support. The establishment of this as a first priority was particularly necessary in the neurological and communicative disorder science areas; this was especially true in the clinical sciences, since historically these disciplines had not received meaningful support from the limited resources available to teaching institutions. For example, the "average" medical school neurological teaching budget in 1950 was $12,983; because of the stimulus of federal assistance, it was $361,475 in 1965. Despite the large size of the United States population afflicted with neurological and communicative disorders and the long-term consequences of these diseases, in the past the neurological and communicative clinical disciplines generally had been assigned responsibilities primarily of a consultative or service nature by the usual medical school, teaching hospital, or clinic. The limited re-sources available to teaching institutions usually were invested in "major" disciplines such as internal medicine, general surgery, and pediatrics; the other disciplines, including the neurological and communicative clinical sciences had to look elsewhere for support.

In 1950 medical neurology usually was relegated as a minor part of a department of medicine or psychiatry. Although medical neurology has had a substantial historical tradition in research, during the years following World War II it received comparatively little attention from teaching institutions for the development of needed research and training facilities, and the recruitment and training of skilled full-time personnel. Otolaryngology and neurological surgery were usually part of the department of surgery; there they were often considered primarily service disciplines, often having to rely on part-time personnel from the surrounding medical community for teaching and research purposes. Speech pathology and audiology also were usually considered service disciplines, with little opportunity or tradition for research; they were housed for administrative purposes in otolaryngology, graduate school divisions, or community speech and hearing clinics. Neurological and sensory basic sciences such as neuroanatomy and neurophysiology, although identified often as specific academic disciplines with unique characteristics and problems, were part of general preclinical departments such as gross anatomy or physiology; the general departments, because of the many pressures and inadequate resources available to them, could give these specialized disciplines only limited attention, not the specific consideration commensurate with the unusually complex and lengthy training required of candidates in these areas.

In order to overcome these historical difficulties of lack of attention and inadequate resources, the Institute found it needed to develop nearly *de novo* centers of training excellence; this was necessary so that viable and productive teaching-research units would be available to serve as the critical base for the recruitment and training of needed teacher-investigators and, in selected areas, specialized clinicians of superior quality. In order to achieve these centers of training excellence, training programs at developmental levels of achievement were established to serve as the means of both altering the nature of the training to be offered and improving its quality. The graduate training grant mechanism was identified by the Institute as the instrument of choice to accomplish this; included in the grant was the provision of funds for: salaries so research and skilled teaching personnel from preclinical and clinical disciplines could devote themselves to teaching in these areas; the purchase of specialized equipment for the use of trainees so they could learn the rapidly developing technology of modern medical science; and the development of modern curricula for the recruitment and preparation of promising candidates for careers as future clinician-scientists, teacher-investigators, and, in special areas of need, clinical specialists. Not as a primary objective, but rather as a derivative of nearly equal consequence, these superior training environments in the clinical science disciplines also served to raise the entire level of teaching to all medical students and clinical residents in these and related clinical disciplines. This "side effect" was particularly important in the neurological and communicative disorders since the only foreseeable hope of beginning to meet the minimal clinical needs of the future in these highly specialized areas was through the training of both family physicians in the special skills required and the recruitment and training of a critical mass of clinical specialists prepared to deal with the enormously complex problems of disorders of the brain, the nervous system, and human communication. The training grant thus became a "pipeline" by means of which the latest information was disseminated to those preparing for careers in academic and clinical practice.

Stipend Support of Trainees

Although the Institute clearly had the legislative authority, the executive authority, and the responsibility for training clinical service personnel, the overwhelming shortage of teacher-investigators dictated that first priority had to be given to increasing the number of academicians so that the necessary number and quality of training units could be made available for all purposes. Therefore the Institute provided stipend support generally only to those

persons preparing for careers as academicians; the exception to this general policy was a congressionally mandated pilot program for the preparation of specialists and family physicians to care for patients with cerebrovascular disease. In addition, the Institute always insisted that it share with the training institution responsibility for the support of trainees, and not assume its total burden. For example, during fiscal year 1969, of a sample of 1,046 persons receiving postdoctoral training in the clinical and basic neurological sciences in training programs receiving NINDS training grant support, only 415 received any portion of their stipend support from the NINDS; comparable figures in the communicative sciences are 225 out of a sample of 475 persons receiving training. Trainees received full stipend support from NINDS training grants only when they were engaged full time in training essential to academic careers. Trainees previously budgeted from institution funds generally received only partial support from NINDS training grants, raising their stipends to levels commensurate with NIH and institutional policy, and permitting them to participate to a greater extent than previously in academic pursuits; this policy usually resulted in the training institution being able to increase the number of trainees beyond those previously budgeted. In any case, with the exception of the pilot cerebrovascular clinical training program, only those trainees who were designated as preparing for careers in academic medicine or research received any personal support from NINDS training grant, fellowship, or special traineeship funds.

In addition to superior quality clinical training, the clinical teacher-investigator requires training in research if he is to meet successfully his career objectives as an academician. This research training must be entered on early in his training program and carried out in parallel with his clinical training if he is to learn to utilize research techniques and approaches meaningfully. This has usually resulted in NINDS trainees in the clinical sciences having either to take longer periods of training than their colleagues preparing for clinical careers (often one or two additional years) or utilizing elective time in academic pursuits rather than service training. NINDS stipend support either through the training grant or special traineeship was utilized for recruiting academic trainees in addition to those generally recognized by the institution as necessary for service responsibilities. Through this cost-sharing principle the NINDS was able to supplement and increase institutional efforts, rather than replace them.

Levels of Training

The NINDS focused its attention primarily on postdoctoral and advanced postdoctoral training, utilizing part-time student traineeships as a method of introducing medical and graduate students during their free time to the possibilities of academic careers in the areas of NINDS responsibility. In selected areas of special need and priority, predoctoral stipends were made available on graduate training grants for advanced graduate students at the level of the master's degree or above. This predoctoral support was particularly important and utilized in the clinical science areas of audiology and speech pathology as well as in the highly specialized neuroscience areas of neuroanatomy, neurophysiology, neurochemistry, and neurobiology.

NINDS TRAINING SUPPORT

A summary of the support for NINDS training appears in Table 1.

CURRENT NINDS TRAINING PROGRAMS (FISCAL YEARS 1974 AND 1975)

The National Research Service Award Act of 1974 (Public Law 93–348) terminated all previous training authorities of the NINDS and substituted for them authority for a program of research fellowships and institutional fellowship grants. As in the past, research fellowships continue to be defined as specific fellowship awards to an individual, the individual being selected by the NIH on the basis of national competition; institutional fellowship grants are defined as competitive awards to an institution, the award including funds for fellowships to applicants selected by the grantee institution. The programs of research career development awards and teacher-investigator awards have

TABLE 1. *Summary of NINDS training support (fiscal years 1952 to 1974)*

	Number	Amount (thousands)
Research fellowships	1,122	$ 11,466
Special traineeships	1,699	32,648
Research career development awards	199	19,259
Teacher-investigator awards	17	1,097
Graduate training grants	446	191,035
Full-time trainees	6,300	
Part-time trainees	4,000	

been continued but as part of the Institute's research grant program.

The National Research Service Award Act also stipulates that research training programs be conducted only in those specific areas in which research personnel are needed as decided by the secretary of the Department of Health, Education, and Welfare. For fiscal years 1974 and 1975, specific research training areas have been designated by the secretary for NINDS training support; for future years this designation of specific areas of training for NINDS support will be dependent on studies of research manpower needs conducted by the National Academy of Sciences and other organizations.

SUMMARY

During the period 1950 to 1973, the training programs of the NINDS focused on the recruitment and training of individuals preparing for careers as basic and clinical scientists and as teacher-investigators. During the first half of this period, special emphasis was given to the development of training environments to serve as national centers of training excellence. In most respects the initial goals of the Institute's programs have been successfully achieved with the establishment of centers of teaching excellence in nearly all academic institutions. The future goals of the program continue to be the recruitment and training of basic and clinical scientists but will focus on those selected research disciplines and research areas of projected future priority and national need.

Introduction and Overview

Dominick P. Purpura

Neuroscience is primarily concerned with general principles underlying the development, organization, and operations of nervous systems ranging in complexity from simple invertebrate nerve nets to the human brain. *The neurosciences,* on the other hand, comprise a variety of disciplines, some with roots in antiquity (e.g., neuroanatomy), others of more recent vintage (e.g., neuroimmunology). *Neuroscience* is a way of thinking about approaches to the understanding of Brain; the *neurosciences* provide the ways and means for exploring this most formidable terra incognita of Man's Inner-Space.

Neuroscientists generally share the view that the next spectacular advances in the life sciences will be in the elucidation of neural mechanisms subserving different varieties of behavior. The ultimate expectation is the prospect of Brain comprehending Itself, a conceptual pheromone that has attracted outstanding molecular biologists, geneticists, and physicists to Neuroscience, with remarkably salutary effects. This optimism is by no means illusory as will be evident to even the most casual reader of this volume, for the past 25 years have witnessed the most extraordinary advances in neuroscience knowledge at all levels of neural organization, from excitable membrane to animal behavior.

It is a matter of record that advances in the neurosciences were greatly facilitated by research and research training programs of the NINCDS. The genesis of the present Golden Age of Neuroscience may be traced to the period just prior to the impact of these programs on neuroscience research. Thus by the early 1950's the ionic basis of the action potential was defined, excitatory and inhibitory synaptic actions were characterized, axoplasmic flow was discovered, and, somewhat later, the fine structural criteria for identification of synapses and the nature of myelin and the process of peripheral myelination were elucidated. During this period morphophysiological techniques for nerve tissue culture studies were elaborated, and methods were described for the isolation of proteins, lipids, and other complex biochemical constitutions of neurons and glia. Also by the early 1950's concepts concerning the organization of the brain were revolutionized by the discovery of diffusely projecting neuronal systems of the brainstem, and pharmacological studies of changes in brain biogenic amines associated with behavioral alterations dealt a mortal blow to dualistic hypotheses of Mind as distinct from Brain.

This volume in effect chronicles the present status of the most important basic neuroscience research areas that have evolved from the foregoing seminal investigations. This collection of relatively brief essays prepared by outstanding neuroscientists has been developed historically and with a view toward emphasis on the most significant features of the latest advances in different disciplines. The emergent theme is that intense pursuit of lines of inquiry concerning fundamental mechanisms and structure-function relations in nervous systems is the only rational approach to the understanding, management, control, and prevention of neurological disorders. Several of the present and future extrapolations of these lines of inquiry are summarized here to illustrate the wide spectrum of subjects considered.

Electron microscopic studies of junctional membrane structure have been greatly facilitated by the application of freeze-fracture etching (FFE) methods for cleaving membranes and thereby revealing different spatial arrangements of intramembranous components. These investigations have now provided suitable criteria for distinguishing, along morphological lines, different functional types of junctional complexes, i.e., gap junctions, tight junctions, and desmosomes. That some of the intramembranous components demonstrated by FFE and X-ray diffraction methods are protein macromolecules seems likely as indicated by several of the contributions in this volume. It may be anticipated that future studies will provide the morphological evidence required to satisfy the fluid mosaic model of the membrane which represents a significant modification of the unit membrane model that has enjoyed considerable success for several decades.

Freeze-fracture techniques have also permitted visualization of possible transmitter release sites in presynaptic membranes and of receptor sites in postsynaptic membranes. There is also a strong suggestion that calcium-binding sites in synaptic vesicles have now been identified. The extent to which present electron microscopic studies of synaptic operations complement and supplement earlier physiological views on mechanisms of chemical synaptic transmission is especially noteworthy.

The functional architecture of excitable membranes is now amenable to analysis by a host of pharmacological and electrophysiological techniques, particularly those employed for measuring gating currents in ionic channels. Not too long ago measurement of the impedance drop in nerve during the passage of an impulse was correctly hailed as an outstanding technological achievement. Today the claim can be made for complete characterization of the ionic channel for sodium in squid axon! There is even the suggestion that the channel is an oxygen-lined pore, 3×5 Å across, that acts like a selectivity filter at least according to one interpretation of tetrodotoxin-binding studies. As indicated in the chapters on these subjects, the individual sodium and potassium channels of axons may soon be available for analysis by protein chemists. Clearly this would be an extension of a line of inquiry on postsynaptic and extrajunctional receptors in neuronal membrane that has employed putative transmitters and ligands for isolation and characterization of different receptors. It will be of importance to define the characteristics of different types of postsynaptic receptors operated by a single transmitter such as serotonin in view of studies reported in this volume to the effect that receptors for this neurotransmitter in molluscan neurons are linked to a variety of ionic conductance increase and decrease mechanisms. Studies of acetylcholine receptors as well as the receptors for glycine, glutamate, and gamma-aminobutyric acid in the central nervous system herald a new wave of pharmacologicalhisto-

chemical studies employing immunocytological methods for identification and localization of receptor sites. The discovery of opiate-receptor sites in the brain has already generated new concepts of pain and morphine analgesia; and it seems likely that further studies of receptors for Substance P and the indolealkylamines may also provide new clues to operation of synaptic systems involved in somatic sensation as well as the analgesic effects of brainstem and dorsal column stimulation.

Perturbations of the excitable plasma membrane of neurons characterize one class of information-transfer processes required for rapid signalling in neuronal subsystems. The earlier discovery of axoplasmic flow identified a second class of transfer processes involving intraneuronal movement of macromolecular components and other biochemical constituents. The several reports dealing with current investigations of axoplasmic transport processes emphasize the operation of a variety of kinetic mechanisms subserving the anterograde and retrograde transfer of endogenous as well as exogenous materials. The role of microtubules in these transport processes is particularly intriguing since disorders of microtubule assembly may be of significance in the pathogenesis of the presenile and senile dementias. Studies of microtubule proteins and axoplasmic transport illustrate the convergence of two lines of basic neurobiological inquiry on an important and possibly preventable class of neurological and behavioral disorders.

Apart from the impetus that axoplasmic transport studies have given to the analysis of metabolic signalling in neuron-neuron and neuron-glia intercellular relations, such studies have had a powerful influence on the development of current neuroanatomical investigations. Retrograde transport of horseradish peroxidase (HRP) taken up by presynaptic terminals and transported to the neuron cell bodies and dendrites now permits identification of afferent projection systems to the site of HRP injection. Intracellular injection of HRP is also a useful method for identifying single cells impaled in electrophysiological studies. Uptake of labeled amino acids or sugars by neurons is followed by incorporation of the label into proteins or glycoproteins and anterograde transport to axonal terminals. Under appropriate conditions release of the labeled macromolecule at nerve endings and subsequent re-uptake by postsynaptic elements can be demonstrated. In this fashion synaptically related systems can be revealed with the accuracy of an electrophysiological investigation of monosynaptic connections. As described in this volume, the application of these new neuroanatomical methods to studies of projection systems in the vertebrate brain has called-up for reexamination of some of the most "established" neuroanatomical connections (for example, the projection of the fornix to the hypothalamus). Contrary to traditional teachings it seems likely from recent studies in the rat that this projection does not arise from the hippocampus proper but from the subiculum! Whether the same is true in the primate brain is not known. What is at issue here is the anatomical reality of the "Papez circuit," a neuronal system that has figured so prominently in hypotheses concerning the neuroanatomical substrate of emotion for several decades.

Perhaps no area of neurobiology is more intriguing than that concerning the factors determining the specificity of neuronal connections. How do neurons recognize each other? What processes influence connectivity patterns? To what extent are nervous systems modifiable by use, disuse, and abuse? Studies reported in several of the following chapters focus upon the probable nature of cell-surface 'recognition' factors in interneuronal relations and the manner in which these factors are regulated. The fact that some of the most exciting work in this area of cellular recognition has been concerned with adhesion molecules in sponges and slime molds emphasizes the broad scope of the inquiry and the extraordinary range of interests and activities of neuroscientists in general.

The development of neuronal subsystems involves more than the proper interaction of 'recognition molecules' on neuronal cell surfaces. The role of specialized glial elements such as those that span embryonic cortical structures and act as guidelines for migrating neurons are now well established. Other modulating agents such as nerve growth factor must also play a crucial role in the development of some varieties of neuronal connections as described in this volume. Apropos of this there is now evidence for a very early development of catecholamine

and indolealkylamine pathways in the mammalian brain, as indicated by histofluorescence studies. Other investigations involving the biochemical determination of biogenic amines have now yielded a wealth of data on the role of norepinephrine, dopamine, serotonin, and probably epinephrine in virtually all brain functions. It is remarkable how many regulatory processes in neuronal operations have now been identified in relation to biogenic amine systems. Induction of synthesizing enzymes, activation of adenylate cyclase, and feedback inhibition of transmitter synthesis are but a few of the processes influenced by biogenic amines. And this says nothing about possible interactions between catecholamine and other putative transmitters such as acetylcholine and gamma-aminobutyric acid in the corpus striatum.

It will be appreciated that the original discoveries in the early 1950's of "biogenic amine depletion" produced by tranquilizers such as chlorpromazine and reserpine was little more than the opening major chord of a complex but as yet unfinished symphony. To the early qualitative histochemical fluorescence surveys of biogenic amine pathways in the mammalian brain have been added quantitative biochemical and immunocytological methods that have led to extensive reinterpretation of earlier findings. Indeed, few of the hypotheses that seemed so attractive a few years ago concerning the role of biogenic amines in behavior have survived intact to the present writing. Nevertheless it is encouraging that those who have contributed most to the field of biogenic amine biology have been among the first to caution against premature speculation and careless extrapolation to problems of clinical neurology and psychiatry. It is important to define the remarkable progress that has been made in the general area of the biogenic amines but it is equally important to emphasize current dilemmas. Such a balanced presentation is included in this volume.

A decade ago we learned that dopamine played a role in the pathogenesis of the dyskinesias. The impact of this discovery on the clinical management of parkinsonism and other movement disorders is now a matter of record. If we have made little progress in defining more precisely the role of dopamine in the organization of motor sensory processes, then this can only reflect the complexity of the problem, not the inadequacy of the effort. After all, aspirin has been with us much longer than dopamine but only recently has the triple action of aspirin (analgesic, antipyretic, and anti-inflammatory) been susceptible to pharmacological analysis at the biochemical level since the discovery of the ubiquitous prostaglandins. Hopefully the rapidly developing field of receptology will provide the methodological approaches for the further definition of the molecular pharmacology of dopamine and other transmitter and 'synapse-modulating' agents. There can be no question but that the general field of 'Neuro-receptology,' combining immunology, molecular biology, and biochemical pharmacology, will undergo the most impressive growth spurt of all the neurosciences in the next decade. The reasons for this are clearly indicated in this volume in studies on morphine receptors, hypothalamic releasing factors, amino acid transmitters, acetylcholine, and biogenic amine receptors.

The nature of membrane receptors is but a small aspect of the concern for the general biochemistry of neuronal and glial membranes. Closely related to this area of inquiry are the lysosomal storage diseases and the immunopathological disorders which include multiple sclerosis and myasthenia gravis. Characterization of precise enzymatic deficiencies in a number of the neurolipidoses has been one of the most outstanding achievements in neurobiology during the past 15 years. Some of the fundamental biochemical studies of lipids, proteolipids, and glycolipids and glycoproteins that have contributed to these successes are considered in this volume. The discovery of an actomyosin-like system in neurons that may function in the release of transmitter from synaptic vesicles or in dendritic and axonal growth cone operations is only one of the many neurochemical advances of the past decade that are likely to generate entirely new approaches to structure-function relations.

Not too long ago the first studies linking protein synthesis to the establishment of 'memory traces' were published, and received mixed reactions from the scientific community. Today, after considerable effort to separate fact from fantasy, it is reasonably certain that biochemical mechanisms involving protein synthesis underlie the establishment of some varieties of memory and learning. The description

of the latest research in this area summarizes one of the most fascinating adventures of modern biology, the quest for the nature of Memory.

One of the central dogmas of Neuroscience is that *neurons make synapses and synapses make behavior.* Up to this point this Introduction has considered essays that deal largely with advances in understanding neuronal and synaptic processes at molecular, macromolecular, and membrane levels of organization. But a broader canvas is portrayed here upon which the fundamental elements of neurons and synapses (and extraneuronal factors) are combined to provide the forms and features of neuronal subsystems operations in specific macrostructures. The vertebrate retina has long been considered a key macrostructure for unlocking the fundamentals of structure-function relations in the brain. Such an expectation is admirably justified by the chapter on the retina which first considers the synaptic organization of inner and outer plexiform layers and then attempts to assign specific functional characteristics of vision to different elements within these layers. Another extension of brain macrostructure, the olfactory bulb, is similarly treated in an essay dealing with one of the most complex sensory information processing problems: the encoding of odors.

Life is synonymous with Movement, the projection of self into extrapersonal space. Sherrington long ago recognized Movement as a major evolutionary pressure for nervous system specializations in general. Little wonder that he devoted virtually his entire scientific career to the elucidation of elementary as well as integrative aspects of Movement control. It is possible to trace a direct line of progress from his early studies of spinal reflexes to current concerns for the integrative operations of identifiable spinal interneurons. What is particularly impressive about present studies is the extent to which analysis of the organization of locomotion is currently being pursued at microphysiological and pharmacological levels. The essays concerned with spinal and cerebral mechanisms of movement control succinctly summarize a wealth of new data that draw ever closer to an understanding of *how* and perhaps even *where* in the brain the signals for movement originate. No doubt an integral component of the motor sensory control system resides in the cerebellum whose neural elements individually and collectively have yielded some of the most important clues to the morphophysiological organization of cortical structures.

Based on current rates of progress it is safe to predict that the next few years will see the development of a major theory of movement control as judged from data obtained in studies of vestibular-ocular reflexes and their modification in animals and man. Furthermore the role of the cerebellum in motor learning mechanisms will be a central feature of this theory as is already evident from several chapters in this volume. But this is only one aspect of the progress in Neuroscience that is directly attributable to recent studies of cerebellar structure and function. Analyses of spike generation and propagation in Purkinje cell dendrites have provided new dimensions of the integrative properties of dendritic systems. The discovery of locus coeruleus-cerebellar projections that liberate norepinephrine and produce long-lasting suppression of Purkinje cell discharges indicates that inhibitory output from the cerebellar cortex may in itself be modulated by 'inhibitory' synaptic events that are distinct from the ionic conductance increase mechanisms subserving inhibitory postsynaptic potentials in the mammalian brain. The mechanisms of drug-induced tremor and the nature of synchronized, inferior olivary input to Purkinje cells contribute further to the understanding of brain mechanisms in normal and abnormal states of functional activity.

The last chapter of this volume is prologue to the neurobiology of behavior. Invertebrate nervous systems provide opportunities for precise definition of pathways involved in clearly identifiable behaviors, some of which may be modifiable by genetic and environmental perturbations. Such studies permit exploitation of the full range of methods, techniques, and approaches that collectively comprise the basic neurosciences. Taken together with the other approaches summarized in this volume it is reasonable to expect that neuroscientists will soon understand *how* and perhaps even *why* simple nervous systems work the way they do.

The foregoing survey has traced the strategies and tactics required for the final ascent to the acme of the biological evolution, the human brain. Both the urgency and hazards of the mission are clear, for there will be few easy victories of understanding. Disorders of brain function are among the most devastating and tragic of human conditions and this is reason enough to mount the enormous effort demanded for the task ahead. However uncertain the initial steps along the way may be it is comforting to know that *even the lowly turtle must stick its neck out to make progress!*

The Nervous System, Donald B. Tower, Editor-in-Chief. *Vol. 1: The Basic Neurosciences.* Raven Press, New York, 1975.

Junctional Membrane Structure

Norton B. Gilula

The plasma membranes of most metazoan cells are differentiated to enable the cells to regulate their internal and external environments as well as to interact with other cells. The membrane specializations that are involved in cellular interactions are generally termed cell-to-cell contacts or cell junctions (1). The primary purpose of this chapter is to review briefly the structural and functional properties of some of the well-characterized junctional membranes.

DESCRIPTION OF JUNCTIONAL MEMBRANE STRUCTURES

The Gap Junction

Approximately 18 years ago, the electrotonic synapse was first described by Furshpan and Potter (2) between neurons in the crayfish central nervous system. Since that time, the electrotonic synapse, or a low-resistance cell-to-cell pathway, has been described in a variety of both excitable and nonexcitable tissues (3–5). Subsequently a phenomenon termed "metabolic cooperation between cells" was described by Subak-Sharpe et al. (6). This phenomenon involves the cell-to-cell transfer of a small metabolite. Recently it was demonstrated that both electrotonic and metabolic transmission can take place between cells simultaneously (7,8). Furthermore Gilula et al. (7) found that a specific structural pathway, the gap junction, was necessary for both of these phenomena to occur between cells in culture. This type of cell-to-cell interaction, conveniently referred to as intercellular communication (3), is epitomized by the electrical synapse that is responsible for the beat synchronization of cells in the myocardium (9).

In 1962 Dewey and Barr (10) described an intimate junctional interaction between muscle cells. In electron microscopic thin sections, this structure had a pentalaminar appearance and the authors described it as the nexus. Thus the nexus was often confused with another pentalaminar junctional element, the zonula occludens (11), for the following 5 years. In 1967 Revel and Karnovsky (12) provided the basis for a clear distinction between a pentalaminar and a septilaminar junctional structure. They demonstrated that a certain kind of pentalaminar junction could be penetrated with the electron-dense extracellular tracer lanthanum hydroxide, whereas other junctions could not be penetrated. The septilaminar structures were comprised of two unit membranes that were separated by a 20- to 40-A space or "gap." Thus the term gap junction appeared in the literature to distinguish the septilaminar structure from the pentalaminar one. With the application of the freeze-fracture technique to junctional membrane studies (13–16), the gap junction was rapidly characterized in a wide variety of tissues (1,17,18). To date, in virtually every adequately characterized system, gap junctions have been demonstrated to coexist with electrotonic cell coupling (for reviews see refs. 1,2,5).

In thin sections the gap junction can be resolved as a septilaminar (seven-layered) structure that is comprised of two 75-Å-thick unit membranes separated by a 20- to- 40-Å space or gap (Figs. 1 and 6). The width of the structure is 150 to 190 Å, or a maximum of 40 Å greater than the combined thickness of two unit membranes. When electron-opaque tracers, such as colloidal lanthanum hydroxide, are used, the 20- to 40-Å gap is penetrated by the electron-dense material (12). A polygonal lattice of 70- to 80-A subunits can be resolved in *en face* views of lanthanum-impregnated gap junctions (12,15). A similar polygonal lattice has been described with permanganate fixation (19) and negative staining of isolated membranes (20).

In freeze-fracture replicas, each junctional membrane is split into two complementary internal membrane halves or fracture faces

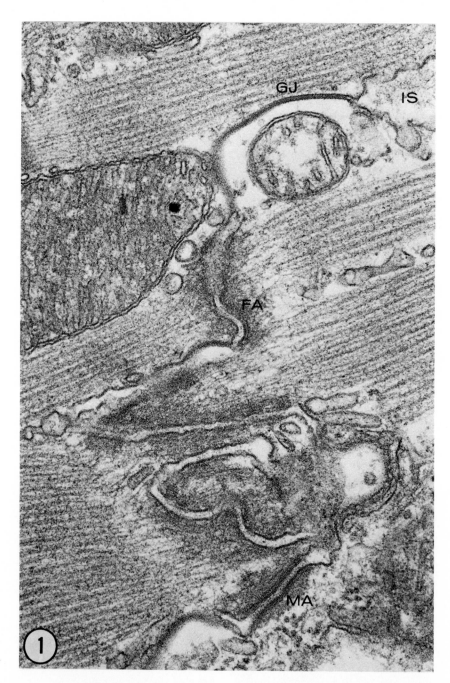

FIG. 1. Thin-section appearance of the intercalated disc joining mouse myocardial cells. The disc is comprised of several intercellular contacts: the gap junction (**GJ**), the fascia adhaerens (**FA**), and the desmosome or macula adhaerens (**MA**). The normal intercellular space (**IS**) is modified in the region of the disc. × 135,000.

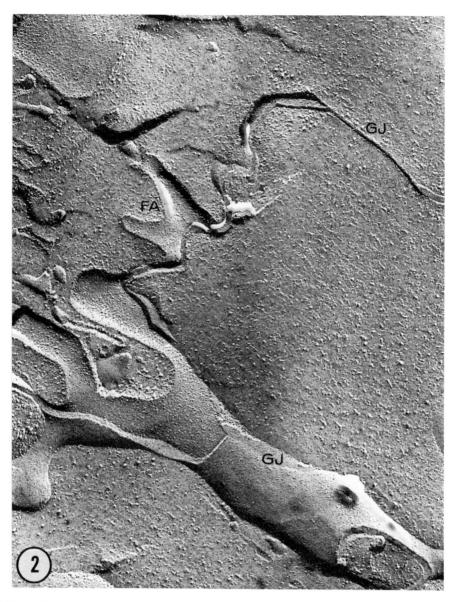

FIG. 2. Freeze-fracture image of the intercalated disc in mouse myocardium. The intramembrane specializations associated with both the gap junction (**GJ**) and the fascia adhaerens (**FA**) are indicated in this micrograph. × 60,000.

(14,15). The two fracture faces can be distinguished on the basis of their relationship to the cytoplasm and the extracellular space. They are commonly referred to as the inner membrane fracture face (face A, Fig. 3), which is adjacent to the cytoplasm, and the outer membrane fracture face (face B, Fig. 3), which is adjacent to the extracellular space. At the site of the gap junction, the A face is specialized into a plaque of polygonally arranged particles that have a 90- to 100-Å center-to-center spacing (Figs. 2 and 3). The B face contains a similar arrangement of complementary pits or depressions (Fig. 3). Gap junctions can occur in a

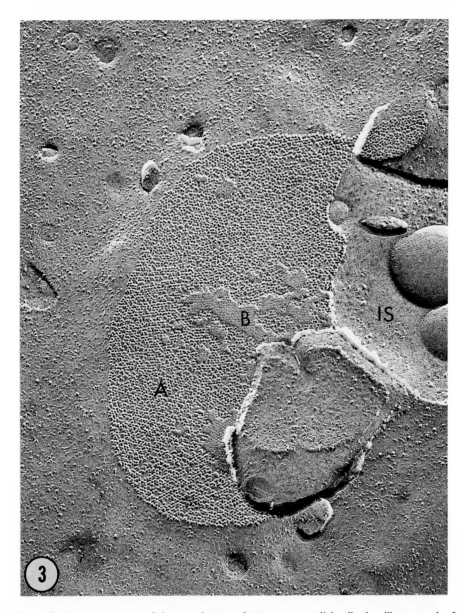

FIG. 3. Freeze-fracture appearance of the sarcolemma of mouse myocardial cells that illustrates the fracture face components of the gap junctional membrane. The gap junction is present as a plaque between adjacent cells. Fracture face **A** contains a polygonal packing of 80- to 90-Å intramembrane particles, whereas fracture face **B** contains a complementary arrangement of pits or depressions. × 100,800.

variety of pleiomorphic forms (1), and one of these forms is represented by a loose packing of the junctional particles (Fig. 4).

A major gap junctional pleiomorphism is present in arthropod tissues (1). This pleiomorphism is best illustrated by freeze-fracture examination (Fig. 5). In the arthropod gap junc-

tion, the junctional particles are usually located on the outer fracture face (B), whereas the complementary depressions are on the A face. The particles are large (110 Å in diameter), often heterogeneous in size, and they are generally present in an irregular, nonpolygonal packing. This junctional pleiomorphism is most

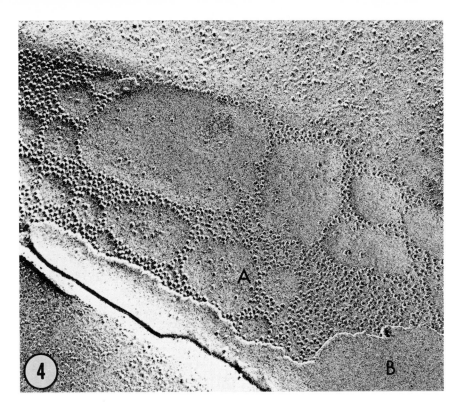

FIG. 4. Gap junctional membrane fracture faces between horizontal cell processes in the outer plexiform layer of the rabbit retina. Note that the **A** face junctional particles are not closely packed, and the complementation (**B** face) is difficult to detect. × 96,000. (From work with Dr. Elio Raviola.)

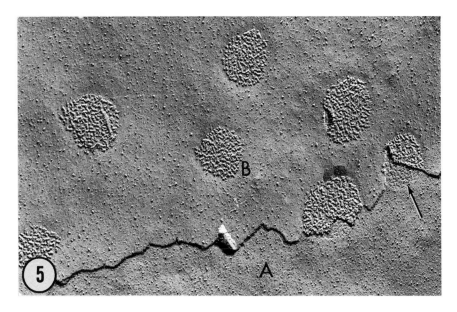

FIG. 5. Arthropod gap junctions from the nervous system of *Limulus*. The particles in these gap junctions are primarily associated with the **B** face, whereas the complementary depressions are located on face **A** (arrow). × 61,800. (From work with Fulton Wong.)

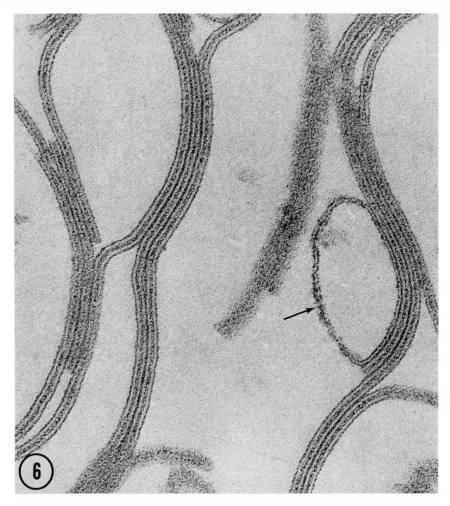

FIG. 6. Subcellular fraction of gap junctions isolated from rat liver. The junctions are aggregated to produce a myelin-like appearance. Note that some nonjunctional membrane (arrow) is contaminating the fraction. × 204,000.

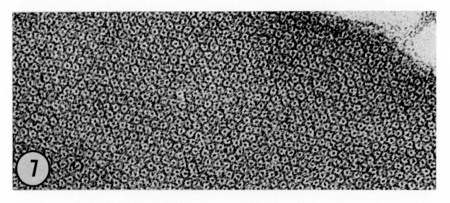

FIG. 7. Negative-stain of an isolated gap junction from rat liver (*en face* view). The junction is comprised of a paracrystalline lattice of particles (80 to 85 Å in diameter). The central region of the particles is penetrated by the stain to produce a 15- to 20-Å electron dense dot. × 360,000.

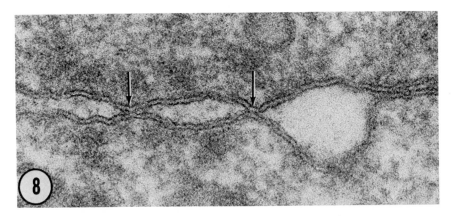

FIG. 8. Thin section of the tight junction between rat hepatocytes. The points of fusion (arrows) between the plasma membranes of adjacent cells are interconnected to form a complete belt or zonula around the cells. × 247,500.

significant because much of the physiological information about intercellular communication has been obtained from arthropod tissues.

The gap junction with a septilaminar appearance in thin sections has now been described between practically all metazoan animal cells (1,17,18). The notable exceptions include mature skeletal muscle cells and circulating blood cells.

The Tight Junction

The tight junction was described as the zonula occludens by Farquhar and Palade in 1963 (11). This structure is present between almost all vertebrate epithelial cells. In thin sections the structure is characterized by a true fusion of the membranes of adjacent cells (Fig. 8). The junction is about 140 to 150 Å thick at the site of the fusion. A series of interconnected fusions effectively provides a complete belt-like (zonula) element that is capable of occluding the diffusion of large molecules between cells (11,13,16,22). Tracer substances, such as lanthanum, are not capable of penetrating the points of fusion in the tight junctional structure.

In freeze-fracture replicas, the tight junctional membranes are characterized by a complementary series of A face ridges and B face grooves (Fig. 9). The A face ridges are interconnected into a zonula that provides an effective occluding barrier. The ridges represent the points of

membrane fusion that are observed in thin sections (23,24).

Several different studies (25–27) have indicated that the tight junction may be involved in transcellular permeability regulation in addition to its apparent role as a diffusion barrier between cells (11,12,16).

The Desmosome

Desmosomes are specialized cell contacts that are primarily involved in cell-to-cell adhesion (11,17,18). These structures are particularly prominent in tissues that are under unusual mechanical stress, such as cardiac muscle (Fig. 1) and stratified squamous epithelium. There are several different types of desmosomes in both vertebrate and invertebrate tissues; however, the most common type is generally called the desmosome or macula adhaerens (11).

In thin sections, the macula adhaerens is a bipartite structure characterized by a dense plaque along the surface of the desmosomal membranes and a crystalline modification of the intervening intercellular space (Fig. 1). Filaments are inserted into the dense surface plaque, and the intercellular space is approximately 250 to 350 Å wide. In some desmosomes the freeze-fractured membranes contain a nonpolygonal arrangement of closely packed particles (80 to 100 Å in diameter) and short

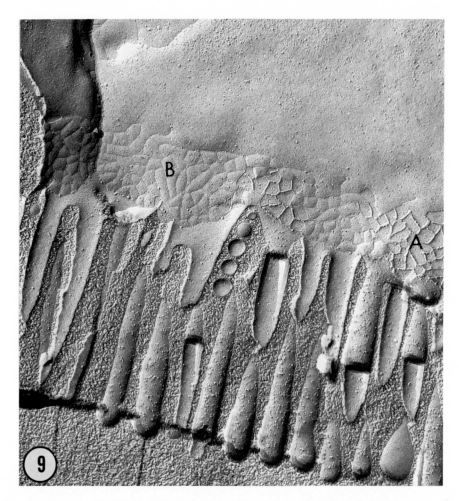

FIG. 9. Freeze-fracture of the tight junction (zonula occludens) between epithelia cells, in the rat small intestine. The tight junctional membranes are comprised of interconnected ridges on the **A** face, and a complementary arrangement of grooves on the **B** face. × 60,000. (From Friend and Gilula, ref. 16, Fig. 21. Reprinted with permission from the Rockefeller University Press.)

filamentous segments on both the A and B faces (17).

Other Cell Junctions

In addition to these cell junctions, many others have been described in a variety of vertebrate and invertebrate tissue. Because of space limitations, they will not be considered in this chapter. Several extensive reviews are available that can provide a useful introduction to the various other junctional elements (1,17,18).

STRUCTURAL AND CHEMICAL PROPERTIES OF ISOLATED GAP JUNCTIONS

Gap junctions have been isolated as subcellular fractions from rat liver, mouse liver, and the goldfish brain (20,28–32). These different fractions vary in purity; however, some fractions have been obtained that are pure enough to provide some meaningful biochemical information (28,31).

Since the gap junctions are specialized regions of plasma membranes, they can be found in subcellular fractions of plasma membranes from a variety of tissues. Gap junctions were first isolated as a relatively enriched subfraction of the plasma membrane fraction from rat liver by Benedetti and Emmelot in 1968 (20). This material was obtained as a detergent-resistant (deoxycholate) fraction from the total plasma membrane fraction. After the deoxycholate treatment, the gap junctions lose the gap (septilaminar) appearance, and consequently they were described as tight junctions (pentalaminar) (20). More recently, Evans and Gurd (30) and Goodenough and Stoeckenius (28) have independently isolated enriched gap junctional fractions from mouse liver. Both fractions were obtained using the anionic detergent Sarkosyl to eliminate most of the nonjunctional elements in the plasma membrane fraction. The fraction obtained by Goodenough and Stoeckenius has an exceptionally high degree of purity, whereas the fraction from Evans and Gurd contains a significant amount of contamination by nonjunctional material.

The subcellular fractionation of gap junctions is extremely difficult work because the procedure requires several days, the yields are very small, and the fraction must be assayed rigorously with ultrastructural techniques (since no endogenous activity has been detected in the fraction). From work on rat liver (31), approximately 100 μg of junctional protein is obtained from 500 g of liver. This fraction contains structurally intact gap junctions by both thin-section (Fig. 6) and negative-stain (Fig. 7) characterizations.

The isolated gap junctional membranes have been structurally characterized with electron microscopic techniques. With negative staining, the junctional membranes contain a paracrystalline arrangement of homogeneous 80- to 90-Å particles (Fig. 7) (20,28,32). These particles presumably represent the same particulate complexes that are exposed with freeze-fracturing (Fig. 3). An electron-dense dot is present in the central region of the junctional particles. This central region may represent the physical location for a low-resistance pathway (5). This pathway should be comprised of hydrophilic material because of the physiological nature of cell-to-cell communication.

Goodenough and Stoeckenius have reported that there are three protein components on

sodium dodecyl sulfate-polyacrylamide gels from mouse liver gap junctions. The most prominent component is around 20,000 daltons. More recently, Goodenough has reported that the same fraction contains two proteins of approximately 10,000 daltons after treatment with sodium dodecyl sulfate and reduction (29). In addition to protein, there is some neutral lipid and some phospholipid (tentatively phosphatidyl choline and phosphatidyl ethanolamine) in this fraction.

We have found two prominent protein components in a gap junctional fraction from rat liver. The two proteins have mobilities of about 25,000 and 18,000 daltons. The 25,000-dalton protein has a low polar amino acid content, whereas the 18,000-dalton protein has a high polar amino acid content. If the proteins are involved in the molecular mechanism for low resistance, then the 18,000 dalton protein could be involved in a channel region, and the 25,000-dalton protein could provide hydrophobic insulation for the channel and interact with the membrane lipids. Thus far no carbohydrate has been detected in the rat liver fraction.

FUTURE APPROACHES FOR STUDYING INTERCELLULAR COMMUNICATION

Physiological

Intercellular communication has already been demonstrated to be a biologically relevant cell-to-cell interaction in excitable tissues. This interaction is equivalent to an electrical synapse between neurons and myocardial cells (2,3,5,9). The electrical synapse is a site of low resistance that permits the movement of current in the form of ions, such as Na^+ and K^+. In the case of metabolic cooperation, a small metabolite, possibly a nucleotide, is transferred between cells (J. D. Pitts, *unpublished observations*). Therefore, if ions and small molecules (such as nucleotides, sugars, and amino acids) can be transmitted between cells, then the potential regulatory role of intercellular communication is most significant. This phenomenon could be exceedingly important during development and differentiation. There are already some preliminary indications that electrical synapses may be involved in the process of muscle differentiation (myoblast fusion) (33) and neuromuscular junction formation (34).

In the future, it will be important to characterize fully the physiological parameters that control cell-to-cell communication and to develop new probes that can be used to study the qualitative and quantitative properties of the low-resistance channels. With regard to the former, Loewenstein and his collaborators (35) have provided extensive evidence for a central role of calcium in regulating communication in arthropod tissue.

Structural

Practically all of the gap junctions that have been characterized with electron microscopic techniques have basically similar structural features. A major exception is the arthropod gap junction.

Future structural studies will have to rely on novel technical advances or different approaches in order to resolve new details about the junctional structure. One attempt has already been made to examine gap junctions with X-ray diffraction (28), and others are currently in progress. The major goal of future structural studies must be to try to resolve, in detail, the elements in the lattice that are responsible for the cell-to-cell transfer of molecules. In this regard it will be extremely important to know the precise arrangement of the lipid and protein within the junctional framework.

Biochemical

Even though gap junctions are difficult to isolate for biochemical studies, it is fortunate that there are very few protein and lipid components in the junctional membranes. This fact makes it reasonable to consider utilizing microanalytical techniques, together with labeling reagents, to characterize the biochemical components as well as their precise location within the junctional lattice. Thus it is quite conceivable to obtain biochemical information that can provide a molecular mechanism for cell-to-cell transfer of ions and small molecules. Future studies must also include attempts to reconstitute the junctional proteins or subunits into lipid systems so that their conductance properties can be examined.

Immunological

A useful approach for studying the biological relevance of communication will rely on the development of junction-specific antisera. Such an antisera (if inhibitory) could provide a means to rapidly examine the significance of gap junctions in a variety of cellular interactions that take place *in vivo* and in culture.

In future studies on gap junctions and intercellular communication, efforts should be made to focus on the biological relevance of this phenomenon. With the exception of the electrical synapse in excitable tissues, there is no biological system where gap junctions have been demonstrated to provide a significant function. It may be useful to focus on the biogenesis of communication, as some workers have done recently (36), in order to try and understand the functional significance of intercellular communication in nonexcitable tissues.

ACKNOWLEDGMENTS

The author gratefully acknowledges the technical assistance of Asneth Kloesman, Eleana Sphicas, and Frederick Wedel. These studies were supported by the Irma T. Hirschl Trust, the Andrew Mellon Fund, and U.S. Public Health Service Research Grant HL 16507.

REFERENCES

1. Gilula, N. B. (1974): Junctions between cells. In: *Cell Communication*, edited by R. P. Cox, pp. 1–29. Wiley, New York.
2. Furshpan, E. J., and Potter, D. D. (1957): Mechanism of nerve-impulse transmission at a crayfish synapse. *Nature*, 180:342–343.
3. Loewenstein, W. R. (1966): Permeability of membrane junctions. *Ann. N.Y. Acad. Sci.*, 137:441–472.
4. Furshpan, E. J., and Potter, D. D. (1968): Low-resistance junctions between cells in embryos and tissue culture. In: *Current Topics in Developmental Biology, Vol. 3*, edited by A. A. Moscona and A. Monroy, pp. 95–127. Academic Press, New York.
5. Bennett, M. V. L. (1973): Function of electrotonic junctions in embryonic and adult tissues. *Fed. Proc.*, 32:65–75.
6. Subak-Sharpe, J. H., Burk, R. R., and Pitts, J. D. (1969): Metabolic cooperation between biochemically marked mammalian cells in tissue culture. *J. Cell Sci.*, 4:353–367.
7. Gilula, N. B., Reeves, O. R., and Steinbach, A.

(1972): Metabolic coupling, ionic coupling, and cell contacts. *Nature,* 235:262–265.

8. Azarnia, R., Michalke, W., and Loewenstein, W. R. (1972): Intercellular communication and tissue growth. VI. Failure of exchange of endogeneous molecules between cancer cells with defective junctions and noncancerous cells. *J. Memb. Biol.,* 10:247–258.

9. Weidmann, S. (1966): The diffusion of radiopotassium across intercalated disks of mammalian cardiac muscle. *J. Physiol.,* 187:323–342.

10. Dewey, M. M., and Barr, L. (1962): Intercellular connection between smooth muscle cells: the nexus. *Science,* 137:670–672.

11. Farquhar, M. G., and Palade, G. E. (1963): Junctional complexes in various epithelia. *J. Cell Biol.,* 17:375–412.

12. Revel, J. P., and Karnovsky, M. J. (1967): Hexagonal array of subunits in intercellular junctions of the mouse heart and liver. *J. Cell Biol.,* 33:C7–C12.

13. Goodenough, D. A., and Revel, J. P. (1970): A fine structural analysis of intercellular junctions in the mouse liver. *J. Cell Biol.,* 45:272–290.

14. Chalcroft, J. P., and Bullivant, S. (1970): An interpretation of liver cell membrane and junction structure based on observations of freeze-fracture replicas of both sides of the fracture. *J. Cell Biol.,* 47:49–60.

15. McNutt, N. S., and Weinstein, R. S. (1970): The ultrastructure of the nexus. A correlated thin-section and freeze-cleave study. *J. Cell Biol.,* 47:666–687.

16. Friend, D. S., and Gilula, N. B. (1972): Variations in tight and gap junctions in mammalian tissues. *J. Cell Biol.,* 53:758–776.

17. McNutt, N. S., and Weinstein, R. S. (1973): Membrane ultrastructure at mammalian intercellular junctions. *Prog. Biophys. Mol. Biol.,* 26:45–101.

18. Staehelin, L. A. (1974): Structure and function of intercellular junctions. *Int. Rev. Cytol.,* 39:191–283.

19. Robertson, J. D. (1963): The occurrence of a subunit pattern in the unit membranes of club endings in Mauthner cell synapses in goldfish brains. *J. Cell Biol.,* 19:201–221.

20. Benedetti, E. L., and Emmelot, P. (1968): Hexagonal array of subunits in tight junctions separated from isolated rat liver plasma membranes. *J. Cell Biol.,* 38:15–24.

21. Satir, P., and Gilula, N. B. (1973): The fine structure of membranes and intercellular communication in insects. *Ann. Rev. Entomol.,* 18:143–166.

22. Brightman, M. W., and Reese, T. S. (1969): Junctions between intimately apposed cell membranes in the vertebrate brain. *J. Cell Biol.,* 40:648–677.

23. Wade, J. B., and Karnovsky, M. J. (1974): The structure of the zonula occludens. A single fibril model based on freeze-fracture. *J. Cell Biol.,* 60:168–180.

24. Staehelin, L. A. (1973): Further observations on the fine structure of freeze-cleaved tight junctions. *J. Cell Sci.,* 13:763–786.

25. Erlij, D., and Martinez-Palomo, A. (1972): Opening of tight junctions in frog skin by hypertonic urea solutions. *J. Memb. Biol.,* 9:229–240.

26. Wade, J. B., Revel, J. P., and DiScala, V. A. (1973): Effect of osmotic gradients on intercellular junctions of the toad bladder. *Am. J. Physiol.,* 224:407–415.

27. DiBona, D. R., and Civan, M. M. (1973): Pathways for movement of ions and water across toad urinary bladder. I. Anatomic site of transepithelial shunt pathways. *J. Memb. Biol.,* 12:101–128.

28. Goodenough, D. A., and Stoeckenius, W. (1972): The isolation of mouse hepatocyte gap junctions. Preliminary chemical characterization and X-ray diffraction. *J. Cell Biol.,* 54:646–656.

29. Goodenough, D. A. (1974): Bulk isolation of mouse hepatocyte gap junctions. *J. Cell Biol.,* 61:557–563.

30. Evans, W. H., and Gurd, J. W. (1972): Preparation and properties of nexuses and lipid-enriched vesicles from mouse liver plasma membranes. *Biochem. J.,* 128:691–700.

31. Gilula, N. B. (1974): Isolation of rat liver gap junctions and characterization of the polypeptides. *J. Cell Biol.,* 63:111a.

32. Zampighi, G., and Robertson, J. D. (1973): Fine structure of the synaptic discs separated from the goldfish medulla oblongata. *J. Cell Biol.,* 56:92–105.

33. Rash, J. E., and Fambrough, D. (1973): Ultrastructural and electrophysiological correlates of cell coupling and cytoplasmic fusion during myogenesis *in vitro. Dev. Biol.,* 30:166–186.

34. Fischbach, G. D. (1972): Synapse formation between dissociated nerve and muscle cells in low density cell cultures. *Dev. Biol.,* 38:407–429.

35. Loewenstein, W. R. (1973): Membrane junctions in growth and differentiation. *Fed Proc.,* 32:60–64.

36. Johnson, R., Hammer, M., Sheridan, J., and Revel, J. P. (1974): Gap junction formation between reaggregated Novikoff hepatoma cells. *Proc. Natl. Acad. Sci. USA,* 71:4536–4540.

The Nervous System, Donald B. Tower, Editor-in-Chief. *Vol. 1: The Basic Neurosciences.* Raven Press, New York, 1975.

An Essay on Neurocytology

Sanford L. Palay

During the past two decades, a distinct change has occurred in the emphasis of morphological studies of the nervous tissue. Before this time, neuroanatomical research meant hodology, the tracing of pathways and the working out of connections between one part of the nervous system and another. Although a few investigators maintained an interest in cytological problems, most neuroanatomists concerned themselves with the results of ablations and tract sections. Except for research into pathological changes, the structure of neurons and their organization within the gray matter were largely ignored. It was apparently considered that cellular studies had been carried as far as they could go by Ramón y Cajal and his coevals at the turn of the century and that the subject had no interesting problems that could be solved with the methods at hand. Cytological approaches to the nervous system, of course, fell under the same opprobrium that all histological work suffered from during the first half of the 20th century. Nevertheless, there were a few attempts, notably by members of the Chicago school, to resolve the outstanding question of continuity across synaptic junctions and to decide whether or not Nissl bodies and neurofibrillae were artifacts (1). There were even some important cytological discoveries during this time, neurosecretion and axoplasmic flow being two that come easily to mind; but the methods at the disposal of investigators at that time could not deliver convincing answers and the subject remained fallow.

Curiously, a method already existed—and in fact antedated all the common histological methods of the time—that was quite suitable for the cellular analysis of the central nervous system at the light microscope level. This method was the Golgi technique, first used in 1873 and the source of intensive research at the end of the nineteenth century. Because of its unpredictable successes and the uncertain interpretation of its products, the method fell

into such disfavor that by the end of the second World War its practitioners could be counted on the fingers of one hand. As a result the efforts of a whole generation of neuroanatomists were devoted to hodological problems, while neglecting a superb method for analyzing the composition and organization of the gray matter.

These remarks are not intended to belittle the importance of hodology, without which neither neuroanatomy nor neurology could advance, but to deplore a lost opportunity, which, had it been exploited, would have made current efforts with newer methods more rapidly fruitful than they have been. Nevertheless enormous strides have been taken in the field of traditional neuroanatomy during the past two decades, largely because of the development of efficient new methods for recognizing preterminal and terminal degeneration (2) and for producing reliable small lesions in the central nervous system. These advances, taken together with the rapid development of electrophysiological techniques for single unit recording, have immeasurably increased the need for taking the next step in morphology, the cellular analysis of the gray matter itself.

The shift in emphasis in morphological studies of the nervous system during the past 20 years has come about in the process of taking this next step. It has involved the creation of a new subdiscipline, neurocytology, which evolved from the application of electron microscopy and cytological methods to neuroanatomical problems. The development of neurocytology has had the effect of restoring neuroanatomy to the mainstream of biology, by revitalizing its cellular foundations. Consequently, the morphology of the nervous system has resumed its rightful place at the forefront of cytological research. Parenthetically it may be remembered in this connection that, among the cytoplasmic organelles, the ergastoplasm, the mitochondria, and the Golgi apparatus were first recognized in neurons. The effect of this development on neuroanatomy has been a return to the fundamental problems of the nervous system—how it is constructed and how it is organized at a cellular and unitary level (3).

The origin of the term *neurocytology* as a name for the new discipline deserves some comment. It was first used by Wilder Penfield in 1925 when he established a Laboratory of Neurocytology at the Presbyterian Hospital in New York (4). This was a laboratory devoted to pathological diagnosis and research with the staining methods that Penfield had learned in Cajal's laboratory in Madrid. It was more a laboratory of neuropathology and experimental neurology than the title would suggest nowadays. However, the laboratory was short-lived, as Penfield migrated to Montreal, and the name disappeared. It was reinvented in 1955 and 1956 by William F. Windle, when he established a Section of Neurocytology in the new Laboratory of Neuroanatomical Sciences which he organized in the then National Institute of Neurological Diseases and Blindness in Bethesda. This bold step was intended to take advantage of the new directions opened up by electron microscopy and the rekindled enthusiasm for cytological research that followed on the first successes of fine structural studies. This time the term entered into general usage among neuroscientists and became as securely established as its older counterparts.

Work in fine structure began with a repetition of the early history of the nerve cell. The first task was to recognize and identify the neuron and its parts in electron-microscopic preparations. With the guidance of the light microscope, this goal was achieved in a short time in so far as the large nerve cells were concerned (1,5). It took longer to identify the parts of smaller cells and to separate thin unmyelinated fibers from dendrites and neuroglial processes.

One of the first successes of neurocytology was the visualization of the lamellar substructure of the myelin sheath (6), followed quickly by the surprising discovery that the lamellae form a continuous spiral rather than concentric layers. In short order, the continuity of the myelin layers with the plasmalemma of the myelin-forming cell was revealed (7), and, in one of the most satisfying discoveries in all of neurocytology, the morphogenesis of the myelin sheath was elucidated (8). Although the story of the myelin sheath was by no means completed with these early studies and they exposed many more questions than they solved, they provided a firm biophysical and embryological footing for much of the subsequent work in ultrastructure.

Another early achievement was the recognition of nerve terminals and synaptic junctions in the mammalian central nervous system (9), which in one stroke confirmed the Neuron Doctrine and opened the possibility of using the electron microscope to study the organization of the nervous system. Such studies rapidly cleared away a century of accumulated speculation and muddled interpretations of observations in the optical microscope, replacing them with sharper definitions, distinctly outlined cells, and intercellular junctions that were previously invisible.

The neuroglial cells proved to be a more vexatious problem, and it was not until improved methods for the preservation of neural tissue came into general use that agreement was reached on the identification of astrocytes and oligodendrocytes. Indeed adequate fixation was always a serious problem for fine structural studies of the nervous system. All through the nineteenth century, it was an obstacle at the light microscope level to the acquisition of a clear idea of the nervous system, and for electron microscopy it posed a hurdle that had to be surmounted before a study of the organization of the nervous system could even begin. The first success came after the demonstration that fixation by vascular perfusion of the living animal was essential for adequate preservation of the central nervous system (10). At first osmium tetroxide was used, but after the introduction of primary fixation with aldehydes, glutaraldehyde, or a mixture of formaldehyde and glutaraldehyde, has become the standard perfusion medium (11).

Upon the solution of the problem of fixation, it became possible to analyze almost all parts of the central nervous system at the fine structural level. Electron microscopy became a necessary tool in neuroanatomical research. It became possible to imagine that one day a complete description of any nucleus in the brain would include a topographic map of each nerve cell, indicating the identification and disposition of all of its afferent terminals. There were two reasons for this optimism. First, electron microscopy was the first (and only) method that could unequivocally identify the synapse, since it alone had the power to visualize the surface membrane of cells and their intercellular junctions. Second, the method exposed a variety of differences among terminals, not only in their sizes and shapes but also in their contents and in their junctional features. This variety has been correlated with the variety of nerve cell types and of inputs generated by different nerve cells, with the distribution of different neurotransmitters, and with different functions. It has turned out in addition that the location of any particular synapse is characteristic of the two participating cells and that particular synapses are distributed with reliable precision over particular parts of the postsynaptic cell (3,11). These findings have vitiated many presumptions of model builders and the speculations of embryological theorists that require randomness and equivalence of interneuronal connections. But they make the problem of constructing a real nervous system more challenging.

The necessity of knowing the three-dimensional form of nerve cells in order to identify them in the electron microscope, and subsequently to recognize their parts in thin sections, revived interest in the Golgi method, the only reliable method for visualizing whole cells in the central nervous system. Since very little work with this method had been carried out since the peak of Cajal's career at the beginning of the twentieth century, the information necessary for electron-microscopic analysis could not be culled from existing publications but had to be worked out afresh. The existing practitioners of this art found themselves much in demand, and many laboratories began to use the method, with more success than they had been led to expect by the established experts. The lateral geniculate body took on new complications. The basal ganglia and the spinal cord, the red nucleus and the olfactory bulb, the dorsal column nuclei and the central cerebellar nuclei had to be reinvestigated at the light microscope level. A new interest was evinced in the cerebellar and cerebral cortices. It was as if the value of the light microscope were discovered all over again, and the old hands could be forgiven their bitter amusement at the rediscovery of facts that they already knew (but never published) or that Cajal had brought to light 70 years before. It was obvious that a combination of the Golgi method with electron microscopy would be useful, and methods have been developed for examining selected cells or their processes in the electron microscope after impregnation by the Golgi method. These procedures have not been so productive as it was hoped since the deposit of silver chromate obscures the junctional details at synapses or falls out leaving an unstable hole, or the preservation leaves much to be desired. Clearly this is a technological area, that would repay attention.

Just preceding the rise of neurocytology, a very important technical advance had been made in the traditional field of hodology. A method for selectively staining the preterminal portions of nerve fibers had been developed by Nauta and his colleagues (see ref. 12). This method permitted the tracing of degenerating nerve fibers into the gray matter close to the terminal field. It still did not reveal the synapses themselves but it came closer than any previous method to permitting the precise identification of synaptic end-stations with certain afferent bundles or with their sources. The method enormously amplified the amount of detail that could be garnered at the light microscope level concerning the projections of cell groups and pathways. Nauta's method underwent several modifications and improvements, the last of which, by Fink and Heimer, evidently does reveal the distribution of terminals (12). Even this modification, however, does not demonstrate the synapse itself but indicates the location of terminals and preterminal fibers within the postsynaptic field. These methods stimulated a prodigious burst of investigative work along the traditional hodological lines, which reevaluated almost all of the previously established connections between parts of the central nervous system and vastly increased the catalogue of known interconnections. These studies emphasized the precision with which the central nervous system is organized. For example, the retention of topographic order as the synaptic links were followed from level to level became more and more impressive. It became progressively clearer that a knowledge of the broad outlines of connections between parts would not suffice for an understanding of the operation of the nervous system. It would be necessary to know how individual cells are linked, and this anatomical knowledge would have to be correlated with single unit physiology.

The successes of the Nauta methods were soon transplanted to the electron microscope level. It was first established that the degeneration of nerve endings could be recognized and the progress of degeneration timed. One surprising result from these studies was the rapidity with which degenerating endings disappeared. One or two days could be sufficient to eliminate completely any trace of nerve endings after they had been disconnected from their parent cell bodies. There are, of course, certain dangers in the fine structural approach. Before undertaking an experimental study it is necessary to be thoroughly familiar with the normal organization of the region. Degeneration can occur spontaneously or at least from nonexperimental causes, and terminals in various states of disintegration can confuse the picture. Sometimes examination of the normal animal can be almost uninformative because of the subtle distinctions between profiles in electron micrographs. Analyses based on the classification of nerve cells and nerve endings according to their fine structure can be misleading even when carefully compared with Golgi preparations. For this reason, all the means at our disposal must be brought to bear on any region when analysis of organization is undertaken.

Recently two new methods have been added to the armamentarium: autoradiography and the uptake of horseradish peroxidase. In the first, an amino acid labeled with tritium is injected into a cellular region and, after it has been taken up into the cell bodies, incorporated into protein, and transported down their axons, the terminals are identified by autoradiography. In the second method, horseradish peroxidase is injected into the region of the terminal arborizations. It is taken up into the nerve endings and transported retrogradely to the cell bodies by way of the agranular reticulum, which thus becomes labeled by an exogenous enzymatic activity of known provenance. Although both of these methods were developed for light microscopy, they have both been extended to electron microscopy, on which they depend for their ultimate usefulness and precision. Such methods can be refined by making use of the specific uptake systems which many nerve cells and fibers have for neurotransmitter compounds and their analogues. Both nerve endings and nerve cells can be specifically marked with tritium-labeled transmitters, e.g., catecholamines or indolamines, and located by autoradiography. In this way nerve cells or nerve endings can be identified not only according to their location and connections but also according to their chemical specificities. Again both light and electron microscopy can be used with these methods, but the latter provides the opportunity to identify a particular transmitter with a particular group of morphological features.

As has already been mentioned, the development of neurocytology has coincided with a remarkable development in neurophysiology, which has arisen largely independently and with little collaboration with neuromorphology. This new aspect of neurophysiology is the analysis of the responses of single nerve cells to natural stimuli such as light, touch, changes in position, and muscular tension. Its development derives from the same source as neurocytology, i.e., the drive to know how the nervous system operates at a cellular level, how organized behavior, perception, and other coherent activities emerge from the coordinated behavior of individual cells. Unitary analysis requires a background of precise morphological information. The geometry of the cellular unit itself must be characterized. The afferent fibers to a cell must all be identified; their distribution over the surface of the cell must be mapped; the types of synaptic interface, their size, number, distribution, and other characteristics must be described; the internal structure of the terminals must be described; and the chemical transmitters must be identified and localized. Electrical coupling sites must be found and characterized. In addition relationships with neighboring nerve cells and with the neuroglia and the orientation of the cell within the neuropil must be known. Such data can be supplied by means of the methods currently at our disposal, although with real difficulties and impediments. In principle, at least, the possibilities for successful coordination of physiological and anatomical research in the nervous system are brighter now than ever before.

Considerable progress has already been made

in this direction in a few selected regions of the central nervous system. The reports on this subject are so numerous that only a few examples can be given. Analysis of the cerebellar cortex is probably the most advanced (see, for example, refs. 11 and 13). But work on the red nucleus, the lateral vestibular nucleus, and the inferior olive, although much less complete, has nevertheless made a substantial beginning. A comprehensive analysis of the cerebellar dentate nucleus shows the power of the morphological methods to point the way for physiology (14,15). The visual pathway, especially the retina and the lateral geniculate body, has received a great deal of attention, but the cochlear nuclei and other centers in the acoustic pathway have hardly been touched. The same is true of the basal ganglia and the thalamus, aside from the lateral geniculate body. The olfactory bulb has received sporadic attention but has not yet been systematically analyzed. Several investigators have started work on the cerebral cortex, but the results are still fragmentary and much more intensive research must be done before the architecture of this region can be understood. These examples are only indications of the starts that have been made. Vast areas of the central nervous system remain to be explored, for example, the entire spinal cord, the reticular formation, and hundreds of other centers both well known and obscure. Furthermore the scope of the exploration has to be expanded to include detailed comparative studies of homologous regions in different species and, most important, the ontogeny of the region at the fine structural level.

Thus the development of neurocytology has focused the efforts of neuromorphologists on the *organization* of the central nervous system. By *organization* is meant the detailed plan of the projections of one nerve cell upon another, their locations, sources, and effects, with some appreciation of their relative weights in the activity of the recipient cell and of the transmitter mechanism involved. This new level of analysis is complementary to and an extension of the older level of investigation into the interconnections between regions and the distribution of somatotopic representations, which continues to be pursued with the aid of the light microscope. But the higher resolution of neurocytology makes it possible to realize the ulti-

mate implications of the cellular fabric of the nervous system. For it is morphological information at this fine level that is fundamental to both physiological and theoretical analyses of how the nervous system functions.

ACKNOWLEDGMENTS

The support of research grant NS03659 and training grant NS05591 from the National Institute of Neurological and Communicative Disorders and Stroke is gratefully acknowledged.

REFERENCES

1. Peters, A., Palay, S. L., and Webster, H. deF. (1976): *The Fine Structure of the Nervous System*. Second edition, Saunders, Philadelphia.
2. Nauta, W. J. H., and Ebbesson, S. O. E. (Eds.) (1970): *Contemporary Research Methods in Neuroanatomy*. Springer-Verlag, New York.
3. Palay, S. L. (1967): Principles of cellular organization in the nervous system. In: *The Neurosciences*, edited by G. C. Quarton, T. Melnechuk, and F. O. Schmitt, pp. 24–31. Rockefeller University Press, New York.
4. Pool, J. L. (1975): *The Neurological Institute of New York, 1909–1974, With Personal Anecdotes*, pp. 8–10. Lakeville Journal, Inc., Lakeville, Connecticut.
5. Palay, S. L., and Palade, G. E. (1955): The fine structure of neurons. *J. Biophys. Biochem. Cytöl.*, 1:69–88.
6. Fernandez-Morán, M. (1950): Electron microscope observations on the fine structure of the myelinated nerve fiber sheath. *Exp. Cell Res.*, 1:143–149.
7. Robertson, J. D. (1955): The ultrastructure of adult vertebrate peripheral myelinated nerve fibers in relation to myelinogenesis. *J. Biophys. Biochem. Cytol.*, 1:271–278.
8. Geren, B. B. (1954): The formation from the Schwann cell surface of myelin in the peripheral nerves of chick embryos. *Exp. Cell Res.*, 7:558–562.
9. Palay, S. L. (1956): Synapses in the central nervous system. *J. Biophys. Biochem. Cytol.*, 2(*Suppl.*):193–202.
10. Palay, S. L., McGee-Russell, S. M., Gordon, S., and Grillo, M. A. (1962): Fixation of neural tissues for electron microscopy by perfusion with solutions of osmium tetroxide. *J. Cell Biol.*, 12:385–410.
11. Palay, S. L., and Chan-Palay, V. (1974): *Cerebellar Cortex, Cytology and Organization*. Springer-Verlag, New York.
12. Heimer, L. (1970): Selective silver-impregnation of degenerating axoplasm. In: *Contemporary Research Methods in Neuroanatomy*, edited by

W. J. H. Nauta and S. O. E. Ebbesson, pp. 106–131. Springer-Verlag, New York.

13. Eccles, J., Ito, M., and Szentágothai, J. (1967): *The Cerebellum as a Neuronal Machine*. Springer-Verlag, New York.

14. Chan-Palay, V. (1973): Neuronal circuitry in the nucleus lateralis of the cerebellum. *Z. Anat. Entwicklungsgesch.*, 142:259–265.

15. Chan-Palay, V. (1976): *Organization of the Cerebellar Dentate Nucleus in the Rat and Monkey*. Springer-Verlag, New York.

The Nervous System, Donald B. Tower, Editor-in-Chief. *Vol. 1: The Basic Neurosciences.* Raven Press, New York, 1975.

Ultrastructural Basis of Synaptic Transmission

George D. Pappas

The National Institute for Neurological and Communicative Disorders and Stroke was established 25 years ago as a separate body within the National Institutes of Health. This was during the period when physiological techniques for intracellular recordings and the isolation of subcellular fractions were coupled with meaningful results from the new biology based on electron microscopy, setting the basis for the modern discipline of neurobiology.

At that time, based largely on the work of Ramón y Cajal, the neuron was accepted as the structural, functional, genetic, and trophic unit of the nervous system. However, there was no direct proof for the neuron theory's premise that the nervous system was composed of distinct cellular compartments that establish intimate contact with each other. The other and older concept, the reticular theory championed by Camillo Golgi, held that the nervous system was a reticular network of anastomosing processes. In other words, it was a complex network of neurons in a syncytium having cytoplasmic continuity with each other. While the events of the new era of modern cell biology have substantiated the neuron theory, nevertheless, the reticular theory has made a contribution to our understanding of dynamic aspects of the nervous system as an integrated tissue.

In order to understand the structure of similar cells in concert forming a tissue, we must have some understanding of the function or activity of these cells. The basic concept of neurons as separate discrete entities delimited by their individual plasma membranes could not be resolved with the microscopes available at the turn of the century when Sherrington assumed that a "surface of separation" must exist between neurons. Sherrington, on physiological grounds, accounted for the characteristic differences between conduction in nerve trunks and reflex arcs. He introduced the term synapse, which in Greek means to come face-to-face with or to join. In other words, on purely functional grounds, Sherrington could not have a cyto-plasmic syncytium. The developments in the past decades continue to demonstrate a give-and-take between an understanding of physiological events within the structural limits of the nervous system.

Studies with the electron microscope demonstrate clearly that neurons at synapses are separated by an extracellular space of approximately 200 Å. Furthermore, the functional polarity, the signal from neuron to neuron, is reflected by a parallel morphological or structural asymmetry. It was about 25 years ago that the controversy was resolved as to whether synaptic transmission in the central nervous system was electrically or chemically mediated. Just when the mode of chemical transmission was no longer controversial and universally accepted, electrical transmission was unequivocally demonstrated at a few sites. Electron microscopic examination of electrotonic synapses show that these junctions have a morphological symmetry and that the extracellular space between the opposing membranes is greatly attenuated. We can now designate structurally as well as physiologically the two classes of synapses as chemical or electrotonic.

The selected and far from inclusive brief description that follows, pertaining to the fine structure of chemical and electrotonic synapses, is presented, hopefully, to complement and advance our understanding of how synapses work. There is no priority, however, as to morphological versus physiological data. An understanding of the morphological substrates cannot take place without some comprehension of the functional state, and vice versa. Hence, we must approach the biology of synapses with a morphophysiological attitude. Of course, this is the true meaning of neurobiology, a field that has had its birth during this past quarter-century.

CHEMICALLY TRANSMITTING SYNAPSE

Less than 5% of the gray matter of the brain is composed of neuronal and glial cell bodies.

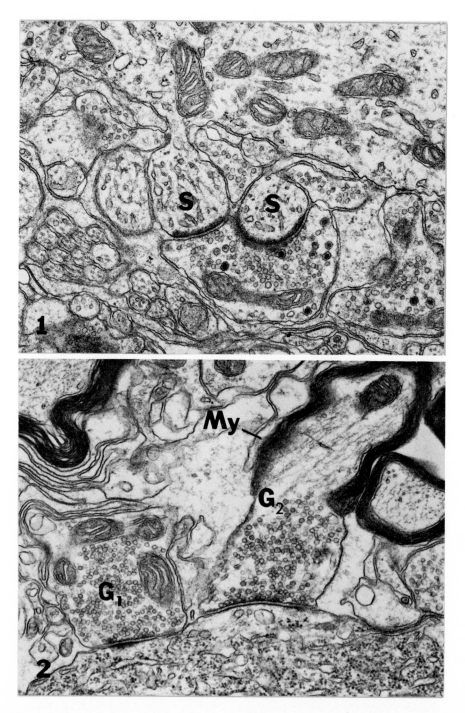

FIG. 1. Electron micrograph of a section from flounder cerebellum. An ending containing clear and dense-core presynaptic vesicles forms synaptic junctions with two dendritic spines (S) of a Purkinje cell dendrite. × 26,000

FIG. 2. Two axosomatic synapses in the spinal cord of the toadfish. Such synapses are sometimes classified as Gray Type 1 (G1) and Gray Type 2 (G2) synapses. My, myelin. × 29,500

Previous to the advent of electron microscopy, the structure of the neuropil was not resolved. Early studies by Wyckoff and Young (1) showed that the neuropil is made up of compact neuronal and glial processes and that is where most of the synapses occur. Studies have shown that neuronal and glial cells and their processes are closely packed in the central nervous system (CNS) and can be shown with the electron microscope to have an extracellular space of about 200 Å. This 200-Å space between the pre- and postsynaptic membranes has been demonstrated to contain a material of intermediate density, the so-called synaptic gap substance. Basic protein and carbohydrate in the form of mucopolysaccharides and glycoprotein have been demonstrated by a variety of histochemical methods at the electron microscope level of resolution. Three important functions have been postulated for the synaptic gap substance (2): (a) it may physically bind or hold together the pre- and postsynaptic membranes; (b) the presence of polyionic substances in the synaptic cleft may play a role in the movement of ions or transmitter molecules and may impede diffusion of the transmitter from the junction; and (c) glycoproteins on membranes are known to be the most immunologically active substances. Glycoprotein in the synaptic cleft may play an important role in intercellular recognition and may thus be implicated in the highly specific synaptic connections formed during synaptogenesis.

Electron microscopic examination of thin sections of pre- and postsynaptic membranes reveal the same basic unit membrane structure as other regions of neuronal and glial plasma membranes. The application of freeze-fracture techniques in electron microscopy has been a recent and important development, for it allows examination of the internal morphology of membranes. Consequently one can now begin to characterize what are interpreted to be receptor sites in the postsynaptic membrane and release sites in the presynaptic membrane. In both the pre- and postsynaptic processes closely associated on the cytoplasmic face of the opposing membranes, there is dense material, apparently rich in basic protein. When preparations are treated with phosphotungstic acid, this dense material may appear to be fibrillar (3). In the presynaptic process of some synapses, the dis-

tribution of this dense material may be in the form of a pattern. Akert and his co-workers (4) have called this the synaptic grid. The distribution of the membrane-associated cytoplasmic dense material may be greater in the postsynaptic than in the presynaptic process, or it may be the same in both processes. Gray has classified these as Type 1 and 2, respectively (3). These types are not always easily distinguished as many intermediate forms are often found. Nevertheless it has served as a useful shorthand to morphologists in describing their findings (see Figs. 1 and 2).

Presynaptic Specializations

The identification of synapses with the light microscope depends primarily on metallic impregnation of bulbous-like *bouton termineaux* or a mesh-like ending (as in the motor end plate). Other synaptic stains are based on the presence of mitochondrial clusters in endings. Electron microscopic examination of thin sections correlates well with light microscopic identification of synapses, although in thin sections only a few profiles of mitochondria are seen. The most important criterion for the identification of synaptic endings with the electron microscope is the presence of vesicles clustered close to the presynaptic membrane. It is the almost universal presence of vesicles only in the presynaptic process that gives the chemical synapse its asymmetric appearance (5,6).

Synaptic vesicles are membrane-bound organelles, which may migrate as such from the cell body to the terminals or may form from smooth tubular endoplasmic reticulum and pinch off near the presynaptic ending. Transmitter release may closely resemble the secretory process of other tissues in that the substances to be secreted are segregated in membrane-bounded granules. Conditions that promote secretion of products synthesized by cells (e.g., hormones, histamine, zymogen) also cause release of neurotransmitters. For example, calcium has been shown to play an essential role in the release of neurotransmitters and hormones. Calcium-binding sites have recently been identified in the synaptic vesicle membrane and implicated in transmitter release (7).

Synaptic vesicles are of various kinds de-

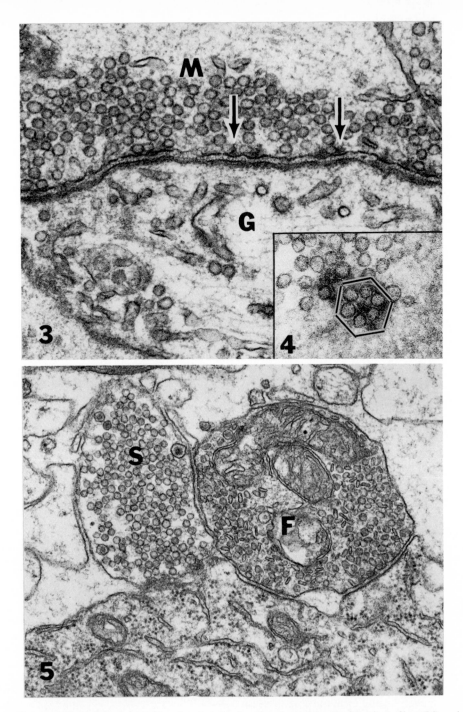

FIG. 3. Electron micrograph of a portion of a synaptic junction formed by the Mauthner fiber (M) and giant fiber (G) in the hatchet fish. Note that cytoplasmic dense material is closely associated with the presynaptic membrane (*arrows*). × 61,000

FIG. 4. A tangential section of a presynaptic ending taken from the toadfish sonic muscle motor endplate. Note that the dense material which is closely associated with the presynaptic membrane (not visible) is surrounded by six vesicles (outline). × 75,000

FIG. 5. Section of two axosomatic synapses in the medulla of the toadfish. Note that one ending has round vesicles (S) whereas the other has a more pleomorphic variety, many of which appear flattened (F). × 42,000

pending on their size, shape, and contents (Figs. 3–5). The identification of acetylcholine (ACh) as the transmitter at neuromuscular junctions has been correlated with the presence of clear round vesicles 400 to 800 Å in diameter. The isolated vesicles from cholinergic synapses from the *Torpedo* electric organ contain almost half of the ACh of the tissue (8).

Vesicles that have dense cores (some are small, around 500 Å in diameter, and others large, up to 2,000 Å in diameter) have been shown by electron microscopic autoradiography that tritiated norepinephrine is localized in terminals containing dense-core vesicles. The demonstration of catecholamines and serotonin with the semiquantitative method of fluorescence histochemistry has shown that neurons and their processes that contain these transmitters can be readily identified. It has been estimated that the norepinephrine content in sympathetic ganglion cell bodies is $\frac{1}{10}$ that in the axon, which, in turn, is $\frac{1}{5}$ of that in the terminal where the dense-core vesicles are concentrated (10).

In addition to the size and contents of synaptic vesicles, the shape of the vesicles is also involved in function. It has been suggested that flattened vesicles having electron-lucent contents may characterize inhibitory synapses (11). Indeed, it has been shown, in the mammalian spinal cord and in a number of invertebrate junctions, that inhibitory postsynaptic potentials occur at sites where flattened presynaptic vesicles may be seen. Often vesicles may appear to be pleomorphic in shape, and sometimes flattened vesicles are found at known excitatory synapses. It appears that the shape of the synaptic vesicles may be determined by the buffers and fixatives used. The morphological identification of flattened vesicles does not directly indicate that the synapse is inhibitory (2). In addition, Gray's Type 1 and Type 2 synapses have been correlated with excitation and inhibition, respectively. However, as in the case of vesicle shape, there are too many exceptions to warrant a hard-and-fast generalization. Excitation and inhibition are after all postsynaptic events, and one would not predict a priori that a presynaptic specialization would be evident. Indeed, excitatory and inhibitory postsynaptic potentials have been recorded where the presynaptic input was from different branches of a single cholinergic neuron (12).

Akert and his co-workers (4), at a number of sites in the CNS, have demonstrated with the use of metallic salts, such as uranyl, bismuth iodide, and lead, a kind of regular pattern of dense material forming a "presynaptic vesicular grid." At many sites even though an orderly grid-like organization is not seen, areas of focal densities associated with the presynaptic membrane can be found, and in some cases in long rows as in the motor end plate (13). The presence of this focal dense material supposedly precludes the release of the synaptic vesicle contents. It has been noted that the clustering of synaptic vesicles at active zones or sites is usually adjacent to the focal cytoplasmic densities on the presynaptic membrane. Gray (14) has proposed that the entire area of the presynaptic process containing the clusters of vesicles has, in the ground cytoplasm, a well-organized, fibrous network, or cytonet to which the synaptic vesicle membranes are somehow attached. It has been suggested recently by Berl and his co-workers (15) that an actin-like protein is present in synaptosomes (isolated synaptic junctions). However, it would be presumptuous at this time to hastily make the obvious construct of the presynaptic ending based on these preliminary reports.

Prominent dense material, the synaptic ribbon, which is organized perpendicular to the presynaptic membrane and surrounded by vesicles, is present in all presynaptic endings of sensory receptor cells. Synaptic ribbons are considered to be a further specialization of the presynaptic dense material described above. The function of synaptic ribbons is not understood. They can be correlated with the fact that cells that have them are not spike generating and that synaptopore sites can be seen closely associated with these presynaptic densities (see the next section).

The Fine Structure of the Pre- and Postsynaptic Membranes

Electron microscopy of thin-section presynaptic membranes have established that unit membrane structure is similar to that found in nonjunctional membranes. Electron microscopic examination of the presynaptic membrane following freeze-fracture reveals pits or invaginations. These pits or synaptopores are apparently arranged next to the areas of the membrane that contain the closely applied cytoplasmic dense material. Synaptopores then outline the pattern followed by the dense material of the synaptic grid (4). Synaptopores are found along the length of the presynaptic membrane and bordering on the synaptic ribbon of receptor cells. In the motor end plate the synaptopores are apparently concentrated in rows next to the areas that contain the cytoplasmic densities. These are considered to be the release sites (16). In addition to pits or invaginations of the presynaptic membrane, there are particles embedded in the lipid bilayers (see Robertson, *This Volume*).

As in the case of the presynaptic membrane, thin sections of the postsynaptic membrane examined with the electron microscope show a regular unit membrane structure. Some investigators have suggested that the extracellular synaptic gap substance is continuous with the postsynaptic cytoplasmic dense material. No direct evidence can be found for this in careful examination of very thin sections. That is, postsynaptic membrane shows unit membrane structure that is not traversed by fibers or filaments. This is true for desmosomes and other specialized junctions in neurons as well as other cells. Freeze-fracture preparations often reveal large particles embedded in the postsynaptic membrane. These are considered to be proteins, which may be the receptor sites. At the present time, such particles in the postsynaptic membrane have not always been demonstrable, and it has been suggested that they may be absent, particularly at inhibitory synapses.

Cytoplasmic dense material is often very closely associated with the postsynaptic membrane. It is found at areas opposing the presynaptic active zones and often is more prominent than the presynaptic dense material. Sometimes in the peripheral nervous system and the CNS, just below the membrane-associated cytoplasmic dense material, there may be a row of dense particles or a continuous bar. Nothing is known about the function of these postjunctional bodies. Indeed nothing is known about any of the cytoplasmic dense material associated with the postsynaptic membrane.

It has been suggested that this material accumulates during the maturation of synaptic contacts (17).

Synaptic Pathways and Metabolic Specificity

Synaptic pathways have traditionally been mapped by degeneration methods and more recently by the use of opaque markers and radioactive substances. Grafstein (18) has demonstrated that after injection of radioactive leucine into the vitreous of the eye, the label can be detected preferentially in the contralateral visual cortex, indicating that specific synaptic pathways can also serve as metabolic pathways. More recently, in an elegant study from Hubel and Wiesel's laboratory (19), it was shown that transsynaptic transport of radioactive fucose and proline injected into the eye not only confirmed the earlier findings of Grafstein (i.e., transsynaptic transport to the visual cortex) but also further demonstrated the high specificity of this transport. They believed that the preferential distribution of the marker demonstrated the occular dominance columns of the striate cortex in layer 4 of the visual cortex. It is not surprising then, that at synaptic junctions, morphological correlates exist for these specific metabolic pathways. It has been noted by Pappas and Waxman (2) that morphological evidence of pinocytosis is 50-fold greater at synaptic junctions than at nonjunctional sites. Injection of electron-opaque marker substances in the neuropil shows that they are taken up both pre- and postsynaptically by vesicles that may or may not be coated. Furthermore, it has been shown that there is an increase in uptake of extracellular markers at synapses during evoked increase in synaptic activity (20,21).

Distribution and Types of Synaptic Junctions

With the advent of intracellular recording techniques, it has been made abundantly clear that differences in physiological parameters are closely related to the distribution and types of synapses encountered. One of the most important morphological confirmations that electron microscopy has contributed to our understanding of the "wiring" of the cortex was made in 1959 by Gray (3), who showed that the dendritic spines are always associated with synaptic junctions, as was assumed by Cajal. In the cerebral cortex, for example, only approximately 2% of the synapses are on cell bodies and large dendritic trunks, whereas 50% are on dendritic spines and virtually all of the rest are on the fine dendritic processes. Dendrites have been demonstrated to exhibit spike electrogenesis and in some neurons, more than one site of spike initiation can occur. It should be emphasized that up to the early 1950s the mechanism of synaptic activity and synaptic activation of different parts of the same neuron was not known. The relatively remote location of synapses on dendrites may allow, depending on the geometry of the synaptic input, linear and nonlinear summation of axosomatic and axodendritic synaptic potentials. The synaptic input to dendrites and spines and the predominance of axodendritic synapses over axosomatic ones, in addition to the complex and branching dendritic patterns, allows for enormous flexibility in information processing (22).

In addition to axodendritic and axosomatic synapses, axoaxonic synapses have been described at a number of sites in the vertebrate nervous system. The most common type is that of synaptic input onto the axon hillock. The distribution of multiple synapses especially where sensory afferent inputs are found, are seen to be in clusters or glomeruli. These synapses are often seen to contain at least three processes. One process is presynaptic to a second, and the second, in turn, is presynaptic to a third. At first it was considered that these were axoaxonic junctions where the second postsynaptic axon forms contact with a dendrite or cell body. And it was suggested that such a synaptic organization could be the basis of understanding presynaptic inhibition. In areas such as the thalamic nuclei, where such serial synapses exist, presynaptic inhibition apparently does not occur, but postsynaptic inhibition does. However, it has recently been shown that in triadic synaptic arrangements, dendrites can be presynaptic. Synaptic clusters or glomeruli have been described in areas of the CNS receiving a major sensory input. Recent studies of serial sections of synaptic glomeruli in rat somatosensory thalamus (23) and the monkey lateral geniculate nucleus (24) have shown that in triadic synaptic arrangements the sensory input axon terminal is presynaptic both to a dendrite of an interneuron (Golgi Type II) and to a dendrite (and occasionally the cell body) of the principal neuron (Golgi Type I). In turn the dendrite of the interneuron is presynaptic to the principal neuron. The functional significance of the Golgi Type II interneuron has been interpreted as playing the role of lateral inhibition (24).

Earlier findings of dendrodendritic synapses were essentially confined to the olfactory bulb where dendrodendritic junctions occur between mitral and granule cells. Most of these synapses are of the reciprocal type in that the dendrites are both pre- and postsynaptic to one another (25). The presence of dendrodendritic synapses on cells that lack axons may be expected, such as between amacrine and bipolar cells of the retina. It is clear, however, that small neurons, whose dendrites can be presynaptic elements in the somato-sensory afferent areas of the brain, have axons (23). Dendrodendritic synapses further complicate our understanding of neuronal function in that information processing can occur as a local intrinsic function along elements of the dendritic tree and without involving the cell body or the axon. Dendrodendritic synapses (and other such combinations, e.g., dendrosomatic, somasomatic) may function as substrates for local intrinsic organization of information processing.

Morphological Changes in Relation to Synaptic Activity

The first electron microscopic observations showing clusters of vesicles in the presynaptic process were published about the same time that the release of transmitter was described as occurring in discrete quantal units (see ref. 26). It was quickly assumed that a vesicle may package a quantum of neurotransmitter and that calculating the amount of quanta released could be directly translated into the number of synaptic vesicles released. Up to approximately 5 years ago, most reports correlating structural with functional changes at synapses have been equivocal. Apparently, under conditions that characterize the physiological parameters of a given site, no striking morphological changes can be discerned (see ref. 2).

Preparations that allow recording of the postsynaptic events at monosynaptic sites have been used recently to correlate morphological changes with synaptic activity. By and large, two preparations having cholinergic synapses have been used in most studies: the neuromuscular junction and sympathetic ganglia preparations. Longenecker et al. (27) have shown that the addition of black widow spider venom to a frog neuromuscular preparation causes the nerve ending to discharge transmitter. When miniature end-plate potentials could no longer be recorded and the preparation was examined by electron microscopy, no synaptic vesicles were found. This report correlates release of transmitter in relation to synaptic vesicles. The effect of the venom is irreversible, for the preparation is no longer viable. Therefore the loss of vesicles could be interpreted as a specific structural "lesion" not directly related to the normal release of transmitter.

Nerve terminal size and mean quantum content (i.e., of releasable transmitter) appear not to vary greatly in many cholinergic endings. Estimates have been made of the number of synaptic vesicles present and the amount of ACh present at rest in both the frog neuromuscular junction and the cat sympathetic ganglia preparations (28). It appears that 85% of the ACh could be stored in the vesicles. The rate of synthesis of transmitter may be coupled to the rate of release. If a quantum is packaged within a vesicle as a precondition for its release, then under normal physiological parameters, a steady state may exist in either the formation of new vesicles or in replenishing transmitter in discharged ones. Several recent reports indicate that when high rates (10/sec and higher) of presynaptic stimulation is applied for short periods (2 to 30 min) and the preparation is then examined with the electron microscope, there is a marked depletion of synaptic vesicles (20,21,32). Following a period of rest, a normal population of vesicles can be found. On the other hand, other reports indicate that synaptic vesicles may play an indirect role in the quantal release of transmitter (28). The sampling of tissue for electron microscopy for the evaluation of the morphological parameter of function is crucial in this or any morphophysiological study. Some of the previously mentioned reports have stressed the importance of using preparations where the physiological recordings can accurately measure postsynaptic potentials

to determine the amount of transmitter released. It follows then, that the ideal morphological study should be made on the same synapse where these measurements were made. Such morphophysiological studies on identical synapses should better define the relationship of presynaptic vesicles to transmitter release.

THE ELECTROTONIC SYNAPSE

As in the case of chemically transmitting synapses, electrically transmitting synapses have a distinct morphological substrate (2). The electrotonic synapse has two features that distinguish it from the chemical synapse: (a) there is no 200-Å synaptic cleft between junctional membranes (Fig. 6) and (b) the area of close apposition appears symmetrical. Usually no functional or morphological features exist for distinguishing the pre- and postsynaptic cells. Functionally speaking, electrotonic synapses show no synaptic delay in contrast to chemical synapses and allow for the spread of current from cell to cell, i.e., electrical coupling. The close apposition of the apposing membranes of electrotonic synapses in very thin sections shows a 20- to 40-Å extracellular space and is described as a gap junction (Fig. 7). Direct correlation of electrical coupling and the presence of gap junctions has been established in many more sites than has the direct demonstration of chemical transmission at the morphologically identifiable chemical synapses. The ubiquitous presence of chemical synapses in the invertebrate and vertebrate nervous system, however, in contrast to the very occasional occurrence of electrotonic synapses, indicates that chemical transmission is the predominant mode of communication between neurons. On the other hand, gap junctions are not limited to excitable tissue. In addition to neurons and muscle (but not skeletal muscle), electrical coupling has been demonstrated in many, if not most, other tissues.

Fine Structure of the Electrotonic Synapse

The use of lanthanum has further elucidated the fine structure of the gap junction. Lanthanum is electron-opaque and has been used as an extracellular marker. It can be seen to enter into the 20- to 40-Å space or gap between the

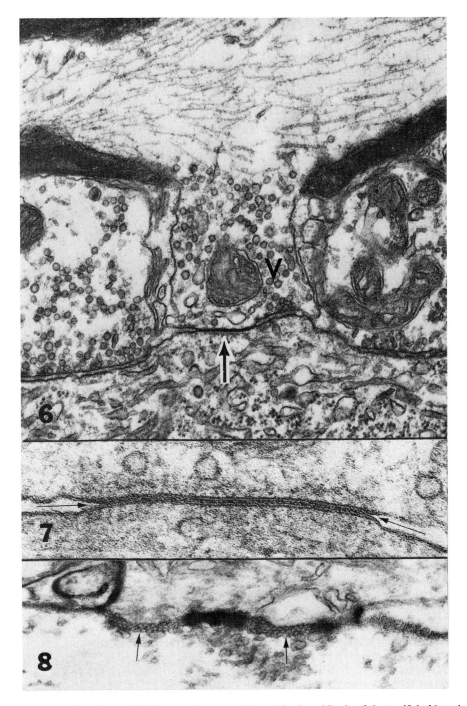

FIG. 6. A section through a nodal electrotonic synapse (*arrow*) in the midbrain of the toadfish. Note that the presynaptic process forms what appears to be a structurally mixed synapse, as clusters of vesicles (**V**) can be seen in one area where the apposing membranes are separated by a 200-Å space. There is no physiological evidence for bimodal transmission. × 36,500

FIG. 7. A high magnification of the junction of two membranes forming an electrotonic synapse. Typical of gap junctions, a 20- to 40-Å space (at *arrows*) can be seen between the two unit membranes forming this electrotonic synapse. × 177,000

FIG. 8. An *en face* section of an electrotonic synapse of the crayfish between the lateral septate and the motor giants fibers. Lanthanum was applied extracellularly outlining regular arrays of facets (*arrows*) or subunits where the intercytoplasmic pathways may exist in gap junctions. × 40,000

apposing junctional membranes. Very oblique or *en face* profiles of gap junctions reveal that the 20- to 40-Å extracellular space is not a continuous one but is confined to a honeycomb network of interlacing channels. These extracellular channels outline and delineate areas, subunits or facets (Fig. 8).

Low molecular weight substances, when injected intracellularly, will pass between the cytoplasm of electrically coupled cells. Dyes such as fluorescein, Procion yellow, and neutral red, as well as sucrose and various hydrated ions, have been shown to enter into adjacent electrically coupled septate axons in the ventral nerve cord of the crayfish. The only likely site for intracellular channels mediating such passage would be areas of the gap junction that are not accessible to the extracellular markers. The intercellular channels should then be located in the facets outlined by the extracellular honeycomb grid (2). Hexagonal packing of particles characterizes gap junctions in freeze-fracture preparations. These particles, ~ 100 Å center-to-center, correspond well to the subunits or facets found in sectioned junctions and may represent the substrate for the intercytoplasmic pathway (29).

Types of Electrotonic Synapses

There are two principal ways in which neurons are electrically coupled (2). The cell bodies or their processes can be readily identified to form gap junctions with each other. However, at many sites, electrically coupled neurons do not form gap junctions with each other. They are coupled by way of a prefiber. Axons have been demonstrated forming gap junctions with at least two cells, hence coupling them. Spinal motor neurons of fish that fire synchronously have been shown to form gap junctions directly with each other or to form gap junctions with the same axon of another neuron type.

It is now well established that synaptic transmission can be resolved in that both modes, electrical and chemical, take place in the nervous system. The distinct morphological substrates for these modes of transmission have been outlined above. Only one clearly established case of dual chemical and electrical transmission has been described to be in the chick

ciliary ganglion (30). The morphological substrate shows gap junctions between apposing membranes and separation of apposing membranes and clusters of vesicles in the presynaptic calyx ending. At many sites where axons form at least one or both parts of the electrotonic synapse, clusters of vesicles somewhat similar to presynaptic vesicles may be found. Nothing is known about the function of these vesicles. Often a morphologically mixed synapse may be seen having the structural characteristics of both electrically transmitting and chemically transmitting synapses (Fig. 6). At some of these sites, there is convincing evidence for purely electrotonic transmission with no chemical component (31). Nothing is known, nor have any plausible theories been advanced about the functional significance of mixed synapses.

SUMMARY

The following salient morphological features can serve as a basis for our current understanding of synaptic function.

1. There are distinct morphological differences between chemically or electrically transmitting synapses. Chemical synapses by far outnumber the less common electrotonic synapses.

2. The vast majority of the synaptic complexes in the CNS are found in the neuropil.

3. Most synaptic activity occurs in relation to dendrites, and dendritic spines are recognized to be the important component of the synaptic input in the brain cortex.

4. Dendrodendritic synapses occur in regions of the CNS noted for their sensory input. Dendrites and even cell bodies of interneurons (Golgi Type II) may be presynaptic to dendrites or cell bodies of the principal neurons (Golgi Type I). Furthermore, interneurons may form dendrodendritic synapses with each other.

5. The pathways and terminals that contain catecholamines and serotonin can be readily identified with fluorescence histochemical techniques.

6. Some morphological criteria may be utilized to distinguish excitatory from inhibitory chemical synapses.

7. Presynaptic vesicles play a role in the storage and release of neurotransmitters. The

precise nature of the mechanisms involved in these events is not well elucidated at this time.

8. Two basic modes of electrotonic coupling of neurons may occur. Neurons may form electrotonic synapses directly with each other or they may be coupled by way of prejunctional fibers.

ACKNOWLEDGMENTS

The electron micrographs included in this paper were taken from the on-going collaborative studies with my colleagues Dr. Pat G. Model and Joe S. Keeter.

This work is supported, in part, by U.S. Public Health Service Grants NS 11431 and NS 07512 and by the Alfred P. Sloan Foundation.

REFERENCES

1. Wyckoff, R. W. G., and Young, J. Z. (1956): The motorneuron surface. *Proc. R. Soc. [Biol.],* 144:440–450.
2. Pappas, G. D., and Waxman, S. G. (1972): Synaptic fine structure – morphological correlates of chemical and electrotonic transmission. In: *Structure and Function of Synapses,* edited by G. D. Pappas and D. P. Purpura. Raven Press, New York.
3. Gray, E. G. (1959): Axo-somatic and axo-dendritic synapses in the cerebral cortex: an electron microscope study. *J. Anat.,* 93:420–433.
4. Akert, K., Pfenninger, K., Sandri, C., and Moor, H. (1972): Freeze etching and cytochemistry of vesicles and membrane complexes in synapses of the central nervous system. In: *Structure and Function of Synapses,* edited by G. D. Pappas and D. P. Purpura. Raven Press, New York.
5. De Robertis, E. D. P., and Bennett, H. S. (1955): Some features of the submicroscopic morphology of synapses in frog and earthworm. *J. Biophys. Biochem. Cytol.,* 1:47–58.
6. Palay, S. L. (1956): Synapses in the central nervous system. *J. Biophys. Biochem. Cytol.,* 2:193–202.
7. Politoff, A. L., Rose, S., and Pappas, G. D. (1974): The calcium binding sites of synaptic vesicles of the frog sartorius neuromuscular junction. *J. Cell Biol.,* 61:818–823.
8. Whittaker, V. P., and Zimmerman, H. (1974): Biochemical studies on cholinergic synaptic vesicles. In: *Synaptic Transmission and Neuronal Interaction,* edited by M. V. L. Bennett. Raven Press, New York.
9. Wolfe, D. E., Potter, L. T., Richardson, K. C., and Axelrod, J. (1962): Localizing tritiated nor-epinephrine in sympathetic axons by electron microscopic autoradiography. *Science,* 138:440.
10. Hall, Z. W. (1972): The storage, synthesis and inactivation of the transmitters acetylcholine, nor-epinephrine and gamma-aminobutyric acid. In: *Structure and Function of Synapses,* edited by G. D. Pappas and D. P. Purpura. Raven Press, New York.
11. Uchizono, K. (1965): Characteristics of excitatory and inhibitory synapses in the central nervous system of the cat. *Nature,* 207:642–643.
12. Gerschenfeld, H. M. (1973): Chemical transmission in invertebrate central nervous systems and neuromuscular junctions. *Physiol. Rev.,* 53:1–119.
13. Couteaux, R., and Peco-Dechavassin, M. (1970): Vesicules synaptiques et poches au niveau des zones actives' de la jonction neuromusculaire. *C. R. Acad. Sci. (Paris) D,* 271:2346–2349.
14. Gray, E. G. (1973): The cytonet, plain and coated vesicles, reticulosomes, multivesicular bodies and nuclear pores. *Brain Res.,* 62:392–435.
15. Berl, S., Puszin, S., and Nicklas, W. J. (1973): Actinomycin-like protein in brain. *Science,* 179:441–446.
16. Heuser, J. E., Reese, T. S., and Landis, D. M. D. (1974): Functional changes in frog neuromuscular junctions studied with freeze-fracture. *J. Neurocytol.,* 3:109–131.
17. Bloom, F. E. (1972): The formation of synaptic junctions in developing rat brain. In: *Structure and Function of Synapses,* edited by G. D. Pappas and D. P. Purpura. Raven Press, New York.
18. Grafstein, B. (1971): Transneuronal transfer of radioactivity in the central nervous system. *Science,* 172:177–179.
19. Wiesel, T. N., Hubel, D. H., and Lam, D. (1974): Autoradiographic demonstration of ocular dominance columns in the monkey striate cortex by means of transsynaptic transport. *Brain Res.,* 79:273–279.
20. Heuser, J. E., and Reese, T. S. (1973): Evidence for recycling of synaptic vesicle membrane during transmitter release at the frog neuromuscular junction. *J. Cell Biol.,* 57:315–344.
21. Ceccarelli, B., Hurlbut, W. P., and Mauro, A. (1973): Turnover of transmitter and synaptic vesicles at the frog neuromuscular junction. *J. Cell Biol.,* 57:499–524.
22. Purpura, D. P. (1972): Intracellular studies of synaptic organizations in the mammalian brain. In: *Structure and Function of the Synapse,* edited by G. D. Pappas and D. P. Purpura, Raven Press, New York.
23. Špaček, J., and Lieberman, A. R. (1974): Ultrastructural and three-dimensional organization of synaptic glomeruli in rat somatosensory thalamus. *J. Anat.,* 117:487–516.
24. Hamori, J., Pasik, T., Pasik, P., and Szentágothai, J. (1974): Triadic synaptic arrangements and their possible significance in the lateral geniculate nucleus of the monkey. *Brain Res.,* 80:379–393.
25. Reese, T. S., and Shepherd, G. M. (1972): Dendro-dendritic synapses in the central nervous system. In: *Structure and Function of the Syn-*

apse, edited by G. D. Pappas and D. P. Purpura. Raven Press, New York.

26. Eccles, J. C. (1964): *The Physiology of Synapses.* Academic Press, Inc., New York.

27. Longenecker, H. E., Jr., Hurlbut, W. P., Mauro, A., and Clark, A. W. (1970): Effects of black widow spider venom on the frog neuro-muscular junction; effects on endplate potential, miniature endplate potential and nerve terminal spike. *Nature,* 225:701–703.

28. Birks, R. I. (1974): The relationship of trans-mitter release and storage to fine structure in a sympathetic ganglion. *J. Neurocytol.,* 3:133–160.

29. Gilula, N. B. (1974): Junctions between cells. In:

Cell Communication, edited by R. P. Cox. Wiley, New York.

30. Martin, A. R., and Pilar, G. (1963): Dual mode of synaptic transmission in the avian ciliary ganglion. *J. Physiol. (Lond.),* 168:443–463.

31. Bennett, M. V. L. (1971): A comparison of electrically and chemically mediated transmis-sion. In: *Structure and Function of Synapses,* edited by G. D. Pappas and D. P. Purpura. Raven Press, New York.

32. Model, P. G., Highstein, S. M., and Bennett, M. V. L. (1975): Depletion of vesicles and fatigue of transmission at a vertebrate central synapse. *Brain Res. (in press).*

The Nervous System, Donald B. Tower, Editor-in-Chief. *Vol. 1: The Basic Neurosciences*. Raven Press, New York, 1975.

Changing Uses of Nerve Tissue Culture 1950–1975

Richard P. Bunge

When the National Institute of Neurological Diseases and Stroke was founded in 1950, an abstract appeared in the Anatomical Record (1) noting that, under favorable tissue culture conditions, myelin sheaths could be observed to form in relationship to axons of chick sensory neurons maintained for several weeks in tissue culture. This observation, reported in full by Peterson and Murray in 1955 (2), established a new trend in the art of nerve tissue culture, a trend characterized in a 1965 review by Murray (3) as correcting an earlier tendency toward "too great an emphasis on growth and too little attention to organization" by substituting "an organized culture pattern in which growth and migration . . . are minimized." This shift of emphasis to achieve a higher degree of organization signaled a fundamental change from the efforts of an extended earlier period in nerve tissue culture.

This earlier period (for review, see refs. 3–5) extended from the early work of Harrison through that of Weiss, and included substantial contributions by Lewis and the Italian histologist Levi. Emphasis during this period was particularly on axon activity and growth; it is understandable that the opportunity to study axon interaction with supporting cells should be a significant divergent step. Indeed, this desire to attain a high degree of complexity in nerve tissue cultures became, for a time, a rivalry based on the degree of "organotypic" organization achieved. Thus, in the period from 1955 to 1968, the art of nerve tissue culture entered briefly into what might be termed a baroque interval. The zealots of this period proclaimed the beauty of their preparations; the detractors questioned their scientific usefulness.

That a baroque era should follow a classical period is perhaps not surprising, just as it is not surprising that the work of artisans of this period (particularly Bornstein, Hild, Murray, Peterson, and Pomerat) was inevitably to spur a younger generation to reverse the trend and to attempt to take apart the whole into its component cells. As exemplified by the efforts of Varon and Raiborn in 1969 (6), this diversion was initially to be short-lived because normal neurons separated from their supporting cells generally did not survive more than several days in culture. It was not unexpected then, that a subschool of this approach should take the stage by the use of tumor-derived cells of both neuronal and glial types. By this approach, extended viability and proliferation were assured. Although the distortion of form was substantial, this "cubist" approach could readily be undertaken by relatively untrained artisans. But, of course, what its admittedly flawed figures had to say about reality needed constant question.

Recently, a culture art form has appeared which, in the judgment of this author, is appealing and clearly realistic. I refer to the fledgling successes in maintaining several neuronal, muscle, and supporting cell types, derived from normal tissues, in isolation in extended culture. This newest approach allows the parts to be established separately or in recombination with the clear promise of gaining unique insight into the realities of systems difficult to know in the whole.

It is the purpose of this brief chapter to discuss some of the uses of these various forms of nerve tissue culture over the past 25 years. It is not possible in the space available to review the literature extensively; fortunately, this has recently been done admirably by Nelson (5). To allow an overview herein, most references given will be to recent reviews. In addition, it is my purpose to provoke the reader into considering that, if it is possible to isolate and establish normally functioning cells outside the body, we may also be able to do so inside the body to correct cellular deficiencies. Whereas neurological diseases may not be the most amenable to this type of therapeutic approach, certain possibilities seem worthy of consideration and are discussed at the conclusion of this chapter.

OF THE CLASSICAL AND THE BAROQUE

The early efforts in nerve tissue culture reviewed by Weiss in 1955 (7) and by Murray in 1965 (3) (see also refs. 8 and 9) had established that (a) the "growth cone" of the growing nerve fiber was an actively ameboid structure, (b) axon elongation occurred only on solid surfaces as this ameboid activity carried the growth cone forward, (c) this activity at the tip included active uptake of medium components by pinocytosis, and (d) the direction of axon growth was most directly determined by the nature of the substrate in or on which this active movement occurred, i.e., by what Weiss termed contact guidance. Later contributions included the demonstration that (a) fibrillar masses (neurofibrils) could be demonstrated within living neurons, (b) the neuronal cytoplasmic component so prominently seen after basic staining procedures, classically termed the Nissl body, could be shown to preexist as a phase-dense region in living neuronal cytoplasm, (c) the myelin "clefts" first described by Schmidt and Lanterman were clearly visible on cultured living nerve fibers and thus were not artifacts of preparatory procedures (as had been often suggested), (d) the myelin supporting cells (Schwann cells and oligodendrocytes) have an innate pulsatile activity in culture, and (e) active movements of particulate cytoplasmic inclusions can be directly visualized in both neuronal somas and processes.

These cytological observations clearly indicated the advantages of the opportunity for direct observations of neurons and supporting cells in culture; but for many biologists, the crucial proof of the expression of characteristic neuronal function was the demonstration of the ability of the cultured neuron to generate action potentials. This proof was provided for peripheral nerve tissue in 1956 by Crain (10) in studies of chick sensory ganglion cells, and for central tissues in 1962 by Hild and Tasaki (11) in a study of cultured cat and rat cerebellum. Thus, save for the demonstration of synaptic interaction in culture (vide infra), most known in vivo characteristics of neurons had been demonstrated in vitro by the early 1960s. Considering also the many demonstrations of the impressive degree of organization of neurons and supporting cells in culture, the general fidelity of nervous tissue in vitro could be considered established at this time.

In addition to this general cytological fidelity, the ability of portions of the CNS to retain a characteristic cytoarchitectonic pattern in tissue culture was also established. Nelson (5) has summarized the extensive literature on this subject for cultures of sensory and autonomic ganglia, spinal cord, cerebellum, neocortex, and other supraspinal structures. Of these, the culture of spinal cord provides one of the most impressive achievements. Transverse sections of embryonic rodent spinal cord allowed to mature in culture may (a) develop clearly defined dorsal and ventral regions with large motor neurons demonstrable in the latter, (b) develop a discrete pair of ventral roots, (c) contain both CNS myelin sheaths in the explant and PNS myelin in the outgrowth, (d) contain numerous large and small interneurons along with a variety of neuroglia, (e) contain a variety of synaptic interrelationships, (f) possess the ability to establish connectivity with adjacent spinal cord or brainstem explants, and (g) exhibit complex bioelectric activity interpreted as indicative of multisynaptic neuronal networks. Perhaps the only additional function one would ask to be expressed is the ability of spinal cord motor neurons to innervate striated muscle and autonomic ganglia in coculture; this has been accomplished in a variety of culture situations (vide infra).

Considering that both neurons and supporting cells were known to express certain normal functions in culture and that a high degree of organization could be attained, many new types of study became feasible. Of these, the study of the myelin sheath gained special prominence during the decade between 1955 and 1965. This was, it should be noted, the era during which the electron microscope provided the first clear definition of myelin organization and mechanisms of formation. The use of tissue culture in the study of the organization, development, and pathology of the peripheral nervous system has been recently reviewed (12) and may be partially summarized as follows. The myelinated sensory ganglion frequently used in this type of study provides a miniature replica of the

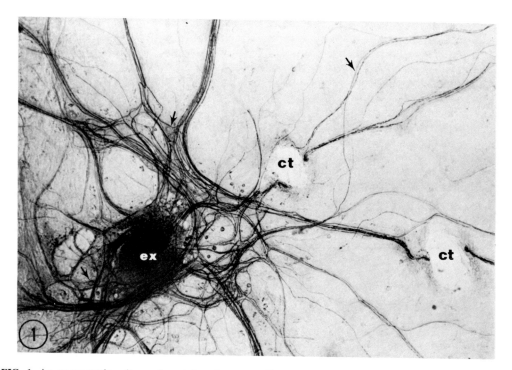

FIG. 1. An organotypic culture of a rat dorsal root ganglion (DRG) prepared by explanting a fetal rat DRG and allowing it to mature for 6 weeks or more in culture. The culture originally contained only the explant (ex) from which numerous nerve fiber bundles grew along with a background of connective tissue cells. Starting in the third week, the culture began to myelinate and in time fascicles of myelinated nerve fibers became the most prominent feature of the outgrowth (which also contains many unmyelinated nerve fibers). This is a control culture from an experiment on nerve fiber degeneration. Two of the outgrowing fascicles were severed at the points marked ct. Distal to these cuts, the myelin segments are seen in the process of degeneration. At the arrow (upper right) a normal myelinated nerve fiber which circumvents the cut is seen coursing with several degenerating fibers. This type of preparation has recently been used (Schlaepfer and Bunge, 1973, *J. Cell Biol.,* 59:456) to demonstrate that the process of Wallerian degeneration is significantly retarded if calcium ion concentrations are reduced in the immediate environment of the damaged axon. In this preparation, most of the neuronal cell bodies are confined in the explant region; in this culture, several neurons (arrows on left) are located outside the ganglion mass and among the myelinated nerve fibers. Sudan black stain after osmium fixation. × 25.

peripheral sensory nervous system (Fig. 1); the cultured ganglion contains both small and large neuronal types and both unmyelinated and myelinated fibers (although the latter represent only the smallest diameter myelinated fibers and shortest myelin segments present in peripheral nerve *in vivo*). As referenced in the review cited above (12), studies with this type of culture have established that (a) Wallerian degeneration occurs after axonal amputation, as *in vivo*, but its onset may be retarded by lowering calcium ion levels in the culture medium, (b) diphtherial toxin produces segmental demyelination as *in vivo*, (c) Schwann cells related to unmyelinated nerve fibers are particularly susceptible to X-irradiation. (d) trypsin

application to the myelinated nerve fiber causes damage (partially reversible) to the paranodal myelin sheath, as do lowered calcium ion concentrations, (e) the sequence of changes during the degeneration of unmyelinated nerve fibers includes an early transient focal swelling phase attributable to failure of ion pumping mechanisms prior to the complete loss of selective permeability of the axolemma, (f) both lymph node and buffy coat cells and (less effectively) serum from animals with allergic neuriti cause the breakdown of myelin sheaths in tissue cultures of sensory ganglion, whereas antiserum to immunoglobulin inhibits the cell mediated demyelination of these cultures, (g) both buffy coat cells and serum from patients with Guillain-Barré syndrome cause demyelination in cultures of peripheral nerve tissues, clearly establishing this syndrome as an autoimmune phenomenon, and (g) brief exposure of sensory ganglion cultures to chlorpromazine causes a substantial but transient increase in lysosomal elements within neurons and supporting cells. In addition to these observations, studies have appeared describing the responses of cultured peripheral neurons to, among other agents, thallium, cyanide, Na azide, thiamine deficiency, colchicine, chloroquine, ouabain, and heavy water. Organized cultures of peripheral tissues have also been useful in studies of the cytopathic effects of several types of viruses (for review, see ref. 5).

Methods of preparing cultures containing CNS myelin were first published in 1957 (13), and many experiments have been reported in which CNS myelin formation was inhibited, or formed myelin was altered by experimental attack. Work with myelinated CNS tissue culture preparations in the study of experimental allergic encephalomyelitis (and human diseases of possibly similar etiology) has provided less consistent results than have experiments with PNS tissues. This may derive from the fact that CNS myelin is more susceptible to capricious deterioration subsequent to subtle changes in media or culture conditions. (For a discussion of the sometimes conflicting recent results, see refs. 14 and 15.) There seems little doubt that experimental variables can be brought under adequate control, that the variety of possible antigens in CNS myelin and their precise mode of exposure in myelin membrane will be systematically sorted out, and that a fuller understanding of the mechanisms of CNS demyelination will be possible.

THE SYNAPSE IN CULTURE

Mentioned only briefly in Murray's 1965 review (3), the synapse was to replace the myelin sheath (from 1965 to 1970) as the hallmark of "organotypacity" in nerve tissue culture. Whereas it is likely that some of Harrison's earliest culture preparations contained functioning neuromuscular junctions, clear evidence for the presence of synapses in tissue cultures first became available from physiological experiments in 1963 and from electron-micro-

scopic observations published in 1965. (For details, see refs. 16–20.) Synaptic development has been observed in culture within small explants of CNS tissues and between (a) tissues established as separate explants, (b) neurons originally dissociated and then allowed to reaggregate, (c) spinal cord neurons and striated muscle, (d) spinal cord neurons and autonomic neurons, and (e) autonomic neurons and target tissues.

In more recent studies, observations on developing nerve tissue cultures have allowed demonstration that synapses may develop under conditions where action potential generation and neurotransmitter release are prevented by continued exposure to xylocaine or Mg^{2+}. As discussed by Crain and Peterson (18), synaptic development in culture may also include the appearance of complex bioelectric discharges believed to originate in elaborate synaptic networks; evidence has also been presented that these networks must include arrays of both excitatory and inhibitory synapses with characteristic pharmacological sensitivities.

This writer has discussed in some detail elsewhere (20) the question of whether or not synapses formed in tissue culture systems conform to the anatomical and physiological forms found *in vivo*. A strong argument is made there that the anatomical form of synapses in culture, the site specificity expressed, the neurotransmitters released, and the pharmacological sensitivities demonstrable are as expected from *in vivo* observations. An example is the synapse formed between spinal cord and autonomic ganglion neurons in cultures containing both of these tissues. Foreign neurons, e.g., from cerebral cortex, were shown not to form this synapse. Recent work by C. P. Ko and H. Burton (*submitted for publication*) on cultures containing explants of spinal cord grown with dissociated autonomic neurons has established this as a nicotinic cholinergic synapse which is blocked by hexamethonium and mecamylamine but not by low concentrations of atropine or by phantolamine. No effects on the activity of this synapse were observed on exposure to the adrenergic blocking agent phenoxybenzamine. On electron-microscopic observation, this ending contains the uniform round vesicles, without demonstrable dense cores, which characterize this synapse *in vivo*.

A masterpiece of baroque culture art worthy of viewing in this context is the recent demonstration by Crain and Peterson (21) of synaptic connectivity in explant clusters containing dorsal root ganglia connected to spinal cord which in turn was juxtaposed to explants of brainstem and medulla. Electrophysiological studies indicated that dorsal root ganglion neurites not only established characteristic sensory synaptic network functions in the dorsal region of the attached spinal cord explants but that these neurites grew through the cord tissue, crossed a region of collagen substrate, and made functional synaptic connections in a localized zone of a nearby medulla explant. In some cases, these sensory neurites were observed to grow through a midbrain region and to establish connectivity only in one discrete zone in a more distally located medulla explant; this zone was judged to be that portion of the medulla normally receiving this input *in vivo*. In addition to this expression of regional specificity, these authors found physiological characteristics and pharmacological sensitivities similar to those found in this sensory system *in vivo*. This type of explant mosaic has been prepared within the limited confines of the Maximow culture assembly. Should this art be undertaken on a larger canvas, how many more figures might be added?

The primary example of the usefulness of tissue culture in studying synaptic development and function is presently provided by the now extensive work on the neuromuscular junction *in vitro* (for review, see refs. 18,22–26). This period in the recent history of nerve tissue culture began in 1968 with the anatomical demonstration of nerve endings on skeletal muscle cells grown in juxtaposition to spinal cord tissue. The art was substantially refined in 1972 (22) with a demonstration that long-term cultures of very low cellular density could be obtained by the judicious use of antimitotic agents. Thus it was possible to seed dissociated neurons from chick spinal cord among developing striated muscle cells in culture and to demonstrate electrophysiological interaction by using intracellular microelectrodes placed within both pre- and postsynaptic elements. This type of preparation, benefiting from advances in both muscle and nerve culture techniques, has allowed a clear solution to one of the long-debated

questions regarding neuromuscular junction development. Tissue culture studies have demonstrated that receptor clustering on the muscle fiber membrane may precede nerve fiber contact with the developing muscle cell. This approach offers every hope of additional key contributions in the near future (especially in regard to trophic interactions; see refs. 18,24, 25). The use of this type of culture preparation should be especially valuable in assessing causative factors in muscular dystrophy, for example. Unfortunately, such studies have in recent years been sharply contradictory, perhaps because of genetic differences in the laboratory animals used as tissue sources (see discussion in ref. 26).

1969 AND THE CUBISTS

In 1969, articles appeared on methods of both CNS (6) and PNS (27) cell dissociation which allowed isolated neurons essentially without supporting cells to be obtained for tissue culture. It was clear from this work that some separation of normal cell types was possible; but it was also clear that, after separation, the viability of the cells was poor (several days at best). Concomitantly, it was reported that neuronal tumors could provide "functional" clonal lines of neurons (28,29) and that certain of these cells were capable of generating action potentials (30) (Fig. 2). This was not the first report on malignant neurons in culture (see, for example, ref. 31). However, these reports (regarding the availability and uses of tumor-derived cells in culture), along with that of Lightbody et al. (32) the following year (regarding "biochemically differentiated" clonal human glial cells in long-term replicating cultures), spurred an increasing interest in the use of tumor-derived cells. Thus the present "cubist" era in nerve tissue culture was born. Especially when considered in the light of the reported poor survival of normal dissociated cells in culture, it is not surprising that work with established cell lines gained rapid acceptance. It is certainly true that, as of this writing, more papers have been published on tumor-derived neurons and glia (during these last 6 years) than have been published on cultures of normal neurons or supporting cells during the entire earlier history of nerve tissue culture. Re-

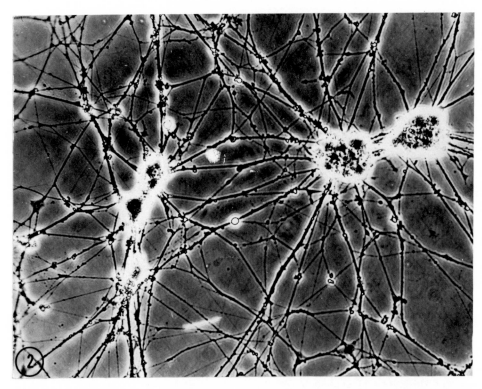

FIG. 2. These cells are from a human ganglioneuroblastoma established in primary culture for 9 days. These small groups of neurons have elaborated a complex network of neurites during this period. Note absence of other cell types. (Photomicrograph provided by Dr. M. Goldstein from culture prepared and carried in his laboratory.) × 175.

cently, Schubert and colleagues (33) generated a substantial number of additional neuronal and glial cell lines from tumors induced by the administration of nitrosourea to pregnant rats. From their observations on the behavior of these cells in tissue culture, they have concluded that (a) tumor cells may be classified as neuronal or glial on the basis of their ability to extend long processes in serum-free medium, (b) certain neurotransmitters are synthesized by cell lines classified as glial, (c) some clonal nerve cell lines synthesize more than one neurotransmitter, and (d) the nervous system proteins designated S100 and 14–3–2 are found in various combinations in both nerve and glial cell lines.

In general, the rapidly developing recent work with tumor-derived cells has been engendered by the vision that this approach will be useful in understanding normal functioning of the nervous system, rather than by the ob-

jective of controlling tumor generation or growth. Certainly, neuronal or glial functions expressed in tumor-derived cell lines (e.g., the generation of an action potential) can be studied in these preparations with the hope of establishing the precise molecular mechanisms involved. The substantial debate about their usefulness regards, at least in part, their use in studying mechanisms of regulation (e.g., enzyme regulation), for the basic regulatory deficiencies of these cells cannot be denied. Work with tumor-derived cells of neural origin in tissue culture has been extensively reviewed (34–36; Nirenberg, *this volume*).

CULTURES OF ISOLATED CELLS FROM NORMAL TISSUES

In 1970, Bray (37) provided both experimental evidence that, as axons elongate, new surface material is added at the growing tip, and details of a method for obtaining autonomic neurons from rat superior cervical ganglion as isolated cells in culture. By using a mechanical dissociation procedure, a medium of high viscosity, a very low CO_2 level, and substantial amounts of nerve growth factor (NGF), Bray obtained neurons free of both connective tissue components and Schwann cells. If maintained in culture several weeks, these neurons grew in size and, via a rich arborization of processes, formed a complex network with neighboring cells. It is now known that the nonneural cells which tend to proliferate during this period of neuronal maturation can be controlled by adjusting the culture medium or employing antimitotic agents; it is thus possible to obtain cultures containing only principal autonomic neurons (Figs. 3 and 4). These can be maintained for at least several months and require no supporting cell population.

Detailed biochemical (38), anatomical (39), and physiological studies (40) have been undertaken on these neurons. In summary, it has been shown that these neurons from the (largely) adrenergic population of the sympathetic trunk (a) have the ultrastructural characteristics of adrenergic neurons, (b) synthesize norepinephrine, (c) maintain resting potentials, (d) generate action potentials, and (d) generally function as would be expected from their class of neurons *in vivo*. These essentially "normal" aspects of their functional expression in culture have tended to be overshadowed by the observation that the neurons make cholinergic synapses with one another (40). As is discussed in some detail elsewhere (20,41), this observation may be explained by the innate propensity of the autonomic neuron to adjust its transmitter synthesis to its environment. According to this explanation, autonomic neurons are capable of synthesizing both acetylcholine and norepinephrine and focus their synthetic activity in response to environmental clues. Similar mechanisms of neurotransmitter selection may be operative during normal embryogenesis (41). However, a basic problem remains: Do certain culture (and embryonic) conditions select for a specific kind (cholinergic or adrenergic) of autonomic neuron, or does the entire population shift its transmitter synthetic capacity, the machinery for synthesis of both transmitters being present in all cells?

This work with the isolated autonomic ganglion neuron in culture is the most developed of the isolated normal neuron cultures reported. Certain sensory neurons have also been grown in complete isolation (42); and several types of central neurons have been grown in relative isolation (e.g., refs. 43,44).

The finding of synapses of unexpected coinage among isolated autonomic neurons in culture should not detract from the basic accomplishment. Neurons from normal tissues can mature and be maintained in culture for extended periods without supporting cells of any type. It should be noted that, during their maturation period in culture, serum must be present in the culture medium. We have observed, however, that after maturation these networks can be maintained (in satisfactory but not showcase condition) for periods of over one month in a completely defined medium of Eagle's minimum essential medium, added glucose, and purified NGF. This accomplishment of culturing entirely isolated neurons undoubtedly derives from the fact that the essential trophic agent (NGF) for this neuron is known and available in substantial amounts. It would appear that trophic factors essential for the long-term survival of other neuronal types may become known and may permit long-term maintenance of other neuronal populations of specific type in isolation. In the interim, these "trophic" factors are generally provided, as in the past, by maintaining some glial component and some degree of cellular aggregation in culture preparations.

It may be useful to comment here on the question of how neurons may survive in complete isolation in culture when it has generally been observed in neuroanatomical and neuroembryological studies that neurons deprived of targets for their synaptic endings do not survive. To this writer, the most attractive hypothesis is that, in general, neurons, during some stage in their development, acquire a critical defect in some vital function (e.g., their ability to transport certain nutrients). This deficiency must be corrected by an outside agent—a trophic factor—if the neuron is to survive and function. This trophic factor may be provided to the neuron from its synaptic input and/or by supporting glia and/or by contact with target tissues. If we provide adequate glial support or target

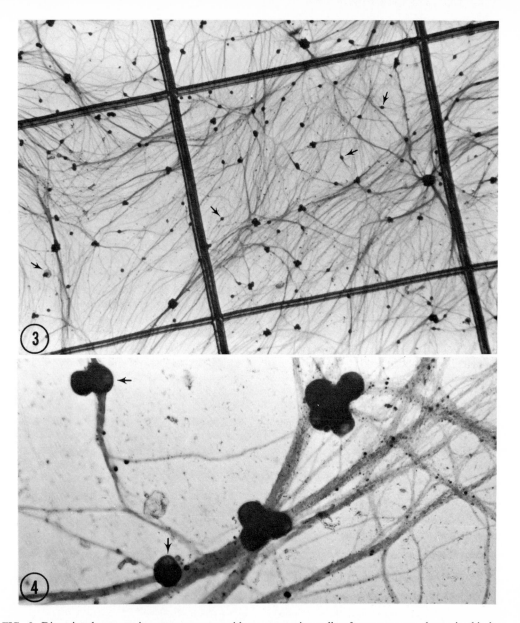

FIG. 3. Dissociated autonomic neurons grown without supporting cells of any type are shown in this low-power light micrograph. The neurons occur either as single cells (3 arrows in center square) or as small aggregates. The outgrowing processes of the neurons have formed a complex network over the surface of the culture dish. Neurons prepared by this method sometimes exhibit large vacuoles within their cytoplasm (arrow to the left). This culture dish was marked prior to preparing the culture with a series of squares (each measuring approximately 2 mm) to allow quantification of the number of neurons present. Sudan black stain after osmium fixation. × 35.

FIG. 4. Higher-magnification light micrograph of the network shown in Fig. 3. A single neuron, as well as groups of 2, 3, and 4, are present along with part of the complex network of neuronal processes formed by these neurons. This network is entirely free of supporting cells and the background is free of fibroblasts. In the absence of these supporting cell types, a substantial amount of debris is found in the culture. The neuronal cell bodies, when growing in the absence of supporting cells, are globular in form and thus appear very dense. In several cell bodies (arrows) the nucleus and nucleolus can be seen. These neurons have survived for approximately 2 months in complete isolation from any supporting tissue. They are known to maintain normal resting potentials (for this cell type) and to generate action potentials as well as form synapses with one another (see text). Sudan black stain after osmium fixation. × 300.

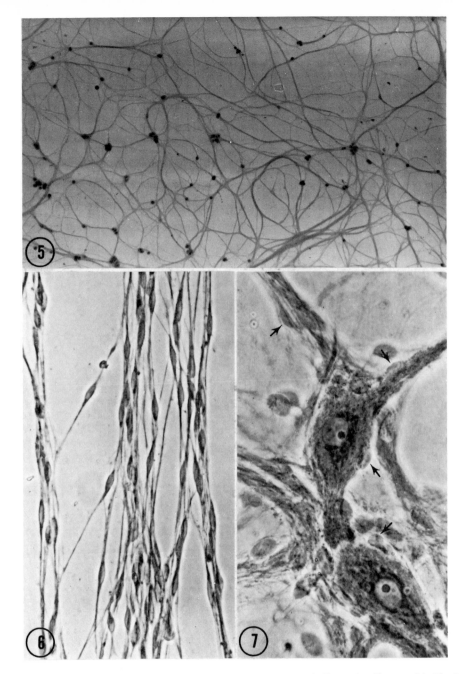

FIG. 5. Light micrograph of a network of isolated autonomic neurons similar to that illustrated in Fig. 3 except that, in this case, the neurons have been grown with Schwann cells. The Schwann cells are not apparent at this magnification for they are located within the nerve fiber fascicles and adjacent to the neuronal cell bodies. Note that there is no background cell component between these elements. In the presence of Schwann cells, the network is more fasciculated (than in Fig. 3) and the neurons are less globular. Sudan black stain after osmium fixation. × 35.

FIG. 6. Preparation containing only Schwann cells. The methods used for obtaining this type of preparation have recently been submitted for publication by Dr. P. Wood. In the absence of neurites, these cells are quiescent but will respond by thymidine incorporation and mitosis if neurites are allowed to grow among them (Wood and Bunge, 1975, *Nature, in press*). The linear configuration of the Schwann Cell is retained even in the absence of a neurite population. Note the absence of other cell types. Sudan black stain after osmium fixation. × 360.

FIG. 7. Isolated autonomic neurons with accompanying Schwann cells (from the network pictured in Fig. 5). Lower two arrows, lightly stained nuclei of two of the Schwann cells surrounding the neuron cell body; upper two arrows, Schwann cell nuclei associated with nerve fascicles. Note that, in the presence of Schwann cells, the neuron cell bodies are more flattened and do not often assume the globular configuration shown in Fig. 4. Sudan black stain after osmium fixation. × 300.

tissue the neuron may survive in culture, even though the specific agent or agents being provided by these cells to correct its deficiencies are not known. If the trophic factor is known (and NGF is certainly such a factor), then the neuron can be maintained indefinitely in complete isolation. Thus, even as Levi-Montalcini (45) was demonstrating the dependence of adrenergic autonomic neurons on the presence of NGF in the culture medium, Murray and colleagues (3) were growing autonomic neurons (with their attendant supporting cells) for long periods in premier condition without NGF addition to the culture medium. This explanation would appear to be supported by the work of Varon and associates (46) who demonstrated the ability of nonneuronal cells to substitute for NGF in the support of neurons during their first hours in culture.

In at least one instance, culture of a specific supporting cell free of other cell types has also been accomplished (Figs. 5–7). A recent report (47) indicates that essentially pure Schwann cell populations may be obtained from rat sensory ganglion explants. Using special methods of explant preparation and application of antimitotic agents, it is possible to prepare explants in which the outgrowth contains only neurites and accompanying Schwann cells. The explant is then excised leaving outgrowth which (after the amputated neurites degenerate) contains only Schwann cells. In this type of preparation, the number of Schwann cells stabilizes after several days; but their number may be increased by exposure to growing neurites. This type of experimental preparation has allowed the demonstration that the growing, unsheathed sensory neurite provides a mitogenic signal for Schwann cells (47). If the nature of this signal could be identified, or a substitute signal found, then it might be possible to obtain normal Schwann cells in large numbers.

There are many reports of success in culturing mixed glial populations from diverse normal sources, as well as substantial literature on culture of tumor-derived central and peripheral supporting cells (35). The culture of "pure" populations of normal Schwann cells is emphasized here because this system appears to provide both the possibility for delineating those functions and properties unique to this specific cell type, and a candidate for use in the type of "cellular therapy" briefly discussed below.

CONCLUSION

The brevity of this chapter has not allowed discussion of several substantive recent developments in nerve tissue culture. Among these are the recent reports of successful cultivation of invertebrate nervous tissue, the description of the fine structure and experiments on the mechanisms of motility and uptake by the growth cone, the use of a variety of culture systems for the study of propagation and cytopathic effects of viruses, the detailed physiological observation available on a number of neuronal types in culture, and the demonstration that certain enzyme activities are expressed only when neurons are allowed a degree of reaggregation in culture.

It seems clear from the accumulated evidence that neurons and glial cells express their native capabilities well in culture. This fact has implications beyond the obvious conclusion that experimental results from cultures can be considered useful in extending our understanding of *in vivo* systems. If we have normal cell types available in culture and if a nervous system disease stems from an absence or deficiency of one of these cell types, then it is an obvious step to transfer cultured cells into the diseased animal to attempt to correct the deficiency. Whereas at present this would not seem practical for many types of neurons, it may be practical for supporting cells (e.g., Schwann or glial).

Lest this appear a possibility of only modest interest, it should be pointed out that the terrain which regenerating peripheral nerves preferentially follow is provided by Schwann cells aligned in the connective tissue framework of the nerve segment distal to the cut. Similarly, in species where in certain situations CNS regeneration is known to occur (48), glial cells may provide a bridge over which the regenerating nerve fibers pass. The possibility may now exist for the construction of a type of cellular bridge for use in vertebrates without the native capacity for this activity in response to injury. Experiments of this type are practical now in highly inbred rodents where the problem of rejection may be circumvented. Whether or not this type of "cellular therapy" can be demonstrated to be useful in animals is a prime challenge of the coming decades; whether or not it might some day be practical in humans is one possible goal for the second 25 years of the NINCDS.

ACKNOWLEDGMENTS

Work in the author's laboratory has been supported from 1962 to the present by grants from the National Institutes of Health, National Institute for Neurological and Communicative Disorders and Stroke, and from the National Multiple Sclerosis Society.

REFERENCES

1. Peterson, E. R. (1950): Production of myelin sheaths *in vitro* by embryonic spinal ganglion cells. *Anat. Rec.*, 106:232.
2. Peterson, E. R., and Murray, M. R. (1955): Myelin sheath formation in culture of avian spinal ganglia. *Am. J. Anat.*, 96:319–355.
3. Murray, M. R. (1965): Nervous tissue *in vitro*. In: *Cells and Tissues in Culture, Vol. 2*, edited by F. M. Willmer, pp. 373–455. Academic Press, New York.
4. Lumsden, C. E. (1968): Nervous tissue in culture. In: *The Structure and Function of Nervous Tissue, Vol. I*, edited by G. H. Bourne, pp. 68–140. Academic Press, New York.
5. Nelson, P. G. (1975): Nerve and muscle cells in culture. *Physiol. Rev.*, 55:1–61.
6. Varon, S., and Raiborn, C. W. (1969): Dissociation, fractionation, and culture of embryonic brain cells. *Brain Res.*, 12:180–199.
7. Weiss, P. (1955): Neurogenesis. In: *Analysis of Development*, edited by B. Willier, P. Weiss, and V. Hamburger, pp. 346–392. Haffner, New York.
8. Pomerat, C. M., Hendelman, W. J, Raiborn, C. W., Jr., and Massey, J. F. (1967): Dynamic activities of nervous tissue *in vitro*. In: *The Neuron*, edited by H. Hyden, pp. 119–178. Elsevier, New York.
9. Nakai, J. (1964): The movements of neurons in tissue culture. In: *Primitive Motile Systems in Cell Biology*, edited by R. D. Allen and N. Kamiya, pp. 377–385. Academic Press, New York.
10. Crain, S. M. (1956): Resting and action potentials of cultured chick embryo spinal ganglion cells. *J. Comp. Neurol.*, 104:285–330.
11. Hild, W., and Tasaki, I. (1962): Morphological and physiological properties of neurons and glial cells in tissue culture. *J. Neurophysiol.*, 25:277–304.
12. Bunge, R. P., and Bunge, M. B. (1975): Tissue culture in the study of peripheral nerve pathology. In: *Peripheral Neuropathy*, edited by P. Dyck, P. Thomas, and E. Lambert. Saunders, Philadelphia. (*In press.*)
13. Hild, W. (1957): Myelinogenesis in cultures of mammalian nervous tissue. *Z. Zellforsch.*, 46:71–95.
14. Seil, F., Smith, M., and Leiman, A. (1975): Myelination inhibiting and neuroelectric blocking factors in experimental allergic encephalomyelitis (EAE). *Science*, 187:951–953.
15. Bornstein, M. (1973): The immunopathology of demyelinative disorders examined in organotypic cultures of mammalian central nerve tissues. In: *Progress in Neuropathology, Vol. II*, edited by H. Zimmerman, pp. 69–90. Grune and Stratton, New York.
16. Crain, S. M. (1966): Development of "organotypic" bioelectric activities in central nervous tissues during maturation in culture. *Int. Rev. Neurobiol.*, 9:1–43.
17. Crain, S. M., Peterson, E. R., and Bornstein, M. B. (1968): Formation of functional interneuronal connections between explants of various mammalian central nervous tissues during development *in vitro*. In: *Ciba Found. Symp. on Growth of the Nervous System*, edited by G. Wolstenholme and M. O'Connor, pp. 13–31. Churchill, London.
18. Crain, S. M., and Peterson, E. R. (1974): Development of neural connections in culture. In: *Trophic Functions of the Neuron*, edited by D. B. Drachman, vol. 228, pp. 6–33. *Ann. NY Acad. Sci.*
19. Bunge, M. B., Bunge, R. P., and Peterson, E. R. (1967): The onset of synapse formation in spinal cord culture as studied by electron microscopy. *Brain Res.*, 6:728–749.
20. Bunge, R. P. (1975): The expression of neuronal specificity in tissue culture. In: *Neuronal Recognition*, edited by S. Barondes. Plenum Press, New York. (*In press.*)
21. Crain, S. M., and Peterson, E. R. (1975): Development of specific sensory evoked synaptic networks in fetal mouse cord-brainstem cultures. *Science*, 188:275–278.
22. Fischbach, G. (1972): Synapse formation between dissociated nerve and muscle cells in low density cell cultures. *Dev. Biol.*, 28:407–429.
23. Shimada, Y., and Fischman, D. A. (1973): Morphological and physiological evidence for the development of functional neuromuscular junctions *in vitro*. *Dev. Biol.*, 31:200–225.
24. Fambrough, D., Hartzell, H. C., Rash, J. E., and Ritchie, A. K. (1974): Receptor properties of developing muscle. In: *Trophic Functions of the Neuron*, edited by D. B. Drachman, vol. 228, pp. 47–61. *Ann. NY Acad. Sci.*
25. Fischbach, G., Henkart, M., Cohen, S., Breuer, A., Whysner, J., and Neal, F. (1974): Studies on the development of neuromuscular junctions in cell culture. In: *Synaptic Transmission and*

Neuronal Interaction, edited by M. V. Bennett, pp. 259–283. Raven Press, New York.

26. Parsons, R. (1974): Expression of the dystrophia muscularis (dy) recessive gene in mice. *Nature,* 251:621–622.

27. Sensenbrenner, M., Lodin, Z., Treska, J., Jacob, M., Kage, M., and Mandel, P. (1969): The cultivation of isolated neurons from spinal ganglia of chick embryo. *Z. Zellforsch.,* 98:538–549.

28. Augusti-Tocco, G., and Sato, G. (1969): Establishment of functional clonal lines of neurons from mouse neuroblastoma. *Proc. Natl. Acad. Sci. USA,* 64:311–315.

29. Schubert, D., Humphreys, S., Baroni, C., and Cohen, M. (1969): *In vitro* differentiation of a mouse neuroblastoma. *Proc. Natl. Acad. Sci. USA,* 64:316–323.

30. Nelson, P., Ruffner, W., and Nirenberg, M. (1969): Neuronal tumor cells with excitable membranes grown *in vitro. Proc. Natl. Acad. Sci. USA,* 64:1004–1010.

31. Goldstein, M. N., and Pinkel, D. (1958): Long-term tissue culture of neuroblastomas. *J. Natl. Cancer Inst.,* 20:675–689.

32. Lightbody, J., Pfeiffer, S. E., Kornblith, P. L., and Herschmann, H. (1970): Biochemically differentiated clonal human glial cells in tissue culture. *J. Neurobiol.,* 1:411–417.

33. Schubert, D., Heinemann, S., Carlisle, W., Tarikas, H., Kimes, B., Patrick, J., Steinback, J. H., Culp, W., and Brandt, B. L. (1974): Clonal cell lines from the rat central nervous system. *Nature,* 249:224–227.

34. McMorris, F. A., Nelson, P. G., and Ruddle, F. H. (1973): Clonal systems in neurobiology. *Neurosci. Res. Program,* 11:412–536.

35. Sato, G. (Ed.) (1973): *Tissue Culture of the Nervous System.* Plenum Press, New York.

36. Steinbach, J. H. (1974): Synapse formation *in vitro.* In: *Frontiers in Neurology and Neuroscience Research,* edited by P. Seeman and G. Brown, pp. 133–141, University of Toronto Press, Toronto.

37. Bray, D. (1970): Surface movements during the growth of single explanted neurons. *Proc. Natl. Acad. Sci. USA,* 65:905–910.

38. Mains, R. E., and Patterson, P. H. (1973): Primary cultures of dissociated sympathetic neurons. (3 parts). *J. Cell. Biol.,* 59:329–366.

39. Rees, R., and Bunge, R. (1974): Morphological and cytochemical studies of synapses formed in culture between isolated superior cervical ganglion neurons. *J. Comp. Neurol.,* 157:1–12.

40. O'Lague, P. H., Obata, K., Claude, P., Furshpan, E. J., and Potter, D. P. (1974): Evidence for cholinergic synapses between dissociated rat sympathetic neurons in cell culture. *Proc. Natl. Acad. Sci. USA,* 71:3602–3606.

41. Patterson, P., and Chun, L. (1974): The influence of non-neuronal cells on catecholamine and acetylcholine synthesis and accumulation in cultures of dissociated sympathetic neurons. *Proc. Natl. Acad. Sci. USA,* 71:3607–3610.

42. Okun, L. M. (1972): Isolated dorsal root ganglion neurons in culture: Cytological maturation and extension of electrically active processes. *J. Neurobiol.,* 3:111–151.

43. Lasher, R. S. (1974): The uptake of ^{3}H-GABA and differentiation of stellate neurons in cultures of dissociated postnatal rat cerebellum. *Brain Res.,* 69:235–254.

44. Nelson, P., and Peacock, J. (1973): Electrical activity in dissociated cell cultures from fetal mouse cerebellum. *Brain Res.,* 61:163–174.

45. Levi-Montalcini, R., and Angeletti, P. U. (1963): Essential role of the nerve growth factor in the survival and maintenance of dissociated sensory and sympathetic embryonic nerve cells *in vitro. Dev. Biol.,* 7:653–659.

46. Burnham, P., Raiborn, C., and Varon, S. (1972): Replacement of nerve-growth factor by ganglionic non-neuronal cells for the survival *in vitro* of dissociated ganglionic neurons. *Proc. Natl. Acad. Sci. USA,* 69:3556–3560.

47. Wood, P., and Bunge, R. (1975): Evidence that sensory axons are mitogenic for Schwann cells. *Nature,* 256:662–664.

48. Reier, P. J., and Webster, H. (1974): Regeneration and remyelination of xenopus tadpole optic nerve fibers following transection or crush. *J. Neurocytol.,* 3:591–618.

The Nervous System, Donald B. Tower, Editor-in-Chief. *Vol. 1: The Basic Neurosciences.* Raven Press, New York, 1975.

Membrane Models: Theoretical and Real

J. David Robertson

A number of qualitatively different membrane models have been presented by various authors in recent years, but only two will be considered here. These are the unit membrane model proposed by the author (1–3) and the fluid mosaic model proposed by Singer and Nicholson (4,5). These two models differ significantly in some important details, and it seems worthwhile to try to reconcile these differences in the hope that a better understanding of the rules of how biological membranes are constructed molecularly may emerge. There are a number of important new facts about biological membranes that have appeared in recent years that need to be incorporated into any model to make it useful, and it is one purpose of this chapter to examine some such new facts and to show how they may be added to bring the unit membrane model up to date. None of these facts was excluded by the original unit membrane model and therefore can be easily included without conflicting with its basic tenets. Some features of the fluid mosaic model, however, cannot be incorporated because they conflict with some of the evidence. It is hoped that these areas of conflict can be made clear but perhaps the most constructive point is to try to illustrate how the models are stimulating new experimental approaches to decide about points of disagreement. This, of course, is the *raison d'être* of all membrane models.

THE UNIT MEMBRANE AND THE FLUID MOSAIC MODEL

The evidence on which the unit membrane model was based has been reviewed recently (1). We need here only to state what the theory said and how it resembles and differs from the fluid mosaic model. The unit membrane model proposed that all biological membranes are constructed molecularly with a single continuous bilayer of lipid as their core with the lipid polar heads pointing outward and associated in some unknown way with protein and other nonlipid molecules. It proposed that there was a chemical asymmetry at least in some membranes caused by the presence of carbohydrate moieties among the proteins of the external surface. This is all the theory said. It said nothing about the particular molecular species involved, nothing about conformation of nonlipids nor the kinds of bonding that might hold the nonlipid and the lipid together nor did it include nor exclude fluidity. It also did not exclude penetration of the lipid bilayer by protein, although it did place some constraints on the extent of this. Thus, as far as it went, the unit membrane theory was correct in the light of what we know today.

How then does the unit membrane model differ from the fluid mosaic model? It differs mainly in quantitative terms. In essence the fluid mosaic theory also visualizes the membrane as a continuous lipid bilayer, but it has all of the protein aggregated into separated clumps of varying size (generally globs 4 to 10 nm thick) that are embedded to varying degrees in the lipid bilayer penetrating partway or all the way through. It also leaves half or more of the lipid polar surfaces of the bilayer that separate the protein moieties exposed directly to the medium on both sides of the membrane. It emphasizes fluidity to an extreme degree.

In its extreme form the fluid mosaic model is misleading. If there were as large a fraction of lipid polar groups directly exposed in the surfaces of the bilayer, surely the mechanical properties of all membranes would be the same as model lipid bilayers and this is not the case. Furthermore, at least some of the many soluble proteins inevitably in contact with the membrane in any living cell would be expected to spread and adsorb on it as they do at any such surface in aqueous model systems of lipid and protein (11). Finally if membranes were as fluid as this model implies, it would be difficult to control the positions of any molecules in the surface. They would all be randomly distributed unless brought together by some outside agency such as antibodies. However, even then only varying sized clumps would be produced that would remain randomly distributed. There is ample evidence in studies of capping and clustering phenomena (6,7) alone to show that this is not so. Furthermore, the experiments of Tamm and Tamm (8) show that whereas selected parts of a given single cell plasma membrane may be quite fluid other regions in the same cell may not be.

Perhaps the most telling argument against the extreme version of the fluid mosaic model is the experiment reported by Mudd and Mudd in 1931 (9). In this study a fresh droplet of human blood was deposited on a glass slide in Locke's solution beside a droplet of one of several different oils. A coverslip was applied and the oil and water phases came together, setting up an oil-water interface. It was observed by light microscopy that some red blood cells entered the oil phase and seemed to be wetted by the oil. White cells never behaved in this way. We have repeated this experiment. Figure 1 shows a group of erythrocytes that are present in the oil phase to the top right of the oil-water interface that runs across the lower left corner. This experiment implies that the erythrocyte membrane can sometimes be wetted by oil. This could hardly occur if most of the surface is made of closely packed hydrophilic lipid bilayer polar heads and the rest of very hydrophilic protein moieties. This latter must be true of all the membrane proteins depicted in the Singer-Nicholson model.

The unit membrane model can easily accommodate the Mudd experiment. All one needs is to postulate that the bilayer surface is completely covered by protein and carbohydrate and that there is a delicate balance between the hydrophilic and hydrophobic groups of the protein components pointing toward the outside. In some cases, perhaps with aging, the balance might shift toward relative hydrophobicity, and the surface might then become wettable by oil.

Another experiment that may be cited along these lines is the classical one of Chambers (10) showing that *Arbacia* egg membranes can be wetted by oil. Chambers in 1938 also pointed out that his results meant that the *Arbacia* egg

membrane was fluid. Incidentally it is interesting that the general idea of fluidity in membranes as well as the idea of a fluid mosaic of lipid and protein was commonly discussed in the 1930s and 1940s (11).

In any case the above experiments provide good reasons to regard the fluid mosaic model as misleading in some important respects. It does, however, serve the useful purpose of reemphasizing the old idea of membrane fluidity and by emphasizing penetration of the bilayer by protein it has again served a useful purpose since both these features of membranes were not dealt with by the original unit membrane theory. However, since neither of these features was excluded by the theory, it can only be said that the theory was incomplete, a fact that was completely appreciated when it was advanced.

Thus it seems that these two views of membrane structure can be reconciled. The principal contribution of the unit membrane theory was the unequivocal establishment of the ubiquity of the lipid bilayer and the concept of chemical asymmetry. Both these ideas are generally accepted. We must now add the fact that hydrophobic polypeptide chains, although not yet resolved, may sometimes penetrate the lipid bilayer and hold together two moieties of a single protein molecule. The experiments of Whiteley and Berg (12) and Ruoho and Kyte (13) established this point, which had been suggested earlier by Bretscher (14), Steck et al. (15), and Marchesi et al. (16). The unit membrane theory must now incorporate this fact. It has also become clear that some proteins may have hydrophilic moieties that lie in the surface of the bilayer with hydrophobic moieties that extend for some distance into the bilayer. Cytochrome b-5 (17) and perhaps cytochrome oxidase (18) are examples of such proteins. There is thus no doubt that the hydrophobic core of the bilayer may contain protein components. The question is how much. The fluid-mosaic model calls for too much. What is needed now is much careful experimentation to determine precisely how some specific biological membranes are constructed in molecular terms so that this question can be answered quantitatively. In our laboratory we are attempting to do this by studying several kinds of biological membranes mainly with the electron

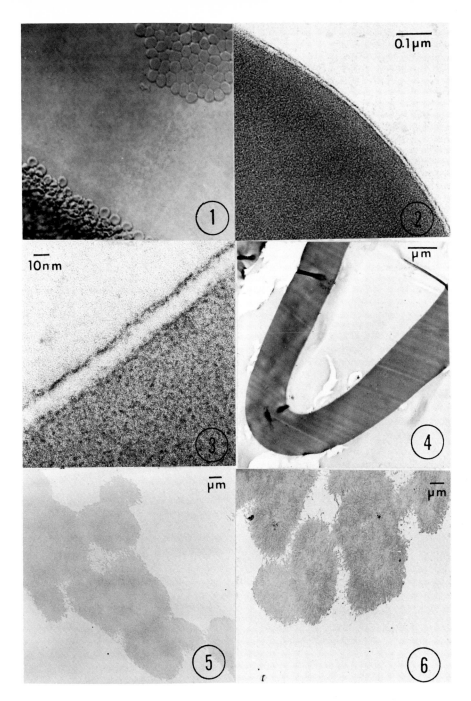

FIG. 1. Interface between Locke's solution containing blood and glyceryl tricaprylate. The water phase is to the lower left and the oil phase is to the upper right. Note the group of red blood cells that is contained in the oil phase. The red blood cells are about 8 μm in diameter.

FIG. 2. Thin section of edge of GACH embedded human red blood cell stained with uranyl and lead. $\times 98{,}000$.

FIG. 3. Higher magnification micrograph of same preparation as Fig. 1. $\times 563{,}900$.

FIG. 4. Catalase fixed with glutaraldehyde, embedded in GACH, and stained with uranyl and lead. $\times 8{,}500$.

FIG. 5. Specimen of polytryptophan fixed with glutararaldehyde and embedded in Epon. Unstained. $\times 3{,}400$.

FIG. 6. Same specimen as Fig. 5 but section was placed in 90% acetone for 18 hr then exposed to OsO$_4$ vapor for 40 min and stained with uranyl and lead. $\times 3{,}400$.

microscope but also by X-ray diffraction and direct chemical analysis.

In this chapter we deal mainly with some studies of model systems designed to see to what extent electron microscopic studies of thin sections may be expected to yield clear-cut information about the molecular organization of unit membranes. The advancement of the fluid mosaic model provided the direct stimulus for much of the work to be reported here, for it seemed to us that if protein molecules 4 to 10 nm in diameter were as frequently embedded in the lipid bilayer of membranes as depicted in the diagram of Singer and Nicholson we should be able to see them in thin sections. We have therefore devised a series of experiments to test this proposition and some of these are reported here in preliminary form.

The triple-layered pattern of the unit membrane as seen with the electron microscope first in 1954 is demonstrable today in all biological membranes by any of the various techniques that are now considered standard. The latest new technique that shows it up clearly is the polyglutaraldehyde-embedding method of Pease and Peterson (19) and of Heckman and Barrnett (20). Here, the tissue is fixed with glutaraldehyde and or formaldehyde. It is then transferred to increasingly concentrated glutaraldehyde, which is caused to polymerize into a hard block. The residual water is extruded and thin sections can be cut and examined by electron microscopy. Contrast can be added by heavy metal staining. Chemical analysis of the resulting tissue blocks show that over 90% of the lipids and proteins present in the native tissue are retained. Figure 2 is an electron micrograph of a portion of a washed human red blood cell prepared in this way and Fig. 3 shows a high magnification view. These cells were fixed with Karnofsky's glutaraldehyde-paraformamide mixture and embedded in polyglutaraldehyde (20). If examined directly such preparations show very little contrast, although cells can be recognized. If the sections are stained with uranyl and lead, the contrast is greatly enhanced and the triple-layered pattern of the unit membranes is essentially the same as that seen with earlier techniques, except that the light central core is wider, making the membrane appear thicker.

The freeze-fracture-etch (FFE) technique (21,22) shows that within the lipid bilayer of almost all membranes there are present particles that generally measure approximately 8 to 10 nm in diameter and appear roughly spherical. Such particles are not seen in FFE preparations of pure lipid (23) or nerve myelin (24). It is assumed that such smooth fracture faces represent the replicated hydrophobic carbon chains of the lipid molecules. It is also assumed by most that the particles present in intact biological membranes represent protein macromolecules. This was supported by the findings of Branton (22), that if erythrocyte ghosts are treated with pronase the particles disappear, and those of Hong and Hubbell (25), that if purified rhodopsin is added to pure phospholipid vesicles particles appear in the fracture faces that were not present before. These pieces of evidence are taken by most as showing that the ubiquitous intramembrane particles are in fact protein macromolecules. It was proposed by Singer and Nicholson (5) that membranes are generally constructed in a manner whereby roughly spherical or oblate protein macromolecules were visualized as floating in a sea of lipid, either extending all the way through the lipid bilayer, or half way, or a little more than half way through.

This general concept of the presence of large amounts of protein completely traversing the bilayer, residing within its center, or embedded in it to varying degrees took hold and gained ground steadily. This is an attractive concept because it provides a very ready explanation for many membrane phenomena that otherwise require more subtle explanations. However, there are definite weaknesses in this concept. For instance, if the particles consist of a specific protein-lipid complex with the protein in the outer part, destroying the protein should destroy the particles and adding such protein to a suitable lipid bilayer should produce new particles. Furthermore, Tanford and Reynolds (26) have pointed out that even the most hydrophobic of membrane proteins still contain relatively large numbers of hydrophilic amino acids. Our findings show that hydrophilic amino acids may be expected generally to stain uranyl and lead and that at least some of the hydrophobic amino acids are also reactive. Added together one would expect these reactivities to make even very hydrophobic proteins stainable. Also

Deamer and Yamanaka (27) have recently reported that the ~8-nm-diameter intramembrane particles in sarcoplasmic reticulum membranes do not change appreciably in number or size after treatment with proteolytic enzymes. They showed that this treatment had reduced all proteins present to molecular weights no larger than 10,000 to 15,000 daltons, and concluded that high molecular weight polypeptides were not required for particles to be produced in membrane fracture faces.

Vergara et al. (28) and Hicks et al. (29) independently have isolated placques from urothelial cell membranes in which there are close-packed hexagonal arrays of intramembrane B face particles spaced at ~15 nm. Even though these particles make up almost 50% of the volume of the bilayer region of the membrane, these membranes are 65% lipid by weight. If the intramembrane particles were simply protein macromolecules, this would be unlikely. Therefore, there is reason to doubt the widely accepted notion that intramembrane particles are protein macromolecules lying within the lipid bilayer. Finally a major problem that arises in interpreting the nature of the intramembrane particles is the fact that the particles never have been detected in thin sections with the electron microscope regardless of the technique.

How can one reconcile the conflicting interpretations? Is it possible to detect by electron microscopy single protein macromolecules of the size implied in the fluid mosaic model in thin sections of biological membranes by utilizing heavy metal staining techniques? This question can be answered unequivocally. Protein particles in the surfaces of urothelial cell membranes (28) and of suckling rat ileum (30) < 10 nm in diameter are clearly seen in frontal views of suitably stained thin sections, and it is even possible to see substructures ~3 nm in diameter in the urothelial cell membrane particles. Furthermore protein filaments such as neurofilaments show up very clearly in longitudinal views in sections as do actin filaments and the individual myosin cross bridges of muscle fibers in very thin sections. Furthermore ribosomes, albeit somewhat larger (~15 nm), show up very clearly indeed in sections of ~100 nm or more. Another important point is the fact that the bilayer region of membranes

containing closely packed arrays of intramembranous particles such as the urothelial cell membranes and synaptic discs (gap junctions) show no evidence in polyglutaraldehyde embedded material of stainable elements that are meaningful. Careful searches of many sections such as those in Figs. 2 and 3 has failed to reveal any particles that could correspond to the intramembrane particles revealed by the FFE technique. To be sure, there are some dense spots in the bilayer region (Fig. 3), but similar dense spots occur randomly in the background. Since the FFE particles are quite numerous, this seems to say that the material making up the intramembrane particles has the same staining properties as the lipids of the lipid bilayer.

We have been trying for some time to reconcile the conflicting evidence outlined above. One question was whether or not hydrophobic amino acids can be expected to take up the heavy metal compounds used to stain sections. We have examined fixed, embedded, and sectioned hydrophilic and hydrophobic proteins and the hydrophilic proteins all stain avidly like the specimen of catalase in Fig. 4. One may thus state unequivocally that hydrophilic proteins generally show up in stained sections, even if only single molecules are present. But what is the probability of seeing a very small hydrophobic protein molecule within the bilayer core of a membrane in a section 30 to 50 nm thick? This is very difficult to answer unequivocally without direct experimental evidence.

EXPERIMENTAL MEMBRANE MODELS

We are presently conducting experiments with the aim of constructing lipid bilayers of known composition in which hydrophobic protein moieties can be placed in precisely known relationships. We hope eventually to be able to define exactly what can be seen by electron microscopy in sections of membranes.

It was necessary first to determine the relative reactivities of hydrophobic and hydrophilic amino acid moieties to the staining procedures. We used selected hydrophobic polyamino acids as test substances. Sections of polytryptophan in GACH, even without staining, give fairly good contrast (Fig. 5). After treatment with heavy metals, the contrast reaches almost the same level as catalase after staining (Fig. 6). Similar results were obtained with several other hydrophobic polyamino acids in Epon after OsO_4 fixation although they did not stain further with uranyl and lead. We conclude that even proteins comprised entirely of a mixture of hydrophobic amino acids should take up heavy metal stains and hence be rendered visible in electron micrographs. The fact that all known membrane proteins contain more than 30 mole % hydrophilic amino acids (26) lends further support to the expectation that they should be visible inside the bilayers of membranes, if they are present in significant amounts.

To test further the detectability of various components of lipid bilayers we performed a series of experiments utilizing multilayers of various lipids prepared by the Langmiur-Blodgett dipping methods as illustrated in Fig. 7. In 1965 Schidlovsky (31) reported on some such experiments. He chose to use as his test substance behenic acid and its barium salts. He made substrates of thin rectangular sheets of methacrylate, which he dipped through a compressed monolayer of either barium behenate or behenic acid in succession. By this means he made multilayer sandwiches with successive layers laid down in controlled and known order. He reported that he was able in sections of the multilayer complexes to see repeating dense and light strata at a period of about 6 nm in the parts containing barium behenate and no contrast in the parts containing only behenic acid.

Robertson and Costello (32) first repeated Schidlovsky's experiments but using Epon. Barium behenate was lifted at 18 dynes/cm from a subsolution of barium chloride adjusted to pH 8.5. Figure 8a–f is a record of one experiment.

We found that fixation embedding and staining were completely unnecessary for imaging of the multilayer arrays with the electron microscope. We simply cut sections of the untreated multilayer arrays onto water. The arrays held together quite well, and we could readily distinguish the Epon from the multilayers and the barium behenate bilayers from the behenic acid bilayers. Figure 9 is a low-power electron micrograph of a complex like that prepared in Fig. 8. The multilayers of barium behenate appear much more dense than

the Epon to the left. The behenic acid multilayers produce very little contrast but one can detect a dense stratum in the middle of the behenic acid zone, which represents the single bilayer of barium behenate that was laid down. The outermost multilayers of barium behenate again produce sharp densities. Figure 10 is a higher power micrograph of a similar complex. The barium behenate bilayers show up as repeating dense and light strata with a period of ~5.4 nm. The dense strata each measure down to 2 nm in thickness. The behenic acid does not produce sufficient contrast to give any intimation of layering, but the overall thickness of the multilayer complex infers the presence of a lamellar structure even though the individual bilayers are not seen. The single bilayer of barium behenate placed in the middle of the behenic acid is readily visible as a dense band somewhat less than 2.5 nm thick, which appears sharp in those places in which it is oriented precisely perpendicular to the electron beam.

During the early stages we used OsO_4 and embedded in Epon. The only effect of the OsO_4 was staining of the Epon. It had no apparent effect on the barium behenate or on behenic acid. In all the embedded material, the complexes very largely dissolved and only scattered patches could be seen. Nevertheless, in Fig. 11 we see a fragment of such a multilayer complex, which is quite revealing. Here only a few multilayers of barium behenate are seen upon an Epon surface. The Epon is clearly delineated below by the fact that it has been stained with OsO_4 and appears dense. The layers of barium atoms in the polar regions of the lipid bilayers appear quite dense, whereas the lipid carbon chains themselves have low electron density. The microdensitometer trace in Fig. 12, which was made by running a light source along a line between the arrows, clearly shows that the light unstained zone next to the Epon is about half as thick as the light zone between the succeeding dense strata representing barium atoms. It seems quite clear that the successive monolayers of barium behenate were indeed deposited on the Epon surface as the surface tension records indicated. Clearly the first monolayer was laid down with its nonpolar carbon chains pointing toward the hydrophobic Epon surface. Perhaps more importantly for our purposes the experiment quite conclusively

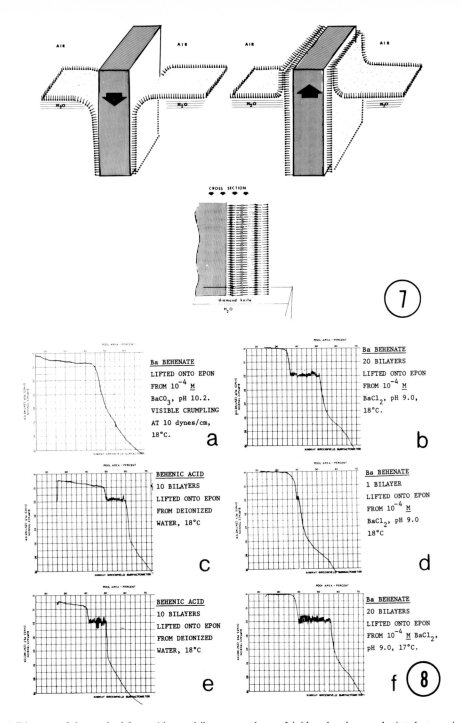

FIG. 7. Diagram of the method for making multilayer complexes. Lipid molecules are depicted at an air-water interface being deflected downward by an Epon block **(1)** being lowered through the compressed monolayer. In (2) the Epon block is raised and the second monolayer is lifted onto the block. **Bottom:** The production of a thin section through the face of the block. The section is being cut with a diamond knife onto a water surface. As indicated in the diagram, different kinds of bilayers can be deposited in various sequences this way.

FIG. 8. a: Surface tension record of a control experiment in which a monolayer was compressed to the collapse point ($\sim$8 dynes/cm). *Abscissa:* The percent area of the trough with 100% to the left and none to the right. *Ordinate:* Surface tension values with none at the top and 72 dynes/cm (pure water) at the bottom. The monolayer was compressed by a Teflon barrier moving from left to right. Twenty bilayers of barium behenate were deposited at a fairly constant surface tension of $\sim$18 dynes/cm **(b)**. Ten bilayers of behenic acid were then added **(c)** and one bilayer of barium behenate was laid down **(d)**. Another ten bilayers of behenic acid were then added **(e)**. Finally twenty bilayers of barium behenate were laid down to complete the multilayer coded array **(f)**.

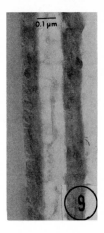
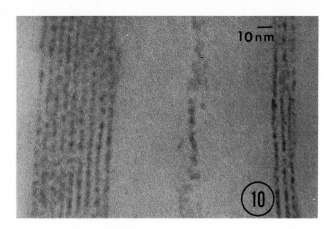

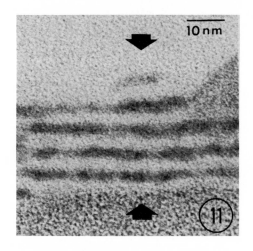

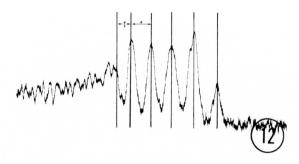

FIG. 9. Section of a multilayer complex like that described in Fig. 7. × 51,725.

FIG. 10. Higher magnification micrograph of an experiment similar to that in Fig. 9. × 418,000.

FIG. 11. High-magnification micrograph of a small part of a multilayer complex of barium behenate on Epon. The Epon block which appears at the bottom of the figure, was exposed to OsO_4 vapor before embedding and is stained. The microdensitometer tracing in Fig. 12 was taken between the arrows. × 990,000.

FIG. 12. A microdensitometer trace through the multilayer complex shown in Fig. 11.

shows that the saturated lipid carbon chains of barium behenate produced low electron scattering under these conditions despite exposure to OsO_4 vapor. The only components that significantly scattered electrons were the metal atoms associated with the polar heads of the lipid molecules. One important point to be made here is that when stainable material, in this case Epon, occupies half of a lipid bilayer, its presence is readily detectable because it can be seen directly.

Figure 13 shows another interesting preparation. In this case the fragment that was sectioned contains only two bilayers of barium behenate. Note that the polar strata of the bilayers are clearly seen only in the region in which they are sectioned exactly perpendicular to the direction of the electron beam. When tilted only 12° off axis they become quite fuzzy and smeared out. One interesting aspect of this micrograph is that where the two bilayers are in apposition down the center of the structure the dense stratum that is produced appears much denser than the nonopposed barium head groups. This observation is consistent with the fact that fatty acid polar heads are known from X-ray studies to be packed in fatty acid crystals in a staggered fashion. If the polar heads were completely interpolated so that they all lay exactly in the same plane, one would not expect to see any difference in scattering between the strata containing only one layer of barium atoms and the strata containing two because there would be the same number of atoms included in the section in either case. This assumes of course maximum close packing of all the polar heads and acyl chains. Thus the electron microscope in this case gives us information about the detailed arrangement of the barium atoms in the strata that hitherto could only be inferred from X-ray diffraction studies. This micrograph is included to illustrate the kinds of information that we can expect to obtain from thin sections of Epon or other plastic embedded material containing lipid bilayers with atomic groupings capable of producing enough electron scattering to produce an image. It also shows the effect of slight tilt of sections. Similar tilt effects occur in sections of unit membranes and if not taken into account can lead to great confusion.

A major aim of these experiments with multilayer complexes was originally to determine precisely what could be seen by electron microscopy by direct imaging of bilayers of known physical and chemical composition. The above shows that it is possible to resolve in thin sections the location of planes of single scattering atoms each constituting a part of a fatty acid head group. So far we have not determined precisely how thin the section may be in order to detect these atomic layers. Some of the sections examined, however, have been gray sections and thus may be safely considered to be less than 50 nm in thickness. These still display approximately the same scattering. We have not yet defined the limits of the method, but we have reason to believe that we can get similar results at thicknesses of 10 nm or less. This comes from examining single bilayers of barium behenate formed over holes in a carbon film grid and examined directly in face view with the electron microscope. Folds occasionally occur in these bilayers and present bilayer profiles of the same appearance as seen in transverse sections. We say with complete certainty that we can distinguish superimposed dense scattering atoms in the polar regions of fatty acid bilayers.

In some preliminary experiments in which we have attempted to insert hydrophobic polyamino acids into the core of the lipid bilayer, this has proven to be very difficult and thus far our success has been very limited. We have succeeded in producing only one multilayer complex that seems to accomplish our aim. We have not been able to repeat this experiment, and it therefore can be presented here only as a highly preliminary, although significant, observation. In this case multilayers of barium behenate were built up on an Epon block and the block was then dipped successively through a monolayer of poly-beta-benzyl aspartic acid (PBBA). An effort was made to put down the monolayers of barium behenate and PBBA in alternate succession but for the most part the polyamino acid did not deposit evenly, and the result was an irregular mass of complexes. Nevertheless, after staining with uranyl and lead, it was possible to find in sections of some regions periodic complexes in which the repeat period was increased from 5.4 to 12.6 nm. This periodic structure is shown in Fig. 14. Figure 15 is a microdensitometer tracing through the complex.

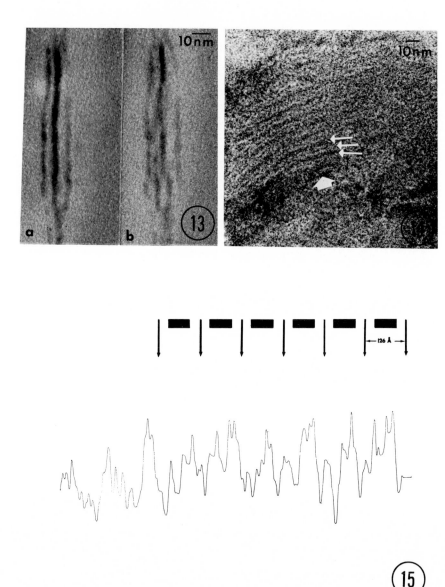

FIG. 13. Fragment of two bilayers embedded in Epon as described in the text. (**A**) The two bilayers are sectioned perpendicularly. (**B**) The section was tilted 12° on the vertical axis of the figure. × 550,000.

FIG. 14. Complex of poly-β-benzyl-L-aspartic acid and barium behenate showing a region with a repeat period of 12.6 nm. The arrows designate the periodic structure. The large block arrow pointing upward indicates the direction of the microdensitometer trace in Fig. 15. × 214,000.

FIG. 15. Microdensitometer trace through the periodic structure in Fig. 15. Tracing was made in the direction of the bottom block arrow.

The repeating unit consists of a thin, dense stratum <2.5 nm thick followed by a light stratum approximately 3 nm wide followed by a dense band about 4 nm wide as indicated by the arrows in Fig. 14. This is succeeded by a light zone about 3 nm wide and then the structure repeats. Sighting along the direction of the arrows by tilting the image brings out the layers

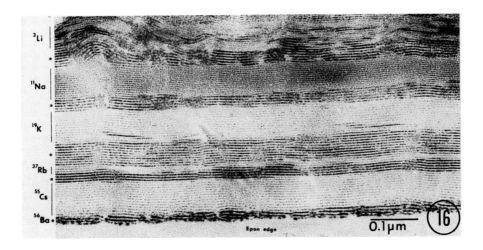

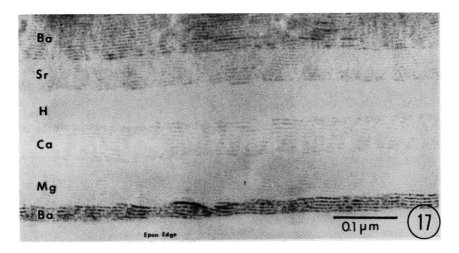

FIG. 16. Micrograph of multilayer complex of the Group 1 metal salts of behenic acid as described in the text. (*) Multilayers of barium, which serve as markers. × 121,000.

FIG. 17. Multilayer complex of behenic acid (**H**) and its Group 2 salts. × 177,000.

clearly. This periodic structure is very clearly displayed and it is difficult to imagine how it could have come about except by the formation of patchy complexes between the barium behenate and the monolayers of PBBA. Thus, in this particular instance, we may have succeeded in placing a hydrophobic polyamino acid in the middle of a succession of bilayers of barium behenate where the polyamino acid forms the hydrophobic core of a bilayer. This preliminary experiment suggests that, if a large amount of hydrophobic proteinaceous material is present within a lipid bilayer, it can be detected in thin sections by electron microscopy.

In some very interesting experiments in building up multilayer complexes R. Waldbillig has been able to show that various monovalent and divalent cations can be substituted for barium and lifted in successive bilayers alongside barium behenate bilayers. These cations in such multilayer complexes have less electron-scattering power and thus can be distinguished from barium behenate layers. Figure 16 is a multilayer complex of periodic table Group 1 metals prepared by Waldbillig. Again it should be reemphasized that the sections were made from the untreated Epon blocks directly onto water and not fixed, embedded, or stained. The complex was made by interspersing multilayers of different behenic acid salts between multilayers of barium which serve as markers. The cations in the successive layers and their atomic numbers are indicated in the figure. The multilayers nearest the Epon are quite regular, although the outermost layers, including lithium behenate, became irregular and mixed up with the barium behenate marker layers. Nevertheless one can see quite clearly the succession of dense and light strata representing each of the different cationic head groups.

We have also examined the periodic table Group IIa metals. The multilayer complex resulting from laying down the Group IIa behenates and their salts along with behenic acid (H) is shown in Fig. 17. Here we see the succession of Epon, ^{56}Ba, ^{12}Mg, ^{20}Ca, behenic acid, and ^{38}Sr.

Waldbillig has recently found that the relative scattering power of successive multilayers with a particular ionic head group is pH and concentration dependent, and therefore we believe that the differences in scattering power indicated between both the Group 1 and 2 elements depend on the relative numbers of metal atoms that are packed per unit volume in the sections. The important point we wish to stress is that it is possible by this technique to detect ionic head groups of atomic numbers less than 12 directly. Sodium is certainly visualized and we think that lithium can be seen. It is important to stress again that we are dealing here with sections of the pure untreated multilayer complexes; no heavy metal stain of any kind has been used.

We have recently begun to work with phospholipids and have succeeded in lifting phosphatidyl serine (PS) in a sandwich between layers of barium behenate. We were unable to see significant scattering from the unstained phospholipid. In fact, the multilayers of PS looked exactly like the multilayers of behenic acid in Figs. 10 and 17. Since there is one phosphorus atom per phospholipid molecule, in this case we can only conclude that it is the packing density that is responsible for the failure to scatter electrons sufficiently to produce a visible density. The area per molecule in a compressed monolayer of phospholipid molecules is two to three times larger than that for a behenic

acid salt, and it may well be that the resultant dilution factor in the multilayer complex sections gives rise to enough reduction in scattering to lead to the results. Another factor may be that the exact positioning of the phosphate groups within the multilayer array may be irregular as compared to the fatty acid soaps. These two factors may operate to produce less effective electron scattering. However, when these sections were treated with OsO_4 vapor for approximately 1 hr the phospholipid region became very dense and the polar heads became more dense than the nonpolar carbon chains. The sample of PS that we used was from bovine brain extract and is presumably unsaturated. Figure 18 is a section of such a complex treated with OsO_4 vapor, and Fig. 19 is a microdensitometer trace through the bordering layers of barium behenate and the phospholipid multilayers. The spacing of the phospholipid multilayers (~3.8 nm) is significantly smaller than that of the barium behenate (~5.4 nm). In Fig. 19 it can be seen that the overall density of the phospholipid multilayer region is increased markedly over that of the barium behenate and that the sharp peaks can only be interpreted as being the polar heads. One can decide this because there is a regular succession of sharp symmetrical peaks of density in the transition region between the barium behenate and the PS. This provides an independent proof of one of the basic experiments on which the unit membrane theory was based, i.e., that phospholipids after treatment with OsO_4 display dominant densities in sections that correspond to the polar heads of the lipid molecules rather than the nonpolar carbon chains.

We are now correlating our model experiments with X-ray diffraction studies of the multilayer arrays. T. McIntosh is obtaining X-ray diffraction patterns from various multilayer complexes produced by Waldbillig. One of McIntosh's X-ray diffraction patterns recorded on film is shown in Fig. 20. This pattern was obtained from barium brassidate, which is an analogue of barium behenate having one trans double bond in the lipid carbon chain in the 12–13 position. Only one half of the diffraction pattern is shown. The origin is to the right and there are 11 orders of a 5.8-nm period visible. Because of the nature of the multilayer experiments it is possible to vary the head

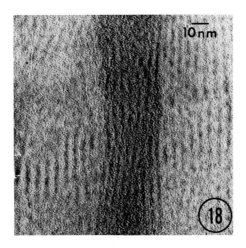

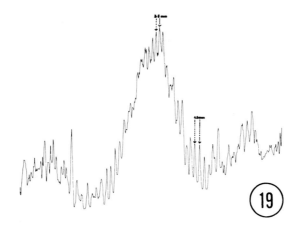

FIG. 18. Multilayer complex of barium behenate (**right**) and with phosphotidyl serine (**left**). The PS is in the middle part of the figure and appears denser. Its period is less than that of the barium behenate. The microdensitometer trace in Fig. 19 was taken in a direction running from left to right in the figure. × 460,000.

FIG. 19. Microdensitometer trace from Fig. 18 showing the density peaks of the polar regions of the barium behenate to the right and left and of the phosphotidyl serine in the middle. Note the relatively high overall density in the PS region. Measurements are given in the text.

group of the particular molecule that is being laid down with each monolayer, which makes it possible to do an isomorphic replacement experiment for each particular set of experiments. This means unequivocal determination of phases is possible. McIntosh has therefore been able to plot the electron-density distribution across one bilayer of barium brassidate as in Fig. 21. Note the sharp dip in density at the center of the bilayer presumably due to the high ordering of the terminal —CH_3 groups. A multilayer complex of barium brassidate was then exposed to bromine vapor for a short time and another X-ray diffraction pattern obtained. This

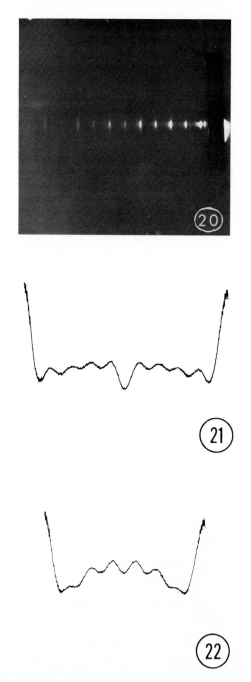

FIG. 20. X-ray diffraction pattern from barium brassidate multilayer complex recorded on film.

FIG. 21. Electron-density plot for a single bilayer of barium brassidate constructed from Fig. 20. The repeat period is 5.8 nm.

FIG. 22. Electron-density plot from barium brassidate after bromination. Note that the central dip in density, presumably due to the CH_3 groups in the middle of the bilayer, is preserved but that there is an overall increase in the density of the hydrocarbon chain regions with a peak symmetrically located about midway along the chains. The period here is 4.4 nm.

caused a reduction of the repeat period from 5.8 to 4.4 nm. The electron-density plot of the brominated brassidate (Fig. 22) shows a rise in density in the region of the hydrocarbon tails between the barium head groups. There is also a rise in density in the terminal methyl groups region presumably due to disordering.

Similar patterns have been obtained from barium behenate, behenic acid, and other metal soaps of this general type. They are also now being obtained from phospholipids and various combinations of monolayers of metallic soaps utilizing fatty acids of different chain lengths. These X-ray results show that we can produce consistent electron-density plots at a resolution of 4.5 Å. We are proceeding now to insert various proteins into these complexes and study the results by both electron microscopy and X-ray diffraction. It should be possible by this means to obtain a very good correlation between what can be determined to be present by the X-ray method and what can be seen by electron microscopy.

CONCLUSIONS

It should be clear from the above that the original unit membrane model for the molecular organization of biological membranes was correct in its broad outlines. The general theory specified that all biological membranes have a lipid bilayer at their core and that protein and other nonlipid materials are concentrated mainly around the polar heads of the lipid molecules in the bilayer. It also introduced the idea of chemical asymmetry. All of these general ideas have been amply confirmed by all that has been learned since the original theory was advanced. Unfortunately the original theory has been interpreted too literally, and some have come to believe that it called for a rigorous exclusion of protein from the core of the bilayer and a rigid membrane structure that could not be fluid. The discussion in this chapter is intended to indicate in part that this represents a misinterpretation of the theory (see ref. 3, Conclusion). It is now abundantly clear that protein does penetrate the bilayer in some membranes to some degree. It now seems very likely that polypeptide chains, perhaps in the form of α-helices, traverse the bilayer from one side to the other connecting hydrophilic moieties of

protein molecules, which may be located in the opposite surfaces of a given membrane. It is also clear that some protein molecules may extend hydrophobic polypeptide chains in some unknown conformations for unknown depths into the lipid bilayer. The nature of the ubiquitous intramembrane particles that are seen in FFE preparations of biological membranes remains, however, a mystery. On the basis of the evidence that has been presented it seems very improbable that all of the ~8- to 10-nm particles seen in various membranes could literally represent protein macromolecules of this size, primarily because of the failure of the thin-section technique to reveal any densities within the lipid bilayer that could reasonably correspond to such structures. It is, of course, possible that the intramembrane particles may have something to do with protein penetrating the bilayer. Conceivably the particles represent regions where polypeptide chains cross the bilayer and pieces of the membrane are torn out of one side during the fracturing process because of a polypeptide chain traversing the bilayer. In this case a much larger piece of material would apparently reside within the bilayer than would exist in the native membrane. This could account for the discrepancy between the sectioning results and the FFE results.

To be sure there are other ways in which to account for the presence of apparent particles of such dimensions within the lipid bilayer. One might assume that a special lipid is segregated out of the bilayer by the protein and that this lipid is perhaps more concentrated, has longer chains, is more saturated or less saturated or in some way significantly different from the surrounding lipid. If this is so, then it might very well act rather like the bristles of a molecular paint brush to cast a shadow, accumulate metal, and resemble an intramembrane particle. This is one plausible explanation for the intramembrane particles. In any case we believe that the experimental approach we are using will yield results in our quest to solve the riddle of the nature of the intramembrane particles. It seems fair to say, however, that on the basis of present evidence we do not believe that the intramembrane particles can be generally identified unequivocally with solid spherical protein macromolecules inserted within the bilayer in the manner depicted by the Singer fluid mosaic model. Much more work is required before any conclusions of this sort can be reached.

REFERENCES

1. Robertson, J. D. (1972): The structure of biological membranes. *Arch. Int. Med.*, 129:202–228.
2. Robertson, J. D. (1959): The ultrastructure of cell membranes and their derivatives. *Biochem. Soc. Symp.*, 16:3–43.
3. Robertson, J. D. (1960): The molecular structure and contact relationships of cell membranes. In: *Progress in Biophysics*, edited by B. Katz and J. A. V. Butler, pp. 343–418. Pergamon Press, New York.
4. Singer, S. J. (1974): The molecular organization of membranes. *Ann. Rev. Biochem.*, 43:805–833.
5. Singer, S. J., and Nicholson, G. L. (1972): The fluid mosaic model of the structure of cell membranes. *Science*, 175:720–731.
6. Ryan, G. B., Borysenko, J. Z., and Karnovsky, M. J. (1974): Factors affecting the redistribution of surface-bound concanavalin A on human polymorphonuclear leukocytes. *J. Cell Biol.*, 62:351–365.
7. Unanue, E. R., Karnovsky, M. J., and Engers, H. D. (1973): Ligand-induced movement of lymphocyte membrane macromolecules III. Relationship between the formation and fate of anti-Ig-surface Ig complexes and cell metabolism. *J. Exp. Med.*, 137:675–689.
8. Tamm, S. L., and Tamm, S. (1974): Direct evidence for fluid membranes. *Proc. Natl. Acad. Sci. USA*, 71:4589–4593.
9. Mudd, S., and Mudd, E. B. H. (1931): The deformability and the wetting properties of leukocytes and erythrocytes. *J. Exp. Med.*, 53:733–750.
10. Chambers, R. (1938): The physical state of protoplasm with special reference to its surface. *Am. Naturalist*, 72:141–159.
11. Höber, R., Hitchcock, D. L., Bateman, J. B., Goddard, D. R., and Fenn, W. O. (1945): *Physical Chemistry of Cells and Tissues.* Blakiston, Philadelphia.
12. Whiteley, N. M., and Berg, H. C. (1974): Amidination of the outer and inner surfaces of the human erythrocyte membrane. *J. Mol. Biol.*, 87:541–561.
13. Ruoho, A., and Kyte, J. (1974): Photaffinity labeling of the ouabain-binding site on (Na⁺ + K⁺) adenosinetriphosphatase. *Proc. Natl. Acad. Sci. USA*, 71:2352–2356.
14. Bretscher, M. S. (1973): Membrane structure: some general principles. *Science*, 181:622–629.
15. Steck, T. L., Fairbanks, G., and Wallach, D. F. H. (1971): Disposition of the major proteins in the isolated erythrocyte membrane. Proteolytic dissection. *Biochemistry*, 10:2617–2624.
16. Marchesi, V. T., Tillack, T. W., Jackson. R. L., Segrest, J. P., and Scott, R. E. (1972): *Proc. Natl. Acad. Sci. USA*, 69:1445.
17. Strittmatter, P., Rogers, M. J., and Spatz, L. (1972): *J. Biol. Chem.*, 247:7188.
18. Maniloff, J., Vanderkooi, G., Hayashi, H., and Capaldi, R. A. (1973): Optical analysis of electron micrographs of cytochrome oxidase membranes. *Biochem. Biophys. Acta*, 298:180–183.
19. Pease, D. C., and Peterson, R. G. (1972): Polymerisable glutaraldehyde-urea mixtures as polar water containing embedding media. *J. Ultrastruc. Res.*, 41:133–159.
20. Heckman, C. A., and Barnett, R. J. (1973): GACH: a water-miscible, lipid retaining embedding polymer for electron microscopy. *J. Ultrastruc. Res.*, 42:156–179.
21. Moor, H., Mühlethaler, K., Waldner, H., and Frey-Wyssling, A. (1961): A new freezing ultra-microtome. *J. Biophys. Biochem Cytol.*, 10:1–13.
22. Branton, D. (1971): Freeze-etching studies of membrane structure. *Phil. Trans. R. Soc. Lond.* [*Biol.*], 261:133–138.
23. Pinto da Silva, P. (1971): Freeze-fracture of dipalmitoyl lecithin vesicles. *J. Microscop.*, 12:185–192.
24. Deamer, D. W., and Branton, D. (1967): Fracture planes in an ice-bilayer model membrane system. *Science*, 158:655–657.
25. Hong, K., and Hubbell, W. L. (1972): Preparations and properties of phospholipid bilayers containing rhodopsin. *Proc. Natl. Acad. Sci.*, 69:2617–2621.
26. Tanford, C., and Reynolds, J. A. (1975): *The Proteins, Vol. 4,* edited by Hans Neurath and Robert L. Hill. Academic Press, New York.
27. Deamer, D. W., and Yamanaka, N. (1975): Freeze-fracture particles in protease treated membranes. *Biophys. J.*, 15:110a.
28. Vergara, J., Zambrano, F., Robertson, J. D., and Elrod, H. (1974): Isolation and characterization of luminal membranes from urinary bladder. *J. Cell Biol.*, 61:83–94.
29. Hicks, R. M., Ketterer, B., and Warren, R. C. (1974): The ultrastructure and chemistry of the luminal plasma membrane of the mammalian urinary bladder: a structure with low permeability to water and ions. *Phil. Trans. R. Soc. Lond.*, [*Biol.*], 268:23–38.
30. Knutton, S., Limbrick, A. R., and Robertson, J. D. (1974): Regular structures in membranes. I. Membranes in the endocytic complex of ileal epithelial cells. *J. Cell Biol.*, 62:679–694.
31. Schidlovsky, G. (1965): Contrast in multilayer systems after various fixations. *Lab. Invest.*, 14:475–495.
32. Robertson, J. D. and Costello, M. J. (1974): In: *Electron Microscopy 1974, Vol. II*, pp. 218–219. Australian Academy of Science, Canberra.

The Nervous System, Donald B. Tower, Editor-in-Chief. *Vol. 1: The Basic Neurosciences*. Raven Press, New York, 1975.

Recent Advances in Neuroanatomical Methodology

W. Maxwell Cowan

The quarter-century since the founding of the National Institute of Neurological and Communicative Disorders and Stroke has witnessed perhaps the most remarkable series of technical developments in the history of neuroanatomy. Beginning in the early 1950s with the introduction of what have come to be known as the "Nauta methods" and the application of the electron microscope to the study of neural tissue, the morphological analysis of the nervous system has, in recent years, been given added impetus by the development and perfection of a number of new methods of considerable promise. Since to a considerable extent the development and evaluation of these methods have taken place in laboratories supported by the NINCDS, it is fitting that they should be reviewed in a volume commemorating the 25th anniversary of the Institute.

In concentrating on the more recent developments in this field, I do not wish either to deprecate the achievements of the past or to exaggerate the merits and usefulness of the newer methods. It is evident to anyone surveying the history of neuroanatomy that each successive generation of workers has built on the technical successes and trials of its predecessors. Indeed very often the stimulus for new methodological developments has come from the perception of some distinct advantage of an existing technique, which was ripe for further exploitation, or from the recognition of the limitations and practical disadvantages of the methods of the past. Since the usefulness of the degeneration methods and the unique advantages inherent to the electron microscopic study of neural tissues have been discussed elsewhere (see, for example, the volume "Contemporary Research Methods in Neuroanatomy"), I shall confine myself in this chapter to a consideration of four relatively recent approaches to the anatomical study of the central nervous system. These include: (a) a

group of techniques based on the anterograde and retrograde transport of various marker molecules; (b) the intracellular labeling of identified neurons or neural pathways; (c) various methods for the cytochemical identification of pathways associated with specific neurotransmitters; and (d) a number of quantitative methods involving the application of small digital computers to neuroanatomical studies. These four developments have been selected because, at the time of writing, they appear to offer the greatest promise for unraveling the complexities of neuronal organization and because they presage a new era in neuroanatomy, in which it should be possible to chemically characterize specific neural pathways and to quantitatively analyze the form of individual neurons and the organization of the afferent and efferent connections of whole neuronal populations. Rather more attention will be given to the methods based on axonal transport than to the others, partly because I am more familiar with the development and use of these techniques, but mainly because at present they appear to be most generally useful for experimental neuroanatomical studies.

TECHNIQUES BASED ON THE INTRAAXONAL TRANSPORT OF VARIOUS MARKER MOLECULES

The Autoradiographic Method for Tracing Connections

Although the notion that the nerve cell body serves as the trophic center for the maintenance of the axon and all its collateral and terminal branches is implicit in the rationale of all the neuroanatomical methods based on the Wallerian degeneration of the axon (1), it was not until comparatively recently that direct experimental evidence in support of this hypothesis was forthcoming. As much of this evidence has been reviewed elsewhere in this volume, it will suffice to note here that Paul Weiss (whose now classic experiments with Hiscoe in 1948 opened up the whole study of axonal transport) was quick to recognize that it might be possible to exploit the phenomenon of axoplasmic transport to trace neuronal pathways. During the ensuing decade several successful attempts were made to apply this approach (see ref. 2 for review). The most convincing of these was the demonstration by Lasek et al. (3) that the central connections of the dorsal root ganglion cells could be as clearly delineated by labeling the ganglia with a tritiated amino acid and, after an appropriate survival period, preparing the spinal cord for autoradiography, as by any of the degeneration methods.

Lasek and his colleagues did not apply the method to the study of pathways arising within the central nervous system, but they did discuss some of the advantages that this might present. Chief among these was the possibility that if the labeled precursors were only taken up and synthesized into transportable macromolecules by the perikarya at the site of the injected label, the concomitant involvement of fibers of passage, which for so long has bedeviled the degeneration techniques that are based on the placement of destructive (and, usually, wholly nonspecific) lesions in the tissue could be obviated. About the same time Hendrickson (4) in this country and Cuénod and his colleagues (5) in Switzerland showed rather clearly that much of the material that was transported somatofugally in what had become known as the "rapid phase of axonal transport" with a transport velocity in excess of 100 mm/day, accumulated preferentially (but by no means exclusively) within the region of the axon terminals. This led to the suggestion that it might be possible, by the appropriate selection of the precursor and with the optimum postlabeling survival period, to more-or-less selectively delimit the sites of termination of the axons arising within a given area from their projection pathways. With this in mind, in 1970 I and a group of my colleagues at Washington University, together with Dr. Anita Hendrickson of the University of Washington, undertook a systematic evaluation of this approach.

The findings of our study and the formal protocol we developed for studies based on the intraaxonal transport of labeled proteins or glycoproteins, have been published *in extenso* (6) and need only be briefly summarized here. Essentially this method involves the injection (either by pressure or iontophoretically) of a small amount (approximately 20 to 50 nl) of a highly concentrated solution of a tritiated (^{3}H) amino acid, or a mixture of ^{3}H-amino acids containing about 1 to 20 μCi. The injections are made stereotaxically either through a 30-gauge needle or a micropipette, and if done slowly enough are often confined to a roughly spherical region about 200 to 300 μ in diameter. After an appropriate survival period (which is determined, in part by the length of the pathway to be studied, but mainly by whether one wishes to demonstrate principally the terminal projection field or the entire course of the pathway), the animal is perfused with a 10% solution of neutral formalin, and the brain or spinal cord prepared for autoradiography. We have found empirically that postinjection periods of 1 to 2 days are adequate for materials transported in the rapid phase of axonal transport even in long projection pathways in monkeys and have often used periods as short as 4 or 6 hr in our neuroembryological studies (7). With longer survival periods (of the order of 4 to 10 days), appreciably greater amounts of material are exported from the cell somata, and, since much of this more slowly transported material is distributed along the length of the axons, the entire course of the pathway can be readily displayed. The preparation of serial autoradiographs by the method of Kopriwa and Leblond (8), using either frozen or paraffin sections, which are subsequently stained with thionine (through the nuclear emulsion), permits one to accurately localize the labeled neurons, their axons, and axon terminals with respect to other identifiable cell masses or fiber pathways. With appropriate procedural modifications the method can be adapted for electron microscopy, which has the unique advantage that it enables one to establish the location of labeled presynaptic processes without altering their morphology.

This method has several advantages over the other techniques that have been used for the anterograde tracing of neural connections. I have already remarked on what is perhaps the most significant of these, namely that its interpretation is not confused by the involvement of fibers of passage. Although axons at the site of the isotope injection are capable of taking up the label, in the absence of the necessary biosynthetic machinery they are incapable of incorporating it into a transportable macromolecular form. This means that several regions of the central nervous system whose connections have until now been extremely difficult to investigate, such as the nuclei of the hypothalamus and the brainstem, are now patent of study; and the success with which some areas have already been analyzed by this method encourages one to believe that within a relatively short time the connections of many hitherto inaccessible areas will be examined. It is likely that a number of generally accepted views concerning neuronal connectivity will need to be reviewed after reexamination with this method. For example I might cite a recent wholly unexpected finding that, in the rat at least, the projection of the fornix to the hypothalamus arises not from the fields of the Ammon's horn (as has been taught for more than a century), but rather from the retrohippocampal fields of the subiculum and presubiculum (9).

A second major advantage of this method is that it can be applied as readily to the study of developing neural pathways as to the adult nervous system. In the past 3 years, my colleagues and I have used it extensively to map the development of the retinotectal projection in the chick and frog and to follow the ingrowth of the commissural and entorhinal afferents to the rat hippocampus and dentate gyrus. The study of developing neural pathways with conventional neuroanatomical methods has always been extremely difficult, but with the autoradiographic method we may anticipate a major thrust in this direction in the near future.

A third advantage of this method is its unusual sensitivity. We, and others, have repeatedly found that pathways that have proved intractable to study by degeneration methods, such as the retinohypothalamic projection, or the projection of the cerebellum upon the inferior olive, are quite easily revealed by the autoradiographic procedure (10–12). By taking advantage of the fact that some percentage of the transported label is released from the terminals of the axons and is available for uptake by the postsynaptic cells (13), it has even been possible to examine second-order projec-

tions. This approach has been used with singular success by Wiesel and his colleagues (14) to directly demonstrate the eye dominance columns in the monkey striate cortex and by Drager (15) to show the differences in the crossed and uncrossed retinal input to the visual cortex in pigmented and albino mice. Although the form in which the label is transsynaptically transferred is not known, and although the situation may be somewhat obscured by the nonspecific diffusion of label from the terminals, the empirical use of this phenomenon may have much to offer.

The last advantage to be mentioned is that this method lends itself particularly well to quantitative analysis. The silver grains, which are actually observed with this method, are readily counted, and in certain cases estimates of the numbers of grains in different regions may provide not only objective evidence for the existence of a connection but also such useful ancillary information as the relative numbers of inputs from the same or different sources, the precise distribution of terminals in particular regions, and changes in the numbers of inputs following partial deafferentation (2).

The autoradiographic method is, of course, not without its limitations. It is sometimes difficult to define precisely the extent of the labeled region since the injected label may diffuse for some distance from the intended site of the injection. This usually makes the analysis of short axonal connections difficult or even impossible. The tracing of pathways containing relatively few fibers is also difficult, especially after short survival periods, although the current use of dark-field optics has significantly helped in this regard. Autoradiography is considered by many investigators to be a complicated and irksome procedure, and certainly electron microscopic autoradiography, for which extremely long exposure periods (up to 6 months) are required, is a rather exacting technique. But perhaps the most serious criticism of this method is that one does not directly observe the labeled axons or axon terminals, only the exposed silver grains in the overlying emulsion. Because of the low penetrance of the β-emissions from tritium, one can only observe the radioactivity in the most superficial 2 or 3 μm of the section. One possible way to circumvent this limitation in the autoradiographic procedure is to use other markers that are anterogradely transported along axons. One of these is the enzyme horseradish peroxidase, which is more commonly used for retrograde transport studied, but under some (as yet undefined) circumstances may also be transported in the anterograde direction (16). The procedure involves the injection of a concentrated solution of the enzyme into the population of neurons whose efferent projection is to be studied, and after an appropriate survival period (say 24 to 48 hr) examining frozen sections of the tissues treated by the method of Graham and Karnovsky (17) for the histochemical localization of the enzyme. Although in many cases that have been studied, little or no evidence of anterograde axonal transport has been found under these circumstances, in others the full extent of the projection pathway can be readily visualized, and since relatively thick sections (up to 50 μm) are used, often the entire terminal arborization of the axons can be seen (18).

The Retrograde Transport of Horseradish Peroxidase and Other Proteins

That individual proteins and even larger molecular aggregates, such as certain neurotrophic viruses, can be taken up (presumably endocytotically) by axon terminals and selectively transported back to the region of the perikaryon, has been known for some years (see ref. 19 for review). However, it was not until comparatively recently that the possibility of using this phenomenon to map the origin of neural pathways was realized. In the earliest experiments of this kind, Evans-blue-labeled albumin was injected into various muscles of neonatal or very young mice and was subsequently found to have accumulated in the corresponding spinal or cranial motoneurons (20). That the same approach could be used in the central nervous system was demonstrated the following year by the LaVails (21), using the avian visual system as an experimental model. Since the publication of their seminal paper and the more complete account of their technique (22), the "HRP method," as it has come to be known, has been promptly applied to more neural systems than almost any new method in recent years with quite remarkable results.

In essence, the method involves injecting small volumes of a solution containing a high concentration of horseradish peroxidase (0.5 mg in 1 μl is commonly used) by pressure or iontophoretically into the area where afferents are to be studied. Some of the injected material is rapidly taken up by axon terminals at the site of the injection and transported retrogradely to their parent somata at a rate of approximately 50 to 100 mm/day. After a suitable survival period (periods of 4 to 24 hr are generally used), the brain is fixed by perfusion with a buffered glutaraldehyde/formaldehyde mixture and the tissue processed in the manner described above for the anterograde transport of the enzyme. The retrogradely transported enzyme is visualized (by its reaction product) as a collection of dense, brown-staining granules in the perikaryon and the larger dendrites of the labeled cells. The refractility of the granular deposits makes them particularly suitable for examination by dark-field optics, and this provides a quick and effective method for mapping the distribution of the labeled neurons. Since it is desirable to define the location of the labeled cells in relation to other cytoarchitectonic features, the sections are usually counterstained by one of the conventional Nissl methods.

As the LaVails (23) have shown, the reaction product can also be readily seen in the electron microscope, where it appears initially in various-sized vesicles or tubular organelles, and at a later stage in lysosomes. There are undoubtedly occasions when electron microscopic analysis is essential, but for the tracing of pathways the method will be principally used at the light microscopic level.

The advantages of this approach (where it can be successfully applied) are manifold, and the number of new findings that have already emerged since its application is striking. Since space does not permit a review of even a small fraction of these findings, it will suffice to say that the method has been used to study such diverse topics as the origin of the various efferent pathways from the cerebral cortex (including corticocortical, corticothalamic, corticotectal, etc.), the origin of the projections to the second sensory areas of the cortex, the origin of the neurons projecting into the hypophysiotrophic area of the hypothalamus, the origin of the retinogeniculate and retinotectal projections, and a number of neuroembryological problems. Although a number of technical difficulties in the use of the method remain to be worked out (e.g., for some reason certain known pathways, such as the projection of the cerebral cortex upon the corpus striatum, have proved refractory to analysis by this approach), it is decidedly superior to the retrograde cell degeneration technique and thus represents a major addition to the neuroanatomist's armamentarium.

INTRACELLULAR LABELING OF PHYSIOLOGICALLY IDENTIFIED NEURONS

Until recently, most of our knowledge about the three-dimensional morphology of neurons was based on the random staining of cells in different parts of the nervous system by the original Golgi method or one of its several variants. Unfortunately this method, even in the best hands, is notoriously capricious, and in any given preparation large sections of the tissue may be quite free of impregnated cells. In the last decade, we have seen a remarkable series of technical developments that promise to combine many of the advantages of the Golgi method (and especially the ability to view individual nerve cells in their entirety) with the possibility of first identifying the neurons to be studied and determining their functional properties (24). Although this has long been one of the major goals of neuroanatomy, it was not until 1968, when Stretton and Kravitz (25) published an account of their method using the dye Procion yellow, that a technique became available that was sufficiently reliable as to find widespread usage. Essentially their technique consists of impaling neurons (either before or after establishing their functional properties) with fine micropipettes, through which the fluorescent dye could be passed either iontophoretically or by pressure. After fixation and the appropriate histological procedures, the tissue is examined in a fluorescence microscope, in which the labeled cells can be readily identified (24). Since the dye binds rather slowly to the neuronal proteins, it tends to spread rather widely throughout the perikaryon and dendrites, but seldom for any great distance into the axon. Although in some respects Procion yellow is not an optimal dye for these purposes, in practice it has proved to be extremely useful, as evidenced by the large number of studies in which it has been used. These include not only studies of readily impaled cells in the nervous systems of a variety of invertebrates, but also in the mammalian central nervous system and in the retinae of a variety of vertebrates (see ref. 24 for bibliography). Several other dyes have been used in addition to Procion yellow; of these, perhaps the most promising is Procion brown, principally because, at present, it is the most easily identified in the electron microscope. This feature should permit one to follow the processes of the labeled cells in ultrathin sections and to identify the synaptic contacts made upon them.

Since this whole approach has been the subject of a recent excellent monograph (24), it need not be elaborated upon here, but an interesting variant of this method should be mentioned. This involves the intracellular injection of labeled metabolic precursors, such as ^{3}H-amino acids, ^{3}H-fucose, and ^{3}H-nucleotides, and has been used extensively by Kreutzberg and his colleagues (26) for the study of what may be termed "the cell biology of neurons." After incorporation, the location of the labeled material is demonstrated in serial autoradiographs and in these it is usually possible to not only display the full extent of the cell and its processes, but also to examine many of the neuron's dynamic properties, including the rate of incorporation of the label, the rate at which it is transported within the axon and dendrites, its rate of turnover, and its ultimate fate. This method has only one serious drawback, and that is that the injected cells can only be studied in autoradiographs. This means that in order to visualize the entire neuron one must serially reconstruct the cell from several sections, which can be no more than just a few microns in thickness (because of the limited penetrance of the β-emissions). Moreover, the image of the labeled cells that one sees in the autoradiographs is that of a dense aggregation of silver grains in the overlying emulsion, rather than the complete filling which one obtains with the dye injection methods. Despite this drawback, this technique has a great deal to offer and we may confidently look forward to its being rigorously exploited in the coming decade.

A less direct method for the intracellular staining of neurons, which has the advantage that it does not necessitate the impalement of the cells, is that based on the retrograde filling of neurons from their axons, either by diffusion or by the retrograde transport of appropriate dyes or metallic salts. At present the most widely used substance for staining cells in this manner is a solution of cobaltous chloride which is reacted with ammonium sulfide to form a black precipitate of cobalt sulfide within the cell (27). However, a variety of dyes, including Procion yellow, and several other markers, including horseradish peroxidase, have been used in the same way. The exact mechanism whereby the marker molecules are transferred along the axon has not yet been determined, but empirically it has been found that if the cut end of the axon is exposed to the marker, it will not only fill the axon but extend beyond it into the perikaryon and out to all the dendritic processes. To date, this approach has been used most successfully for studying peripherally directed axons in various invertebrate ganglia (28) and in the mammalian spinal cord. In general the method seems less readily applicable to the study of central neural pathways, but even here it has been shown that on occasion cells may be retrogradely filled and their three-dimensional appearance fully demonstrated (29).

The principal advantage of all these methods is that they permit one to view the cell in its entire three-dimensional form. And already they have been used effectively to determine not only the location of particular neurons of known functional properties, but also to determine the degree of consistency in the branching pattern of the dendrites of the same type and to examine the changes that occur in neurons following various experimental manipulations, such as deafferentation. Since they are not subject to the capriciousness of the Golgi technique, nor to its random and wholly unpredictable staining of cells, they clearly promise much for the future study of neuronal geometry.

METHODS FOR THE CYTOCHEMICAL IDENTIFICATION OF TRANSMITTER-SPECIFIC NEURAL PATHWAYS

Most of the neuroanatomical techniques in common use are relatively nonspecific, in the sense that they either reveal all the pathways arising or terminating within a given area or, as in the case of the Golgi method, only a small percentage of the cells is stained in an apparently random manner. This has long been recognized as a serious limitation in neuroanatomical methodology, and accordingly a number of attempts have been made to develop techniques that selectively reveal certain cytochemically distinct pathways. This has been done in the hope that we will be able not only to provide a more complete account of the pathways in the brain and spinal cord but also, in time, to develop a fairly complete picture of the chemical architecture of the central nervous system. That this might be possible was suggested some years ago by the empirical finding that certain pathways, such as the hypothalamo-hypophysial tract, could be selectively stained by such methods as the chrome alum hematoxylin technique, but it was not until relatively recently that significant progress was made toward the development of well-defined cytochemical methods. Since this field is in a state of considerable flux, with new methods being described more rapidly than they can be effectively evaluated, it will only be possible in this section to give a rather general account of the approaches that are currently being explored and those that seem, at this time, to be the most promising.

The most widely used cytochemical methods are the various fluorescence techniques for the demonstration of monoamine-containing neurons and their axons. This approach was first used in the 1950s by Eränko to stain the cells in the adrenal medulla (30), but it was not until the development of the method now commonly referred to as the "Falck-Hillarp technique" in 1962 that it came into widespread use (31). This method is based on the finding that most biologically active amines condense with formaldehyde to yield strongly fluorescent products. The tissue to be studied is either freeze-dried or, if whole mounts are used, dried in air, and then exposed to formaldehyde vapor. During this process the amines are converted into highly fluorescent compounds, which can be readily visualized in a fluorescence microscope. Although there has been some debate about the specificity of the reaction and the certainty with which different monamines can be distinguished on the basis of their fluorescence, there is now fairly general agreement that, when carefully used, this approach permits one to recognize the cell bodies and the axon terminals of the relevant neurons in both the central and peripheral nervous systems. In general the method is less satisfactory for tracing axons over long trajectories, and for this the more recently developed glyoxylic acid technique is recommended (32). The pretreatment of the tissue in glyoxylic acid is said to significantly improve the sensitivity of the method so that even the relatively small amounts of the amine present in the axons (as opposed to the axon terminals) can be clearly visualized. The distinction between the various biogenic amines with these methods depends on relatively slight differences in their fluorescence when condensed by formaldehyde.

A more rigorous approach to this issue is that based on the immunofluorescence of a labeled antibody specific to one of the enzymes involved in the biosynthesis of the amines (33) or to one of the associated carrier proteins (34). The former is probably the method of choice and presages the development of a whole new spectrum of methods that should be highly specific and readily applicable to potentially all pathways where synaptic transmission is chemically mediated. As the development and evaluation of this method has recently been reviewed at length by Geffen (35), it will suffice here to say that it is based on the isolation of an antibody specific to the enzyme dopamine-β-hydroxylase. To this enzyme a fluorescent label is attached, and the labeled antibody is reacted with frozen sections of the tissue, and viewed in the usual way in a fluorescence microscope (33). The striking demonstration that this method has given of the norepinephrine-containing neurons in the locus coeruleus and of their extensive axonal ramifications (36) marks it as one of the most powerful new tools in neuroanatomy. Currently a number of attempts are being made to apply the same principle to pathways involving other known neurotransmitters. Several laboratories are actively working to produce a suitable antibody to the enzyme choline acetyltransferase (37,38), and Roberts and his colleagues (39) have already had considerable success with the immunocytochemical localization of L-glutamate decarboxylase, the enzyme that forms γ-aminobutyric acid (GABA).

A quite different approach to this problem is based on the finding that neurons that act by the release of a particular chemical transmitter also have a high-affinity uptake system for that transmitter. Thus, when exposed to a concentrated solution of the transmitter that has been labeled (say, with tritium), the presence of the transmitter in the relevant neurons and in their axon terminals can be readily detected. To date this approach has been used most effectively to identify neurons in the cerebellar cortex and elsewhere that are thought to use GABA as their transmitter (40), but it has also been used quite effectively in the mammalian spinal cord for the identification of glycine-containing interneurons and their terminals, which are thought to be inhibitory upon motoneurons (41). Interestingly, in the latter situation, the uptake of the ^{3}H-glycine appears in electron micrographic autoradiographs to be confined to presynaptic processes, which in aldehyde-fixed material contain flattened or pleiomorphic vesicles. Loading tissues with norepinephrine, or more commonly with 5-hydroxydopamine, has similarly been used to identify norepinephrine-containing axon terminals, either by increasing the number and density of the dense-core vesicles that they contain or, if a ^{3}H-norepinephrine is used, by the accumulation of the radioactive label in the terminals.

As more neurotransmitters are identified, we can expect to see this approach used increasingly, not only for the morphological identification of the appropriate neurons and their processes, but also for dynamic studies of transmitter synthesis, utilization, and regulation.

SOME COMPUTER APPLICATIONS IN NEUROANATOMY

Although neuroanatomy, like most morphological sciences, has been traditionally descriptive rather than quantitative in its emphasis, increasing interest has been directed in recent years to the development of rigorous quantitative methods for the analysis of certain types of neuroanatomical data. Unfortunately the methods available for the collection of quantitative data have, with few exceptions, been of limited accuracy and, at the same time, extremely tedious. The remarkable success with which computers have been used in other areas of neurological research has prompted several groups of investigators to attempt to develop computer systems for the collection, collation, and analysis of a variety of neuronal parameters such as cell number, cross-sectional areas of neuronal perikarya, diameters of axons, and, more ambitiously, the three-dimensional reconstruction of neurons impregnated by the Golgi method or filled intracellularly by an appropriate dye. Limitation of space precludes a full consideration of each of these topics; instead I shall briefly describe some applications of small digital computers to these and certain related problems with which I and some of my colleagues at Washington University have been associated.

The Three-Dimensional Reconstruction of Neurons

Because of the inherent optical difficulties involved in examining very thick tissue sections and whole-mount preparations, our view of neuronal structure has, until recently, been largely two-dimensional and almost entirely nonquantitative. This, despite the fact that we have known for almost a century that in certain types of neurons (the cerebellar Purkinje cells are a good example), the orientation and extent of the cells' processes are critical determinants of their function. Various strategies have been suggested to circumvent some of these difficulties, but it was not until Glaser and Van der Loos (42) showed how a small analog computer might be interfaced with a microscope in order to analyze the dendritic organization of Golgi-impregnated cells that this came to be seen as a realistic possibility. Since then several computer systems have been developed for the three-dimensional reconstruction of neurons impregnated by the Golgi method or filled by one of the intracellular methods described above. The most ambitious of these systems are fully automated and are said to involve minimal operator intervention (43). However, until they have been operational for some time, it will be difficult to evaluate how effectively they deal with such problems as the overlap of processes from adjoining cells, and the elimination of various artifacts,

which are present in almost every histological preparation. In practice it seems that the systems that have been most useful are those that may best be described as semiautomated, with the observer making all decisions regarding image-identification while the computer is used to collate, store, and analyze the quantitative data that is collected. One such system was developed at Washington University by Wann et al. (44). This employs a PDP-12 computer with a modified Zeiss Universal microscope with a motor-driven stage, and a computer-controlled fine-focus mechanism. As this system has already proven itself to be extremely effective for the analysis of such key neuronal parameters as total dendritic length, lengths of individual dendritic segments and branches, growth changes in dendrites, etc., its operation merits a brief description.

Having selected the neuron to be analyzed, the operator brings its soma into focus in the center of the field of view (using a pair of cross hairs in one eyepiece as the reference point). The position of the soma in three-dimensional space is then signaled to the computer and serves as the zero reference position from which all subsequent measurements are made. Then, using a joy-stick to direct the movements of the stage of the microscope in the X and Y dimensions and a toggle-switch control for the fine focus mechanism (both of which act through the computer), the origins of each dendrite to be studied are, in turn, brought into focus in the center of the field and their location signaled to the computer (in the form of an x-y-z triplet). This is followed by the tracking and logging of data from the first dendrite. At intervals of approximately 7 to 20 μm (depending on the regularity of the process) the three-dimensional structure of the dendrite is signaled to the computer and stored for subsequent reconstruction. When a branch point is encountered, this is signaled by a separate topological identifier, as is the end of the branch. When the end of the branch is reached, the computer automatically returns the stage and fine focus position to the location of the last branch point, in readiness for the logging of that branch. When its endpoint has been reached and its location signaled and stored in triplet form, the stage and fine focus controls are again activated by the computer and the penultimate branch point is brought into focus in the center of the field. The process of data logging is repeated until all the branches of the first dendrite have been examined, and then the computer automatically brings the origin of the next dendrite into view. The process is then repeated until all the dendrites have been logged, by which time the computer has stored in memory a complete set of data for the three-dimensional reconstruction and display of the cells' entire dendritic tree.

One of the major features of systems such as this is their ability to provide a visual display of the reconstructed cell (as a stick-figure rather than with all the morphological pecularities of the dendrites) and by rotating the displayed image, to view the cell from any spatial angle. Thus a neuron reconstructed from, say, a frontal section of the brain can be readily viewed as it might appear in sagittal or horizontal sections, and various programming features enable one to highlight specific processes, or parts of a process, during the dynamic rotation of the cell.

Recently the programming of this system has been extended in several directions, one of the most promising of which enables one to follow a process through adjoining serial sections. For this a series of key topological landmarks are provided to the computer as reference points, and when the adjoining sections are examined the necessary translational and rotational adjustments are made so that the end-points of the branches (actually the truncated cut ends) are automatically identified and serially brought into view. As further programming features are developed, it should be possible to provide a fairly complete picture of the reconstructed cells, including information about the number and location of dendritic spines, dendritic diameters, volume and surface areas, and the clustering of small populations of neurons that are, or might be, functionally interrelated.

Automatic Grain-Counting in Autoradiographs

The development of the autoradiographic method for tracing connections, which was described in the first section of this chapter, has prompted the development of an automated system for determining grain densities in autoradiographs (45). Using essentially the same hardware as was used for the three-dimensional reconstruction of nerve cells, together with a Plumbicon-type TV camera, it has been possible to accurately count the numbers of silver grains in small areas of tissue on a fully automated basis and using a program for the automatic advancement of the slide to relatively quickly determine the silver grain density over areas as large as 4 or 5 mm². Since the details of this system have been described in full elsewhere, I shall only give a general account of its configuration and mode of operation.

The operator first selects the total area of the autoradiograph that is to be scanned and enters into memory certain key topographical landmarks (such as nuclear boundaries, cortical laminae, etc.). With this data it is later possible to accurately relate the grain densities to the critical morphological features of the tissue. After this the system operates largely in the automatic mode, with the computer controlling field selection, stage advance, focusing, grain counting, data logging, and print-out.

Beginning at one corner of the area to be counted, the entire population of silver grains in the emulsion layer overlying an area about 80×80 μm are counted. This is done first by determining the optimum plane of focus within the emulsion layer and then scanning the field of view on a raster basis, the x and y locations of each grain being stored in memory and subsequently printed out as a single number, representing the grain density in that field. When the first field has been scanned in this way, the stage is advanced exactly one field diameter and the process repeated until the entire area to be scanned has been covered. Using dark-field optics, this system has been improved to the point that it can now effectively determine the grain densities over an area of 4 mm² in as little as 2 to 3 hr, with considerable accuracy and with none of the tedium inherent in visual grain counting.

A Simple System for Measuring Cell and Nuclear Areas

One of the most practically usfeul systems we have developed involves the use of an acoustical data tablet interfaced with a small computer for measuring various neuronal parameters such as the cross-sectional areas of the perikarya and nuclei of nerve cells, the diameters of axons, and the linear dimensions of various processes (46). The simplicity of the system, both in its design and in its use, has made it extremely useful for a variety of morphometric studies, including the growth of neurons during development, the effects of various experimental manipulations (e.g., axotomy, deafferentation, etc.), the morphometric identification of various cell types, and estimates of axonal and synaptic vesicle diameters.

The system consists essentially of a data tablet with a pair of directionally sensitive strip microphones along its left and upper edges, a pen that emits an acoustical spark, and a pair of counters that are activated at the moment the pen contacts the tablet surface. The objects to be measured can be traced directly from a microscope (with the aid of a camera-lucida or similar drawing apparatus), from a projector, from drawings or photomicrographs. On contacting the tablet, a small stationary window is opened, and as the outline of the cell or other structure is traced, the area enclosed within the outline is integrated, or its linear dimension computed, the time of arrival of the sound wave at the two microphones being converted into x and y spatial dimensions. When the pen re-enters the stationary window, the measurement is automatically terminated and the appropriate area, length, or equivalent diameter computed and printed out.

In practice it has been possible to measure cells at a rate of about 6 to 10/min with this system, which is about an order of magnitude more rapid than can be achieved with most conventional morphometric methods for measuring cell or nuclear sizes. This has meant that several problems, which in the past would have been considered too formidable to be undertaken can now be done with little hesitation. In addition the system can be readily adapted for a number of other purposes, of which perhaps the most generally useful is the reconstruction of neurons or their processes from serial light or electron micrographs.

There are, of course, several other applications of computers to neuroanatomical studies, and in selecting the above developments it is not my intention to exaggerate their significance or to diminish that of others. It is evident, for example, that systems for the three-dimensional reconstruction of neurons and neuronal processes from electron micrographs like that de-

veloped by Levinthal and his associates (47) provide the greatest possible information about neural organization at the synaptic level. The usefulness of their system for developmental and genetic studies is only now being exploited, but it is already apparent that for "small nervous systems," or restricted portions of the nervous systems of higher organisms, this type of approach is both essential and definitive.

CONCLUSION

It should be evident from even this rather cursory survey of the subject, that the past quarter-century has seen the development of a number of neuroanatomical techniques of considerable promise, which may well change our entire approach to the study of central neural structure. Perhaps the most exciting aspect of these new developments is that they are not limited to the study of the more "static" features of the nervous system, but open up a whole new vista that extends well beyond the "jurisdictional" boundaries that for so long have separated neuroanatomy from its related disciplines of neurophysiology and neurochemistry. If the years between now and the turn of the century should prove as fruitful in the development of new approaches as the past 25 years have been, we may confidently look forward to fulfillment of what has long been the goal of neuroanatomical studies, namely, to provide a secure morphological basis for our understanding of normal and disturbed behavior.

ACKNOWLEDGMENT

I should like to take this opportunity to acknowledge, with gratitude, the continued support that my work has received from the National Institutes of Health. This most recent contribution was supported in part by U.S. Public Health Service Grant NS-10943 from the National Institute of Neurological Diseases and Stroke.

REFERENCES

1. Cajal, S. Ramón y (1928): *Degeneration and Regeneration of the Nervous System,* translated by R. M. May. Oxford University Press, London.
2. Cowan, W. M., and Cuénod, M. (1975): The use of axonal transport for the study of neural con-

nections: A retrospective survey. In: *The Use of Axonal Transport for Studies of Neuronal Connectivity*, edited by W. M. Cowan and M. Cuénod. Elsevier, Amsterdam.

3. Lasek, R. J., Joseph, B. S., and Whitlock, D. G. (1968): Evaluation of a radioautographic neuroanatomical tracing method. *Brain Res.*, 8:319–336.

4. Hendrickson, A. E. (1969): Electron microscopic radioautography: Identification of origin of synaptic terminals in normal nervous tissue. *Science*, 165:194–196.

5. Schonbach, J., Schonbach, C., and Cuénod, M. (1971): Rapid phase of axoplasmic flow and synaptic proteins: An electron microscopical autoradiographic study. *J. Comp. Neurol.*, 141:485–498.

6. Cowan, W. M., Gottlieb, D. I., Hendrickson, A. E., Price, J. L., and Woolsey, T. A. (1972): The autoradiographic demonstration of axonal connections in the central nervous system. *Brain Res.*, 37:21–51.

7. Crossland, W. J., Cowan, W. M., Rogers, L. A., and Kelly, J. P. (1974): The specification of the retino-tectal projection in the chick. *J. Comp. Neurol.*, 155:127–164.

8. Kopriwa, B. M., and Leblond, C. P. (1962): Improvements in the coating technique of radioautography. *J. Histochem. Cytochem.*, 10:269–284.

9. Swanson, L. W., and Cowan, W. M. (1975): Hippocampo-hypothalamic connections: Origin in the subicular cortex not Ammon's horn. *Science*, 189:303–304.

10. Moore, R. Y., and Lenn, N. J. (1972): A retino-hypothalamic projection in the rat. *J. Comp. Neurol.*, 146:1–14.

11. Hendrickson, A. E., Wagoner, N., and Cowan, W. M. (1972): An autoradiographic and electron microscopic study of retino-hypothalamic connections. *Z. Zellforsch.*, 135:1–26.

12. Graybiel, A. M., Nauta, H. J. W., Lasek, R. T., and Nauta, W. J. H. (1973): A cerebello-olivary pathway in the cat: an experimental study using autoradiographic tracing techniques. *Brain Res.*, 58:205–211.

13. Grafstein, B. (1971): Transneuronal transfer of radioactivity in the central nervous system. *Science*, 172:177–179.

14. Wiesel, T. N., Hubel, D. H., and Lam, D. M. K. (1974): Autoradiographic demonstration of ocular-dominance columns in the monkey striate cortex by means of transneuronal transport. *Brain Res.*, 79:273–279.

15. Dräger, U. C. (1974): Autoradiography of tritiated proline and fucose transported transneuronally from the eye to the visual cortex in pigmented and albino mice. *Brain Res.*, 82:284–293.

16. Lynch, G., Gall, C., Mensah, P., and Cotman, C. W. (1974): Horseradish peroxidase histochemistry: A new method for tracing efferent projections in the central nervous system. *Brain Res.*, 65:373–380.

17. Graham, R. C., and Karnovsky, M. J. (1966): The early stages of absorption of injected horseradish peroxidase in the proximal tubules of mouse kidney in ultrastructural cytochemistry by a new technique. *J. Histochem. Cytochem.*, 14:291–302.

18. Scalia, F., and Colman, D. R. (1974): Aspects of the central projection of the optic nerve in the frog as revealed by anterograde migration of horseradish peroxidase. *Brain Res.*, 79:496–504.

19. Kristensson, K. (1975): Retrograde axonal transport of protein tracers. In: *The Use of Axonal Transport for Studies of Neuronal Connectivity*, edited by W. M. Cowan and M. Cuénod. Elsevier, Amsterdam.

20. Kristensson, K., and Olsson, Y. (1971): Retrograde axonal transport of proteins. *Brain Res.*, 29:363–365.

21. LaVail, J. H., and LaVail, M. M. (1972): Retrograde axonal transport in the central nervous system. *Science*, 176:1416–1417.

22. LaVail, J. H., Winston, K. R., and Tish, A. (1973): A method based on retrograde intra-axonal transport of protein for identification of cell bodies of origin of axons terminating within the CNS. *Brain Res.*, 58:470–477.

23. LaVail, J. H., and LaVail, M. M. (1974): The retrograde intraaxonal transport of horseradish peroxidase in the chick visual system: A light and electron microscopic study. *J. Comp. Neurol.*, 157:303–357.

24. Kater, S. B., and Nicholson, C., Eds. (1973): *Intracellular Staining in Neurobiology*. Springer-Verlag, New York.

25. Stretton, A. O. W., and Kravitz, E. A. (1968): Neuronal geometry: determination with a technique of intracellular dye injection. *Science*, 162:132–134.

26. Kreutzberg, G., and Schubert, P. (1975): The cellular dynamics of intraneuronal transport. In: *The Use of Axonal Transport for Studies of Neuronal Connectivity*, edited by W. M. Cowan and M. Cuénod. Elsevier, Amsterdam.

27. Pitman, R. M., Tweedle, C. D., and Cohen, M. J. (1972): Branching of central neurons: intracellular cobalt injection for light and electron microscopy. *Science*, 276:412–414.

28. Pitman, R. R., Tweedle, C. D., and Cohen, M. J. (1973): The form of nerve cells: determination by cobalt impregnation. In: *Intracellular Staining in Neurobiology*, edited by S. B. Kater and C. Nicholson, pp. 83–97. Springer-Verlag, New York.

29. Llinas, R. (1973): Procion yellow and cobalt as tools for the study of structure-function relationships in vertebrate central nervous systems. In: *Intracellular Staining in Neurobiology*, edited by S. B. Kater and C. Nicholson, pp. 211–224. Springer-Verlag, New York.

30. Eränko, O. (1955): Histochemistry of noradrenaline in the medulla of rats and mice. *Endocrinology*, 57:363–368.

31. Falck, B., Hillarp, N. A., Thieme, G., and Torp, A. (1962): Fluorescence of catecholamines and related compounds condensed with formal-

dehyde. *J. Histochem. Cytochem.*, 10:348–354.

32. Lindvall, O., Björklund, A., Nobin, A., and Stenevi, U. (1974): The adrenergic innervation of the rat thalamus as revealed by the glyoxylic acid fluorescence method. *J. Comp. Neurol.*, 154:317–348.

33. Hartman, B. K. (1973): Immunofluorescence of dopamine β-hydroxylase: Application of improved methodology to the localization of the peripheral and central noradrenergic nervous system. *J. Histochem. Cytochem.*, 21:312–332.

34. Geffen, L. B., Livett, B. G., and Rush, R. A. (1969): Immunohistochemical localization of protein components of catecholamine storage vesicles. *J. Physiol. (Lond.)*, 204:593–606.

35. Geffen, L. (1975): Biochemical and histochemical methods of tracing transmitter specific neuronal molecules (with special reference to adrenergic neurons). In: *The Use of Axonal Transport for Studies of Neuronal Connectivity*, edited by W. M. Cowan and M. Cuénod. Elsevier, Amsterdam.

36. Swanson, L. W., and Hartman, B. K. (1975): The central adrenergic system. An immunofluorescent study of the location of cell bodies and their efferent connections in the rat utilizing dopamine β-hydroxylase as a marker. *J. Comp. Neurol. (in press)*.

37. McGeer, P. L., McGeer, E. G., Singh, V. K., and Chase, W. H. (1974): Choline acetyltransferase localization in the central nervous system by immunohistochemistry. *Brain Res.*, 81:373–379.

38. Eng, L. F., Uyeda, C. T., Chao, L. P., and Wolfgram, F. (1974): Antibody to bovine acetyl cholinetransferase and immunofluorescent localization of the enzyme in neurones. *Nature*, 250:243–245.

39. McLaughlin, B. J., Wood, J. G., Saito, K., Barber, R., Vaughn, J. E., Roberts, E., and Blu, J. Y. (1974): The fine structural localization of glutamate decarboxylase in synaptic terminals of rodent cerebellum. *Brain Res.*, 76:377–391.

40. Iversen, L. L., and Schon, F. (1973): The use of autoradiographic techniques for the identification and mapping of transmitter-specific neurones in CNS. In: *New Concepts in Transmitter Regulation*, edited by A. Mandel and D. Segal, pp. 153–193. Plenum Press, New York.

41. Matus, A. I., and Dennison, M. E. (1971): Autoradiographic localization of tritiated glycine at 'flat-vesicle' synapses in spinal cord. *Brain Res.*, 32:195–197.

42. Glaser, E. M., and Van der Loos, H. (1965): A semi-automatic computer microscope for the analysis of neuronal morphology. *IEEE Trans. BME*, 12:22–31.

43. Llinás, R., and Hillman, D. E. (1975): A multipurpose tridimensional reconstruction computer system for neuroanatomy. In: *Golgi Centennial Symposium Proceedings*, edited by M. Santini, pp. 71–79. Raven Press, New York.

44. Wann, D. F., Woolsey, T. A., Dierker, M. L., and Cowan, W. M. (1973): An on-line digital computer system for the semi-automatic analysis of Golgi-impregnated neurons. *IEEE Trans. BME*, 20:233–247.

45. Wann, D. F., Price, J. L., Cowan, W. M., and Algunek, M. A. (1974): An automated system for counting silver grains in autoradiographs. *Brain Res.*, 81:31–58.

46. Cowan, W. M., and Wann, D. F. (1973): A computer system for the measurement of cell and nuclear sizes. *J. Microscop.*, 99:331–348.

47. Levinthal, C., Macagno, E., and Tountas, C. (1974): Computer-aided reconstruction from serial sections. *Fed. Proc.*, 33:2336–2340.

The Nervous System, Donald B. Tower, Editor-in-Chief. *Vol. 1: The Basic Neurosciences*. Raven Press, New York, 1975.

Cytology of Mechanoreceptors in Oral Mucosa and Facial Skin of the Rhesus Monkey

Bryce L. Munger

Current concepts regarding the cytologic organization and function of mechanoreceptors have been largely derived from studies on general somatic glabrous or hairy skin. The oral area is known to be exquisitely sensitive as defined by two-point tactile discrimination, and representation of trigeminal sensory afferents in the brainstem and cerebral cortex of primates is extensive (1). The coordination of sensory input from the oral area is important not just for feeding (including suckling in the newborn) but in man it is also critical for speech (1). Although the central projections of the trigeminal system are similar as one compares lower mammals with primates, important differences do exist, and extrapolation from cat to rhesus monkey or from rhesus monkey to man must be done with great caution. Considering the importance of the oral sensory system, it is surprising that the nature of sensory receptors within the oral mucosa or associated facial skin has not been systematically explored in primates. This chapter attempts to define the repertoire of mechanoreceptors that are present in the oral area of the rhesus monkey and that are likely to be involved in the transduction of tactile stimuli. The superficial or mucosal receptors are considered here, whereas taste buds, teeth, and deep receptors of joints are not discussed.

The descriptive material concerning the nature of sensory receptors in primate oral mucosa has been derived from an ongoing study of the differentiation of sensory receptors in the primate oral area. Tissue for analysis was harvested following vascular perfusion with dilute paraformaldehyde-glutaraldehyde fixative, and tissue was prepared for light and electron microscopy as described in detail elsewhere (2,3). For light microscopy paraffin sections were stained with a neurofibrillar silver impregnation, and corresponding areas of oral mucosa were prepared for electron microscopy.

ORAL MUCOSA

The oral mucous membrane of the rhesus monkey contains a distinctive array of sensory receptors, including corpuscular receptors, presumptive free nerve endings, and intraepithelial nerve terminals.

Corpuscular Receptors

Numerous types of corpuscular receptors have been described in the oral mucosa by light microscopy (1,4,5). Corpuscular receptors include a somewhat bewildering array of discrete entities as described by light microscopy, and they usually carry eponymic designations that pose a significant conceptual problem in terms of correlating structure and function. In an attempt to simplify this complicated nomenclature, I use the term "corpuscular" to denote a sensory terminal that is discrete within the general vascular connective tissue stoma as visualized by light microscopy, and this terminal may or may not be truly encapsulated (2,3,6,7). Two distinctive corpuscular receptors have been defined to date in rhesus monkey oral mucosa by light and electron microscopy— Meissner and glomerular corpuscles (2) (Fig. 1).

Meissner corpuscles have been repeatedly described by light microscopy in primate (including human) oral mucosa (1,4,5,8). On the basis of electron microscopy as well as light microscopy, Meissner corpuscles, identical in every respect to Meissner corpuscles of primate glabrous digital skin, have been identified in palatal (3), lingual (2), and lip mucosa. These sensory receptors are characterized by a regular winding back and forth of the terminal neurite

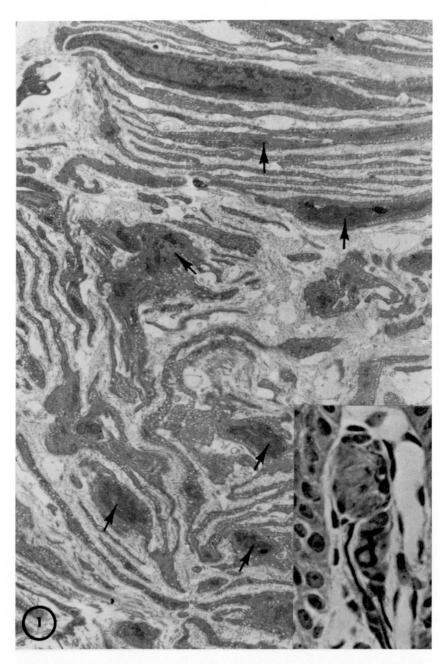

FIG. 1. A portion of a Meissner corpuscle (*top*) and a glomerular corpuscle (*bottom*) are illustrated in this electron micrograph taken from rhesus palatal mucosa. A corresponding area is seen by light microscopy in the insert. The Meissner corpuscle has many thin cytoplasmic lamellae separating the flattened neurite profiles (*upper two arrows*). The glomerular corpuscle in the bottom half of the micrograph has a larger diameter neurite (*lower four arrows*), which courses in an irregular manner through the connective tissue. A delicate basal lamina envelops the lamellae. **Inset:** An equivalent area is seen in a light micrograph of a silver-stained section. The Meissner corpuscle (*upper*) has very thin neurite profiles, and the (*lower*) glomerular corpuscle has a loosely coiled terminal neurite. Electron micrograph × 8,000; light micrograph × 640.

separated by many stacks of thin cytoplasmic lamellae derived from the lamellar cell of the receptor core. The lamellar cell is regarded as a specialized Schwann cell probably derived from neural crest elements (9). The lamellar cell of the receptor core is characterized by the presence of a delicate basal lamina, and its cytoplasm repeatedly projects from the cell body in thin sheets. The thin, flat cytoplasmic plates, referred to as lamellae, are closely applied to one another, separated by thin compartments of connective tissue. The stacks of flattened lamellae of the receptor core in many respects resemble the inner core of Pacinian corpuscles (6,7). These thin cytoplasmic lamellae are also enveloped by basal lamina, and characteristically contain myriads of pinocytotic vesicles. The terminal neurite, as it courses between the stacks of lamellae, is sandwiched between two contiguous lamellae. The neurite and its pair of associated lamellae bear a striking resemblance to the flattened neurite and associated flattened Schwann cell processes present in lanceolate endings on hairs (6,10,11). This similarity has been discussed in more detail previously (6).

The role of the complex ultrastructural organization of Meissner corpuscles (i.e., stacks of lamellae and winding neurite) in the transduction process and/or adaptive properties of this receptor is not known. In glabrous digital skin, these receptors are usually regarded as rapidly adapting mechanoreceptors (6,7,11). Direct proof for this conclusion is not available. If the presence of numerous pinocytotic vesicles in a given cell implies an active transport of extracellular fluid, the inner core of many corpuscular receptors is the site of intense transport activity. The lamellae and lamellar cells of Pacinian, Meissner, glomerular, and simple corpuscles (12), as well as genital end bulbs (6) and lanceolate endings on hairs (10), share the cytologic characteristic in that numerous pinocytotic vesicles are present. Certainly a significant transport of ions in the core of corpuscular receptors could affect electrical events at the level of the terminal neurite. Such an event would be especially profound, if such transport is highly ordered in space and the stacks of lamellae could provide such spatial order. Based on the available physiologic evidence, these corpuscular receptors are all

thought to be rapidly adapting mechanoreceptors and should thus be regarded as a functionally related group. The common denominator in cytologic terms is the presence of lamellae within the core of the corpuscle. The geographic separation of Meissner corpuscles in primate palatal (3) and lingual (2) mucosa could provide a system for analyzing the events in mechanical transduction as well as definitively assessing the adaptive characteristics of Meissner corpuscles.

A second corpuscular receptor present in lingual but less frequently in palatal mucosa has been designated a glomerular corpuscle (2) (Fig. 1). This terminal is distinct from Meissner corpuscles in that the terminal neurite resembles a tangled skein of yarn by light microscopy and, by electron microscopy, lacks the characteristic stacks of cytoplasmic lamellae separating the terminal arborizations of the neurite, a characteristic feature of Meissner corpuscles. Glomerular corpuscles are commonly seen in the dorsum of the tip of the rhesus tongue (2). The terminal neurite retains its large diameter (3 to 8 μm) in glomerular corpuscles, whereas in Meissner corpuscles the terminal neurite becomes very thin as it courses back and forth in the corpuscle and is relatively difficult to impregnate with silver (Fig. 1). Glomerular corpuscles as defined above, in my opinion, would thus include Krause end bulbs, genital end bulbs, Dogiel end bulbs, and mucocutaneous end organs (6,7).

Other corpuscular receptors have been described especially in relationship to the bones and joints of the face including Pacinian, Golgi-Mazzoni, and Ruffini corpuscles (see below). Golgi-Mazzoni corpuscles have been described in physiological terms (13) in the periosteum of the mandible but the ultrastructure of this receptor has not been elucidated. In summary only two types of corpuscular receptors have been defined to date in the superficial mucosa of the rhesus oral cavity, a conclusion supported by Kadanoff and Gürowski (4) in their study by light microscopy on the nature of sensory terminals in human oral mucosa.

Free Nerve Endings

The characterization of free nerve endings in oral mucosa poses the same problem as encountered in skin (6); i.e., the precise definition of a free terminal is almost impossible using cytologic techniques (light and electron microscopy). Furthermore the functional parameters have not been defined in neurophysiologic terms. Although a free ending can be seen in special situations such as raccoon glabrous digital skin (12), such terminals are infrequently seen in situations where the *end* of the neurite can be defined. In the case cited (raccoon digital skin) (12), nerve fibers approach the epidermis perpendicular to the skin surface and repeatedly branch, terminating loosely in the connective tissue of the dermis. If the course of such a fiber were not unique but rather haphazardly arranged in the connective tissue, the recognition of any one branch as distinct from small unmyelinated axons (? autonomic or somatosensory) would be impossible. Thus the definition in cytologic terms of free nerve endings is a difficult if not impossible task. Throughout the oral mucosa, single unmyelinated neurites are present in Schwann cells, but verification of the nature of such neurites remains an unsolved problem. Since these presumptive terminals are often implicated in the transduction of painful and/or thermal stimuli, their importance cannot be overemphasized. Certainly the precise definition of thermal and nociceptive receptors remains an important area for future study.

Merkel Cell-Neurite Complexes

Intraepithelial neurites have been repeatedly described in oral mucosa (4,5) by light microscopy (excluding the innervation of taste buds). Our studies to date verify an extensive intraepithelial innervation in oral mucosa, and furthermore this intraepithelial innervation consists chiefly of numerous Merkel cell-neurite complexes (6,7,14). Not only are isolated Merkel cell-neurite complexes present, but clusters of these units can be encountered resembling the Merkel rete papillae of raccoon glabrous digital skin (15).

Merkel cell-neurite complexes encountered in the rhesus monkey oral mucosa (Fig. 2) resemble those previously described in a wide variety of species (6,7,11,16) including man (17, and McGavran, cited in ref. 18). At a cytologic level, Merkel cells have a remarkably constant

appearance. A large epidermal cell contains numerous secretory granules polarized in the cytoplasm toward a contiguous large diameter neurite. The Merkel cell can be regarded conceptually as an epidermal cell because numerous desmosomes are present between the Merkel cell and contiguous cells of the stratified squamous epithelium. The presence of desmosomal connections clearly differentiates the Merkel cell from the melanocyte population of skin. In the present author's previous studies on Merkel cell-neurite complexes (6,7,14,15), junctional complexes were not observed between the neurite and its associated Merkel cell. Andres (10), on the other hand, described membrane specializations in the neurite and clusters of secretory granules in the Merkel cell oriented to the membrane specialization (10,11). In our recent studies on primate oral mucosa, membrane thickenings have been repeatedly observed (Fig. 2) in Merkel cell-neurite complexes (3). In some cases the neurite contains clusters of vesicles at the site of a membrane specialization. Our cytologic observations to date do not exactly conform to the idealized drawing of Andres and von Düring (11). In their experience a membrane thickening is present only on the neurite plasma membrane. As can be seen in Fig. 2, the apposed plasmalemmae of Merkel cell and neurite appear to have corresponding areas of membrane thickening. The nature of such membrane specializations is not known at the present time. The available cytologic evidence would not justify the designation of such areas as synapses, but would implicate a potential for interaction between neurite and associated Merkel cell.

A peculiar feature of oral innervation is the relative absence of Merkel cell-neurite complexes in primate lingual mucosa; at least they have not been encountered in material studied to date (2). By way of contrast, clusters of Merkel cell-neurite complexes (similar to Merkel rete papillae in the raccoon glabrous digital skin) (15) are prominent in mucosa of lip and hard palate (3). This regional variation in the distribution of sensory receptors has no explanation at the present time.

Merkel cell-neurite complexes are usually regarded as the anatomic substrate of slowly adapting mechanoreceptors (6,7,12,15–17), but the actual function of Merkel cells is speculative.

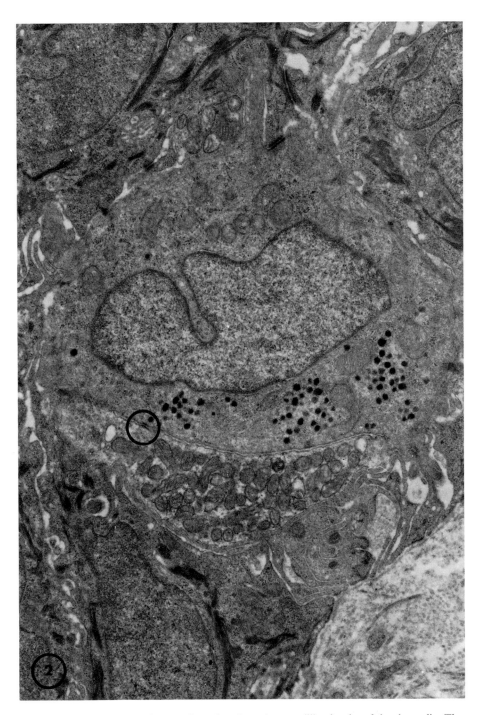

FIG. 2. Part of a Merkel cell-neurite complex taken from the vermillion border of the rhesus lip. The neurite profile contains numerous mitochondria. The Merkel cell secretory granules are polarized in the cytoplasm toward the neurite. The circle delineates an area of thickening of the plasma membrane in both Merkel cell and apposed neurite. × 17,000.

The hypothesis that these cells are transducers, as proposed originally by Merkel (19), has not been verified by any direct experimental evidence. In fact the chemical nature of the secretory granules, the characteristic cytoplasmic specialization of these cells, is still a mystery (6,14,17,20). Various functions for Merkel cells have been proposed, including: (a) cellular transduction, i.e., conversion of mechanical to electrical activity, perhaps involved in the production of a generator potential similar to that present in Pacinian corpuscles; (b) modulating the activity of a mechanoreceptor, i.e., a sensory neurite (mechanoreceptor) would be altered by the secretory activity of Merkel cells to become slowly adapting in a physiologic sense; and (c) trophic activity, i.e., secretory activity (tissue-tissue interactions) of the epidermis could modify the growth of peripheral neurites by controlling the entry of such neurites into the stratified squamous epithelium or for that matter into superficial dermis. While all of these options are speculative, the function of Merkel cells and the events involved in mechanical transduction at a cellular level remain major areas for future research. One conclusion appears justified at this time: Merkel cells can be implicated as a site for interaction between stratified squamous epithelium (skin and oral mucosa) and the nervous system. The importance of the nervous system in the pathogenesis of dermatalogic disorders is an accepted fact, and the Merkel cell is the only documented cellular link between the two systems.

HAIRY SKIN OF LIP AND CHEEK

As one proceeds from the vermillion border of the lip to the hairy skin of the lip and cheek, one encounters epidermis and associated appendages typical of body skin. In the rhesus monkey the lip contains a profusion of vibrissae in addition to conventional hairs, and the sensory innervation is profuse (1). The mechanoreceptors present in hairy skin are usually regarded as consisting of the following: (a) Haarscheibe (21) or touch domes (16), (b) free nerve endings, (c) innervated hairs, and (d) vibrissae, present only in nonhuman primates and other mammals.

The first two categories will be considered only in passing since the specific receptors have been discussed above with respect to oral mucosa.

Haarscheibe (17,21) or touch domes (16) are dome-like elevations of epidermis containing numerous Merkel cell-neurite complexes. Since these elevations can be seen grossly, the precise correlation of structure and function is possible, and they represent slowly adapting mechanoreceptors (16,17). Since Merkel cell-neurite complexes have already been discussed with respect to oral mucosa, their cytology and function will not be discussed further. The term "Haarscheibe" as coined by Pinkus (21) connotes a dome-like elevation of the epidermis associated with a hair. Depression of a hair could activate the Haarscheibe by touching the top of the dome. Even though Pinkus (21) described Haarscheibe in great detail, including their involvement in human dermatologic disorders, the importance of these structures has only relatively recently been appreciated as a result of the elegant studies of Iggo and his co-workers (16). Haarscheibe, present in the hairy facial skin of primates, represent an exquisitely sensitive tactile transducer.

The presence of free nerve endings in hairy skin has been described (18) but the problems as noted above with respect to oral mucosa still exist. The precise definition of an ending is very difficult (6).

Conventional hairs are innervated with a regular array of lanceolate endings (6,7,10) arranged as a collar around the hair shaft below the level of the sebaceous gland. These receptors are usually regarded as rapidly adapting in a physiologic sense (6,7). The cytology of lanceolate endings is similar among the various animals studied to date and has been reviewed in detail elsewhere (6,7,11). The rhesus monkey conforms to this established pattern.

The lip of the rhesus monkey is richly endowed with large and extremely small vibrissae in addition to conventional hairs. A small vibrissa at first glance can often be confused with a conventional hair.

The problem of correlating the cytology of sensory receptors in hairy skin with presumptive function has recently been complicated by the conclusion by Gottschaldt et al. (22), on the basis of studying vibrissae, that a lanceolate ending is a slowly adapting mechanoreceptor. This conclusion, based on circumstantial evi-

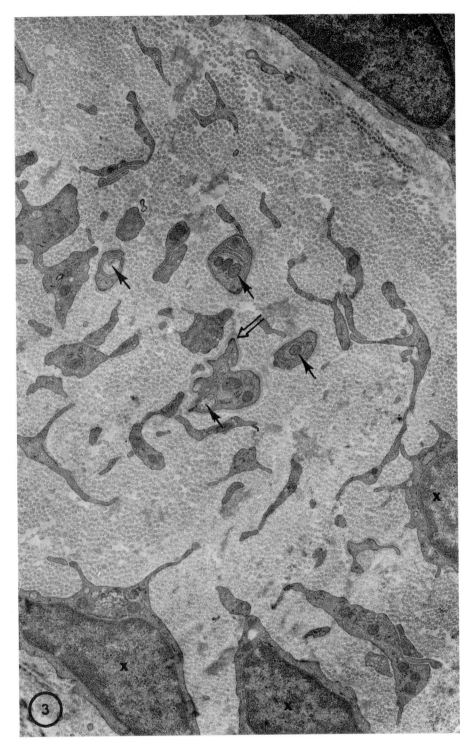

FIG. 3. A portion of a pilo-Ruffini complex. Small branches of a terminal neurite (*solid arrows*) are enveloped by thin extensions of Schwann cell cytoplasm. A delicate basal lamina (*open arrow*) envelops the Schwann cell and its stellate processes. A second cell (nuclei labeled x), termed a septal cell, also has numerous stellate processes compartmentalizing parallel bundles of collagen fibrils cut in cross section. The septal cell lacks a basal lamina. The shaft of the hair follicle is not depicted, but this micrograph is a cross section of the corpuscle which envelops the hair shaft circumferentially. × 8,000.

dence in terms of location, is exactly opposite to the consensus noted above, that lanceolate endings on conventional hairs are rapidly adapting. These authors also attribute some rapidly adapting characteristic in these vibrissae to Golgi-Mazzoni corpuscles. In many animals, including the rhesus monkey, in our experience, distinct corpuscular receptors are not presently associated with facial vibrissae.

Vibrissae are known to contain Merkel cell-neurite complexes as well as conventional lanceolate endings (6,10), and these receptors are usually regarded as the source of the slowly and rapidly adapting responses, respectively, that are characteristic of vibrissae (6,7). Gottschaldt et al. (22) found two types of slowly adapting mechanoreceptors in cat vibrissae similar to the two types of slowly adapting mechanoreceptors described in physiologic terms in glabrous digital skin (11,25). The necessity of having two slowly adapting mechanoreceptors led to the conclusion that lanceolate endings were slowly adapting. A recently described sensory receptor associated with nonsinus (conventional) hairs (23) may resolve this apparent discrepancy. This receptor, termed a pilo-Ruffini complex, is a Ruffini corpuscle wrapped circumferentially around the hair shaft (Fig. 3). The receptor is characterized by a highly ordered association of (a) bundles of parallel, circumferential collagen fibrils, (b) extremely small diameter branches of a terminal neurite associated with (c) stellate Schwann cells, and (d) a stellate, nonneural septal cell, all arranged circumferentially around the hair. The receptor closely resembles in cytologic pattern the Golgi tendon organ as described by Schoultz and Swett (24). As a matter of fact, the resemblance is striking at an ultrastructural level. Whereas a Ruffini corpuscle has recently been described as a slowly adapting receptor in physiologic terms by Chambers et al. (25), ultrastructural cytologic documentation is lacking as to the cellular nature of the receptor. The pilo-Ruffini complex is also a slowly adapting mechanoreceptor in that the hair when moved adapted slowly (23). Thus nonsinus hairs may be innervated by lanceolate endings (rapidly adapting) or a Ruffiini corpuscle (slowly adapting). The possible presence of Ruffini corpuscles in primate vibrissae could explain the presence of two

slowly adapting mechanoreceptors in vibrissae (22) and avoid the necessity of identifying lanceolate endings as slowly adapting mechanoreceptors.

In summary facial hairy skin in the rhesus monkey appears to contain the same spectrum of sensory receptors present within general somatic skin, with the possible exception of pilo-Ruffini complexes. This terminal has not been identified to date in general somatic skin, but it provides still another type of specific sensory terminal that can perhaps begin to explain the complex but specific nature of sensory data perceived by the nervous system.

ACKNOWLEDGMENT

This study was supported in part by U.S. Public Health Service Grant NIH-NIDR-72-2401 from the National Institute of Dental Research.

REFERENCES

1. Darian-Smith, I. (1973): The trigeminal system. In: *Handbook of Sensory Physiology, Vol. 2,* edited by A. Iggo, pp. 271–314. Springer, New York.
2. Munger, B. L. (1973): Cytology and ultrastructure of sensory receptors in the adult and newborn primate tongue. In: *Fourth Symposium on Oral Sensation and Perception, Development of the Fetus and Infant,* edited by J. F. Bosma, pp. 75–95. DHEW Publ. (NIH) 73–546, U.S. Govt. Printing Office 1747–0008, Washington, D.C.
3. Munger, B. L. (1975): Specificity in the development of sensory receptors in primate oral mucosa. In: *Development of Upper Respiratory Form and Function; Implications for Sudden and Unexpected Infant Death,* edited by J. F. Bosma. U.S. Govt. Printing Office, Washington, D.C.
4. Kadanoff, D., and Gürowski, A. (1963): *Morphologic der Rezeptoren des Atmungs—und Verdaungssystem beim Menschen.* G. Fisher, Jena.
5. Grossman, R. C., and Hattis, B. F. (1967): Oral mucosal sensory innervation and sensory experience. In: *Oral Sensation and Perception,* edited by J. F. Bosma, pp. 5–62. Charles C Thomas, Springfield, Ill.
6. Munger, B. L. (1971): Patterns of organization of peripheral sensory receptors. In: *Handbook of Sensory Physiology, Vol. 1,* edited by W. R. Loewenstein, pp. 523–556. Springer, Berlin.
7. Munger, B. L. (1971): The comparative ultrastructure of slowly and rapidly adapting mech-

anoreceptors. In: *Oral-Facial Sensory and Motor Mechanisms,* edited by R. Dubner and Y. Kawamura, pp. 83–103. Appleton-Century-Crofts, New York.

8. Kadanoff, D. (1971): Die eingekapselten sensibler Nervenendapparate der Haut und der Schleimhäute bei den Primaten vom Standpunkt der Stammesgeschichte. *Anat. Anz.,* 128:302–313.

9. Saxod, R. (1973): Developmental origin of the Herbst cutaneous sensory corpuscle—Experimental analysis using cellular markers. *Dev. Biol.,* 32:167–178.

10. Andres, K. H., (1966): Über die Feinstruktur der Rezeptoren an Sinushaaren, *Z. Zellforsch.,* 75:339–365.

11. Andres, K. H., and von Düring, M. (1973): Morphology of cutaneous receptors. In: *Handbook of Sensory Physiology, Vol. 2,* edited by A. Iggo, pp. 3–28. Springer, Berlin.

12. Munger, B. L., and Pubols, L. M. (1972): The sensorineural organization of the digital skin of the raccoon. *Brain, Behav., Evol.,* 5:367–393.

13. Sakada, S. (1971): Response of Golgi-Mazzoni corpuscles in the cat periostea to mechanical stimuli. In: *Oral-Facial Sensory and Motor Mechanisms,* edited by R. Dubner and Y. Kawamura, pp. 105–122. Appleton-Century-Crofts, New York.

14. Munger, B. L. (1965): The intraepidermal innervation of the snout skin of the opossum. A light and electron microscopic study, with observations on the nature of Merkel's *"Tastzellen." J. Cell Biol.,* 26:79–97.

15. Munger, B. L., Pubols, L. M., and Pubols, B. H. (1971): The Merkel rete papilla—A slowly adapt-

ing sensory receptor in mammalian glabrous skin. *Brain Res.,* 29:47–61.

16. Iggo, A., and Muir, A. R. (1969): The structure and function of a slowly adapting touch corpuscle in hairy skin. *J. Physiol. (Lond.),* 98:163–178.

17. Smith, K. R. (1970): The ultrastructure of the human Haarscheibe and Merkel cell. *J. Invest. Dermatol.,* 54:150–159.

18. Cauna, N. (1963): Light and electron microscopical structure of sensory end organs in human skin. In: *The Skin Senses,* edited by D. R. Kenshalo, pp. 15–29. Charles C Thomas, Springfield.

19. Merkel, F. (1880): Über die Endigungen der sensiblen Nerven in der Haut der Wirbeltniere, Schmidt, Rostock.

20. Winkelman, R. K., and Breathnach, A. S. (1973): The Merkel cell, *J. Invest. Derm.,* 60:2–15.

21. Pinkus, F. (1905): Über Hautsinnesorgane neben dem menschlichen Haar (Haarscheiben) und ihre vergleichend-anatomische Bedeutung, *Arch. Mikr. Anat.,* 65:121–179.

22. Gottshaldt, K. M., Iggo, A., and Young, D. W. (1973): Functional characteristics of mechanoreceptors in sinus hair follicles of the cat. *J. Physiol. (Lond.),* 235:87–315.

23. Biemesderfer, D., Dubner, R., and Munger, B. L. (1975): The pilo-Ruffini complex: A new sensory receptor in primate hairy skin. *In preparation.*

24. Schoultz, T. W., and Swett, J. E. (1972): The fine structure of Golgi tendon organs. *J. Neurocytol.,* 1:1–26.

25. Chambers, M. R., Andres, K. H., von Düring, M., and Iggo, A. (1972): The structure and function of the slowly adapting type II mechanoreceptor in hairy skin. *Quart. J. Physiol.,* 57:417–445.

The Nervous System, Donald B. Tower, Editor-in-Chief. *Vol. 1: The Basic Neurosciences*. Raven Press, New York, 1975.

Structure and Function of the T-System of Vertebrate Skeletal Muscle

Lee D. Peachey

The existence of the T-system or transverse tubules in skeletal muscle cells has been known for almost 20 years. During this time there has been a gradual improvement in our knowledge of its particular morphology in a variety of types of muscle cells of both vertebrates and invertebrates. We also have obtained information on the T-system's association with the cell surface and with the sarcoplasmic reticulum (SR), on its quantity in the muscle fiber, and on its apparent electrical properties. These are the subject of this chapter.

The discovery of the T-system of skeletal muscle should be credited to Porter and Palade (1). The electron microscope preparation methods of the time limited them in their visualization of the structures we now call transverse tubules, but they correctly described membrane-limited structures that were associated closely and specifically with the terminal cisternae of the sarcoplasmic reticulum. These associations were in structures that Porter and Palade called triads and that were located primarily near the Z-lines of the myofibrils in amphibian skeletal muscles. A few years later Andersson-Cedergren (2) demonstrated, with serial thin sections in the electron microscope, the transverse continuity of this membrane organelle and provided us with its present name. Since that time it has further been shown that the T-system in amphibian muscle fibers invaginates from the fiber surface membrane and remains in continuity with it. Thus the T-system represents an invasion of a sort of extracellular space into the confines of the fiber outline. Furthermore it provides an extensive augmentation of the surface area of the fiber and plays an important part in the bioelectric behavior of the fiber.

STRUCTURE OF THE T-SYSTEM

The development and recent state of our knowledge of the structure of the T-system was very capably reviewed 2 years ago (3), and I will not repeat that material here, beyond what has already been said. Instead I will attempt to emphasize quantitative data, some recent results and trends in the study of the structure of the T-system, and briefly mention some new experimental approaches to the study of its function in the muscle cell.

The generally held morphological view of the T-system of vertebrate skeletal muscles as revealed by thin sections in the electron microscope is that of networks of tubules encircling myofibrils and lying in planes oriented roughly transverse to the fiber axis. Tubular dimensions can be measured when a tubule is cut transversely to its own axis. The total length of tubule in a transverse plane across the muscle fiber can be estimated by measuring the total fibril perimeter or by estimating the total length of interfibrillar space from the average fibril size and fiber size. These figures can be used to compute T-system surface area and volume for a given amount of muscle fiber. For a frog skeletal muscle of the twitch type (4), this gives a figure of 0.3% for the volume of the transverse tubules, expressed as percent of total fiber volume. The corresponding surface area, expressed as a ratio of T-system surface area to the outer surface area of a fiber 100 μm in diameter, is 7. Recent results on the same muscle using electron microscopic stereology have confirmed these figures (5). By comparison a recent estimate of the quantity of transverse tubules in slow fibers of the frog cruralis muscle, derived from high-voltage electron micrographs, gives lower figures of 0.06% for T-system volume as a percent of fiber volume, and a T-system area to outer surface area of the fiber ratio of 1, for fibers 50 μm in diameter. There clearly is less T-system in the slow fibers than in the faster contracting twitch fibers.

Similar quantitative data on the T-system have been obtained by Nag (6) for two kinds of twitch fibers (white and red) from the caudal musculature of a fish (trout, *Salmo gairdneri*). The volume fraction for the T-system is 0.4 and 0.1% for white and red fibers, respectively, in the same range as for frog fibers. The surface area ratios are 5.3 for white fibers and 1.3 for red fibers in these fish muscles, values that are smaller than for frog twitch fibers largely because of the smaller diameter of the fish muscle fibers.

Stereological analysis of red skeletal muscle fibers of a mammal (guinea pig soleus) gives values of 0.14% for T-system fractional volume and 0.5 for surface area ratio (7). White fibers from the vastus muscle of the guinea pig have a larger quantity of T-system (8). The volume fraction for these fibers is 0.27% and the T-system surface to fiber surface ratio is 1.5.

Looked at together these figures indicate a tendency for faster contracting fibers to have more T-system and for more slowly contracting fibers to have less T-system. This is in agreement with the idea that the T-system functions in muscle cells as a rapid transmission system for the excitatory impulse from the fiber surface throughout the fiber interior, down to the most centrally located myofibrils.

A few other data of this kind are available, but it seems unfortunate that extensive data do not exist on other types of muscle, especially on other muscles of mammals, muscles in diseased states, muscles during development or regeneration, etc. Most electron microscopic descriptions of membrane systems in muscle cells are qualitative only, and this makes comparison difficult and uncertain. Progress in the study of neuromuscular diseases affecting muscle cell structure will be inhibited, perhaps seriously, by the lack of such data until more becomes known.

HIGH-VOLTAGE ELECTRON MICROSCOPY OF THE T-SYSTEM

Most of what has been discussed above about the structure of the T-system has been obtained by electron microscopic study of thin sections of muscle tissue, as shown in Fig. 1. The power of this method is the ease with which it resolves the approximately 10 nm thick membranes forming the usually 30 to 100 nm diameter tubules comprising the T-system: the weakness of the thin-section method is the very small amount of tissue and even smaller amount of T-system that is present in the small areas of thin sections examined. For example a typical electron micrograph at 20,000 magnification shows less than 2×10^{-13} g tissue, of which less than 1% will be T-system elements. The microscopist is obliged to examine a large number of micrographs showing small samples of the T-system in different orientations and then to deduce what its overall, three-dimensional structure is like. The result, when care is taken, can be quite an accurate and informative idea of what a typical portion of the T-system might be like, and this can be extrapolated to a sort of averaged view of all the T-system of a muscle fiber. This extrapolation is possible and reasonable because the T-system is a network that, although not truly crystalline in its regularity, has considerable regularity and repetitiveness both longitudinally and transversely. It must be emphasized again, however, that thin sections do not show very large expanses of any one portion of the T-system. More recent studies using high-voltage electron microscopes (HVEM) to look at relatively thicker slices of tissue are now beginning to show considerable expanses of T-system network and offer a much improved approach toward visualization of the T-system across the entire transverse width of a muscle fiber.

A key point in the preparation of thick slices of tissue for imaging the T-system by HVEM is selective staining of the T-system tubules so that they will stand out in the images in spite of the considerable amount of cell structure lying above and below them in the thickness of the slice. A useful stain for this purpose is the exogenous peroxidase method (9), which deposits a dense precipitate in the T-system lumen and other extracellular space in the muscle (see Fig. 2 legend).

Figure 2 shows a typical low-magnification HVEM image of a transverse slice of a frog twitch skeletal muscle fiber stained by the peroxidase method. This is a view of the T-system that could not have been obtained by conventional electron microscopic procedures

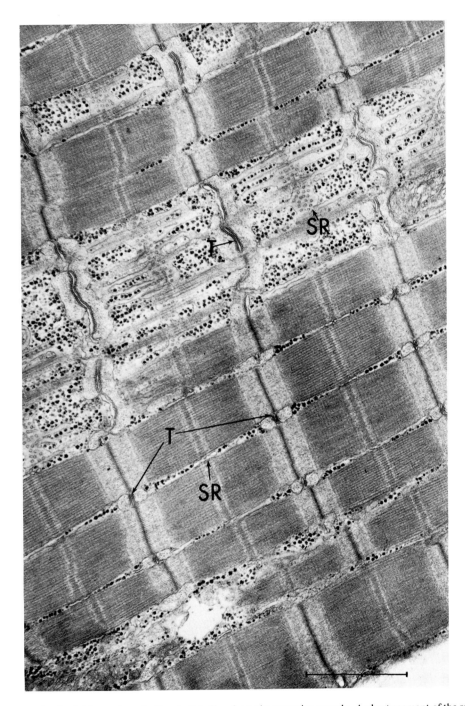

FIG. 1. Longitudinal thin section of a frog twitch fiber from the sartorius muscle. A short segment of the surface of the fiber is at the lower right. T-system (T) and sarcoplasmic reticulum (SR) appear between the fibrils and, in a band just above center, sectioned in face view where the plane of the section coincides with the interfibrillar space. Scale 1 μm.

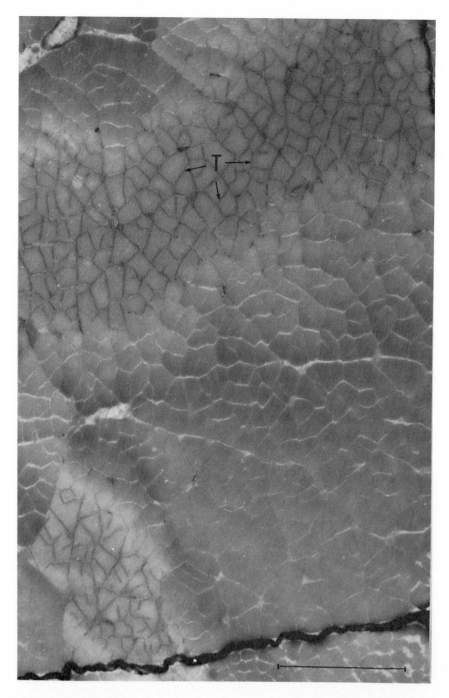

FIG. 2. Low magnification HVEM of a 0.7 μm thick transverse slice of a frog twitch fiber. This preparation was stained selectively for the T-system by soaking bundles of muscle fibers in horseradish peroxidase and incubating according to the method of Graham and Karnovsky (9). This method deposits a dense precipitate in the T-tubules and in the extracellular space. A broad band of T-system network (T) appears near the top of the figure. Another patch of T-system network is seen at the lower left, near the extracellular space between two fibers. Scale 1 μm.

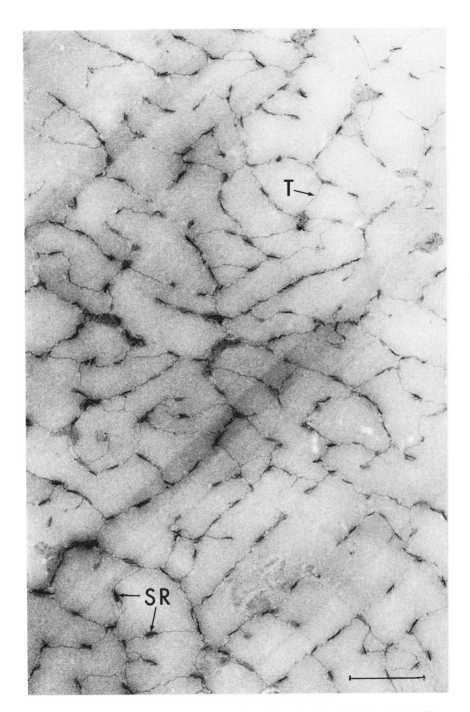

FIG. 3. Low magnification HVEM of a 1.0 μm thick slice of frog slow fiber. The fine tubules (T) are segments of the T-system, where it is not in contact with the SR. The dense patches along the tubules are where contact with the SR is made. Staining similar to that for Fig. 2. Scale 1 μm.

using thin sections. Two broad expanses of T-system are seen in this one micrograph. Figure 3 is a similar view, but of a frog slow fiber, also stained by the peroxidase method. The transverse tubules have a smaller caliber than those of twitch fibers, and associate with SR only in small regions that appear as dense patches along the tubules in the micrograph.

An immediate result of this kind of image is the ability to analyze the network parameters of the T-system more realistically than has been done previously with thin sections. Since an area of network considerably broader than the mesh size of the network is present in these HVEM images, one can count and measure reliably such parameters as the number of branches per node, and the distances between nodes in the network (10). This information may be useful for future models for the electrical properties of the T-system. The results for frog twitch fibers show that most commonly there are three branches per node, with four, five, and six branches at a single node or branch point being less common. The average value is about 3.5 branches per node. These studies also show that the average branch length between nodes is about 1 μm. Whereas the network certainly is in fact more irregular than previously assumed in models of the T-system used in theoretical analyses as electric cables

(11,12), it does not appear to be drastically different from what was expected from thin section studies. It remains to be seen how much difference the new structural information will make when incorporated into theoretical models.

An unexpected result of these HVEM studies of frog twitch fibers is the finding that two T-system networks adjacent to each other in the longitudinal direction are not structurally independent, as previously thought, but are interconnected by "ramps" of T-system (13). The result is that large regions of T-system (several successive networks in the longitudinal direction at least) are connected together in a sort of spiral arrangement (Fig. 4). The extent to which this is a common or constant feature of muscle cell structure has not yet been determined, although Tiegs reported some years ago (14) that spiral bands were common in a large variety of muscle types from many different species. The physiological implications of this spiral arrangement of T-system, if any, are not yet clear. It seems unlikely that it has any major effect on the inward spread of the T-system action potential leading to activation of contraction, since two longitudinally adjacent T-system networks must be synchronized with each other to within about 1 μsec given the relatively high velocity of longitudinal conduction of the action

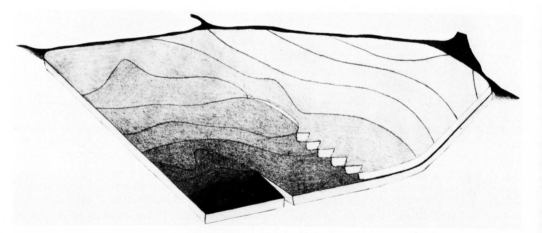

FIG. 4. Sketch to show the spiral disposition of the striations and T-system as reconstructed from serial transverse slices in the HVEM. The sketch shows the complete transverse area of one fiber. The lines across the fiber area are the boundaries of T-system networks seen in one particular slice, that is they represent where the T-system network passes from one slice to the next serial slice. As indicated in the sketch, the network spirals around a dislocation near the center of the fiber. Another dislocation, at the left, front edge, is a simple tear in the network plane, and not another spiral dislocation.

potential at the surface of the fiber (approximately 200 cm/sec). There would be very little electrical potential gradient longitudinally along the T-system "ramps" in the spiral, and thus propagation would not be expected to take place along the spiral from one T-system level to the next. Such propagation along the spiral might, however, be a possible explanation for the relatively slowly propagating waves of contraction observed by Natori (15) and by Costantin and Podolsky (16) in fibers with their outer membranes stripped off. The velocities of these waves along the fiber, about 1 mm/sec, would be consistent with propagation at about 5 cm/sec around a spiral path with a diameter of 40 μm and a pitch of 2.5 μm. These figures are in the range of measured velocities of conduction in the T-system of frog muscle (17) and the diameters of spirals observed in several frog fibers by HVEM. It must be noted, however, that this apparent agreement may be fortuitous and this idea needs to be checked experimentally after more structural information has been obtained on the T-system spiral arrangement.

One could summarize the present state and trends in structural studies of the T-system of striated, skeletal muscle fibers by saying that we know quite well the general structure and topology of the T-system that seems to be common to all fibers, but that we understand less well than we would like to the variation among fiber types and pathological states in different muscles. We desire to have more quantitative information so that comparisons can be meaningful. HVEM of thick tissue slices may provide a quicker route than thin-section studies toward obtaining the desired information.

ELECTRICAL ACTIVITY OF THE T-SYSTEM

Parallel to structural studies of the T-system have been studies of its electrical activity and role in excitation-contraction coupling. An important advance in our understanding of the electrical activity of the T-system was the demonstration by Costantin (18) that the T-system conducts a propagated action potential from the surface to the center of the fiber. In earlier studies of the inward spread of activation, under experimental conditions where the surface membrane was controlled with a voltage clamp, tetrodotoxin was included in the external medium bathing the fibers, and the T-system appeared to be passive (11,12). In Costantin's experiments, when tetrodotoxin was not used, active inward spread of activation was observed. The active spread depended on the presence of at least about half the normal extracellular sodium concentration, thus supporting the idea of an action potential in the T-system similar to the one known to operate on the cell surface. This study was followed by the demonstration that such a mechanism in the T-system could be used in computation of action potentials on the surface of the muscle fiber and in the T-system that seemed reasonably consistent with observed rates of conduction and that gave potential changes at the center of the fiber that reasonably would be expected to activate contraction of axial fibrils (19).

Figure 5 shows two examples of such computed action potentials. When the T-system tubules are considered as passive cable elements (no sodium- or potassium-active conductance changes), the depolarization of the tubules at the center of the fiber is relatively small and might not be expected to activate contraction there (Fig. 5A). When the tubules are considered as containing sodium- and potassium-activation mechanisms in their membranes similar to those present in the surface membrane of the fiber, the center depolarization, although delayed, is similar in magnitude to that of the surface (Fig. 5B). It can be concluded that this kind of action potential conducting system in the transverse tubules could account for rapid activation of centrally located myofibrils.

One further recent development in electrophysiological study of the T-system is noteworthy and will be discussed briefly here. A more complete discussion will have to await further work and more complete publication by the workers engaged in these studies.

The electrical capacitance of cells has always been thought to be constant in value, with all measurements consistent with estimates of surface area and a value for specific capacitance of about 1 μF/cm^2. The cellular capacitance has always been thought to be linear, that is the specific capacitance does not change with voltage. Recently two groups of workers (20,21) have detected nonlinear capacitance in frog

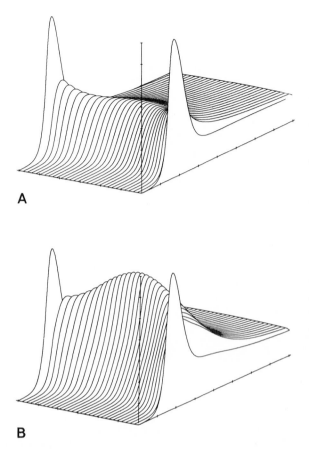

A

B

FIG. 5. Computed action potentials for a frog muscle fiber with a radius of 50 μm at 20°C. The vertical axis is membrane potential, with the resting potential of −95 mV at the base of the figure and with each mark on the axis representing 20 mV in the positive direction. The scale to the left is radial distance across the fiber, from one surface to the diametrically opposite surface. The scale to the right is time in units of 1 msec. **A:** The T-system was treated as a passive cable. The potential change at the center of the fiber is considerably smaller than that at the surface. **B:** The T-system was given activation parameters similar to those for the surface, but reduced in magnitude, and the center depolarization is increased. (From Adrian and Peachey, ref. 19.)

muscle cells depolarized to the region of the mechanical threshold, about −50 mV. These nonlinearities, equivalent to an extra charge moving across the membrane when the transmembrane potential enters or leaves a critical region, are detected only by a rather involved procedure of comparing pulses to potentials within the critical region with equivalent pulses outside the critical region. It is tempting to think that these charge movements are an expression of an event in the T-system membrane that is a step between the T-system action potential and the activation of calcium release from the SR. The proof of this idea, and further speculation, will be left for the future.

In summary, it seems that structural studies are continuing to refine our knowledge of the T-system and that HVEM may represent a new era in these studies. Subtle electrophysiological signals, possibly representing charge movements in the T-system, may be showing us the way to a further closing of the gap in our knowledge of the events linking action potentials with calcium release.

ACKNOWLEDGMENTS

The research reported in this chapter was supported by grants from the Muscular Dystrophy Association of America, Inc. and the National Institutes of Health (HL-15835). A Research Resource at the University of Colorado and supported by the National Institutes of Health was used for high-voltage electron microscopy (No. RR-592).

REFERENCES

1. Porter, K. R., and Palade, G. E. (1957): Studies on the endoplasmic reticulum. III. Its form and distribution in striated muscle cells. *J. Biophys. Biochem. Cytol.,* 3:269.
2. Andersson-Cedergren, E. (1959): Ultrastructure

of motor and plate and sarcoplasmic components of mouse skeletal muscle fiber as revealed by three-dimensional reconstructions from serial sections. *J. Ultrastruct. Res.,* Suppl. 1:1.

3. Franzine-Armstrong, C. (1973): Membranous systems in muscle fibers. In: *The Structure and Function of Muscle, Vol. II,* edited by G. Bourne, p. 531. Academic Press, New York.

4. Peachey, L. D. (1965): The sarcoplasmic reticulum and transverse tubules of the frog's sartorius. *J. Cell Biol.,* 25:209.

5. Mobley, B. A., and Eisenberg, B. R. (1975): Sizes of components in frog skeletal muscle measured by methods of stereology. *J. Gen. Physiol.,* 66:31.

6. Nag, A. C. (1972): Ultrastructure and adenosive triphosphatase activity of red and white muscle fibers of the caudal region of a fish, *Salmo gairdneri. J. Cell Biol.,* 55:42.

7. Eisenberg, B. R., Kuda, A. M., and Peter, J. B. (1974): Stereological analysis of mammalian skeletal muscle. I. Soleus muscle of the adult guinea pig. *J. Cell Biol.,* 60:732.

8. Eisenberg, B. R. (1975): *J. Ultrastr. Res. (in press).*

9. Graham, R. C., and Karnovsky, M. J. (1966): The early stages of absorption of injected horseradish peroxidase in the proximal tubules of mouse kidney: Ultrastructural cytochemistry by a new technique. *J. Histochem. Cytochem.,* 14:291.

10. Eisenberg, B. R., and Peachey, L. D. (1975): The network parameters of the T-system in frog muscle. *Proc. Thirty-Third Annual Electron Microscope Society of America Meeting.*

11. Adrian, R. H., Chandler, W. K., and Hodgkin, A. L. (1969): The kinetics of mechanical activation in frog muscle. *J. Physiol.,* 204:207.

12. Adrian, R. H., Costantin, L. L., and Peachey, L. D. (1969): Radial spread of contraction in frog muscle fibres. *J. Physiol.,* 204:231.

13. Peachey, L. D., and Eisenberg, B. R. (1975): The T-systems and striations of frog skeletal muscle are spiral. *Biophys. J.,* 15 (2):253a.

14. Tiegs, O. W. (1955): The flight muscles of insects —Their anatomy and histology with some observations on the structure of striated muscle in general. *Phil. Trans.,* B238:221.

15. Natori, R. (1965): Propagated contractions in isolated sarcolemma-free bundle of myofibrils. *Jikei Med. J.,* 12:214.

16. Costantin, L. L., and Podolsky, R. J. (1967): Depolarization of the internal membrane system in the activation of frog skeletal muscle. *J. Gen. Physiol.,* 50:1101.

17. Gonzalez-Serratos, H. (1971): Inward spread of activation in vertebrate muscle fibres. *J. Physiol.,* 212:777.

18. Costantin, L. L. (1970): The role of sodium current in the radial spread of contraction in frog muscle fibers. *J. Gen. Physiol.,* 55:703.

19. Adrian, R. H., and Peachey, L. D. (1973): Reconstruction of the action potential of frog sartorius muscle. *J. Physiol.,* 235:103.

20. Schneider, M. F., and Chandler, W. K. (1973): Voltage dependent charge movements in skeletal muscle: A possible step in excitation-contraction coupling. *Nature,* 242:244.

21. Almers, W. (1975): Observations on intramembrane charge movements in skeletal muscle. *Proc. Roy. Soc. [Biol.] (in press).*

The Nervous System, Donald B. Tower, Editor-in-Chief. *Vol. 1: The Basic Neurosciences*. Raven Press, New York, 1975.

The Vertebrate Retina

John E. Dowling

Over the past two decades significant progress has been made in furthering our understanding of the anatomy and physiology of the vertebrate retina. This progress has come about largely through the use of newer techniques, such as electron microscopy and intracellular recording, in studies on the retina. In this paper I briefly review current views on the functional organization of the vertebrate retina, stressing in particular studies from our laboratory. A fuller account of much of this material has been presented in recent review articles (1,2).

CELLULAR ORGANIZATION

The vertebrate retina consists of five types of neurons and one type of glial cell. The perikarya of the retinal cells are organized into three nuclear layers, whereas the retinal synapses are confined almost exclusively to two synaptic zones, the outer and the inner plexiform layers. In each plexiform layer the processes of three cell types synaptically interact.

Most of the information we have concerning the cell types in the vertebrate retina, the extent and distribution of their processes, has come from light microscopic studies of retinal tissue processed by the method of Golgi (3–5). The many variants of this silver impregnation technique have been used profitably for a century and are today still providing critical information. Figure 1 depicts schematically the principal cell types found in the vertebrate retina by the Golgi method and some of their characteristics.

In the distal retina processes from the bipolar

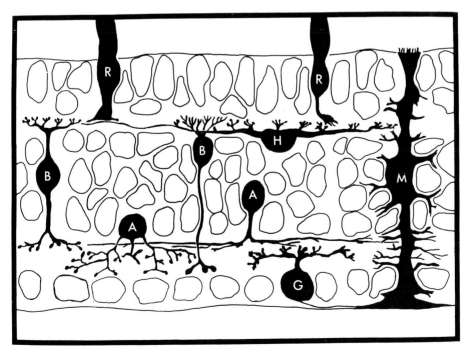

FIG. 1. Principal cell types found in the vertebrate retina. Drawing is based on observations of cells in the mudpuppy retina impregnated by the Golgi method. See text for description of cells. R, receptors; H, horizontal cell; B, bipolar cells; A, amacrine cells; G, ganglion cell; M, Muller (glial) cell. (From Dowling, ref. 1.)

and horizontal cells extend through the outer plexiform layer to the level of the receptor terminals, where they receive input from the receptors. Horizontal cells in most species extend processes widely in the outer plexiform layer, and this has long been interpreted to mean that horizontal cells mediate lateral interactions in the outer plexiform layer (3,4).

The bipolar cells are the vertical pathways carrying visual information from the outer to the inner plexiform layer. In the inner plexiform layer, processes from the bipolar, amacrine, and ganglion cells synaptically interact. The processes of some amacrine cells extend laterally for considerable distances, along discrete strata in the inner plexiform layer, and these are often the longest processes found in the retina. The processes of other amacrine cells spread diffusely throughout the thickness of the inner plexiform layer. The dendrites of the ganglion cells also may be either stratified or diffuse, depending on the type of ganglion cell from which they originate. The axons of the ganglion cells run along the inner margin of the retina and through the optic disc to form the optic nerve.

The Müller (glial) cells extend vertically through the retina. Fine processes that envelop, at least partially, all the nearby neurons extend laterally from the prominent column of glial cell cytoplasm that runs from the external to the internal limiting membranes.

SYNAPTIC ORGANIZATION

Electron microscopy provides the resolution necessary to examine the synaptic contacts between retinal neurons. Current views concerning the synaptic interactions in the vertebrate retina are summarized in Fig. 2. This summary diagram was originally drawn to illustrate synaptic contacts of the frog retina (6); it now appears that it can be generalized to summarize synaptic contacts in many vertebrate retinas.

Outer Plexiform Layer

The most obvious junctions seen at the level of the outer plexiform layer are the ribbon synapses of the receptors. In almost all species, these synapses occur within invaginations in the receptor terminals (7–9). Three or more

processes extend into a single invagination and appear related to the synaptic ribbon that overlies the invagination. It is generally assumed that all the processes in an invagination receive input from the receptor via the ribbon synapse.

In most species there is a precise arrangement of processes in the invaginations. Two deeply inserted processes are positioned on either side of the synaptic ribbon, whereas one to three processes lie centrally and more superficially. Studies of retinas from a variety of species have demonstrated that the deeper lateral elements are invariably horizontal cell processes, whereas the central elements are bipolar cell dendrites (8,10).

In addition to the invaginated ribbon synapses, a superficial, flat, or basal contact has been described between the receptor terminals and the dendrites of certain bipolar cells (the flat bipolars) (8–10). Not much synaptic specialization is seen at these contacts in most species. For example no ribbon or cluster of synaptic vesicles is usually observed associated with these contacts, which are distinguished only by some membrane densification on both sides of the contact and by occasional filamentous material extending across the extracellular space. However, since it has been shown that the flat bipolars make only this type of contact with the receptors, it is generally assumed that these contacts are also synaptic.

In many species synaptic contacts made by horizontal cell processes have been observed (6,11). These contacts, marked by an aggregation of vesicles on the presynaptic side and some membrane densification on both pre- and post-synaptic membranes at the site of the junction, have been termed conventional synapses. These synapses have been observed on adjacent bipolar cell dendrites or other horizontal cell processes. A horizontal cell synapse has never been observed feeding back onto a receptor terminal, and so it has been generally assumed that horizontal cell processes mediate lateral interactions in the outer plexiform layer by acting principally on the bipolar cell dendrites (12). [Recent physiological evidence, however, suggests that in some species horizontal cells do interact with receptors (13). Junctions that might mediate such interaction have not been identified.]

Although horizontal cell synapses onto bi-

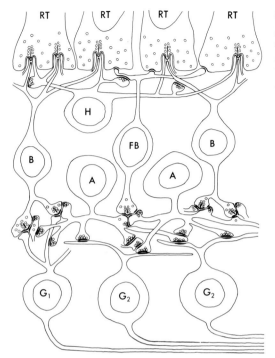

FIG. 2. Summary diagram of the arrangements of synaptic contacts found in vertebrate retinas. In the outer plexiform layer, processes from bipolar (B) and horizontal (H) cells penetrate into invaginations in the receptor terminals (RT) and terminate near the synaptic ribbons of the receptors. The processes of flat bipolar cells (FB) make superficial contacts on the bases of some receptor terminals. Horizontal cells make conventional synaptic contacts onto bipolar dendrites and other horizontal cell processes (not shown). Since horizontal cells usually extend further laterally in the outer plexiform layer than do bipolar dendrites, distant receptors can presumably influence bipolar cells by way of the horizontal cells. In the inner plexiform layer, two basic synaptic pathways are suggested. Bipolar terminals may contact one ganglion cell (G_1) dendrite and one amacrine cell (A) process at the ribbon synapses (*left*) or two amacrine cell processes (*right*). When the latter arrangement predominates in a retina, numerous conventional synapses between amacrine cell processes (serial synapses) are observed, and the ganglion cells (G_2) are contacted mainly by amacrine processes (*right*). Amacrine processes in all retinas make synapses of the conventional type back onto bipolar terminals (reciprocal synapses). (From Dowling, ref. 6.)

polar cell dendrites have been described in several species, the total number of horizontal-bipolar synapses is so low in all species thus far studied that it seems questionable whether horizontal-bipolar cell interactions occur only at these synaptic points. Thus, it has been suggested that the unusual, invaginated synaptic complexes in the receptor terminals could also allow for interactions between horizontal and bipolar cell processes in some way not presently understood (9). For example the deeply inserted horizontal cell processes are strategically positioned in the invaginations to regulate transmitter flow from receptor to bipolar cell dendrite.

To summarize, electron microscopic observations of the outer plexiform layer suggest that bipolar cells are directly activated by nearby receptors and are also influenced by distant receptors via the horizontal cells. The horizontal-bipolar cell interaction may occur at the conventional synapses observed between horizontal and bipolar cell processes or, perhaps, within the receptor terminal invaginations.

Inner Plexiform Layer

In all vertebrate retinas, the inner plexiform layer is considerably thicker than the outer plexiform layer. Many more synaptic contacts per unit area are seen, and a greater variety of synaptic contacts is observed. Differences between species are much more apparent in the inner plexiform layer than in the outer plexiform layer (6,14).

The bipolar terminals contact amacrine cell processes and ganglion cell dendrites at ribbon synapses (Fig. 2). In all species studied, two postsynaptic elements are observed associated with the synapse. This synaptic arrangement has been termed a dyad (9). The postsynaptic elements at a dyad consist most often of a ganglion cell dendrite and an amacrine cell process, or two amacrine cell processes (6). Which of these two principal pairings predominates in a retina is species dependent. For example, monkey and cat retinas have the amacrine-ganglion cell pairing at about 80% of their dyads, whereas the frog has two amacrine cell processes at about 75% of its dyads (6). In the mudpuppy and rabbit, approximately 50% of the dyads are amacrine-amacrine; the other 50% are amacrine-ganglion (12).

Abundant synapses of the amacrine cells (of the conventional type) are seen in the inner plexiform layer of all species. Such amacrine cell synapses are observed on bipolar terminals, ganglion cell dendrites, and other amacrine cell processes (6,9).

Two types of synaptic arrangements entered into by amacrine processes are unusual and deserve special comment. First, at many dyads of the bipolar terminals, the participating amacrine cell process is observed to make a nearby synapse back onto the bipolar terminal. This arrangement has been termed a reciprocal synapse; it suggests that a local feedback interaction may occur between bipolar terminals and amacrine processes near the ribbon synapses (6,9).

The second noteworthy synaptic arrangement in the inner plexiform layer involves mainly amacrine processes. When an amacrine process is observed to make a synapse on an adjacent amacrine process, occasionally the second amacrine process is seen to make a nearby synapse on a third element. This arrangement has been termed a serial synapse and suggests the possibility of very local interactions between amacrine processes (6,14). The third element in the series may be a ganglion cell dendrite, a bipolar terminal, or yet another amacrine process. In species with numerous amacrine cell synapses, the serial synapses observed in a single section may involve as many as four consecutive synapses (6).

Observations indicating alternate synaptic pathways in the inner plexiform layer have come from comparative studies of vertebrate retinas whose ganglion cell physiology has been extensively examined. For example the receptive field organization of the ganglion cells in the monkey and cat has been termed "simple" in the sense that their fields can be satisfactorily mapped using static spots of light projected onto the retina. These receptive fields are organized into two concentric and antagonistic zones, such that stimulation of one zone excites or inhibits firing of the cell; stimulation of the other zone elicits the opposite response in the cell (15,16).

On the other hand, the receptive field organization of animals such as the frog and pigeon has been termed complex in the sense that more than simple static spots of light are needed to map adequately most of their receptive fields (17). That is, many receptive fields in these species respond best to spots, bars, or edges of light moving through the receptive field in a specific direction. When stimulated with static spots of light, receptive fields of such cells respond with short, transient, on- and off-bursts of impulses to stimulation anywhere in the field.

When the anatomy of these various species is compared, it is found that the retinas with the simple receptive field organization (monkey and cat) have most of the dyad pairings consisting of one amacrine and one ganglion cell process, a relatively low number of amacrine synapses per unit area, and few serial synapses. On the other hand, the retinas with the more complex receptive field organization (the frog and pigeon) have dyad pairings consisting mostly of two amacrine cell processes, abundant amacrine synapses per unit area, and many serial synapses. Retinas with numerous examples of both types of receptive fields (rabbit, ground squirrel, or mudpuppy) show about equal numbers of amacrine-ganglion cell and amacrine-amacrine pairings at the dyads, and intermediate numbers of amacrine synapses, and serial synapses per unit area (6.14).

The comparative observations indicate two things; (a) in the retinas where the simple type of receptive field organization is predominant, bipolar terminals make numerous direct contacts with ganglion cell dendrites; in the retinas where the complex type of receptive field organization is predominant, relatively few, direct, bipolar-ganglion cell contacts occur; and (b) there are significantly more amacrine synapses and amacrine-amacrine interactions in retinas with complex receptive fields as compared with retinas with simpler receptive fields. The amacrine cells, therefore, would appear to be the cell type mediating complex interactions, such as motion detection and directional selectivity, in the inner plexiform layer. A further implication of the above data is that in the retinas with more complexly organized receptive fields, amacrine cells may be interposed between the bipolar terminals and ganglion cell dendrites. In such a pathway, there may be a four-neuron chain through the retina; receptors to bipolars to amacrines to ganglion cells. Recent work on the ground squirrel retina has now shown that some ganglion cells do receive their input entirely from amacrine cells, in confirmation of this notion (18).

In the inner plexiform layer, therefore, two different synaptic pathways to the ganglion cells are suggested. The first consists mainly of direct bipolar-ganglion cell connections. In the second pathway the bipolar terminals contact mainly the amacrine cells. The amacrine cell processes interact among themselves and provide the primary input into the ganglion cells.

These ideas are summarized in the lower half of Fig. 2. The left-hand side of the drawing represents the simpler inner plexiform organization (i.e., typical of cat and monkey); the bipolar terminals connect directly with the ganglion cell dendrites. The right-hand side represents the more complex inner plexiform layer organization (i.e., typical of frog and pigeon); bipolars feed into the amacrine processes, and these processes synapse among themselves and onto the ganglion cell dendrites. This suggests two basic types of ganglion cells in the vertebrate retina: one that receives direct input from bipolar cells (G_1); another that receives its input mainly from the amacrine cells (G_2).

INTRACELLULAR RESPONSES

Although it has been possible to study synaptic organization anatomically in a great variety of vertebrate species, only in a few species has it been possible to record intracellular responses from all the types of retinal cells (19–21). The mudpuppy is one such species that has particularly large cells, and this feature makes it particularly advantageous for intracellular recordings.

Figure 3 shows responses from each of the neuronal types in the mudpuppy retina elicited with a spot of light about 100 μm in diameter focused on the electrode, or with centered annuli of 250 or 500 μm radius. The responses were assigned to their respective cell types after intracellular staining with Niagara sky blue, which permitted identification of the perikaryon shape and its location in the retina by light microscopy (19). More recent intracellular staining in the retina has employed the dye Procion yellow which has the great advantage of diffusing throughout the cell into both dendritic and axonic processes (20,21). Thus identification of retinal cell types after Procion yellow staining is usually unequivocal.

These records represent typical examples of about 80% of the recordings made in mudpuppy; the cellular origin of the other 20% of record-

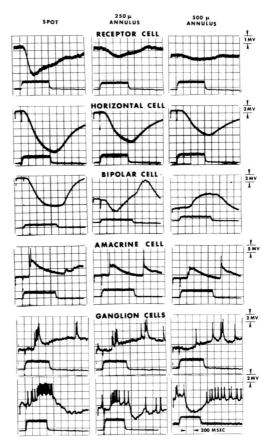

FIG. 3. Intracellular recordings from neurons in the mudpuppy retina. Responses were elicited with a spot of light focused on the electrode (*left*) and with a small and large annulus (*center* and *right*). See text for discussion of receptive field properties of the various neurons. (From Werblin and Dowling, ref. 19.)

ings could not be firmly established (19). Since this work was done, Muller (glial) cell potentials in the mudpuppy retina have been identified and characterized (22). Also it appears from recent work that there is a second type of amacrine cell response in some species that is more sustained than the amacrine cell responses described here (23). The amacrine cells in goldfish that respond in a more sustained fashion are differentially sensitive to color. Few cells differentially sensitive to color (such as C-type S-potentials) have been found as yet in mudpuppy, and this may explain why sustained-type amacrine cell responses have not been identified in this species.

The more distal neurons—the receptors, horizontal cells, and bipolar cells—respond to retinal stimulation with sustained potentials, which are graded with intensity. Nerve impulses have never been seen associated with these responses. The neurons in the proximal retina respond with mostly depolarizing and transient potentials, on which there are superimposed nerve impulses. The absence of impulses in the distal retina is of considerable interest and may be explained by the fact that these are neurons with relatively short processes that do not need to transmit information over long distances. Thus electrotonic spread of slow potentials is probably sufficient for information to reach the furthest extension of these cells.

The other finding of unusual interest is that these distal neurons respond mostly with hyperpolarizing potentials. In spike-generating neurons, hyperpolarization is associated with inhibition. Here, however, no impulses are fired by the cells, and presumably excitation can be signalled by hyperpolarization of the cells. That all vertebrate photoreceptors so far recorded hyperpolarize when excited by light (24) would appear to be compelling evidence that excitation can be signaled by hyperpolarizing potentials in the distal retina.

With spot and annular stimulation, it is possible to characterize the responses of each cell type and describe its receptive field organization. For example receptors in mudpuppy give large responses to spot illumination, but only small responses when small and large annuli are presented. The small responses evoked by the annular stimulation are believed to be caused by stray light. Experiments using spot and annular stimuli together show only small differences when compared with spot stimulation alone. This suggests that receptors in mudpuppy are not substantially affected by surrounding illumination. The same appears to be true for goldfish receptors (23), but in turtle it has been shown that large annuli can depolarize receptors, apparently by feedback from horizontal cells (13). Evidence for feedback from horizontal cells onto receptors has been obtained also in Gekko retinas (28), but such feedback appears to be absent in marine toad rods (29).

In turtle and marine toad, it has further been shown that adjacent receptors sum activity, probably by way of electrotonic junctions between receptors (13,27). In turtle cones, the summation area is only about 50 μm in diameter; but in toad, rods sum over an area of about 800 μm. The functional significance of receptor summation is unclear at the present time (27).

Horizontal cells in mudpuppy respond with large hyperpolarizing potentials over a retinal area several hundred microns in diameter. Thus both spot and annular stimulation evoke sizable potentials and when spots annuli are presented together, their effects are summed. It has been shown that horizontal cells in dogfish are electrically coupled to one another (28), and in several species electrical-type junctions between horizontal cells have been demonstrated anatomically (29).

In mudpuppy, virtually all horizontal cells hyperpolarize only in response to light, regardless of stimulus intensity, wavelength, and configuration. In other species, particularly those with color discrimination, horizontal cells may both hyperpolarize and depolarize depending on the wavelength of the stimulus (30,31). Such horizontal cells have been termed C-type cells; horizontal cells that only hyperpolarize are called L-cells. In mudpuppy, only one C-cell has so far been recorded in our laboratory.

Two physiological types of bipolar cells have been found in the mudpuppy and in all other retinas in which bipolar responses have been recorded (20,21). One type hyperpolarizes in a sustained fashion to central spot illumination (Fig. 3). The other type depolarizes to spot illumination. With either cell type, annular illumination added while the central region is illuminated antagonizes or reduces the sustained potential produced by the central spot. In mudpuppy annular illumination does not drive the membrane potential back beyond the resting potential of the cell, so that to see the effects of the surrounding illumination, central illumination must be present. At the bipolar cell level, therefore, an antagonistic center-surround receptive field organization is observed, such that with appropriate stimulus conditions, potentials of opposite polarity may be obtained from the bipolar cell (Fig. 3). In other species annular stimulation alone may polarize the cell (20,21), but in most other respects bipolar cell responses are remarkably similar between species.

In mudpuppy, amacrine cells respond predominantly transiently to retinal illumination regardless of the configuration of stimulus used, or where in the receptive field of the amacrine cell the stimulus is presented. The amacrines are the first cell type along the visual pathway to respond primarily in a transient fashion, and they usually give on- and off-responses to illumination anywhere within their receptive fields. Some differences between amacrine cells in the relative sizes of the on- and off-components are observed, and these differences usually depend on the geometry and position of stimulation used. For example, Fig. 3 illustrates a cell that gives a large on-response to central spot illumination, whereas with annular illumination, the off-responses are enhanced and are comparable in size to the on-responses.

Nerve impulses are often observed superimposed on the transient depolarizing responses of the amacrine cells. However, in mudpuppy seldom are more than two spikes observed riding on the transient depolarization, regardless of intensity or configuration of the stimulus. Thus it is unclear whether it is the slow potential part of the response or the spikes which is the most important component for signal transmission by the amacrine cells.

As noted earlier, sustained amacrine cell responses have been observed in other species (23,32). Such cells may either hyperpolarize or depolarize to light, and the response polarity may depend on wavelength. Intracellular amacrine responses that combine both transient and sustained components have also been observed in several species (32).

Two basic types of ganglion cell responses are found in the mudpuppy retina, which appear to relate to the activity of one or the other of the cell types providing input to the ganglion cells (i.e., amacrine and bipolar cells). One ganglion cell type strongly resembles the amacrine cell response, giving transient responses at both the onset and cessation of stimulation (Fig. 3). Differing amounts of on- and off-contributions may be evoked with different stimulus configurations, as is observed with amacrine cell responses. The ganglion cell responses differ from the amacrine cell responses in having numerous spikes riding on the transient depolarization, and in that the number of spikes fired appears closely related to the amount of depolarization.

The second type of ganglion cell (lowermost

records, Fig. 3) has a receptive field organization that more closely resembles that of the bipolar cells. With central illumination a sustained slow potential and steady discharge of spikes are evoked from the cell. With some central illumination maintained, large annular illumination hyperpolarizes the cell and inhibits firing in a sustained fashion.

A Model of the Synaptic Organization Retina

How the various potentials and receptive field properties of the neurons may be produced by synaptic interactions in the vertebrate retina is suggested in Fig. 4. This drawing correlates a

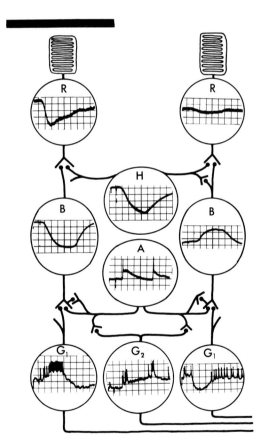

FIG. 4. Summary figure correlating the synaptic organization of the vertebrate retina with the intracellularly recorded responses of the neurons. R, receptors; H, horizontal cell; B, bipolar cells; A, amacrine cell; G, ganglion cells. A flash of light is presented to the receptor on the left (indicated by the bar above the receptor). (From Dowling, ref. 1.)

wiring diagram of the synaptic pathways in the vertebrate retina (based on the connections suggested in Fig. 2) with the potentials recorded from the neurons in the mudpuppy (Fig. 3). To obtain the illustrated responses in the neuronal array, a flash of light is presented to the receptor on the left.

As already noted, receptors in mudpuppy respond relatively autonomously. There is no anatomical evidence of any feedback from horizontal cells onto the receptors, and substantial surrounding illumination does not alter significantly the receptor response in the mudpuppy. Thus a large response is observed only in the illuminated receptor; the adjacent (nonilluminated) receptor shows only a tiny response, which is probably caused by stray light or, possibly, by weak input from the illuminated receptor.

Horizontal cells sum inputs from a wide retinal area. Latencies of horizontal cell responses closely match the latencies of bipolar cell responses, suggesting that both are driven by the receptors. The anatomy also suggests that bipolar dendrites and horizontal cell processes are activated together at the synaptic ribbon synapses in the invaginations along the bases of the receptors.

The bipolar cells are polarized strongly in a graded, sustained fashion by direct receptor-bipolar cell contacts (Fig. 4, left). Sustained, bipolar cell polarization is antagonized by horizontal cells acting on bipolar cell dendrites (Fig. 4, right). Anatomical evidence suggests that such horizontal-bipolar cell interactions could occur at horizontal-bipolar cell synapses, or perhaps within the receptor terminal invaginations, or both.

Since horizontal cells usually have a greater lateral extent in the outer plexiform layer than do the bipolar cells, a center-surround receptive field organization is therefore observed in the bipolar cell response. The central response appears mediated by the direct receptor-bipolar cell junctions; the antagonistic surround response by the receptor-horizontal-bipolar cell pathway. In the mudpuppy, the bipolar cell receptive-field center matches closely the dendritic spread of the bipolars in area, whereas the surround approximates the lateral spread of the horizontal cells. The only other cell type in the mudpuppy retina spreading far enough laterally to account for the antagonistic surround in the bipolar cell response is the amacrine cell, which also synaptically contacts the bipolar cells. The mudpuppy amacrine cells, however, respond transiently to retinal illumination at both on and off. The surround inhibition observed in the bipolar cell response is, on the other hand, graded and sustained and has the approximate form of the horizontal cell response.

Amacrine cells respond transiently at both the onset and cessation of static illumination placed anywhere in the receptive field. How the sustained responses of the distal retinal cells are converted to transient responses at the level of amacrine cells is not known, but the anatomy of the bipolar-amacrine cell synaptic complex provides the basis of a suggestion. That is, the reciprocal synapses of the amacrine cell processes back onto the bipolar terminals just adjacent to the bipolar ribbon synapses could conceivably turn off the bipolar excitation locally, and a transient response in the amacrine could result.

The two types of ganglion cell responses found in the mudpuppy retina appear to be related to the primary type of input into each type of cell. For example one type of ganglion cell (G_1) has a receptive field organization quite similar to the bipolar cells (left and right sides of Fig. 4). Central illumination depolarizes the cell in a sustained fashion; surround illumination inhibits the activity of the cell in a sustained fashion. This type of ganglion cell would appear to receive most of its synaptic input directly from the bipolar terminals.

The second type of ganglion cell (G_2) (Fig. 4, center) responds transiently to retinal illumination much as the amacrine cells do. This type of ganglion cell presumably receives its major synaptic input from the amacrine cells. Evidence has recently been provided that such on- and off-type ganglion cells respond very well to motion, and many may show directionally selective responses (33). This suggests, as does the anatomy, that the amacrine cells are the neurons in the retina most responsible for mediating complex ganglion cell activity, such as motion and direction selectivity. Recent experiments showing that the bipolar and more distal neurons show no directionally selective responses provide more direct evidence that the amacrine cells must play such a role (33).

How amacrine cell interactions might account for directionally selective responses is yet to be determined. The amacrine responses, by being transient in nature and occurring at both the onset and cessation of illumination, seem well suited for mediating the motion-sensitizing responses. For example amacrine cells respond in a similar fashion to a bright spot on a light background or a dark spot on a light background, a feature of many motion-sensitive and directionally selective cells (34).

In conclusion, the outer plexiform layer of the vertebrate retina appears concerned mainly with the static or spatial aspects of the illumination of the receptors. The neurons contributing processes to the outer plexiform layer respond primarily with sustained, graded potentials, and the neuronal interactions in the outer plexiform layer accentuate contrast in the retinal image by forming an antagonistic center-surround organization at the level of the bipolar cells.

The inner plexiform layer, on the other hand, appears concerned with the more dynamic or temporal aspects of illumination on the receptors. Amacrine cells accentuate the changes in retinal illumination and respond vigorously to moving stimuli. For example interactions in the inner plexiform layer probably account for the motion- and direction-selective responses of the ganglion cells.

SUMMARY

Research over the past two decades has provided us with a broad outline of how the vertebrate retina is synaptically organized, and it has given us some clues as to how and where in the retina ganglion cell receptive field properties are mediated. For example, both anatomical and physiological evidence suggests that the outer plexiform layer operates much the same way in all species. By the level of the bipolar cells, an antagonistic center-surround organization is established. The center response appears to be mediated by direct receptor-bipolar cell interactions, while the surround response appears to be provided by an antagonistic horizontal cell input. In some species, the antagonistic horizontal cell effect is observed at the receptor level, and in all species it is observed in the bipolar cell response.

Both anatomical and physiological studies also indicate that the inner plexiform layer of the retina is a more complexly organized neuropil than is the outer plexiform layer. All the evidence points to the amacrine cell as playing the key role in mediating the complex response properties expressed at the level of the ganglion cells. Beyond this, however, we can say little of substance at present about the mechanisms involved. Amacrine cell responses in the same and different species vary in waveform, exhibiting often both transient and sustained components. It appears virtually certain that additional significant features of amacrine cell responses will be discovered as more detailed recordings are made. The synaptic relationships of the amacrine cells are also complicated. Amacrine cells appear capable of forming both reciprocal and serial synaptic arrangements with each other and with bipolar terminals in all retinas, but the details and functional significance of the synaptic pathways from bipolar terminals through amacrine cell processes to the ganglion cells are obscure. The observations that the inner plexiform layer in some species may be more simply organized may provide us with experimental situations with which to learn more about the complexity of intraretinal interactions. To understand in depth how complex ganglion cell-receptive field properties are formed would appear to require a much greater understanding of the amacrine cells and their synaptic organization.

REFERENCES

1. Dowling, J. E. (1970): Organization of vertebrate retinas. *Invest. Ophthal.*, 9:655–680.
2. Dowling, J. E., and Werblin, F. S. (1971): Synaptic organization of the vertebrate retina. *Vision Res.*, 3:1–15.
3. Cajal, S. R. (1894): *Die Retina der Wirbelthiere,* Translated by R. Greeff. Bergmann, Wiesbaden.
4. Polyak, S. L. (1941): *The Retina.* University Press, Chicago.
5. Boycott, B. B., and Dowling, J. E. (1969): Organization of the primate retina: Light microscopy. *Phil. Trans. [Biol.]*, 255:109–184.
6. Dowling, J. E. (1968): Synaptic organization of the frog retina: an electron microscopic analysis comparing the retinas of frogs and primates. *Proc. Roy. Soc. [Biol.]*, 170:205–227.
7. Sjostrand, F. S. (1958): Ultrastructure of retinal rod synapses of the guinea pig eye as revealed by three-dimensional reconstructions from serial sections. *J. Ultrastruct. Res.*, 2:122–170.

8. Missotten, L. (1965): *The Ultrastructure of the Retina*. Arscia Uitgaven, Brussels.
9. Dowling, J. E., and Boycott, B. B. (1966): Organization of the primate retina: electron microscopy. *Proc. Roy. Soc. [Biol.]*, 166:80–111.
10. Kolb, H. (1970): Organization of the outer plexiform layer of the primate retina: electron microscopy of Golgi-impregnated cells. *Phil Trans. [Biol.]*, 258:261–283.
11. Dowling, J. E., Brown, J. E., and Major, D. (1966): Synapses of horizontal cells in rabbit and cat retinas. *Science*, 153:1639–1641.
12. Dowling, J. E., and Werblin, F. S. (1969): Organization of retina of the mudpuppy. *Necturus maculosus*. I. Synaptic structure. *J. Neurophysiol.*, 32:315–338.
13. Baylor, D. A., Fuortes, M. G. F., and O'Bryan, P. M. (1971): Receptive fields of single cones in the retina of the turtle. *J. Physiol.* (Lond.), 214:265–294.
14. Dubin, M. (1970): The inner plexiform layer of the vertebrate retina: a quantitative and comparative electron microscopic analysis. *J. Comp. Neurol.*, 140:479–506.
15. Kuffler, S. W. (1953): Discharge patterns and functional organization of mammalian retina. *J. Neurophysiol.*, 16:37–68.
16. Hubel, D. H., and Wiesel, T. N. (1960): Receptive fields of optic nerve fibers in the spider monkey. *J. Physiol.* (Lond.), 154:572–580.
17. Maturana, H. R., Lettvin, J. Y., McCulloch, W. S., and Pitts, W. H. (1960): Anatomy and physiology of vision in the frog (*Rana pipiens*). *J. Gen. Physiol.*, 43:129–175.
18. West, R., and Dowling, J. E. (1972): Synapses onto different morphological types of retinal ganglion cells. *Science*, 178:510–512.
19. Werblin, F. S., and Dowling, J. E. (1969): Organization of the retina of the mudpuppy, *Necturus maculosus*. II. Intracellular recording. *J. Neurophysiol.*, 32:339–355.
20. Kaneko, A. (1970): Physiological and morphological identification of horizontal, bipolar, and amacrine cells in the goldfish retina. *J. Physiol.* (Lond.), 207:623–633.
21. Matsumoto, N., and Naka, K. I. (1972): Identifi-

cation of intracellular responses in the frog retina. *Brain Res.*, 42:59–71.
22. Miller, R. F., and Dowling, J. E. (1970): Intracellular responses of the Müller (glial) cells of the mudpuppy retina: their relation to b-wave of the electroretinogram. *J. Neurophysiol.*, 33:323–341.
23. Kaneko, A. (1971): Physiological studies of single retinal cells and their morphological identification. *Vision Res. (Suppl.)*, 3:17–26.
24. Tomita, T. (1970): Electrical activity of vertebrate photoreceptors. *Quart. Rev. Biophys.*, 3:179–222.
25. Kleinschmidt, J. (1973): Adaptation properties of intracellularly recorded Gekko photoreceptor potentials. In: *Biochemistry and Physiology of Visual Pigments*, edited by H. Langer, pp. 219–228. Springer-Verlag, New York.
26. Brown, J. E., and Pinto, L. H. (1974): Ionic mechanism for the photoreceptor potential of the retina of *Bufo marinus*. *J. Physiol.* (Lond.), 236:575–592.
27. Fain, G. L. (1975): Quantum sensitivity of rods in the toad retina. *Science*, 188:270–273.
28. Kaneko, A. (1971b): Electrical connexions between horizontal cells in the dogfish retina. *J. Physiol.* (Lond.), 213:95–105.
29. Stell, W. K. (1972): The morphological organization of the vertebrate retina. In: *Handbook of Sensory Physiology. Vol. VII/2, Physiology of Photoreceptor Organs*, edited by M. G. F. Fuortes, pp. 111–213. Springer-Verlag, Berlin.
30. MacNichol, E. F., and Svaetichin, G. (1958): Electric responses from the isolated retinas of fishes. *Am. J. Ophthal.*, 46:26–46.
31. Tomita, T. (1963): Electrical activity in the vertebrate retina. *J. Opt. Soc. Am.*, 53:49–57.
32. Toyoda, J., Hashimoto, H., and Ohtsu, K. (1973): Bipolar-amacrine transmission in the carp retina, *Vision Res.*, 13:295–307.
33. Werblin, F. S. (1970): Response of retinal cells to moving spots: Intracellular recording in Necturus maculosus. *J. Neurophysiol.*, 33:342–351.
34. Barlow, H. B., and Levick, W. R. (1965): The mechanism of directionally selective units in the rabbit's retina. *J. Physiol.* (Lond.), 178:477–504.

The Nervous System, Donald B. Tower, Editor-in-Chief. *Vol. 1: The Basic Neurosciences*. Raven Press, New York, 1975.

Neurotoxins: Pharmacological Dissection of Ionic Channels of Nerve Membranes

Toshio Narahashi

It has been well established that excitation of nerve membranes takes place as a result of changes in ionic permeabilities. The original analyses by Hodgkin, Huxley, and Katz established the basis of the ionic theory, which can describe almost any phenomena associated with nerve excitation. However, the physical and chemical nature of ionic channels remains largely to be seen, and a variety of approaches and techniques have been utilized including voltage clamp, isolation of membrane macromolecules, artificial lipid membranes, photometric techniques, and model simulation. It should be emphasized that these approaches are not mutually exclusive and that they should be integrated at a high level to achieve the goals. Because of complexity of the problem, one-sided studies can no longer give a definitive answer to the question.

Use of chemicals as tools to characterize the physiological function of the nervous system is by no means a new idea. During the late nineteenth century, Langley took advantage of the action of nicotine to stimulate and then paralyze the ganglia for the purpose of mapping the autonomic nervous system. Curare has long been used to study the mechanism of neuromuscular and ganglionic transmission. However, it was not until the 1960s that the advantage of use of chemicals as tools was fully appreciated. The debut of tetrodotoxin (TTX) has certainly stimulated studies along this line. Several other neurotoxins have since been demonstrated to have potent and specific actions on various parameters associated with nerve excitation and synaptic transmission.

This chapter describes some highlights of "pharmacological dissection" of ionic channels using toxins as tools. It is not intended to give a comprehensive review but rather to rationalize this approach to characterization of ionic channels. Although TTX is one of the most impor-

tant toxins for such purposes, it will be described only briefly since there are already several review articles on the subject (1,2).

TTX

Mode of Action

Chemistry and pharmacology of TTX (Fig. 1) have been extensively studied in Japan since the beginning of this century, because the toxin is contained in the ovary and liver of the puffer fish, one of the fish regarded as most delicious among Japanese. A number of accidental deaths occur yearly in Japan as a result of ingestion of TTX, which blocks nerve and muscle conduction even at low doses, with death resulting from respiratory paralysis.

The potential usefulness of TTX as a tool in the study of excitable membranes was recognized when the selective blockage of the sodium conductance increase was first suggested (4). Widespread use of TTX was initiated as soon as this concept was clearly demonstrated by voltage clamp experiments (5). Further characterization of TTX action has strengthened its usefulness (6–8).

The action of TTX on nerve membranes may be summarized as follows. It reversibly blocks the sodium conductance increase at nanomolar concentrations without affecting the potassium conductance increase. The kinetics of the sodium conductance is not affected, and only $\bar{g}_{Na}$ of the Hodgkin-Huxley formulation is decreased. The block is independent of ionic species passing through the sodium channel and independent of the direction of ion current. It is effective only from outside of the nerve membrane, and interacts with the sodium channels on a one-to-one stoichiometric basis. Thus it is clear that TTX interacts directly with either the sodium channel itself or nearby macro-

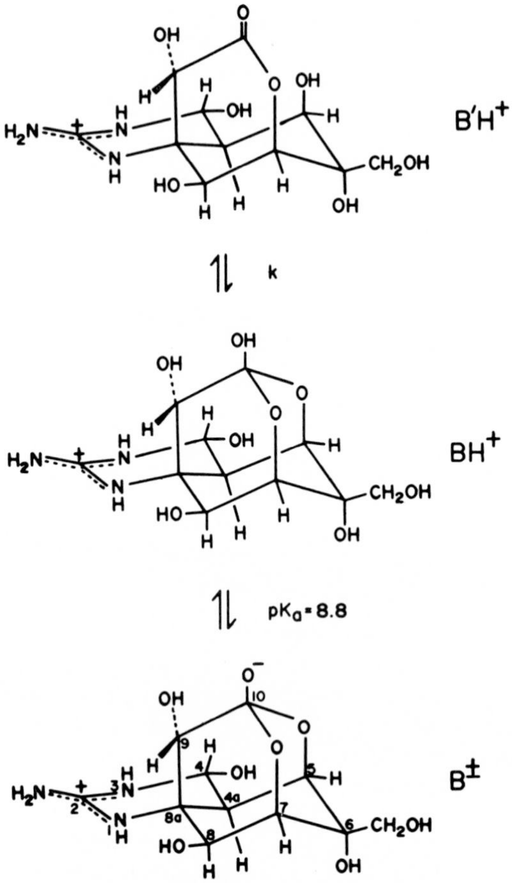

FIG. 1. Structures of tetrodotoxin. (From Narahashi, Moore, and Frazier, ref. 3.)

molecule that controls the opening of the sodium channel. It should be emphasized that many other nerve-blocking agents (e.g., local anesthetics) do not have such specific actions on the sodium mechanism (7,9,10). Saxitoxin (STX) has essentially the same effect as TTX (11).

Sodium Channels as Analyzed by TTX

One of the early attempts to use TTX for analysis of sodium channels was to estimate the density of TTX binding sites in nerve membranes. The first such experiment was performed by bioassay using the walking leg nerve of the lobster. Binding of TTX to the nerve membrane was estimated by measuring the decrease in TTX concentration in a small amount of bathing medium, which had been repeatedly applied to several nerve preparations (12). To great surprise, the density of TTX binding sites was extremely low being $13/\mu m^2$ of the membrane at most. Since TTX binds to the receptor site on a one-to-one stoichiometric basis (13,14), the density of sodium channels should be equally low. Such measurements have since been repeated with other preparations using bioassay or tritiated TTX with the results of 3 to 500 binding sites/μm^2 of the membrane (1,15). It is clear that the sodium channels are separated widely and that sodium current flows through these discrete sites during excitation.

The gating current has recently been recorded from the squid giant axon (15,16). It is of special interest that TTX and STX have essentially no effect on this current (15).

In vitro binding of TTX to membrane components has recently been studied. The rationale of these studies is to isolate, purify, and identify the components of membrane that exhibit a high affinity for TTX. Homogenate of garfish olfactory nerves is able to bind tritiated TTX, and the dissociation constant (8.3×10^{-9} M) and the number of binding sites ($3.9/\mu m^2$ of membrane) agree with those obtained .with intact nerves (17). Similar agreement between the data with homogenate and those with intact preparation was obtained with lobster walking leg nerves (18). Several enzymes were tested for their effect on TTX binding in nerve membrane homogenate (19). TTX binding was inhibited by trypsin, α-chymotrypsin, and pronase, and the inhibitory action was enhanced by pretreatment with phospholipase A. These observations suggest that TTX binding sites are proteins embedded in a phospholipid environment.

An attempt to solubilize TTX binding component has also been made (19,20). The rate of dissociation of solubilized TTX-receptor complex (0.95 min^{-1}) is almost the same as the rate of reversal of TTX inhibition of sodium conductance (0.82 min^{-1}). The binding rate constant is also the same in the solubilized preparation and in the intact nerve (20–22). However, it should be borne in mind that such solubilized membrane preparations are extremely heterogeneous and that further separation and purification of TTX binding components are absolutely necessary to identify their chemical nature. Some experiments have been performed along this line, and there are at least four to five major components of proteins in garfish olfactory nerves (23). However, no functional identification has been made for any of these protein components.

It is of interest that certain monovalent, divalent, and trivalent cations compete with STX for the binding site (21). The dissociation constant is approximately 10^{-3} M for trivalent cations, 1 to 3×10^{-2} M for divalent cations, and over 0.5 M for monovalent cations. Thallous ion (Tl^+) has an unusually low dissociation constant of 2×10^{-2} M. The apparent dissociation constants of these ions to inhibit sodium current are of the same order of magnitude. These observations may be taken to support the notion that STX and TTX block the sodium channel by plugging mechanism, probably by virtue of its guanidinium group (7,24,25).

TTX is being used for many other types of experiments (1). For instance its extreme usefulness has been proved in the study of the development of sodium channels in cultured or developing muscles, the mechanism of synaptic and neuromuscular transmission, the mechanism of excitation of giant neurons, skeletal muscles, smooth muscles, cardiac muscles and sensory receptors, and the mechanisms of action of other neuroactive agents.

GRAYANOTOXINS, BATRACHOTOXIN, AND VERATRIDINE

Sources and Chemistry

Grayanotoxins (GTXs) are contained in the leaves of the plants that belong to the family Ericaceae, including *Leucothoe, Rhododendron, Andromeda,* and *Kalmia*. There are three major components, i.e., GTX I, GTX II, and GTX III (Fig. 2) (1).

Batrachotoxin (BTX) is one of the toxic principles contained in the skin secretion of the Colombian arrow poison frog, *Phyllobates aurotaenia*. It is a steroidal compound with several unique chemical moieties, i.e., a 3α, 9α-hemiketal linkage, a seven-membered 14β-heterocyclic ring and a Δ^{16} unsaturation (Fig. 3) (27,28). The LD_{50} for mice is about 2 $\mu g/kg$, a value fivefold more toxic than TTX.

Veratridine is one of the active ingredients contained in the alkaloids from *Veratrum, Zygadenus,* and *Schoenocaulon*. Veratrum alkaloids are steroidal compounds composed of the C_{27} alkamines. They are divided into two

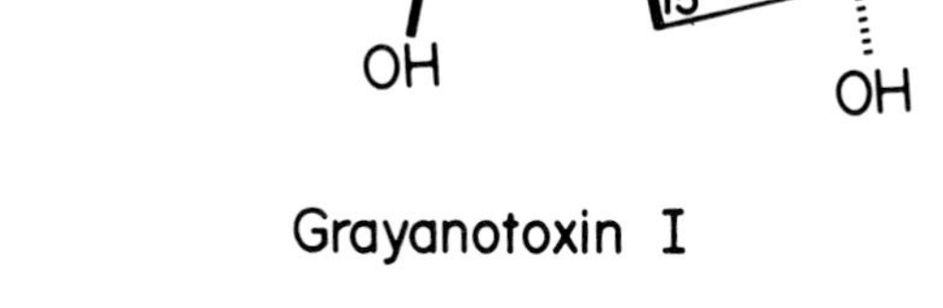

Grayanotoxin I

FIG. 2. Structure of grayanotoxin I. (From Narahashi and Seyama, ref. 26.)

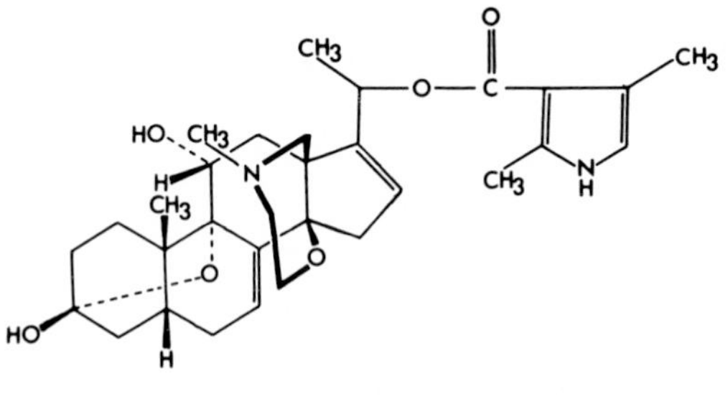

FIG. 3. Structure of batrachotoxin. (From Narahashi, ref. 29.)

groups, the jerveratum group with a secondary nitrogen, and the ceveratum group with a tertiary nitrogen. Veratridine belongs to the latter and is the ester of the alkamine veracevine and veratroyl (Fig. 4) (30,31).

Mode of Action on Nerve Membranes

Effect on Membrane Potential

Batrachotoxin, GTXs, and veratridine have one action in common, i.e., depolarization of nerve membranes. The depolarization has been demonstrated to be caused by the specific increase in resting sodium permeability. Since the effects of the three compounds are basically the same, the study with GTX I (26) is described here. Any significant differences among the three are pointed out.

When applied to the squid giant axon, either externally or internally, GTX I causes a

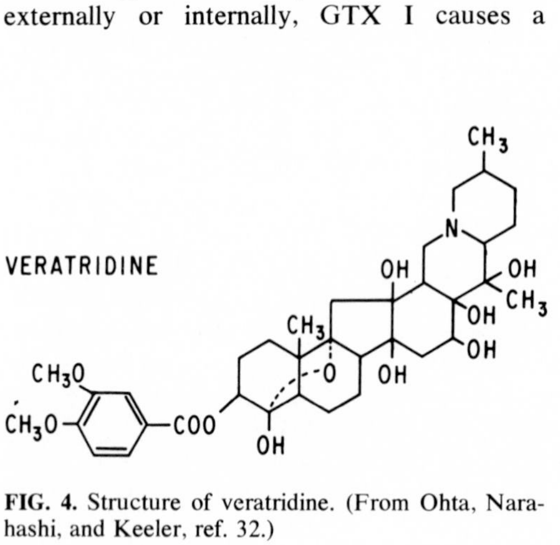

FIG. 4. Structure of veratridine. (From Ohta, Narahashi, and Keeler, ref. 32.)

sizable depolarization of the membrane (Fig. 5). The depolarization proceeds faster with internal application than external application and finally attains a steady-state level that is determined by the concentration. The effect is reversible by washing the axon with GTX-free media. Since the GTX-induced depolarization is so large—sometimes reaching or exceeding the zero membrane potential—that an increase in resting sodium permeability is suspected as the major cause of action. In support of this, a drastic decrease in external sodium concentration from 449 to 1 mM by substituting Tris for sodium results in a quick hyperpolarization of the membrane to a level that exceeds the control membrane potential obtained in 1 mM Na prior to GTX application (Fig. 5). It is of interest that TTX also restores the membrane potential in the presence of GTX I (Fig. 5). However, it should be emphasized that this experiment does not exclude other possibilities such as a decrease in potassium permeability or an increase in chloride permeability, which may occur concurrently with an increase in sodium permeability.

In order to examine these possibilities, the following experiments have been performed. The membrane potential (E_m) may be described by the constant field equation (33):

$$E_m = \frac{RT}{F} \ln \frac{P_K(a_K)_o + P_{Na}(a_{Na})_o + P_{Cl}(a_{Cl})_i}{P_K(a_K)_i + P_{Na}(a_{Na})_i + P_{Cl}(a_{Cl})_o},$$

$$(1)$$

where R, T, and F represent the gas constant, absolute temperature, and Faraday constant, respectively, (a_K), (a_{Na}), and (a_{Cl}) represent the activities of K, Na, and Cl, respectively, with subscripts o and i referring to outside and inside phases of the axon, respectively, and P_K, P_{Na}, and P_{Cl} are permeability coefficients for K, Na, and Cl, respectively. The simplest way to test the notion that only P_{Na} is increased by GTX I would be to examine the membrane potential in the axon with the sodium terms of both denominator and numerator eliminated. This condition can easily be established with internally perfused squid axons by eliminating sodium ions from both external and internal perfusates. Such experiments have clearly shown that no depolarization is produced by application of GTX I. Thus it can be concluded

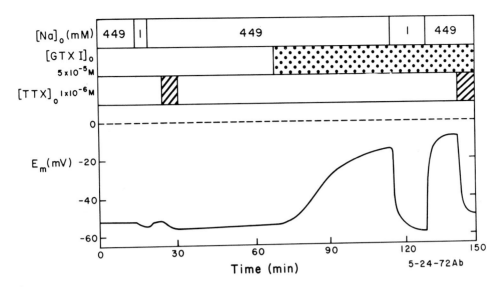

FIG. 5. Changes in resting membrane potential (E_m) of an intact squid axon produced by external application of 5×10^{-5} M grayanotoxin I (GTX I). Decrease of external sodium concentrations ($[Na]_o$) to 1 mM hyperpolarizes the membrane in GTX I. Externally applied tetrodotoxin (TTX) also reverses depolarization. (From Narahashi and Seyama, ref. 26.)

that GTX I increases the resting sodium permeability in a highly specific manner.

Similar experiments have been performed with α-dihydrograyanotoxin II (α-2H-GTX II) (34), BTX (35), and veratridine (32). All of them have basically the same effect as GTX I, depolarizing the membrane by a specific increase in resting sodium permeability. However, two differences are noted: (a) the effect of BTX is irreversible, whereas the effects of the other compounds are reversible; and (b) the relative potency in terms of the reciprocal of the effective concentration is BTX > α-2H-GTX II > GTX I > veratridine.

Quantitative Measurements of Sodium Permeability Increase

The experiments described in the preceding section do not show the degree of increase in sodium permeability under the influence of GTX I. Quantitative measurements have been made by means of voltage clamp techniques (26). The ionic compositions of both external and internal perfusates were modified to make the equilibrium potentials for potassium and chloride (E_K and E_{Cl}) equal to each other (e.g., −70 mV). If the membrane is voltage clamped at this level, the holding current should be carried by ions other than potassium and chloride. Since GTX I increases the sodium permeability exclusively, any increase in the holding current caused by application of GTX I is carried by sodium ions, and the resting sodium conductance can be calculated.

An example of the result of such an experiment is illustrated in Fig. 6. Prior to application of GTX I the holding ionic current is very small reflecting a small value for the resting sodium conductance. The membrane potential under unclamped conditions and the membrane ionic current under clamped conditions can be recorded alternately by using an electronic switch. After introduction of GTX I to the internal perfusate, the membrane starts depolarizing and at the same time the holding ionic current starts increasing in inward direction. This current is carried mostly by sodium ions. The resting sodium conductance is calculated to be 0.9 mmho/cm².

Decrease in external sodium concentration has been found to change the holding sodium current in a predicted manner (Fig. 6). As the sodium concentration is lowered, both the GTX-induced depolarization and the holding sodium current decrease in magnitude. In order to describe sodium current (I_{Na}) in low external sodium concentrations, sodium perme-

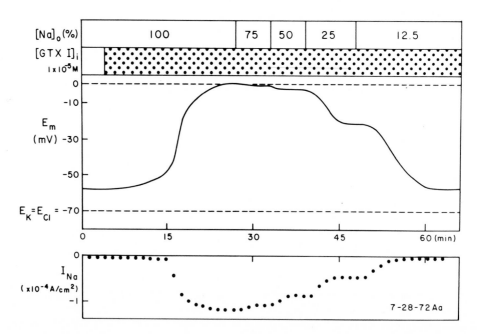

FIG. 6. Changes in resting membrane potential (E_m) and holding membrane current carried by sodium (I_{Na}) by internal perfusion of 1×10^{-5} M GTX I. Current with a minus sign denotes an inward current. External sodium concentration ($[Na]_o$) is 449 mM in normal artificial sea water, and reduced sodium concentrations are expressed as percentages of that solution. The membrane potential was voltage clamped for 7 sec at 90-sec intervals at −70 mV, which was made equal to the equilibrium potentials for potassium (E_K) and chloride (E_{Cl}) by alteration of the ionic composition of internal perfusate. (From Narahashi and Seyama, ref. 26.)

ability has been calculated from the constant field equation (33):

$$I_{Na} = P_{Na} \frac{-F^2 E_m}{RT} \frac{[Na]_o - [Na]_i e^{-E_m F/RT}}{1 - e^{-E_m F/RT}} \quad (2)$$

where $[Na]_o$ and $[Na]_i$ refer to the external and internal sodium concentrations. Calculations indicate that, although sodium current is decreased by a decrease in external sodium concentration, the sodium permeability remains almost constant except at the lowest sodium concentration used (56.1 mM) in which it is greatly decreased. No clear explanation is afforded for the decrease, but the direct effect of the sodium substitute choline cannot be excluded. These measurements indicate that GTX I opens the sodium channels.

The average value for the sodium permeability in the axons internally perfused with 1×10^{-5} M GTX I is estimated to be 1.31×10^{-6} cm/sec. This represents a 90-fold increase compared with the value of normal squid axons (1.5×10^{-8} cm/sec) (36,37). Since the apparent dissociation constant of GTX I in increasing

sodium permeability is estimated to be 4×10^{-5} M, the increase in sodium permeability by high concentrations of GTX I should exceed 100-fold.

Dose-response relation for the action of GTX I in increasing the sodium permeability can be fitted by a curve based on one-to-one stoichiometric interaction between GTX I and the receptor. However, if one plots the amount of depolarization as a function of the logarithm of GTX I concentration, a different curve is obtained with a different value of the apparent dissociation constant (1×10^{-5} M). Such a plot does not give an accurate estimate, because depolarization is the final product of a chain of events; an increase in sodium permeability causes a depolarization, which in turn increases potassium permeability, and the potassium permeability increase tends to hyperpolarize the membrane.

TTX Antagonism

The effect of TTX in reversing the depolarization produced by GTX I was described in a previous section. The measurements of resting sodium conductance in GTX I by the voltage clamp technique enable us to study the mechanism of TTX antagonism in a more precise manner. As discussed in the preceding section, the depolarization produced by GTX I cannot be taken as a reliable parameter. It is essential to measure the primary action of GTX, i.e., increase in resting sodium permeability.

The resting sodium current was measured after internal application of various concentrations of GTX I in the presence and absence of 3×10^{-8} M TTX externally (26). Data were analyzed by the Lineweaver-Burk plots. TTX antagonizes the action of GTX I in a noncompetitive manner. The inhibition constant of TTX is estimated to be 4.1×10^{-8} M.

The noncompetitive antagonism of TTX is compatible with the proposed sites of action of TTX and GTX. The onset of GTX-induced depolarization and the recovery after washing are faster when GTX is applied internally. In addition GTX III is much more effective from inside than from outside. Collectively these observations support the idea that GTX acts from the internal membrane surface. On the other hand, TTX is effective only from outside. Thus, GTX and TTX presumably act on different sites in the membrane, so that the antagonism is expected to occur in a noncompetitive manner.

It should be noted that the inhibition constant of TTX to antagonize the GTX-induced depolarization is one order of magnitude larger than that to block sodium current during activity. This supports the notion that the sodium channels that undergo a conductance increase during excitation are operationally different from the resting sodium channels in the presence of GTX.

Effects on Voltage-Dependent Ionic Conductances

In spite of the large increase in resting sodium conductance in the presence of GTX, the voltage-dependent sodium and potassium conductances still undergo a near-normal increase upon depolarizing stimulation provided that the membrane potential is brought back to the normal level by anodal current (34). However, the activity of the voltage-dependent con-

ductances gradually deteriorates during a prolonged application of α-2H-GTX II (Starkus and Narahashi, *unpublished observation*). In the BTX-treated axon, the voltage-dependent conductances are also maintained active for some time (35).

These observations are not very surprising if consideration is given to the actual values for sodium conductance. The resting sodium conductance in normal squid axons is of the order of 0.015 mmho/cm². The sodium conductance is increased to a maximum of 100 mmho/cm² during depolarizing stimulation. Thus the net increase in sodium conductance in normal axons is 99.985 mmho/cm². In GTX I the resting sodium conductance is increased to 1.3 mmho/cm². Thus, even after treatment with GTX I, there still is a large fraction of sodium conductance that can be increased to the normal maximum value of 100 mmho/cm².

Voltage Dependency of GTX-Induced Resting Sodium Conductance

In an attempt to characterize the GTX-induced sodium conductance, its dependency on the membrane potential has been studied by voltage clamp (ven den Bercken and Narahashi, *unpublished observation*). Squid axons were externally and internally perfused with media in which all potassium ions were replaced by cesium ions. Thus the holding membrane currents measured at various membrane potentials should contain sodium, chloride, and other ionic components present in the media. Measurements of the holding current were made before and after applications of GTX I, and the difference between the two currents was plotted as a function of the membrane potential. Since GTX I increases only sodium permeability, and since no potassium current is involved, which is otherwise the major component in normal conditions, the resultant plot represents the sodium current-voltage relationship in the GTX-treated axons. There is a clear negative conductance in the membrane potentials ranging from -100 to -50 mV, the region where no such negative conductance is observed for the sodium conductance responsible for nerve excitation. Thus this observation is not compatible with the idea that the sodium conductance that undergoes an increase during depolarizing stimulation and the resting sodium conductance are the same entity.

Ionic Permeability Sequence

The permeabilities of the resting membrane to various cations have recently been measured before and after application of GTX I (38). The squid axon membrane was voltage clamped at −70 mV, which was made equal to the potassium and chloride equilibrium potentials by changing the ionic compositions of internal perfusate. Holding membrane currents were measured first in standard external solution whose major cation was sodium and then in test solutions in which test cations were substituted for sodium.

To our great surprise, the resting membrane is highly permeable to formamidine and guanidine, the permeabilities to sodium and these two organic cations being of the same order of magnitude. Methylamine is rather poorly permeable. A similar permeability sequence has been obtained before and after exposure to GTX I, suggesting that the sodium channel in GTX I is basically the same as that of normal membrane. These high permeabilities to formamidine and guanidine are in contrast with rather poor permeabilities to these ions during peak transient current (25). These results are easily accounted for if one assumes separate resting and active sodium channels in nerve membranes.

Binding of GTX to Membrane Components

Binding of tritiated α-2H-GTX II to various membranes has been measured by equilibrium dialysis (39). Extensive binding was found to membrane preparations obtained from lobster nerves, *Torpedo* electroplax, housefly head, and rat brain, kidney, and liver. However, no saturation of binding was detected with any of these preparations. This suggests that α-2H-GTX II binds to the membrane in a nonspecific manner.

Nature of Resting Sodium Channel as Studied by GTXs

The aforementioned results with GTXs are suggestive in interpreting the nature of resting sodium channels. The fact that TTX antagonizes the GTX-induced sodium permeability increase in a noncompetitive manner implies different sites of action of these two toxins. The inhibition constant of TTX in antagonizing GTX action is about one order of magnitude higher than that in blocking sodium conductance increase produced by stimulation. This result is not compatible with a single sodium channel concept. The difference in the cation permeability sequence in resting sodium channel and that in active sodium channel is too large to regard these two sodium channels as the same entity. The membrane potential ranges where sodium conductance exhibits a negative slope are different in the resting and active sodium channels, supporting the above-mentioned notion.

All of these observations tend to support separate resting and active sodium channels in squid axon membranes. However, these results should not be taken as conclusive, since none of them clearly excludes the other possibility, or clearly demonstrates the proposed notion. Despite such uncertainty, GTXs, BTX, and veratridine will continue to serve as useful and powerful tools to analyze the properties of sodium channels.

SUMMARY AND CONCLUSION

Certain neuroactive toxins have been demonstrated to serve as useful tools for the study of ionic channels. TTX blocks the sodium conductance increase normally occurring upon depolarization at very low concentrations, and has been extensively used for characterizing the sodium channel. It appears that TTX either directly binds to the sodium channel at its external opening or binds to the nearby macromolecule that controls the sodium gating mechanism.

GTXs, BTX, and veratridine depolarize the nerve membrane by a specific increase in resting sodium permeability. Detailed analyses with GTX I indicate that the increase amounts to 100-fold or more, and that the resting sodium channel in the toxin behaves in a manner different from the sodium channel that undergoes a conductance increase during excitation. These observations tend to support the notion that the resting sodium channel and the active sodium channel are different entities. However, no conclusive evidence has so far been obtained, and these toxins will continue to serve as powerful tools for characterization of sodium channels.

ACKNOWLEDGMENTS

This research was supported by U.S. Public Health Service Grant NS10823. The unfailing secretarial assistance of Mrs. Frances Bateman and Mrs. Gillian Cockerill is greatly appreciated.

REFERENCES

1. Narahashi, T. (1974): Chemicals as tools in the study of excitable membranes. *Physiol. Rev.,* 54:813–889.
2. Kao, C. Y. (1966): Tetrodotoxin, saxitoxin and their significance in the study of excitation phenomena. *Pharmacol. Rev.,* 18:997–1049.
3. Narahashi, T., Moore, J. W., and Frazier, D. T. (1969): Dependence of tetrodotoxin blockage of nerve membrane conductance on external pH. *J. Pharmacol. Exp. Ther.,* 169:224–228.
4. Narahashi, T., Deguchi, T., Urakawa, N., and Ohkubo, Y. (1960): Stabilization and rectification of muscle fiber membrane by tetrodotoxin. *Am. J. Physiol.,* 198:934–938.
5. Narahashi, T., Moore, J. W., and Scott, W. R. (1964): Tetrodotoxin blockage of sodium conductance increase in lobster giant axons. *J. Gen. Physiol.,* 47:965–974.
6. Moore, J. W., Blaustein, M. P., Anderson, N. C., and Narahashi, T. (1967): Basis of tetrodotoxin's selectivity in blockage of squid axons. *J. Gen. Physiol.,* 50:1401–1411.
7. Narahashi, T., Anderson, N. C., and Moore, J. W. (1967): Comparison of tetrodotoxin and procaine in internally perfused squid giant axons. *J. Gen. Physiol.,* 50:1413–1428.
8. Takata, M., Moore, J. W., Kao, C. Y., and Fuhrman, F. A. (1966): Blockage of sodium conductance increase in lobster giant axon by tarichatoxin (tetrodotoxin). *J. Gen. Physiol.,* 49:977–988.
9. Taylor, R. E. (1959): Effect of procaine on electrical properties of squid axon membranes. *Am. J. Physiol.,* 196:1071–1078.
10. Shanes, A. M., Freygang, W. H., Grundfest, H., and Amatniek, E. (1959): Anesthetic and calcium action in the voltage clamped squid giant axon. *J. Gen. Physiol.,* 42:793–802.
11. Narahashi, T., Haas, H. G., and Therrien, E. F. (1967): Saxitoxin and tetrodotoxin: comparison of nerve blocking mechanism. *Science,* 157:1441–1442.
12. Moore, J. W., Narahashi, T., and Shaw, T. I. (1967): An upper limit to the number of sodium channels in nerve membrane? *J. Physiol. (Lond.),* 188:99–105.

13. Cuervo, L. A., and Adelman, W. J., Jr. (1970): Equilibrium and kinetic properties of the interaction between tetrodotoxin and the excitable membrane of the squid giant axon. *J. Gen. Physiol.,* 55:309–335.
14. Hille, B. (1968): Pharmacological modifications of the sodium channels of frog nerve. *J. Gen. Physiol.,* 51:199–219.
15. Keynes, R. D., and Rojas, E. (1974): Kinetics and steady-state properties of the charged system controlling sodium conductance in the squid giant axon. *J. Physiol. (Lond.),* 239:393–434.
16. Armstrong, C. M., and Bezanilla, F. (1974): Currents related to movements of the gating particles of the sodium channels. *Nature,* 242:459–461.
17. Benzer, T. I., and Raftery, M. A. (1972): Partial characterization of a tetrodotoxin-binding component from nerve membrane. *Proc. Natl. Acad. Sci. USA,* 69:3634–3637.
18. Barnola, F. V., Villegas, R., and Camejo, G. (1973): Tetrodotoxin receptors in plasma membranes isolated from lobster nerve fibers. *Biochim. Biophys. Acta,* 298:84–94.
19. Benzer, T. I., and Raftery, M. A. (1973): Solubilization and partial characterization of the tetrodotoxin binding component from nerve axons. *Biochem. Biophys. Res. Comm.,* 51:939–944.
20. Henderson, R., and Wang, J. H. (1972): Solubilization of a specific tetrodotoxin-binding component from garfish olfactory nerve membrane. *Biochemistry,* 11:4565–4569.
21. Henderson, R., Ritchie, J. M., and Strichartz, G. R. (1973): The binding of labelled saxitoxin to the sodium channels in nerve membranes. *J. Physiol. (Lond.),* 235:783–804.
22. Schwarz, J. R., Ulbricht, W., and Wagner, H. H. (1973): The rate of action of tetrodotoxin on myelinated nerve fibres of *Xenopus laevis* and *Rana esculenta. J. Physiol. (Lond.),* 233:167–194.
23. Grefrath, S. P., and Reynolds, J. A. (1973): Polypeptide components of an excitable membrane. *J. Biol. Chem.,* 248:6091–6094.
24. Kao, C. Y., and Nishiyama, A. (1965): Actions of saxitoxin on peripheral neuromuscular systems. *J. Physiol. (Lond.),* 180:50–66.
25. Hille, B. (1971): The permeability of the sodium channel to organic cations in myelinated nerve. *J. Gen. Physiol.,* 58:599–619.
26. Narahashi, T., and Seyama, I. (1974): Mechanism of nerve membrane depolarization caused by grayanotoxin I. *J. Physiol. (Lond.),* 242:471–487.
27. Tokuyama, T., Daly, J., and Witkop, B. (1969): The structure of batrachotoxin, a steroidal alkaloid from the Colombian arrow poison frog, *Phyllobates aurotaenia* and partial synthesis of batrachotoxin and its analogs and homologs. *J. Am. Chem. Soc.,* 91:3931–3938.
28. Albuquerque, E. X., Daly, J. W., Witkop, B. (1971): Batrachotoxin: Chemistry and pharmacology. *Science,* 172:995–1002.
29. Narahashi, T. (1973): Drugs affecting axonal

membranes. In: *Fundamentals of Cell Pharmacology,* edited by S. Dikstein, pp. 395–424. C. C. Thomas, Springfield, Ill.

30. Benforado, J. M. (1968): The veratrum alkaloids. In: *Physiological Pharmacology,* edited by W. S. Root and F. G. Hofmann, pp. 331–398. Academic Press, New York.

31. Kupchan, S. M., and Flacke, W. E. (1967): Hypotensive veratrum alkaloids. In: *Antihypertensive Agents,* edited by E. Schlittler, pp. 429–458. Academic Press, New York.

32. Ohta, M., Narahashi, T., and Keeler, R. F. (1973): Effects of veratrum alkaloids on membrane potential and conductance of squid and crayfish giant axons. *J. Pharmacol. Exp. Ther.,* 184:143–154.

33. Hodgkin, A. L., and Katz, B. (1949): The effect of sodium ions on the electrical activity of the giant axon of the squid. *J. Physiol. (Lond.),* 108:37–77.

34. Seyama, I., and Narahashi, T. (1973): Increase in sodium permeability of squid axon membranes by α-dihydrograyanotoxin II. *J. Pharmacol. Exp. Ther.,* 184:299–307.

35. Narahashi, T., Albuquerque, E. X., and Deguchi, T. (1971): Effects of batrachotoxin on membrane potential and conductance of squid giant axons. *J. Gen. Physiol.,* 58:54–70.

36. Brinley, F. J., and Mullins, L. J. (1965): Ion fluxes and transference numbers in squid axons. *J. Neurophysiol.,* 28:526–544.

37. Baker, P. F., Blaustein, M. P., Keynes, R. D., Manil, J., Shaw, T. I., and Steinhardt, R. A. (1969): The ouabain-sensitive fluxes of sodium and potassium in squid giant axons. *J. Physiol. (Lond.),* 200:459–496.

38. Hironaka, T., and Narahashi, T. (1975): Ionic permeability profile of the resting axon membrane as affected by grayanotoxin I. *Fed. Proc.,* 34:360.

39. Soeda, Y., O'Brien, R. D., Yeh, J. Z., and Narahashi, T. (1975): Evidence that α-dihydrograyanotoxin II does not bind to the sodium gate. *J. Memb. Biol.,* 23:91–101.

The Nervous System, Donald B. Tower, Editor-in-Chief. *Vol. 1: The Basic Neurosciences*. Raven Press, New York, 1975.

Synthetic Machinery and Axoplasmic Transport: Maintenance of Neuronal Connectivity

Bernard Droz

The information flow in the nervous system is processed by a complex network of cellular expansions that allows neurons to build up specific connections and thereby to communicate with each other. The differentiation of neuronal processes gives rise to dendrites and axons. The branching of the dendritic arborization greatly enhances the receptive field of input signals impinging on a neuron. The axon, which frequently extends a long distance from the perikaryon, is specialized for the propagation of nerve impulses. The transmission of nerve impulses from the axon to another cell is mediated by presynaptic axon terminals. Each

function of the neuron, e.g., reception of multiple signals at the surface membrane of dendrites, conduction of spike trains along the axon or synaptic transmission of nerve impulses, requires rapid changes of molecular conformation in neuronal membranes. In the course of transitional changes, the possibility that proteins cannot recover their functional structure must be considered; moreover the electrical stimulation of nerve has been reported to increase neuronal proteolysis and catabolic processes. According to Lajtha and Marks (1), proteinases and peptide hydrolases are indeed present in sufficient amount in the nervous

TABLE 1. *Turnover of protein and glycoprotein in various parts of neurons*

Nerve cell bodies	Tracer	Half-lives (days)		References
Purkinje cells (rat)	^{3}H-leucine	1.0	9.5	(9)
Pyramidal cells of the hippocampus (rat)	^{3}H-leucine	0.6	12.0	(9)
Ganglion cell of the semilunar ganglion (mouse)	^{3}H-arginine	0.8	9.5	(9)
Spinal motoneurons (rat)	^{35}S-methionine	2.2 2.8[a]	27.0 38.0	Jakoubek et al. (1968)
Axons				
Preganglionic axons of the ciliary ganglion (chick)	^{3}H-lysine ^{3}H-fucose	3.5[b]	15.2	(7) Bennett et al. (1973)
Nerve endings				
Ciliary ganglion (chick)	^{3}H-lysine ^{3}H-fucose	0.5 7.0	10.0	(7) Bennett et al. (1973)
Optic lobe (pigeon)	^{3}H-leucine	0.5–4[a]	18.0[b]	Cuénod and Schonbach (1971)
	^{3}H-fucose	3.0[a]	38	Marko and Cuénod (1973)
Lateral geniculate body (rabbit)	^{3}H-leucine	1.0[a]	9.6	Karlsson and Sjöstrand (1971)

The data have been obtained from decay curves of radioactivity measured in radioautographs.

[a] Calculated from cell fractions.

[b] Calculated from the reported data.

system, including nerve endings, to completely break down neuronal proteins to peptides and amino acids. However, it would be essential to determine whether the breakdown of neuronal macromolecules results either from a specific recognition of worn-out protein or from a random process. A supplementary loss of protein occurs in chemical synapses: during stimulation the release of the neurotransmitter is accompanied by the release of proteins associated with synaptic vesicles.

Thus the various parts of neurons are the sites of a continual loss of proteins. The rates of disappearance range from hours to weeks (Table 1). The intense turnover of protein in all parts of neurons reflects, therefore, the need of new macromolecules to replace the lost ones.

SOURCES OF NEURONAL MOLECULES

To supply the neurons with new molecules, three main sources must be considered.

Local Synthesis of Molecules

Each part of the neuron is capable of synthesizing protein, but the producing rates and the spectrum of molecular species vary to a large extent if we consider the perikaryon, the dendrites, the axon, or its presynaptic terminals. The synthesis of neuronal proteins takes place mainly in the perikaryon and the large dendritic shafts. Both structures contain Nissl bodies made of numerous polyribosomes, either free in the neuroplasm or attached to endoplasmic reticulum membranes. Electron microscopic autoradiography has pointed to the rough endoplasmic reticulum as the major site for protein synthesis in neurons and to a lesser extent to free polyribosomes dispersed in the cytoplasmic matrix (2). Cerebral microsomes, obtained after cell fractionation of rat brain, allowed Roberts et al. (3) to specify that the synthetic activity was indeed initiated on polyribosomes. In contrast the axon and its presynaptic terminals, which are poor in or devoid of cytoplasmic polyribosomes, display only a rather discrete capacity to incorporate labeled amino acids.

Special attention has been paid to isolated nerve endings. It was decisively demonstrated by Gambetti et al. (4) that a slight synthesis of

protein takes place in synaptosomes; nonetheless the part taken by the presynaptic mitochondria and plasma membranes in the synthesis of a limited number of membrane polypeptides is still a matter of discussion. At most the local synthesis in axon terminals accounts for less than 2% of the rapidly renewed synaptic proteins. Although nerve endings are somewhat unapt to renew their own proteins, the presynaptic regions of the axons are the sites of an intense metabolic activity that is linked with the secretory process of chemical synaptic transmission. To ensure the synthesis, storage, and release of the neurotransmitter, the axon terminals must be supplied with specific enzymes and proteins arrayed in a highly organized structure. As emphasized by Couteaux (5), the cooperation of these mechanisms in a compact area reflects a strategic advantage, which reduces delay in the supply of neurotransmitter. The remarkable autonomy of axon terminals to purvey for neurotransmitter singularly contrasts with the complete dependence on the supply of enzymes controlling the synthesis of the neurotransmitter, the constituents of synaptic vesicles ensuring its storage and the specific macromolecules allowing its release at the presynaptic plasma membrane.

Importation of Molecules from Microenvironment

The neuronal membrane possesses high-affinity transport mechanisms, which permit the reuptake and presynaptic reutilization of neurotransmitters (e.g., norepinephrine) or metabolites (e.g., choline). When exogenous macromolecules, such as horseradish peroxidase, are introduced into the intercellular spaces of the nervous system, some of them are transferred into the neurons by endocytotic processes (6).

The intercellular exchange of informative molecules between glia and neuron should promote the functional coupling of these cells. However, the transfer of macromolecules from the surrounding glial cells can hardly supply qualitatively or quantitatively the axonal need of specific proteins, at least in vertebrates.

There is evidence that radioactive substances accumulated in axons or nerve terminals may be transferred to other neurons, which in turn become radioactive. It is important to ascertain whether the intercellular transfer of label corresponds to an exchange of radioactive macromolecules or small molecules. In other words, does the appearance of label in postsynaptic structures result from a transsynaptic delivery of radioactive proteins or from a release of amino acids followed by a reincorporation into nascent proteins synthesized in postsynaptic elements? This question may be answered after the local application of an inhibitor of protein synthesis, which prevents the reutilization of free labeled amino acids. The results indicate that most of the radioactivity found in the postsynaptic neurons is caused by the passage of low molecular weight molecules (7). Such an interneuronal transfer of small molecules allows adjacent neurons to spare metabolites; if the cooperation between pre- and postsynaptic elements is initiated and maintained by an exchange of larger molecules playing an informative role, their neuronal uptake seems to be a rather limited process.

Intraneuronal Migration of Macromolecules

The development of our present concept of axonal transport has depended largely on improvements in nuclear tracer methodology and more specifically in their autoradiographic localization. If one goes back to the early studies of Remak in 1838, Waller in 1850, Scott in 1906, and Marinesco in 1909, it was proposed that the nerve cell body acts as a trophic center ensuring the growth and the maintenance of the axonal process. A few years later, Ramón y Cajal (1928), in agreement with the views of Heidenhain (1911), opposed the concept of proximodistal convection of material along the axon to that of local process of assimilation and growth of the axon. On the basis of a controversial observation, he believed that Wallerian degeneration evolves simultaneously along the entire course of the distal segment after a nerve transsection; for this reason, he held the view that the axons "are not influenced by material or chemical reserves of the soma or nucleus of the neurones" and that "the trophic influence exercised by the central neurones is of a dynamic and not of a material nature." The theory of a somatofugal flow of material from the nerve cell body to the axon was put forth again by Gerard in 1932, Parker in 1933, and remarkably explicited by Weiss and Hiscoe (8) in their famous 1948 paper on the mechanism of nerve growth. Their experiments were based on the following principle: if the axonal growth proceeds from the neuronal perikaryon, then constriction of peripheral nerves should impede the flow of material along the axon and produce damming of the axoplasm. The subsequent removal of the constriction should allow the axoplasm to resume its somatofugal movement. Both phenomena were indeed observed by Weiss and Hiscoe, but the part represented by the local nerve injury was difficult to estimate. An experimental approach that does not damage the nerve was needed. This aim was achieved by the advent of tritium-labeled amino acids, which help localize labeled protein in individual axons by means of autoradiography. Taking advantage of this method, Droz and Leblond (9) in 1963 demonstrated that proteins migrate from nerve cell bodies into and along intact axons and dendrites of various neurons in the central and peripheral nervous system. Later the use of cell fractionation and biochemical analyses allowed McEwen and Grafstein (10) in 1968 to specify that different molecular species are conveyed at different rates of transport to different parts of neurons. Such a heterogeneous behavior of the transported material raises a crucial question: does the dispatch of newly synthesized proteins to their various operative sites result from a pure random process or from compartmentalized channels present in the neuronal cytoplasm? In other words, how are different molecules (e.g., receptors, ionophores, tubulin, vesiculin, choline acetyltransferase, or succinodehydrogenase) selectively driven and guided to their strategic sites? Questions of this kind remained unanswered for many years and gave rise to controversial arguments, which can be resolved now by new technical developments.

SMOOTH ENDOPLASMIC RETICULUM AND FAST AXONAL TRANSPORT

Today it is common knowledge that the neuronal cytoplasm is compartmentalized; intraneuronal channels called rough endoplasmic reticulum, Golgi apparatus, and smooth endoplasmic reticulum are insulated from the

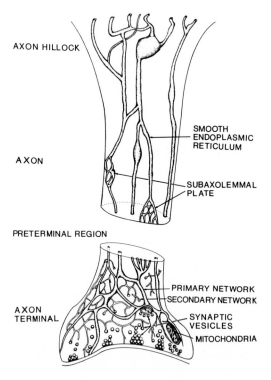

AXON HILLOCK

AXON

SMOOTH
ENDOPLASMIC
RETICULUM

SUBAXOLEMMAL
PLATE

PRETERMINAL REGION

AXON
TERMINAL

PRIMARY NETWORK
SECONDARY NETWORK

SYNAPTIC
VESICLES

MITOCHONDRIA

FIG. 1. Diagrammatic representation of the axonal smooth endoplasmic reticulum. The axonal endoplasmic reticulum appears as a continuous system of channels extending from the perikaryon to the axon terminal. The convoluted tubules of the smooth endoplasmic reticulum enter the initial segment of the axon and run parallel to its long axis. They are loosely anastomosed and give rise to subaxolemmal plates made up of smaller tubules. In the preterminal region of the axon, the large tubules of the smooth endoplasmic reticulum anastomose peripherally and form the primary network. The well developed "secondary network," caged within the primary network, is composed of smaller elements originating from the wide tubules. Thin and wide tubules of the smooth endoplasmic reticulum appear occasionally to be closely apposed to the axolemmal and presynaptic membrane. It is postulated that the exchange of fast axonally transported macromolecules takes place at the contact between the subaxolemmal plate or tubules. The synaptic vesicles, which are appended like blebs at the tip of thin tubular branches, visualize their fission from or their fusion with the smooth endoplasmic reticulum. (From Droz et al., ref. 26.)

surrounding neuroplasmic matrix by a well-developed system of intracellular membranes. The smooth endoplasmic reticulum is the only one to be represented in the axon. In his pioneer electron microscopic studies, Palay

(1958) had suspected that the smooth endoplasmic reticulum forms a continuous structure connected by thin canaliculi with synaptic vesicles in nerve endings. The recent advent of high-voltage electron microscopy made it possible to elucidate the tridimensional configuration of the intracellular channels in 1 to 2 μm thick sections. Under these conditions, the smooth endoplasmic reticulum appears as a continuous system channeling the whole length of the axon from the cell body to terminals (Fig. 1). In the perikaryon, the smooth endoplasmic reticulum consists of a network connected with the rough endoplasmic reticulum and the Golgi apparatus on the one hand and with tubular channels entering the axon on the other hand. The tubules of the smooth endoplasmic reticulum run along the axon and occasionally enlarge to give rise to subaxolemmal plates closely apposed underneath the surface of the plasma membrane (Fig. 2). In the preterminal regions, the tubules of the smooth endoplasmic reticulum resolve into a primary network that gives rise to a secondary network made of thinner canaliculi (Fig. 3). Frequently synaptic vesicles are budding at the tip of thin canaliculi whereas other canaliculi approach the presynaptic plasma membrane (Figs. 1 and 4). Does this complex system of intraneuronal plumbing play a role in the selective transport of macromolecules? To solve this problem, let us consider the results collected from neurochemical investigations and high-resolution autoradiographic studies.

All the biochemical data listed by Grafstein in her comprehensive review (11) indicate that proteins, glycoproteins, phospholipids, and membrane-bound enzymes, which are conveyed with the fast phase of the axonal transport (Table 2), are associated primarily with particulate rather than soluble fractions. The use of electron microscope autoradiography has provided a deeper insight into the sequence of the intracellular events, which precede the insertion of these macromolecules in their operative sites (2,7).

The results may be summarized as follows. The synthesis of protein starts first in the Nissl bodies; polypeptide chains, which are released from polyribosomes into the lumen of the rough endoplasmic reticulum, are eventually transferred to the Golgi apparatus (Fig. 5). In the course of their translocation from the rough endoplasmic reticulum to the Golgi apparatus, carbohydrate groups may be successively added to the nascent protein moiety and give rise to glycoprotein. Newly formed proteins and glycoproteins, following the channels of the smooth endoplasmic reticulum, enter the axon and move along its length (Figs. 5 and 6). In the axon, the axolemma is supplied with the major part of fast-transported constituents (Figs. 6 and 7); they are presumably yielded to the axolemma by means of the subaxolemmal plates (Figs. 1, 2, and 6). A minor part of fast-transported macromolecules accumulates in the axon terminals (Figs. 5 and 8); there they are mainly distributed to synaptic vesicles and presynaptic plasma membranes, and to a lesser extent to mitochondria (Figs. 5 and 8). The transfer of protein and glycoprotein to these synaptic elements is presumably mediated by the tubules and canaliculi of the primary and secondary network of the presynaptic endoplasmic reticulum (Figs. 3 and 4). It is likely that the bulging of vesicles at the ends of thin canaliculi (Fig. 4) visualizes recycling or biogenesis of synaptic vesicles exchanging macromolecules rapidly transported with the axonal endoplasmic reticulum (5).

The fact that many molecular species are transported rapidly in the smooth endoplasmic reticulum (Table 2) raises several questions.

1. Are given specific proteins transported in a determined channel of the smooth endoplasmic reticulum or are all protein species intermingled during their fast transport? The answer is not yet known, but only suggested. An experiment performed by Anderson and McClure (see review in ref. 12) led to the conclusion that proteins dispatched from spinal ganglion cell bodies to the central or peripheral axon terminals correspond to different molecular species. In the case of hydrolytic enzymes, the sequestration is rendered necessary to prevent the breakdown of the material during its transport. In spite of some uncertainties, it appears that the compartmentalization of the fast transport results from a compartmentalization of the protein synthesis in the Nissl body. Moreover the need for specialized channels of the axonal endoplasmic reticulum becomes obvious when it is admitted that material secluded in tubules of the axonal endoplasmic reticulum may also be conveyed

in a retrograde direction from the axon terminals to the cell body. La Vail and La Vail (6) showed that the retrograde transport of horseradish peroxidase occurs only in some of the axonal tubules of the smooth endoplasmic reticulum. It is therefore probable that the axon possesses different channels specialized for the transport of material from the cell body to the axon terminals and from the axon terminals to the nerve cell body.

2. Do the molecules transported with the fast phase of the axonal transport migrate at the same rate? The answer to this question is still pending, since several intermediary rates or even a wide spectrum has been found in the optic system and in various peripheral nerves (11). However, if we consider a homogeneous population of neurons, in which the axons display identical characteristics of length, diameter, and synapses, a single rate of fast axonal transport could be measured, that is 280 ± 50 mm/day (7).

3. Does the fast-transported material migrate within the lumen of the axonal endoplasmic reticulum or does it flow with the membrane components themselves along the channel wall? To solve this problem, the fast transport of labeled protein was arrested by exerting a slight compression of a nerve. Within a few hours, a simultaneous accumulation of labeled proteins and profiles of the smooth endoplasmic reticulum was observed in compressed axons. The contorted and dilated tubules of the smooth endoplasmic reticulum exhibited an increase of their luminal content; this indicates that one part of the transported material is probably conveyed within the endoplasmic reticulum (the intraluminal material corresponds probably to hydrolytic enzymes or soluble proteins such as those enclosed in synaptic vesicles). Another part, which consists of membrane components, would be integrated as building blocks of the endoplasmic reticulum membranes. This latter possibility is supported by the accumulation of phospholipids in front of an axonal interruption (Fig. 9). Since fast-transported phospholipids are a major membrane component, this finding indicates that the membrane of the smooth endoplasmic reticulum as well as its content shifts rapidly toward nerve endings.

4. What is the propelling mechanism responsible for the fast transport of material?

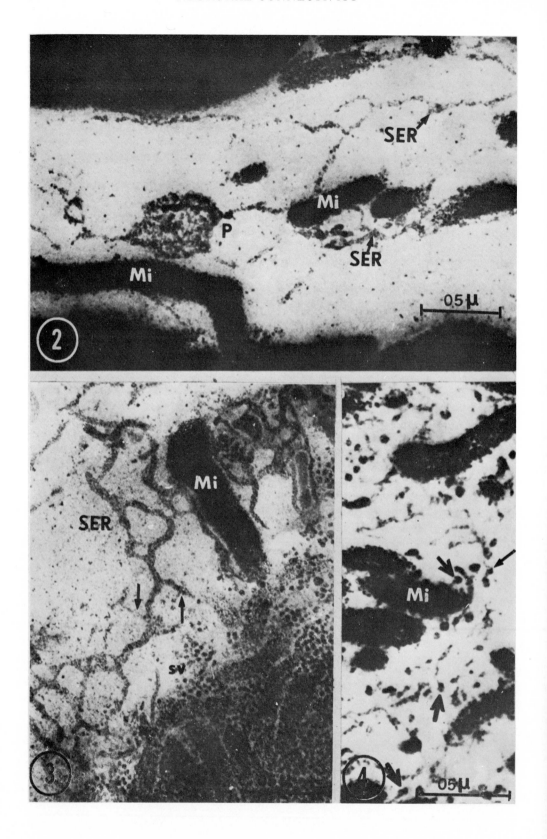

It has been proposed that the fast axonal transport would result from interactions of the microtubule-neurofilament system with either sliding vesicles or with intraaxoplasmic channels. Hence the microtubule-neurofilament system would transduce the free energy released from mitochondrial metabolism into axonal translation (13). According to the Curie-Prigogine principle, such a coupling between scalar and vectorial processes requires an anisotropic medium; this is carried out by the membrane interfaces of the axonal smooth endoplasmic reticulum. Thus, the cooperation of the smooth endoplasmic reticulum with other axonal organelles such as mitochondria and the microtubule-neurofilament system would allow new macromolecules to be translocated from their perikarial sites of synthesis to their axonal sites of utilization.

5. Since the major part of the fast transported material is destined to replace membrane constituents of the axon and presynaptic terminals, does the blockade of the fast axonal transport affect nerve impulse conduction and transmission? The most revealing result was obtained by Cuénod et al. (14) who, after inhibition of the fast axonal transport by means of colchicine, showed that the nerve impulse conduction was at most slightly decreased whereas the synaptic transmission was deeply depressed. Correlatively the synapses exhibited degenerative changes with the appearance of large vesicles, numerous filaments, and abnormal mitochondria. Contrary to the effects of a nerve constriction, the electrophysiological and ultrastructural alterations were followed by a recovery of both synaptic structures and functions. These obser-

TABLE 2. *Nature of the material presumably transported in axonal compartments*

Smooth endoplasmic reticulum
Membrane protein and glycoprotein
Acetylcholinesterase
Dopamine hydroxylase
Chromogranine
Adenylcyclase
Hydrolases (lysosomal enzymes)
Some mitochondrial proteins
Sulfated mucopolysaccharides
Gangliosides
Phospholipids

Axoplasm
Soluble proteins
Tubulin
Neurofilament subunit
Choline acetyltransferase
Tyrosine hydroxylase
Phosphodiesterase
Lactate dehydrogenase
Phosphoglucuronic dehydrogenase

Mitochondria
Monoamine oxidase
Cytochromes
Succinodehydrogenase

vations provide positive evidence for the supply of material by the fast axonal transport to ensure the maintenance of axonal membranes and mainly of synaptic structures.

In summary, the axonal smooth endoplasmic reticulum forms a continuous system of channels ensuring a rapid shuttle of molecules between the cell body and the axon terminals (Fig. 5). Some channels are involved in the rapid translocation of newly synthesized material from the perikaryon up to nerve endings; con-

←

FIG. 2. Axon in 1 μm thick sections of chick ciliary ganglion after impregnation with uranyl and lead. The myelinated axon exhibits tubules of the smooth endoplasmic reticulum (SER) which run parallel to the long axis. Subaxolemmal plates (*P*), which are made up of thin anastomosed canaliculi, correspond to vesicular profiles frequently encountered underneath the axolemma in thin sections (see Fig. 6). Mitochondrial profiles (Mi) are seen in contact with the smooth endoplasmic reticulum. (From Droz et al., ref. 26.)

FIG. 3. Presynaptic terminals in 1 μm thick sections of chick ciliary ganglion after impregnation with uranyl and lead. The peripheral region of axon terminals shows a well developed smooth endoplasmic reticulum (SER) forming the primary network. Only rare segments of thin canaliculi forming the secondary network are visible (*arrow*). Note the close association between the smooth endoplasmic reticulum and mitochondria (Mi). In the lower right corner, numerous synaptic vesicles (sv) are clustered. (From Droz et al., ref. 26.)

FIG. 4. Presynaptic terminals of chick ciliary ganglion after impregnation with uranyl and lead. The central region of axon terminals exhibits the thin canaliculi of the secondary network. Many connections between the thin canaliculi and synaptic vesicles (*arrow*) are shown in this thin section. (From Droz et al., ref. 26.)

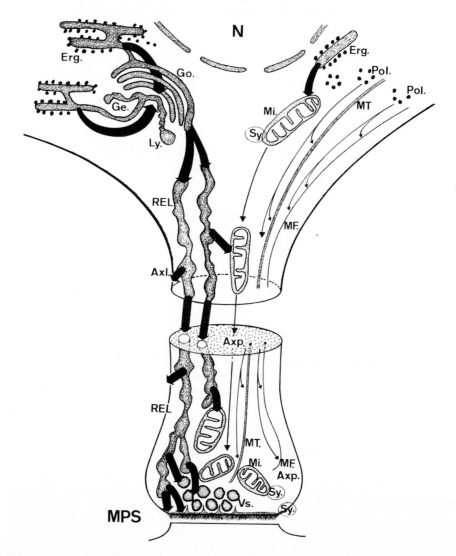

FIG. 5. Diagrammatic representation of the contribution of the axonal migration of macromolecules to the maintenance of nerve cell processes and synapses. On the left side, the thick arrows indicate the part taken by the fast transport. Polypeptide chains synthesized in the ergastoplasm of the Nissl body (Erg) are transferred to the Golgi apparatus (Go) and give rise to protein and glycoprotein sequestered in the smooth endoplasmic reticulum (REL). Passing into the axon with the axonal endoplasmic reticulum, they are transported at a high speed and yield new membrane components to the axolemma (Axl) and mitochondria (Mi). They accumulate in the terminal part of the axon and ensure the renewal of constituents of synaptic vesicles (Vs) and presynaptic plasma membranes (MPS). Thus the fast transport purveys with new membrane components the logistical support of the conduction and mainly of the transmission of nerve impulses. On the right side, the thin arrows point to the elements transported with the slow axonal flow. Polypeptide chains are released from free poly-ribosomes (Pol) into the neuronal cytoplasm and migrate slowly into the axoplasm (Axp). They may assemble as protein subunits giving rise to microfilaments (MF) and microtubules (MT). Mitochondria receive by transfer the great majority of their own proteins; these organelles are displaced along the axon and continue to exhibit a slight synthesis of hydrophobic polypeptides (Sy). The retrograde axonal transport has not been represented in this figure. (From Droz et al., ref. 27.)

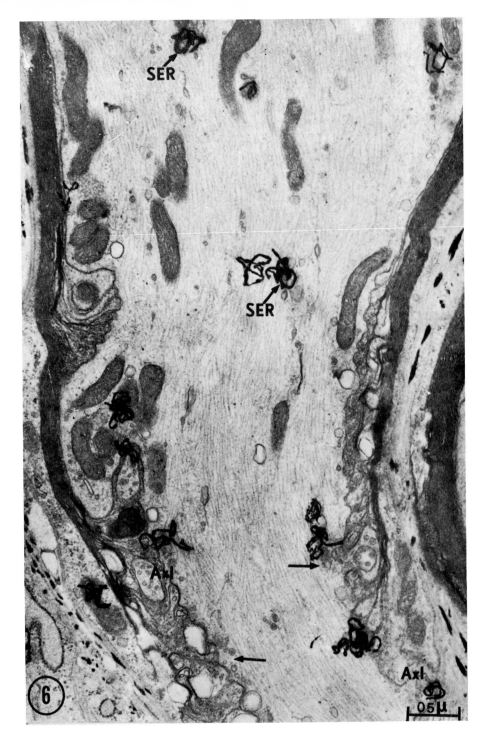

FIG. 6. Arrival of fast-transported glycoprotein at the last node of Ranvier, in the preterminal region of the axon. Three hours after the intracerebral injection of ^{3}H-glucosamine, the preganglionic axons of the ciliary ganglion of chick (located 10 mm farther) exhibit silver grains, which are distributed over profiles of the smooth endoplasmic reticulum (SER) and the axolemma (Axl). The vesicular profiles seen underneath the axolemma (*arrow*) probably correspond to sectioned subaxolemmal plates (see Fig. 2).

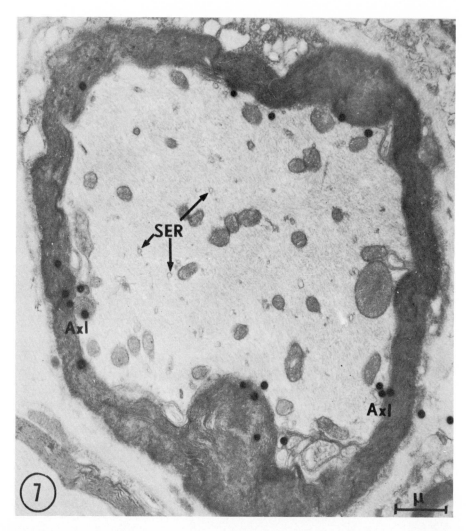

FIG. 7. Fate of fast-transported glycoprotein in the axon. Six days after the fast flow of ^{3}H-fucosylglycoprotein, the smooth endoplasmic reticulum (SER) is free of radioactivity. The silver grains located over the axolemmal region (Axl) point to the axonal plasma membrane as the main beneficiary of the transferred glycoprotein.

versely other channels are probably involved in driving back molecules from synapses to the cell body. Since a membrane flow of the endoplasmic reticulum seems to occur along the axon, it is probable that the smooth endoplasmic reticulum acts like a travelator: first, the smooth endoplasmic reticulum is loaded with new material in the perikaryon and unloaded along its axonal course to nerve endings; second, the smooth endoplasmic reticulum is probably reloaded with disused material, which is then carried back to the cell body and there broken down by the numerous lysosomes. Small molecules produced by the hydrolysis of disused material could be reutilized in the perikaryon for building new macromolecules. If this molecular recycling bears on a large number of metabolites, it would represent an advantageous feature for the neuronal economy.

AXOPLASM AND SLOW AXONAL TRANSPORT

Around the channels of the smooth endoplasmic reticulum, the axoplasm forms a huge compartment extending from the perikaryon to

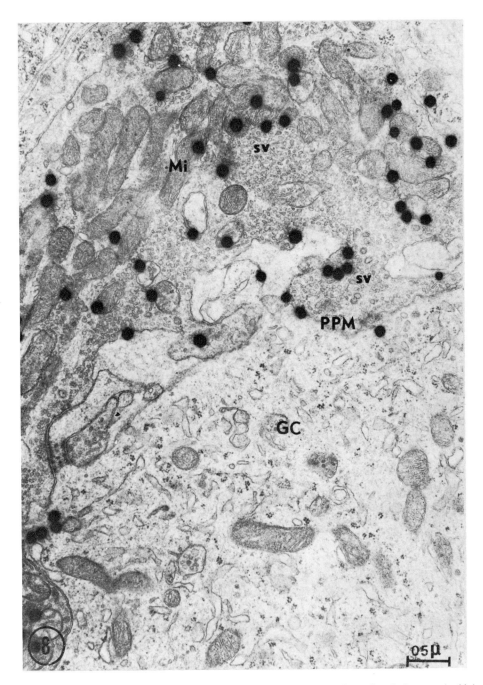

FIG. 8. Accumulation of labeled protein transported to nerve endings. Two days after the intracerebral injection of ^{3}H-lysine, one fraction of the fast-transported protein persists in the axon terminal, whereas the first slowly migrating protein begins to arrive. In the giant nerve ending of the ciliary ganglion of the chick, silver grains are distributed over areas occupied by the presynaptic plasma membrane (PPM), synaptic vesicles (sv) and mitochondria (Mi). The postsynaptic perikaryon of the ganglion cell (GC) is almost free of label.

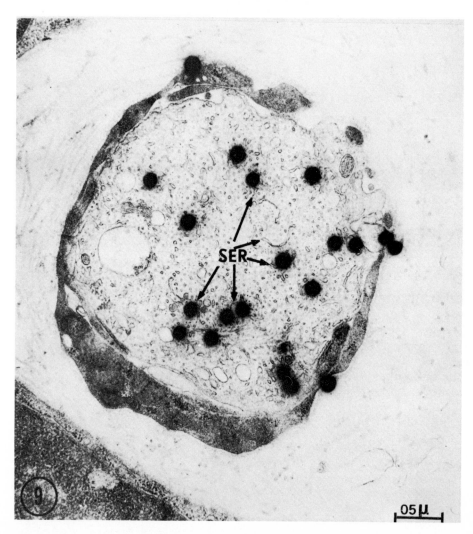

FIG. 9. Accumulation of phospholipids and smooth endoplasmic reticulum in an axon, 1 hr after the nerve section. Phospholipids, which were synthesized in the nerve cell body from ^{3}H-glycerol, pile up in the proximal stump (and none in the distal one); silver grains are found only in axons characterized by a concommitant increase of the number of smooth endoplasmic profiles (SER).

the axon terminals. The axoplasmic matrix contains most of the so-called soluble proteins that are recovered after cell fractionation. The neurofilaments and the microtubules that are embedded in the axoplasmic matrix result from the aggregation of polymeric protein subunits. In the presynaptic region, enzymes controlling the synthesis of neurotransmitters, e.g., tyrosine hydroxylase for catecholamines or choline acetyltransferase for acetylcholine, accumulate in the axoplasm embedding the synaptic vesicles. Besides glycogen particles, protein is almost the exclusive macromolecular component of the presynaptic axoplasm.

The axoplasmic proteins are submitted to a continuous turnover (Table 1). The synthesis takes place in the polyribosomes of the perikaryon either located in the Nissl body or scattered among neurofilaments and microtubules (Fig. 5). After release in the perikaryal cytoplasm, the newly formed polypeptides and proteins slowly invade the axon hillock and the initial segment of the axon; they migrate toward nerve endings at rates ranging between 1 and

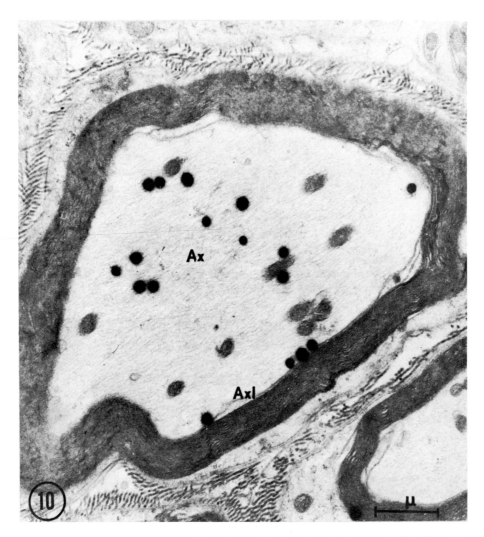

FIG. 10. Slowly transported protein in a myelinated axon. Six days after the intracerebral injection of ^{3}H-lysine to a chick, numerous silver grains are distributed over the preganglionic axons. Most of the radioactivity is found in the axoplasm (Ax); only a few silver grains persist over the axolemma (Axl) after the fast flow of protein. An unlabeled postganglionic axon is partially visible in the right lower corner.

10 mm/day as has been observed in a homogenous population of axons (7). Little is known about the mechanism responsible for the slow axoplasmic transport. Weiss (15) has proposed a peristaltic propulsion of the axon as a whole. However, the progressive longitudinal spread of the radioactive wave reflects a gradual dispersion of the migratory proteins along the axon; once arrived in presynaptic regions, the slowly migrating proteins gather again. Hence the slow convection of the axoplasmic components does not fit the requirements for a bulk transport of the axon.

The slow axoplasmic transport contributes to the renewal of the largest part of the axonal proteins (Fig. 10 and Table 2): the total amount of slowly transported proteins is about four times as great as that of the fast-transported ones. Only a small fraction of the slowly transported proteins reaches the axon terminals; the great majority is slowly catabolized in the axon (7).

The steady state of this system would be

preserved as long as the migration of axo-plasmic proteins goes on to rejuvenate the axoplasm. This is a general phenomenon, which occurs in neurons of the central nervous system, as well as in peripheral nerves. In young growing animals, there is a lengthening of nerve fibers as well as an increase of the axonal diameter. Hence the migrating axo-plasmic proteins might have been used not only for renewal but also for growth (9). If it were the case, the amount of protein transported per unit of time through the axon should be in-creased in growing neurons as compared with neurons in steady state. Measurements carried out in growing neurons indicate indeed an en-hanced output of newly synthesized proteins in the perikaryon and an enhanced migration rate, which is at least twice as rapid in growing as in steady-state neurons (9,16). In neurons regenerating transsected axons, conflicting results have been obtained; the axoplasmic transport of slowly migrating proteins appears to be increased in some neurons and decreased in others (11,17). This discrepancy would re-flect the different ability of nerve cells to adapt their metabolism to the axonal growth after in-jury of peripheral nerves. All the studies under-taken in the central nervous system insist on the role played by the axoplasmic transport for maintaining the integrity of neuronal connec-tions. In the course of reparative processes in the central nervous system, the slow axoplasmic transport carries the material required to pro-mote the collateral sprouting, which permits the establishment of functional synapses with newly deafferented neurons. It is important to emphasize that regenerative processes in the central nervous system are not impeded by a defect of the axoplasmic transport but by other factors such as degenerating axons and glial reactions (see review in ref. 12).

In view of all these findings, it seems that the slow axoplasmic transport conveys most of the material required for growth, maintenance, and regeneration of axonal processes. Whereas the transit time does not exceed a few days to travel along short axons, the axoplasmic trans-port of proteins lasts probably several months to cover one meter in the axons of a human sciatic nerve. This presents a so far unanswered challenge to prevent the breakdown of the migratory proteins that reach the remotest part of the axons.

An attractive application of the axoplasmic transport has emerged to trace neuronal path-ways in the central nervous system (18). By taking advantage of the possibility to administer a labeled amino acid into or beside nerve cell bodies, the newly formed radioactive proteins are used as endogenous tracer to visualize auto-radiographically the axonal pathways and the synaptic junctions of intact neurons. In this respect the use of axoplasmic transport for studies of neuronal connectivity constitutes a decisive step toward disentangling the most complex neuronal pathways (19).

THE MITOCHONDRIAL COMPARTMENT OF THE AXON

The mitochondrial population of the axon constitutes a series of intraaxoplasmic com-partments scattered between the perikaryon and the synaptic terminals. If we consider mito-chondria located in the perikaryon, that is, close to the machinery synthesizing proteins, and those confined to nerve endings, that is, em-bedded in a cytoplasm devoid of polyribosomes, their natural environment is completely dif-ferent. Now the mitochondria are almost en-tirely dependent upon cytoplasmic polyribo-somes for the synthesis of mitochondrial en-zymes. Under the peculiar conditions existing in the axon, it is important to determine what is the part taken by the autonomous protein syn-thesis in mitochondria, the transfer of protein to these organelles and the axoplasmic transport of mitochondria as a whole.

The autonomous synthesis of protein takes place in mitochondria located in the perikaryon, the axon, and synaptic terminals. This synthetic capacity is restricted to the manufacture of strongly hydrophobic polypeptides, which seem to promote the assembly of enzymatic supra-molecular aggregates in cristae. Attardi et al. (21) suggest that the autonomous protein synthesis plays a key role in modulating the mitochondrial activity in response to phys-iological stimuli.

The transfer of protein from cytoplasmic polyribosomes to mitochondria represents the major source of protein, especially of enzymes. In the perikaryon there is a rapid exchange of newly formed protein between the rough endo-plasmic reticulum and mitochondria (2). In the axon and nerve endings, the situation is completely different. Our studies indicate that fast-moving proteins conveyed along the smooth endoplasmic reticulum contribute to the replacement of mitochondrial components (7). This transfer of protein is probably facilitated by the frequent contacts existing between the smooth endoplasmic reticulum and mitochondria (Figs. 1 and 3).

The axonal transport of mitochondria, which has been formerly shown by Barondes (21), displays speed characteristics which are similar to those of the slow axoplasmic transport, but when mitochondria are directly observed in living axons, they are animated by rapid bidirectional motions. In fact the net displacement of mitochondria along the axon corresponds to the slow rate of the axoplasmic transport. Thus mitochondria, which have grown in the cell body and are laden with new components, enter the axon and sweep down slowly to nerve endings (7).

In the course of their slow migration, the axonal mitochondria are aging; once arrived at synaptic endings, they frequently disclose some failure of their enzymatic activities. This would indicate that neither the autonomous protein synthesis, nor the fast axonal transport of mitochondrial components compensate for the re-'placement of some worn out enzymatic function (22). Contrary to Weiss's statement (15), the spontaneous degeneration of mitochondria seems to be such a rare event that it can hardly account for the disappearance of mitochondrial components. An early but reversible alteration of synaptic mitochondria has been found by Cuénod et al. (14) after blockade of the fast transport with colchicine. This observation would indicate that components of axonal and synaptic mitochondria are replaced mainly by a balanced influx and efflux of macromolecules.

REGULATION OF THE MAINTENANCE OF NEURONAL CONNECTIVITY

The continuous renewal of macromolecular constituents making up axons and dendrites is a corollary of the perennial life of the neurons. The cellular expansions that are integrated in a neural circuit by means of synapses are submitted to a molecular wear and tear. The efflux of macromolecules must be exactly balanced by a corresponding influx. The regulation of the dynamic state of protein in neurons remains a

challenging problem. Several mechanisms are likely to control the maintenance of neuronal expansions and to adapt the turnover of protein to physiological conditions. First, Roberts et al. (3) have emphasized that the synthesis of polypeptide chains on polyribosomes of the nervous tissue is unusually sensitive to factors, e.g., the level of free amino acids, which qualitatively modulate protein synthesis. Moreover certain messenger ribonucleic acid-polyribosome complexes are extremely unstable; their easy dissociation may qualitatively prevent the synthesis of specific proteins and promote the synthesis of others. Second, the proximodistal axoplasmic transport may be adapted to axonal requirements; Lux et al. (23) have shown that neuron stimulation produces a tremendous increase of the amount of material transported per unit of time. A third mechanism acts upon the disappearance of axonal and synaptic macromolecules. Besides the enzymatic breakdown of protein which takes place in the whole axon (1), a secretory process of specific protein occurs at synapses when the transmitter is released from cathecholaminergic (24) or cholinergic (25) nerve endings. Unused presynaptic macromolecules, which are probably associated with membranes, are removed from axon terminals by retrograde axonal transport along the smooth endoplasmic reticulum and broken down in the cell body by lysosomes (6); metabolic products may influence in turn the nuclear transcription and the ribosomal translation (1,3). Thus it appears that every step of protein metabolism may contribute to the control of the steady state in neurons. However, in some cases, these delicate regulatory mechanisms seem to fail. Axons may undergo degenerative processes such as neuroaxonal dystrophy. In the huge ballooning of the altered axon terminals, the accumulation of membranous elements may result either from an overflow or from an inefficient removal of material. Until now the studies on the axonal transport in experimentally induced neuropathies did not permit a decisive conclusion. Future research should define the defecting regulatory process.

CONCLUSION

Maintenance of neuronal connectivity requires that two contradictory properties — integrity and adaptability of the synaptic junctions — must be conciliated (2). Only dynamic structures, which are continuously renewed by a flux of macromolecules, make it possible both to repair altered components in aging synaptic terminals (maintenance of integrity) and to revamp synaptic junctions by collateral sprouting (promotion of adaptability). To carry out this dynamic design, the neuron has to cope with a paradoxical situation. On one hand, the synaptic terminal synthesizes, stores, and releases the neurotransmitter; on the other hand, the metabolism of the neurotransmitter is controlled by specific proteins that are genetically programmed in the nucleus and synthesized by the perikaryal machinery. Thus to replenish the axon terminal, the neuron has to dispatch new enzymes, membrane components, and mitochondria; simultaneously, disused synaptic constituents have to be cleared up. Such a diversified and compartmentalized activity of the neuron could be considered as a molecular waste of information, energy, and structure; but at the integrated level of neural circuits, the expenses resulting from the dynamic condition of neuronal constituents are largely compensated by the unique advantage which is offered by the ability to maintain the functional integrity of interneuronal communication.

ACKNOWLEDGMENTS

I wish to thank Drs. G. Bennett, L. Di Giamberardino, H. L. Koenig, and A. Rambourg who have greatly contributed to our research project. I also express my gratitude to Mrs. J. Boyenval and R. Hässig for their appreciated assistance in the preparation of electron microscopic autoradiographs and illustrations. Drs. P. Gambetti and L. Autilio-Gambetti are especially acknowledged for their suggestions in writing the manuscript.

REFERENCES

1. Lajtha, A., and Marks, N. (1971): Protein turnover. In: *Handbook of Neurochemistry, Vol. 5B, Metabolic Turnover in the Nervous System,* edited by A. Lajtha, pp. 551–629. Plenum Press, New York.
2. Droz, B., and Koenig, H. L. (1970): Localization of protein metabolism in neurons. In: *Protein Metabolism of the Nervous System,* edited by A. Lajtha, pp. 93–108. Plenum Press, New York.
3. Roberts, S., Zomzely, C. E., and Bondy, S. C.

(1970): Protein synthesis in the nervous system. In: *Protein Metabolism of the Nervous System,* edited by A. Lajtha, pp. 3–37. Plenum Press, New York.
4. Gambetti, P., Autilio-Gambetti, L. A., Gonatas, N. K., and Shafer, B. (1972): Protein synthesis in synaptosomal fractions. Ultrastructural radioautographic study. *J. Cell Biol.,* 52:526–535.
5. Couteaux, R. (1974): Remarks on the organization of axon terminals in relation to secretory process at synapses. In: *Advances in Cytopharmacology, Vol. 2, Cytopharmacology of Secretion,* edited by B. Ceccarelli, F. Clementi, and J. Meldolesi, pp. 369–379. Raven Press, New York.
6. La Vail, J. H., and La Vail, M. M. (1974): The retrograde axonal transport of horseradish peroxidase in the chick visual system: A light and electron microscopic study. *J. Comp. Neurol.,* 157:303–358.
7. Droz, B., Koenig, H. L., and Di Giamberardino, L. (1973): Axonal migration of protein and glycoprotein to nerve endings. I. Radioautographic analysis of the renewal of protein in nerve endings of chicken ciliary ganglion after intracerebral injection of ^{3}H lysine. *Brain Res.,* 60:93–127.
8. Weiss, P., and Hiscoe, H. L. (1948): Experiments on the mechanism of nerve growth. *J. Exp. Zool.,* 107:315–396.
9. Droz, B., and Leblond, C. P. (1963): Axonal migration of proteins in the central nervous system and peripheral nerves as shown by radioautography. *J. Comp. Neurol.,* 121:325–346.
10. McEwen, B. S., and Grafstein, B. (1968): Fast and slow components in axonal transport of protein. *J. Cell Biol.,* 38:494–508.
11. Grafstein, B. (1975): Axonal transport: The intracellular traffic of the neuron. In: *The Handbook of the Nervous System, Vol. 1: Cellular Biology of Neurones,* edited by E. R. Kandel. American Physiology Society, Washington, D.C.
12. Guth, L. (1974): Axonal regeneration and functional plasticity in the central nervous system. *Exp. Neurol.,* 45:606–654.
13. Ochs, S. (1972): Fast transport of materials in mammalian nerve fibers. *Science,* 176:252–260.
14. Cuénod, M., Boesch, J., Marko, P., Perisic, M., Sandri, C., and Schonbach, J. (1972): Contributions of axoplasmic transport to synaptic structures and functions. *Int. J. Neurosci.,* 4:77–87.
15. Weiss, P. A. (1970): Neuronal dynamics and neuroplasmic flow. In: *The Neurosciences — Second Study Program,* edited by F. O. Schmitt, pp. 840–850. The Rockefeller University Press, New York.
16. Hendrickson, A. E., and Cowan, W. M. (1971): Changes in the rate of axoplasmic transport during postnatal development of the rabbit's optic nerve and tract. *Exp. Neurol.,* 30:403–422.
17. Frizell, M., and Sjöstrand, J. (1974): The axonal transport of slowly migrating ^{3}H leucine labelled proteins and the regeneration rate in regenerating

hypoglossal and vagus nerves of the rabbit. *Brain Res.*, 81:267–283.

18. Lasek, R. J., Joseph, B. S., and Whitlock, D. G. (1968): Evaluation of a radioautographic neuroanatomical tracing method. *Brain Res.*, 8:319–336.

19. Cowan, W. M., and Cuénod, M. (1975): *The Use of Axonal Transport for Studies of Neuronal Connectivity.* Elsevier, Amsterdam.

20. Attardi, G., Costantino, P., England, J., Lederman, M., Ojala, D., and Storries, B. (1973): Mitochondrial protein synthesis in HeLa cells. *Acta Endocrinol.*, Suppl. 180:263–293.

21. Barondes, S. H. (1966): On the site of synthesis of the mitochondrial protein of nerve endings. *J. Neurochem.*, 13:721–727.

22. Hajos, F., and Kerpel-Fronius, S. (1973): Comparative electron cytochemical studies of presynaptic and other neuronal mitochondria. *Brain Res.*, 62:425–429.

23. Lux, H. D., Schubert, P., Kreutzberg, G. W., and Globus, A. (1970): Excitation and axonal flow: Autoradiographic study on motoneurons intracellularly injected with a ^{3}H-amino acid. *Exp. Brain Res.*, 10:197–204.

24. De Potter, W. P., De Schaepdryver, H., Moerman, E., and Smith, A. D. (1969): Evidence for the release of vesicle proteins together with noradrenaline upon stimulation of the splanchnic nerves. *J. Physiol.* (Lond.), 204:102–104.

25. Musick, J., and Hubbard, J. I. (1972): Release of protein from mouse motor nerve terminals. *Nature,* 237:279–281.

26. Droz, B., Rambourg, A., and Koenig, H. L. (1975): The smooth endoplasmic reticulum: Structure and role in the renewal of axonal membrane and synaptic vesicles by fast axonal transport. *Brain Res.,* 93:1–13.

27. Droz, B., Koenig, H. L., and Di Giamberardino, L. (1974): *Actualités Neurophysiologiques, Vol. 10,* edited by A. M. Monnier, pp. 236–260. Masson, Paris.

The Nervous System, Donald B. Tower, Editor-in-Chief. *Vol. 1: The Basic Neurosciences*. Raven Press, New York, 1975.

Toward a Molecular Basis of Neuronal Recognition

Samuel H. Barondes

The recognition processes that determine intercellular associations in all tissues are probably most highly developed in the nervous system. Embryological studies have provided some insight into the rules for specification of neuronal connections (1-3). However, to fully understand cellular recognition, it will be necessary to isolate and characterize the specific molecules that mediate this process. This might be particularly difficult in the nervous system, where cellular interactions appear to be so complicated. Therefore, studies with simpler biological systems seem preferable to lay the ground work. Additional rules may be required to assure the graded specifications required for precise interneuronal interactions, but it is likely that the general rules followed in simpler systems will be conserved.

Present knowledge about cellular recognition is extremely limited. Most of the work on this subject is guided by some general ideas, which can be traced to proposals by Tyler (4) and Weiss (5). These ideas can be paraphrased as follows.

1. There are specific molecules on the surface of different cells that recognize each other.

2. The recognition molecules on the surface of two cells that recognize each other are probably complementary; i.e., the association is like that of an antigen with an antibody.

3. One or both of the recognition pair are probably proteins because of the many specific recognition sites that can be created with proteins.

In addition to these ideas, several others are also fairly widely held, although they are even more conjectural.

1. Carbohydrates on the cell surface are involved in cellular recognition. More specifically cellular recognition occurs by a specific association between an oligosaccharide receptor (in glycoprotein or glycolipid) on the surface of one cell with a protein specific for this oligosaccharide on the surface of another cell. I have,

in the past, reviewed the reasons for the appeal of this hypothesis (6).

2. Some of the recognition molecules, although associated with membranes, are, in Singer's terminology (7), "peripheral proteins" that can be readily isolated in aqueous solution without detergents. This is supported by some of the literature that will be reviewed below. However, it remains likely that some recognition molecules are "integral proteins" (7) that will not be solubilized from membranes without detergents.

3. The association between the complementary molecules involved in cell recognition is not always a simple binding association but may also involve enzymatic action of one of the components that thereby modifies the receptor. Roseman (8) proposes that a glycosyl transferase on the surface of one cell recognizes an oligosaccharide receptor on the other cell, which stabilizes their association. Upon transfer of a sugar residue to the oligosaccharide receptor from a sugar nucleotide, the cells may separate and a specific modification of the receptor may be achieved.

Each of these ideas has some experimental support. The purpose of this chapter is to review work that bears on the molecular basis of cellular recognition, briefly describe recent work from my laboratory on cellular recognition, and consider the implications of this work for neuronal recognition. A recent book (9) contains a more detailed discussion of many of these points.

STUDIES WITH SIMPLE METAZOA AND MICROORGANISMS

Sponge

The pioneering studies on cellular recognition were done with sponges. It was observed early in this century that when sponges are dissociated mechanically the cells will come together and reform an organism. Furthermore when cells from two species of sponge (that are distinguishable by their color) are mixed, the cells reassociate in a species-specific manner. Therefore, species-specific cellular recognition exists in this simple organism. Humphreys (10) and Moscona (11) showed that when sponges are dissociated in a sea water medium from which magnesium and calcium have been removed, the cells reassociate poorly. However, addition of a soluble factor from the medium plus divalent cations leads to cell association. The soluble factor from *Microciona parthena* has been shown to be a proteoglycan with an apparent molecular weight of about one million which consists of approximately 50% protein and 50% carbohydrate (12). The soluble factors from different species of sponge preferentially agglutinate the parent species (12). In one species of sponge, the agglutination mediated by the soluble sponge factor can be blocked by addition of glucuronic acid (but not other uronic acids) to the medium (13), suggesting that a molecular component of the association is dependent on macromolecular glucuronic acid, which is found in the soluble sponge factor. The major conclusions from this work are that there are species-specific proteoglycans in sponge that play a role in specific cellular adhesion, that the adhesion factors can be isolated in soluble form, although they are large macromolecular complexes, that the molecules are rich in carbohydrate, and that carbohydrates may play a role in some aspect of the cell adhesion process.

Chlamydomonas

These unicellar organisms have mating types. The mating types of each species associate specifically before transfer of genetic material. In a series of studies reviewed by Wiese (14), it has been shown that in some cases treatment of one mating type with proteolytic enzymes inactivates the type-specific mating reaction, whereas treatment of the other mating type has no effect. Conversely, glycosidase treatment inactivates only the mating type that is insensitive to the proteolytic enzymes. The inference is that mating involves association between a protein on one mating type with a carbohydrate receptor on the other mating type. Studies with yeast also show that glycoproteins are involved in this type of recognition phenomenon (15).

VERTEBRATE TISSUES

Adhesion Molecules from Vertebrate Tissues

Moscona (16) has recently reviewed work on soluble factors from vertebrate tissues which promote the aggregation of dissociated cells from the parent tissue. For example, Garber and Moscona (17,18) have shown that there are soluble macromolecules in the medium of cultures of embryonic cerebrum or cerebellum that can augment the association of dissociated cerebral or cerebellar cells, respectively. The substances are considered tissue specific (16), since only the substance from the homologous tissue augments cell association; but they do not appear to be cell specific (16) since both cerebral and cerebellar tissue contain many cell types, all of which associate in the mixed aggregate that is formed. Another example is a factor from neural retinal cells identified by Lilien, which augments the association of neural retinal cells but not brain cells (19). Balsamo and Lilien (20) found that aggregation-enhancing factors from chick neural retina and cerebrum, each labeled *in vivo* with radioactive glucosamine, bind respectively to neural retinal or cerebral cells. Since the factors are labeled with radioactive glucosamine, they are presumably glycoproteins. None of these substances has been completely purified so that their nature as well as the mechanism of promotion of cell association is presently unclear.

Specific Substances on Cell Surfaces and Cell Membranes

In pioneering studies Moscona and colleagues showed that mixtures of dissociated embryonic cells from two tissues reassociate in a tissue-specific way when rotated on a gyratory shaker (16). This suggests that there are substances on the surface of the cell membranes that mediate tissue-specific recognition. Using alternative assays Roth (21) and Walther et al. (22) have demonstrated similar findings. Merrel and Glaser (23) and Gottlieb et al. (24) have begun studies of the effects of membrane fragments obtained from chick neural retina, cerebellum, or tectum on specific association of cells from these tissues. They have shown that radioactive membranes obtained from neural retina bind preferentially to neural retinal cells as opposed to cerebellar cells, and that cerebellar membranes bind preferentially to cerebellar cells as opposed to neural retinal cells. They have also shown that the homotypic membrane fragments block adhesion and aggregation formation of the homotypic cells presumably by covering cell surface-binding sites. The membrane specificities change strikingly with development of the tissues. For example membranes from 7-day chick embryo retinal cells react strongly with 7-day retinal cells but not with 8- or 9-day retinal cells. Of particular interest for development of interneuronal relationships is the report by Barbera at al. (25) of specific association of dissociated retinal cells from one half of the retina with the half of the optic tectum where these cells would normally send their nerve terminals.

Cell Surface Glycosyl Transferases

Considerable evidence has been presented that there are glycosyl transferases on the surface of mammalian cells (reviewed in ref. 8). Glycosyl transferases on the surface of platelets apparently play a role in their adhesion to collagen (26). Recent evidence indicates that the mating types of a species of *Chlamydomonas* may contain specific receptors for glycosyl transferases of the opposite mating type (27).

Changes in Oligosaccharides on the Cell Surface of Mammalian Cells with Differentiation or Neoplastic Transformation

There has been considerable work in this general area. Two types of studies are done. In one type the cells are labeled with a radioactive sugar precursor (e.g., radioactive glucosamine) and the surface glycopeptides are released with a proteolytic enzyme. The glycopeptides (sometimes after more digestion) are then fractionated (e.g., by gel filtration). As an example of this approach, the surface glycopeptides obtained from neuroblastoma cells which are derived from clones that form neurites were compared with those of other clones that do not form neurites. The glycopeptide profiles of these two clones were discriminable (28). Another more popular approach is to study receptors on the surface of different cell types by determining if lectins, a class of plant agglutinins, bind to or agglutinate cells. There are many studies that indicate that neoplastic transformation of cells leads to alterations in agglutinability by various lectins. Changes in lectin interactions during cell maturation have also been observed. For example, Kleinschuster and Moscona (29) found that concanavalin A, a plant lectin, agglutinated retinal cells from early embryos but was less effective in agglutinating retinal cells from later stages of development. Studies of this type indicate that there are cell-surface changes with maturation either in the number of cell-surface receptors for the lectin or in their accessibility to lectins or their mobility in the membrane (30).

Inferences from This Work

It seems clear that there are discriminable recognition sites on the surface of different cells and of cells at different stages of maturation. There is recurrent evidence that substances that contain oligosaccharides may play a role in specific cellular associations and that the oligosaccharides themselves may specifically participate. Although many strategies of investigation are presently being pursued, the overall field is in a preliminary stage of development. One gets the sense that similar things are happening in the specific cellular associations found with simple eukaryotes and with vertebrate cells; but this impression will require much more substantial confirmation.

ADVANTAGES OF CELLULAR SLIME MOLDS FOR STUDIES OF CELL RECOGNITION

There are a number of advantages in using cellular slime molds for studies of specific cellular associations. (a) A large number of identical cells can be raised in culture; therefore cellular heterogeneity which would plague any studies of cellular recognition in a complex tissue are obviated. (b) The culture conditions resemble the natural environment of these organisms more closely than in culture of cells from metazoa. (c) The cells can be isolated in a vegetative (noncohesive) and a cohesive form. As long as the cells are grown on bacteria (which they eat), they do not aggregate into multicellular colonies; but when bacteria are removed the cells become cohesive and form multicellular aggregates within 9 to 12 hr. (d) When the cells from different species of slime mold are mixed they sort out into separate colonies each composed of slime mold cells of a single species (31,32). They therefore display species-specific cellular association.

Beug et al. (33–35) have emphasized the usefulness of cellular slime molds for studies of cellular association. They compared vegetative slime mold amoebae that are grown in the presence of bacteria and that show only weak intercellular associations (that can be blocked with appropriate concentrations of EDTA) with slime molds deprived of bacteria that are cohesive (not blocked by the same concentrations of EDTA). They raised antibodies to cohesive slime mold cells and adsorbed the antibodies with vegetative slime mold cells. The antibodies that did not bind to vegetative cells were degraded to a univalent form (Fab fragments) and were shown to block cohesion. This indicates that new antigens have appeared on the surface of cohesive slime molds and that these antigens presumably mediate cell cohesion. Because the antibodies specific for the cohesive cells are a heterogeneous mixture, it was not possible to use them as an analytical tool for isolation of the specific proteins involved in cohesion. Despite this limitation, the work demonstrated that discrete substances (identified as antigens) appear on the surface of cells as they become cohesive, and that these substances play a role in cohesiveness.

CARBOHYDRATE-BINDING PROTEINS MAY MEDIATE RECOGNITION IN CELLULAR SLIME MOLDS

In the past few years we have attempted to determine the precise mechanism for species-specific cellular association in cellular slime molds. This work, still in progress, will be summarized briefly here. Details are to be found in published papers, although some preliminary studies will also be mentioned. All the work supports the general hypothesis that species-specific carbohydrate-binding proteins and oligosaccharide receptors on the surface of cellular slime molds mediate cellular recognition.

Synthesis of Carbohydrate-Binding Proteins in Cellular Slime Molds as They Become Cohesive

As the cellular slime molds *Dictyostelium discoideum* (36) and *Polysphondylium pallidum* (37) differentiate from a vegetative to a cohesive state, they synthesize proteins that agglutinate erythrocytes. Formalinized erythrocytes of appropriate type are generally used for agglutination assays, since they are more stable than fresh erythrocytes. The agglutinins are carbohydrate-binding proteins, since the agglutination can be blocked by specific sugars. For example the agglutination of formalinized sheep erythrocytes by an agglutinin from *D. discoideum* was inhibited by 50% upon addition of 2 mM *N*-acetyl-D-galactosamine (36). Higher concentrations of this monosaccharide could completely inhibit agglutination. Several other monosaccharides, including D-galactose, also inhibited agglutination, but were less potent inhibitors. Still others (e.g., *N*-acetyl-D-glucosamine) were totally inactive when tested at concentrations up to 150 mM. This suggested that the agglutinin was like the carbohydrate-binding proteins called lectins (38) that have previously been observed in animal and vegetable tissues. Because of its affinity for D-galactose, the agglutinin from *D. discoideum* was adsorbed by a Sepharose column (made up of polymers of alternating D-galactose and 3,6-anhydro-L-galactose), whereas all the other proteins in the extracts were not adsorbed. The adsorbed agglutinin could then be eluted in pure form by washing the column with D-galactose (39). The purified protein was named discoidin.

Agglutinins from *D. discoideum* and *P. pallidum* Are Different

Agglutination activity from extracts of *P. pallidum* was also inhibited by specific saccharides (37). However, the relative potency of the saccharides as inhibitors was different from that observed with discoidin (37,40). Of the saccharides that affected *P. pallidum* agglutinin, lactose was the most potent. N-acetyl-D-galactosamine, the most potent inhibitor of discoidin, was a relatively weak inhibitor of *P. pallidum* agglutinin. The relative potencies of a number of other simple sugars also discriminated these agglutinins, which indicated that their carbohydrate-binding sites were different. These differences were also found after the agglutinin from *P. pallidum* was purified by an affinity adsorption procedure in which agglutination activity was quantitatively adsorbed onto formalinized erythrocytes and then eluted with D-galactose (37,41). The single pure protein that was recovered was named pallidin. Pallidin and discoidin differed in molecular weight, subunit molecular weight, isoelectric point, and amino acid composition (41). Further chemical characterization of the proteins and evaluation of the heterogeneity of discoidin are in progress (41a). Evidence for similar but discriminable agglutinins from four other species of cellular slime mold was recently presented (40).

The Agglutinins Present on the Cell Surface

Discoidin's presence on the cell surface was first shown by the finding that formalinized sheep erythrocytes formed rosettes around cohesive slime mold cells, which could be blocked by N-acetyl-D-galactosamine but not by N-acetyl-D-glucosamine (36). In subsequent studies an antibody raised to discoidin was shown to distribute on the surface of cohesive *D. discoideum* cells using immunofluorescent and immunoferritin techniques (42). The antibody did not bind to vegetative *D. discoideum* cells. A subcellular fraction from cohesive pallidin cells that is believed to be enriched in plasma membranes has recently been shown to be highly enriched in pallidin (*unpublished*).

Slime Mold Cohesion Can Be Blocked by Specific Sugars

When cohesive *P. pallidum* cells are heated under appropriate conditions, the cells retain cohesiveness as measured by formation of aggregates in a gyratory shaker and determination of aggregate formation using a Coulter Electronic Particle Counter (37). This cohe-siveness could be blocked by lactose or D-galactose (for which pallidin has a relatively high affinity) but not by identical concentrations of D-mannose or D-glucose. With further heat treatment, cohesiveness is diminished, but the heat-treated cells are agglutinable with pallidin. Again specific sugars block this reaction, whereas others do not (37). Recent experiments show that under appropriate conditions the cohesion of *D. discoideum* cells can be blocked by specific sugars and that glutaraldehyde-fixed *D. discoideum* cells can be agglutinated by discoidin and this agglutination is blocked by specific sugars.

Evidence for Specific Cell-Surface Receptors

Preliminary experiments (42a) indicate that glutaraldehyde-fixed vegetative *D. discoideum* cells are agglutinated only by high concentrations of discoidin, whereas cohesive cells fixed in the same manner are agglutinated much more effectively and with much lower concentrations of discoidin. Appearance of increased agglutinability roughly parallels the development of cohesiveness. Furthermore, fixed vegetative *D. discoideum* cells adsorb very little discoidin, whereas fixed cohesive *D. discoideum* cells adsorb much more. Preliminary studies also suggest that the affinity of glutaraldehyde-fixed cohesive *D. discoideum* cells for discoidin is about an order of magnitude greater than it is for pallidin and conversely that the affinity of glutaraldehyde-fixed *P. pallidum* cells for pallidin is about an order of magnitude greater than it is for discoidin.

Summary of Findings with Cellular Slime Molds

All the findings with cellular slime molds are consistent with the hypothesis that in differentiating from a vegetative to a cohesive state the cell surface is modified by addition of carbohydrate-binding proteins and molecules that contain oligosaccharide receptors. Both the carbohydrate-binding proteins and the receptors appear to be species-specific. Although considerable additional work is required, it appears that cellular recognition in cellular slime molds is mediated by specific carbohydrate-protein interactions at the cell surfaces. This provides strong support for previous speculations that similar reactions might occur in complex tissues (reviewed in ref. 6).

CONCLUSIONS

Whereas work on cellular recognition in the nervous system appears formidably complex, there is a growing body of work on the general problem of cellular recognition that will hopefully be relevant. The published work is all consistent with the hypothesis that specific cellular interaction is due to a reaction between complementary substances on the surface of adjacent cells. Much of the work is also consistent with the hypothesis that, at least in some cases, the complementary interaction is between a protein on one cell and an oligosaccharide receptor on the adjacent cell. It remains distinctly possible that other types of interactions may also be employed.

Assuming that these suggestions are substantiated, how could reactions of this type mediate specific interneuronal recognition? As inferred from studies of retinal-tectal connections (1–3) specification of both the retina and the tectum appear to be graded so that appropriate cells from any small region of the retina go to appropriate cells in a small region of the tectum. One way in which this might be achieved is by specifying each cell in the retina and tectum to synthesize a unique cell-surface protein that could interact only with the unique complementary protein. This seems unlikely since there are millions of retinal and tectal cells, which exceeds the number of genes for specific proteins in vertebrate DNA (unless there were some type of genetic splicing like that sometimes proposed to explain antibody diversity). A more likely possibility is that a gradation of relative affinities produces specific retinal-tectal associations (1,6). One way to think of this is in terms of an inductive gradient that spreads from the midline of an embryo and sets up a graded signal across both the retina and tectum that is highest near the midline and lowest most laterally. The signal could either be the concentration of the inductive substance or a secondary change that it produces. Systematic variation in the intensity of signal could lead to a permanent graded expression of a gene that controls a property of the cell surface. For example there could be graded expression of a gene that controls synthesis of the polypeptide backbone of a glycoprotein. The cells close to the midline during the inductive gradient would therefore have a large amount of the putative glycoprotein on their surface, whereas those very far from the midline would have very little. The cells might then associate in a manner whereby nerve endings rich in this glycoprotein preferred target cells that were poor in this substance, and conversely. In this way cells in the retina close to the midline during the inductive gradient would make synapses with cells in the optic tectum relatively far from the midline during the time of the inductive gradient. Similar inductive gradients could also determine the synthesis of another cell surface protein in another dimension (e.g., dorsal-ventral).

Clearly this hypothesis is highly speculative. Even if correct, it leaves other questions unanswered (e.g., why do retinal cells migrate to the tectum rather than elsewhere?). Again slime molds may offer an answer since specific chemotactic signals have been shown to orient and elicit the migration of slime mold cells toward an aggregation center (43,44). In the case of D. discoideum, the chemotactic signal is cyclic AMP (43,44), but different substances may be used in other species of slime molds. In a like manner, a diffusible chemotactic signal from the tectum might orient retinal cells and ensure their migration to the tectum; thereafter specific cellular associations could be mediated by graded cell surface changes like those proposed above.

ACKNOWLEDGMENTS

The research from my laboratory reported in this chapter was supported by U.S. Public Health Service Grant MH18282 from the National Institute of Mental Health and by a grant from the Alfred P. Sloan Foundation.

REFERENCES

1. Sperry, R. W. (1965): Embryogenesis of behavioral nerve nets. In: *Organogenesis*, edited by R. L. DeHaan and H. Ursprung, pp. 161–186. Holt, Rhinehart and Winston, New York.
2. Jacobson, M. (1970): *Developmental Neurobiology*. Holt, Rhinehart and Winston, New York.
3. Gaze, R. M. (1970): *The Formation of Nerve Connections*. Academic Press, New York.

4. Tyler, A. (1946): An auto-antibody concept of cell structure, growth and differentiation. *Growth,* 10:7–19.

5. Weiss, P. (1947): The problem of specificity in growth and development. *Yale J. Biol. Med.,* 19:235–278.

6. Barondes, S. H. (1970): Brain glycomacromolecules and interneuronal recognition. In: *The Neurosciences, Second Study Program,* edited by F. O. Schmitt, pp. 747–760. Rockefeller University Press, New York.

7. Singer, S. J. (1974): The molecular organization of membranes. *Ann. Rev. Biochem.,* 43:805–834.

8. Roseman, S. (1974): Complex carbohydrates and intercellular adhesion. In: *The Cell Surface in Development,* edited by A. A. Moscona, pp. 255–271. Wiley, New York.

9. Barondes, S. H., editor (1975): *Neuronal Recognition.* Plenum Press, New York.

10. Humphreys, T. (1963): Chemical dissolution and *in vitro* reconstruction of sponge cell adhesions. I. Isolation and functional demonstration of the components involved. *Dev. Biol.,* 8:27–47.

11. Moscona, A. A. (1963): Studies on cell aggregation: demonstrations of materials with selective cell-binding activity. *Proc. Natl. Acad. Sci. USA,* 49:742–747.

12. Henkart, P., Humphreys, S., and Humphreys, T. (1973): Characterization of sponge aggregation factor. A unique proteoglycan complex. *Biochemistry,* 12:3045–3050.

13. Kuhns, W. J., Weinbaum, G., Turner, R., and Burger, M. M. (1974): Sponge aggregation: a model for studies on cell-cell interactions. *Ann. N.Y. Acad. Sci.,* 234:58–74.

14. Wiese, L. (1974): Nature of sex specific glycoprotein agglutinins in *Chlamydomonas. Ann. N.Y. Acad. Sci.,* 234:383–395.

15. Crandall, M. A., and Brock, T. D. (1968): Molecular aspects of specific cell contact. *Science,* 161:473–475.

16. Moscona, A. A. (1964): Surface specification of embryonic cells: Lectin receptors, cell recognition and specific cell ligands. In: *The Cell Surface in Development,* edited by A. A. Moscona, pp. 67–99. Wiley, New York.

17. Garber, B. B., and Moscona, A. A. (1972): Reconstruction of brain tissue from cell suspensions. I. Aggregation patterns of cells from different regions of the developing brain. *Dev. Biol.,* 27:217–234.

18. Garber, B. B., and Moscona, A. A. (1972): Reconstruction of brain tissue from cell suspensions. II. Specific enhancement of aggregation of embryonic cerebral cells by supernatant from homologous cell cultures. *Dev. Biol.,* 27:235–243.

19. Lilien, J. E. (1968): Specific enhancement of cell aggregation *in vitro. Dev. Biol.,* 17:657–678.

20. Balsamo, J., and Lilien, J. (1974): Embryonic cell aggregation: kinetics and specificity of binding of enhancing factors. *Proc. Natl. Acad. Sci. USA,* 71:727–731.

21. Roth, S. (1968): Studies on intercellular adhesive selectivity. *Dev. Biol.,* 18:602–612.

22. Walther, B. T., Ohman, R., and Roseman, S. (1974): A quantitative assay for intercellular adhesion. *Proc. Natl. Acad. Sci. USA,* 70:1569–1573.

23. Merrell, R., and Glaser, L. (1973): Specific recognition of plasma membranes by embryonic cells. *Proc. Natl. Acad. Sci. USA,* 70:2794–2798.

24. Gottlieb, D. I., Merrell, R., and Glaser, L. (1974): Temporal changes in embryonal cell surface recognition. *Proc. Natl. Acad. Sci. USA,* 71:1800–1802.

25. Barbera, A. J., Marchase, R. B., and Roth, S. (1973): Adhesive recognition and retino-tectal specificity. *Proc. Natl. Acad. Sci. USA,* 70:2482–2486.

26. Jamieson, G. A., Urban, C. L., and Barber, A. J. (1971): Enzymatic basis to platelet: collagen adhesion as the primary step to haemostasis. *Nature New Biol.,* 234:5–7.

27. McLean, R. J., and Bosmann, H. B. (1974): Cell recognition: glycosyltransferases on the surface of *Chlamydomonas* gametes. *J. Cell Biol.,* 63:218a.

28. Glick, M. C., Kimhi, Y., and Littauer, U. Z. (1973): Glycopeptides from surface membranes of neuroblastoma cells. *Proc. Natl. Acad. Sci. USA,* 70:1682–1687.

29. Kleinschuster, S. J., and Moscona, A. A. (1972): Interaction of embryonic and fetal neural retina cells with carbohydrate-binding phytoagglutinins: cell surface changes with differentiation. *Exp. Cell. Res.,* 70:397–410.

30. Nicolson, G. L. (1974): The interactions of lectins with animal cell surfaces. *Int. Rev. Cytol.,* 39:89–190.

31. Raper, K. B., and Thom, C. (1941): Interspecific mixtures in the *Dictyosteliaceae. Am. J. Botany,* 28:69–78.

32. Bonner, J. T., and Adams, M. S. (1958): Cell mixtures of different species and strains of cellular slime moulds. *J. Embryol. Exp. Morphol.,* 6:346–356.

33. Beug, H., Gerisch, G., Kampff, S., Riedel, V., and Cremer, G. (1970): Specific inhibition of cell contact formation in *Dictyostelium* by univalent antibodies. *Exp. Cell. Res.,* 63:147–158.

34. Beug, H., Katz, F. E., Stein, A., and Gerisch, G. (1973): Quantitation of membrane sites in aggregating *Dictyostelium* cells by use of tritiated univalent antibody. *Proc. Natl. Acad. Sci. USA,* 70:3150–3154.

35. Beug, H., Katz, F. E., and Gerisch, G. (1973): Dynamics of antigenic membrane sites relating to cell aggregation in *Dictyostelium discoideum. J. Cell Biol.,* 56:647–658.

36. Rosen, S. D., Kafka, J., Simpson, D. L., and Barondes, S. H. (1973): Developmentally-regulated, carbohydrate-binding protein in *Dictyostelium discoideum. Proc. Natl. Acad. Sci. USA,* 70:2554–2557.

37. Rosen, S. D., Simpson, D. L., Rose, J. E., and Barondes, S. H. (1974): Carbohydrate-binding protein from *Polysphondylium pallidum* im-

plicated in intercellular adhesion. *Nature*, 252:128, 149–151.

38. Lis, H., and Sharon, N. (1973): The biochemistry of plant lectins (phytohemagglutinins). *Ann. Rev. Biochem.*, 42:541–574.

39. Simpson, D. L., Rosen, S. D., and Barondes, S. H. (1974): Discoidin, a developmentally regulated carbohydrate-binding protein from *Dictyostelium discoideum:* purification and characterization. *Biochemistry*, 13:3487–3493.

40. Rosen, S. D., Reitherman, R. W., and Barondes, S. H. (1975): Distinct lectin activities from six species of cellular slime molds. *Exp. Cell Res., in press.*

41. Simpson, D. L., Rosen, S. D., and Barondes, S. H. (1975): Pallidin: characterization of a carbohydrate-binding protein from *Polysphondylium pallidum* implicated in intercellular adhesion. *Biochim. Biophys. Acta, in press.*

41a. Frazier, W. A., Rosen, S. D., Reitherman, R. W., and Barondes, S. H. Purification and comparison of two developmentally regulated lectins from *Dictyostelium discoideum:* Discoidin I and II. *J. Biol. Chem., in press.*

42. Chang, C. M., Reitherman, R. W., Rosen, S. D., and Barondes, S. H. (1975): Cell surface localization of discoidin, a developmentally regulated carbohydrate-binding protein from *Dictyostelium discoideum. Exp. Cell Res., in press.*

42a. Reitherman, R. W., Rosen, S. D., Frazier, W. A., and Barondes, S. H. Cell surface species-specific high affinity receptors for discoidin: Developmental regulation in *D. discoideum. Proc. Natl. Acad. Sci. USA, in press.*

43. Bonner, J. T., Hall, E. M., Noller, S., Oleson, F. B., Jr., and Roberts, A. B. (1972): Synthesis of cyclic AMP and phosphodiesterase in various species of cellular slime molds and its bearing on chemotaxis and differentiation. *Dev. Biol.*, 29:402–409.

44. Robertson, A., and Grutsch, J. (1974): The role of cyclic AMP in slime mold development. *Life Sci.*, 15:1031–1043.

The Nervous System, Donald B. Tower, Editor-in-Chief. *Vol. 1: The Basic Neurosciences*. Raven Press, New York, 1975.

Axoplasmic Transport

Sidney Ochs

The commemoration of the 25th anniversary of the National Institute of Neurological and Communicative Disorders and Stroke is a particularly suitable occasion on which to give an account of axoplasmic transport. Over approximately this same period of time the concept of a material movement in nerve has been revitalized to become an accepted aspect of nerve function. On the basis of our present understanding of the molecular events underlying the nerve impulse, we require a supply of enzymes, structural proteins, and other components required to maintain the ionic asymmetry on which excitability depends. Some required component supplied by the cell body was indicated long ago by the loss of excitation and Wallerian degeneration of nerve fibers cut off from their cell bodies.

TECHNIQUES OF STUDY AND CHARACTERISTICS OF TRANSPORT

The swellings seen in the fibers above constrictions made in nerves were interpreted by Weiss and Hiscoe (1) to mean that all of the axoplasm moves or grows as a whole down the individual nerve fibers at a rate of approximately 1 to 3 mm/day. With the introduction of radioactive isotopes as tracers, the labeled precursor ^{32}P as orthophosphate was injected systemically into rats by Samuels and co-workers (2), so that, after its uptake by the nerve cell bodies and incorporation, the outflow of labeled components in the nerve could reveal such transport. In later studies the labeled precursor was injected by means of micropipettes into the nervous system either into the lower lumbar segments of the spinal cord of cats, the dorsal root ganglia, or applied to the brain. By this means the blood-brain barrier was bypassed and a high level of uptake and incorporation of labeled materials in the cell bodies was ensured. With this method a regular outflow of labeled components was seen in the roots and sciatic nerves and in the vagus or phrenic nerves as a declining exponential curve. A shift in the curves with time gave rates variously estimated as a few millimeters per day to 50 to 75 mm/day (3,4). Amino acids labeled with ^{3}H or ^{14}C were later employed. These were of particular interest, because it was recognized that the neuron is a cell with a high level of protein synthesis. A slow outflow of labeled proteins at a rate of several millimeters per day was seen by Droz and Leblond (5) using radioautography showing that the outflow was intracellular. Later, a fast transport of proteins of several hundred millimeters per day was found (6–12). Using the longer lengths of nerve available in the sciatic nerves of cats, the rate of fast axoplasmic transport could be definitely established by a crest of labeled proteins. The crest was seen to be moving outward in the fibers at a regular rate of 410 mm/day (9). Fast axoplasmic transport was found to be independent of myelinated nerve fiber diameter and the same rate was found in nonmyelinated fibers (9,11). The same fast rate was found in a wide variety of mammalian species and, interestingly, also in nonmammalian species, such as the garfish olfactory nerve (13) and frog nerve (14) when a temperature correction to the mammalian body temperature of 38°C was made.

Another technique of study introduced by Lubińska (4) and her colleagues was the use of ligations to study the transport of a normally present constituent, acetylcholinesterase (AChE). The pattern of accumulation of the enzyme above nerve ligations and its depletion within double-ligated segments showed in later studies that the transport of AChE in the fibers occurs at a fast rate. The transmitter norepinephrine (NE) was similarly studied in double-ligated adrenergic nerves by Dahlström (10). NE is seen as a fluorescent material which was correlated in electron micrographs with the dense granules or filled vesicles found in the sympathetic nerve terminals where it has a neurotransmitter function.

A related technique that depends on an accumulation of components at nerve terminals in the goldfish tectum was exploited by Grafstein (6). The precursor ³H-leucine or, better, ³H-proline is injected into one eye and, after uptake by the retinal ganglion cells and incorporation into proteins, is transported in optic nerve fibers to accumulate at the terminals ending in the tectum (fish) or lateral geniculate (rat, mouse). The curves of accumulation indicated the presence of both fast and slow rates.

It is possible to catalog the various components carried down the fibers at fast and slow rates. Using ³H-glucosamine, ³H-fucose, or ³⁵SO₄ as precursors, a fast transport of glycoproteins and glycolipids was found (12). A fast rate for phosphatidyl choline was reported using ³H-leucine, ³H-choline, or both as precursors (15). This observation suggests the fast transport of membrane-bound or membrane-forming substances.

When an amino acid such as ³H-leucine is used as a precursor for uptake by L7 dorsal ganglion cells or motoneuron cells, a wide variety of proteins and polypeptides are found labeled in the nerves. This was shown by the homogenization and differential centrifugation of nerves taken at various times after an injection of the precursor followed by a time allowed for downflow. The nerves are removed, homogenized, and subjected to differential centrifugation. Gel filtration and other procedures were used to separate various components in the high-speed supernatant (9). At early times, corresponding to fast axoplasmic transport, a higher proportion of the protein incorporated activity transported was found present in the small particulate fraction. A smaller amount of high and low molecular weight proteins, polypeptides, and some free leucine was also found present. At later times, corresponding to slow transport, a higher proportion of labeling was found in the high molecular soluble protein fraction and a lesser amount in other components.

In spite of the identification of some components with fast and slow transport, the inference that there are two different transport mechanisms in the fibers has recently come under question and further consideration of this point will be taken up after a discussion of the models proposed for the fast transport mechanism.

TRANSPORT MODELS

Fast-transported materials still move down the nerve at the same rate after the destruction of the nerve cell bodies. This shows that a local process in the fibers underlies transport. A similar behavior has also been shown for the garfish olfactory nerve by Gross and Beidler (13). Such observations have turned attention away from nonspecific forces, a diffusion or a peristaltic pumping of the fiber, as a driving force for axonal contents. Following the recognition of the important role played by microtubules in many different cells by K. Porter (16) and others, microtubules have been implicated as playing an important role in axoplasmic transport.

In one model where vesicles were the only constituent considered to be specifically carried down the fibers, a series of attachments of the vesicular surface to binding sites on the microtubules was visualized (8). These bonds were considered to be rapidly made and broken, thus allowing the vesicles to "roll" down the microtubules. This model did not take into account the wide range of components known to be transported in the fibers by fast axoplasmic transport, which in addition to vesicles or particules includes high molecular weight proteins, polypeptides, and free amino acids. All these components were seen in studies with Sabri to be transported at the same fast rate. In the "transport filament" hypothesis these components are considered to be bound to transport filaments which are moved down along the microtubules by means of cross-bridges, the requisite energy for cross-bridge action supplied by ATP (9).

In a later extension of the model, a unitarian view was advanced to account also for slow-transported components (17). These are considered to be less firmly bound to the transport filaments than fast-transported materials and to come off the transport filaments more readily to become locally incorporated into nerve fiber structures. On this basis we can account for the outflow patterns seen in the plateau region behind the crest and as well the shifts with time in the declining exponential curve of slow transport. The unitary view can account for the various transport rates reported for the mitochondrion. Using dark-field or Nomarski optics microscopy, a fast forward and as well a fast retrograde movement of mitochondria has been observed (18). Yet, on the basis of accumulation studies (19–21) a net slow transport of mitochondria was seen. In the unitarian view, this can be explained by the repeated binding and unbinding of the mitochondria to transport filaments that move along two sets of microtubules, one directing movement down the fiber in the orthograde direction, the other in the retrograde direction back toward the cell body.

ENERGETICS OF TRANSPORT

An important aspect of the transport filament hypothesis is that a supply of energy is required for the movement of the transport filament. A dependence of fast axoplasmic transport on $\sim P$ [combined ATP + creatine phosphate] was found (9). With nerves transporting labeled components *in vitro,* a block of oxidative phosphorylation by N_2 anoxia or the addition of cyanide, dinitrophenol, or azide all caused a block of fast axoplasmic transport within approximately 15 min. At that time the level of $\sim P$ fell to half, from about 1.2 $\mu M/g$ to 0.6 $\mu M/gm$. When the citric acid cycle was blocked with fluoracetate, transport failed after approximately 1 hr and with glycolysis blocked by iodoacetate (IAA), in approximately 1.5 hr. In all cases $\sim P$ also fell to half at the time when axoplasmic transport was blocked. The utilization of ATP would require an ATPase present at the crossbridges. An actinomyosin-like Mg,Ca-ATPase similar to that found in brain by Berl et al. (22) was found in cat sciatic nerve in studies with Khan (23). Its localization is as yet unknown.

Using the fast transport of mitochondria visualized in chicken nerve by Nomarski optics microscopy, N_2 anoxia and the metabolic blocking agents CN, DNP, and IAA were all shown to be analogous in their block of movement to the blocking effects of those agents on the downflow of labeled proteins (18). The presence of glucose as an exogenous metabolite was not needed to maintain *in vitro* transport for hours in the microscopical studies indicating, as in experiments on labeled protein transport, that an adequate supply of endogenous metabolite is present within the nerve fibers.

MEMBRANE-TRANSPORT MECHANISM RELATIONSHIPS

The evidence that fast axoplasmic transport depends on ATP requires that we consider the nature of the supply of ATP to both the transport mechanism and to the sodium pump. A common pool of ATP seems to be involved. This was indicated by studies made in chambers where action potentials could be elicited from the same nerves in which fast axoplasmic transport was also going on. When anoxia was initiated by replacing the O_2 in the chamber with N_2, both action potentials and axoplasmic transport were blocked in about 15 min, at the time when $\sim P$ fell to half its control level.

An excitable membrane is not, however, a necessary condition for the continued operation of the fast axoplasmic transport mechanism. With procaine present to block excitability, fast axoplasmic transport was unchanged (9). Similarly, lidocaine and halothane were found to block excitability without effecting fast axoplasmic transport. Only at higher concentration do these two agents block transport by an action inside the fibers. Tetrodotoxin (TTX) blocks excitability by blocking Na channels and has little effect on transport. However, batrachotoxin (BTX), which blocks excitability by keeping Na channels in an open state, was recently found by Ochs and Worth (24) to block fast axoplasmic transport in very low concentrations, at less than 0.2 μM. That work has suggested the possibility that BTX acts on the transport mechanism itself.

A coupling between the membrane and the transport mechanism was looked for by stimulating nerves *in vitro* at high rates while transport was going on. No changes in rate (25) had been seen by Lubińska and her colleagues in the fast transport of AChE. In work with Smith (26), a small 10% decrease was reported. However, recent studies with Worth showed stimulation at rates up to 350 pps to have no effect on transport. Small apparent changes were traced to a temperature difference and other factors not related to transport *per se.* High rates of stimulation also did not change the level of ATP and CP indicating a sufficient supply of $\sim P$ to the pump mechanism in the membrane and the transport mechanism within the fiber.

MICROTUBULES AND TRANSPORT

Evidence that microtubules play a role in axoplasmic transport has come from studies of colchicine and the vinca alkaloids vinblastine and vincristine. These agents are known to block the division of cells by causing a disassembly of the microtubules forming the spindles. They act by binding to the protein subunit of the microtubules, the tubulin. The mitotic blocking agents were also shown to interrupt fast axoplasmic transport first by Dahlström (27) and Kreutzberg (28) and more recently by Austin and Banks and their associates (29, 30). However, a disassembly of microtubules into their tubulin subunits may not account for the block of transport seen in all nerves. Colchicine can cause block of transport in crayfish ventral cord axons without a disruption of microtubular morphology, as shown in electron micrographs (31). On the other hand, studies of other nerves have shown a reduced number of microtubules indicative of disassembly after treatment with colchicine (32). After exposure to vincristine the disassembled tubulin may be reaggregated into a lattice pattern, as seen in electron micrographs.

Microtubules are disassembled at low temperatures as indicated by the reduction of microtubules in electron micrograph preparations in toad nerves by Rodriguez-Echandia and Piezzi. In mammalian nerves fast axoplasmic transport *in vitro* is blocked by bringing the nerves to temperatures below 11°C, as shown by studies with Smith (33). This cold-block persists indefinitely and it could very well be due to a disassembly of the microtubules. After a period of cold-block lasting some 12 to 18 hr, a return of the nerves to a temperature of 38°C results in a resumption of fast axoplasmic transport. Therefore, if the microtubules do in fact disassemble as a result of cold-block, they apparently can reassemble within some 0.5 to 1.0 hr on rewarming. The transport filaments which come free in the axoplasm on disassembly would have to find their way back onto the reassembled microtubules to resume transport.

The turnover of protein in the microtubules is of considerable interest. Microtubules do not rapidly grow into the fiber. Most probably the microtubules undergo a continual partial disassembly and reassembly all along their length. Some recent studies of purified tubulin caused to assemble show, however, a coiling of the growing chains making up the wall of the microtubules with addition of the subunits at the ends of the chains. Further studies of microtubular assembly and disassembly in purified systems should help reveal the process of microtubular assembly and help our understanding of how this occurs in the nerve fiber.

DIFFERENTIAL ROUTING IN NERVE BRANCHES

In the monkey, where the dorsal roots are sufficiently long, the rate of fast transport was determined by the position of the crests of outflow in the roots as well as in the nerve. These studies revealed similar rates but a three- to fivefold greater amount of labeled activity in the crest moving down the peripheral nerve as compared to the dorsal root (9). The neurons of the L7 dorsal root ganglion branch in T-fashion with one branch entering the root, the other branch the sciatic nerve. The asymmetry of downflow seen after L7 ganglion injection with ^{3}H-leucine cannot be simply accounted for by a difference in the diameters of the fiber branches entering the nerves as compared to the root, as was shown in studies with Erdman (34). The numbers of microtubules or neurofilaments in comparable fibers of the two branches of the L7 dorsal root ganglion neurons were also found to be closely similar, so that the disparity in the amounts of labeled components transported cannot be ascribed to that factor. These findings lead therefore to consideration of a separate routing of components into the two branches of the same neuron. On the basis of the transport filament hypothesis, different sets of transport filaments move down along the microtubules, one set passing down into the root branch, the other set along microtubules leading into the nerve branch. By such routing, the cell can exert a control over the amount and, perhaps more important, the type of materials destined for each branch. We would expect that different materials are required to supply the sensory terminals of the peripheral branch and the branch entering the cord ending as presynaptic terminals to effect synaptic transmission.

RETROGRADE TRANSPORT

Various hypotheses have been advanced to account for the phenomenon of chromatolysis seen in the cell bodies starting a week or so after an interruption of their fibers and lasting several months. The most likely hypothesis is that the chromatolysis comes about through the failure of some signal substance, which normally continuously ascends along the fibers to reach the cell body and there to regulate the level of protein synthesis. If, as seems likely, the signal material acts as a negative feedback control, its lack as a result of nerve interruption would result in an increased protein synthesis in the cell body.

A retrograde transport of material was first shown for the nerve by Lubińska (4), who found an accumulation of AChE below ligations made in the nerve as well as above such ligations. Lubińska and Niemierko (35) have shown that AChE has a fast rate of transport, and in studies with Ranish (36) a still faster rate was found, one close to that of axoplasmic transport measured by labeled proteins. In both studies the rate of retrograde movement was found to be approximately half that of the forward rate. A retrograde transport was also shown for horseradish peroxidase (37,38). The enzyme is taken up by the nerve terminals, and then it appears soon after in the nerve cell bodies. LaVail and LaVail (39) indicate that its retrograde rate of movement is over 84 mm/day, but the rate has not as yet been definitively measured. In the older literature, toxins and viruses have been reported as moving upward within nerve fibers, and recent studies by Kristensson et al. (40) showing a retrograde movement of herpesvirus appear to substantiate the phenomenon. No doubt a number of other viral and toxic agents will be investigated again in the light of what is now known of retrograde transport.

During chromatolysis the rate of axoplasmic transport has been reported as being increased, decreased, or unchanged. Most of these studies were based on the accumulation of materials at ligations or terminals as a measure of rate. Using crest outflow in the sciatic nerve to measure the rate of fast transport, no change in the rate was seen in the fibers of chromatolytic cells, as compared to normal controls. Studies of transport in newborn kittens where the level of protein synthesis of neurons is higher than that of the mature animals have also shown little difference in the rate of fast axoplasmic transport as compared to the rate in mature animals. Such findings indicate that the mechanism responsible for fast axoplasmic transport in the fibers is relatively independent of those processes underlying synthesis of materials in the cell body or its overall level. This may be termed provisionally as the independence principle of axoplasmic transport. It is too early, however, to exclude definitely the possibility that some regulatory substances continually produced either in the cell body or substances passing from the nerve terminals may have some effect in regulating the rate of transport within the fiber.

TRANSPORT IN CNS NERVE FIBERS

On entering the cord, a branch of the dorsal root fibers ascends within the dorsal columns of the spinal cord. After L7 ganglion injection with ^{3}H-leucine, a crest of incorporated activity is seen in the dorsal columns to move at a rate close to that found for peripheral nerve (9). Such studies make it appear likely that the same fast axoplasmic transport mechanism is present in other CNS fibers, although this has not been confirmed by crest movement in other long tract systems. Other techniques, however, have shown axoplasmic transport in neurons of the brain and cord. By making cuts at various points in the brainstem and cortex and finding an accumulation in the fibers facing the cell body of origin with their depletion in fibers distal to the cut, cholinergic and three well-defined monamine systems of neurons have been discovered in the brain. Such systems and their properties are described by Bloom (elsewhere in this volume).

NERVE TERMINALS—TRANSMITTER AND TROPHIC SUBSTANCES

At the neuromuscular junction, the transmitter acetylcholine (ACh) is hydrolyzed by AChE located in the postsynaptic membrane, and the choline hydrolyzed from ACh is taken back into the motor nerve terminal to be resynthesized to ACh. The question as yet unresolved is how much transmitter is being carried down the nerve fibers and how much ACh is locally reconstituted. This pertains also to the adrenergic nerves where NE and dopamine are known to be transported down the fibers as well as dopamine-β-hydroxylase and tyrosine hydroxylase, enzymes involved in the synthesis of transmitter locally within the nerve terminals (41).

Some components other than transmitter may be required for the maintenance of neurotransmission. Miledi and Slater (42) found that the loss of miniature end-plate potential (MEPP) activity some time following nerve section occurred sooner on cutting the nerve close to the muscle than it did at a higher level. The estimated time of movement of some factor in nerve maintaining transport was 360 mm/day, a rate close enough to the 410 mm/day rate found for the movement of labeled proteins in rat nerves to consider that the same fast transport system is responsible.

The glycoproteins found located in the synaptic cleft are likely to play an important role in transmission. It is of interest that glycoproteins are carried down the nerve fiber by fast axoplasmic transport, presumably followed by their translocation into the synaptic cleft (43).

Direct evidence for a translocation of materials from the nerve to the postsynaptic cell is limited. Korr and his colleagues (44) indicated an entry of labeled material from motor nerves to muscle using radioautography, and Grafstein (45) reported a movement of labeled material from retina through the lateral geniculate accumulated in the striate cortex. At present, however, it is uncertain whether this evidence represents a specific transfer of material or a nonspecific spread of labeled components from the nerve terminals.

Trophic substances transported in the nerve fibers are released from their terminals to enter the postsynaptic cell and to modify its functional state. This is suggested by the changed excitability, contractility, metabolism, and eventual overall size of muscle fibers, which follows at various times after section of its nerve supply (46). This is also indicated by the conversion of fast-contracting to slow-contracting muscle and slow-contracting to fast-contracting muscle after cutting their nerves and cross-innervating

the muscles, so that after nerve regeneration the muscles receive a new nerve input. The cross-innervated muscles become changed in accord with their new nerve supply, most likely due to their different supply, as shown by Buller et al. (47).

The various trophic factors so far studied act at different times after nerve section. The lag in the onset of metabolic changes of muscle seen when the nerve supply is cut far from the muscle and close to it was shown for metabolic changes by Gutmann (48) and the appearance of fibrillation by Luco and Eyzaguirre (49) to be relatively slow, compared to the rapid appearance of TTX-resistant action potentials in denervated muscle found by Harris and Thesleff (50) and the decrease in the level of resting membrane starting at the end-plate region by Albuquerque et al. (51). These time differences support the concept that different trophic materials move down the nerve.

The synthesis of ACh receptor protein, which normally in the mature animal is found predominantly in the end-plate region, appears to be under the control of a trophic substance supplied by the nerve. On denervation, ACh sensitivity was seen some days later to spread out into the muscle membrane from the end-plate region by Thesleff (52) and by Miledi (53). Actinomyosin D blocks the formation of new receptor protein indicating that the trophic substance likely acts by repressing the level of receptor protein synthesis at the DNA level.

The possibility that changed muscle states occur as a result of nerve activity was studied by the chronic application of local anesthetics applied through cuffs placed around the nerve in order to block nerve impulse conduction. A block of nerve activity may not, however, be the only effect produced when certain local anesthetics, such as lidocaine, are used (54). This agent can enter the fibers to effect at least a partial block of axoplasmic transport. At certain concentrations, muscle changes were seen after chronic application of colchicine or vinblastine without the nerves losing their excitability or the ability to discharge neurotransmitter distal to the block (55). In other cases, as shown by Persic and Cuenod (56) and by Pilar and Landmesser (57), transmission was blocked. Thus colchicine, the vinca alkaloids, and certain local anesthetics that can enter the fibers may selectively interfere with the transport of some, but not all transported components depending on the concentration and the time the agents have been applied to the nerve. A transport of such agents down to the terminal to interfere with the release of some substances and not others is also possible. An explication of this phenomenon should have important consequences for our understanding of the mechanisms of transmission and could perhaps serve as a useful tool to produce a selective block of some and not of other components.

SUMMARY AND FUTURE EXPECTATIONS

At various points in this review, possible future studies to extend our information or to test the implications of ideas so far developed

have been noted. It will be useful here to consider the information that has been gained and to use it in a framework with which to suggest expected new advances.

The main point to be made is that the neuron must now be seen as an integrated entity. This view of nerve integration is shown in the diagram of Fig. 1. In Fig. 1A, the cell body region, protein synthesis takes place as indicated at the ribosomes, the nucleus controlling the kinds of proteins made. The compartment indicates the storage of some types of proteins, which only later are transported into the axon, as is shown after a pulse of labeled precursor is presented to the cell. The timing and release of substances from the cell for export into its own axon should be a fertile field of future investigation. The release of incorporated materials from the cell into the axon appears to be

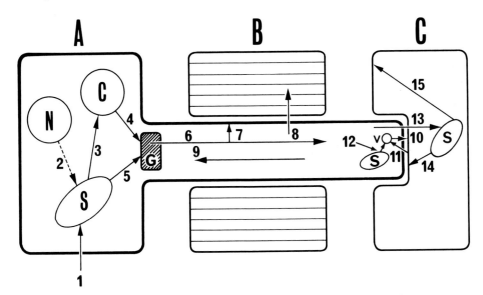

FIG. 1. Diagrammatic representation of the neuron. Cell regions indicated are: **(A)** cell body, **(B)** nerve fiber, and **(C)** terminal region with a synapse on a muscle fiber. **(A)** Upon entry of precursor (1), the nucleus (N) controls (2) the level and type of synthesis (S) with arrow (3) showing a compartmentalization (C) of synthesized materials. From the synthetic site and the compartment, materials move at different times into the axon (4, 5) with (G) the Golgi apparatus controlling egress into the axon. The transport system moving materials down the nerve fiber is shown by (6). Arrows to the membrane (7) show an insertion of components into the axonal membrane and components passing to the Schwann cell (8), the latter having a control over the myelin sheath (horizontal lines) form and function. A retrograde axoplasmic transport in the axon is indicated by an arrow directed back to the cell body (9). In the terminal region C, vesicles (V) involved in synaptic transmission are shown (10) passing contents to the synaptic cleft with also a local reconstitution of transmitter in vesicles (11). Synthesis of transmitter and transmitter-related components within the terminal is indicated by (S) with a contribution of transported components or control materials by (12). An arrow from the nerve terminal entering the postsynaptic cell, in the example the muscle fiber (13), indicates the movement of trophic materials. One of these control synthesis (S) of receptor protein is inserted into the membrane in the end-plate region normally (14) and, if the trophic control is lost, into new receptor sites outside the end-plate region (15).

controlled by a gate which could be the Golgi apparatus. The gate may perhaps be the site where some transported components are packaged or perhaps bound on to the transport filaments for transport down the fiber.

In region B, the axoplasmic transport system in the axon is indicated which, on the unitary concept, accounts for both fast and slow transport. In the latter case, components more readily come off the transport filaments for local incorporation. The membrane has recently been viewed by Singer as a phospholipid bilayer with globular proteins embedded in it. Some of these proteins probably confer a selective permeability to the membrane, e.g., act as channels for Na^+ and K^+ and other ions on which excitability depends. A number of proteins, including the enzyme Na,K-ATPase which moves down slowly as shown in studies with Iqbal, must be inserted into the membrane. These proteins as they are turned over are replaced by the transport system as part of a continuous process. The isolation and identification of the various enzymes and components required to maintain the form and function of the nerve are vitally needed.

The Schwann cells of the axon region also require some control material by the axon, as indicated by the Wallerian degeneration seen in the distal part of a transected nerve. A specification of that substance, or substances, would be of great interest with respect to our understanding and control of the demyelinating diseases.

The retrograde transport system present in the axon is considered to carry a signal substance back to the cell body to regulate the level of proteins synthesized in the cell body. A knowledge of the nature of this signal substance and how its control is accomplished within the cell would greatly advance our knowledge of the processes controlling protein metabolism throughout the nervous system.

Finally, in region C, the nerve terminal, the mechanisms of synthesis or translocation of transmitter in synaptic vesicles would be advanced by a better knowledge of what control and supply materials are carried down to the terminals by the transport mechanism. Sensory transduction will probably also depend on such mechanisms.

Several trophic materials move from the nerve terminal into the postsynaptic cell to modify the function of the postsynaptic cells. This includes some trophic control over the synthesis of receptor protein and other materials leading to changed membrane excitability and overall metabolism changes in the postsynaptic cell. An identification and specification of the range of trophic substances so far indicated would be of obvious fundamental importance.

As part of the immediate program of future research, the mechanism of transport requires further study. The transport filament model is a hypothesis that requires further substantiation. An isolation and identification of the transport filaments is a goal much to be desired.

There seems little doubt that on the basis of what has been gained so far, a better understanding of the mechanism and the properties of axoplasmic transport will bring about a better understanding of the nervous system. We can now visualize the neuron as an integrated unit and, through trophic control, an integrating element of the nervous system. A further understanding of those processes will no doubt lead to a new therapy of long-standing clinical problems.

REFERENCES

1. Weiss, P., and Hiscoe, H. B. (1948): Experiments on the mechanism of nerve growth. *J. Exp. Zool.*, 107:315–395.
2. Samuels, A. J., Boyarsky, L. L., Gerard, R. W., Libet, B., and Brust, M. (1951): Distribution exchange and migration of phosphate compounds in the nervous system. *Am. J. Physiol.*, 164:1–15.
3. Miani, N. (1963): Analysis of the somato-axonal movement of phospholipids in the vagus and hypoglossal nerves. *J. Neurochem.*, 10:859–874.
4. Lubińska, L. (1964): Axoplasmic streaming in regenerating and in normal nerve fibers. In: *Mechanisms of Neural Regeneration. Progress in Brain Research, Vol. 13*, edited by M. Singer, and J. P. Schade. Elsevier, Amsterdam.
5. Droz, B., and Leblond, C. P. (1963): Axonal migration of proteins in the central nervous system and peripheral nerves as shown by radioautography. *J. Comp. Neurol.*, 121:325–346.
6. Grafstein, B. (1967): Transport of protein by goldfish optic nerve fibers. *Science*, 157:196–198.
7. Lasek, R. J. (1970): Protein transport in neurons. *Int. Rev. Neurobiol.*, 13:289–324.
8. Schmitt, F. O. (1968): Fibrous proteins-neuronal organelles. *Proc. Natl. Acad. Sci. USA*, 60:1092–1101.
9. Ochs, S. (1974): Systems of material transport in nerve fibers (axoplasmic transport) related to

nerve function and trophic control. *Ann. N.Y. Acad. Sci.*, 228:202–223.

10. Dahlström, A. (1971): Axoplasmic transport with particular respect to adrenergic neurons. *Phil. Trans. R. Soc. [Biol.]*, 261:325–358.

11. Byers, M. R., Hendrickson, A. E., Fink, B. R., Kennedy, R. D., and Middaugh, M. E. (1973): Effects of lidocaine on axonal morphology, microtubules, and rapid transport in rabbit vagus nerve in vitro. *J. Neurobiol.*, 4:125–143.

12. Barondes, S. H., and Dutton, G. R. (1972): Protein metabolism in the nervous system. In: *Basic Neurochemistry*, Chapt. 12, edited by R. W. Albers, G. J. Siegel, R. Katzman, and B. W. Agranoff. Little, Brown and Co., Boston.

13. Gross, G. W., and Beidler, L. M. (1973): Fast axonal transport in the C-fibers of the garfish olfactory nerve. *J. Neurobiol.*, 4:413–428.

14. Edström, A., and Hanson, M. (1973): Temperature effects on fast axonal transport of proteins *in vitro* in frog sciatic nerves. *Brain Res.*, 58:345–354.

15. Abe, T., Haga, T., and Kukokawa, M. (1973): Rapid transport of phosphatidylcholine occurring simultaneously with protein transport in the frog sciatic nerve. *Biochem. J.*, 136:731–740.

16. Porter, K. R. (1966): Cytoplasmic microtubules and their functions. In: *Principles of Biomolecular Organization*. Ciba Foundation Symposium, edited by G. E. W. Wolstenholme and M. O'Conner, pp. 308–356. Little, Brown, Boston.

17. Ochs, S. (1975): A unitary concept of axoplasmic transport based on the transport filament hypothesis. *Third International Congress on Muscle Diseases*. Newcastle upon Tyne, edited by W. G. Bradley, D. Gardner-Medwin, and J. N. Walton.

18. Kirkpatrick, J. B., Bray, J. J., and Palmer, S. M. (1972): Visualization of axoplasmic flow *in vitro* by Nomarski microscopy. Comparison to rapid flow of radioactive proteins. *Brain Res.*, 43:1–10.

19. Barondes, S. H. (1966): On the site of synthesis of the mitochondrial protein of nerve endings. *J. Neurochem.*, 13:721–727.

20. Jeffrey, P. L., James, K. A. C., Kidman, A. D., Richards, A. M., and Austin, L. (1972): The flow of mitochondria in chicken sciatic nerve. *J. Neurobiol.*, 3:199–208.

21. Khan, M. A., and Ochs, S. (1975): Slow axoplasmic transport of mitochondria MAO and lactic dehydrogenase in mammalian nerve fiber. *Brain Res., in press.*

22. Berl, S., Puszkin, S., and Nicklas, W. (1973): Actomyosin-like protein in brain. *Science*, 179:441–446.

23. Khan, M. A., and Ochs, S. (1974): Magnesium or calcium activated ATPase in mammalian nerve. *Brain Res.*, 81:413–426.

24. Ochs, S., and Worth, R. (1975): Batrachotoxin block of fast axoplasmic transport in mammalian nerve fibers. *Science*, 187:1087–1089.

25. Jankowska, E., Lubińska, L., and Niemierko, S. (1969): Translocation of AChE-containing particles in the axoplasm during nerve activity. *Comp. Biochem. Physiol.*, 28:907–913.

26. Ochs, S., and Smith, C. (1971): Effect of temperature and rate of stimulation on fast axoplasmic transport in mammalian nerve fibers. *Fed. Proc.*, 30:665.

27. Dahlström, A. (1968): Effect of colchicine on transport of amine storage granules in sympathetic nerves of rat. *Eur. J. Pharmacol.*, 5:111–113.

28. Kreutzberg, G. W. (1969): Neuronal dynamics and axonal flow. IV. Blockage of intra-axonal enzyme transport by colchicine. *Proc. Nat. Acad. Sci. USA*, 62:722–728.

29. James, K. A. C., Bray, J. J., Morgan, I. G., and Austin, L. (1970): The effect of colchicine on the transport of axonal protein in the chicken, *Biochem. J.*, 117:767–771.

30. Banks, P., Mayor, D., Mitchell, M., and Tomlinson, D. (1971): Studies on the translocation of noradrenaline-containing vesicles in post-ganglionic sympathetic neurons *in vitro*. Inhibition of movement by colchicine and vinblastine and evidence for the involvement of axonal microtubules. *J. Physiol.*, 216:625–639.

31. Fernandez, H. L., Huneeus, F. C., and Davison, P. F. (1970): Studies on the mechanism of axoplasmic transport in the crayfish cord. *J. Neurobiol.*, 1:395–409..

32. Samson, F. E. (1971): Mechanism of axoplasmic transport. *J. Neurobiol.*, 2:347–360.

33. Ochs, S., and Smith, C. (1975): Low temperature slowing and cold-block of fast axoplasmic transport in mammalian nerves *in vitro*. *J. Neurobiol.*, 6:85–102.

34. Ochs, S., and Erdman, J. (1974): "Routing" of fast transported materials in nerve fibers. *Abst. Soc. Neurosci.*, 4:359.

35. Lubińska, L., and Niemierko, S. (1970): Velocity and intensity of bidirectional migration of acetylcholinesterase in transected nerves. *Brain Res.*, 27:329–342.

36. Ranish, N., and Ochs, S. (1972): Fast axoplasmic transport of acetylcholinesterase in mammalian nerve fibers. *J. Neurochem.*, 19:2641–2649.

37. LaVail, J., and LaVail, M. (1972): Retrograde axonal transport in the central nervous system. *Science*, 176:1416–1417.

38. Kristensson, K., and Olsson, Y. (1971): Retrograde axonal transport of protein. *Brain Res.*, 29:363–365.

39. LaVail, J., and LaVail, M. (1974): Intra-axonal transport of horseradish peroxidase following intravitreal injections in chicks. *Abst. Soc. Neurosci.*, 4:299.

40. Kristensson, K., Lycke, E., and Sjöstrand, J. (1971): Spread of herpes simplex virus in peripheral nerves. *Acta Neuropathol.*, 17:44–53.

41. Geffen, L. B., and Livett, B. G. (1971): Synaptic vesicles in sympathetic neurons. *Physiol. Rev.*, 51:98–157.

42. Miledi, R., and Slater, C. R. (1970): On the degeneration of rat neuromuscular junctions after nerve section. *J. Physiol.*, 207:507–528.

43. Karlsson, J. O., and Sjöstrand, J. (1971): Rapid intracellular transport of fucose-containing glyco-

proteins in retinal ganglion cells. *J. Neurochem.*, 18:2209–2216.

44. Korr, I. M., Wilkinson, P. N., and Chornock, F. W. (1967): Axonal delivery of neuroplasmic components to muscle cells. *Science*, 155:343–345.

45. Grafstein, B. (1971): Transneuronal transfer of radioactivity in the central nervous system. *Science*, 172:177–179.

46. Drachman, D. B., editor (1974): Trophic functions of the neuron. *Ann. N.Y. Acad. Sci.*, 288: 1–423.

47. Buller, A. J., Eccles, J. C., and Eccles, R. M. (1960): Differentiation of fast and slow muscles in the cat hind limb. *J. Physiol.*, 150:399–416.

48. Gutmann, E. (1964): Neurotrophic relations in the regeneration process. In: *Mechanisms of Neural Regeneration. Progress in Brain Research, Vol. 13*, edited by M. Singer, and J. P. Schade, pp. 72–112. Elsevier, Amsterdam.

49. Luco, J. V., and Eyzaguirre, C. (1955): Fibrillation and hypersensitivity to acetylcholine in denervated muscle: Effect of length of degenerating nerve fibres. *J. Neurophysiol.*, 18:65–73.

50. Harris, J. B., and Thesleff, S. (1972): Nerve stump length and membrane changes in denervated

skeletal muscle. *Nature New Biol.*, 236:60–61.

51. Albuquerque, E. X., Schuh, F. T., and Kauffman, F. C. (1971): Early membrane depolarization of the fast mammalian muscle after denervation. *Pflugers Arch.*, 328:36–50.

52. Thesleff, S. (1960): Effects of the motor innervation on the chemical sensitivity of skeletal muscle. *Physiol. Rev.*, 40:734–752.

53. Miledi, R. (1960): The acetylcholine sensitivity of frog muscle fibres after complete or partial denervation. *J. Physiol.*, 151:1–23.

54. Lømo, T., and Rosenthal, J. (1972): Control of ACh sensitivity by muscle activity in the rat. *J. Physiol.*, 221:493–513.

55. Albuquerque, E. X., Warnick, J. E., Tasse, J. R., and Sansone, F. M. (1972): Effects of vinblastine and colchicine on neural regulation of the fast and slow skeletal muscles of the rat. *Exp. Neurol.*, 37:607–634.

56. Perisic, M., and Cuénod, M. (1972): Synaptic transmission depressed by colchicine blockade of axoplasmic flow. *Science*, 175:1140–1142.

57. Pilar, G., and Landmesser, L. (1972): Axotomy mimicked by localized colchicine application. *Science*, 177:1116–1118.

The Nervous System, Donald B. Tower, Editor-in-Chief. *Vol. 1: The Basic Neurosciences.* Raven Press, New York, 1975.

The Eyes Have It: Axonal Transport and Regeneration in the Optic Nerve

Bernice Grafstein

The visual system has a number of features that make it especially suitable for studies of axonal transport by the use of radioactive tracers. The eye is readily accessible for tracer injection, can accept a relatively large amount of injected material, and limits the dispersal of this material to a reasonably constant volume. Tracer injected into the eye has easy access to the perikarya of the retinal ganglion cells, the axons of which emerge from the eye in the optic nerve, a clearly delimited fiber bundle ending in an identifiable group of brain nuclei. Some of the outflow pathways from these nuclei, particularly the connection from the lateral geniculate body to the cerebral cortex in the mammal, are well known. Tissue samples can be easily obtained from the site of tracer application (i.e., the retina), from the transport pathway (optic nerve) and its terminal field (e.g., optic tectum in lower vertebrates, lateral geniculate body or superior colliculus in mammals), as well as from the terminal field of the second-order neurons (striate cortex). These advantages have made it possible to use this system for reproducible quantitative studies of both axonal transport in the optic axons and the transfer of axonally transported material from these axons to adjacent neurons. Also, since the terminal field of the optic axons is accessible for injection, this system has been equally convenient for studies of retrograde transport, i.e., from the axon terminals to the ganglion cell bodies. Finally, since the optic axons in lower vertebrates are capable of regeneration, this system has served for studies of the morphological and metabolic aspects of the response to axotomy in a central neuron with proven regenerative capacity. In general, the principles of axonal transport established by studies on the optic nerve have been found to be valid also for other axonal pathways, although the precise values for the rates of transport differ somewhat in different nerves (see chapter by Ochs, *this volume*).

EVIDENCE FOR ANTEROGRADE AXONAL TRANSPORT

The suitability of the visual system for studying axonal transport was first perceived by Taylor and Weiss (1), who introduced the technique of injecting a labeled metabolic precursor into the vitreous humor of the eye. They showed that tritiated leucine injected in this way becomes incorporated into labeled protein in the retinal neurons, particularly the retinal ganglion cells, which constitute the innermost cellular layer of the retina and hence receive the highest concentration of the precursor. Quantitative analysis of autoradiographs of the optic nerves revealed that the labeled protein moves along the optic axons with a displacement of about 1 mm per day.

In a comparable experiment in the goldfish, Grafstein (2) found evidence for the axonal transport of protein in the optic axons at a similar rate (although somewhat slower because of lower body temperature). This rate of transport, however, was not adequate to account for the rapidity with which labeled protein appeared in the terminals of those axons in the optic tectum. On the other hand, the slowly moving material, although detectable in the axon trunks, did not seem to penetrate into the axon terminals. The conclusion from these experiments was that there are two qualitatively different components of axonal transport. Subsequently, both a fast and a slow rate of transport have been identified in the optic nerves of many different species, such as mouse (3), rabbit (4,5), pigeon (6,7), chick (8), and monkey (9). The maximum rate of transport for the fast component has been calculated to be 70 to 100 mm per day in the goldfish, and 150 to 250 mm per day in the various mammalian and avian species; the rate of the slow component is about 0.5 mm per day in the goldfish and 1 to 3 mm per day in mammals and birds. Karlsson and Sjöstrand (4) have recognized two intermediate components as well, but the status of these has not yet been completely clarified.

EVIDENCE FOR RETROGRADE AXONAL TRANSPORT

Retrograde transport in the optic axons has been demonstrated by LaVail and LaVail (10), who injected an exogenous marker protein, horseradish peroxidase, into the optic tectum of goldfish or chick, and then used a histochemical method to reveal the appearance of the peroxidase in the retinal ganglion cell bodies. The applied protein presumably enters the axon terminals by endocytosis, and is then transported within membrane-bound vesicles at a rate of about half that of the anterograde fast transport.

NATURE OF THE TRANSPORTED MATERIAL

The identification of the materials involved in the various components of anterograde axonal transport has proceeded through the use of three principal techniques: separation of the proteins contained in homogenates prepared from tissues containing labeled axonally transported protein; selection of radioactive precursors to label specific compounds undergoing axonal transport; and morphological identification of the cellular structures that become labeled in the course of transport.

Protein Separation Technique

The idea that the fast and slow components of axonal transport are qualitatively different was confirmed by studies on the goldfish nerve, in which McEwen and Grafstein (11) showed that the fast component consists almost entirely of particulate proteins, whereas most of the soluble protein is associated with the slow component. In both components a whole array of proteins can be demonstrated by gel electrophoresis, but the proteins in each component are distinct. Willard et al. (12) detected the presence

of 43 different axonally transported proteins, 23 of them associated specifically with the fast component and the remainder distributed among the slow component and two components of intermediate rate. One of the proteins in the slow component has been identified as tubulin, the microtubule protein (13).

Precursor Selection Technique

Although a number of different amino acids have by now been used as precursors in axonal transport studies, there has been no indication that any of them becomes incorporated preferentially into one or the other component of transport. However, from the study by Forman et al. (14) in which radioactive glucosamine, a precursor of glycoproteins and glycolipids, was used, it is clear that in this case the transported material is associated only with the fast component. A similar result was obtained by Elam and Agranoff (15) when ^{35}S was used to label sulfated mucopolysaccharides and glycoproteins. Glycoproteins labeled with radioactive fucose are also confined to the fast component (16), although synthesis of the transported material continues for a prolonged period after the injection of the fucose into the eye. Protein synthesis inhibitors have no effect on axonal transport itself (11) but when they are applied to the retina they have an immediate effect in reducing the amount of glycoprotein made available for transport (14,16). This shows that in order for the sugar moiety to be transported, it has to be attached to a newly synthesized polypeptide.

When labeled glycerol was used as a precursor for phospholipids in the goldfish, the maximum amount of labeled material transported to the optic tectum was seen at a time intermediate between the usual fast and slow components of axonal transport (17). Although this might be taken as an indication of an intermediate rate of transport, it was evident from the results of a number of experimental manipulations that a fast rate of transport is involved, but that the transported material is released from the cell body over a prolonged period of time. As in the case of the glycoproteins, the transport of phospholipid depends on the availability of newly synthesized polypeptide, but the transported phospholipid itself need not be newly synthesized. In all likelihood, the phospholipid is transported in association with protein in an assembled membrane structure.

Colchicine, which is not a metabolic precursor, has been useful in the analysis of axonal transport because it becomes bound to microtubule protein. In the goldfish, the rate of transport of labeled colchicine has been found to be equivalent to that of the slow component of transport (18), indicating that microtubule protein is one of the constituents of this component, in confirmation of the protein separation experiments described above.

With the use of RNA precursors (e.g., uridine, guanosine, orotic acid), evidence has been sought for the axonal transport of RNA. After injection of the precursor into the eye, labeled RNA could be detected along the course of the optic axons, and its time course of appearance in the optic terminals suggested a rate of transport related to the slow component (19). However, the appearance of labeled RNA at any point along the nerve was preceded by the appearance of a substantial quantity of labeled precursor, and autoradiography showed that most of the labeled RNA was in glial cells (20) and in neurons adjacent to the axon terminals. There is a very good possibility, therefore, that much of the labeled RNA that appears in the nerve is synthesized in cells in contact with the labeled axons from precursor that they receive from these axons. A small proportion of the RNA, nevertheless, may be axonally transported, particularly in regenerating or developing axons (19,21).

Morphological Identification

Grafstein's (2) original assertion that the two components differ in their disposition within the axon has been borne out in experiments in which electron microscopy was used to identify the labeled cell organelles. Hendrickson (9) showed that the proteins transported in the fast component are localized mainly, though not exclusively, in the terminals of the optic axons, whereas the slow component makes a greater contribution to the axon trunks. Schonbach et al. (6) found that the structures labeled in association with the fast component include the plasma membrane and agranular endoplasmic reticulum in the axons, and mitochondria and synaptic

vesicles in the terminals. During the arrival of the slow component, the axoplasm, microtubules, neurofilaments, and axonal mitochondria become labeled, but in the wake of this component there is increased labeling of some of the structures associated with the fast component (7). Thus, although the two components differ with respect to the kind of protein that is transported, it is possible that both may eventually contribute to some of the same membranous structures.

Summary of Component Composition

Each component of axonal transport contains a unique assortment of materials. The fast component consists primarily of membranous structures that have glycoproteins, glycolipids, mucopolysaccharides, and phospholipids. This component makes a large contribution to the mitochondria and synaptic vesicles in the axon terminals, and to the plasma membrane and agranular endoplasmic reticulum in the axon trunks.

The slow component of transport, on the other hand, contains most of the soluble proteins of the axoplasm. Tubulin is associated with this component, and some RNA may be axonally transported at the slow rate. The cell constituents labeled by the slow component include the axoplasm, microtubules, neurofilaments, and axonal mitochondria.

FACTORS INFLUENCING AXONAL TRANSPORT

The cellular mechanisms underlying the various components of axonal transport are still unknown, but it is clear from the fact that the fast and slow components respond so differently to various influences that different mechanisms must be involved. As Karlsson et al. (22) have shown, the fast component can be nearly completely arrested by microtubule-disrupting drugs such as colchicine, and this has led to the suggestion that the microtubules may be active participants in this kind of transport (see Ochs, *this volume*). The fast component shows a temperature sensitivity appropriate for an oxidative process (23), and its rate is not influenced by axon length (24) or by the level of electrical activity in the axon

(3). In young animals the rate of fast transport is slower than in adults (5,8).

The slow transport, by contrast, is more resistant to the effects of colchicine (22). Its rate is faster in longer axons (24), and possibly also in axons with a higher level of electrical activity (3). In younger animals the rate is faster than in adults (5,8).

TRANSNEURONAL TRANSFER OF TRANSPORTED MATERIAL

Specht and Grafstein (25) found that in the mammal some of the radioactivity that is axonally transported in the optic axons to the lateral geniculate body can subsequently be detected in the terminals of the geniculocortical axons in the striate cortex. Some of the transported material must therefore be transferred from the optic axons to the geniculate neurons. This transfer is not confined to neurons that are synaptically linked with the optic axons, since neurons that are merely contiguous with the labeled terminal field also become labeled. Another indication that a synaptic process is not involved is that the amount of transferred radioactivity appears to be independent of the rate of physiological activity in the optic axons. There are some indications that the transfer involves whole macromolecules rather than small molecular weight breakdown products, and glycoproteins may be of particular importance, since fucose is a specially good precursor for demonstrating the transneuronal transfer. It appears, therefore, that a significant proportion of the axonally transported material may be relatively freely liberated from the nerve cell surface, and it is possible that the liberated material might have a trophic effect on appropriately susceptible neurons nearby.

REGENERATION

The remarkable regenerative capacity displayed by the goldfish optic axons generates a special interest in how the retinal ganglion cells respond to axotomy, particularly in comparison to mammalian retinal ganglion cells, which are incapable of regeneration. The status of axonal transport in the regenerating cells is particularly interesting, since it would regulate the supply of materials required for axonal outgrowth.

After section of the optic axons the earliest alteration in the goldfish ganglion cells, as detected by Murray and Grafstein (26), is an increase in RNA synthesis, first seen at 3 days after the lesion. This is followed about a day later by an increase in protein synthesis and still later by an increase in cell body size. Axonal outgrowth can be detected in many of the axons at 4 to 6 days after the lesion, but the slow component of axonal transport remains unchanged until 6 to 8 days, when it begins to increase in rate (27). The changes develop in intensity until they reach a peak at the time that the growing axons reconnect with the optic tectum, at 3 to 4 weeks after the lesion. The net effect of these changes is to greatly increase the amount of protein delivered to the axon tip during the period of active outgrowth. The changes in synthesis are not initiated by the axon outgrowth, since they are activated before outgrowth begins, but the increase in transport rate might conceivably be a consequence of the outgrowth.

SUMMARY

Studies of axonal transport in the optic nerve have demonstrated the presence of two qualitatively different components of anterograde transport, one fast and one slow, with rates (in mammals) of approximately 200 and 2 mm per day, respectively. Some intermediate rate components probably also exist but have been less clearly characterized, and a retrograde transport has been demonstrated as well. Each component of anterograde transport contains a distinctive array of proteins. The fast component, which consists almost entirely of membrane-bound material, mainly contributes constituents to the nerve terminals, whereas the slow component, which contains microtubule protein and most of the soluble proteins of the axoplasm as well as the bulk of the mitochondria, mainly contributes materials to the axon trunks. The two components may be differentially modified by various factors such as the action of microtubule-disrupting agents, the length of the axon, and the age of the animal, which suggests that different mechanisms are involved. During regeneration of the optic axons in the goldfish there is an increase in the rate of the slow transport, possibly induced by axonal outgrowth.

ACKNOWLEDGMENT

This research was supported by U.S. Public Health Service Research Grant NS-09015 from the NINDS.

REFERENCES

1. Taylor, A. C., and Weiss, P. (1965): Demonstration of axonal flow by the movement of tritium-labeled protein in mature optic nerve fibers. *Proc. Natl. Acad. Sci. USA,* 54:1521–1527.
2. Grafstein, B. (1967): Transport of protein by goldfish optic nerve fibers. *Science,* 157:196–198.
3. Grafstein, B., Murray, M., and Ingoglia, N. A. (1972): Protein synthesis and axonal transport in retinal ganglion cells of mice lacking visual receptors. *Brain Res.,* 44:37–48.
4. Karlsson, J. O., and Sjöstrand, J. (1971): Synthesis, migration and turnover of protein in retinal ganglion cells. *J. Neurochem.,* 18:749–767.
5. Hendrickson, A. E., and Cowan, W. M. (1971): Changes in the rate of axoplasmic transport during postnatal development of the rabbit's optic nerve and tract. *Exp. Neurol.,* 30:403–422.
6. Schonbach, J., Schonbach, C. H., and Cuénod, M. (1971): Rapid phase of axoplasmic flow and synaptic proteins: An electron microscopical autoradiographic study. *J. Comp. Neurol.,* 141:485–498.
7. Schonbach, J., Schonbach, C., and Cuénod, M. (1973): Distribution of transported proteins in the slow phase of axoplasmic flow. An electron microscopical autoradiographic study. *J. Comp. Neurol.,* 152:1–16.
8. Marchisio, P. C., and Sjöstrand, J. (1972): Radioautographic evidence for protein transport along the optic pathway of early chick embryos. *J. Neurocytol.,* 1:101–108.
9. Hendrickson, A. E. (1972): Electron microscopic distribution of axoplasmic transport. *J. Comp. Neurol.,* 144:381–398.
10. LaVail, J. H., and LaVail, M. M. (1974): The retrograde intraaxonal transport of horseradish peroxidase in the chick visual system: A light and electron microscopic study. *J. Comp. Neurol.,* 157:303–358.
11. McEwen, B. S., and Grafstein, B. (1968): Fast and slow components in axonal transport of protein. *J. Cell Biol.,* 38:494–508.
12. Willard, M., Cowan, W. M., and Vagelos, P. R. (1974): The polypeptide composition of intra-axonally transported proteins: Evidence for four compositionally distinct phases of transport. *Proc. Natl. Acad. Sci. USA,* 71:2183–2187.
13. McEwen, B. S., Forman, D. S., and Grafstein, B. (1971): Components of fast and slow axonal transport in the goldfish optic nerve. *J. Neurobiol.,* 2:361–377.
14. Forman, D. S., McEwen, B. S., and Grafstein, B. (1971): Rapid transport of radioactivity in goldfish optic nerve following injections of labeled glucosamine. *Brain Res.,* 28:119–130.
15. Elam, J. S., and Agranoff, B. W. (1971): Transport of proteins and sulfated mucopolysaccharides in the goldfish visual system. *J. Neurobiol.,* 2:379–390.
16. Forman, D. S., Grafstein, B., and McEwen, B. S. (1972): Rapid axonal transport of [³H]fucosyl glycoproteins in the goldfish optic system. *Brain Res.,* 48:327–342.
17. Grafstein, B., Miller, J. A., Ledeen, R. W., Haley, J., and Specht, S. C. (1975): Axonal transport of phospholipid in goldfish optic system. *Exp. Neurol.,* 46:261–281.
18. Grafstein, B., McEwen, B. S., and Shelanski, M. L. (1970): Axonal transport of neurotubule protein. *Nature,* 227:289–290.
19. Ingoglia, N. A., Grafstein, B., McEwen, B. S., and McQuarrie, I. G. (1973). Axonal transport of radioactivity in the goldfish optic system following intraocular injection of labeled RNA precursors. *J. Neurochem.,* 20:1605–1615.
20. Gambetti, P., Autilio-Gambetti, L., Shafer, B., and Pfaff, L. (1973). Quantitative autoradiographic study of labeled RNA in rabbit optic nerve after intraocular injection of [³H]uridine. *J. Cell Biol.,* 59:677–684.
21. Bondy, S. C. (1972): Axonal migration of various ribonucleic acid species along the optic tract of the chick. *J. Neurochem.,* 19:1769–1776.
22. Karlsson, J. O., Hansson, H. A., and Sjöstrand, J. (1971): Effect of colchicine on axonal transport and morphology of retinal ganglion cells. *Z. Zellforsch.,* 115:265–283.
23. Grafstein, B., Forman, D. S., and McEwen, B. S. (1972): Effects of temperature on axonal transport and turnover of protein in goldfish optic system. *Exp. Neurol.,* 34:158–170.
24. Murray, M. (1974): Axonal transport in the asymmetric optic axons of flatfish. *Exp. Neurol.,* 42:636–646.
25. Specht, S., and Grafstein, B. (1973): Accumulation of radioactive protein in mouse cerebral cortex after injection of ³H-fucose into the eye. *Exp. Neurol.,* 41:705–722.
26. Murray, M., and Grafstein, B. (1969). Changes in the morphology and amino acid incorporation of regenerating goldfish optic neurones. *Exp. Neurol.,* 23:544–560.
27. Grafstein, B. (1971): Role of slow axonal transport in nerve regeneration. *Acta Neuropathol.,* Suppl. 5:144–152.

The Nervous System, Donald B. Tower, Editor-in-Chief. *Vol. 1: The Basic Neurosciences*. Raven Press, New York, 1975.

Physiology of Electrogenic Excitable Membranes

Harry Grundfest

THE GENERALIZED EQUIVALENT CIRCUIT

Hodgkin and Huxley (1) modeled their ionic theory of spike electrogenesis with an equivalent circuit that remains an adequate paradigm for many of the spike generating cells that have been studied in the ensuing quarter century. However, other varieties of data on the same and other cells have necessitated formulation of a more elaborate equivalent circuit (Fig. 1). It adopts the assumption of the Hodgkin and Huxley theory, that the excitable membrane incorporates relatively permselective ionic channels that are gated into either open or closed states by appropriate stimuli. The sum of the conductances of individual open channels of a given species is the conductance (G_x) for that ion and the current across the membrane carried by that species is $I_x = G_x (E_M - E_x)$, where E_x is the Nernst potential for the species and E_M is the membrane potential. Much recent work has led to acceptance of the general validity of the assumption.

The equivalent circuit of Fig. 1 accounts for most, although not all, electrophysiological manifestations of excitable membranes. Its salient features are given below.

(a) Inclusion of the electrically inexcitable (voltage-insensitive) electrogenic processes that predominate at the input membrane of neurons, muscle fibers, and sensory and secretory cells. The gates for electrically inexcitable channels are operated by chemical, mechanical, photic, or thermal energy changes, whereas electrostatic forces must open or close gates of electrically excitable (voltage-sensitive) channels.

(b) The primary response to an appropriate excitation may be closure of a gate (inactivation) or its opening (activation). Obviously the detection of a change in conductance depends on the initial state of the gates and on the proportion of gates that undergo a change of state.

(c) The electrically excitable gates may be opened or closed by hyperpolarization as well as by depolarization.

The equivalent circuit of Fig. 1 is a generalization. Not all the elements represented there occur in any particular excitable cell. Furthermore, the various elements assort differently in different membranes. For example, the membrane of crayfish muscle fibers incorporates depolarizing and hyperpolarizing Ca activation, depolarizing K activation, depolarizing and hyperpolarizing K inactivation, and hyperpolarizing Cl activation. The latter is insignificant in lobster muscle fibers, and the difference is reflected in different conditions for eliciting a regenerative hyperpolarizing inactivation response.

Membranes differ also with respect to the passive or "leak" components that may affect significantly the inside-negative resting potential. These channels may be exclusively or predominantly permselective for K. E_M then is at or close to E_K. Other cells at rest may have an appreciable proportion of channels that are permselective for Cl or Na or Ca and the resting potential may deviate considerably from E_K. For example, medial giant axons of crayfish at rest are permeable to Na, Ca, and Cl, as well as to K, but the permeabilities to these ions are low. Their contributions to the resting potential are small and evidenced only by special procedures. Squid axons, which are impermeable to Cl, are rather permeable to Na (and perhaps to Ca) at rest, so that the resting potential is considerably positive to E_K and the I-E relation is nonlinear even close to the resting potential. Many, but probably not all, muscle fibers are quite permeable to Cl. In crustacean muscle fibers, the Cl permeability seems to be predominantly in the transverse tubules, whereas in frog fibers the Cl-channels are in the surface membrane.

The membrane is also the seat of various active transport systems, the best-known of which is the ATPase-energized Na-K pump (2). Pumps

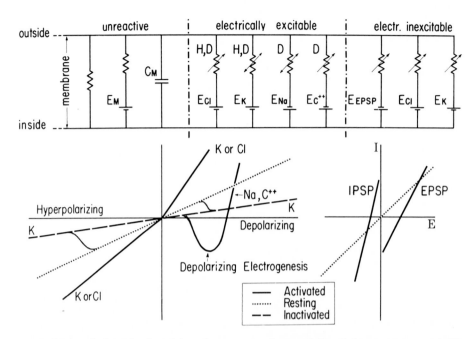

FIG. 1. Generalized equivalent circuit and the voltage-current characteristics of a heterogeneous excitable membrane with a variety of ionic batteries. **Above:** Equivalent circuit diagram. Electromotive forces (emf) contributed by electrogenic ion pumps are omitted. **Below:** Current-voltage (I-E) characteristics of electrically excitable components (*left*) and of electrically inexcitable (*right*) in voltage clamp presentations. Origins are set at resting potential (E_M).

Membrane capacity (C_M) and the invariant conductive component represent major, unreactive portions of the membrane. The conductive component is subdivided into an ion permselective element with E_M as the average emf and a nonselective element symbolized by a resistance without emf. Reactive components are represented by selectivities for specific ions. E_K and E_{Cl} in general are close to E_M, but E_{Na} and E_C^{++} (usually Ca) are shown as inside positive. Permselective electrically excitable channels respond to depolarizing (D) and/or hyperpolarizing (H) stimuli with activation ($\nearrow$) or inactivation ($\swarrow$). Hyperpolarizing Ca-activation has been demonstrated since the diagram was made. The excitability of the E_C^{++} channel should therefore be designated with letters H and D. Electrically inexcitable depolarizing electrogenesis of receptive and synaptic membrane is indicated by an inside-positive battery (E_{EPSP}). Inhibitory synaptic electrogenesis involves increased conductance for either Cl (E_{Cl}) or K (E_K). The conductances of synaptic or sensory receptor membranes may be decreased in responses to specific stimuli. The electrically inexcitable channels therefore should be shown with double-headed arrows, like the electrically excitable E_K and E_{Na} channels.

The unreactive channels and the resting electrically inexcitable electrogenic components have linear (ohmic) I-E characteristics, but activation of reactive electrically inexcitable components by specific stimuli increases the slope (indicating higher conductance in voltage clamp presentation). Depolarizing electrogenesis translates the characteristic to the right. The diagram shows inhibitory electrogenesis (IPSP) as hyperpolarizing and the characteristic translated to the left. As the membrane is polarized by applied currents, the resting and active characteristics approach a crossing beyond which the sign of the recorded electrically inexcitable response is reversed relative to the steady membrane potential. The reversal potential approximates the equilibrium (Nernst) potential of ionic batteries that cause the electrogenesis.

The I-E characteristics of electrically excitable components exhibit nonlinearities that result from transition of the resting membrane conductance to higher or lower values. Only the conductance increase caused by Na or C^{++} activation shifts the characteristic significantly along the voltage axis. Three nonlinear regions with negative slope characteristics are shown. They mark transitions from E_M to E_{Na} or E_C^{++} by activation processes and from the resting conductance to lower conductance by depolarizing and hyperpolarizing K inactivation, respectively. (From Grundfest, ref. 35.)

may be symmetrical and electroneutral or asymmetrical and electrogenic (3). Pump electrogenesis may contribute to the resting potential, but demonstration of this electrogenesis may require special methods (4).

PERMSELECTIVITY, CHANNELS, AND GATES

Permselectivity and the capacity to change this are no longer regarded as exclusively the attributes of living cells. Nonliving membranes, e.g., ion-sensitive glass electrodes, exhibit degrees and patterns of selectivity which also occur in cells. A major determinant arises from the energy barriers of charged sites interacting with hydrated ions (5; *cf.* 6). The orders of selectivities for monovalent cations, divalent alkaline earth ions, and monovalent anions can change depending on the electrostatic energy of the charged sites. Conformational changes in the macromolecules of the cell membrane might be responsible for such transitions, which are basic to the electrogenic manifestations of living cells.

Lipid bilayer membranes, which are "doped" by addition of traces of various proteinaceous macromolecules, are capable of changes in conductance and those that become electrically excitable are of particular relevance (7–9). Doped with excitability-inducing material (EIM) the conductance increases by many orders of magnitude from that of the undoped membrane ($> 10^{-8}$ mho/cm^2) and the membrane is unselectively permeable to monovalent cations. The conductance decreases when a current is applied across the membrane, the effect resembling the inactivation processes depicted in Fig. 1. The kinetics of the conductance changes indicate that they result from voltage-sensitive all-or-none transitions between two stable—open and closed—states of cation-permeable channels (10). When it is open, each channel has a conductance of about 10^{-10} to 10^{-11} mho. Channels remain electrically excitable but can become anion-permeable when the EIM-doped membrane is further treated with polyanions. The interplay of the two voltage-sensitive conductance systems can give rise to changes in membrane potential that are similar, except for their kinetics, to various types of repetitive responses of cells (11).

Other doping agents (e.g., alamethicin, monazomycin) confer electrical excitability by a different mechanism. The conductance is low until a sufficient potential difference is applied across the membrane. The conductance channels probably develop by movement of the doping monomers into the hydrophobic region of the membrane, where they aggregate into macromolecular tubular complexes, which form aqueous channels through the membrane. The circumference and diameter of the tube may vary depending on the number of monomers in the aggregate, so that the conductance of a single channel may vary in a step-wise fashion (12,14). With alamethicin as the channel-forming translocator (9), the conductance increases more or less symmetrically when the exciting current is in either direction across the membrane. The conductance rises in response to current flow in only one direction when monazomycin is the translocator. The *I-E* characteristic exhibits rectification like that of many living membranes that respond with increased conductance for K or Cl only to depolarizing stimuli (Fig. 1).

Other agents (e.g., valinomycin) induce a high degree of selectivity as well as high permeability on the bilayer membranes, but the latter remain electrically inexcitable. The transport of the ions is probably caused by selective combination of the ion and the agent, acting as a carrier that shuttles across the hydrophobic interior of the membranes (8,9). Carriers are probably involved in numerous transfer processes of cell membranes, including ion-specific pumps, but not in the electrogenic changes which arise from changes in conductance. The latter very probably arise exclusively in preformed channels, like those that are believed to be formed by EIM. However, formation of new channels like those believed to occur in monazomycin- or alamethicin-treated bilayers is not ruled out for some cases.

The energetically determined selectivity of preformed channels is presumably derived from negatively charged oxygens at cation-selective sites and the anion selectivity from positive charges contributed by quaternary ammonium or amino groups. Selectivity is also conferred by dimensional factors. Hille (14) has suggested that Na channels have an orifice of about 3×5 Å lined with oxygen ions. Some ions that might not fit the opening (e.g., hydroxylammonium) can move through the Na channels probably by hydrogen-bonding whereas an ion of similar dimension but lacking the hydroxyl (e.g., methylammonium) cannot. Thus, by its chemical composition and physical dimensions, the orifice behaves as a selectivity filter. The cross-section of the channel need not be uniform.

Agents that are attracted energetically to the channel but cannot pass may act as pharmacological inactivators by blocking the orifice. TTX and STX are attracted strongly to the external orifice of the Na channel, but not the internal, and once attached are not driven off by applied currents which would move the ions out

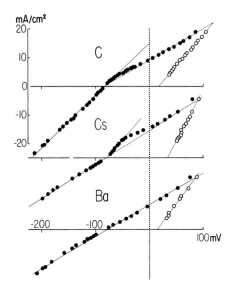

FIG. 2. *I-E* characteristic of an eel electroplaque bathed in control saline (C), with mM Cs present, and with 2.5 mM Ba present. The conductance in the hyperpolarizing quadrant of C is the sum of $G_L + G_K$ (ca. 0.21/mho/cm²). Depolarizations evoke spikes whose peaks are shown by the open circles. The slope is $G_L + G_{Na}$ (ca. 0.29 mho/cm²). The filled circles now represent the steady-state conductance G_L (ca. 0.12 mho/cm²) since the K channels have closed by depolarizing K-inactivation. Both Cs and Ba reduce the conductance in the hyperpolarizing quadrant to G_L alone, since both cations block the reactive K channels to inward current. These channels remain closed in the presence of Ba, but when Cs is the blockader the outward current sweeps the Cs out of the K channels, so that the conductance returns to its higher value ($G_L + G_K$) until the depolarization closes the K gates.

of the channel. A relatively simple case of pharmacological K-inactivation is the effect of Cs, Rb, or Ba on eel electroplaques (15). The electrically excitable reactive K-channels are blocked for inward currents (Fig. 2). They are also blocked for outward currents by Ba, but not by Cs or Rb. We have suggested that the external orifice of these K channels attracts the cations by its negative charge, but that Ba with a smaller ionic radius enters and attaches more strongly with its double positive charge and cannot be driven off by outward currents as are Cs or Rb. Block of K channels of squid axons by intracellular Cs is eliminated by inward currents. Rb eliminates anomalous rectification in frog muscle fibers (ref. 16, Fig. 13). The *I-E* characteristic becomes linear for a range of at least ±80

mV, like the steady-state characteristic of Ba-treated eel electroplaques (Fig. 2). I have designated these effects, where the channels are plugged by foreign agents, as pharmacological inactivation because the mechanism and phenomenology differ from the inactivation caused by closure of electrically operated gates. (For further discussion and references, see refs. 17–19).

The density of the channels may be estimated from data on conductance of single channels (ca. 10^{-10} to 10^{-11} mho) and the conductance of a given membrane (ca. 0.15 to 0.3 mho/cm²) when either Na or K activation is at its peak. Hille (17) has estimated the density of Na channels at about 270/μm², 7,200/μm², and 7,500/node in squid, lobster and frog axons, respectively. Other estimates range rather widely (18). The density of K channels may be of the same order. In eel electroplaques there are three distinctive channels (leak, K, and Na) of approximately the same maximum conductance (ca. 0.15 mho/cm²). If the conductances of individual channels are similar to those in squid or frog axons, there should be about 300 channels of each type/μm².

There is, however, a very interesting difference between K channels in eel electroplaques and the more widely studied axons. In frog axons, for example (Fig. 3), the steady-state *I-E* characteristic has two branches each of constant positive slope. They become progressively separated by a negative-slope region, which grows deeper as $[K]_0$ is increased. The branch in the hyperpolarized quadrant has the low conductance (leak) characteristic of the resting membrane, whereas the right branch has the high conductance of the activated K channels. Thus, the number of K channels appears to be constant for all values of $[K]_0$. This is not the case for eel electroplaques (Fig. 4). While the leak conductance g_L remains essentially constant (rising from about 0.12 mho/cm² for $K_0 = 0$ to about 0.2 mho/cm² for $K_0 = 220$ mM) the K conductance g_K is strongly dependent on $[K]_0$. It is essentially zero when $K_0 = 0$, rises linearly with log K_0 and begins to saturate at $K_0 > 50$ mM. The difference may perhaps be related to the fact that the K channels of eel electroplaques are open at the resting potential, whereas they are nearly all closed in the frog axon.

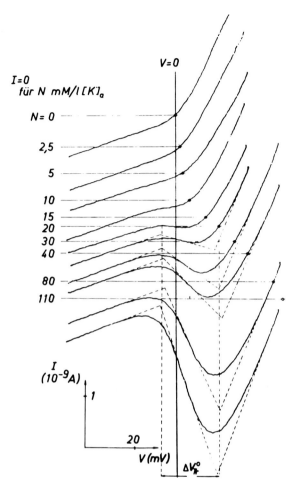

I=0
für N mM/l [K]ₐ

N= 0

2,5

5

10
15
20
30
40

80
110

I
$(10^{-9}A)$

20

V (mV)

V=0

FIG. 3. *I-E* characteristics of a voltage clamped frog node of Ranvier in different $[K]_0$. The successive curves are spaced proportional to log $[K]_0$. The dots on the curves represent the membrane potentials (E_K) for $I = 0$ and they are connected by thin lines to column on left, where $[K]_0$ values are given. The heavy vertical line passes through the resting potential for $K_0 = 0$. The negative slope region, which develops and becomes steeper as E_K shifts toward inside positivity, arises from the relation: $dI/dE = dG/dE(E - E_K) + G$. The two branches with positive slope are nearly parallel for all the curves, indicating that the conductance is relatively independent of $[K]_0$ and is dominated by the membrane potential. Note that the negative slope region allows K-spikes to be generated when the membrane is held in the low conductance state and is excited by a brief depolarization. Note also that applying an inward current to the depolarized axon causes a regenerative hyperpolarizing inactivation response as the characteristic shifts across the negative slope region, from right to left. (From Muller-Mohnssen, ref. 36.)

The control of ionic permeability in electrically excitable channels must depend upon some change in charged particles (1) effected by the applied electric field. The particles may be side chains of the macromolecules that form the channels and their reorientation might lead to conformational changes that would change the electrostatic conditions in charged membrane sites. The selectivity of the channels would then shift from one to another of the sequences observed in nonliving charged membranes (5,6). Changes in the permeability sequence could account for closure of channels as well as for their opening.

Small displacement currents, distinct from the current that charges the membrane capacity, have been observed flowing outward preceding the inward Na current in squid giant axons and inward when the Na current is turned off by hyperpolarization (18,20). They appear to be the electrical signs of the *m* gating process and among other characteristics are distinguished by their insensitivity to TTX. The insensitivity probably arises from the mechanism of block by TTX, since the agent occludes the orifice of the Na channel and need not affect the flow of displacement current. The kinetics of the Na gates are clearly independent of the ion that flows through the channels (Fig. 5).

The electrically excitable K gates appear to possess a wider variety of voltage-sensitivity. They are closed in the range of the resting potential in many cells, but a proportion may be open in other cells. The extreme case is that of eel electroplaques, where there is a large number open at the resting potential. The dependence of G_K on $[K]_0$ indicates that the gates of the K channels in eel electroplaques

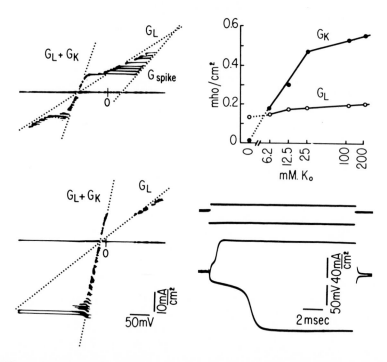

FIG. 4. The different K-permselective channels in an electroplaque. **Left:** Steady-state characteristics as measured with currents that cause different degrees of change in the membrane potential. **Upper graph:** Cell in the standard saline; **lower,** after replacing all Na with K. At rest the conductance is the sum of two components, contributed by the unreactive leak channels, G_L and the reactive channels G_K. The latter close when the membrane potential is displaced beyond certain values. Elimination of G_K causes the membrane potential to shift regeneratively to larger $I \cdot R$ values. In the control saline, suprathreshold depolarizing currents evoked spikes, the peaks of which are registered as the points on the extreme right. The G_K component of the resting cell is increased markedly in high K, as denoted by the steeper slope of the characteristic **(lower left)** and in the graph for another cell **(upper right).** G_L is increased relatively little, however. Note also (Fig. 2) that G_L is unaffected by Cs or Ba, which block the G_K channels. The negative slope during the transition from the high conductance $(G_L + G_K)$ to low conductance (G_L) in either direction is accentuated, creating a forbidden zone of instability. The records **(lower right)** show the inactivation responses evoked in high K by depolarizing and hyperpolarizing currents. Note that the threshold for depolarizing inactivation was lower than that for hyperpolarizing inactivation. This difference is also seen in the characteristic curves **(lower left).** The records on the right also show that the development of hyperpolarizing K inactivation was much slower, despite the higher applied inward current. (Modified from Ruiz-Manresa, ref. 37.)

open as $[K]_0$ is increased, giving rise to the increase in G_K observed in Fig. 4. As the number of open channels is increased by raising $[K]_0$ more Ba is required to plug them and the relation is a competitive one (15).

The kinetics of K gates have not been studied as yet. There are, however, indications that once opened the gates in some membranes may remain open for a considerable time. Depolarizing K-activation in frog slow muscle fibers induces a hyperpolarizing electrogenesis which may last for more than 1 sec (ref. 21, Fig. 11). The K-spikes of *Tenebrio* muscle fibers may last for 10 sec or more (ref. 21, Fig. 8B) and

those of puffer neurons may last almost 1 min (ref. 21, Fig. 7). The long-lasting increases in K conductance signify that depolarizing K inactivation is relatively insignificant or is absent and that once the K gates are opened they close spontaneously at a slow rate.

Opening of K gates by hyperpolarizing K activation is seen in frog muscle fibers bathed in physiological saline (ref. 16, Fig. 14) and forms the basis of anomalous rectification when depolarizing K activation is abolished (ref. 16, Fig. 13).

K-gates may be closed by depolarizing and/or hyperpolarizing currents. The decreased con-

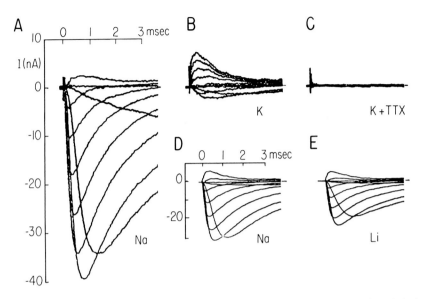

FIG. 5. Currents carried by Na, K, or Li in Na channels of frog nodes. TEA (6 mM) eliminated the late current. Membrane was clamped at 10 steps of 15 mV increments in each set of records. Currents became outward at highest depolarizations. **A:** Node in control saline. **B:** All Na replaced with K. The permeability of the channels to K was more than 10% of Na permeability. Note the brief durations of the currents, indicating that the closing of Na channels is independent of the species of ions moving through them. **C:** TTX (150 μM) added. The Na channels were blocked to K-flux. **D, E:** Another node. The Na channels are only about 10% less permeable to Li (**E**) than to Na (**D**). (Modified from Hille, ref. 14.)

ductance with increasing currents thus gives rise to negative slope regions in the characteristic (Fig. 1), and a regenerative change in membrane potential (Fig. 4). The relatively simple responses seen in Fig. 4 indicate that only K-channels are involved. A similarly simple hyperpolarizing response is observed in frog axons that are depolarized in high K_0 (ref. 11, Fig. 29).

Where few, if any, K channels are open at the resting potential, hyperpolarizing inactivation responses can be elicited by first opening the channels with depolarization by K. The shift to inside negativity with an applied current then traverses the negative slope region (Fig. 3) from right to left. Regenerative inactivation responses of this type are observed in many cells (11,16). Inactivation responses, whether induced by depolarization or hyperpolarization, result from the increased IR drop across the higher resistance of the inactivated membrane. Therefore they are not sustained responses, but terminate when the current is withdrawn. Hyperpolarization can increase the conductance for other ions (Fig. 1), so that hyperpolarizing

responses may take on a rather complicated appearance. The response of crayfish muscle fibers bathed in physiological saline (i.e., Cl is present) to hyperpolarizing currents generates only a characteristic that exhibits delayed rectification (ref. 11, Fig. 26). The conductance increase is abolished by removing Cl_i (11, Fig. 27), and the cell now exhibits a regenerative "upside-down" spike (Fig. 6). The large negativity is reduced, however, while the current is maintained constant, in still another manifestation of delayed rectification. When the current is terminated, the membrane develops a small after-depolarization, which is associated with an increased conductance. The plateau is accompanied by contraction of the muscle fiber and a further contraction may develop on removing the current. The plateau, the after-depolarization, and the contraction are blocked or reduced with Mn. The increased conductance during the current thus must be caused by hyperpolarizing Ca activation and the after-depolarization to persistence of open Ca channels.

The occurrence of excitable channels for Ca

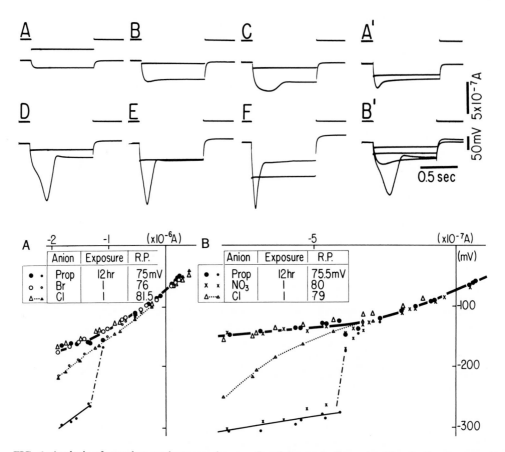

FIG. 6. Analysis of complex conductance changes. Crayfish muscle fibers. **A′:** Muscle fiber in control saline shows only delayed rectification in response to hyperpolarizing currents. **B′:** Replacement of Cl in the solution with NO_3. A regenerative upside-down spike is produced. Reduction in hyperpolarization while the current is maintained indicates an increase in conductance. This change in membrane potential is accompanied by a strong contraction of the muscle fiber. Further contraction occurs during the small after-depolarization when the current is terminated. **A–E:** Cl replaced with propionate. Sequence of records for successively increasing inward currents. The peak of the upside-down spike increases relatively little with larger currents, but its duration is shortened, signifying a more rapid onset of the hyperpolarizing Ca-activation. Note also that the plateau changes little with increasing currents.

Graphs: *I-E* relations. Smaller symbols represent potentials at peaks of hyperpolarizing responses, larger symbols the plateau potentials. **A:** Preparation in propionate saline for 12 hr to reduce Cl_i. Regenerative increase in E indicated by broken line. Replacement of propionate with Br or Cl eliminated regenerative response. Note delayed rectification. **B:** Another preparation. Note expanded scale of abscissa. Regenerative change occurred in NO_3 as well as in propionate. After 1 hr in Cl saline regenerative change was eliminated, but considerable increase in resistance is still evident. These data indicate therefore the interplays of hyperpolarizing Cl activation and hyperpolarizing K inactivation, both fairly rapid, and a slower higher threshold Ca activation. The latter persists for some time after the current is terminated and contributes a small after-depolarization. There is Ca influx during both the plateau and the after-depolarization.

is now widely recognized (22). In crustacean muscle opening of Ca channels by depolarizing currents results in spikes or graded responses, depending on the relative kinetics of the Ca and K gates. In many cells the depolarization induced by Ca influx is severely reduced by the nearly simultaneous increase in K efflux, so that only small graded responses are observed. Agents that depress or block K efflux (e.g., procaine, D_2O) can thus expose the spike of Ca electrogenesis. The spikes are rather prolonged, indicating that once opened the Ca gates close slowly. Ca can also move through Na channels, but the permeability is probably only about 1% of that to Na.

Depolarizing activation of Cl channels is the mode of spike electrogenesis of the fresh water algae *Chara* and *Nitella,* in which the Cl-gradient is inside-positive. Cl-activation also occurs in the skate electroplaque (ref. 16, Figs. 8–10), in which the Cl-gradient is inside-negative. The channels opened by depolarization appear to be only Cl-permeable and the conductance increases about 10- to 15-fold above the resting value. Cl-spikes lasting more than 1 sec may be evoked by substituting Cl_0 with an impermeant anion to reverse the gradient for Cl.

Electrically inexcitable channels must be gated by still other means. A particularly fruitful model would seem to be the acetylcholine receptor, which has been studied in a variety of ways (23). Karlin (24) has suggested that the receptor of eel electroplaques has two reactive sites (S-S; Θ) approximately 12 Å apart when the synaptic channels are closed. When acetylcholine or a mimetic combines with the two sites their distance is decreased to about 9 Å. Presumably there is a conformational change in the membrane and a redistribution of charges, which opens the synaptic channel.

A receptor that reacts with acetylcholine or its mimetics may increase conductance for Cl, K, or for the complex of ions subsumed under E_{EPSP} in Fig. 1. If the receptor-transmitter interaction is considered as a gate the channel structure, characterized by the selectivity of the channel, must be distinct from the gating element. The same conclusion applies to other receptor systems, as well. This is reinforced by the recent finding (25) that acetylcholine can activate three distinctive electrophysiological processes in *Aplysia* neurons: an EPSP and two IPSPs, the IPSPs involving increased conductance for Cl and K, respectively. Despite the fact that the three synaptic responses are initiated by the same transmitter, their time courses are very different, the rise and fall of the K-conductance being particularly prolonged.

The slow rise and persistence of the K-generated hyperpolarization may be a secondary effect mediated by a stimulus that increases intracellular Ca and thereby increases K conductance. Two example of such electrogenesis

have been described recently. The outward-facing (lumenal) membrane of skate electroreceptors in the lateral line canal system is electrically excitable, a long-lasting depolarization arising from Ca activation, with entry of Ca from the external medium. The Ca then diffuses through the cytoplasm to the inner side of the serosal surface. The latter membrane is electrically inexcitable but Ca induces an increased conductance, probably for K, since the increase is accompanied by repolarizing electrogenesis and the membrane potential returns to the resting state (38). Intracellular release of Ca is implicated in the light-induced hyperpolarization of some giant neurons in *Aplysia.* The hyperpolarization arises from an increased K conductance. The cells contain pigmented granules that release Ca on illumination. Injection of a buffer to maintain Ca at or below 10^{-8} M eliminated the K current (39).

Even more complex is the effect of 5-hydroxytryptamine on the synapses of molluscan neurons where six different conductance changes are observed (26). Thus the changes in the membrane that induce the changes in conductance must have very different kinetics and must be independent of the persistence of the transmitter agent. A similar conclusion has been deduced for the EPSP of eel electroplaques (27). The time constant of the membrane is about 100 μsec, but the falling phase of the EPSP lasts 10 to 15 msec. The electroplaques are very rich in acetylcholinesterase and it is unlikely that acetylcholine released from the nerve terminals persists throughout this period.

Synaptic transmitters may cause a decrease in conductance (26,28). This may be regarded as the phenomenological analogue of inactivation processes that are induced by electrical stimuli in electrically excitable channels (Fig. 1), although the mechanisms may be very different. A related finding may be the decreased conductance effected by quinine in taste buds (29). Other stimuli (salt, sweet, acid) cause an increased conductance in the same cells.

Although the conductance changes of input membrane are not initiated by electrical stimuli, some degree of responsiveness of the electrically inexcitable channels to such stimuli is also known. The kinetics of the decay of end-plate currents of frog muscle are modified by a change in membrane potential (see ref. 30 for references). The effect is small, a change of 50 mV in the potential causing approximately 1.5-fold change in the rate constant of the closing of the channels. The synaptic channels of eel electroplaques are closed rapidly by strong depolarization (27), but the kinetics of this change have not been studied. The changes in conductance might result from an electrical effect on the receptor-transmitter interaction, which is the chemosensitive gate, or it might develop from an electrostatic effect within the channels themselves, like the gating of electrically excitable channels. In the latter case it is possible that the conformational change, which presumably causes activation of the synaptic channels, renders them electrically excitable to a degree.

Some new information on the chemosensitive gating of channels is coming from analysis of the fluctuations in the current of the postsynaptic membrane, which is depolarized by acetylcholine or its mimetics (31). Anderson and Stevens (30, which should also be consulted for further literature) have carried out similar measurements in voltage clamped end-plates. A unitary channel gate opened by ACh has a conductance range of about 2×10^{-11} to 10^{-10} mho. The increase lasts about 1 msec at 20°C and contributes about 0.3 μV to the depolarizing electrogenesis. The conductance increases evoked by some other agents may be shorter or longer, probably indicating the different kinetics of interaction of the drugs with the receptors. Anderson and Stevens (30) have developed an analysis of the kinetics of the gating processes.

THE SYNAPTIC CHANNELS

The electrogenesis of orthodox inhibitory synapses is generated by the conductance increase of a single channel permeable either to Cl or K. Both types of channels may be present in the same cell and may be activated by the same or different agents. As already noted, the Cl and K channels in *Aplysia* neurons, which respond to acetylcholine, have very different kinetics, the first giving rise to fast, brief IPSPs and the second to slowly rising and prolonged IPSPs. The relative selectivity of the Cl channels follows one or another of the

sequences for halides predicted by Eisenman (6). In lobster muscle fibers, the inhibitory synaptic channels are also somewhat permeable to propionate as well. The structure of the K channels in *Aplysia* neurons appears to be similar to that of electrically excitable K channels in the same and other cells, since the slow IPSPs are blocked by intracellularly applied TEA or Cs (25). Thus, the difference in gating mechanisms does not preclude similar dimensional and electroenergetic characteristics of the channels.

The depolarizing (excitatory) electrogenesis (generator potential, EPSP) of receptive or postsynaptic membranes involves an increased conductance for Na in most if not all cases. However, the maximum (reversal) potential of the ionic battery (E_{EPSP}, Fig. 1) is not E_{Na}, but some value that is usually approximately midway between E_K and E_{Na}, indicating that the electromotive forces of both these batteries contribute to E_{EPSP}. The absolute value of E_{Na} is usually somewhat smaller than that of E_K so that E_{EPSP} is often somewhat negative. In eel electroplaques, however, E_{Na} is about 100 to 200 mV, whereas E_K is about -80 mV and E_{EPSP} is about 30 to 50 mV inside-positive (15).

The depolarizing electrogenesis appears to arise from a simultaneous increase in permeability to both Na and K. There are only a few reports of the independent modification of the conductance for one or the other cation (for discussion, see ref. 23), and it is generally assumed that the two-ion species flow either in a single type of channel or in a system of closely coupled pairs of ion-selective channels. In either case the energetic and dimensional characteristics differ markedly from those of electrically excitable channels as is evidenced by different pharmacological properties. The inward movement of Na is not blocked by TTX or STX (32). Agents that block efflux of K in the inhibitory synapses as well as in electrically excitable K channels do not affect EPSPs (15,25).

The ionic selectivity of the channels for the depolarizing electrogenesis has not been studied extensively. The channels are somewhat permeable to some organic cations in the crayfish stretch receptor (32). The synaptic membrane of eel electroplaques is somewhat permeable to Ca and Mg (15).

The foregoing account has concentrated on the nature and properties of the ionic channels that satisfy the conceptual framework of the Hodgkin and Huxley theory and its subsequent developments. We already know numerous modifications of the various electrogenic components and of the electrophysiological consequences of these changes. The framework will undoubtedly be enriched in the near future by ongoing studies that seek to combine classical electrophysiological and pharmacological methods with those of several other disciplines — anatomy, biochemistry, genetics, immunochemistry, physics, and physical chemistry.

Among the most interesting and pioneering of these developments is the application of tissue culture and genetics to produce cells with membranes of unusual properties (33). Results of optical (primarily fluorescence) studies have been summarized by Cohen et al. (34). Space precludes references to the numerous recent conferences and symposia on growth, differentiation and reconstitution of membranes and on the interactions between nerve cells and other cell types.

ACKNOWLEDGMENTS

Work in this laboratory is supported in part by grants from the Muscular Dystrophy Associations of America, Inc.; by Public Health Service Research Grant NS 03728 and Training Grant NS 05328 from the National Institute of Neurological Diseases and Stroke and from a grant from the National Science Foundation (GB 31807X).

REFERENCES

1. Hodgkin, A. L., and Huxley, A. F. (1952): A quantitative description of membrane current and its application to conduction and excitation in nerve. *J. Physiol. (Lond.)*, 117:500–544.
2. Skou, J. C. (1974): The ($Na^+ + K^+$) activated ensyme and its relationship to transport of sodium and potassium. *Quart. Rev. Biol.*, 7:401–434.
3. Thomas, R. C. (1972): Electrogenic sodium pump in nerve and muscle cells. *Physiol. Rev.*, 52:563–594.
4. Akiyama, T., and Grundfest, H. (1971): The hyperpolarization of frog skeletal muscle fibres induced by removing potassium from the bathing medium. *J. Physiol. (Lond.)*, 217:33–60.
5. Eisenman, G. (1962): Cation selective glass electrodes and their mode of operation. *Biophys. J.*, 2:259s–323s.
6. Diamond, J. M., and Wright, E. M. (1969): Biological membranes: The physical basis of ion and non-electrolyte selectivity. *Ann. Rev. Physiol.*, 31:581–646.
7. Mueller, P., and Rudin, O. (1968): Resting and action potentials in experimental bimolecular lipid membranes. *J. Theor. Biol.*, 18:222–258.
8. Mueller, P., and Rudin, D. O. (1969): Translocators in bimolecular lipid membranes: Their role in dissipative and conservative bioenergy transductions. *Curr. Top. Bioenerg.*, 3:157–249.
9. Haydon, D. A., and Hladky, S. B. (1972): Ion transport across thin lipid membranes: a critical discussion of mechanism in selected systems. *Quart. Rev. Biophys.*, 5:187–282.
10. Ehrenstein, G., Blumenthal, R., Latorre, R., and Lecar, H. (1974): Kinetics of the opening and closing of individual excitability-inducing material channels in a lipid bilayer. *J. Gen. Physiol.*, 63:707–721.
11. Grundfest, H. (1966): Comparative electrobiology of excitable membranes. In: *Advances in Comparative Physiology and Biochemistry, Vol. 2,* edited by O. E. Lowenstein, pp. 1–116. Academic Press, New York.
12. Finkelstein, A., and Holz, R. (1973): Aqueous pores created in thin lipid membranes by the polyene antibiotics nystatin and amphotericin B. In: *Membranes, a Series of Advances, Vol. 2,* edited by G. Eisenman, pp. 377. Marcel Dekker, New York.
13. Boheim, G. (1974): Statistical analysis of alamethicin channels in black lipid membranes. *J. Memb. Biol.*, 19:277–303.
14. Hille, B. (1972): The permeability of the sodium channel to metal cations in myelinated nerve. *J. Gen. Physiol.*, 59:637–658.
15. Ruiz-Manresa, F., and Grundfest, H. (1973): Ionic pharmacology of the electrically excitable potassium conductance system (g_K) of eel electroplaque. *J. Gen. Physiol.*, 61:268.
16. Grundfest, H. (1966): Heterogeneity of excitable membrane: Electrophysiological and pharmacological evidence and some consequences. *Ann. N.Y. Acad. Sci.*, 137:901–949.
17. Hille, B. (1970): Ionic channels in nerve membranes. *Prog. Biophys.*, 21:3–32.
18. Armstrong, C. M. (1974): Ionic pores, gates and gating currents. *Quart. Rev. Biophys.*, 7:179–209.
19. Narahashi, T. (1974): Chemicals as tools in the study of excitable membranes. *Physiol. Rev.*, 54:813–889.
20. Keynes, R. D., and Rojas, E. (1974) Kinetics and steady-state properties of the charged system controlling sodium conductance in the squid giant axon. *J. Physiol. (Lond.)*, 29:393–434.
21. Grundfest, H. (1971): The varieties of excitable membranes. In: *Biophysics and Physiology of Excitable Membranes,* edited by W. J. Adelman, Jr., pp. 477–504. Van Nostrand Reinhold, New York.

22. Reuter, H. (1973): Divalent cations as charge carriers in excitable membranes. *Prog. Biophys. Mol. Biol.* 26:1–43.

23. Rang, H. P. (1974): Acetylcholine receptors. *Quart. Rev. Biophys.,* 7:283–399.

24. Karlin, A. (1969): Chemical modification of the active site of the acetylcholine receptor. *J. Gen. Physiol.,* 54:245s–264s.

25. Kehoe, J. (1972): Three acetylcholine receptors in *Aplysia* neurones. *J. Physiol. (Lond.),* 225:115–146.

26. Gerschenfeld, H. M., and Paupardin-Tritsch, D. (1974): Ionic mechanisms and receptor properties underlying the responses of molluscan neurones to 5-hydroxytryptamine. *J. Physiol. (Lond.),* 243:427–456.

27. Ruiz-Manresa, F., and Grundfest, H. (1971): Synaptic electrogenesis in eel electroplaques. *J. Gen. Physiol.,* 57:71–92.

28. Weight, F. F., and Padjen, A. (1973): Slow synaptic inhibitions: evidence for synaptic inactivations of sodium conductance in sympathetic ganglion cells. *Brain Res.* 55:219–224.

29. Ozeki, M. (1971): Conductance change associated with receptor potentials of gustatory cells in rat. *J. Gen. Physiol.,* 58:688–699.

30. Anderson, C. R., and Stevens, C. F. (1973): Voltage clamp analysis of acetylcholine produced end-plate current fluctuations at frog neuromuscular junctions. *J. Physiol. (Lond.),* 235:655–691.

31. Katz, B., and Miledi, R. (1972): The statistical nature of the acetylcholine potential and its molecular components. *J. Physiol. (Lond.),* 224:665–699.

32. Grundfest, H. (1971): The general electrophysiology of input membrane in electrogenic excitable cells. In: *Handbook of Sensory Physiology, I. Principles of Receptor Physiology,* edited by W. R. Loewenstein, pp. 135–165. Springer-Verlag, Berlin.

33. Nelson, P. G. (1975): Nerve and muscle cells in culture. *Physiol. Rev.,* 55:1–61.

34. Cohen, L. B., Salzberg, B. M., Davila, H. V., Ross, W. N., Landowne, D., Waggoner, A. S., and Wang, C. H. (1974): Changes in axon fluorescence during activity: Molecular probes of membrane potential. *J. Memb. Biol.,* 19:1–36.

35. Grundfest, H. (1967): Synaptic and ephaptic transmission. In: *The Neurosciences. A Study Program,* edited by G. C. Quarton, T. Melnechuck and F. O. Schmitt, pp. 353–372. Rockefeller University Press, New York.

36. Müller-Mohnssen, H. (1967): *Stationärer Negativer Widerstand Und Verstärkerfunktion des Ranvierschen Schnürrings.* Institut für Biologie, Münich.

37. Ruiz-Manresa, F. (1970): *Electrogenesis of Eel Electroplaques. Conductance Components and Impedance Changes During Activity.* Ph.D. Thesis, Columbia University, New York.

38. Clusin, W., Spray, D., and Bennett, M. V. L. (1974): Activation of a voltage-insensitive conductance by inward calcium current. *Biol. Bull.,* 147:472.

39. Brown, A. M., Baur, Jr., P. S., and Tuley, F. H. Jr. (1975): Phototransduction in *Aplysia* neurons: Calcium release from pigmented granules is essential. *Science,* 188:157–160.

The Nervous System, Donald B. Tower, Editor-in-Chief. *Vol. 1: The Basic Neurosciences.* Raven Press, New York, 1975.

Organization of the Ionic Channels in Nerve Membranes

Richard D. Keynes

ACTIVE AND PASSIVE TRANSPORT

The primary purpose of this chapter is to consider recent evidence on the functioning of the sodium and potassium channels responsible for the electrical excitability of nerve fibers. It must not be forgotten, however, that the fibers depend for maintenance of the high internal potassium and low sodium on the presence of an active transport system operating in parallel with the excitability channels, which brings about a coupled, or at any rate a partially coupled, transfer of sodium and potassium against their respective concentration gradients. There is insufficient space here to discuss the sodium pump in detail, but some of its properties are covered by Table 1, which summarizes the evidence for believing that the active and passive ion movements take place through entirely separate pathways.

THE HODGKIN-HUXLEY EQUATIONS

The changes in the sodium and potassium conductances of the membrane during excitation have been described by Hodgkin and

TABLE 1. *Evidence of the independence of the sodium pump from the Na and K excitability channels*

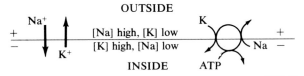

	Na and K Channels	Na Pump
Direction of ion movements	Down the electrochemical gradient	Against the electrochemical gradient
Source of energy	Preexisting concentration gradient	ATP
Voltage dependence	Regenerative link between potential and Na conductance	Independent of potential
Blocking agents	TTX blocks Na at 10^{-8} M; tetraethylammonium blocks K at 10^{-3} M	TTX and tetraethylammonium have no effect
	Ouabain has no effect	Ouabain blocks at 10^{-7} M
External calcium	Increase in [Ca] raises threshold for excitation; decrease lowers threshold	No effect
Selectivity	Li not distinguished from Na	Li pumped much more slowly than Na
Effect of temperature	Rate of opening and closing of channels has large temperature coefficient, but maximum conductances are unaffected	Velocity of pumping greatly slowed by cooling
Number of channels or pump sites	Rabbit vagus has 27 TTX-binding sites per μm^2; squid axon has 500/μm^2	Rabbit vagus has 750 ouabain-binding sites per μm^2; squid axon has 4,000 per μm^2
Maximum rate of movement of Na$^+$	10^{-8} mole/cm^2 sec during rising phase of spike	6×10^{-11} mole/cm^2 sec at room temperature
Metabolic inhibitors	No effect; electrical activity is normal in axon perfused with pure salt solution	CN (1 mM) and DNP (0.2 mM) block as soon as ATP is exhausted

Huxley (1) in terms of five equations relating them to time and voltage:

$$g_{Na} = \bar{g}_{Na} m^3 h \qquad [1]$$

$$\frac{dm}{dt} = \alpha_m(1 - m) - \beta_m m \qquad [2]$$

$$\frac{dh}{dt} = \alpha_h(1 - h) - \beta_h h \qquad [3]$$

$$g_K = \bar{g}_K n^4 \qquad [4]$$

$$\frac{dn}{dt} = \alpha_n(1 - n) - \beta_n n \qquad [5]$$

where $\bar{g}_{Na}$ and $\bar{g}_K$ are constants representing the peak conductances per unit area of membrane, and m, h, and n are dimensionless variables obeying the first-order differential equations [2], [3], and [5], in which the αs and βs are forward and backward rate constants whose magnitude is determined by the instantaneous value of the membrane potential. Although originally developed for the squid giant axon, these equations also apply reasonably well to frog muscle (2), to *Myxicola* giant axons (3) and to the node of Ranvier in myelinated fibers from *Xenopus* (4,5), except that m^2 and n^2 may sometimes fit the data better than m^3 and n^4. They have stood the test of time remarkably well and need relatively little modification to accommodate more recent experimental findings. It does now appear, however, that, as first noted by Cole and Moore (6) for the potassium conductance of the squid giant axon, if the membrane potential is initially held at a level much more negative than the normal resting value, then the rise in ionic current on depolarization of the membrane is no longer well fitted by the expression

$$I = I_\infty \left[1 - \exp\left(-\frac{t}{\tau}\right) \right]^a \qquad [6]$$

with $a = 4$, but the power to which the exponential term is raised needs to be about 25 in order to obtain the observed delay in the rise of g_K. A similar, although smaller, delay has been reported for g_{Na} by Keynes and Rojas (7), amounting to 50 to 100 μsec at 6°C for a holding potential of -150 mV. It would also seem from the observations of Narahashi (8), Adelman and Palti (9), Chandler and Meves (10), Goldman and Schauf (11), and Rudy (12) that the kinetics of inactivation of the sodium conductance are not always perfectly described in terms of an independent h variable obeying a first-order equation, and that there are relatively slow inactivation effects not taken into account by Hodgkin and Huxley's (1) equations.

NUMBER OF CHANNELS

It has sometimes been suggested that it is not necessary to postulate the existence of separate channels for sodium and potassium, and that there might be a single set of channels whose selectivity varied appropriately with time. This idea can now be dismissed, since it is incompatible with the widely reported finding that the sodium conductance can be reduced to zero by the application of tetrodotoxin (TTX) without any perceptible change in the time course or voltage dependence of g_K, while the same is true for g_{Na} when the potassium conductance is blocked by quaternary ammonium ions. There is thus no doubt that the sodium and potassium channels are functionally distinct entities. From studies of the high-affinity or specific binding of tritiated TTX, the density of the sodium channels has been estimated as varying from 2.5/μm^2 in garfish olfactory nerve, and 16 and 27/μm^2 in the slightly larger nonmyelinated fibers of lobster and rabbit vagus nerve, respectively (13), to 550/μm^2 in the squid giant axon (14). The figure for squid is satisfactorily consistent with counts of the channels based on determinations of the rate of blocking and unblocking of the sodium conductance by TTX and saxitoxin (15), with measurements of ionic current noise (16), and with measurements of the total charge displacement in gating current experiments (17,18). Hodgkin (19) has calculated that numbers of this order are to be expected in squid if a maximum velocity of conduction of the impulse is to be achieved. In the absence of a really high-affinity blocking agent for the potassium channels, there is relatively little evidence as to their density, but Conti et al. (16) have estimated that it is nearly an order of magnitude smaller than the figure for sodium.

THE MECHANISM OF IONIC SELECTIVITY

From an examination of the relative permeability of the sodium channels in myelinated nerve fibers to a series of organic cations, Hille

(20) has suggested that their selectivity is achieved through a good fit between the dimensions of the penetrating ion and the disposition of hydrogen-bonding groups in the negatively charged walls of the channel. Thus he explained his results on geometrical grounds by assuming that the sodium channel was an oxygen-lined pore about 3×5 Å in cross section, one pair of oxygens being an ionized carboxylic acid group. When tested with the same series of cations, the sodium channels in the squid giant axon behave in a closely similar fashion (21). The portion of the selectivity filter into which TTX is such a remarkably good fit, with $K_m = 3$ nM, certainly faces outward, since the toxin is ineffective when applied internally. However, the equally high affinity observed for saxitoxin and TTX despite their quite different molecular structures still has no explanation in terms of the detailed arrangement of bonding groups in the mouth of the channel. The facts that the selectivity does not vary while the channels are opening and closing and that the behavior of the gating current is not obviously affected by the presence or absence of TTX (17) suggest that the filter operates in series with and to a large extent independently of the voltage-controlled gating mechanism. Studies of the blocking effect of quaternary ammonium ions at the node of Ranvier and in squid axons (22,23) suggest a more complex structure for the potassium channels. Both types of nerve have a receptor accessible only from the inside after the opening of the voltage-activated gate; at the node there is in addition an external receptor with rather different properties. Hille (24) has proposed that the narrowest part of the potassium channel is a circle of oxygen atoms approximately 3 Å in diameter with a low electrostatic field strength.

THE SODIUM GATING CURRENT

We come now to a consideration of recent evidence on the nature of the voltage-sensitive gating mechanism. As was pointed out by Hodgkin and Huxley (1) at the outset, the existence of any such mechanism carries the implication that operation of the gate involves some transfer of charge across the membrane preceding the passage of ionic current. They were unable to detect what has come to be known as the gating current, because they had no means of reducing the ionic current sufficiently to unmask it. But with the advent of TTX to block the sodium channels and using cesium or tetraethylammonium to block the potassium channels, observation of gating currents has now become possible both in the squid giant axon (17,18,25) and at the node of Ranvier (26). The basic phenomenon is illustrated in Fig. 1, which shows the asymmetry of the displacement current recorded on application of ±120 mV voltage-clamp pulses to a squid axon in which the ionic current had been almost completely abolished. Graphical addition of the two single-sweep records to eliminate the symmetrical capacity transient reveals the presence of an asymmetrical component of the membrane current that flows outward at the start of the depolarizing pulse and inward at the finish, pursuing an exponential time course with a relaxation time of a few hundred microseconds. The typical family of records seen in Fig. 2, which was obtained with the help of a signal averager, shows further that the gating current time constant varies with potential, decreasing progressively as the voltage during the pulse becomes more positive, but remaining roughly constant for the restoration of a fixed holding potential at the end of the pulse. In this axon, as was often the case, there was some rectification of the leakage current during the pulse, which resulted in the superimposition of a rectangular pedestal on the exponential tails. On other occasions, what appeared to be a variation of the leakage current with time was observed, giving rise to a sloping pedestal and appreciably complicating the search for any slow components of the gating current.

The fundamental criteria for regarding the sharply rising and exponentially declining components of the asymmetrical displacement current as originating from the movement of mobile charged particles or dipoles that constitute an integral part of the membrane are that (a) the total transfers of charge in each direction at the beginning and end of the pulse should be exactly equal, i.e., $Q_{on} = Q_{off}$; (b) the charge displacement should reach a ceiling or saturation level Q_∞ when large enough pulses are applied; (c) Q_∞ should not be temperature-dependent.

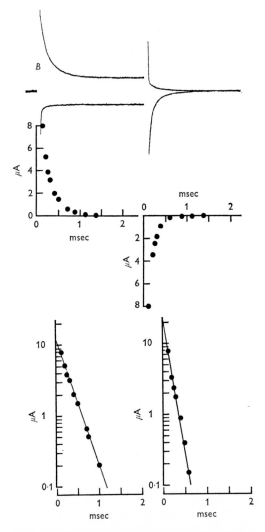

FIG. 1. Asymmetry of the displacement current on application of equal and opposite voltage-clamp pulses to a squid axon perfused with 300 mM CsF and bathed in Na- and K-free saline containing 1,000 nM TTX. The *top traces* are single-sweep records of the membrane current for ±120 mV pulses, applied at a holding potential of −100 mV. The difference between them is plotted beneath on linear and logarithmic scales. (From Keynes and Rojas, ref. 17.)

For short pulses, there seems no doubt that these conditions are satisfied to within the accuracy of the measurements, but when the period of depolarization is prolonged, there are indications (27; and Meves, and Keynes and Rojas, *unpublished*) that an appreciable fraction of the charges may return to their

original configuration rather slowly on restoration of the holding potential, giving rise to an apparent reduction in the ratio Q_{off}/Q_{on}. This marked modification of the relaxation time or mobility of some of the gating particles would appear likely to be related in a manner not yet understood to the process of inactivation of the sodium channels.

At least for experiments conducted at a fairly high holding potential, a detailed comparison of the behavior of the gating current with the properties of the sodium conductance system, defined in terms of Hodgkin and Huxley's (1) m and h parameters, strongly supports the identification of the mobile charges responsible for generation of the gating current with the hypothetical m gating particles. Thus the time constant τ_{Ig} of the asymmetrical displacement current agrees very well both in absolute magnitude and in voltage dependence with the m system time constant τ_m, which equals $(1/\alpha_m + \beta_m)$ (7,17,28). If the mobile charges had nothing to do with the sodium conductance, it seems most unlikely that both systems would have precisely the same relaxation time over such a wide range of experimental conditions. However, some further comment is necessary on the problem of reconciling the observed time constant for shutting off the sodium conductance at the end of a short pulse, $\tau_{Na,off}$, with the prediction of m^3 kinetics that it should exactly equal $\frac{1}{3}(\tau_m)$, which has been reported both by Armstrong and Bezanilla (25) and by Keynes and Rojas (17) not to hold well. In this connection we must also account for the lengthening of the gating current tails with increasing pulse size (17,18), and explain why heavy water should slow down the sodium conductance change but not the gating current (18). A careful comparison between $\tau_{Na,off}$, measured with low sodium in the external medium to minimize errors from incomplete compensation for the electrical resistance in series with the membrane, and $\tau_{Ig,off}$ measured in the same axons, has shown (Keynes and Rojas, 7) that for large pulses there is actually rather little disagreement in size between $\tau_{Na,off}$ and $\frac{1}{3}(\tau_{Ig,off})$. But since $\tau_{Na,off}$ is independent of pulse size, whereas $\tau_{Ig,off}$ is not, the discrepancy remains as far as small pulses are concerned. I suggest that this behavior could readily be explained by the type of scheme illustrated in Fig. 3. Here

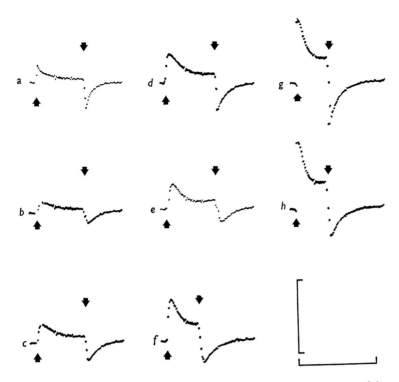

FIG. 2. A family of gating current records obtained by summation with a signal averager of the membrane currents for 60 positive and 60 negative pulses, which started and finished at the arrows. The axon was perfused with 55 mM CsF, and bathed in Na- and K-free saline containing 300 nM saxitoxin. Pulse amplitude **a–h**, 40–110 mV; holding potential, −70 mV; vertical bar, 5.56 μA; horizontal bar, 2,500 μsec; membrane area, 0.06 cm²; temperature, 7°C. (From Keynes and Rojas, ref. 17.)

the main voltage-dependent steps, which are those that give rise to the gating current, are A → B, B → A, B* → A*, and C → A**. If it is supposed that the relatively rapid interaction between the gating particles that opens the channel for the passage of ions involves a conformational change B → B* that can take place *only after all three* of the particles have first reached state B, and that this affects the subsequent relaxation time making $\tau_{B^* \to A^*}$ appreciably greater than $\tau_{B \to A}$, then for a small pulse in which few of the channels are opened and few of the particles reach state B*, $\tau_{Ig,off}$ will approximate to $\tau_{B \to A}$. For a large pulse, on the other hand, the majority of the particles will achieve state B*, and $\tau_{Ig,off}$ will therefore approach $\tau_{B^* \to A^*}$ in size. Whatever the potential during the pulse, $\tau_{Na,off}$ will remain equal to $\frac{1}{3}(\tau_{B^* \to A^*})$ as

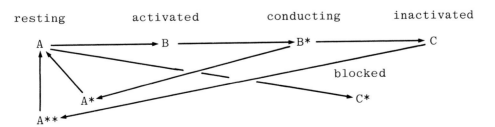

FIG. 3. A possible sequence of events during the application of a depolarizing voltage-clamp pulse.

observed experimentally. A further argument in support of this scheme is that if the conformational change B → B* involves hydrogen bonding, then—unlike the purely voltage-dependent steps—it might be slowed by heavy water; since $\tau_{Na,on} = \tau_{A \to B} + \tau_{B \to B^*}$, this would go some way toward explaining the observations of Meves (18).

Let us next compare the data for the steady-state distribution of the mobile charges with the curves relating sodium conductance and the parameter m to membrane potential. From a number of measurements of the dependence of peak sodium conductance on membrane potential, made in perfused axons at a large negative holding potential, the midpoint of the curve for $(g_{Na}/\bar{g}_{Na})^{1/3}$ was found to fall at approximately -34 mV (7). This is satisfactorily close to the value of -35 mV for the midpoint of the m_∞ curve given by Hodgkin and Huxley (1). The midpoint for the steady-state charge distribution curve in comparable axons was -26 mV (7). When the external calcium was changed, or the internal ionic strength was lowered, both curves were shifted along the voltage axis by amounts that agreed well with the data of Frankenhaeuser and Hodgkin (29) and Chandler et al. (30). Hence, over a rather wide range of experimental conditions, the midpoints of the charge

distribution curve and of the m_∞ curve coincided to within approximately 10 mV. A similar conclusion was reached by Nonner et al. (26) for the node of Ranvier. The residual discrepancy may be attributable to imperfect corrections for junction potential differences in the two sets of experiments, or if the scheme of Fig. 3 is valid, it may arise because the step $B \to B^*$ is governed to a limited extent by potential.

MODELS OF THE SODIUM GATING MECHANISM

The slope of the steady-state charge distribution curve at its steepest point corresponded to 19 mV for an e-fold change (17,18). Since for a singly charged particle displaced through the whole of the electric field the figure would be 25 mV for an e-fold change, the effective valency of the individual gating particles is $25/19 = 1.3$, this being the actual charge multiplied by the fraction of the electric field acting on the particle. There is at present no means of distinguishing between the cases of a single dipole moving through the greater part of the field, and of a molecule carrying a number of charged groups each of which moves through a small fraction of the field. Thus the two quite different models shown in Fig. 4, and no doubt

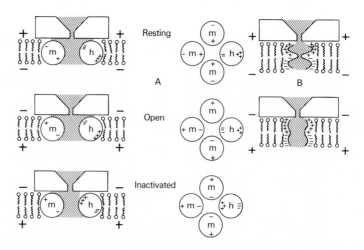

FIG. 4. Two possible models of the sodium channel. **A:** Based on a proposal by Rojas (34), the gating particles are shown as globular dipoles that rotate through 180° when the electric field changes. The channel conducts only when the negative charges on all three *m* particles and the *h* particle are in a position close to the aqueous pathway. **B:** The gating particles are seen as helical structures carrying positive and negative charges arranged in such a way that depolarization stretches them out and opens a pathway between them. In the inactivated state (not shown) the particles would be supposed to undergo a further conformational change that would close the pathway again.

many other arrangements of the charges, could have the same effective valency. Thus if the charges on the globular dipoles of Fig. 4A spanning the 25-Å membrane were separated by 23 Å, and if they rotated through 180° at 45° to the plane of the membrane, the effective valency would be $2 \times (23/25) \sin 45 = 1.3$. Equally the helix of Fig. 4B, carrying, say, 20 singly charged groups moving through an average of 3.25 Å at 30° to the plane of the membrane, would have an effective valency of $20 \times (3.25/25) \sin 30 = 1.3$. The only positive statement that can be made is that the total charge cannot be less than 1.3.

This uncertainty does not prevent the calculation of the number of separate gating particles that have to make the transition to the gate-open position (or configuration B* in Fig. 3) in each channel. The change in sodium conductance with potential is much steeper than the change in charge distribution, only 6.5 mV being required for an e-fold change (7). The most straightforward explanation for the difference would be that several particles are involved in the operation of the gate, the number in the squid giant axon being $19/6.5 = 3$. It is satisfactory that the quite different approach of seeking for the best fit of the initial rise in g_{Na} to Eq. (6) should yield the same figure (1,7). At the node of Ranvier, the change in sodium conductance is slightly less steep, but the charge distribution curve is steeper, so that the number of particles is $14.9/7.1 = 2$ (26), again in excellent agreement with the kinetic approach (4).

INACTIVATION OF THE SODIUM CONDUCTANCE

The discussion has so far been confined to activation of the sodium conductance. The inactivation process and the question of h-gating current must now be considered. It can be calculated from the data for h_∞ and τ_h of Hodgkin and Huxley (1), that if each channel incorporated a single independent h particle as well as the three m particles, then a pulse taking the membrane to the vicinity of 0 mV would reveal a second slow component of the gating current with an initial amplitude about 25% of the main one. Clearly there is no such component in the record shown in Fig. 1, which is

wholly typical in that it falls to 1% with a single time constant. There seems no doubt that normally the whole population of mobile charges has the same relaxation time, and although more slowly displaced ones must surely be present, they form no more than 2 or 3% of the total. Since no contribution to the gating current displaying the kinetics of the h system has yet been detected, the conclusion has to be that inactivation does not in fact involve the displacement of the separate and independent h particle portrayed in Fig. 4A. If instead the transition B* $\rightarrow$ C in the scheme of Fig. 3 were a time- rather than a voltage-dependent process, it would not be accompanied by any easily measurable passage of gating current. The mathematics of a three-state system have recently been explored by Goldman (31), and

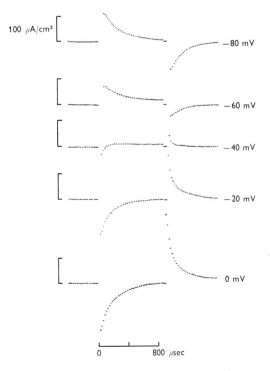

FIG. 5. The effect of varying the holding potential on the records of net displacement current obtained by summation of the membrane currents for equal and opposite voltage-clamp pulses. Axon perfused with a CsF solution of low ionic strength, and bathed in acetate saline containing 300 nM tetrodotoxin. Pulse size ± 150 mV. The membrane potential was held for several minutes at the level indicated to the right of each record. (From Keynes et al., ref. 37.)

shown to be fully compatible with Hodgkin-Huxley kinetics for the sodium conductance. It would appear that it is a system of this general type, in which activation and inactivation are not independent, with which we must deal.

Although there should be no difficulty in reconciling with the observed kinetics the conclusion that inactivation involves a purely time-dependent conformational change in the gating particles, it raises an awkward problem in relation to the steady-state characteristics. As has been seen, the midpoints of the m_∞ and charge distribution curves lie at around -25 mV. Why then should the midpoint of the h_∞ curve fall close to -60 mV (1)? A displacement in a nega-

tive direction of the curve for the degree of inactivation of the sodium conductance is to be expected because of the cubing operation that is involved, but this cannot account for a difference of 35 mV. An observation that seems rather likely to be related to this question is illustrated in Fig. 5. Here it is seen that when the holding potential is progressively lowered, the gating current records made by the technique of adding together the displacement currents for equal and opposite voltage-clamp pulses become inverted at a potential in the region of -50 mV. Very similar records have been obtained by Meves (18). This certainly does not mean that the direction of flow of the displacement current is reversed, as will be

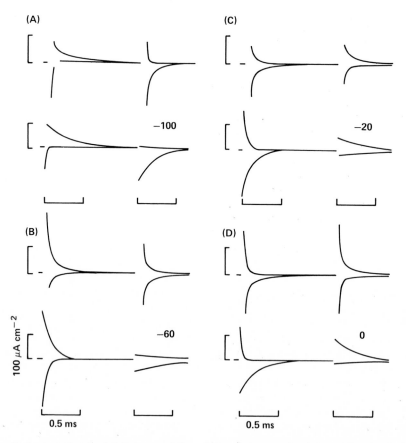

FIG. 6. The effect of varying the holding potential on single-sweep records of the unidirectional displacement current. The actual traces are shown above, and the calculated time course of the displacement current after subtraction of the capacity transient is shown below. Axon perfused with high ionic strength CsF solution and bathed in Na- and K-free isethionate saline containing 300 nM tetrodotoxin. Temperature 6.4°C. The holding potential in millivolts is given next to each group of records. Vertical calibration bars, 100 μA/cm²; horizontal bars, 0.5 msec. (From Rojas and Keynes, ref. 28.)

clear from the single-sweep records shown in Fig. 6, but simply that the midpoint of the charge distribution curve has somehow moved from −25 to −50 mV. At the same time it appears that the total amount of charge displaced by a large pulse may become appreciably smaller, recovery from this effect being a relatively slow process (18,27; and Bezanilla and Armstrong, reference 38). Much more information is needed about the rate of inception of these changes before their precise relationship to the mechanism of inactivation can be decided. In the meantime it may very tentatively be suggested that maintained depolarization results in the blocking of a certain proportion of the sodium channels because one of the three gating particles adopts a configuration indicated as C* in Fig. 3 in which it renders the other two incapable of displacement from state A. It would also seem necessary to suppose that depolarization alters either the electric field seen by the individual particles or their internal structure and hence their effective charge, thus changing both the steady-state distribution curve and the relaxation time. A similar suggestion may apply in relation to the action of zinc, which cuts down both the amplitude of the gating currents and the sodium conductance (32; H. Meves, *personal communication*).

THE POTASSIUM GATING CURRENT

The argument that the existence of a voltage-sensitive control mechanism implies the occurrence of gating currents has the same strength for potassium as it does for sodium. It will therefore be asked whether the potassium gating current has yet been recorded. The answer is in the negative, but this is not unexpected, since Hodgkin and Huxley's (1) data for the *n* system, taken with Conti et al.'s (16) evidence for the relatively low density of potassium channels in the membrane, suggests that the *n* particles might well contribute no more than 1% of the total gating current. If this were indeed the case, it would be very difficult to disentangle the potassium gating current from the slow component or components of the sodium gating current, and from the vagaries of any time-dependent variation in the leakage current.

CONCLUSIONS

It is evident that although a dim outline of the organization of the sodium channel is beginning to emerge, the details of its chemical structure are still wholly obscure. It may be presumed that it is a protein molecule that like other membrane proteins has a central section that is at home in the low-dielectric constant environment provided by the hydrocarbon chains of the lipid matrix. The irradiation inactivation studies of Levinson and Ellory (33), using TTX binding as an index of the intactness of the molecule, have yielded a molecular weight of about 230,000; but it is not clear that this measurement applies strictly to the whole channel, since there is some degree of functional independence between the TTX binding site and the gating mechanism. The gating current studies have provided rather strong support for the idea, originally put forward in Hodgkin and Huxley's (1) penetrating analysis of the kinetics of the conductance changes, that the voltage sensitivity derives from a displacement of and interaction between three charged subunits, although the new evidence also suggests that after the channel has opened, its subsequent closure involves further conformational changes within these same three subunits rather than the delayed displacement of a fourth subunit responsible for inactivation. It is for protein chemists to judge the relative plausibilities of the type of model proposed by Rojas (34) and shown in Fig. 4A, in which the passage of ions through a preexisting aqueous channel is controlled by the rotational movement of globular dipoles, and of the alternative mechanism of Fig. 4B, in which appropriate changes in the structure of three basically helical subunits open up a passage through the aqueous channel between them. The experimental evidence available does not yet provide an adequate basis for choosing between these possibilities. There is, however, a good prospect that future comparisons between the detailed behavior of the gating current and of the sodium conductance during treatment with agents like pronase (35) that selectively destroy inactivation, and others that may act by shifting the m_∞ and h_∞ curves (36), will help to solve the problem. Another respect in which measurement of the gating current bids fair to provide an important new tool is for elucidation of the mechanism of action of local anesthetics. It has been shown by Keynes and Rojas (17) that procaine reversibly reduces both the changes in sodium conductance and the amplitude of the gating currents, and at the same time irreversibly reduces the relaxation time. It will be most interesting to see how far it is the properties of the gating particles themselves that are affected by anesthetics and how far the interaction that presumably takes place between the particles and the surrounding lipids is also involved.

REFERENCES

1. Hodgkin, A. L., and Huxley, A. F. (1952): A quantitative description of membrane current and its application to conduction and excitation in nerve. *J. Physiol.* (Lond.), 117:500–544.
2. Adrian, R. H., Chandler, W. K., and Hodgkin, A. L. (1970): Voltage clamp experiments in striated muscle fibres. *J. Physiol.* (Lond.), 208:607–644.
3. Goldman, L., and Schauf, C. L. (1973): Quantitative description of sodium and potassium currents and computed action potentials in *Myxicola* giant axons. *J. Gen. Physiol.*, 61:361–384.
4. Frankenhaeuser, B. (1960): Quantitative description of sodium currents in myelinated nerve fibres of *Xenopus laevis. J. Physiol.* (Lond.), 151:491–501.
5. Frankenhaeuser, B. (1963): A quantitative description of potassium currents in myelinated nerve fibres of *Xenopus laevis. J. Physiol.* (Lond.), 169:424–430.
6. Cole, K. S., and Moore, J. W. (1960): Potassium ion current in the squid giant axon: dynamic characteristic. *Biophys. J.*, 1:1–14.
7. Keynes, R. D., and Rojas, E. (1975): The temporal and steady state relationships between activation of the sodium conductance and movement of the gating particles in the squid giant axon. *J. Physiol.* (Lond.), *in press.*
8. Narahashi, T. (1964): Restoration of action potential by anodal polarization in lobster giant axons. *J. Cell. Comp. Physiol.*, 64:73–96.
9. Adelman, W. J., and Palti, Y. (1969): The effects of external potassium and long duration voltage conditioning on the amplitude of sodium currents in the giant axon of the squid, *Loligo pealei. J. Gen. Physiol.*, 54:589–606.
10. Chandler, W. K., and Meves, H. (1970): Slow changes in membrane permeability and long-lasting action potentials in axons perfused with fluoride solutions. *J. Physiol.* (Lond.), 211:707–728.
11. Goldman, L., and Schauf, C. L. (1972): Inactivation of the sodium current in *Myxicola* giant axons. *J. Gen. Physiol.*, 59:659–675.
12. Rudy, B. (1975): Slow recovery of the inactivation of sodium conductance in *Myxicola* giant axons. *J. Physiol.* (Lond.), 249:22P.
13. Colquhoun, D., Henderson, R., and Ritchie, J. M. (1972): The binding of labelled tetrodotoxin to nonmyelinated nerve fibres. *J. Physiol.* (Lond.), 227:95–126.
14. Levinson, S. R., and Meves, H. (1975): The binding of tritiated tetrodotoxin to squid giant axons. *Phil. Trans. R. Soc. Lond.* [*Biol.*], 270:349–352.
15. Keynes, R. D., Bezanilla, F., Rojas, E., and Taylor, R. E. (1975): The rate of action of tetrodotoxin on sodium conductance in the squid giant axon. *Phil. Trans. R. Soc. Lond.* [*Biol.*], 270:365–375.
16. Conti, F., de Felice, L. J., and Wanke, E. (1975): Potassium and sodium ion current noise in the membrane of the squid giant axon. *J. Physiol.* (Lond.), 248:45–82.
17. Keynes, R. D., and Rojas, E. (1974): Kinetics and steady-state properties of the charged system controlling sodium conductance in the squid giant axon. *J. Physiol.* (Lond.), 239:393–434.
18. Meves, H. (1974): The effect of holding potential on the asymmetry currents in squid giant axons. *J. Physiol.* (Lond.), 243:847–867.
19. Hodgkin, A. L. (1975): The optimum density of sodium channels in an unmyelinated nerve. *Phil. Trans. R. Soc. Lond.* [*Biol.*], 270:297–300.
20. Hille, B. (1971): The permeability of the sodium channel to organic cations in myelinated nerve. *J. Gen. Physiol.*, 58:599–619.
21. Rojas, E. (1975): Currents carried by various cations through the membrane of the giant axon of *Loligo. Pflügers Arch.*
22. Armstrong, C. M. (1971): Interaction of tetraethylammonium ion derivatives with the potassium channels of giant axons. *J. Gen. Physiol.*, 58:413–437.
23. Armstrong, C. M., and Hille, B. (1972): The inner quaternary ammonium ion receptor in potassium channels of the node of Ranvier. *J. Gen. Physiol.*, 59:388–400.
24. Hille, B. (1973): Potassium channels in myelinated nerve. Selective permeability to small cations. *J. Gen. Physiol.*, 61:669–686.
25. Armstrong, C. M., and Bezanilla, F. (1974): Charge movement associated with the opening and closing of the activation gates of the Na channels. *J. Gen. Physiol.*, 63:533–552.
26. Nonner, W., Rojas, E., and Stämpfli, R. (1975): Displacement currents in the node of Ranvier. Voltage and time dependence. *Pflügers Arch.*, 354:1–18.
27. Bezanilla, F., and Armstrong, C. M. (1975): Inactivation of gating charge movement. *Biophys. J.*, 15:163a.
28. Rojas, E., and Keynes, R. D. (1975): On the relation between displacement currents and activation of the sodium conductance in the squid giant axon. *Phil. Trans. R. Soc. Lond.* [*Biol.*], 270:459–482.

29. Frankenhaeuser, B., and Hodgkin, A. L. (1957): The action of calcium on the electrical properties of squid axons. *J. Physiol.*, 137:218–244.

30. Chandler, W. K., Hodgkin, A. L., and Meves, H. (1965): The effect of changing the internal solution on sodium inactivation and related phenomena in giant axons. *J. Physiol.* (Lond.), 180: 821–836.

31. Goldman, L. (1975): Quantitative description of the sodium conductance of the giant axon of *Myxicola* in terms of a generalized second-order variable. *Biophys. J.*, 15:119–136.

32. Bezanilla, F., and Armstrong, C. M. (1974): Gating currents of the sodium channels: three ways to block them. *Science*, 183:753–754.

33. Levinson, S. R., and Ellory, J. C. (1973): Molecular size of the tetrodotoxin binding site estimated by irradiation inactivation. *Nature New Biol.*, 245:122–123.

34. Rojas, E. (1975): Gating mechanism of sodium currents in nerve membranes. *Pflügers Arch., in press.*

35. Armstrong, C. M., Bezanilla, F., and Rojas, E. (1973): Destruction of the sodium conductance inactivation in squid axons perfused with pronase. *J. Gen. Physiol.*, 62:375–391.

36. Narahashi, T. (1974): Chemicals as tools in the study of excitable membranes. *Physiol. Rev.*, 54:813–889.

37. Keynes, R. D., Rojas, E., and Rudy, B. (1974): Demonstration of a first-order voltage-dependent transition of the sodium activation gates. *J. Physiol.* (Lond.), 239:100–101P.

38. Bezanilla, F., and Armstrong, C. M. (1975): Inactivation of gating charge movement. *Biophys. J.*, 15:163a.

The Nervous System, Donald B. Tower, Editor-in-Chief. *Vol. 1: The Basic Neurosciences.* Raven Press, New York, 1975.

Evolution of Theories of Nerve Excitation

Ichiji Tasaki

In this chapter, a brief survey is made of the evolution of hypotheses and theories proposed to explain the process of nerve excitation. The objective of this survey is to show the experimental facts from which the basic concepts and ideas adopted by previous and recent investigators in this field were derived. There have been very few articles published in which a historical and comparative approach has been taken toward the problem of nerve excitation; the following reasons may be cited for this situation.

The modern scientific community is highly competitive. Even in a limited field of investigation, the volume of literature published yearly is so great that it is difficult to keep abreast of the events in the field. In addition, new methods and techniques are frequently introduced into the field, and it is very difficult for traditionally trained investigators to understand the full significance of the newly acquired results. To sustain research activities on public funds, investigators are under constant pressure to publish their results, emphasizing the novelty and the originality of their own views. These investigators would have little time to pay attention to what has happened many years ago. In many respects, the social environment for scientists at present is very different from that at the time when Mendel's law was rediscovered.[1]

In spite of this trend, there seems little doubt that a historical and comparative approach can greatly facilitate a full, factual understanding of the problem of nerve excitation. Presentation of one particular theory inevitably leads to an overemphasis of a particular set of experiments. As in other fields of investigation, there are many cases in which "new" theories are not altogether new. They simply represent a revival or recombination of old ideas. It is not surprising that an inquiry into old theories and forgotten facts frequently furnishes useful hints for new ideas. No one would doubt that a reasonable prediction of the future of the field is possible only on the basis of a careful study of the course of evolution in that field.

Among the living tissues studied by biologists, the structure of an axon is relatively simple. Nevertheless, experimental studies on axons are manifold, and the results obtained are quite complex. Although experiments carried out under well-defined conditions are highly reproducible, it is extremely difficult (if not impossible) to describe the significance of these experimental results objectively. Precautions are taken in this chapter to distinguish clearly between experimental facts and their interpretations.

NERNST'S SEMIPERMEABLE MEMBRANE THEORY

In 1908, Walther Nernst (1) published his theory, the physicochemical basis of which is quite sound; the manner in which he treated the experimental data could be regarded as exemplary of quantitative biological research. Since this was the first theory of this kind, its impact on physiologists at that time must have been very great. Even in the 1930s, several professors of physiology in Japan were dedicating their entire effort to extending Nernst's approach.

At the time his theory was formulated, the foundation of electrochemistry was well established. Both the ion theory of Arrhenius (1883) and the dilution law of Ostwald (1888) were already fully accepted, and Planck (1890) had just published his mathematical solutions of electrodiffusion problems including the constant-field equation.

Nernst started his theory by pointing out that

---

[1] Gregor Mendel's article "Versuche über Pflanzen-Hybriden" was published in 1866 and his death came in 1884. The famous rediscovery took place 16 years after his death.

high-frequency alternating current (a.c.) is far less effective as a stimulus to nerves than low-frequency a.c. He showed that an electric current passing through a homogeneous electrolytic solution causes no change in the ionic composition. (Note that the number of ions entering into every volume element at any moment is equal to that of the same ion species leaving the same volume element.) He argued that a semipermeable membrane that prevents free diffusion of ions is responsible for the maintenance of the difference in electrolyte composition inside and outside the nerve. When a current penetrates this semipermeable membrane, a change is brought about in the electrolyte composition in the vicinity of the membrane.

Nernst did not specify the ion species that penetrate the semipermeable membrane. Of course, he did not have any idea about physicochemical properties of the nerve membrane. Nevertheless, he predicted that the passage of a current through such a membrane brings about a rise in the salt concentration of one side and a fall (or desalination) on the other side. (The term salt concentration, and not ion concentration, was used throughout.) The rate of salt accumulation is proportional to the current intensity. The salt accumulated on the surface of the membrane is carried by diffusion away from the surface of the membrane.

The equation describing this diffusion process is

$$\frac{\partial c}{\partial t} = k\,\frac{\partial^2 c}{\partial x^2}$$

where c, the salt concentration, is a function of time (t) and distance (x) from the membrane; k is the diffusion coefficient (determined by the mobilities of the anions and cations involved). The boundary condition (at $x = 0$) is

$$-k\,\frac{\partial c}{\partial x} = vi$$

where i is the current density and v the proportionality constant. At $x = \infty$, c is constant and equal to c_o. When the current intensity varies sinusoidally with time, namely, when

$$i = a \sin nt$$

n being the circular frequency and a the amplitude, the solution of the diffusion equation is given by

$$c = c_0 + \frac{av}{(nk)^{1/2}} \sin\left(nt + \frac{\pi}{4}\right)$$

For the current to be effective in exciting the nerve, the salt concentration at the membrane surface must exceed a certain critical value. From this consideration, it follows that the relationship between the frequency of the a.c. ($2\pi m = n$) and threshold strength i is given by

$$i(m)^{1/2} = \text{constant}$$

When rectangular current pulses are used for stimulation, the following relationship was obtained between the threshold strength and the duration t:

$$i(t)^{1/2} = \text{constant}$$

Nernst made an extensive comparison between the theoretical results and the experimental data (obtained by his own collaborators and by other physiologists). He obtained excellent agreement between the theory in the range of frequency higher than 100 Hz and experiment. Table 1 shows an example of the results quoted in his paper. With rectangular current pulses, a good agreement was within a limited range of duration. He attributed the deviation observed with pulses of long duration to accommodation (see below).

Soon after the publication of this paper, Hill (2) derived an equation for the strength-duration relation under the condition that the two boundaries (membranes) were separated by a short

TABLE 1.

m	i Observed	i Calculated	Difference	$i(m)^{1/2} \cdot 10^2$
105	−.81	0.78	−4.2%	78
136	0.88	0.92	+4.6%	75
785	2.16	2.21	+2.3%	77
960	2.41	2.47	+2.9%	77
2230	3.85	3.73	−3.1%	81

distance. Hill did not specify the location of his two membranes in the nerve fiber. However, since his equation contains three adjustable parameters, good agreement was obtained with observation in a wider range of pulse durations. Lucas (3) examined the significance of these three parameters in Hill's equation by determining *i-t* relations under a variety of experimental conditions.

In spite of the fantastic simplicity and beauty of these highly mathematical treatments, the quantitative aspects of these theories are now completely abandoned.[2] Nernst's basic assumption about the semipermeability of the nerve membrane is still considered correct.

LOEB'S COLLOID THEORY

Jacques Loeb's theory was formulated on the basis of his own experiments in which the effects of various ions on excitable tissues were compared with their effects on various biocolloids. At that same time, Ringer (1880 to 1886) and Locke (1894) had already published their recipes for saline solutions that are favorable for maintaining the excitability of excised muscles and nerves. To explain the effects of Ca ions on excitable tissues, Loeb introduced the concept of ion-antagonism. Although Loeb's theory is qualitative, I believe that the basis of his idea is quite sound and has been exploited, often unknowingly, by many recent investigators. The following paragraphs are taken directly from his monograph (4) published in 1906, summarizing his ideas published earlier.

> The salt, or electrolytes in general, do not exist in living tissues as such exclusively, but are partly in combination with proteids or fatty acids. The salts or electrolytes do not enter into this combination as a whole, but through ions. The great importance of these ion-proteid compounds (or soaps) lies in the fact that, by the substitution of one ion for another, the physical properties of the proteid compound change. We thus possess in these ion-proteid or soap compounds essential constituents of living matter, which can be modified at desire, and hence enable us to vary and control the life phenomena themselves [*p. 78*].

> Life phenomena, and especially irritability, depends on the presence in the tissues of a number of various metal proteid, or soaps (Na, Ca, K and Mg), in definite proportions [*p. 78*].

> The quotient of the concentration of the Na-ions over the Ca-ions, C_{Na}/C_{Ca}, becomes therefore of importance for phenomena of irritability [*p. 79*].

> We know that in general a substitution of Ca for K or Na in colloids favors the formation of more solid or insoluble compounds. In the case of the coagulation of blood or milk, it is also obvious that Ca in moderate quantities favors coagulation [*p. 87*].

> The normal irritability of animal tissues depends upon the presence in these tissues of Na-, K-, Ca-, and Mg-ions in the right proportion; ... any sudden change in the relative proportions of these ion lipoids or ion proteids or ion carbohydrates alters the properties of the tissues and gives rise to an activity or an inhibition of the activity [*p. 95*].

> It is not impossible that a substitution of K for Ca, or vice-versa, in ion colloid actually occurs at the cathode, while a constant current flows through the nerve [*p. 102*].

Loeb's colloid theory was modified to a considerable extent by Höber. He found, on the basis of his experiments on muscles (1904 to 1919), that the magnitude of the effects of ions on the excitability follows Hoffmeister's lyotropic series. The ion effects on the nerve were explained also in terms of the lyotropic series (see ref. 5, p. 659).

It is important to note that, in the experiments carried out by Loeb and Höber, frog nerve-muscle preparations, heart muscles, and other excitable tissues were employed, taking muscular contraction as an index of effective stimulation. Hence the results obtained were frequently confusing. Nevertheless, with slight modifications, Loeb's idea can be used to explain the results of most recent observations on the effects of ions on excitable systems (see below).

---

[2] We now believe that the constant in Nernst's $i(m)^{1/2}$ equation reflects the time constant of the myelin sheath and not the diffusion constant of ions near the nodal membrane.

CHRONAXIE

For many years after the publication of Nernst's paper, many physiologists sustained their enthusiasm for precise measurements of the strength-duration (*i-t*) relations in nerves and muscles. Lapicque's term "chronaxie" was used to characterize these relations (6). (Chronaxie represents the critical duration required for excitation with twice the threshold intensity for a direct current.) At that time, rectangular current pulses were generated mechanically by opening two switches successively with a heavy dendulum. A precise measurement of the chronaxie required an advanced knowledge of electricity. Great satisfaction could have been derived from successful determination of pulse durations of a fraction of a millisecond with a moving-coil galvonometer whose response time was several seconds.[3] Lapicque's monograph (1926) describes the account of chronaxie measurements on a large number of excitable tissues under a variety of experimental conditions. Lapicque believed that the mechanism of neuromuscular transmission could be elucidated by determining the chronaxie of the nerve and muscle. Many physiologists attempted to interpret complex phenomena in the central nervous system on the basis of Lapicque's concept.

It should be noted, however, that even at the peak of the popularity of chronaxie measurements few papers questioned the significance of such measurements. Davis (8), for example, pointed out that the chronaxie of a muscle measured with large electrodes is much longer than the value obtained with a small stimulating cathode. Finally, Rushton (9) put a damper on this popularity; he also stressed the dependence of the chronaxie on the arrangement of the electrodes used for stimulation.

When a current pulse is delivered to a nerve trunk, a change in the potential drop is produced across the nerve membrane. Since the time of Hermann (10), it has been known that the nerve membrane can be represented by a leaky capacitor. It is possible to derive a

strength-duration relation on the assumption that the threshold is reached when this capacitor is charged to a critical level (7). It is not surprising that the strength-duration relation for an excitable tissue is affected to a great extent by the experimental arrangement used to deliver the pulses. There is no doubt that the strength-duration relation offers some information about the electric properties of the excitable tissue. However, measurements with a high degree of precision do not seem to yield highly reliable information about the tissue.

TWO FACTOR THEORIES

During the early 1930s, mathematically oriented physiologists were interested in describing the process of nerve excitation by using one or two differential equations (see ref. 11). The leaders of this approach were Blair, Monnier, Rashevsky, and Hill. These equations describe the behavior of some property (or quantity) produced in the nerve by a stimulating electric current. Monnier and others called this quantity *l'état d'excitation;* Hill and others called it local potential. The physicochemical nature of this quantity was not specified; only the alleged law governing the rise and fall of this quantity was expressed by the differential equations. Different authors employed slightly different mathematical expressions to describe the process. Again it was assumed that threshold was reached when the local excitatory state reached a certain critical level.

Let us follow the formulation developed by Hill (41). The rate of rise of the local potential V is assumed to be proportional to the intensity of the current i. At the same time, V spontaneously decays and the rate of this decay is proportional to $(V - V_0)$, where V_0 is the value of V before the onset of the stimulating current pulse. Thus the law governing the rise and fall of V is described by

$$\frac{dV}{dt} + \frac{(V - V_0)}{k} = bi$$

where b and k are constants. The critical value of V required for excitation of the nerve is U. Furthermore, it was assumed that U rises slowly when long current pulses were used for stimulation (accommodation).

---

[3] Note that cathode-ray oscillographs were not available for most physiologists until about 1930. although Erlanger and Gasser (7) started using them earlier.

$$\frac{dU}{dt} + \frac{(U - U_0)}{\beta} = \frac{(V - V_0)}{\lambda}$$

where β and λ are also constants. This pair of differential equations can be solved for rectangular current pulses (i = constant) and for exponentially decaying (i.e., condenser discharge) pulses. The solutions of these equations were found to adequately describe the observed strength-duration relation when the adjustable constants in the equations were properly chosen.

Why did this pure formalism appear so attractive to physiologists at that time? And why was this approach completely abandoned later? I would like to quote Heilbrunn's opinion (ref. 12, p. 431) on these points.

> Because of their deep admiration of the science of physics, biologists are often too enthusiastic about the application of the mathematical method to problems of excitation. If a mathematical physicist were asked to develop equations for a process involving chemical substances acting in a system whose physical properties are largely unknown, he would presumably feel rather hesitant about making any attempt at mathematical analysis. Some of the mathematicians who have worked in the field of excitation have been but little aware of the complexities of biological material; often enough they have too little understanding of what it is they are trying to explain.

Heilbrunn is right, I am afraid. In spite of the great popularity at that time, the results of precise measurements of the strength-duration relation and of chronaxie did not make any contribution to the progress that took place in the following decades.

RUSHTON'S CONCEPT OF LIMINAL LENGTH OR AREA

A dramatic revival of an old concept in physiology took place shortly before World War II. By applying Hermann's idea of restimulation by local currents, Rushton (13) predicted the existence of a small area of the membrane in the excited state when the stimulating current is subthreshold.

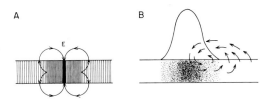

FIG. 1. Diagrams showing the local currents in the nerve. (Diagram **A** is adapted from Hermann, ref. 10; diagram **B** is redrawn from Lillie, ref. 14.)

Figure 1A is adapted from Hermann's handbook of physiology (10) published in 1879. Symbol E in the figure represents the area of the membrane thrown into the excited state by the stimulating current. This area is traversed by an inwardly directed current. In the neighboring zones, there are outwardly directed currents that tend to excite these zones. The inwardly directed current through the primary excited membrane area tends to bring this area back to the resting state. Figure 1B is reproduced from a figure in Lillie's monograph (14) published in 1932, illustrating his conception of the local current flowing between the excited region and the resting area of a frog nerve fiber. He based his entire argument on the similarity in electric behavior between a passive iron wire in nitric acid and a nerve. It is interesting to note that the excited region of the nerve in this figure is represented by discrete stipples.

With this picture in mind, Rushton developed the following argument. The primary excited area is expected to increase with the stimulus intensity. When the area is large enough, a propagated all-or-none action potential is initiated by the stimulus. However, if the stimulating current pulse is weak, the size of the excited area produced by the applied stimulating pulse could be too small to initiate a propagated nerve impulse. Thus the condition for initiation of the nerve impulse is that, to use Rushton's expression, "an action potential should arise over a region great enough to generate an action current sufficient to stimulate the neighbouring region." In other words, if the local currents are acting as a restimulating agent, there should be a small response localized at the site of (subthreshold) stimulation. To facilitate his mathematical analysis, Rushton assumed that the primary excited area is delineated sharply, as shown in Hermann's diagram, by two lines perpendicular to the long axis of the axon. However, there is no reason why the excited area cannot be irregular or patchy, as hinted in Lillie's figure (Fig. 1B). At that time Rushton was convinced that the experiment carried out by the youngest member in his laboratory, Hodgkin, indicated the validity of the local current theory. Soon after Rushton's prediction, Hodgkin actually succeeded in demonstrating the existence of a small, graded response at the site of subthreshold stimulation.

In this connection, it is interesting to note that graded, subthreshold responses can be demonstrated easily in an iron wire model of nerve (Matsumoto). When a subthreshold current pulse is applied to a passive iron wire, small, discrete, "active" patches and spots can be seen to appear on the passive surface. The number of active spots and patches increases with the current strength. (These spots and patches disappear quickly when the applied current is terminated.) When the fraction of the surface covered by these spots and patches reaches a certain critical value, the entire surface of the iron is thrown into the active state. This observation points out the possibility of the existence of active patches and spots in the nerve membrane.[4]

It was realized at about that time that, in analyzing excitation processes in frog nerve fibers, the structural factors arising from the existence of nodes of Ranvier and myelin sheath must be taken into consideration. Tasaki and his collaborators (15) have demonstrated that the myelin sheath is a good electric insulator (particularly to d.c.) and that the process of excitation is localized at nodes of Ranvier. Furthermore, nerve impulses were shown to propagate from one node to the next as the result of restimulation by local currents, the rate of propagation being determined almost exclusively by the cable property of the myelin sheath. When this saltatory nature of impulse propagation in myelinated nerve fibers was revealed, many baffling mysteries that surrounded previous studies of nerve conduction were solved (15). However, it also became very clear that the use of vertebrate nerve fibers for

studies of excitation processes *per se* presents various kinds of difficulties arising from the smallness of these fibers. Soon thereafter neurophysiology entered a new era in which much larger invertebrate nerve fibers were used for analysis of excitation processes.

THE THEORY OF HODGKIN AND HUXLEY

The important effect of the Na ion on the excitability of muscles and nerves was discovered in 1902 by Overton (17). Overton's experiments were mentioned by Höber (5) in his 1926 monograph. However, it is almost impossible to find these results in Bayliss' textbook of physiology published in 1924. Apparently, these results were not publicized as much as his lipoid-solubility theory of narcosis. Since Overton's experiments were carried out on frog muscle-nerve preparations taking muscular contraction as an index of excitation, all the results obtained were of a qualitative nature.

In 1949, Hodgkin and Katz (44, see also refs. 18 and 19) extended Overton's experiment and arrived at a quantitative conclusion as to the role of Na^+ in nerve excitation. They used, instead of frog nerves, squid giant axons introduced to physiologists by Young (20). The diameter of these axons is so large that the membrane potentials can be measured directly by inserting one of the recording electrodes into the protoplasm (42,43).

The results of measurements of action potentials with an internal recording electrode (referred to the electrode in the external medium) have shown that the effect of the external sodium concentration, $[Na]_e$, can be described by

$$E_a = \frac{RT}{F} \ln [Na]_e + \text{constant}$$

where E_a is the potential level at the peak of excitation. Hodgkin and Katz (44) assumed that the colloidal material inside the axon did not affect their potential measurements and concluded that E_a was very close to E_{Na} defined by the Nernst equation for Na^+, namely, by

$$E_{Na} = \frac{RT}{F} \ln \frac{[Na]_e}{[Na]_i}$$

---

[4] Quite recently, electric signs of such active patches have been obtained by using hyperfine microelectrodes placed near the surface of squid giant axons (16).

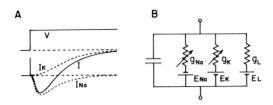

FIG. 2. A: Membrane current I observed under voltage clamp. **B:** The equivalent electrical circuit proposed by Hodgkin and Huxley. (Adapted from Hodgkin, ref. 19.)

$[Na]_i$ being the internal Na^+ concentration.

In the next step of the study of the role of Na ions, the method of voltage clamp with a pair of long internal metal electrodes was employed (45). The method of introducing a long metal electrode longitudinally into a squid axon was invented by Marmont (46); Cole's report (21) describing an example of voltage-clamp experiment had appeared shortly before. By using these new methods, the potential inside an axon could be suddenly raised above the level at rest and maintained for a predetermined period of time. When the potential jump produced by the clamping device was between 30 and 90 mV, the membrane current required to clamp the membrane was found to consist of (a) a fast transient called a capacitative current, (b) an inward current carried mainly by the major external univalent cation, Na^+, and (c) a delayed outward current carried by the major internal cation, K^+.

Figure 2A shows an example of the record obtained by this method. Hodgkin and Huxley assumed that the electric properties of the axon membrane could be represented by the equivalent circuit shown in Fig. 2B, where the electromotive forces (emfs) of the two batteries, E_{Na} and E_K, are defined by the Nernst equation for Na^+ and K^+, respectively. The two variable conductances, g_{Na} and g_K, one fixed resistor, g_L, and a fixed emf, E_L, were so chosen to fit the time course of the observed membrane current. The (total) membrane current under voltage clamp in this circuit is given by

$$I = I_{Na} + I_K + I_L$$

where the component currents are described by

$$I_{Na} = g_{Na}(V - E_{Na})$$
$$I_K = g_K(V - E_K)$$

and

$$I_L = g_L(V - E_L)$$

where both g_{Na} and g_K are assumed to be continuous functions of the voltage V and time t. Separation of I_{Na} from I was achieved by substituting the major portion of the external Na ions with inert choline ions.

The final step of the analysis carried out by Hodgkin and Huxley (47) was to use the empirically determined functions of $g_{Na}(V,t)$ and $g_K(V,t)$ and calculate the time course of the action potential produced under the unclamped conditions (namely, with the total membrane current kept at zero). They found that the action potential obtained by calculation closely followed that of the observed action potential. Based on these results, they concluded that the action potential in the squid axon membrane is produced by a rapid rise in g_{Na} followed by a gradual rise in g_K.

From a purely electrical point of view, the circuit shown in Fig. 2B is equivalent to a simpler circuit with a single battery of which the emf is given by $(g_{Na}E_{Na} + g_K E_K + g_L E_L)/(g_{Na} + g_K + g_L)$ and the internal resistance by $1/(g_{Na} + g_K + g_L)$. As long as V does not exceed the limits set by E_{Na}, E_K, and E_L, it is possible to describe any change in the membrane potential by properly choosing these time- and voltage-dependent conductances. It is also possible to fit the experimental data by introducing more batteries in the circuit (e.g., E_{Ca}, E_{Cl}). In fact, many physiologists explain their experiments by using such a circuit with many batteries.

EFFECTS OF EXTERNAL AND INTERNAL Na IONS

The successful reconstruction of the action potential by using the mathematical formulas for g_{Na} and g_K was (and still is) regarded by all physiologists as a gigantic step forward in our understanding of the process of nerve excitation. This enthusiastic acceptance of the theory brought about a tendency among physiologists to apply the basic concepts of the theory beyond the limit of applicability. Consequently, for investigators who are not dealing directly with squid giant axons, it has sometimes become very difficult to distinguish experimental results from inferences and experimental facts from interpretations. It therefore seems worthwhile to describe a few facts about the effect of Na and K ions on axon excitability for the benefit of non-axonologists.

Dispensability of Na Ions

There are many excitable systems that develop large action potentials in the absence of Na ions in the external medium. Nitella, studied extensively by Osterhout (48), and crustacean muscle fibers, studied by Fatt and Katz (49) and Hagiwara et al. (50), are the best known examples.

It is true that in both squid giant axons and frog nerve fibers the action potential amplitude diminishes rapidly when NaCl in the external medium is replaced with choline chloride. However, when the salts of hydrophilic cations (e.g., hydrazinium, hydroxylamine ion) are used instead of choline or tetraethylammonium ions, there is little or no decline in the action potential amplitude (see ref. 22).

When the action potential amplitude is examined under intracellular perfusion, it is found that the chemical species of both internal cations and anions have a large effect on the amplitude. Anions with low lyotropic numbers (F, phosphate, sulfate) give rise to large action potentials (22). When favorable anions are chosen, it is easy to demonstrate large action potentials in the absence of univalent cations in the external medium. The presence of a divalent cation salt is required in the medium in all these cases. The salt of cations with poor Na-substituting ability in the external medium (choline, tetramethylammonium, tetraethylammonium) produces large action potentials when used internally.

It is now well established that an axon internally perfused with a Na-salt solution is capable of developing all-or-none action potentials

when immersed in a medium containing $CaCl_2$ (16,22–24). Figure 3 shows an example of such observations. Record A was obtained from an axon internally perfused with 30 mM NaF and immersed in a medium containing 100 mM $CaCl_2$. The osmotic balance across the axon membrane was maintained by addition of glycerol to the internal and external media. Note that the concentration gradient for Na^+ is opposite that for normal (internally unperfused) axons immersed in sea water. Records B and C show that addition of NaCl to the external medium brings about a definite increase in the action potential amplitude.

In squid giant axons internally perfused with the solution of a favorable salt [CsF, $N(CH_3)_4F$], it was shown recently (Inoue, *unpublished*) that the dependence of the action potential amplitude on the external Na^+ and Ca^{2+} concentrations is adequately described by the equation

$$E_a = \frac{RT}{2F} \ln \{[Ca^{2+}]_e + Q\ [Na^+]_e^2\} + \text{constant}$$

where constant Q is a constant of the order of 0.05 mM^{-1}. [This empirical equation has been used to describe the behavior of a Ca-sensitive glass electrode in a mixed solution of $CaCl_2$ and NaCl; the dependence of the potential difference across such a glass membrane on Ca^{2+} and Na^+ derives from the cation-exchanger property of the glass phase.] In the absence of Na^+ in the medium, the action potential varies directly with log $[Ca^{2+}]_e$. However, when $[Na^+]_e > [Ca^{2+}]_e$, the effect of Na^+ becomes dominant; $E_a \approx (RT/F) \ln[Na]_e + \text{constant}$.

Influx of Na Ions

It has been stated frequently that influx of Na ions across the normal squid axon membrane is a prerequisite to the development of

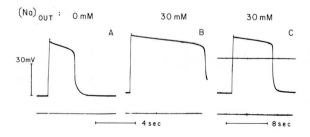

FIG. 3. All-or-none action potentials observed in a squid giant axon internally perfused with a solution containing NaF and glycerol. A: Taken when the external medium contained $CaCl_2$ and glycerol (but no sodium salt). B and C: Recorded after addition of 30 mM NaCl to the external medium. (From Watanabe et al., ref. 25.)

an action potential. This statement is either erroneous or misleading. To illustrate this point, let us consider an axon internally perfused with a K-salt solution and immersed in a medium containing NaCl and $CaCl_2$. To evoke an action potential, let us apply a strong and brief pulse (about 0.1 msec long) of outwardly directed current. When the pulse is strong enough to raise the membrane potential about 120 mV above the resting level, an action potential is evoked immediately. Under these conditions, there is no question that production of the action potential is preceded by an increased transport of K ions into and across the membrane, accompanied by a decrease in Na influx.

When the stimulating pulse is barely above the threshold, the membrane potential rises after the end of the pulse and then reaches the peak of the action potential. In this case also, the direct effect of the stimulating pulse is an increase of K efflux and a decrease of Na and Ca influx. During the rising phase of the action potential, there must be an increase in the Na and Ca influx. However, the question may be raised as to whether or not it is justifiable to call this increased Na influx a *cause* of excitation. According to Rushton's concept of subthreshold response (see section on Rushton's Concept of Liminal Length or Area), a small portion of the axon membrane is already in the excited state. There is an inward membrane current (carried mainly by Na ions in this case) in the excited zone surrounded by the resting area of the membrane. Thus it is possible (and quite natural) to interpret this increased Na influx as being the consequence of (partial) excitation of the membrane.

Tetrodotoxin

In recent literature, tetrodotoxin (TTX) played a significant role in the discussion of the role of the Na ion in the excitation process. Since the effect of this powerful puffer-fish poison is discussed elsewhere in this volume, only one aspect of the TTX effect is described here.

Originally, TTX gained its reputation as an agent capable of blocking Na influx through the membrane. However, it was later found that TTX suppresses action potentials even when there are no sodium ions in the external medium

(24,25). The conclusion drawn from this observation is that TTX cannot be used as a diagnostic tool to determine which ion species is involved in action potential production. A close inspection of the records obtained under the action of TTX reveals that a strong stimulating current pulse produced small, graded responses. Most physiologists accept the existence of two types of ion pores or channels, one more-or-less specific to Na ions and the other to K ions. If this is accepted, it is reasonable to interpret that TTX acts primarily on the early transient (Na) channel of the membrane (see below).

POTASSIUM IONS IN INTERNAL AND EXTERNAL MEDIA

Soon after the method of internal perfusion of squid axons was invented, experiments were carried out designed to examine the relationship between the internal K ion concentration and the resting membrane potential (see refs. 19 and 22). In these experiments, the major portion of the axoplasm was removed and the internal perfusion fluid containing the K salt of a favorable anion was continuously flowing through the axon interior. (Note that the favorability of internal anions falls in the following order: F ~ phosphate > sulfate > glutamate > Cl. . . .) The external medium was sea water, either natural or artificial. It was immediately found that the resting membrane potential is very insensitive to a large change in $[K]_i$. In the range of $[K]_i$ between 50 and 500 mM, the observed change in the membrane potential was roughly 10 mV, which is only approximately one-sixth of the value expected from the Nernst slope.

Two diametrically opposite interpretations were proposed to explain this somewhat unexpected experimental finding. In one interpretation (22), this finding was interpreted as indicating the absence of fixed charges of any appreciable density on the inner side of the axon membrane. In cation-exchanger membranes with a high density of fixed charges, the membrane potential is known to change with an ideal Nernst slope (approximately 58 mV for a 10-fold change in the concentration). The lack of such an effect was taken as indicating the absence of such fixed charges. In the other interpretation proposed by Chandler and Hodgkin

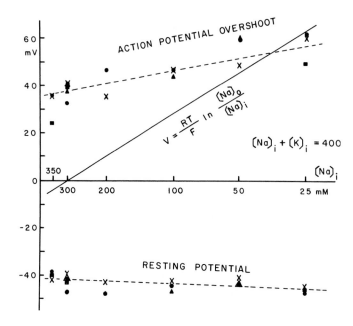

FIG. 4. The effect of changing the internal $K^+ - Na^+$ concentration ratio on the resting and action potentials of a squid giant axon. The sum of $[Na]_i$ and $[K]_i$ was kept constant. (From Tasaki and Takenaka, ref. 49.)

(26), the small concentration-effect of the internal K salt was attributed to the existence of an additional source of emf in series with the axon membrane proper. By assigning a certain type of concentration-dependent emf to this layer, it was argued that the entire experimental results could be explained without modifying the theory explained in the preceding section.

Figure 4 shows the results of an experiment conducted later, in which $[K]_i$ was varied by replacing Na^+ for K^+ without changing the ionic strength. The anions in the perfusion fluid were a mixture of fluoride and phosphate. [If chloride or other less favorable anions are used, a gradual deterioration of the axon sets in; note that NaCl was used in an early experiment (19) yielding a significantly different result.] With

these most favorable anions internally, the excitability of the axon can be maintained during the entire experiment. As can be seen in Fig. 4, there was hardly any appreciable change in the resting membrane potential when $[K]_i$ was varied in a wide range in this manner.

Why then had physiologists believed since the time of Bernstein (27) that the resting membrane potential was determined by K ions? Before the advent of the method of intracellular perfusion, the effect of varying the $[K]_e$ was examined by many investigators (e.g., ref. 18). Figure 5 shows the general character of the effect. In the range between approximately 100 and 500 mM, the membrane potential changes directly with log $[K]_e$, the slope being very close to 58 mV for a 10-fold change. In the range less

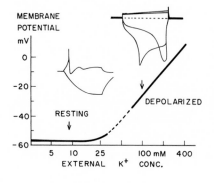

FIG. 5. Diagram showing the dependence of the membrane potential on the external K ion concentration. The potassium ion concentration was varied by replacing NaCl in the artificial sea water with KCl. *Insets*, responses of the axon membrane to rectangular current pulses.

than approximately 20 mM, variation of $[K]_e$ does not affect the membrane potential appreciably. There is the intermediate range, in which the dependence of the membrane potential on $[K]_e$ changes gradually. In a medium with a high $[K]_e$ (i.e., in a depolarized state), the axon is incapable of developing (normal) action potentials. In a low $[K]_e$ medium, the axon is able to develop normal action potentials. In the intermediate range of $[K]_e$ (designated as a mixed state), graded responses may be observed.

In the late 1950s, another important property of the axon membrane in the depolarized state was discovered [Segal, Tasaki, Stämpfli (see ref. 28)]. It was found that the depolarized axon membrane is capable of developing "hyperpolarizing" responses when tested with inwardly directed stimulating currents. (The sign of these responses is, as shown in Fig. 5, opposite to that of a normal, i.e., depolarizing, response.) Hyperpolarizing responses can never be observed in the normal, resting state of the axon membrane. Thus it is clear that a depolarized state of the membrane is quite distinct from a normal resting state. *It is in a depolarized state, and not in a normal resting state, that the membrane potential is dominated by K ions.* In an intact (i.e., internally unperfused) axon immersed in a K^+-rich medium, K^+ is the only predominant cation species inside and outside the membrane. Therefore, the K^+ dependence of the membrane potential under these conditions can reasonably be interpreted as an indication of cation-exchanger properties of the membrane (namely, the existence of ionized carboxylate or phosphate groups).

Since the time of Höber (ref. 5, pp. 640 and 650), physiologists have known that the depolarizing power of alkali metal ions decreases in the following order: $K > Rb > Cs > Na$. Squid axons can be depolarized by any one of these cations if the level of the external Ca-ion concentration is properly chosen. Further evidence is presented showing that a depolarized state of the membrane is distinct from the normal resting state.

EXCITATION BY NONELECTRICAL MEANS

It has long been known that a nerve can be excited by mechanical, osmotic, chemical, or thermal means. Osterhout and Hill (48) found that a *Nitella* cell can be excited by addition of a dilute KCl solution to the external medium. Blinks showed that an action potential can be evoked in a *Nitella* cell by sudden cooling (see ref. 22). Under intracellular perfusion of squid giant axons, it is easy to demonstrate excitation of the axon membrane by these nonelectrical means.

Figure 6A shows an example of the experimental results demonstrating an abrupt depolarization caused by a change in the chemical composition of the external medium. The axon was internally perfused with a dilute CsF solution in this case. Initially, the external medium contained 200 mM $CaCl_2$ only. When KCl was added (by replacing nonelectrolyte with the

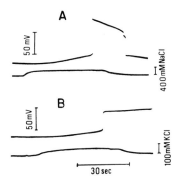
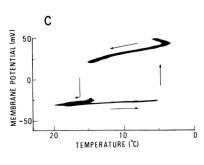

FIG. 6. Triggering abrupt changes in the membrane potential by a change in the univalent-divalent cation concentration ratio in the external medium (**A** and **B**) and by a cyclic change in the ambient temperature (**C**). (From Inoue et al., ref. 50.)

potassium salt), a sudden, large jump in the level of the internal potential was observed at a critical KCl concentration. As in Osterhout's experiments, this sudden jump in the membrane potential is regarded as representing the onset of a prolonged action potential. The critical concentration of KCl required for triggering this transition from the resting to the depolarized (i.e., the excited) state was found to vary with the external $CaCl_2$ concentration; in a high Ca medium, a higher concentration of K ion was required to produce abrupt depolarization. As is well known, the ability of the alkali metal ions to induce depolarization decreases in the following order: K > Rb > Cs > Na. It is possible to produce an abrupt depolarization by addition of NaCl to the medium when a proper level of $CaCl_2$ is chosen (16).

Figure 6C shows an example of the results demonstrating triggering a transition of the axon membrane between the resting and excited (i.e., depolarized) states by changes in the ambient temperature. In this case, the axon used was internally perfused with a dilute NaF solution and was immersed in a medium containing both NaCl and $CaCl_2$. It is seen in the figure that gradual cooling induced an abrupt depolarization and subsequent warming brought about an abrupt repolarization. Note the distinct hysteresis loop produced by a cyclic change in the temperature. Again, other alkali metal ions (such as Cs) can be used instead of Na in this experiment.

Quite recently it was found that similar transitions in the state of the membrane can be induced by changes in (a) hydrostatic pressure, (b) pH, and (c) salinity of the internal perfusion fluid (Inoue, *unpublished*). Initiation of an abrupt depolarization is always preceded by a huge increase in the amplitude of the fluctuation of the membrane potential.

TWO STABLE STATE THEORY

The two stable state theory was proposed originally by me together with a number of colleagues in this laboratory (Hagiwara, Singer, Watanabe, Lerman, Carnay, Kobatake). Various aspects of this theory were discussed from time to time in review articles from this laboratory (e.g., ref. 22). The theory was expanded and modified by several recent investigators (Changeux, Lehninger, Adam). More recently,

further experimental evidence has been obtained in support of this theory. I believe that this theory is now on a firm experimental basis.

We note that cleaned axons are incapable of developing action potentials when immersed in a medium completely free of divalent cations (e.g., in a medium containing EDTA). Based on the experimental facts described in the preceding sections, we accept the old idea (Loeb, Clowes, Heilbrunn, Brink, Tobias) that divalent cations play a crucial role in the process of nerve excitation. To this old idea, an important new notion is added that the macromolecules in the external membrane layer possess two stable conformational states separated by an unstable state. The concept of stability, instability and fluctuations in physical systems has been discussed recently by Prigogine and Glansdorf (29).

Let us consider an axon internally perfused with a solution containing a univalent cation salt and immersed in a medium containing the salts of both univalent and divalent cations, e.g., $CaCl_2$ and NaCl. We note that the univalent-divalent cation concentration ratio in the external medium plays an important role in determining the stability of the membrane macromolecules (Fig. 6). When the Ca ion concentration is high, the macromolecules assume one stable conformational state (resting state). As the univalent cation concentration is raised in the medium, the membrane macromolecules become unstable. Above a certain critical univalent-divalent cation concentration ratio, a different conformational state (i.e., excited or depolarized state) becomes stable.

We may visualize the membrane macromolecules of an axon in a Ca-rich medium as being held together by Ca ions acting as bridges between negatively charged sites. In such a Ca-rich state, the macromolecules are compact and have a low water content. These bridges are broken when the univalent cation concentration in the medium is increased. When a certain fraction of these bridges is broken, the macromolecules become unstable. In the state in which all or most bridges are broken, the macromolecules are stable again. In this univalent cation-rich state, the macromoles are less compact and have a high water content. A formal thermodynamic description of this ion-exchange process is presented elsewhere.

Based on our knowledge of the behavior of

nonbiological cation-exchangers, we assume that the replacement of Na ions for Ca ions bound to the negatively charged sites of the membrane macromolecules is exothermic. Therefore, lowering of the temperature favors substitution of divalent cations with univalent cations.

Under the conditions of the experiments described above (Fig. 6), variations of the membrane potential involve large changes in the phase-boundary potential between the external medium and the membrane. (The reader is reminded of the situation that the potential measured by a pH-sensitive glass-electrode is a reflection of the base-boundary potential rather than the semipermeability of the glass layer.) The membrane resistance is governed primarily by the water content of the membrane macromolecules: the higher the water content, the lower is the membrane resistance. (Note that the statement made above is little more than rephrasing the experimental findings described in the preceding two sections.)

The interior of the axon is free of Ca ions. A strong outwardly directed (i.e., stimulating) current through the membrane in the resting state drives internal univalent cations into the membrane, bringing about the replacement of some of the Ca ions in the membrane with univalent cations. It is important to note that the effect of electric stimulus is additive to the effect of changing the univalent-divalent cation concentration ratio in the medium. This is shown by the fact that the threshold intensity for electric stimulation falls rapidly and approaches zero as the univalent-divalent cation concentration ratio in the medium is brought close to the critical level for initiation of an abrupt depolarization. Thus electric stimuli are considered to bring about abrupt conformational changes by the same univalent-divalent cation-

exchange mechanism. The major difference between electric and nonelectric stimuli lies in the fact that only electric stimuli can bring about cation-exchange processes simultaneously over a wide area of the membrane. Weak electric stimuli are effective only when the state of the membrane macromolecules is not far from the unstable point.

The process of producing a hyperpolarizing response represents a transition from a depolarized (i.e., excited) state of the membrane to the resting. Let us consider an axon of which the membrane is in contact with a medium containing a relatively high concentration of univalent cations and a low concentration of divalent cations. A strong inwardly directed current through the membrane is expected to drive both univalent and divalent cations into the membrane. Because of the large difference in the intramembrane cation mobilities, however, univalent cations are transported through the membrane and divalent cations tend to remain in the membrane. By this mechanism, the membrane can be driven from the depolarized to the repolarized state.

When the axon membrane in the resting state is brought close to the critical point, a small fraction of the membrane may undergo a transition into the excited state. When this occurs, electric currents are generated between the excited and resting parts of the membrane. These currents are inwardly directed through the patches and domains in the excited state and outwardly directed through the resting area of the membrane (Fig. 7A). These currents may be called "ring currents"; they are different from local currents observed at the wave front of a propagated action potential in that ring currents in a macroscopically uniform membrane do not produce any potential drop along the long axis of the axon. The ring currents vanish when the

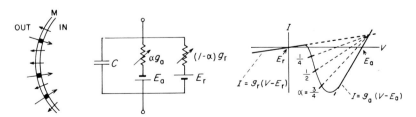

FIG. 7. Left: Diagram showing active patches of the axon membrane surrounded by the membrane area at rest. **Middle:** Equivalent electrical circuit representing a partially excited membrane. **Right:** Diagram showing the relationship between the *I-V* curve and the active fraction of the axon membrane. (Taken from Tasaki, ref. 22.)

axon membrane is either uniformly excited or uniformly resting. In the present theory, this ring current plays a crucial role in creation of cooperativity in the process of nerve excitation. The membrane system with ring currents is associated with an extra dissipation of free energy and is, in general, unstable.

The procedure of voltage clamping is an effective means of suppressing ring currents. Even in a mixed (i.e., nonuniformly excited) state, electric currents tend to flow directly between the internal and external electrodes. As the clamped level of the membrane potential (V) is raised, the fraction of the membrane in the excited state increases. According to Kirchhoff's law applied to the membrane in the partially excited state, the membrane current I is equal to the sum of the component flowing through the patches in the excited state I_a and the component through the resting area I_r, namely, by

$$I = I_a + I_r$$

These components are described by

$$I_a = \alpha\, g_a\, (V - E_a)$$

and

$$I_r = (1 - \alpha)\, g_r\, (V - E_r)$$

where α represents the fraction of the membrane in the excited state, g_a and g_r are the membrane conductances of the membrane in the uniformly excited and resting state, respectively, and E_a and E_r are the emfs in the two states of the membrane (see Fig. 7B). This set of equations is practically equivalent to that proposed by Hodgkin and Huxley (see section on their theory, presented earlier). Since α increases monotonically with the membrane potential V and since $g_a \gg g_r$, the membrane conductance increases monotonically with V. Thus the present theory offers a reasonable interpretation to the experimental finding that the membrane conductance is voltage-dependent. An analogous interpretation was proposed much later by Ehrenstein and Lacar (30).

Instead of inactivation, the term relaxation is used to describe the gradual change in E_a resulting mainly from the enormous enhancement of cation interdiffusion in the excited state of the membrane. When there are only two cation species in the system, one univalent and the other divalent, the rate of cation-interdiffusion

is low; consequently, E_a changes very slowly.

In dealing with the rising phase of an action potential (observed without voltage clamp), the present theory leads to practically the same mathematical treatment as that of Hodgkin and Huxley (note the similarity between Figs. 2B and 7B). From a physicochemical point of view, it is extremely difficult to develop a mathematical theory that deals with the rapidly changing membrane potential and conductance during the falling phase of an action potential. When an axon at rest is thrown into its excited state, the membrane and conductance increase so profoundly that the potential and conductance are no longer membrane-diffusion controlled (see ref. 22, p. 126). There is an appreciable accumulation of K salt in the periaxonal space (31). Unquestionably there is an accumulation of Na and Ca ions in the deeper layer of the axon membrane. Physicochemical theories of membrane phenomena are not yet capable of treating such a complex time-dependent system mathematically. However, there seems to be little doubt that the major factor that brings about a gradual fall in the membrane potential and eventual return to the resting state is enhanced cation interdiffusion across the membrane (see ref. 22, p. 126).

ION-PORE THEORY

Among physiologists, the term "ion channel" is used to denote the pathway of ion across the nerve membrane. Many physiologists interpret the equivalent circuit of Hodgkin and Huxley as suggesting the existence of three spatially distinct ion channels in the axon membrane. There are absolutely no physical means of determining the sites of penetration of these ions through the membrane even in the resting state of the axon. Many physiologists believe that TTX, which is capable of suppressing rapid, cooperative change in the squid axon membrane, can be used as a diagnostic tool for the involvement of Na channels.

On this point, Frankenhaeuser says in an article published in 1968 (ref. 32, p. 103), "Some of the very basic properties of the specific permeabilities are still unclear although indirect evidence accumulates on these points. No findings directly decide whether sodium and potassium are moving through the same or through different sites. Calcium clearly affects both the sodium and potassium systems." In his article in which the effects of anesthetics are explained, Mullins (see ref. 33, pp. 32–33) states: "The sharp pharmacological separation that can be made between sodium and potassium inhibitor has convinced many investigators that sodium channels and potassium channels are distinct and separate entities. While the evidence in this direction is not entirely overwhelming, for the following discussion, it is simpler to treat the experimental observations as if one were dealing with separate sodium and potassium carrying systems."

Notwithstanding the indirectness of the evidence for the existence of separate ion channels in the membrane, physiologists who have unquestioning faith in the equivalent circuit shown in Fig. 2B proceeded to the business of depicting a very precise picture of the Na channels in the nerve membrane. In his article published in 1972, Hille (34) states: "The pore has a rectangular hole 3.1×5.1 Å formed by a ring of oxygen atoms. This hole is both the pathway for ion flow and the selectivity filter which determines which ions can flow. The narrow part of the pore is further supposed to be very short and to bear a single negative charge. The charge attracts cations and repels anions."

Hille's hypothetical pore structure is designed to explain why Na^+ is preferred over other univalent cations in generating a strong inward current under voltage clamp. Based on the observation of intracellularly applied tetraethyl-ammonium ion, a similar hypothetical pore structure of the K channel is considered. This approach was without a doubt warmly encouraged by the discovery of macrocyclic ligands, which can be designed to be selective for particular cations (35). Furthermore, it has been suggested that an electric field could induce transitions between conducting and nonconducting states (36).

Although studies of the behavior of macrocyclic ligands have given a great impetus to the analysis of ion selectivity, prudent caution must be exercised against the overemphasis of the importance of these molecules. According to Williams (37), it is incorrect to conclude that macrocyclic systems only generate a particular cation selectivity. When the negatively charged sites in the membrane derive from weak acid anions (such as carboxylate and phosphate), any order of selectivity is possible, depending on the ion radii and the number of ligands coordinated (see ref. 37, p. 346).

According to the experimental findings stated in preceding sections, the nerve membrane is characterized by its lability. The excitability can readily be suppressed by intracellular application of the salt of unfavorable anions (e.g., Cl^-, Br^-, NCS^-) or cations (e.g., Ca^{2+}). The external surface of an axon is quite insensitive to unfavorable anions, indicating that the ion channels are not simple holes in the membrane. Enzymatic removal of the protein layer on the inner surface of the axon membrane reduces the maximum value of membrane conductance at the peak of excitation. Internal perfusion solutions with a low ionic strength are favorable in the axon interior, whereas an isotonic sugar solution exhibits a strong deteriorative effect on the external membrane surface. These experimental facts, as well as those described previously, are consistent with the idea that the excitable part of the membrane is composed of an asymmetric lipoprotein complex with a high density of negative fixed charges in the outer layer and a low density in the inner membrane layer. It seems very difficult to interpret these experimental facts on the assumption that cations are transported through rigid ion pores across the membrane. No attempt has yet been made to explain any of these experimental facts from the standpoint of the specific ion-pore theory.

The experimental facts that are regarded as indicative of the validity of the ion-pore theory can be reinterpreted on a different theoretical basis. For example, intracellularly administered NEt_4 ions can be considered as being weakly bound to the hydrophobic part of the protein molecules on the inner side of the membrane. These polyatomic cations can easily be displaced by application of a strong inward current but not by an outward current. The increase of the hydrophobicity of the protein layer brought about by these organic cations would reduce the outward current carried predominantly by K^+ under ordinary experimental conditions. Electric currents are carried through a membrane with negative fixed charges mainly by small cations. When the potential difference across such a membrane is displaced by a current from an external source by 25 mV ($=RT/F$) or more, the current is carried predominantly by the univalent cations on the anodal side of the membrane.

The Na-K permeability ratio for the axon membrane in the excited state has been determined by comparing the peak inward membrane current (under voltage clamp) before and after replacement of NaCl in the external medium with KCl. From a physicochemical point of view, this is by no means a simple procedure. Even when the external $CaCl_2$ concentration is kept constant, the univalent-divalent cation concentration ratio in the outer membrane layer is expected to vary (increase) with a change (an increase) in the K-Na ratio in the medium. According to the results of analyses of hyperpolarizing responses of axons in a K-rich medium, the difference in emf between the two (repolarized and depolarized) states of the membrane is only 20 mV or less. The peak intensity of the inward current under voltage clamp is proportional to the difference in emf between the two states of the membrane. Therefore, the observed reduction of the peak inward current brought about by substitution of KCl for NaCl in the external medium does not automatically indicate that the membrane in the excited state is less permeable to K^+. (Note that in the two stable state theory, changes in the phase-boundary potential associated with cooperative univalent-divalent cation exchange plays a dominant role in determining the difference in the membrane potential in the two states.)

Some of the recent theories of nerve excitation (e.g., the one advanced by Urry, ref. 36) have a definite element of the "stable-stable state" concept, as well as the concept of ion-pores. It might be possible both to elaborate such an approach and to explain most of the experimental facts known at present. It is important, however, to note that the threshold membrane potential is only about 25 mV ($\approx RT/F$) above the resting potential level. The amount of energy delivered directly to a membrane macromolecule by such a stimulus would be far smaller than the energy of random thermal motion. (To account for the large change in the membrane property produced by such a stimulus, the concept of cooperativity has been introduced.) Any theory of nerve excitation must account for this fact, as well as for the experimental results described earlier.

OPTICAL AXONOLOGY AND ITS FUTURE

In 1968, Cohen et al. (38) published an article describing changes in turbidity and birefringence of nerve fibers during action potentials. Shortly after this publication, my collaborators and I (39) reported the demonstration of changes in extrinsic fluorescence during the process of nerve excitation. From these early studies, a new field of investigation which may be called "optical axonology" has emerged. Since then, more than a dozen articles have appeared describing the experimental results obtained by the use of these new optical methods.

At the time of the early studies, it was hoped that the changes in the supramolecular structure during the process of nerve excitation would soon be elucidated by these new methods. At present, however, the initial goal of these investigations is almost as far as it was 5 years ago. There is no consensus of opinion among the investigators in the field on how the results obtained should be interpreted.

To illustrate this point, the results of a recent analysis of birefringence signals by Watanabe and Terakawa (40) are described here (see Fig. 8). Figure 8 shows that the change in the birefringence summates when the nerve is repetitively stimulated. (Note that the action potentials never summate under these conditions.) Obviously, this summation derives from the situation that the change in birefringence outlasts the action potential. Based on these and other findings, Watanabe and Terakawa (40) concluded that birefringence signals are produced by an alteration of the protein structure underneath the nerve membrane, possibly re-

A   B

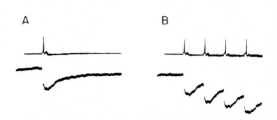

FIG. 8. *Upper traces,* action potentials recorded externally from a crab nerve; *lower traces,* birefringence changes recorded with a d.c. amplifier. The nerve was placed between an analyzer and a polarizer in the crossed position. Note that the intensity of light passing through the nerve remained low after the end of the action potential. (From Watanabe et al., ref. 53.)

sulting from the Ca influx associated with action potentials. This interpretation is in sharp contrast to the view that these signals are caused by the variation of the membrane potential (Kerr effect). It is true that the results obtained by the use of the voltage-clamp technique give strong support to the notion that these signals are voltage-dependent. Nevertheless, it is evident that the result shown in Fig. 8 can not be interpreted in terms of the Kerr effect.

The method of labeling with fluorescent probes has shown that it is possible to determine (a) the absorption and/or excitation spectra, (b) emission spectra, and (c) the orientation of the probe molecules in the nerve membrane at rest as well as during the process of nerve excitation. It is not possible to attribute these changes in the fluorescence spectra and polarization to the direct effect of the electric field on the fluorescent probe molecules. However, the results obtained by the use of the voltage-clamp technique have led to an emphasis of the voltage-dependent aspect of these signals.

In spite of this present-day status of the optical axonology, these new methods have already yielded (and will continue to yield) significant information concerning the molecular organization of the nerve membrane. [Note that purely electrical methods, such as voltage clamping, give us only a macroscopic (i.e., smeared) picture of the membrane.] If we learn much more about the microscopic picture of the nerve membrane, it might eventually be possible to offer reasonable interpretations as to the changes in the averaged quantities of the membrane (such as potential and current changes).

CONCLUSIONS

In the early part of this chapter, the theories of nerve excitation proposed during the first half of this century and their experimental bases are described. It is pointed out that almost all of the physicomathematical parts of these theories are at present almost meaningless. Nevertheless, several definite conclusions are drawn from the experimental studies carried out during this period. First, the semipermeable membrane at the surface of a nerve fiber is shown to play a crucial role in production of action potentials. Next, the importance of the local currents is established. The different roles played by various cations in the process of

nerve excitation have also become very clear. Finally, the properties of the vertebrate nerve fibers in relation to their myelin sheath and nodes of Ranvier are also elucidated during this period.

In the latter part of this chapter, the experimental bases of recent theories of nerve excitation are critically reexamined. First, the resting membrane potential of an excitable nerve fiber is shown to be very insensitive to changes in the K ion concentration on either side of the membrane. The experimental results demonstrating excitation by nonelectrical means are interpreted by this author as indicating the existence of two stable conformational states in the membrane macromolecules. Experimental evidence is presented that transitions between the two states of the membrane macromolecules are brought about by changes in the univalent-divalent cation concentration ratio in the medium. It is suggested that all the known experimental facts can reasonably be interpreted on the basis of the two stable state theory. The connection between this theory and the Hodgkin-Huxley theory is discussed.

REFERENCES

1. Nernst, W. (1908): Zur Theorie des elektrischen Reizes. *Pfluegers Arch. Physiol.*, 122:275–314.
2. Hill, A. V. (1910): A new mathematical treatment of changes of ionic concentration in muscle and nerve under the action of electric currents, with a theory as to their mode of excitation. *J. Physiol. (Lond.)*, 40:190–224.
3. Lucas, K. (1910): An analysis of changes and differences in the excitatory process of muscles and nerves based on the physical theory of excitation. *J. Physiol. (Lond.)*, 40:225–249.
4. Loeb, J. (1906): *The Dynamics of Living Matter*. McMillan and Co., London.
5. Höber, R. (1926): *Physikalische Chemie der Zelle und der Gewebe*. Wilhelm Engelmann, Leibzig.
6. Lapicque, L. (1926): *L'excitabilitéen fonction du temps*. Hermann, Paris.
7. Erlanger, J., and Gasser, H. S. (1937): *Electrical Signs of Nervous Activity*. University of Pennsylvania, Philadelphia.
8. Davis, H. (1923): The relationship of the "chronaxie" of muscle to the size of the stimulating electrode. *J. Physiol. (Lond.)*, 57:1xxxi.
9. Rushton, W. A. H. (1935): The time factor in electrical excitation. *Biol. Rev.*, 10:1–17.
10. Hermann, L. (1879): *Handbuch der Physiologie*. Band II, Theil I. F. C. W. Vogel, Leibzig.
11. Rashevsky, N. (1960): *Mathematical Biophysics. Vol. 1*. Dover Publications, New York.

12. Heilbrunn, L. V. (1938): *An Outline of General Physiology*. Saunders, Philadelphia.
13. Rushton, W. A. H. (1937): The initiation of the nerve impulse. *J. Physiol. (Lond.)*, 90:5.
14. Lillie, R. S. (1932): *Protoplasmic Action and Nervous Action*. University of Chicago Press, Chicago.
15. Tasaki, I. (1953): *Nervous Transmission*. Charles C Thomas, Springfield.
16. Inoue, I., Tasaki, I., and Kobatake, Y. (1974): A study of the effects of externally applied sodium ions and detection of spatial nonuniformity of the squid axon membrane under internal perfusion. *Biophys. Chem.*, 2:116–126.
17. Overton, E. (1902): Beiträge zur allgemeinen Muskel und Nervenphysiologie. II. Uber die Unentbehrlichkeit von Na (oder Li) Ionen für die Contractilität des Muskels. *Pfluegers Arch.*, 92:346–386.
18. Hodgkin, A. L. (1951): The ionic basis of electrical activity in nerve and muscle. *Biol. Rev.*, 26:339–409.
19. Hodgkin, A. L. (1964): *The Conduction of the Nervous Impulse*. Liverpool University Press, Liverpool.
20. Young, J. Z. (1936): Structure of nerve fibres and synapses in some invertebrates. *Cold Spr. Harb. Symp. Quant. Biol.*, 4:1.
21. Cole, K. S. (1968): *Membranes, Ions and Impulses*. University of California Press, Berkeley and Los Angeles.
22. Tasaki, I. (1968): *Nerve Excitation: A Macromolecular Approach*. Charles C Thomas, Springfield.
23. Tasaki, I., Lerman, L., and Watanabe, A. (1969): Analysis of excitation process in squid giant axons under bi-ionic conditions. *Am. J. Physiol.*, 216:130–138.
24. Meves, H., and Vogel, W. (1973): Calcium inward currents in internally perfused giant axons. *J. Physiol. (Lond.)*, 235:225–265.
25. Watanabe, A., Tasaki, I., Singer, I., and Lerman, L. (1967): Effects of tetrodotoxin on excitability of squid giant axons in sodium-free media. *Science*, 155:95–97.
26. Hodgkin, A. L., and Chandler, W. K. (1965): Effect of changes in ionic strength on inactivation and threshold of perfused fibers of Loligo. *J. Gen. Physiol. (Suppl.)*, 48:27–33.
27. Bernstein, J. (1912): *Elektrobiologie*. Braunschweig, Vieweg.
28. Tasaki, I. (1959): Demonstration of two stable states of the nerve membrane in potassium-rich media. *J. Physiol. (Lond.)*, 148:306–331.
29. Glasdorff, P., and Prigogine, I. (1971): *Thermodynamic Theory of Structure, Stability and Fluctuations*. Wiley-Interscience. New York.
30. Ehrenstein, G. (1971): Excitability in lipid bilayer membranes. In: *Biophysics and Physiology of Excitable Membranes*, edited by W. J. Adelman, Jr., pp. 463–476. Van Nostrand-Reinhold, New York.
31. Adelman, W. J., Jr., and Palti, Y. (1972): The role of periaxonal and perineuronal spaces in modifying ionic flow across neural membranes. In: *Current Topics in Membranes and Transport*, edited by F. Bronner and A. Kleinzeller, pp. 199–235. Academic Press, New York.
32. Frankenhaeuser, B. (1968): The ionic currents and the nervous impulse in myelinated nerve. In: *Progress in Biophysics and Molecular Biology*, edited by J. A. V. Butler and D. Noble, pp. 97–105. Pergamon Press, Oxford.
33. Mullins, L. J. (1973): The use of models of the cell membrane in determining the mechanism of drug action. In: *A Guide to Modern Pharmacology-Toxicology. Part I*, edited by R. M. Featherstone, pp. 2–52. Marcel Dekker, New York.
34. Hille, B. (1972): The permeability of the sodium channel to metal cations in myelinated nerve. *J. Gen. Physiol.*, 59:637–658.
35. Pedersen, C. J. (1967): New macrocyclic polyether. *J. Am. Chem. Soc.*, 89:7017.
36. Urry, D. W. (1972): A molecular theory of ion-conducting channels: A field-dependent transition between conducting and non-conducting conformations. *Proc. Natl. Acad. Sci. USA*, 69:1610–1614.
37. Williams, R. J. P. (1970): The biochemistry of sodium, potassium, magnesium and calcium. *Quart. Rev.*, 24:331–365.
38. Cohen, L. B., Keynes, R. D., and Hille, B. (1968): Light scattering and birefringence changes during nerve activity. *Nature*, 218:438–441.
39. Tasaki, I., Watanabe, A., Sandlin, R., and Carnay, L. (1968): Changes in fluorescence, turbidity, and birefringence associated with nerve excitation. *Proc. Natl. Acad. Sci. USA*, 61:883–888.
40. Watanabe, A., and Terakawa, S. (1974): A long-lasting birefringence change recorded from a tetanically stimulated squid giant axon. *J. Neurobiol. (In press.)*
41. Hill, A. V. (1936): Excitation and accommodation in nerve. *Proc. R. Soc. Lond. (Biol.)*, 119:305–355.
42. Hodgkin, A. L., and Huxley, A. F. (1939): Action potentials recorded from inside nerve fibre. *Nature*, 144:710–711.
43. Curtis, H. J., and Cole, K. S. (1940): Membrane action potentials from squid giant axon. *J. Cell. Comp. Physiol.*, 15:147–157.
44. Hodgkin, A. L., and Katz, B. (1949): The effect of sodium ions on the electrical activity of the giant axon of the squid. *J. Physiol. (Lond.)*, 108:37–77.
45. Hodgkin, A. L., Huxley, A. F., and Katz, B. (1952): Measurement of current-voltage relations in the membrane of the giant axon of *Loligo*. *J. Physiol. (Lond.)*, 116:424–448.
46. Marmont, G. (1949): Studies on the axon membrane. I. A new method. *J. Cell. Comp. Physiol.*, 34:351–382.
47. Hodgkin, A. L., and Huxley, A. F. (1952): A quantitative description of membrane current and its application to conduction and excitation in nerve. *J. Physiol. (Lond.)*, 117:500–544.
48. Osterhout, W. J. V., and Hill, S. E. (1938):

Calculations of bioelectric potentials. *J. Gen. Physiol.*, 22:139–146.

49. Fatt, P., and Katz, B. (1973): The electrical properties of crustacean muscle fibers. *J. Gen. Physiol. (Lond.)*, 120:171.

50. Hagiwara, S., Chichibu, S., and Naka, K. (1964): The effect of various ions on resting and spike potentials of barnacle muscle fibers. *J. Gen. Physiol. (Lond.)*, 48:163.

51. Tasaki, I., and Takenaka, T. (1963): Resting and action potential of squid giant axons intra-cellularly perfused with sodium-rich solutions. *Proc. Natl. Acad. Sci. USA*, 50:619–626.

52. Inoue, I., Kobatake, Y., and Tasaki, I. (1973): Excitability instability and phase transitions in squid axon membrane under internal perfusion with dilute salt solutions. *Biochim. Biophys. Acta*, 307:371–377.

53. Watanabe, A., Terakawa, S., and Nagano, M. (1973): Axoplasmic origin of the birefringence change associated with excitation of a crab nerve. *Proc. Japan Acad.*, 47:470–475.

The Nervous System, Donald B. Tower, Editor-in-Chief. *Vol. 1: The Basic Neurosciences*. Raven Press, New York, 1975.

Circulation and Energy Metabolism of the Brain

Seymour S. Kety

The energy requirement of the mammalian brain, and therefore that for oxygen and substrate, is substantial and continuous, and a large number of adaptive mechanisms have evolved for maintaining a constancy in the supply of these materials by way of the cerebral circulation. There are numerous cardiovascular reflexes that operate to maintain the arterial blood pressure under physiological and adverse circumstances and intrinsic mechanisms exist to adjust the perfusion of small regions of the brain to local metabolic requirements. That interplay was first recognized in 1890 by Roy and Sherrington (1), whose relatively crude measurements, fortified by brilliant insights, indicated a responsiveness on the part of the cerebral circulation not only to the arterial blood pressure but also to the important intrinsic mechanisms responsive to regional functional need. Their remarkable deduction, however, went unheeded for a generation and it was not until the first quarter of the present century, in which began the work of Cobb, Forbes, Wolff, Fog, Schmidt, and their collaborators, that the importance of the intrinsic control of this circulation was generally appreciated (2). In the past 25 years, observations on the cerebral circulation in man have adduced information regarding the control of that function under physiological conditions, its response to various drugs, and its alterations in pathological states (3–5).

MEASUREMENT OF THE HUMAN CEREBRAL BLOOD FLOW

The first reliable measurements of blood flow in the mammalian brain were those by Dumke and Schmidt, in 1943, on the rhesus monkey, a species whose cerebral circulation resembled that of man in being readily isolated from the extracerebral blood supply to the head (6). An ingenious bubble flow meter interposed in the arterial supply to the brain yielded quantitative estimates of total cerebral blood flow.

In man so direct a procedure was out of the question. It was thought possible, however, that the Fick Principle, which forms the basis of cardiac output and renal blood flow measurement, could be modified and successfully applied to the cerebral circulation.

Fick stated his important principle in two paragraphs of the *Proceedings of the Würzberg Physikalische-medizinische Gesellschaft* in 1870. It was the simple and, in the wisdom of hindsight, quite self-evident statement that the quantity of oxygen absorbed per minute must be equivalent to the pulmonary blood flow multiplied by the arteriovenous difference for oxygen across the lungs. In animals, and more recently in man, it is possible to measure with considerable precision the necessary components of that equation and to compute the pulmonary blood flow with few assumptions or approximations.

Unfortunately, the brain, unlike the kidney, does not specifically and selectively remove foreign substances from the blood and excrete them for accurate measurement. Furthermore, although it does consume large quantities of oxygen, that consumption cannot independently be measured or even assumed to be constant since it would be expected to vary with activity and disease. The brain does, however, absorb by physical solution an inert gas such as nitrous oxide, which reaches it by way of the arterial blood. It was hoped that the quantity of this gas absorbed by the brain would be independent of the state of mental activity and susceptible to measurement on the basis of physical solubility alone. If this were found to be the case, then the numerator of a Fick equation applied to the brain could be derived.

Studies were begun on the solubility of nitrous oxide in blood and brain. It was eventually found that the solubility of this gas was the same in brain as in blood and moreover that the solubility was the same in the brain of dog and man, in living brain and in dead brain, and was unaffected by a variety of diseases. Experiments were designed to measure the uptake of nitrous oxide by the brains of dogs exposed to low concentrations of this gas for varying lengths of time. It was found that at the end of 10 min the brain was essentially in equilibrium with the venous blood that drained it, and therefore the nitrous oxide concentration in the inaccessible brain could be obtained from its concentration in readily accessible cerebral venous blood. This finding was confirmed in man with the use of a radioactive isotope of the inert gas, krypton, which permitted measurement of its concentration in living human brain by means of an externally placed Geiger-Müller counter.

It was necessary now to derive the denominator of the Fick equation, or the arteriovenous difference in nitrous oxide concentration for the brain during this process of equilibration. More than a decade before, a technique had been devised for obtaining samples of venous blood from the brain by insertion of a needle into the superior bulb of the internal jugular vein at its point of emergence from the skull. Arterial blood samples could be obtained from the femoral or any other convenient artery. Such blood specimens, taken at intervals over a 10-min period of inhalation of 15% nitrous oxide were analyzed for this gas and characteristic concentration curves were obtained. The arteriovenous difference in concentration is not constant but variable, being initially rather large and decreasing progressively as equilibrium is approached. It was necessary to broaden the classical Fick principle, originally designed for a steady state of oxygen uptake, to a more general one embracing the uptake of inert gases by a tissue. Thus a new expression was derived (7):

$$\text{Cerebral blood flow} = \frac{Cu}{\int_0^u (A - V)dt} \quad [1]$$

The denominator of this expression is measured as the area between the arterial and venous curves over a period of time (u), whereas the numerator is equal to the concentration in cerebral venous blood at the end of that time.

Since this represents not a total amount but a concentration of nitrous oxide (quantity per unit weight of brain), the values for flow thus obtained are in terms of flow per minute per unit weight of brain.

Before these values could be accepted as valid measures of cerebral circulation, it was necessary to determine to what extent blood samples obtained from one internal jugular vein were representative of mixed venous blood from the brain arising from extracerebral regions such as the face and scalp. The first of these problems was attacked by simultaneous determinations employing the right and left internal jugular veins (7). It was found that there was no significant difference between the two sides, and it was therefore concluded that, in the average individual, cerebral venous blood is adequately mixed by the time it leaves the brain. Lassen and his associates have pointed out the greater precision to be obtained in individual cases by simultaneous bilateral determinations, but also support the conclusion that in studies on a series of individuals without unilateral disease, mean values obtained from right or left jugular samples are equivalent. No information is available comparing concentration curves in the internal jugulars with other cerebral venous exits such as the emissary veins or the cerebrospinal plexus, although flow in these ancillary channels would be expected to be small in comparison with that in the jugulars under normal circumstances.

In order to determine to what extent blood from extracerebral regions is present in the internal jugular vein at the point of sampling, studies were performed at the operating table in cases where exposure of the carotid bifurcation was necessary. A small quantity of dye (Evan's blue) was injected into the external carotid artery while blood samples were taken from the internal and external jugular veins. By spectrophotometric analysis of these blood samples, it was found that practically all of the injected dye appeared in the external jugular vein, only insignificant amounts of blood of external carotid and therefore extracerebral origin finding their way into the internal jugular samples (8).

As a final evaluation of the nitrous oxide method, experiments were performed in monkeys in which cerebral blood flow was measured simultaneously by this method and directly by means of the bubble flow meter. An excellent correlation was found between the two methods (7).

Evaluation of the quantity of tracer that has accumulated in the brain is a crucial question. The nitrous oxide method offered a resolution of the problem, which is theoretically sound but subject to certain approximations in practice. This was based upon the realization that in the process of equilibration of blood and brain with a constant tension of nitrous oxide in the inspired air, there would be a time, designated *u,* at and beyond which the venous blood emerging from the brain would be in virtual equilibrium with the brain itself with respect to the tension of the gas.

In a process of equilibration extending over several minutes, the limiting factor is not diffusion between capillaries and tissue but the disparities between tissues with different perfusions and the rate at which the tissue with the slowest perfusion comes into virtual equilibrium. For that reason, application of the principle of the nitrous oxide technique to other regions such as the extremities or the splanchnic area is beset with the difficulty that in such regions very slow components (fat, resting muscle) make the time *u* impractically long.

Later measurements of local perfusion rates throughout the brain (9) show a minimum value, in white matter, of 0.23 ml/gm/min in the unanesthetized cat. Similar values for the slow component in normal human brain have been computed by numerous investigators. These data permit one to question whether 10 min is sufficiently long to achieve complete equivalence between the brain and its venous blood for nitrous oxide tension, since calculation shows that it could result in an overestimation of the cerebral blood flow by 5% under normal circumstances and by 10 to 12% in those cases where the flow in white matter is reduced by 50%. Extending the equilibration time to 15 or 20 min has been suggested as one way of minimizing this error.

Another possible source of error is represented by the small fraction of blood in the internal jugular vein, which is derived from extracerebral tissues. To the small contamination

measured by dye injection into the external carotid, must be added the blood derived from the internal carotid but which drains the orbital tissues and the meninges. This admixture of blood from slowly perfused areas together with the slow equilibration of the cerebrospinal fluid with the inert gas results in the addition of several slowly equilibrating components of small magnitude to the more rapid equilibrium occurring in the brain itself. This may result in underestimating the cerebral blood flow in the average case by approximately 10% when the calculation is made at 10 min, the error increasing nearly linearly as that time is extended.

Thus the original nitrous oxide technique is probably subject to two relatively small errors of opposite sign and, at 10 min of equilibration, nearly equal in magnitude. If that is so, extending the equilibration time does not necessarily improve the accuracy.

Aukland has demonstrated the feasibility of measuring molecular hydrogen in blood and tissues by a polarographic technique. If such measurements are applied during a 10- to 20-min period of desaturation immediately following a similar period of saturation with a low tension of gaseous hydrogen, it is possible to minimize the error caused by incomplete equilibration of white matter and that resulting from extracerebral contamination. In addition continuous arterial and cerebral venous curves permit more extensive and accurate computations.

The nitrous oxide technique has two important limitations. Since it requires a period of 10 min for the determination of a single value for cerebral blood flow, it is not applicable to the study of rapid changes in this function as are likely to occur in syncope or in convulsions. Furthermore, since no generally applicable technique is at hand for obtaining venous blood from localized areas, the method yields only an average for the brain as a whole.

Lewis and collaborators demonstrated the feasibility of estimating total cerebral blood flow from Eq. (1) throughout the period of equilibration without assuming any relationship between cerebral tissue and venous blood. The use of a gamma-emitting inert gas (Kr^{79}) made it possible to estimate directly the accumulation of the gas in brain.

MEASUREMENT OF REGIONAL BLOOD FLOW

Considerations of the exchange of inert, diffusible substances between capillary and tissue (10) permitted the development of equations that have been useful in the measurement of regional blood flow in the brain. Concentrations of a tracer, especially if it were radioactive, could readily be obtained for regions of the brain by autoradiography in animals or by collimated external radiation counters in man, but the appropriate venous blood samples would be unavailable. If one assumed, however, that for some tracers diffusion would be sufficiently rapid that each small portion of tissue would reach equilibrium with the blood as it traversed it, it was possible to derive an expression for the accumulation of such a tracer or its clearance from each tissue region in terms of the concentration in the arterial blood, the appropriate partition coefficient, and the blood flow through the tissue:

$$C_i(T) = k_i \lambda_i \exp(-k_i T) \int_0^T A\, \exp(k_i t) dt \qquad [2]$$

where $C_i(T)$ represents the concentration of tracer in an individual tissue at time T, λ_i the tissue:blood partition coefficient for the tracer, A, the arterial concentration of tracer, and k_i the rate of perfusion per solubility-equivalent unit of tissue, $F/\lambda W$.

Where the tissue is being cleared of the tracer in the presence of a negligible arterial concentration, this reduces to:

$$C_i(T) = C_i(T_0) \exp(-k_i T) \qquad [3]$$

The first of these equations permitted the development of autoradiographic techniques for measurement of local cerebral blood flow (9,11), whereas the second is the basis of the clearance methods developed by Ingvar and Lassen (12) using radioactive gases.

How could one be sure that for certain tracers and particular tissues of the brain, diffusion would be sufficiently rapid that each small portion of tissue would reach equilibrium with the blood as it traversed it? Krogh (13) had used a model consisting of parallel capillaries, each with a cylinder of tissue surrounding it, in order to calculate the diffusion processes for oxygen in muscle. Bohr (14) had described the dif-

fusion of oxygen from the alveolus into the pulmonary capillary in terms of diffusion, capillary geometry, blood flow, and the capacity of hemoglobin for oxygen. In a steady state, oxygen gradients are constant but in the case of a nonmetabolized substance these would change with time and introduce another dimension of complexity. With the use of models and reasoning based upon the work of Bohr, it was possible to derive a first approximation to the situation which might hold for an inert but diffusible substance in the flowing capillary blood during its exchange with tissue (10). A constant was derived: $m = 1 - \exp(-D'S/F)$, expressing the degree of equilibration between capillary blood and the external phase in terms of the diffusion coefficient of the tracer (D'), the capillary diffusing surface (S), and the perfusion rate (F).

That derivation was a first approximation, since it made several simplifying assumptions, but rough calculations of m indicated that a substance that diffused through the entire capillary membrane (such as an inert gas) would be limited by blood flow rather than by diffusion in its exchange with tissues of the brain. For a wide range of less diffusible substances that expression became a basis for examining their permeability through the capillary wall (15). Experimental validation of the theory came eventually from studies that indicated that substances as diverse in their molecular weights and diffusion rates as hydrogen, xenon, or trifluoroiodomethane have similar rates of uptake or clearance from the brain (9,16).

The implicit assumption that all the small tissue regions in which measurements have been made are homogeneously perfused, however, is open to serious question. It has been found that in gray matter the clearance of the tracers used often deviates from a single exponential function but may be approximated by the sum of at least two such functions. This suggests that the assumption of homogeneity may not be tenable for a number of regions, although alternative explanations may have to be ruled out. However, Ingvar and Lassen (12) showed mathematically that under appropriate conditions the initial slope of a compound exponential curve, such as is obtained from a heterogeneous tissue, is determined by the average flow and the average partition coefficient of the region in question. This has permitted them to compute average flows for heterogeneous regions under local observation which are compatible for values obtained in the brain as a whole (16).

Significant heterogeneity of the small regions examined by means of the autoradiographic technique, if it occurred, would compromise the accuracy of the values that have been obtained. On the other hand, these measurements made at the end of only 1 min of equilibration are probably sufficiently close to the initial slope to yield a satisfactory average perfusion value on the basis of Ingvar and Lassen's derivation. It is interesting that the weighted average for cerebral blood flow as a whole obtained from such regional measurements agrees well with values obtained by the nitrous oxide method that requires no assumptions regarding the absence of arteriovenous shunts or extremely rapid capillary-tissue equilibrium.

Measurement of cerebral blood flow also permitted the evaluation of two other cerebral functions. One of these is cerebrovascular resistance, a measure of all the factors opposing the cerebral blood flow, most prominent of which is the tone of the vessels themselves. Most important of all, however, is the ability to calculate the rate of cerebral metabolism in terms of oxygen or glucose consumption or, in fact, the utilization or production by the brain of any substance that can accurately be detected in arterial and venous blood. Normal values for these functions were obtained in a series of healthy young men (7, Table 1). The blood flow of the brain was found to represent about $\frac{1}{6}$ of the cardiac output and its oxygen consumption nearly $\frac{1}{4}$ that of the entire body at rest.

The first application of the new method was to the problem of the effects on cerebral circulation of alterations in the oxygen and carbon dioxide tensions of arterial blood. The results confirmed classical experiments on animals that demonstrated that carbon dioxide was a potent cerebral vasodilator as was anoxia, whereas high oxygen tensions and low carbon dioxide pressures produced mild and severe vasoconstriction, respectively. Evidence was acquired in these studies to suggest that the dominant control of cerebral vessels in man was a chemical one, activated by levels of carbon dioxide, oxygen, and hydrogen ion. A study on the role of the cervical sympathetic supply to the brain (17) cast further light on this question of the normal control of the cerebral circulation. It was found that procaine block of both stellate ganglia produced no change in cerebral circulation or resistance, suggesting that the known sympathetic channels to the brain do not exert an appreciable tonic effect on cerebral vessels.

THE REGULATION OF CEREBRAL BLOOD FLOW: CHEMICAL INFLUENCES

The studies in man since that time do not substantiate the earlier belief that cerebral blood flow passively follows changes in arterial blood pressure. Instead they have strengthened the concept that a normal arterial pressure is zealously maintained by numerous homeostatic mechanisms, such as the carotid sinus reflex and the central control of peripheral vascular tone, and that as long as the mean arterial pressure remains above a critical minimum level, cerebral blood flow is actually regulated intrinsically by changes in cerebral vascular resistance. This concept, which has recently been designated as "autoregulation" was first

TABLE 1. *Representative values for cerebral blood flow (CBF) in man in various physiological and pathological states*

Physiological condition	CBF (ml/100g/min)	Pathological state	CBF (ml/100g/min)
Healthy males age 25 yr	54–62[a]	Cerebral hemangioma	164
Healthy males age 71 yr	58	Increased intracranial pressure	34
Infants age 6 yr	106	Primary polycythemia	25
Healthy males, asleep	65	Severe anemia	79
Hyperventilation	34	Cerebral arteriosclerosis	41
Inhalation CO_2 5–7%	93	Essential hypertension	54
Inhalation O_2 85–100%	45	Schizophrenia	54

[a] Range of numerous series employing various modifications of the nitrous oxide technique.

put forth by Roy and Sherrington (1): "We conclude then, that the chemical products of cerebral metabolism contained in the lymph which bathes the walls of the arterioles of the brain can cause variations in the caliber of the cerebral vessels: that in this reaction the brain possesses an intrinsic mechanism by which its vascular supply can be varied locally in correspondance with local variations of functional activity."

The factors involved in this intrinsic mechanism and the contributions of the various chemical products of cerebral metabolism as well as the role of neurogenic factors have been the subject of considerable investigation in recent years. Although changes in the tension of oxygen and of carbon dioxide in arterial blood are undoubtedly capable of altering cerebral vascular resistance acutely, these effects can be overridden by another factor, presumably hydrogen ion concentration in the extracellular fluid which surrounds the arteriole. In chronic emphysema cerebral blood flow may be within the normal range in spite of a chronic and severe elevation of arterial carbon dioxide tension, and in diabetic acidosis cerebral blood flow may be increased although the carbon dioxide tension may be considerably reduced. These observations can be explained by the tissue hydrogen ion concentration, which in the first case may be normal, but in uncompensated metabolic acidosis may be elevated. It is also possible that periarteriolar pH may be a common factor mediating the effects of elevated carbon dioxide and reduced oxygen tensions (18,19).

THE REGULATION OF CEREBRAL BLOOD FLOW: NEUROGENIC FACTORS

The role of neurogenic influences has been more difficult to elucidate, since clear-cut effects of the activation or extirpation of the identified autonomic supply to cerebral vessels has not been easy to elicit under reasonably physiological circumstances. A segmental division of cerebral circulatory control has been suggested in which metabolic products constitute the intrinsic autoregulation, whereas the sympathetic innervation may operate to affect the caliber of the larger cerebral vessels.

Recently, by means of an immunofluorescence technique, noradrenergic nerve terminals have been visualized on small arteries in the brain parenchyma (20). The source of these terminals appears to be the central noradrenergic neurons rather than the peripheral sympathetic nervous system. Citing the observations of Shalit and associates that brainstem lesions abolish the responsiveness of cerebral vessels to arterial carbon dioxide and those of Scheinberg that electrical stimulation of central noradrenergic pathways resulted in increased cortical blood flow, the authors postulate that one of the functions of the central noradrenergic system is concerned with the microregulation of cerebral blood flow (20). Thus a new and entirely intrinsic neurogenic influence on parenchymal vessels in the brain has emerged and appears to be associated with a system that may have important mediating effects on arousal and attention. It is possible that autoregulation depends upon both chemical and neurogenic factors. In the case of muscular exercise, it is now generally accepted that the cardiovascular and respiratory reflexes anticipate the chemical changes, and it is tempting to suggest that similar adaptations apply in the regulation of regional cerebral circulation to functional activity.

CEREBRAL BLOOD FLOW AND METABOLISM IN HUMAN DISEASE

One of the unique values of methods applicable to man is the opportunity thus afforded for studying the pathogenesis of human disease. Several disorders were found to be associated with significant disturbances in cerebrovascular resistance or cerebral blood flow (3). Increase in intracranial pressure as a result of brain tumor was found to produce a progressive rise in cerebrovascular resistance undoubtedly as a result of external compression of the thin-walled vessels of the brain. The cerebral blood flow, however, was not significantly compromised until cerebrospinal fluid pressure exceeded 400 mm of water, a homeostasis achieved by a compensatory increase in blood pressure. Thus Cushing's classical experiments on dogs were completely confirmed by observations on man.

The method was applied to essential hypertension with findings of some interest. There was practically a twofold increase in cerebrovascular resistance, which in the absence of significant changes in intracranial pressure or blood viscosity had to be attributed to vasoconstriction. This change, however, is in exact proportion to the elevation in blood pressure with the result that cerebral blood flow is practically normal. These observations on cerebral vessels were similar to those of other investigators who had studied the vascular beds of the kidneys, extremities, and splanchnic viscera in this disease. The effects of a reduction in the high blood pressure to more normal values are of importance in understanding the nature of the increased cerebrovascular tone and in determining the wisdom of reducing the blood pressure of hypertensive patients. After interruption of the sympathetic outflow to the trunk and lower extremities achieved either by procaine or surgical sympathectomy, evidence was found of a relaxation of the abnormally increased cerebrovascular tone and a tendency to preserve a normal cerebral blood flow. These findings clearly demonstrated the remarkable autoregulatory properties of the cerebral circulation, and contradicted an earlier notion of the dependence of this circulation on arterial blood pressure.

CEREBRAL METABOLISM

A number of disturbances in cerebral metabolism were studied by means of this method. Among the earliest of these was that on diabetic acidosis and coma (21). It was learned that the state of coma, contrary to the prevailing theory, was not the result of a deficient cerebral blood flow—in fact this function was actually somewhat greater than normal—but, rather, was associated with a significant reduction in cerebral oxygen utilization. This occurred in spite of an adequate supply of blood and oxygen to the brain and an oxyhemoglobin dissociation curve that favored the uptake of oxygen by the tissues. The evidence found suggested an intracellular defect possibly on the basis of acidosis or ketosis. The increased cerebral perfusion in the face of a markedly reduced carbon dioxide tension but a low pH was early evidence of the importance of hydrogen ion in the regulation of cerebral blood flow.

In the hypoglycemia and coma of insulin shock therapy were seen the results of a fairly acute reduction in glucose available for cerebral utilization. There was a progressive decrease in cerebral oxygen and glucose consumption as the blood glucose concentration fell. Blood pressure and cerebral blood flow were maintained within normal limits. These observations and the stoichiometric relationships, which exist between cerebral consumption of glucose and oxygen reinforced the importance of glucose as the major substrate for cerebral energy requirements under normal circumstances. Recently it has been demonstrated that in chronic hypoglycemia and ketosis, the brain is able to shift from glucose to the oxidation of ketone bodies (22).

A surprising result was obtained by Sokoloff (22) when it was learned that cerebral oxygen utilization in hyperthyroidism was not increased above the normal level in spite of a marked increase in oxygen consumption by the body as a whole. That interesting finding was the first suggestion that thyrotoxicosis may not represent a generalized acceleration in metabolism of all body cells. It was on the basis of that finding that Sokoloff went on to develop his concept of the major physiological action of thyroid hormone on protein synthesis and demonstrated, early on, an important hormonal control of this process.

In the mental changes associated with increased intracranial pressure, diabetic or hypoglycemic coma, or anesthesia, it is not difficult to discern a cause-effect relationship between a gross defect in cerebral nutrition or metabolism and the alteration in mental activity. In one of the important mental illnesses such a relationship is still tenable. Studies in the psychoses of senility showed a significant reduction in cerebral blood flow and oxygen consumption, presumably on the basis of an increased cerebrovascular resistance, a physiological confirmation of the well-known sclerosis of cerebral vessels often associated with this disorder. A systematic study of the cerebral circulation in various aging populations (23) supported the thesis that a primary reduction in perfusion was responsible for an important component of senile dementia.

In schizophrenia, on the other hand, similar studies revealed no detectable change in the total circulation or oxygen consumption of the brain even in severely affected patients. A similar finding was obtained in normal subjects during the performance of mental arithmetic. In these states involving higher nervous function, Risberg and Ingvar (24) and Ingvar and Lassen (25) have observed interesting regional changes in cerebral blood flow which were not revealed by measurements of the total cerebral circulation.

There were other examples of profound changes in mental function that show no correlation with overall blood flow or oxygen consumption of the brain. A study on normal sleep showed a slight increase in cerebral blood flow and no significant change in cerebral oxygen consumption in this condition. These findings were incompatible with those theories of sleep that were predicated upon an ischemia or a narcosis of the brain and indicated that sleep was a phenomenon quite different from coma. They challenged the prevailing notion of the time of a generalized neuronal inactivity during sleep and anticipated the findings of electrophysiologists that sleep was a highly active neuronal state. In more recent studies, Reivich and his associates have demonstrated a generalized and substantial increase in blood flow in most of the regions of the brain during REM sleep (25).

Studies in man yielded important insights into the pharmacology of the cerebral circulation (5). This is understandable since only in human subjects or clinical disorders can relevant dosages of drugs be used, therapeutic effects studied and possible species differences circumvented. These studies have served to reinforce the characterization of a few of the cerebral dilator drugs but to question the efficacy of many more. They may be expected to play a significant role in the evaluation of new drugs and therapeutic procedures.

RECENT DEVELOPMENTS

The nitrous oxide technique and its various modifications have been of value in elucidating the physiology of the circulation in the normally functioning human brain freed of such constraints as anesthesia or surgical intervention. It has provided information on human cerebral disease, which was previously unavailable, and on the effects of drugs under therapeutic conditions. In the clinical study of the individual patient, more convenient techniques, especially those that can examine specific regions within the brain, are desirable for diagnosis, localization, and evaluation of progress. Here the regional clearance of radioactive gases, as developed by Lassen and Ingvar, or noninvasive techniques, which require only external counting of gamma-ray emitting isotopes such as those developed by Veall or by Obrist should be especially useful. Radioactive oxygen ($^{15}O_2$) has been successfully applied by Ter-Pogossian and his associates to measurement of both oxygen consumption and blood flow within the brain. One of the most exciting recent developments is that of Sokoloff and Reivich of the autoradiographic visualization and measurement of glucose consumption in small regions of the brain (25). The results thus far obtained show a remarkable relationship between glucose uptake and regional neuronal activity and suggest that the technique may be extremely useful in mapping the distribution of functional activity in the brain.

The cerebral circulation is another area that demonstrates the important interaction between fundamental knowledge and clinical application. Measurement of cerebral blood flow in man depended upon accumulated knowledge in basic physiology, chemistry, and physics. In their turn, the studies in man have yielded information regarding the processes involved in the circulation and energy metabolism of the brain and their regulation, which had not been available from studies on lower animals.

REFERENCES

1. Roy, C. S., and Sherrington, C. S. (1890): On the regulation of the blood supply of the brain. *J. Physiol. (Lond.)*, 11:85–108.
2. Cobbs, S., Frantz, A. M., Penfield, W., and Riley, H. A., editors (1938): The circulation of the brain and spinal cord. *Res. Publ. Assoc. Nerv. Ment. Dis.*, 28.
3. Kety, S. S. (1960): The cerebral circulation. In: *Handbook of Physiology, Sect. 1-Neurophysiology, Vol. III*, edited by J. Field, H. W. Magoun, and V. E. Hall, pp. 1751–1760. American Physiological Society, Washington, D.C.
4. Lassen, N. A. (1959): Cerebral blood flow and oxygen consumption in man. *Physiol. Rev.*, 39:183–238.
5. Sokoloff, L. (1959): The action of drugs on the cerebral circulation. *Pharmacol. Rev.*, 11:1–85.
6. Dumke, P. R., and Schmidt, C. F. (1943): Quantitative measurements of cerebral blood

flow in the macacque monkey. *Am. J. Physiol.*, 138:421–428.

7. Kety, S. S., and Schmidt, C. F. (1948): Nitrous oxide method for the quantitative determination of cerebral blood flow in man: Theory, procedure, and normal values. *J. Clin. Invest.*, 27:475–483.

8. Shenkin, H. A., Harmel, M. H., and Kety, S. S. (1948): Dynamic anatomy of the cerebral circulation. *Arch. Neurol. Psychiatry*, 60:240–252.

9. Landau, W. M., Freygang, W. H., Rowland, L. P., Sokoloff, L., and Kety, S. S. (1955): The local circulation of the living brain: Values in the unanesthetized and anesthetized cat. *Trans. Am. Neurol. Assoc.*, 80:125–129.

10. Kety, S. S. (1951): The theory and applications of the exchange of inert gas at the lungs and tissues. *Pharmacol. Rev.*, 3(1):1–41.

11. Reivich, M., Jehle, J., Sokoloff, L., and Kety, S. S. (1969): Measurement of regional cerebral blood flow with antipyrine-^{14}C in awake cats. *J. Appl. Physiol.*, 27:296–300.

12. Ingvar, D. H., and Lassen, N. A. (1962): Regional blood flow of the cerebral cortex determined by krypton[85]. *Acta Physiol. Scand.*, 54:325–338.

13. Krogh, A. (1919): The number and distribution of capillaries in muscles with calculation of the oxygen pressure head necessary for supplying the tissue. *J. Physiol. (Lond.)*, 52:391–408.

14. Bohr, C. (1909): Über die spezifische Tätigkeit der Lungen bei den respiratorischen Gasaufnahme und ihr Verhalten zu der durch die Alveolarwand stattfindenen Gas diffusion. *Skand. Arch. Physiol.*, 22:221–280.

15. Renkin, E. M. (1955): Effects of blood flow on diffusion kinetics in isolated, perfused hindlegs of cats. *Am. J. Physiol.*, 183:125–136.

16. Ingvar, D. H., and Lassen, N. A., editors (1965): Regional cerebral blood flow, an International Symposium. *Acta. Neurol. Scand. Suppl.*, 14.

17. Harmel, M. H., Hafkenschiel, J. H., Austin, G. M., Crumpton, C. W., and Kety, S. S. (1949): The effect of bilateral stellate ganglion block on the cerebral circulation in normotensive and hypertensive patients. *J. Clin. Invest.*, 28:415–418.

18. Ingvar, D. H., Lassen, N. A., Siesjo, B. K., and Skinhøj, E., editors (1968): Cerebral blood flow and cerebro-spinal fluid, Third International Symposium. *Scand. J. Clin. Lab. Invest.*, Suppl. 102.

19. Fieschi, C., and Bozzao, L. (1972): The physiology of cerebral circulation. In: *International Encyclopedia of Pharmacology and Therapeutics, Vol. I, Pharmacology of the Cerebral Circulation*, pp. 1–33. Pergamon Press, Oxford.

20. Hartman, B. K., Zide, D., and Udenfriend, S. (1972): The use of dopamine betahydroxylase as a marker for the central noradrenergic nervous system in rat brain. *Proc. Natl. Acad. Sci. USA*, 69:2722–2726.

21. Kety, S. S. (1957): The general metabolism of the brain *in vivo*. In: *Metabolism of the Nervous System*, edited by D. Richter, pp. 221–237. Pergamon Press, Oxford.

22. Sokoloff, L. (1974): Changes in enzyme activities in neural tissues with maturation and development of the nervous system. In: *The Neurosciences: Third Study Program*, edited by F. O. Schmitt and F. G. Worden, pp. 885–898. MIT Press, Cambridge, Massachusetts.

23. Dastur, D. K., Lane, M. H., Hansen, D. B., Kety, S. S., Butler, R. N., Perlin, S., and Sokoloff, L. (1963): Effects of aging on cerebral circulation and metabolism in man. In: *Human Aging: A Biological and Behavioral Study*. Public Health Service publication No. 986, pp. 59–76. U.S. Government Printing Office, Washington, D.C.

24. Risberg, J., and Ingvar, H. (1971): Increase of blood flow in cortical association areas during memorization and abstract thinking. *Eur. Neurol.*, 6:236–241.

25. Ingvar, D. H., and Lassen, N. A., editors (1975): *The Working Brain: The Coupling of Function, Metabolism and Blood Flow in the Brain*. Munksgaard, Copenhagen.

The Nervous System, Donald B. Tower, Editor-in-Chief. *Vol. 1: The Basic Neurosciences.* Raven Press, New York, 1975.

Analysis of Structure and Function in the Olfactory Pathway

Gordon M. Shepherd, Thomas V. Getchell, and John S. Kauer

Neurobiologists are concerned not only with particular anatomical and physiological studies in different parts of the nervous system, but also, and increasingly so in recent years, with detailed correlations between structure and function, in order to understand the dynamic operations of the systems in question. The olfactory system has been of interest in this regard, by virtue of its stereotyped neuronal structures and its accessibility to experiment. We review in this chapter certain aspects of the studies that have been carried out recently at several successive levels in this system.

OLFACTORY RECEPTORS

Cellular Organization

Portions of the vertebrate nasal cavity are lined with a pseudostratified neuroepithelium termed the olfactory epithelium (2,15,34). It is approximately 150 to 200 μm thick and contains three cell types: olfactory receptor cells, sustentacular cells, and basal cells, with their nuclei forming three distinct strata (Fig. 1). The apical portions of receptor cells (b) and

sustentacular cells (c) are bound together by tight junctions, which presumably serve to isolate the overlying mucus from the interstitial fluid surrounding these cells. The mucus bathing the epithelial surface appears to have two sources: the sustentacular cells and the subepithelial multicellular Bowman gland cells (Fig. 1c). Sustentacular cells with granular inclusions morphologically resemble secretory cells. Their apical surface bears numerous short microvilli, which are less than 10 μm long.

Olfactory receptor cells are the prototype of a bipolar neuron. From the soma, which lies in the intermediate nuclear stratum within the olfactory epithelium, a dendrite approximately 1 to 2 μm in diameter extends distally to the surface (see Fig. 1). There it terminates in a knob, from which project several long cilia (up to 200 μm in length). Proximally the receptor cell axon projects into the lamina propria where it joins with other axons to form the olfactory nerve. The axons have a modal cross-sectional diameter of 0.2 μm and project to the olfactory bulb without axon collaterals or synapses. Low-resistance channels (gap junctions) between adjacent receptor cells are few or absent; hence, it is generally considered that olfactory receptor cells function as independent physiological units (8,26).

Physiological Properties

Two types of stimulus-evoked voltage transients are recorded extracellularly in order to investigate receptor cell function (13). The first type, recorded as a slow monophasic negative voltage change from the surface of the epithelium, is generated by populations of olfactory receptor cells in response to odor stimulation. It is considered to be a summated receptor potential. It was originally termed the electroolfactogram (EOG) (25), and more recently it

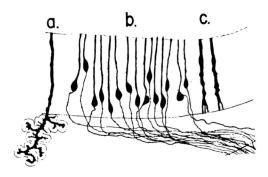

FIG. 1. Elements of the vertebrate olfactory epithelium, as stained in Golgi preparations. (a) Bowman's gland; (b) olfactory receptor cells; (c) sustentacular cells. (From Retzius, 1892.)

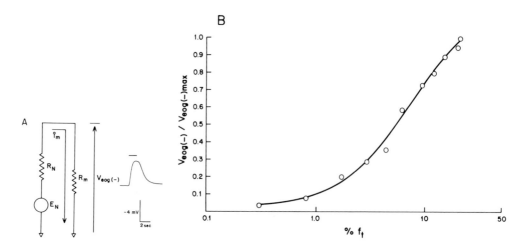

FIG. 2. A: The voltage transient, $V_{\mathrm{eog(-)}}$, measured across R_m is due to a single source (E_N) when activated by an odor. A semilogarithmic plot of $\%$ $V_{\mathrm{eog(-)max}}$ as a function of stimulus flow rate shows the general sigmoid relationship (**B**). (From Getchell, ref. 11.)

has been designated as $V_{\mathrm{eog(-)}}$ (11). If one assumes that the resistance of tight junctions in the apical regions of the receptor and sustentacular cells is less than the resistance of their cell membranes, then $V_{\mathrm{eog(-)}}$ is primarily due to summed current flow (i_m) through the extracellular resistance of the epithelium (R_m) when a single excitatory source (E_N) with its source resistance (R_N) is activated by an odor (see Fig. 2A). The relationship between the relative amplitude of the odor-evoked response, $V_{\mathrm{eog(-)}}/V_{\mathrm{eog(-)max}}$, and the stimulus flow rate, f_t, is sigmoidal, suggesting that $V_{\mathrm{eog(-)}}$ reflects the amount of current flow resulting from molecular activation of olfactory receptors (Fig. 2B) (this approach is further discussed in ref. 11).

Molecular recognition mechanisms of odor molecules by olfactory receptors are similar to those postulated for other systems involving specific molecular interactions such as chemical synapses, hormonal receptors, immunological mechanisms, and drug actions. As a working hypothesis, it is assumed that there are molecular receptors, or active sites of a receptor molecule, in the ciliary and/or apical knob appendages of the olfactory receptor. Recent evidence obtained through the use of group-specific protein reagents, for example N-ethyl maleimide, suggests that receptor molecules are proteins that may interact with more than one molecular species (9). Odors that evoke dis-

tinctly different odor sensations and/or have dissimilar molecular characteristics do not interact with the receptor sites. Whether or not different molecules that evoke similar odor sensations or share common molecular characteristics interact with the same receptor site type is currently under investigation.

It is assumed that the stimulus-receptor complex initiates a series of events that results in ionic current flow into the apical regions of the receptor cell. Hence, if one assumes that a molecular receptor site type is not spatially restricted to a single cilium or ciliary region, then the olfactory knob functioning as a focal current sink is the first site of signal integration in the olfactory system. The current then spreads electrotonically through the dendrite into the receptor soma. The length constant is presumably sufficiently long to allow for this passive spread (27).

The second type of voltage transient is recorded extracellularly as an action potential during an intraepithelial electrode penetration (Fig. 3). An analysis of the three basic voltage conformations displayed by action potentials recorded from the bipolar receptor suggested a hypothesis that describes the underlying receptor events (10). The results are summarized in Fig. 3. Intracellular current, initiated by the stimulus-receptor complex, flowing centripetally into the receptor soma, depolarizes the membrane in the region of spike initiation. An

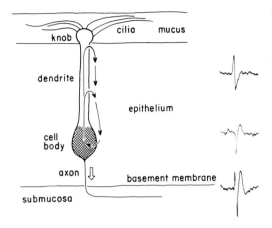

FIG. 3. A schematic diagram to illustrate current flow during depolarization underlying the three types of extracellulary recorded spikes from olfactory receptors. (From Getchell, ref. 10.)

extracellular microelectrode records a diphasic spike with an initial negative voltage component when positioned in the somatic region, suggesting an inward flow of extracellular current. Current associated with spike electrogenesis spreads into the dendrite, at which level a spike with an initially positive diphasic voltage component is recorded extracellularly. Current also orthodromically spreads into the axon where a triphasic, positive-negative-positive voltage sequence spike is recorded with the electrode positioned deep in the olfactory epithelium.

Odor-Evoked Responses

Discrimination among odors by olfactory receptors has been investigated at the unitary level. There appears to be a general consensus that single receptors have relatively broad response spectra to molecules that evoke different odor sensations (8,13). A given odor may or may not evoke an excitatory response in any individual receptor. The lack of an excitatory response when an odor is delivered over a wide concentration range presumably reflects the absence of a receptor site for that compound on the receptor cell.

In order to elucidate receptor mechanisms underlying molecular discrimination, spontaneous activity and excitatory discharge patterns have been investigated using quantitative methods of data analysis (12). For example, spontaneous activity in the frog typically varies over a wide range from 0.07 to 1.8 spikes/sec with intervals ranging from 13.7 to 0.5 sec. It is typically asynchronous, as evidenced by standard deviations, which closely approximate the mean interval calculated for a given unit.

Benzaldehyde evokes a bitter almond odor sensation with a characteristic sweet note in man. In physiological experiments, it has been shown to evoke excitatory responses in certain olfactory receptors in frogs. In the unit illustrated in Fig. 4A, spontaneous activity was monitored for 2.5 min and had a mean discharge rate of 0.3 spikes/sec (Fig. 4A-1). The activity was asynchronous as evidenced by a mean interspike interval of 3.4 ± 5.9 sec (mean $\pm$ SD) and a coefficient of variation of 1.8. An aliquot of 45 nM benzaldehyde did not significantly change the frequency or distribution of intervals and was therefore judged to be below threshold. Increasing the concentration to 0.45 μM evoked an excitatory response (Fig. 4A-3) during which the firing frequency increased to 2.9 spikes/sec. Interspike intervals during the response were quite variable in length ranging from about 100 to 480 msec (Fig. 4B). The mean interspike interval was 0.3 ± 0.2 sec. Compared with the spontaneous activity, the relative variability was reduced to 0.8. When the concentration of benzaldehyde was increased by two log units to 45 μM the firing frequency during the excitatory response (Fig. 4A-4) was increased to 4.2 spikes/sec. The mean interspike interval was further reduced to 0.21 ± 0.04 sec (Fig. 4B). The relative variability in intervals was reduced by nearly a factor of 4 to 0.2. Hence, when stimuli were delivered to olfactory receptors at low concentrations, there was typically a 10-fold increase in the mean rate of discharge over that of the spontaneous activity by the lowest concentration, which was then nearly doubled by a 2-log step increase in concentration. Increasing concentrations of the stimulus not only decreased the mean interspike interval but also reduced the variability in the intervals as evidenced by the decreased coefficient of variations when compared with spontaneous activity.

Each response in this experiment was initiated by a nearly exponential decrease in inter-

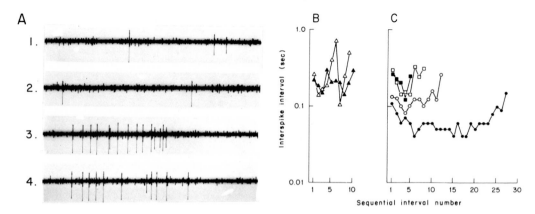

FIG. 4. A: Unitary spikes recorded from frog olfactory receptors showing spontaneous activity (**1**), lack of a response to control (**2**), and excitatory responses evoked by 45 μM benzaldehyde (**3**) and 0.45 μM benzaldehyde (**4**). **B:** Sequential interspike interval analysis; $\triangle$, 0.45 μM benzaldehyde and $\blacktriangle$, 45 μM benzaldehyde. **C:** Different units excited by 0.33 mM o-tolylurea (■) and 0.33 mM p-tolylurea (□); 3.7 μM nitrobenzene (●) and 4.5 μM benzaldehyde (○). (From Getchell, ref. 12, and Getchell and Getchell, ref. 13.)

spike intervals during the initial two to four intervals which ranged from about 250 to 800 msec in total duration. This presumably reflects the initial rapid invasion of generator currents triggered by the stimulus into the site of spike initiation. Quantitative methods of data analysis such as these may be considered as an essential step toward an understanding of the interval timing of impulse generation as well as possible correlations of specific discharge patterns with the molecular characteristics of the stimulus.

OLFACTORY BULB: SYNAPTIC ORGANIZATION

An orientation to the olfactory pathway, in mammals, is provided by the diagram in Fig. 5. The four main components consist of the olfactory epithelium, olfactory nerves, olfactory bulb, and olfactory cortex.

The schematic diagram of Fig. 5 illustrates the main neuronal components of the olfactory bulb. The olfactory axons, arising from the receptors in the olfactory epithelium, project to the surface of the olfactory bulb. The bulb is a spherical protrusion from the brain, containing concentric laminae of cells and their processes. Deep to the superficial nerve layer is a layer of rounded structures, the so-called olfactory glomeruli. All of the olfactory axons terminate within the glomeruli. Also within the

glomeruli are tufts of branches from the dendrites of mitral cells, which are the main output cells from the bulb. The tuft arises from a mitral primary dendrite; other, secondary, dendrites ramify in the external plexiform layer (EPL), but do not reach back to the glomeruli. A few recurrent collaterals from the mitral cell axons also terminate in the EPL. In the EPL are also found cell bodies of tufted cells, which appear in some respects to be smaller versions of mitral cells.

There are two main types of interneuron in the bulb. In the glomerular layer are periglomerular (PG) cells. Each has a dendritic tree confined within a glomerulus and an axon that connects laterally to neighboring glomeruli. It may be regarded as a type of short-axon cell. In deeper layers are found numerous granule cells. Each has a central process and a peripheral process that ramifies extensively within the EPL; the branches are invested with numerous spines. The granule cell has no axon, and the processes have the outward appearance and fine structure characteristic of dendrites in other parts of the nervous system. Also present in the bulb are other examples of short-axon cells, as well as numerous input fibers from the telencephalon, which will not further concern us here.

We now focus on the organization of the two main layers for integrative processing in the bulb—the glomerular layer and the EPL.

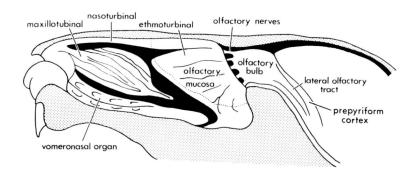

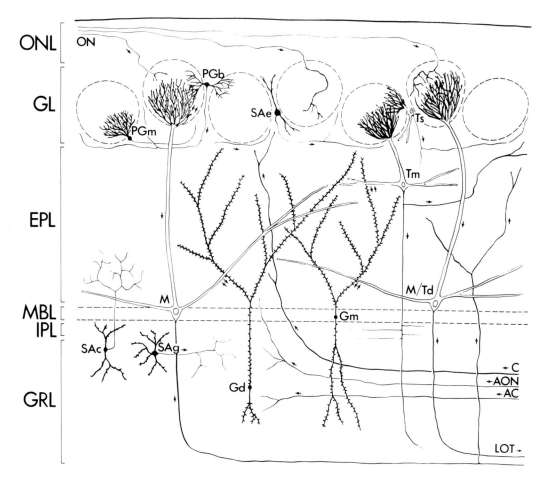

FIG. 5. **Top:** Diagram showing olfactory structures of the rabbit as a representative mammal. **Bottom:** Diagram based on Golgi stains of main types of neurons in mammalian olfactory bulb. ON, Olfactory nerves; PGb, periglomerular cell with biglomerular dendrites; PGm, periglomerular cell with monoglomerular dendrites; SAe, short-axon cell with extraglomerular dendrites; M, mitral cell; M/Td, displaced mitral or deep tufted cell; Tm, middle tufted cell; Ts superficial tufted cell; Gm, granule cell with cell body in mitral body layer; Gd, granule cell with cell body in deep layers; SAc, short-axon cell of Cajal; SAg, short-axon cell of Golgi; C, centrifugal fibers; AON, fibers from anterior olfactory nucleus; AC, fibers from anterior commissure; LOT, lateral olfactory tract. Main layers of bulb are indicated at left. ONL, olfactory nerve layer, GL, glomerular layer; EPL, external plexiform layer; MBL, mitral body layer; IPL, internal plexiform layer; GRL, granule layer. (From Shepherd, ref. 38.)

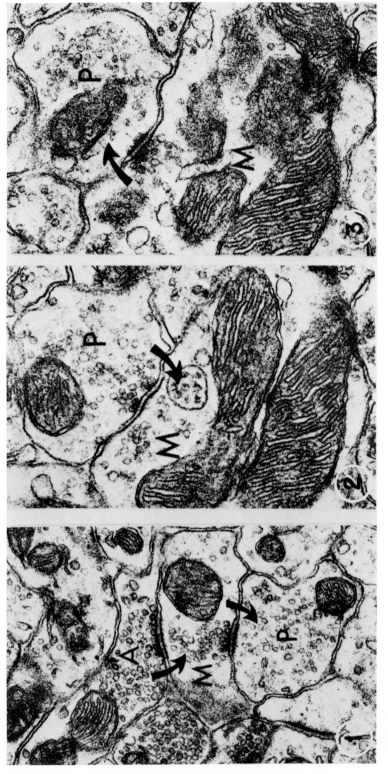

FIG. 6. Electron micrographs of olfactory glomerulus of the rat. A, Olfactory axon terminal; M, presumed mitral cell dendrite; P, presumed periglomerular cell dendrite. Arrows indicate polarity of synapses. ×23,000. (From White, ref. 41.)

Glomerular Layer

The olfactory glomerulus is a complex structure containing the terminals of olfactory axons as well as the dendritic tufts of mitral, tufted, and PG cells. Identification of synaptic terminals has depended on serial reconstructions from electron micrographs and careful comparison with the processes observed in Golgi-impregnated material. On this basis it has been possible to identify some characteristic patterns of synaptic connections (29,40,41).

Olfactory axon terminals are commonly observed making synapses onto mitral or PG cell dendrites. As illustrated in Fig. 6A, the axon terminals are large and contain many spherical vesicles. The synapses they make are characterized by a cluster of vesicles against a region of asymmetrical membrane densities (29,40,41). Mitral (and tufted) cell dendrites contain smaller, variable amounts of vesicles. They commonly make synapses onto other dendritic profiles.

These synapses are also characterized by spherical vesicles and asymmetric membrane densities. Some of the postsynaptic structures are the dendrites of PG cells. The connections are sometimes observed in serial sequences, as in Fig. 6-1. The PG cell dendrites also are presynaptic to other dendrites; the synapse is characterized by flattened vesicles and symmetric membrane densities. A common pattern is a reciprocal relation between a mitral and PG cell dendrite, as in Fig. 6-2,3 (29,40,41).

Electrophysiological evidence for the properties of these synapses has been sought in experiments in which volleys have been set up in the olfactory nerves while recording from single glomerular layer units (see Fig. 7). When a weak test volley, just at threshold for eliciting a spike response from the unit (*cf.* controls in A), is preceded by a weak conditioning volley, evidence has been obtained for facilitation (B) and suppression (C) of the unit recorded from. These effects are not due to refractoriness of

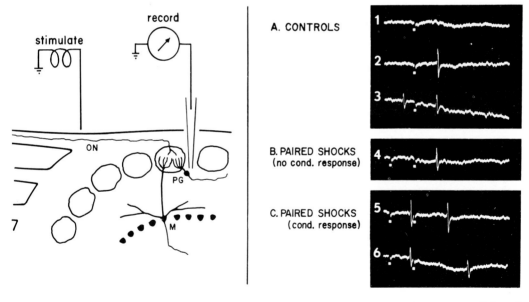

FIG. 7. **Left:** Schematic diagram of experimental set-up in rabbit olfactory bulb. ON, Olfactory nerve; PG, periglomerular cell; M, mitral cell. **Right:** Extracellular unitary recordings from presumed periglomerular cell; depth 324 μm. A: Control responses to single volleys in olfactory nerves. Stimulus duration 0.5 msec; intensity 52 μA, straddling threshold. Representative trials in which unit failed (1) and succeeded (2) in generating a spike response. Stimulus artefact indicated by white dot. In (3) response was preceded by spontaneously generated spike. B: Representative response (4) to test volley when threshold conditioning volley failed to elicit a spike. C: Representative test responses (5 and 6) when conditioning volley elicited a spike. Time interval between shocks: 10 msec; shocks repeated once every 10 sec. Spikes have been retouched. Spikes varied somewhat in size; variations were related to ongoing wave activity, not to afferent volley or type of response. Single unit observed for 40 min. (From Shepherd, ref. 37.)

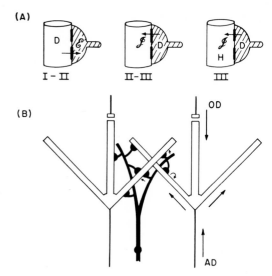

the unit (see A) or to olfactory nerve properties
(T. V. Getchell and G. M. Shepherd, *unpublished observations*). Preliminary analysis has
suggested that the facilitation reflects properties
of excitatory synapses, possibly of olfactory
nerve terminals or of mitral cell dendrites.
Suppression, on the other hand, may reflect
synaptic inhibition by PG cells, through synapses made by their dendrites as well as by
their axons.

Such synaptic actions are identical to those
inferred by electron microscopists from the
morphology of the synapses in the glomerular
layer (see above). Of particular interest is the
postulated inhibitory action of the PG cell; in
this respect it may serve as a model for the
synaptic actions of short-axon cells in other
parts of the central nervous system. No support has been found for the possibility of
excitatory interactions between the PG cells
(see ref. 7).

EPL

The EPL is composed mainly of just two
types of neuronal element: the dendrites of
mitral (and tufted) cells and the peripheral
dendritic trees of granule cells (see Fig. 5).
Most of the volume of the EPL is in fact occupied by the granule cell dendrites (33). The

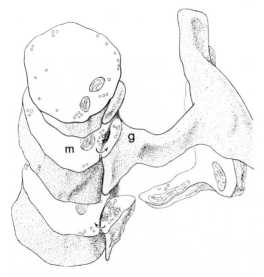

FIG. 8. Serial reconstruction of mitral cell dendrite
(m) and granule cell spine (g), showing side-by-side
reciprocal dendrodendritic synapses (*arrows*). (From
Rall et al., ref. 33.)

FIG. 9. A: Diagrams to illustrate mechanism of dendrodendritic synapses in EPL. Depolarization (D) of
mitral dendrite activates excitatory (E) synapses onto
granule gemmule (*shaded*) (time periods I and early
II). Depolarization of gemmule activates inhibitory
(J) synapse back onto mitral dendrite (periods II and
early III). Inhibitory synaptic activity results in long-lasting hyperpolarization of mitral dendrite (period
III). **B:** Diagram illustrating dendrodendritic synaptic
pathways through granule cells that provide for both
lateral and self-inhibition of mitral cells. Note that
dendrodendritic synapses of mitral secondary dendrites are activated in similar fashion by either orthodromic (OD) or antidromic (AD) impulse activity.
(From Rall and Shepherd, ref. 32.)

mitral and granule cell dendrites are each presynaptic to the other, through reciprocal,
side-by-side synapses that connect granule
cell spines and mitral cell dendrites (33). These
have been thoroughly identified in reconstructions from serial sections, as in Fig. 8. The
mitral-to-granule synapse is characterized by
spherical vesicles and asymmetric membrane
densities; the granule-to-mitral synapse is
characterized by flattened vesicles and symmetric membrane densities (31). Approximately
80% of all synapses in the EPL are members of
these reciprocal pairs.

Electrophysiological studies have taken
advantage of the fact that the mitral axons lie
together in the lateral olfactory tract. An antidromic volley in the axons sets up a sequence of
three main actions in the bulb: (a) antidromic
invasion of the mitral cells; (b) synaptic excitation of granule cells; and (c) synaptic inhibition

of the mitral cells. The antidromic invasion and subsequent recurrent inhibition of mitral cells has been documented in both extracellular and intracellular recordings (24,28,42).

The presence of granule cells in the recurrent inhibitory pathway onto mitral cells was inferred from these physiological studies. A pathway for granule excitation through the mitral secondary dendrites was postulated on the basis of computational models for the mitral and granule cell populations and reconstruction of the summed extracellular potentials evoked in the bulb (32,33). The postulated sequence of synaptic actions is illustrated schematically in Fig. 9A. The implications for pathways for self- and lateral inhibition of the mitral cells are shown in Fig. 9B.

ODOR PROCESSING IN THE OLFACTORY BULB

Both massed-unit (1,23) and single unit (1,3,16,39) recordings from the vertebrate olfactory bulb have shown that different areas of the bulb are preferentially excited depending on the odor used for stimulation. In addition these studies have indicated that individual cells are not activated by only a single odor, but rather are both excited and inhibited by a range of odor compounds. Thus it is assumed that the quality of any one odor is encoded by a pattern of activity occurring in many cells simultaneously. This idea has been formally described as an across-fiber pattern (6).

Since there is no continuum of physical characteristics along which odors may be grouped, as there is for visual and auditory stimuli, the idea of an across-fiber pattern has formed the basis on which several investigators have tried to define similarity between different odors using similarity between neuronal responses. In this way elegant attempts have been made to place odors in groups by comparing responses that different odors elicit from olfactory bulb units (5,14,17,22). Although it was hoped that this course of analysis would provide a framework within which qualitatively different odors could be related, no clear relationships between odors have emerged and the concept of primary odors or the presence of other schemes that have been suggested for relating odors has not been verified.

In studying the olfactory system there have always been problems of adequately insuring spatial and temporal control over the stimulus, in addition to the lack of a framework for defining the relationships between qualitatively different odors. Indeed the multiplicity of response types seen in many studies and the disappointing lack of coherence among odors grouped on the basis of neuronal responses may, at least in part, arise from the difficulty of delivering odor stimuli defined in both space and time. Such control is essential for making meaningful comparisons among responses elicited by different odors in the different neuronal components of the system.

Response Types in Olfactory Bulb Units

Recently it has been possible to effect spatial (19) and temporal (18,20,21,30) control over odor pulses. Using carefully defined stimuli in the concentration, temporal, and spatial domains it has been possible to find reproducible kinds of responses in the hamster (21) and salamander (18) olfactory bulb. In the salamander these responses fall into a small number of

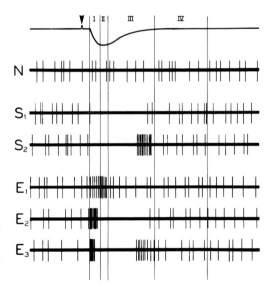

FIG. 10. Responses of salamander olfactory bulb neurons represented schematically relative to phases of the electroolfactogram (I,II,III,IV). Arrow indicates when stimulus delivery valve was switched. N, No response; S_1, S_2, types of suppressive response; E_1, E_2, E_3, types of excitatory response. (From Kauer, ref. 18.)

categories, which have been seen in different units with each of the odors tested and thus are not sufficient in themselves to define an odor type (18). This is consistent with the concept of an across-fiber pattern signaling odor type. These major categories consist of (a) suppression of activity during the odor (termed an S response) (b) excitation during the presence of the odor (E_1); initial excitation followed by suppression (E_2); initial excitation followed by suppression, followed by a second excitation (E_3) (3), and no response to the odor (N) (see Fig. 10).

Responses to Changes in Odor Concentration

Whereas the concept of an across-fiber pattern seems relevant for understanding coding of odor quality, odor quantity (concentration) has been found to correlate with changes in the temporal structure of the excitatory response types in individual cells (18). It was found, when an excitatory response was seen in the mitral/tufted cells of the salamander olfactory bulb, that excitation tended to be maintained for the duration of the odor pulse only if the concentration were also maintained at a certain level (E_1 response). As noted in previous studies (4,5,17), it was found that as the concentration was raised an inhibitory component became evident in the response. That is, there was an initial brief excitation abruptly followed by suppression (E_2). With a further increase in concentration a second excitation followed this suppression (E_3) (see Fig. 11). This phenomenon has been termed concentration tuning (18) and may possibly form the basis on which odor quantity is encoded. Suppressive responses (S), in general, showed no change in their temporal pattern with change in concentration.

Responses to Changes in Odor Duration

Precise temporal control over odor pulses has recently allowed the presentation of relatively square pulses of odor that have been used

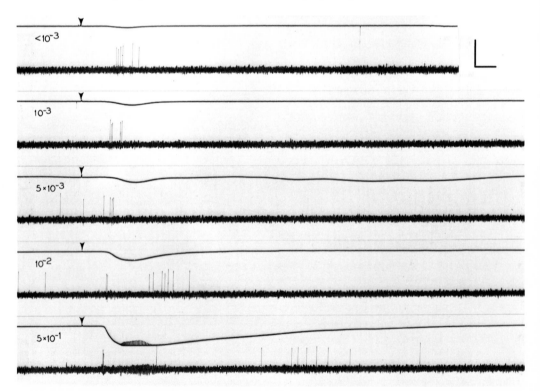

FIG. 11. Responses of a salamander olfactory bulb neuron to five concentrations of pinene. Arrows indicate when the stimulus delivery valve was switched. Calibration marks equal 1 sec and 500 μV and refer to the spike trace. The oscillation of the EOG seen with the highest concentration is commonly observed with very intense stimuli. (From Kauer, ref. 18.)

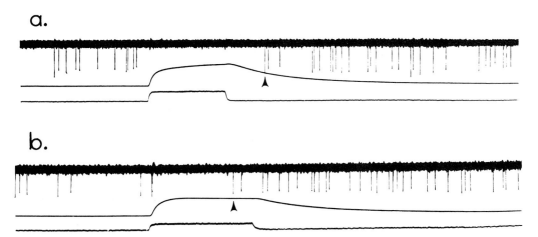

FIG. 12. a: Response of a salamander olfactory bulb unit showing suppression to a 6-sec pulse of 0.1% camphor. Arrow indicates return of spontaneous activity after the end of the pulse. **b:** Response of a different salamander bulb unit to an 8-sec step pulse of 0.1% camphor. Here the unit shows a sequence of a short excitation (two spikes), suppression, and following slight excitation. Arrow indicates that, in this case, firing resumes before the end of the pulse. (From Kauer and Shepherd, ref. 20.)

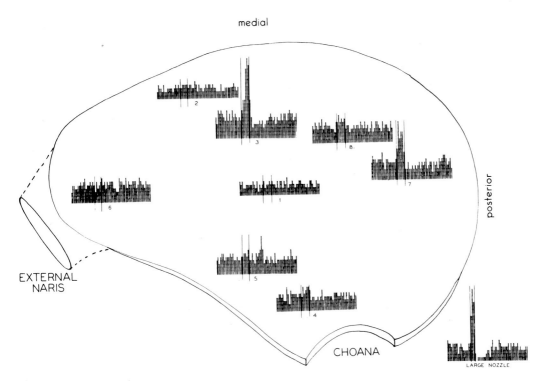

FIG. 13. Histograms of olfactory bulb unit responses showing relationship between response of a single unit to camphor odor and site of stimulus application. Each example of the response is placed on that area of the olfactory receptor sheet which, upon stimulation, elicits the activity shown in the histogram. Large nozzle indicates response to stimulation of entire receptor sheet. (From Kauer and Moulton, ref. 19.)

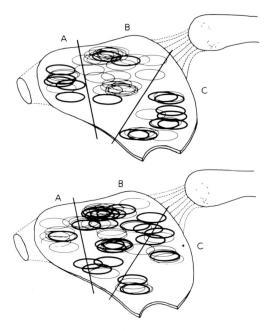

FIG. 14. Compilation of all data gathered for two different odors using punctate odor stimulation with olfactory bulb single unit recording. *Heavy ovals* indicate areas that give maximum excitation in salamander olfactory bulb units. *Light ovals* signify all other areas tested with each odor. **Top:** Amyl acetate; **bottom:** camphor. (From Kauer and Moulton, ref. 19.)

to study both the electroolfactogram (30) and olfactory bulb units (20). In addition a system has been devised for monitoring the odor stimulus during the experiment (20). By using controlled and monitored step odor pulses of different durations, it was found that in most cases suppressive responses tended to last for the entire duration of long pulses (up to 8 sec), whereas the suppression after the short initial burst in excitatory responses ($E_2 - E_3$) did not last for the duration of the pulse (20). This suggested that the suppression in these two response types possibly arose from different sources (see Fig. 12). Further studies are in progress on characterizing these response types with the ultimate aim of relating them to the synaptic organization of the olfactory bulb, as described in the previous section (J. S. Kauer and G. M. Shepherd, *unpublished observations*).

Responses to Changes in Odor Position on the Receptor Epithelium

Control over the spatial extent of odor stimuli has also been achieved. Using a specially

constructed small delivery nozzle, punctate (400 to 500 μm diameter) applications of odor to the olfactory epithelium of the salamander have been made in order to attempt mapping of the receptive fields of the bulbar neurons (19). Using this method, it was found that single unit excitatory responses, elicited by odors delivered to wide areas of the receptor sheet, would be elicited with localized odor presentation only if the odor were delivered to certain areas of the mucosa (see Fig. 13). In addition those areas that were appropriate for giving a response with a certain odor were surprisingly constant for different units in different experimental animals for one odor (see Fig. 14). In contrast to this, suppressive responses elicited by odor application to large mucosal areas were also elicited using punctate odor stimulation to most of the epithelium. Thus when the response was excitation (E) the bulbar units had relatively small, localized receptive fields, and when the response was suppression (S) the bulbar units had relatively large, diffuse receptive fields.

CONCLUSION

Investigation of odor responses from the olfactory bulb has reached the point where preliminary descriptions of the responses of olfactory bulb units to carefully controlled odors have been made. It should now be possible to perform experiments in the olfactory system similar to those in other sensory systems where precise stimulus control has been used. Using these methods it should be feasible to characterize the kinds of responses of the various cell types at all levels of the olfactory system under uniform stimulus conditions and thereby to achieve understanding of the neuronal circuitry underlying these responses. In addition methods of precise stimulus control should allow more detailed comparisons between neuronal responses to be made, in the hope of elucidating the mechanisms by which odors are encoded in the olfactory system.

ACKNOWLEDGMENTS

The research reported here was supported in part by U.S. Public Health Service grants NS-07609 to G.M.S. and NS-11667 to T.V.G.; by NSF research grant GB-28016 to T.V.G.; and

NINDS Special Fellowship NS-02701 to T.V.G.

REFERENCES

1. Adrian, E. D. (1951): Olfactory discrimination. *Ann. Psychol.*, 50:107–113.
2. Bloom, G. (1954): Studies on the olfactory epithelium of the frog and toad with the aid of light and electron microscopy. *Z. Zellforsch.*, 41:89–100.
3. Doving, K. B. (1966): The influence of olfactory stimulation on the activity of the secondary neurons in the burbot. *Acta Physiol. Scand.*, 66:290–299.
4. Doving, K. B. (1966): An electrophysiological study of olfactory discrimination of homologous compounds. *J. Physiol. (Lond.)*, 186:97–109.
5. Doving, K. B. (1966): Analysis of odour similarities from electrophysiological data. *Acta Physiol. Scand.*, 68:404–418.
6. Erickson, R. P., Doetsch, G. C., and Marshall, D. A. (1965): The gustatory neural response function. *J. Gen. Physiol.*, 39:247–263.
7. Freeman, W. J. (1974): A model for mutual excitation in a neuron population in olfactory bulb. *IEEE Trans. Biomed. Eng.*, BME21:350–357.
8. Gesteland, R. C. (1971): Neural coding in olfactory receptor cells. In: *Handbook of Sensory Physiology, Vol. 4, Chemical Senses, Part 1, Olfaction*, edited by L. M. Beidler, pp. 132–150. Springer, New York.
9. Getchell, M. L., and Gesteland, R. C. (1972): The chemistry of olfactory reception: Stimulus specific protection from sulfhydryl reagent inhibition. *Proc. Natl. Acad. Sci. USA*, 69:1494–1498.
10. Getchell, T. V. (1973): Analysis of unitary spikes recorded extracellularly from frog olfactory receptor cells and axons. *J. Physiol. (Lond.)*, 234:533–551.
11. Getchell, T. V. (1974): Electrogenic sources of slow voltage transients recorded from frog olfactory epithelium. *J. Neurophysiol.*, 37:1115–1130.
12. Getchell, T. V. (1974): Unitary responses in frog olfactory epithelium to sterically related molecules at low concentrations. *J. Gen. Physiol.*, 64:241–261.
13. Getchell, T. V., and Getchell, M. L. Signal-detecting mechanisms in the olfactory epithelium: Molecular discrimination. *Ann. N.Y. Acad. Sci.*, 237:62–75.
14. Giachetti, I., and MacLeod, P. (1973): Supériorité du pouvoir discriminateor des cellules mitrales compare a celui des recepteors olfactifs. *J. Physiol. (Paris)*, 6:399–467.
15. Graziadei, P. P. C. (1971): The olfactory mucosa of vertebrates. In: *Handbook of Sensory Physiology, Vol. 4, Chemical Senses, Part 1, Olfaction*, edited by L. M. Beidler, pp. 27–58. Springer, New York.
16. Green, J. D., Mancia, M., and von Baumgarten, R. (1962): Recurrent inhibition in the olfactory bulb. I. Effects of antidromic stimulation of the lateral olfactory tract. *J. Neurophysiol.*, 25:467–488.
17. Higashino, S., Takeuchi, H., and Amoore, J. E. (1969): Mechanism of olfactory discrimination in olfactory bulb of bullfrog. In: *Olfaction and Taste III*, edited by C. Pfaffman, pp. 192–211. Rockefeller University Press, New York.
18. Kauer, J. S. (1974): Response patterns of amphibian olfactory bulb neurones to odour stimulation. *J. Physiol. (Lond.)*, 243:695–715.
19. Kauer, J. S., and Moulton, D. G. (1974): Responses of olfactory bulb neurones to odor stimulation of small nasal areas in the salamander. *J. Physiol. (Lond.)*, 234:717–737.
20. Kauer, J. S., and Shepherd, G. M. (1975): Olfactory stimulation with controlled and monitored step pulses of odor. *Brain Res.*, 85:108–113.
21. Macrides, F., and Chorover, S. L. (1972): Olfactory bulb unit activity correlated with inhalation cycles and odor quality. *Science*, 175:84–87.
22. Meredith, M. (1974): Olfactory coding for aminoacids at the second-order neurone level in goldfish. PhD dissertation, University of Pennsylvania.
23. Moulton, D. G. (1961): Electrical activity recorded by means of chronically implanted electrodes in the olfactory bulb of the rabbit. *Physiologist*, 4:77.
24. Nicoll, R. A. (1969): Inhibitory mechanisms in the rabbit olfactory bulb: Dendrodendritic mechanisms. *Brain Res.*, 14:157–172.
25. Ottoson, D. (1956): Analysis of the electrical activity of the olfactory epithelium. *Acta Physiol. Scand.*, 35 (suppl. 122):1–83.
26. Ottoson, D. (1971): The electroolfactogram. In: *Handbook of Sensory Physiology, Vol. 4, Chemical Senses, Part 1, Olfaction*, edited by L. M. Beidler, pp. 95–131. Springer, New York.
27. Ottoson, D., and Shepherd, G. M. (1967): Experiments and concepts in olfactory physiology. In: *Progress in Brain Research: Sensory Mechanisms, Vol. 23*, edited by Y. Zotterman, pp. 83–138. Elsevier, New York.
28. Phillips, C. G., Powell, T. P. S., and Shepherd, G. M. (1963): The responses of mitral cells to stimulation of the lateral olfactory tract in the rabbit. *J. Physiol. (Lond.)*, 168:65–88.
29. Pinching, A. J., and Powell, T. P. S. (1971): The neuropil of the glomeruli of the olfactory bulb. *J. Cell Sci.*, 9:347–377.
30. Poynder, T. M. (1973): Response of the frog olfactory system to controlled odour stimuli. *J. Soc. Cosmetic Chem. Gt. Brit.*, 5:1–20.
31. Price, J. L., and Powell, T. P. S. (1970): The synaptology of the granule cells of the olfactory bulb. *J. Cell Sci.*, 7:125–155.
32. Rall, W., and Shepherd, G. M. (1968): Theoretical reconstruction of field potentials and dendrodendritic synaptic interactions in olfactory bulb. *J. Neurophysiol.*, 31:884–915.
33. Rall, W. G., Shepherd, G. M., Reese, T. S. and

Brightman, M. V. (1966): Dendrodendritic synaptic pathway for inhibition in the olfactory bulb. *Exp. Neurol.*, 14:44–56.

34. Reese, T. S. (1965): Olfactory cilia in the frog. *J. Cell Biol.*, 25:209–230.

35. Reese, T. S., and Shepherd, G. M. (1972): Dendrodendritic synapses in the central nervous system. In: *Structure and Function of Synapses*, edited by G. D. Pappas and D. P. Purpura, pp. 121–136. Raven Press, New York.

36. Shepherd, G. M. (1963): Neuronal systems controlling mitral cell excitability. *J. Physiol. (Lond.)*, 168:101–117.

37. Shepherd, G. M. (1971): Physiological evidence for dendrodendritic synaptic interactions in the rabbit's olfactory glomerulus. *Brain Res.*, 32:212–217.

38. Shepherd, G. M. (1972): Synaptic organization of the mammalian olfactory bulb. *Physiol. Rev.*, 52:864–917.

39. Walsh, R. R. (1956): Single cell spike activity in the olfactory bulb. *Am. J. Physiol.*, 186:255–257.

40. White, E. L. (1972): Synaptic organization in the olfactory glomerulus of the mouse. *Brain Res.*, 37:69–80.

41. White, E. L. (1973): Synaptic organization of the mammalian olfactory glomerulus: New findings including an intraspecific variation. *Brain Res.*, 60:299–313.

42. Yamamoto, C., Yamamoto, T., and Iwama, K. (1963): The inhibitory system in the olfactory bulb studied by intracellular recording. *J. Neurophysiol.*, 26:403–415.

The Nervous System, Donald B. Tower, Editor-in-Chief. *Vol. 1: The Basic Neurosciences.* Raven Press, New York, 1975.

Activity of Cerebral Neurons in Relation to Movement

Edward V. Evarts

This chapter deals with experiments on the role of three interconnected components of the brain's motor control system: (a) the cerebral motor cortex, (b) the cerebellum, (c) the basal ganglia. Figure 1, taken from a paper by Kemp and Powell (1), illustrates in schematic form some of the anatomic connections between these three structures. At one time the pyramidal system, arising from neurons whose cell bodies are located in the cerebral cortex, was thought of as functioning separately from the extrapyramidal system. Studies carried out by a number of investigators and summarized in the paper by Kemp and Powell (1) now make it clear that the two systems are closely interrelated. The interrelationship is particularly close for the phylogenetically newer components of the pyramidal and extrapyramidal systems. Thus the lateral cerebellar hemispheres, which undergo such an enormous increase in size in relation to the evolution of the cerebral motor cortex in the higher primates and man, actually feed out into motor behavior (via the dentate nucleus, the superior cerebellar peduncle, and the thalamic nucleus ventralis lateralis) by way of the motor cortex and pyramidal system. The basal ganglia, which undergo striking development in subhuman primates and in man, also feed out into motor behavior via the thalamus, motor cortex, and pyramidal system. A central problem in studies of motor control has thus become the elucidation of the

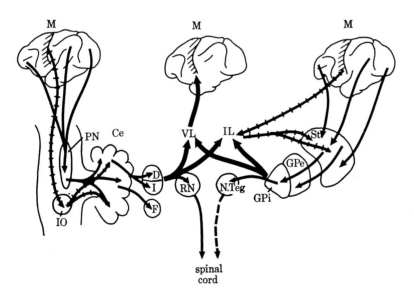

FIG. 1. This figure illustrates the similarity in organization of the cerebral connections of the cerebellum and basal ganglia. Presumed equivalent pathways in the two systems are shown by the same kinds of symbols. Interrupted lines indicate possible connections. Ce, cerebellar cortex; D, dentate nucleus; F, fastigial nucleus; GPe, globus pallidus, external segment; GPi, globus pallidus, internal segment; I, interpositus nucleus; IL, intralaminar nuclei of the thalamus; IO, inferior olive; M, motor cortex; N. Teg., tegmental nuclei; PN, pontine nuclei; RN, red nucleus; St, striatum; VL, ventrolateral nucleus of the thalamus. (Reprinted from Kemp and Powell, ref. 1.)

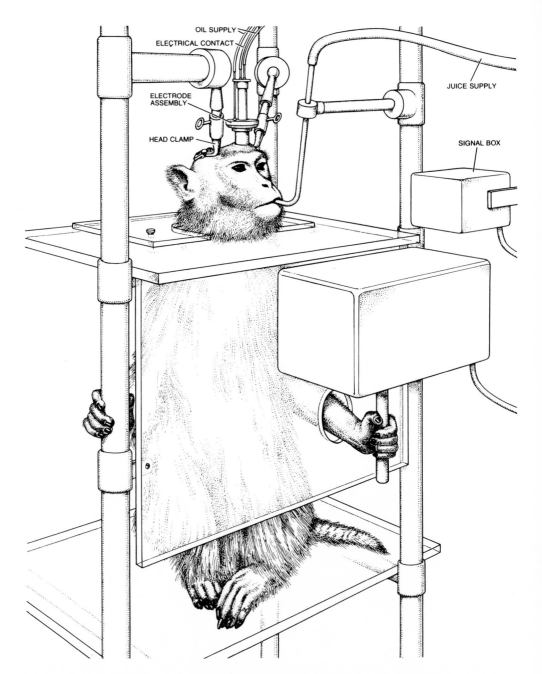

FIG. 2. Recordings of the activity of single nerve cells in the brain are obtained while a monkey performs a learned task in this primate chair. The monkey's head is painlessly immobilized so that the microelectrode in the brain does not change position during the experiment. The monkey can be trained to move the rod either in response to a visual stimulus or when the rod itself is perturbed by a torque motor in the box from which the rod protrudes. In the latter case, the direction in which the handle must be moved is indicated by an instruction (red or green lamp) flashed from the signal box. Thus, the signal box tells the monkey how to move, whereas the handle's movement tells him when to move. If the monkey makes the required movement within a specified time, it receives a reward of fruit juice through the tube in its mouth. Signals from the microelectrode in the brain, along with data from the signal box and transducers connected to the rod, are fed into a computer for analysis. (Reprinted from Evarts, ref. 17.)

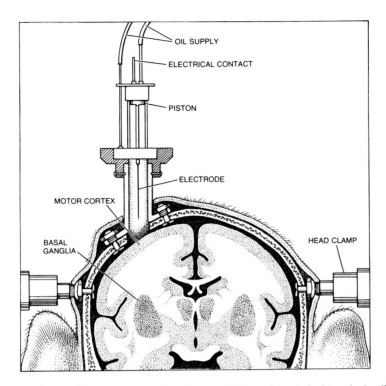

FIG. 3. Microelectrode assembly consists of a fine platinum-iridium wire attached to a hydraulically actuated piston. A stainless steel cylinder permanently attached to the monkey's skull provides access to the brain. The bolts on the sides of the skull are also permanently implanted. They are attached to clamps during the experiment to prevent head movement. After the electrode assembly is bolted to the cylinder, the electrode is lowered by pumping oil into the inlet on the right and raised by pumping oil into the inlet on the left. (Reprinted from Evarts, ref. 17.)

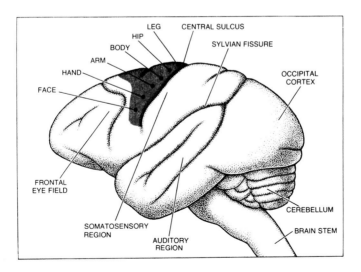

FIG. 4. Cerebral cortex of a monkey's brain. Electrical stimulation of the points indicated on the motor cortex causes involuntary contraction of the corresponding group of muscles on the opposite side of the body. Damage to an area of the motor cortex usually results in paralysis of the muscles controlled by that area. The frontal eye field is involved in eye movements. (Reprinted from Evarts, ref. 17.)

nature of the functional interrelationship between these three major components of the motor control system.

This review will focus on experiments utilizing a technique that has come into general use during the past decade. The technique (Fig. 2) involves recording the activity of single nerve cells in association with natural movements carried out in monkeys. Monkeys are initially trained to carry out certain specified movements in order to receive a reward. The movements necessary to receive the reward may be hand movements (as in Fig. 2) or a variety of other movements (e.g., eye, jaw). With a monkey seated in the primate chair as in Fig. 2, a microelectrode is lowered into the part of the brain under investigation, and the action potential of a single nerve cell is picked up and studied in relation to concurrent movements. Figures 3 and 4 illustrate additional details of the procedure. Figure 3 shows how the microelectrode is lowered into the brain by a hydraulic cylinder. Depending upon where the cylinder is attached to the skull, the microelectrode may be used to pick up activity from motor cortex (Fig. 4), from cerebellum, from basal ganglia, from thalamus, or from other parts of the brain.

TIMING OF BRAIN ACTIVITY IN RELATION TO MOVEMENT

One of the first studies carried out utilizing this technique was designed to determine the time at which cells in the precentral motor cortex of monkeys discharged in association with a simple volitional movement (2). In this experiment monkeys were trained to depress a telegraph key and to watch for the appearance of a light, which came on at unpredictable times. Monkeys were rewarded for releasing the telegraph key promptly following the appearance of the light. The reward was a drop of fruit juice. By simultaneously recording both the brain cell discharges and muscle discharges (Fig. 5), it was possible to determine the temporal relationship between them. In these studies it was found that cells in motor cortex discharged approximately 60 msec prior to the occurrence of muscular contraction in the corresponding part of the body. As one would expect, cells in one hemisphere are related primarily to the movements of the contralateral hand.

The finding that cells in the motor cortex discharged prior to movement was not surprising: it was to be expected from the occurrence of paralysis of movement following lesions of the motor cortex in man. However, information on the timing of activity in relation to movement was not so easily predictable from clinical information for structures such as the cerebellum and basal ganglia. It was in these structures that recordings of neuronal activity have proved particularly valuable.

Thach (3) recorded activity of cerebellar neurons in relation to rapidly alternating arm movements in monkeys, and found clear modifications of cerebellar activity in relation to such movements (Fig. 6). In subsequent studies Thach studied the discharge of cerebellar cells

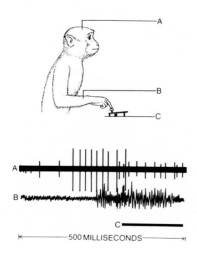

FIG. 5. Temporal relation between the discharge of a nerve cell in the motor cortex and a simple hand movement is shown above. A monkey was trained to depress a telegraph key and then to release it within 350 msec after a light came on. The upper trace (**A**) shows the activity of a single nerve cell in the arm region of the motor cortex, which was recorded by a microelectrode. The trace starts at the onset of the light signal. In a series of trials the nerve cell became active first, usually within 150 msec of the signal. There followed a contraction of arm muscles (**B**), which was detected by an electromyograph. Trace (**C**) shows when the telegraph key opened. (Reprinted from Evarts, ref. 17.)

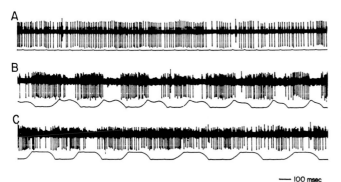

FIG. 6. Discharge of a Purkinje cell in the absence of movement (**A**), and during rapidly alternating movement of the ipsilateral wrist (**B**) and of the ipsilateral shoulder (**C**). *Upper trace,* the unit discharge; *lower trace,* movements of the lever. (Reprinted from Thach, ref. 3.)

— 100 msec

related to prompt movements triggered by the appearance of a light. In such studies it was shown that cerebellar neurons discharged well in advance of volitional movements (Fig. 7). Thus the notion that cerebellar neurons discharged only in relation to feedback from the moving part could be rejected, and clear evidence was presented that the activity of cerebellar neurons was important prior to the movement as well as following.

The axons of the cerebellar nuclear cells project to nucleus ventralis lateralis of the thalamus (VL) which relays information to the motor cortex. Evarts (4) recorded activity of neurons in VL and observed that here, too, neurons were active in advance of movement. VL receives inputs not only from the cerebellum but also from the globus pallidus. Thus VL is a major point of convergence between two of the major divisions of the extrapyramidal system, i.e., the cerebellum and the basal ganglia. DeLong's

studies (5) have shown that, as for the cerebellum, neurons in the basal ganglia also change their discharge prior to the onset of arm movements. The distribution of onset times found by DeLong for pallidal neurons was similar to that for neurons of the arm area of the motor cortex.

The observations reported above, showing that all three major subdivisions of the brain's motor control system (motor cortex, cerebellum, and basal ganglia) discharge prior to movement, support the notion put forward by Kemp and Powell (1) and illustrated in Fig. 1. It is apparent in this figure that the entire cerebral cortex sends fibers both to the basal ganglia and to the cerebellum, and that these two structures in turn send massive connections back to the motor cortex by way of the thalamus. Thus the basal ganglia and cerebellum receive information from the somatosensory, visual, auditory, and associative regions of the cerebral cortex, transform this information and then send a new

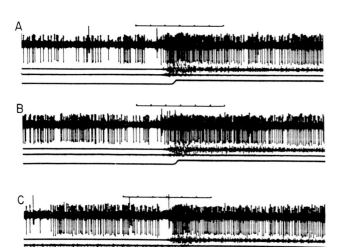

FIG. 7. Discharge of a Purkinje cell during three successive triggered flexions of the wrist. A pause in firing of the simple spike preceded and a burst accompanied the movement. The complex spike also occurred in relation to this movement. (Reprinted from Thach, ref. 3.)

pattern of signals to the motor cortex via the thalamus. Whereas the traditional view of motor organization held that cerebral motor cortex was at the highest level of motor integration and that the subcortical structures were at a lower level, probably operating to control movement on the basis of feedback, it now appears that both cerebellum and basal ganglia are important in the early stages of motor programming. Of course, it must be kept in mind that this statement holds true for only certain parts of the cerebellum and basal ganglia. The cerebellum, for example, is a structure that, although remarkably uniform in its architecture, has vastly different connections depending upon the phylogenetic stage at which the cerebellar part in question developed. Thus there are certain parts of the cerebellum that are dominated by feedback from muscle receptors and sense organs such as the labyrinth, whereas other parts of the cerebellum receive their major inputs from the cerebral cortex and get relatively little direct input from peripheral receptors.

It is of interest to compare these observations on activity of single neurons in monkey to observations on activity of single nerve cells in man that have been obtained over the past decade. Recordings in man have been made available by introduction of microelectrodes into the brain of patients undergoing stereotaxic surgery for the relief of motor disorders, as described by Jasper (6). The many reports that have appeared in the 15 years of such work are too numerous to consider in this review, but have been summarized in a recent paper by Hongell et al. (7). These studies on man show that activity of VL neurons is strikingly related to volitional movements carried out by the patient, whereas passive movements have relatively little effect on VL neuron discharge. Similar observations have been made in monkeys (8). These observations in monkeys and in man are consistent with the view that the activity of VL neurons is of importance in relaying motor programs to the motor cortex, but is relatively uninvolved in simple relay of sensory impulses from the periphery.

BRAIN ACTIVITY IN GETTING SET FOR MOVEMENT

The studies referred to above have been concerned primarily with the circuits that come into play in the initiation of abrupt movements of the type that are commonly used in studying simple reaction time. Another phase of work on motor control has recently been initiated in primates, this phase having to do with the processes that occur during the decision-making period prior to the occurrence of movement. These experiments on the changes in the activity of the brain during a period prior to the decision to move (when the subject is preparing a motor program) were based on observations in man indicating that the intention or set of the subject can profoundly modify motor responses elicited by muscle stretch. Such an observation of the effect of intention on motor activity was described by Hammond (9).

Hammond, using human subjects, found that sudden extension of the elbow (which stretched the biceps muscle) elicited a 50-msec latency biceps response when the subject had been instructed to resist, but not when the subject had been instructed not to resist. Hammond's observations in man have provided the basis for work that is currently being conducted in monkeys to determine the neuronal processes underlying this effect of prior instruction. The consistency and short (50-msec) latency of the response in Hammond's subjects, when instructed to resist, led him to suggest that "a stretch reflex is at work when the arm is forcibly extended." He added, however, that "This must be reconciled with the fact that prior instructions to 'let go' can interfere so rapidly and effectively with the subject's response. It is accordingly suggested that a spinal stretch reflex mechanism can be preset by nervous activity from the brain."

In order to study the central events associated with this phenomenon, monkeys were trained to react to a sudden perturbation of the arm according to a prior instruction. In this training monkeys were required to grasp a handle and maintain it in a certain position for 2 to 4 sec prior to the perturbation of the handle. A white lamp signaled a correct holding position. An instruction was introduced during the holding period. This instruction told the monkey how he should respond to a perturbation of the handle that would occur subsequently. The instruction was a red or green light, which appeared after 2 to 4 sec of correct holding and 0.6 to 2.0 sec prior to the onset of handle perturbation. The times varied unpredictably within these ranges. The red light informed the monkey that he should pull toward himself when the perturbation occurred and the green light meant that he should push away when the perturbation occurred. There were two different directions of perturbation, one being a movement of the handle toward the monkey and the other a movement of the handle away from the monkey. A given instruction called for a movement synergistic with the tendon jerk for one direction of perturbation and antagonistic to this reflex for the other direction of perturbation. When the monkey had learned to perform this task, recordings from individual sensorimotor cortex neurons were obtained during performance of the movement.

Figure 8 shows EMG records from the biceps muscle for the four possible combinations of the two instructions and the two perturbations.

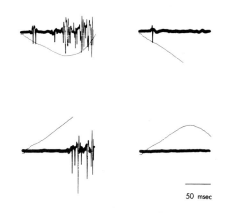

50 msec

FIG. 8. The set-up illustrated in Fig. 2 was used to study biceps activity for different instruction-stimulus combinations. A lamp in the signal box told the monkey what to do and a perturbation of the handle told him when to do it. Instructions to pull or push and perturbations toward or away from the monkey could be combined in four possible ways, as shown in the four pairs of traces in this figure. Each pair of traces shows biceps EMG activity and the output of a potentiometer coupled to the handle, with upward deflection of the potentiometer trace indicating movement of the handle toward the monkey and downward deflection of the potentiometer trace indicating movement of the handle away from the monkey. For the set of traces at upper left, the prior instruction was pull, calling for biceps contraction and the perturbing stimulus (indicated by the potentiometer trace) moved the handle away from the monkey, thereby stretching the biceps. At lower right the instruction was push and the initial perturbation was a movement of the handle toward the monkey, resulting in biceps shortening. For further explanation, see text. (Reprinted from Evarts and Tanji, ref. 18.)

In addition to the EMG records, Fig. 8 shows potentiometer traces indicating movements of the handle grasped by the monkey. Upward deflection of the potentiometer trace indicates movement of the handle toward the monkey (with consequent shortening of biceps) and downward deflection indicates movement away from the monkey (with biceps stretch). Each trace begins at the time when power was applied to a torque motor whose shaft was coupled to the handle. The lag between energization of the torque motor and the beginning of handle displacement was about 4 msec. In the two sets of traces at the top of Fig. 8, the perturbation moved the handle away from the monkey, stretching the biceps, and evoking a short latency EMG response (tendon jerk). In the two sets of traces at the bottom of Fig. 8 the perturbation was a movement of the handle toward the monkey. This perturbation shortened the biceps and there was no tendon jerk. For the two sets of traces at the left of Fig. 8 the prior instruction was pull, which required that the biceps contract. For the two sets of traces at the right of Fig. 8 the prior instruction was push, which did not require biceps contraction. Of these four instruction-perturbation combinations, the one at the upper left of Fig. 8 was associated with maximum biceps activity: the perturbation (involving biceps stretch) elicited a tendon jerk and the instruction called for biceps contraction. Thus the perturbation and prior instruction reinforced each other, both favoring biceps activity. The condition of minimum biceps activity is seen at the lower right in Fig. 8 where neither the perturbation nor the prior instruction called for biceps activity: a perturbation that shortened the biceps was paired with a prior instruction to push. In this situation, as in the first, the perturbation and response reinforced each other, but now both called for biceps quiescence rather than for biceps activity.

For the two remaining parts of Fig. 8, the perturbation and prior instruction were antagonistic. At the lower left is shown the case where the instruction called for biceps contraction but the segmental reflex effects of the perturbation (involving biceps shortening) tended to silence biceps activity. Here the tendon jerk is absent, as one would expect. In addition the biceps contraction called for by the prior instruction has a longer latency than it had had

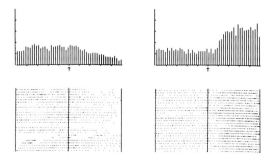

FIG. 9. Instruction-evoked motor cortex activity. This figure shows rasters and histograms corresponding to 2 sec of activity of a precentral PTN. In the rasters the central line represents the time of occurrence of the instruction (red or green light); dots to the left of the central line represent neuronal discharge occurring during 1 sec when the animal was waiting for the instruction. The arrow at the center of each histogram indicates the time of occurrence of the instruction; histogram bin width is 40 msec. About 200 msec after the instruction to push (green), there was an increase in discharge (right raster and histogram). In contrast, after the instruction to pull (red), there was a decrease in discharge (left raster and histogram). (Reprinted from Evarts and Tanji, ref. 18.)

when the perturbation involved biceps stretch.

The last of the four instruction-perturbation pairings is shown at the upper right of Fig. 8, where the perturbation was biceps stretch (tending to elicit biceps contraction) but the prior instruction was push, which did not call for biceps contraction. Here again there is antagonism between the perturbation and the instruction, and this antagonism results in a reduction in the tendon jerk elicited by biceps stretch: the tendon jerk elicited by biceps stretch is smaller when the stretch is coupled with a prior instruction calling for push than when coupled with a prior instruction calling for pull. It is thus apparent that the two different instructions give

rise to differential presetting of spinal cord reflex mechanisms mediating the tendon jerk.

The EMG responses described earlier were triggered by a stimulus to the hand, and, although these EMG responses varied depending on prior instruction, the instruction itself did not evoke any EMG response. For motor cortex neurons, however, the picture was quite different. Recordings of precentral neuron activity revealed that the instructions themselves elicited marked alternations in discharge patterns of both PTNs and non-PTNs in motor cortex. An example of the effect of instruction is shown in Fig. 9. For the neuron whose activity is displayed in this figure, the instruction push was followed by an increase in activity, whereas the instruction pull led to a decrease of neuronal activity. Many precentral neurons were influenced by the instruction, this effect appearing from 200 to 500 msec after the onset of the red or green light. Both PTNs and non-PTNs showed clear responses to the instruction.

A major point of interest in analyses of these responses was the interaction between the short latency perturbation-evoked neural response and prior instruction. Figure 10 illustrates a case of this interaction for a precentral PTN. This neuron was active in association with the push movement, and in addition the neuron discharged in response to externally produced handle movements toward the monkey (S+). The magnitude of the PTN response to handle movement differed considerably depending upon whether the prior instruction had been push or pull. The PTN shown in Fig. 10 had its most intense response when an instruction to *push* was paired with a perturbation that moved the handle toward (S+) the monkey (upper right of Fig. 10), whereas the PTN was almost totally silenced when an instruction to pull was paired

$\longrightarrow$

FIG. 10. Effect of prior instruction on PTN response. This PTN was most active (*upper right*) when a prior instruction to push was triggered by an opposing perturbation, i.e., one that moved the handle toward (S+) the monkey. The effect of prior instruction on this PTN response to perturbation may be seen by comparing *upper right* with *upper left,* where the same handle movement (S+) failed to evoke discharge when there had been a prior instruction to pull. At *lower right,* the instruction (push) but not the perturbation (S−) called for discharge of this PTN, and at *lower left* neither the instruction (pull) nor the perturbation (S−) called for discharge, and the neuron became almost totally silent within 20 msec of the perturbation (S−). The perturbation occurs at the center line in rasters and at the arrow in histograms, and activity is displayed for 500 msec before and after the perturbations. Histogram bin width is 20 msec. The solid line in the right half of each raster-row indicates the completion of the motor response, following which the monkey would return the handle to the central holding zone and await a new instruction. (Reprinted from Evarts and Tanji, ref. 18.)

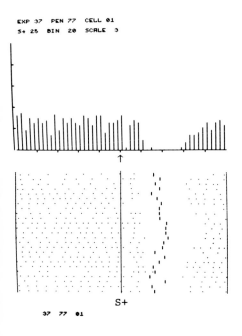

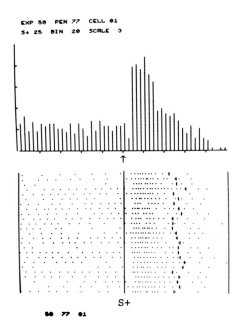

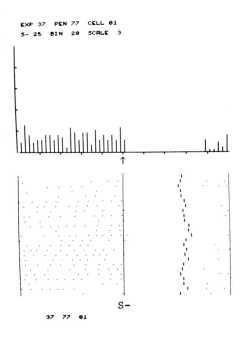

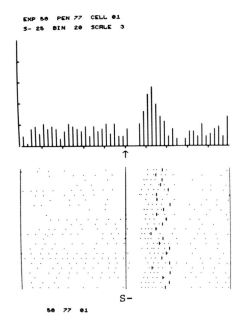

PULL

PUSH

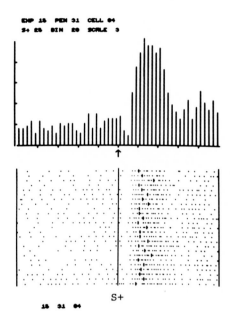
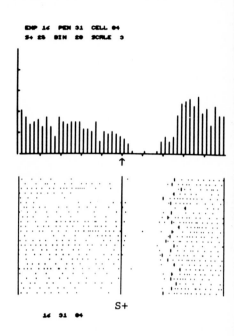
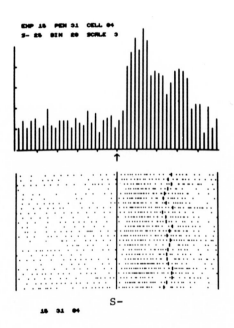
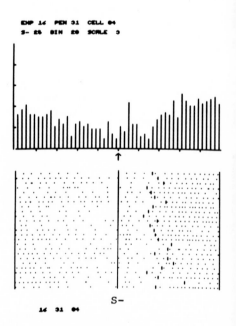

PULL   PUSH

FIG. 11. Effect of prior instruction on non-PTN response. This non-PTN was most active (*lower left*) when a previously instructed pull was triggered by an opposing perturbation (S−). For further details of this figure, see text. (Reprinted from Evarts and Tanji, ref. 18.)

with a stimulus that moved the handle away (S—) from the monkey (lower left of Fig. 10).

Figure 11 shows another motor cortex neuron (a non-PTN) whose activity in the four different perturbation-instruction pairings was analogous to biceps rather than triceps. This cell was active with voluntary pull and was activated by an opposite external perturbation, i.e., a perturbation that moved the arm away from the monkey. Like biceps muscle in Fig. 8, this unit was maximally activated when an instruction to pull was paired with a perturbation that moved the arm away from the monkey. Again in analogy with biceps muscle, the cell was silenced when an instruction to push was paired with a perturbation that moved the arm toward the monkey. In this neuron the reflex response evoked by the excitatory perturbation was enhanced after the excitatory instruction, just as the tendon jerk of a muscle was enhanced after an instruction calling for activation of the muscle.

The results that have now been presented show that both spinal and cerebral responses are modified by prior instruction, and it seems reasonable to conclude that both of these modifications underlie the difference in the later phase of the muscular response, i.e., the phase of muscular response that is responsible for the performance of the movement called for by the instruction. Hammond (9) proposed that the later phase of muscle activity was a spinal reflex that could be preset by nervous activity from the brain. We have observed changes of PTN discharge, which vary depending on the prior instruction, and the ability of motor cortex PTN output to preset spinal reflexes is well documented. Granted that PTNs function in presetting spinal cord reflexes as a result of prior instruction, is it also possible that motor cortex neurons participate in a high-speed loop that actually mediates the later phase of perturbation-evoked muscle activity? Evidence for such cerebral mediation has been provided both by our PTN recordings and by the work of Marsden et al. (10), who obtained latency measurements compatible with a cortical pathway for the later phase of muscle response in man.

Two components of motor cortex PTN discharge are initiated by a movement of a rod held in an animal's hand. The first component of activity is a short latency response dependent in large measure on the nature of the kinesthetic input. The second component of PTN discharge depends primarily on the intended movement and this discharge occurs at latencies as short as 50 msec. Excitation of PTNs in the course of this second phase of discharge presumably involves very different pathways from those involved in the first phase. The second phase of discharge would seem to be the manifestation of a central program, whereas the first phase of activity appears to be more automatic and is thus akin to a reflex. Recordings of activity of neurons in nucleus VL show that these neurons have properties consistent with their playing a role in mediating the second phase of PTN discharge: VL neurons are related to the intended movement and are relatively independent of the specific features of the sensory input that triggers this intended movement.

STUDIES ON CONTROL OF EYE MOVEMENT

The preceding sections of this report have dealt largely with studies on parts of the central nervous system that play a role in the control of limb movements. Another major segment of recent work on motor control has dealt with control of eye movements. The models that investigators have sought to explore in examining the activity of central neurons in association with eye movement have been summarized by Robinson (11). Robinson lists four oculomotor subsystems controlling saccadic, smooth pursuit, vestibular, and vergence eye movements, and points out that almost all eye movements in primates are combinations of the movements produced by each of these subsystems. Neurophysiological investigations of central control of eye movement have focused on isolating the neural substrates for each of these separate aspects of eye movement control. Bizzi (12), for instance, has found that nerve cells in the frontal eye fields of monkey can be separated according to whether they are involved in smooth pursuit or saccadic eye movements. Examples of Bizzi's results are shown in Fig. 12.

Another phase of work on eye movements is concerned with the mechanisms involved in plasticity of reflex control. Prominent in this work is the hypothesis that the cerebellum may be important in changes of reflex gain as a result of experience. Robinson (13) has observed

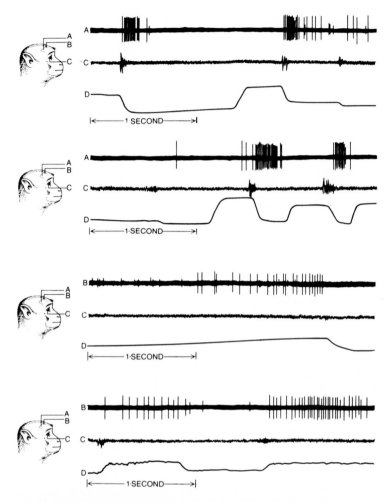

FIG. 12. Recordings of the activity of single nerve cells in the frontal eye field by Emilio Bizzi of the Massachusetts Institute of Technology show that one type of cell (**A**) discharges during voluntary saccadic eye movement and a second type of cell (**B**) discharges during smooth pursuit eye movement and during maintained position. The electromyographic activity of an eye muscle (**C**) and eye movements (**D**) also were recorded. The top traces show a cell (**A**) discharging during saccadic movements. The bottom traces show the discharge of a different cell (**B**) during smooth pursuit (**upper B**) and maintained eye position (**lower B**). (Reprinted from Evarts, ref. 17.)

a loss of plasticity of the vestibulo-ocular reflex as a result of cerebellar lesions, and Ito (*This Volume*) puts forward a theory that the cerebellum functions as a feed-forward control to allow fine adaptive tuning of the vestibulo-ocular reflex.

Studies by Miles (14) have demonstrated that the plasticity of the vestibulo-ocular reflex of the rhesus monkey is adaptive. In these experiments Miles fitted monkeys with telescopic spectacles which either magnified the world by a factor of two or diminished it to half of its normal size. The vestibulo-ocular reflex of monkeys fitted with such spectacles gradually underwent adaptations such that the magnitude of eye movements generated in association with the monkeys' head movements became appropriate to the compensatory eye movement needed to maintain stable retinal images during head movements. The role of the vestibulo-ocular reflex is to maintain a steady retinal image during head turns, and the adaptive plasticity in Miles' experiments helped the reflex to accomplish this purpose.

In addition to studying the plasticity of the vestibulo-ocular reflex, Miles and Fuller (15) have studied single unit firing patterns in vestibular nuclei related to voluntary eye movements and passive body rotation in monkeys. The results of these experiments demonstrate that individual neurons in the vestibular nuclei are points of convergence between impulses representing central eye movement programs and impulses bringing feedback information from the periphery. This convergence between the two sorts of information underlies the automatic eye-head coordination which is a feature of the eye motor control system. This system of automatic eye-head coordination, reviewed by Bizzi (16), provides compensation for the magnitude of the head movements that ordinarily accompany saccadic eye movements.

SUMMARY AND CONCLUSIONS

The experiments that have been reviewed deal with central mechanisms controlling volitional and reflex movements in subhuman primates and in man. These experiments provide information both as to the way in which volitional and reflex factors interact in control of movement and as to mechanisms involved in plasticity of motor behavior. As such studies continue, we can expect to discover the major functional significance of motor control structures that have thus far been so difficult to understand. Thus we may be able to understand the role of motor structures such as the cerebellum and the basal ganglia and to discover how their outputs interact in control of motor behavior.

REFERENCES

1. Kemp, J. M., and Powell, T. P. S. (1971): The connexions of the striatum and globus pallidus: Synthesis and speculation. *Phil. Trans. R. Soc. Lond.* [*Biol.*], 262:441–457.
2. Evarts, E. V. (1966): Pyramidal tract activity associated with a conditioned hand movement in the monkey. *J. Neurophysiol.*, 29:1011–1027.
3. Thach, W. T., Jr. (1970): The behavior of Purkinje and cerebellar nuclear cells during two types of voluntary arm movement in the monkey. In: *The Cerebellum in Health and Disease*, edited by W. S. Fields and W. D. Willis, Jr., pp. 217–230. Warren H. Green, St. Louis.
4. Evarts, E. V. (1971): Activity of thalamic and cortical neurons in relation to learned movement in the monkey. *Int. J. Neurol.*, 8:321–326.
5. DeLong, M. R. (1974): Motor functions of the basal ganglia: Single unit activity during movement. In: *The Neurosciences*, edited by F. O. Schmitt and F. G. Worden, pp. 319–325. MIT Press, Cambridge.
6. Jasper, H. H. (1966): Recording from microelectrodes in stereotactic surgery for Parkinson's disease. *J. Neurosurg. Suppl.*, Part II, 24:219–221.
7. Hongell, A., Wallin, G., and Hagbarth, K. E. (1973): Unit activity connected with movement initiation and arousal situations recorded from the ventrolateral nucleus of the human thalamus. *Acta Neurol. Scand.*, 49:681–698.
8. Strick, P. L. (1974): Activity of neurons in the ventrolateral nucleus of the thalamus in relation to learned movement in the monkey. In: *Abstracts, Fourth Annual Meeting of the Society for Neurosciences*, p. 442.
9. Hammond, P. H. (1956): The influence of prior instruction to the subject on an apparently involuntary neuro-muscular response. *J. Physiol.* (Lond.), 132:17P–18P.
10. Marsden, C. D., Merton, P. A., and Morton, H. B. (1972): Servo action in human voluntary movement. *Nature* (Lond.), 238:140–143.
11. Robinson, D. A. (1968): Eye movement control in primates. *Science*, 161:1219–1224.
12. Bizzi, E. (1970): Single unit activity in the frontal eye fields of unanesthetized monkeys during eye and head movement. *Exp. Brain Res.*, 10:151–158.
13. Robinson, D. A. (1974): The effect of cerebellectomy on the cat's vestibulo-ocular integrator. *Brain Res.*, 71:195–208.
14. Miles, F. A. (1974): Single unit firing patterns in the vestibular nuclei related to voluntary eye movements and passive body rotation in conscious monkeys. *Brain Res.*, 71:215–224.
15. Miles, F. A., and Fuller, J. H. (1974): Adaptive plasticity in the vestibulo-ocular responses of the rhesus monkey. *Brain Res.*, 80:512–516.
16. Bizzi, E. (1974): The coordination of eye-head movements. *Sci. Am.*, 231:100–106.
17. Evarts, E. V. (1973): Brain mechanisms in movement. *Sci. Am.*, 229:96–103.
18. Evarts, E. V., and Tanji, J. (1974): Gating of motor cortex reflexes by prior instruction. *Brain Res.*, 71:479–494.

The Nervous System, Donald B. Tower, Editor-in-Chief. *Vol. 1: The Basic Neurosciences*. Raven Press, New York, 1975.

The Cerebellar Cortex

Rodolfo Llinás

The study of the function of neuronal circuits in the cerebellar cortex, together with the recent knowledge concerning the retina (see Dowling, *This Volume*) and the olfactory bulb (see Shepherd, *This Volume*), has begun a new trend in our attempts at understanding brain function. This trend emphasizes the importance of nerve cell form and connectivity in specifying the functional properties of central nerve nets. Specifically, the efforts provide solid examples that the functional properties of the brain are imbedded in the very structure of the system, from the molecular to the multineuronal level. Furthermore, the results of these studies suggest that the following general tenets are probably correct.

1. In general, the morphological classifiability of neurons with respect to their form, spatial localization, and synaptic connectivity may represent an underlying functional equivalence. This finding allows the formulation of such powerful generalizations as: All Golgi cells in the cerebellar cortex (morphological classification) are inhibitory (functional characterization). Moreover, this type of generalization appears to be holding at ultrastructural and microchemical levels [e.g., all Purkinje cells use γ-aminobutyric acid (GABA) as their synaptic transmitter], implying a rather fundamental correlation between structure and function.

2. Once the different elements are characterized functionally, the physiological properties of the particular center may be described by the sum total of the activities that cells exercise upon each other (i.e., all phenomenology observed is, in principle, explicable on the basis of known types of interactions between known neurons).

This chapter describes the basic morphology of cerebellar circuitry and its functional properties and will suggest ways in which such knowledge may serve as the basis for a more holistic understanding of the function of this center.

THE BASIC CEREBELLAR CIRCUIT AND ITS FUNCTIONAL ORGANIZATION

Our knowledge of cerebellar neurobiology covers not only its evolution and embryogenesis, but also the anatomical connectivity and functional interactivity of all the major types of neurons, from the simplest to the highest vertebrates (1–3). The general concepts regarding its morphology were described to a great extent by Ramón y Cajal (4).

Basically the cerebellar cortex is organized in a rather stereotyped manner (see Fig. 1). It has a single type of output system (the axons of Purkinje cells), two main types of input (the mossy- and climbing-fiber systems), and a set of indigenous neurons (the stellate, basket, Golgi, and granule cells). A third afferent system has recently been discovered (5). This noradrenergic system probably has an important bearing in cerebellar activities during wakefulness and sleep rhythms. At this juncture it is not clear, however, as to how it is related to other functions of the cerebellar circuits.

The Cerebellar Cortex Output System — The Purkinje Cell

The Purkinje cell constitutes the central neuronal element of the cerebellar cortex. These cells are arranged as a continuous sheath, one cell in depth throughout the cortex, thus forming a continuous stratum — the Purkinje cell layer — which serves to demarcate the limits of the molecular layer (the superficial layer) from the deeper stratus or granule cell layer (Fig. 1).

Purkinje cells are among the most complex vertebrate neurons as far as their extent and number of synapses are concerned. Morphologically, one of its remarkable characteristics is the isoplanarity of its dendritic tree, which has been known since the early studies of Henle. The Purkinje cell axons run inward into the white

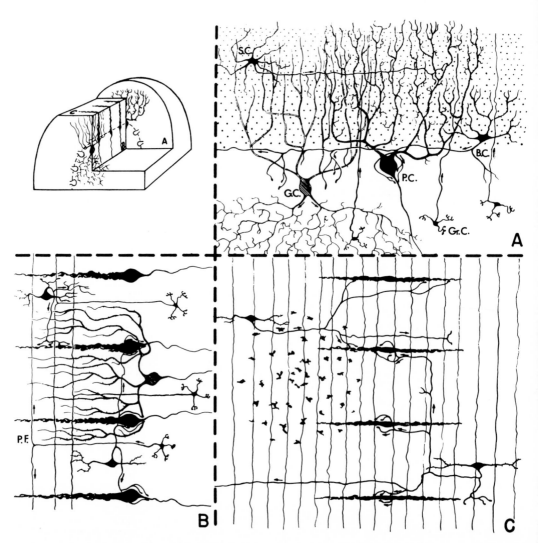

FIG. 1. Detail of the geometrical organization of the neuronal elements of the cerebellar cortex. The drawing demonstrates different sections through a cerebellar folium. **A:** Transverse plane; **B:** saggital plane; **C:** tangential plane. The cellular elements are displayed in drawings **A, B,** and **C,** as though the cerebellar cortex were to be transparent. The orthogonal organization of the parallel fibers, with respect to the isoplanar characteristics of the dendrites of Purkinje cells and basket and stellate cells, are self-explanatory. Note that the axons of the basket and stellate cells run at right angles with respect to parallel fibers and the dendritic tree of Golgi cells is close to cylindrical rather than isoplanar. BC, basket cell; GC, Golgi cell; GrC, granule cell; PC, Purkinje cell; PF, parallel fiber; SC, stellate cell. (From Llinás, ref. 21.)

matter of the cerebellar mass and contact the centrally located cerebellar nuclei.

Integrative Properties of Purkinje Cells

Although the particular morphology that characterizes Purkinje cells has been known since the turn of the century, only recently has information become available regarding the func-

tional properties of the complex spatial organization of this neuron. Among the outstanding features of this cell is its widely branching dendritic tree, which may arise from one or two or, in particular cases, several somatic stems. In reptilia and amphibia, for instance, the dendritic tree arises from a single-stem dendrite that bifurcates repeatedly along its path to the cerebellar surface (6,7), generating the characteristic

Purkinje cell arbor. This particular morphology suggests a specific functional role in neuronal integration. Probably the most strictly organized Purkinje cells, from a structural point of view, are those found in the cerebella of certain teleosts, such as the mormyrid, in which the dendrites of the Purkinje cells are known to stem from basal dendrites situated near the level of the Purkinje cell somas (8). The branches of these main dendrites ascend in an almost perfectly perpendicular course with astonishing regularity and suggest once again a specific functional role for this specialized dendritic organization.

For the most part, past physiological investigations on Purkinje cells did not place much emphasis on the functional properties of the dendritic tree. Most investigations assumed that the dendritic arbor of the Purkinje cell served, as in the case of a motoneuron, as a simple integrating device that transmits synaptic depolarization electrotonically to the cell soma. More recently, however, studies on the alligator cerebellum (9,10) have indicated that the dendritic tree of the Purkinje cell is not simply an apparatus for electrotonic summation of excitatory and inhibitory potentials. Rather it appears as a site of complex integratory mechanisms involving the generation of dendritic local responses and action potentials capable of propagating toward the soma. This new set of data emphasizes the need for reevaluation of the functional properties of dendrites in other neurons.

Dendritic Spike Properties in Purkinje Cells

As opposed to other neurons, the antidromic invasion of the Purkinje cell seems to be blocked at the level of the main dendrites as demonstrated by extracellular field potential analysis and by intradendritic recordings (9,10). On the other hand, orthodromic activation of these cells will generate field potentials indicating large sinks at the superficial level, in contrast to the positivities recorded at the same site during antidromic invasion. These results, together with those from intradendritic recordings, strongly imply that these cells are capable of generating dendritic spikes and that such spikes may be preferentially conducted in a somatopetal direction (Fig. 2). Somatofugal spikes do not actively invade the peripheral half of the

dendritic tree because of the heavy load imposed by the tree on the antidromic action current and by impedance mismatch (9–11). In this manner, a type of "dynamic polarization" is achieved, owing to the electrical properties of the neuron in question. The conduction of dendritic spikes toward the soma is envisaged as occurring in a pseudosaltatory fashion (9). Following synaptic activation of the peripheral dendritic branchlets, a local response is generated in the peripheral smooth dendritic branches, probably at strategically located hot spots. From these sites the spike is conducted passively to the next hot spot until the lower dendritic tree is reached at which moment the initial segment, the axon, and the soma fire in short sequence.

Dendritic Inhibition

Classically it has been assumed that inhibition, in order to be effective, must be located at the soma of the nerve cell in the vicinity of the axon hillock. This location has been assumed to be the most effective in blocking the firing of a neuron since it is known that action potentials are initiated, for the most part, at the axon hillock. In recent years, however, many lines of research strongly suggest that inhibition may be localized at the dendritic level as well and that in some cases such inhibition is the only form present in given neurons. Although such dendritic inhibition would not participate greatly in the blockage of action potentials produced by somatic inputs, it does have two other important regulatory functions. First, it serves as a tonic inhibitory system, and, second, it has a special role in those cells capable of generating dendritic spikes.

An advantage of dendritic inhibition in neurons that generate dendritic spikes is that of "functional amputation" of certain dendritic segments (9,11). Their importance is especially clear when coupled with the view that dendrites can generate action potentials independently from the activity of other dendrites or the soma. Morphological studies of cerebellum (3,12) favor the view of dendritic location of inhibitory synapses in remote dendrites. In the case of Purkinje cells, this distinction is rather significant, especially since the most common excitatory input, the parallel fibers, does not establish synaptic contacts directly with the smooth den-

A

B

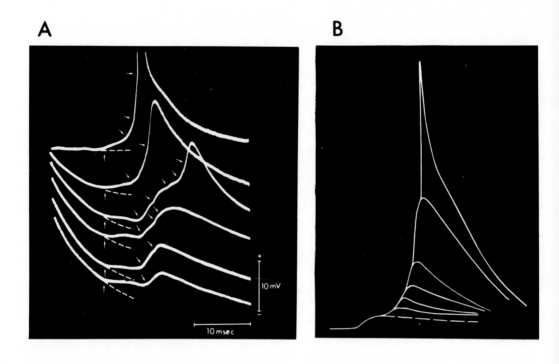

C

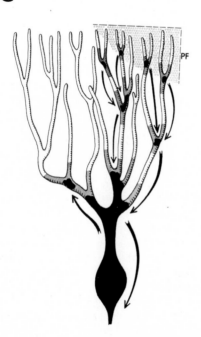

FIG. 2. Intradendritic recording from a Purkinje cell in Caiman sclerops. **A:** Action potentials recorded in a dendrite 200 μm from the surface. Successive hyperpolarizing current injected through the recording electrode revealed that the large dendritic spike shown on the first trace is actually produced by the addition of all-or-none components (*arrows*). This dendritic spike was generated by a dendritic EPSP produced by parallel fiber stimulation (*upward arrow*). As the hyperpolarization is increased, the different all-or-none depolarizing potentials are blocked in a sequential manner. **B:** Reconstruction of the intradendritic action potential showing the six all-or-none components shown in A. **C:** Diagram of mechanism of dendritic spike generation. Each all-or-none component is taken to be generated by a different hot spot (*dark area*) at or near dendritic bifurcation. The action potential is produced by the summation of all-or-none local responses, which finally reach the soma and generate a full outgoing action potential. (Modified from Llinás and Nicholson, ref. 9.)

dritic tree but rather with specialized thorns in the spiny branchlets, which are always peripheral to the smooth dendrites. This form of spiny synapse may be visualized as serving a "current-limiting resistor" function (12), which allows a more linear summation of synaptic potentials at the expense of a reduced efficacy for any particular synapse. The main difference between excitatory and inhibitory terminals in the Purkinje cell is thus their location and the actual form of the synaptic junction. Direct synaptic contact of inhibitory boutons ensures a significant current shunt for all dendritic inputs peripheral to that particular dendritic branch without necessarily affecting integration in other dendrites (12).

CEREBELLAR CORTEX INPUT SYSTEMS: THE MOSSY AND CLIMBING FIBERS

The two main afferent systems, the mossy fibers (MF) and climbing fibers (CF), seem to be present in all cerebella throughout the vertebrate scale and are distributed in all forms over the entire extent of the cerebellar cortex in a precise topological fashion. As will be seen below, however, these two inputs are extremely different from each other. The difference relates to their distribution, ontogenetic development, and connectivity.

THE CF-PURKINJE CELL SYSTEM

The anatomical relationship between these two neural elements is rather unique. Developmentally, the first contacts between the CF and its Purkinje cell occur early in ontogenesis. During development the CF surrounds the body of the Purkinje cell and forms a nest-like structure recognized by Ramón y Cajal (4) and called by him "capuchon." As the molecular layer develops, Purkinje cell dendrites grow outward to this layer, apparently carrying the CF with them (13). For many years it was thought that connectivity of the CF with Purkinje cells was restricted to the smooth parts of the dendritic tree and Purkinje cell. It is now agreed that the CF does contact only the smooth branches but does so through sets of small spines, which are generally organized in groups of four or five processes. The number of such synapses varies with species (300 in the frog and approximately

170 in the alligator). Such calculations are not as yet available in higher vertebrates, but it is reasonable to expect that they would be comparable. The CF system arises for the most part from the inferior olive (IO) (14) although some reports have suggested that they may have other sites of origin. However, it is now agreed that the IO is the main site of origin for CFs as emphasized by studies such as those using the drug harmaline (15,16). The olivo-cerebellar system, which generates the CFs, also contacts other cells in the cortex and in the deep nuclei. Collaterals to Golgi and basket cells have been described, as well as possible collaterals to granule cells (3). At the nuclear level, the olivo-cerebellar system seems to project to all cerebellar nuclei as well as to Deiters' nucleus directly.

Function of the CF-Purkinje Cell Junction

The functional properties of this system have been known for some time (17). The CF exercises a strong excitatory action on Purkinje cells, which appears to be present in all cerebella along the phylogenetic scale (12). The synapse has been determined to be a chemically transmitting junction, having an extremely large quantal content. Since the CF and Purkinje cell have a one-to-one relation, the CF response of the Purkinje cell is an all-or-nothing event, consisting of a stereotyped burst of action potentials (Fig. 3).

Functional Properties of the Olivo-Cerebellar System

Intracellular studies of electrical properties of the IO indicate that the neurons in this system are electrotonically coupled (18). As in previous examples, the demonstration of coupling in these cells is done by indirect electrophysiological means, and the presence of short-latency depolarization (SLD) is observed following antidromic invasion of neighboring neurons. The IO coupling is rather commonly encountered and shows a finely graded SLD. This SLD is often capable of activating the IO cells and tends to synchronize their firing. Among the more interesting possibilities arising from this example of electrical synapse is that of "variable electrotonic coupling." This possibility has been demonstrated in *Navanax* (19) where it is suggested

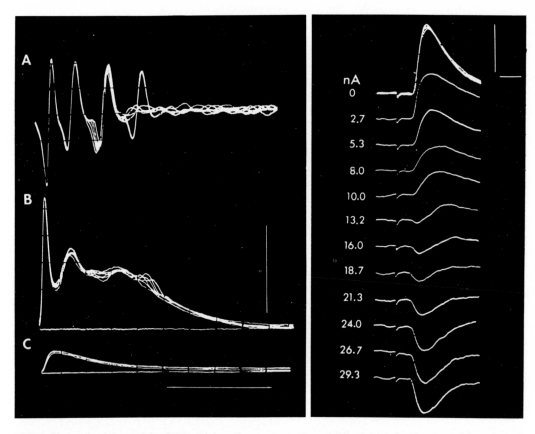

FIG. 3. Electrophysiology of the CF-Purkinje cell synapse. **A:** Extracellular burst of action potentials generated by a Purkinje cell upon stimulation of the CF. Five bursts are superimposed to demonstrate the repeatability of the firing from one activation to the next. **B:** Intracellular recording from the same Purkinje cell. Six spikes are superimposed. The initial action potential is followed by a prolonged and complex late potential, which corresponds in time to the action potentials seen extracellularly. The response is all-or-nothing. The potential in **B** is generated by an all-or-nothing depolarization, a synaptic potential, shown in **C** after the cell has ceased to fire, due to damage. Voltage calibration: 5 mV in **A** and 50 mV in **B** and **C**. Time calibration: 10 msec. **D:** Chemical nature of the CF synapse. The synaptic potential generated by the CF activation (*upper record*) may be reduced and finally reversed in polarity by the artificial modification of the cell's membrane potential. This is achieved by the injection of small d.c. currents (shown in nanoamperes to the left of each record) through the recording microelectrode. Calibration: voltage 10 mV, time 1 msec. (Llinás and Nicholson, *unpublished observations.*)

that shunting may be the basis for dynamic "uncoupling." In the IO, coupling appears to be restricted to the rather specialized inferior olive glomerulus (20). The morphological findings suggest the possibility of a variable coupling since ultrastructurally the gap junctions are located at the center of a glomerulus formed by short dendrites and the glomerulus is surrounded by chemical synaptic terminals (20).

This strategic arrangement of synapses in the glomerulus implies shunting of the charge transference between cells by postsynaptic conductance increase due to chemical synaptic action.

Thus the functional significance of this variable electrotonic coupling would be that of increasing the number of possible electrotonic interaction states between cells in the IO (21) (Fig. 4).

THE MF-GRANULE CELL-PURKINJE CELL SYSTEM

In contrast to the one-to-one monosynaptic input to Purkinje cells, the MF afferent system can be considered among the richest in the brain in regard to the number of synaptic contacts it generates. As opposed to the CF system,

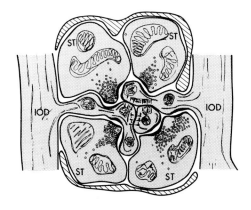

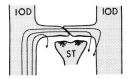

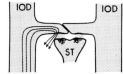

ELECTROTONIC COUPLING   **ELECTROTONIC UNCOUPLING**

FIG. 4. Diagram of the IO glomerulus. (**Upper**) General organization of the IO glomerulus. In the central core, dendritic branches are seen coupled by means of gap junctions (*arrowheads*). The central core is surrounded by synaptic terminals (ST), which establish contact with the core elements. (**Lower, left**) The path of coupling current between two IO neurons. (**Lower, right**) Hypothetical function for the synaptic junction at the glomerulus. When the synapses are activated, the conductance change produced by the synaptic transmitter action on the postsynaptic membrane produces a shunt at the glomerular level which reduces the coupling co-efficient between the cells, since the current tends to be lost across the shunt. (Modified from Llinás, ref. 21.)

the MFs do not terminate directly on Purkinje cells but rather on small neurons, the granule cells, which lie immediately beneath the Purkinje cell layer (4). These granule cells serve as intermediaries between MFs and dendrites of Purkinje cells. The number of granule cells in the cerebellar cortex of man (10^{11}) may be 10 times greater than the number of cells previously estimated for the totality of the brain (22).

The axons of these granule cells are generally unmyelinated and have a T-like distribution in space. The ascending portion of the T brings the axon of the granule cell into the molecular layer where the dendrites of the Purkinje cell are dis-

tributed. The horizontal part of the T forms the so-called parallel fibers that occupy all levels within the molecular layer. One of the most remarkable characteristics of these axons is that they are parallel to each other in all planes (see Fig. 1).

After its bifurcation, the parallel fiber runs between the Purkinje cell dendrites and contacts these cells on spines that emerge in great numbers from the terminal portion of the highly ramified Purkinje cell dendrite, the so-called spiny branchlets (1,23). The junction itself is formed between the head of a spine and a globular expansion of the parallel fiber, which is filled with synaptic vesicles. The actual contact may resemble a ball and joint arrangement, where the spine penetrates the expanded portion of the parallel fiber. For the most part, a parallel fiber contacts Purkinje cells only once or, rarely, twice, and yet most of the input to the Purkinje cells is through the parallel fiber system.

Electrophysiological studies of this afferent system demonstrate the MF-to-granule cell synapse to be excitatory, as is also the parallel fiber-to-Purkinje cell synapse (24).

Functional Properties of the MF Afferents

The MF afferents are organized in a functionally flexible manner where, rather than the stereotyped connectivity found in the one-to-one CF-Purkinje cell synapse, a given fiber relays information to many thousands of glomeruli and, through them, to large numbers of parallel fibers (Fig. 1). The isoplanar character of the Purkinje cell ensures that the cell should see as many parallel fibers as possible within the spread of its dendritic tree (maximum convergence). Each particular parallel fiber establishes one or possibly two synaptic contacts with each Purkinje cell and so these cells receive information from as many parallel fibers as possible (maximum divergence). This maximum convergence with maximum divergence is probably the most characteristic pattern of the parallel fiber Purkinje cell organization and is apparently typical of the Purkinje cell (23). There is, therefore, a totally different arrangement of this input as compared to the CF system. As in the case of the CF system, there are many hypotheses regarding the ultimate functional significance of the MF input (25).

MF afferents have been studied using a variety of physiological stimuli. The results from these experiments suggest that this input is capable of producing a continuously graded activation of the Purkinje cell. This has been shown for vestibular and auditory stimulation, skin proprioception, and during movement generation (26). In any event, it appears clear that the MF input relays sensory information to the cerebellum as well as information regarding the internal functional state of the nervous system in general. This information reaches the cerebellar cortex through all three peduncles and arrives, for the most part, from the spinal cord by way of spinocerebellar systems, from the cortex by way of the pontine system, and from the brainstem through reticulospinal systems, to name only a few. The MF system is thus a far more elaborate and larger system than the CF input. From an evolutionary point of view, it is, in fact, the MF system that has undergone the largest modification. This is apparent when the complexities of the cerebellar circuits are compared at different stages in phylogeny (12). Thus the granule cell layer increases steadily through evolution as do the numbers of dendritic branchlets of the Purkinje cell. Equally important, the inhibitory interneurons of both molecular and granular layers show a marked increase in number and complexity as the cerebellum evolves. Since the interneurons of the cortex are mainly related to the MF-granule cell circuit, they will be described as part of this system.

The Interneurons of the Cerebellar Cortex

Two general categories of short axon neurons are found in the cerebellar cortex: one indigenous to the molecular layer and the other to the granular layer. These two sets of interneurons are, for the molecular layer, the basket and stellate cells and, for the granular layer, the Golgi cells. The basket and stellate cells receive their input from the parallel fibers and their axons contact Purkinje cells. The basket neuron establishes synaptic junctions in the lower dendrites and the soma of this cell (1,3,4,12,23), whereas the stellate cells are more or less confined to the dendrites. The spatial distribution of the axons of both types of interneuron is such that they run at right angles to the direction of the parallel fiber, forming a criss-cross arrangement with them. Functionally these two types of interneurons are inhibitory.

The Golgi cell resides in the granular layer and receives information from the parallel fibers as well as directly through the MFs and CFs (1,3,12,23). The axons of these cells exercise a feedback type of inhibition onto the granule cells and form, together with the MF terminal and the dendrites of the granule cell, a specialized synaptic linkage known as the cerebellar glomerulus. This glomerulus is constituted by a central MF expansion surrounded by dendrites of granule cells, which are in turn surrounded by the inhibitory terminals of the Golgi cells. This glomerulus represents the basic functional unit of the granular layer (3,4,12,23,24).

The actual physiological role of these inhibitory neurons was first assumed to be that of feedforward lateral inhibition for the stellate and basket cells and of a simple feedback inhibition for the Golgi cells (24). Given, however, that Purkinje cells fire repetitively following physiological stimulation (see above), these interneurons are considered today more as modulators of Purkinje cell activity, either directly or indirectly, through granule cell inhibition. The molecular layer interneurons serve more to set the level of excitability and thus to regulate or linearize the dynamic range of the cerebellar cortex rather than to obliterate the activity of particular Purkinje cell groups. The Golgi cells have a central role in the organization of cerebellar function. They probably channel the information reaching the molecular layer and are sensitive to the patterns of MF input.

GENERAL COMMENTS ON THE PHYSIOLOGICAL PROPERTIES OF THE CEREBELLAR CORTEX

Clearly one of the central points in understanding the function of the cerebellar cortex is that of the difference between MF and CF afferents. Several hypotheses have been generated in relation to this point. Basically it has been assumed that MFs and CFs form part of an interactive system, which comes together at the Purkinje cell level (1). Others believe that the two systems represent totally separate channels to the cerebellar cortex. Thus the concept of "time-sharing" (TS) was suggested as applying in this cortex (21). In simple terms the TS hypothesis suggests that the MF system activates, in a graded manner, a large number of Purkinje cells organized spatially along the parallel fiber bundles stimulated. On the other hand, the CF afferent system—not bound by such connectivity—can activate in an all-or-nothing manner particular Purkinje cells with high priority owing to the synaptic potency of this input. This allows the activation of selected individual groups of Purkinje cells, their actual spatial distribution reflecting the patterns of IO activity rather than those of intracerebellar connectivity, as is the case with the MF input.

By time-sharing it is meant, therefore, that a given Purkinje cell may at a certain moment be part of either an MF- or a CF-generated pattern. In addition to the spatial distribution of these two forms of afferent activation, the timing property is rather different. In experiments where IO cells fire synchronously, such as after the administration of harmaline, the IO evokes a fixed pattern of motor responses by activation of the vestibulospinal and reticulospinal systems (15,16). The IO must be considered, therefore, as a motor triggering center. Since groups of cells in the IO distribute their cortical afferents in long sagittal zones (27), the IO clusters may be regarded as organized for particular motor sequences involving the activation of different muscular territories throughout the body.

On the other hand, one may envisage the MF afferents as utilizing the cerebellar cortex as a two-dimensional continuous representation of the functional states and positions of the somatic musculature, joints, and limbs at any given instant, as well as the internal functional state. Thus, when new motor instructions are blended (probably through complex topological functions) with this "state of readiness" in the cerebellar cortex, the ensuing motor command would be modified to be in context with the total motor stance of the animal. From this point of view, therefore, the information received from the periphery via the MF system, rather than being a true feedback, may serve more to reset the state of readiness of the cerebellar cortex into a continuously upgraded mirror of the motor functional state.

ACKNOWLEDGMENTS

This research is supported by U.S. Public Health Grant NS-09916 from the National Institute of Neurological Diseases and Stroke.

REFERENCES

1. Eccles, J. C., Ito, M., and Szentagothai, J. (1967): *The Cerebellum as a Neuronal Machine.* Springer-Verlag, Heidelberg.
2. Llinás, R., editor (1969): *Neurobiology of Cerebellar Evolution and Development.* American Medical Association, Chicago.
3. Palay, S. L., and Chan-Palay, V. (1974): *Cerebellar Cortex: Cytology and Organization.* Springer-Verlag, Heidelberg.
4. Ramón y Cajal, S. (1911): *Histologie du Système Nerveux de l'Homme et des Vertébrés.* Maloine, Paris.
5. Bloom, F. E., Hoffer, B. J., and Siggins, G. R. (1971): Studies on norepinephrine-containing afferents to Purkinje cells of rat cerebellum. I. Localization of the fibers and their synapses. *Brain Res.,* 25:501–521.
6. Hillman, D. E. (1969): Neuronal organization of the cerebellar cortex in amphibia and reptilia. In: *Neurobiology of Cerebellar Evolution and Development,* edited by R. Llinás, pp. 279–325. American Medical Association, Chicago.
7. Sotelo, C. (1969): Ultrastructural aspects of the cerebellar cortex of the frog. In: *Neurobiology of Cerebellar Evolution and Development,* edited by R. Llinás, pp. 327–371. American Medical Association, Chicago.
8. Nieuwenhuys, R., and Nicholson, C. (1969): Aspects of the histology of the cerebellum of mormyrid fishes. In: *Neurobiology of Cerebellar Evolution and Development,* edited by R. Llinás, pp. 135–169. American Medical Association, Chicago.
9. Llinás, R., and Nicholson, C. (1971): Electrophysiological properties of dendrites and somata in alligator Purkinje cells. *J. Neurophysiol.,* 34:532–551.
10. Nicholson, C., and Llinás, R. (1971): Field potentials in the alligator cerebellum and theory of their relationship to Purkinje cell dendritic spikes. *J. Neurophysiol.,* 34:509–531.
11. Llinás, R., and Nicholson, C. (1969): Electrophysiological analysis of alligator cerebellum: A study on dendritic spikes. In: *Neurobiology of Cerebellar Evolution and Development,* edited by R. Llinás, pp. 431–465. American Medical Association, Chicago.
12. Llinás, R., and Hillman, D. E. (1969): Physiological and morphological organization of the cerebellar circuits of various vertebrates. In: *Neurobiology of Cerebellar Evolution and De-*

velopment, edited by R. Llinás, pp. 43–73. American Medical Association, Chicago.

13. Larramendi, L. M. H., and Victor, T. (1967): Synapses on the Purkinje cell spines in the mouse: An electron microscopical study. *Brain Res.,* 5:15–30.

14. Szentágothai, J., and Rajkovits, K. (1959): Ueber den Ursprung der Kletterfasern des Kleinhirns. *Z. Anat. Entwicklungsgesch,* 121:130–141.

15. Montigny, C. de, and Lamarre, Y. (1973): Rhythmic activity induced by harmaline in the olivo-cerebello-bulbar system of the cat. *Brain Res.,* 53:81–95.

16. Llinás, R., and Volkind, R. A. (1973): The olivo-cerebellar system: Functional properties as revealed by harmaline-induced tremor. *Exp. Brain Res.,* 18:69–87.

17. Eccles, J. C., Llinás, R., and Sasaki, K. (1966): The excitatory synaptic action of climbing fibres on the Purkinje cells of the cerebellum. *J. Physiol. (Lond.),* 182:268–296.

18. Llinás, R., Baker, R., and Sotelo, C. (1974): Electrotonic coupling between neurons in the cat inferior olive. *J. Neurophysiol.,* 37:560–571.

19. Spira, M. E., and Bennett, M. V. L. (1972): Synaptic control of electrotonic coupling between neurons. *Brain Res.,* 37:294–300.

20. Sotelo, C., Llinás, R., and Baker, R. (1974): Structural study of the inferior olivary nucleus of the cat. Morphological correlates of electrotonic coupling. *J. Neurophysiol.,* 37:541–559.

21. Llinás, R. (1974): Eighteenth Bowditch Lecture: Motor aspects of cerebellar control. *Physiologist,* 17:19–46.

22. Braitenberg, V., and Atwood, R. P. (1958): Morphological observations on the cerebellar cortex. *J. Comp. Neurol.,* 109:1–34.

23. Fox, C. A., Hillman, D. E., Siegesmund, K. A., and Dutta, C. R. (1967): The primate cerebellar cortex: A Golgi and electron microscopical study. *Prog. Brain Res.,* 25:174–225.

24. Eccles, J. C., Llinás, R., and Sasaki, K. (1966): The mossy fibre-granule cell relay of the cerebellum and its inhibitory control by Golgi cells. *Exp. Brain Res.,* 1:82–101.

25. Llinás, R. (1970): Neuronal operations in cerebellar transactions. In: *The Neurosciences: Second Study Program,* edited by F. O. Schmitt, pp. 409–426. Rockefeller University Press, New York.

26. Evarts, E. V., and Thach, W. T. (1969): Motor mechanisms of CNS: Cerebrocerebellar interrelations. *Ann. Rev. Physiol.,* 31:451–498.

27. Oscarsson, O. (1973): Functional organization of spinocerebellar paths. In: *Handbook of Sensory Physiology, Vol. II (Somatosensory System),* edited by A. Iggo, pp. 339–380. Springer-Verlag, Heidelberg.

The Nervous System, Donald B. Tower, Editor-in-Chief. *Vol. 1: The Basic Neurosciences*. Raven Press, New York, 1975.

Learning Control Mechanisms by the Cerebellum Investigated in the Flocculo-Vestibulo-Ocular System

Masao Ito

Investigations in the past two decades have provided analytical data on the structure and function of the central nervous system (CNS). Elementary neuronal processes have been revealed, and nerve net structures have been determined in many parts of the CNS. Yet, there is still a great deal of uncertainty with regard to extrapolating higher nervous system functions (such as perception, control of complex motions, learning, intellectual faculties, symbolic thought in speech and language) from the presently available data at cellular levels. Important information, probably a great deal, is still missing.

Recent successes in the analyses of structure and function of the cerebellum have provided a constructive approach to studying higher nervous system functions. Through studies of classic physiology and pathology, the cerebellum has been shown (3) to be equipped with a learning capability and to contribute to motor control by providing measures of the body in time and space. The intensive studies on the cerebellum to account for these functions on the basis of our knowledge at cellular levels may be broadly classified into three categories. First, synaptic actions and neuronal connections have been determined in the cerebellar cortex (4). One may speculate on the basis of the neuronal diagram of the cerebellar cortical sheet what kind of information processing occurs there (18). Second, impulse discharges have been recorded from cerebellar Purkinje cells and nuclear cells, while an alert animal is moving (25). One may infer from the recorded activity what sort of information processing actually occurs there. Third, interconnections between parts of the cerebellum and the related subcerebellar centers have been dissected (4,8). One may infer what role is played by the

cerebellum in actual motor control. Each of these three lines of approach has yielded a certain success, yet essential parts of cerebellar mechanisms do not seem to have been uncovered.

Difficulties arise from the following factors. First, electrophysiological analyses of the neuronal circuitry have been performed primarily by electrical stimulation in anesthetized animals. Those components susceptible to anesthesia might be missed, and spatial information contained among parallel elements might be obscured. The recent trend is thus to replace the electric by natural stimuli adequate to the receptors involved and to choose anesthetic drugs that cause minimal impairment or to use no anesthesia at all. Second, the cerebellum is, in general, located remote from both input receptors and output effectors of the animal's body. Further, in classic behavioral and neurological studies, specific functions of cerebellar areas have been defined only vaguely. Therefore, the task of extracting functional meanings from the dissected connections and recorded impulse activities has been very arduous. It would be of great importance to establish a system in which the meanings of its input-output signals and of its overall performance can be defined explicitly.

Recent studies of the cerebellar flocculus have attempted to systematically minimize these difficulties. The flocculus is closely connected with one of the well-established elementary reflexes, i.e., the vestibulo-ocular reflex. The relatively simple construction of this reflex system allows detailed analyses of the neuronal connectivities involved. Specific function of the flocculus can be defined unequivocally in relation with the performance of the vestibulo-ocular reflex which produces compensatory eye movements during head rotation so as to stabilize retinal images of the visual surround. The flocculus occupies a small area of the cerebellar cortex (of the order of 10 mm^2 in rabbits) and so contains a relatively small number of Purkinje cells (ca. 5,000). This facilitates survey of the neuronal events in the flocculus which may readily be correlated with the behavioral execution by the flocculus.

BASIC NEURONAL CIRCUITRY

Figure 1 illustrates the relationship between the cerebellar flocculus and the vestibulo-ocular reflex arc, determined in mammals by histological and electrophysiological techniques. Impulses from the vestibular organ excite second-order vestibular neurons which, in turn, excite or inhibit oculomotor neurons to produce eye movement. The flocculus receives primary afferent signals from the vestibular organ as a mossy fiber input and, as output, sends Purkinje cell impulses to certain second-order vestibular neurons (8). The synaptic action of flocculus Purkinje cells proved to be inhibitory as in other cerebellar areas (4). Thus the flocculus is incorporated in the vestibulo-ocular reflex arc as a sidepath parallel with the primary vestibular projection to second-order vestibular neurons. It is obvious that the flocculus is in a position to influence directly the vestibulo-ocular reflex. Figure 1 also illustrates two visual pathways to the flocculus: one courses through the accessory optic tract and the central tegmental tract, to eventually reach the flocculus via the climbing fibers (15); the other pathway supplies mossy fiber terminals to the rostrodorsal region of the flocculus (Maekawa and Takeda, *personal communication*).

In Fig. 1, vestibular signals arising from five end-organs (three semicircular canals and two otolith organs) are shown together, for convenience. Recent efforts have been devoted to test the validity of Fig. 1 in each component pathway of the vestibulo-ocular reflex arc arising from one end-organ and reaching an eye muscle. With the technique of selectively stimulating individual canals, 12 principal pathways for the rabbit vestibulo-ocular reflexes were identified in terms of the receptor canal, reflex action, relay nucleus and target muscle (9). A specific pattern of the inhibitory

action of flocculus Purkinje cells has thus been revealed; the inhibition is exerted on six of these 12 pathways. Climbing fiber impulses evoked by stimulation of the optic tract caused Purkinje cell inhibition only in two of the six pathways. Both of these pathways originate at the horizontal canal: one excites the medial rectus and the other inhibits the lateral rectus motoneurons for the ipsilateral eye. Hence, Fig. 1 best applies to the reflex arc from the horizontal canal to the ipsilateral eye.

AS A CONTROL SYSTEM

The neuronal diagram similarly obtained for the vestibulospinal reflex arc differs markedly from that shown in Fig. 1 in that the second-order neurons of this reflex arc are not inhibited by those cerebellar areas that receive primary vestibular fibers as a mossy fiber input. This peculiar difference in the neuronal construction between the two vestibular reflex arcs has been correlated to their difference as control systems (8). The vestibulospinal reflex serving to hold the head position constant is a typical feedback control; the "final output" — the head position — readily influences the vestibular organ, i.e., the input of the reflex arc. By contrast, the final output of the vestibulo-ocular reflex is the constancy of retinal images which can be monitored by vision. However, there is no straightforward connection of feedback to return visual signals to the vestibular organ. Hence, superficially the vestibulo-ocular reflex is essentially an open loop control.

It has been hypothesized that the functional role of the flocculus is to assist the open-loop control of the vestibulo-ocular reflex. In engineering systems an open loop control may be simpler in design and easier to operate than a closed loop control because no feedback loop is required. On the other hand, however, the performance of such an open loop system is very susceptible to external disturbances as well as changes in internal parameters. Any misperformance once introduced would remain or become worse unless it is corrected by some device that replaces the feedback. For such a device a computer may be used in engineering systems. The point thus made is that a part of the cerebellar cortex is likewise utilized to assist a reflex system that has the open loop

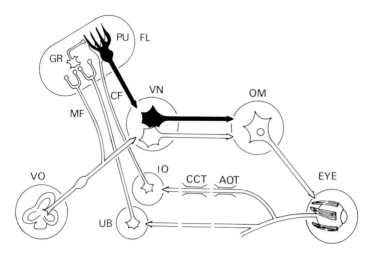

FIG. 1. Basic neuronal circuitry of the flocculo-vestibulo-ocular system. OM, Oculomotor neuron; IO, inferior olive; CTT, central tegmental tract; AOT, accessory optic tract; VO, vestibular organ; FL, flocculus; VN, second-order vestibular neurons; CF, climbing fiber; MF, mossy fiber; GR, granule cell; PU, Purkinje cell. UB, unidentified brainstem nucleus. Inhibitory neurons are filled in black, and excitatory neurons are indicated by hollow structures. Modified from Ito (8).

control performance. This view may be generalized to account for insertion of cerebellar cortical areas into a variety of motor systems. Open loop conditions occur in the following situations. First, the input and output of a system may deal with signals of different modalities, as in the vestibulo-ocular reflex. Second, even if signals are of the same modality, the input and output may be spatially remote from each other, as in the tonic neck reflex. Third, even if there is a feedback pathway, its performance may be incomplete when the control system operates at high speed; the so-called loop time will be the limiting factor. Relevance of the cerebellum to ballistic movements (12) may have such a meaning.

Figure 1 is, of course, an initial skeleton diagram for the flocculo-vestibulo-ocular system that should be elaborated by further investigation. Essential points of the above-stated views, nevertheless, would hold even when such modifications are introduced into the diagram.

OPERATION OF THE VESTIBULO-OCULAR REFLEX

Eye movement induced by head rotation in the absence of visual stimuli represents the net vestibulo-ocular reflex. Manni (17) induced the tonic vestibulo-ocular reflex by tilting the cat's head and found that this reflex became abnormal after floccular lesion. Recently, Carpenter (2) measured the horizontal vestibulo-ocular reflex in decerebrate cats and reported that cooling or removing the cerebellum caused a gain drop and a phase advance at lower frequencies of rotation. Robinson (21), however, maintains on the basis of his experiment on chronic cats that lesion of the flocculus produces a much less significant phase advance, while the gain of the reflex becomes either too low or too high, in comparison with the normal value of unity.

In comparison with cats (21) and human subjects (7), the horizontal vestibulo-ocular reflex of rabbits exhibits a relatively low gain, about 0.5 (1,10). In the very recent investigation by Batini, Ito, Kado, Miyashita, and Yagi (*to be published*), chronic extirpation of the rabbit flocculus resulted in appreciable reduction of this gain, to below 0.2 as measured with 5° (peak-to-peak) head rotation. Yet, frequency characteristics of the reflex were maintained only with a minor change, when tested over the range of frequencies from 0.03 to 0.5 Hz.

The flocculus thus appears to contribute to the net vestibulo-ocular reflex by adjusting the gain and also, to a lesser extent, the phase of the reflex. The adjustment is slight, in the sense that the gross reflex act is executed even without the flocculus. The flocculus functions provide the subtle improvement which maintains the reflex performance within the normal range.

CORRECTION OF THE VESTIBULO-OCULAR REFLEX BY VISION

Flocculus function is further exhibited in the situation where the vestibulo-ocular reflex is affected by vision. Takemori and Cohen (24) demonstrated in monkey that the horizontal vestibulo-ocular reflex provoked by labyrinthectomy, caloric stimulation or administration of alcohol was depressed in light and that this visual effect was removed by extirpation of the cerebellar flocculus. In the experiments on alert rabbits (10), visual stimuli were provided by a movable vertical slit light, placed before the eye under observation (Fig. 3A) which was either held stationary or rotated concentrically with the turntable, with angular amplitude twice as large as that of the turntable. This slit light rotation produces the vision reversal along the horizontal axis which in human subjects (7) and cats (22) was obtained with a Dove prism. The slit light at a fixed position represents the normal situation where the visual environment stays

stationary. As plotted in Fig. 2, the fixed slit light enhanced significantly (by 20 to 110%) the horizontal vestibulo-ocular reflex, while the moving slit light reduced the reflex appreciably (by 20 to 50%). The augmentation and reduction were effected instantaneously with presentation of the slit light and were never exhibited in those rabbits whose flocculus had been chronically destroyed.

The enhancement of the horizontal vestibulo-ocular reflex should have the effect of reducing the slip of the retinal image of the slit light. Likewise, reduction of the horizontal vestibulo-ocular reflex should favor seeing the moving slit light, as the light moves in the direction opposite to the reflex eye movement. Hence, vision modifies the eye movement always in the direction of stabilizing the retinal image during head rotation. The initial postulate that the flocculus refines the open loop control of the vestibulo-ocular reflex by introducing visual feedback is strongly supported.

PROGRESSIVE MODIFICATION OF THE VESTIBULO-OCULAR REFLEX BY VISION

Relevant to the computer action postulated for the flocculus, it may be suggested that when the activity of visual impulses lasts sufficiently

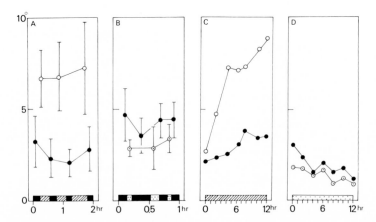

FIG. 2. Horizontal eye rotation in alert rabbits induced by sinusoidal head rotation and its modification during presentation of slit lights in the visual field. **A–D** plot against the time angular amplitudes of the horizontal eye movement measured in four rabbits during continuous head rotation by 10°. Each plotted circle represents the amplitude averaged over 30 to 100 successive rotations. Vertical bars attached to circles in **A** and **B** indicated standard deviation. Visual stimulus conditions at the moments of measuring eye movement are: ●, in darkness; ○, with the fixed light; ⊙, with the moving light. Visual stimulus conditions during continuous rotation are shown on the abscissae: *solid,* without light; *shaded,* with the fixed light; *stippled;* with the moving light. Modified from Ito et al. (10,11).

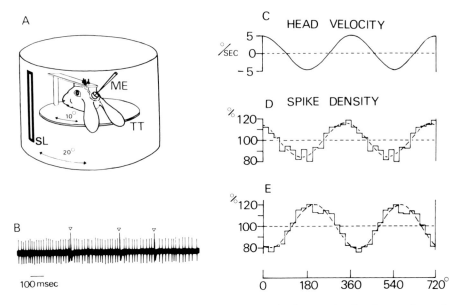

FIG. 3. Recording from Purkinje cells of alert rabbits. **A:** Schematic diagram showing the experimental arrangement. TT, Turntable; SL, slit light; ME, microelectrode. (Note that the body and limbs of the rabbit were omitted for simplicity.) **B:** Spikes recorded from a Purkinje cell of the flocculus. Complex spikes are marked by ▽. **C:** Sine-curve representing the instantaneous head velocity (ordinate) during two successive periods of rotation. Positive values of the velocity are for the ipsilateral rotation and negative ones for the contralateral rotation. **D** and **E:** Spike-density histograms obtained for two flocculus Purkinje cells, during 30 and 40 rotations in darkness, respectively. Ordinates, number of simple spikes recorded per bin, relative to the mean spike number calculated over one period of rotation. Histograms obtained for one period are duplicated to cover two periods, to facilitate visual estimation of the modulation. From Ghelarducci et al. (6).

long, signalling inadequate performance of the vestibulo-ocular reflex, there will be a change in parameters involved in activation of flocculus Purkinje cells so that the system may acquire an improved performance (8). Lorente de Nó (14) previously described that even though newborn rabbits exhibit the vestibulo-ocular reflex before their eyes are open, the performance of the reflex is abnormal. Its final development is achieved about 40 days after birth, and apparently visual influence plays a role in this development. It was a remarkable finding of Gonshor and Melvill-Jones (7) that in human subjects the horizontal vestibulo-ocular reflex was gradually depressed, or even reversed in polarity, if the visual input was kept reversed in the horizontal plane by means of a Dove prism. Robinson (22) demonstrated that the plasticity similarly produced in cats was indeed impaired after the cerebellectomy including the flocculus. Miles and Fuller (19) revealed that vestibulo-ocular responses of the rhesus monkey exhibited adaptive plasticity

when the visual field was enlarged or reduced by means of telescopic glasses.

Occurrence of an adaptive plastic change in the rabbit vestibulo-ocular reflex can readily be demonstrated in the experiments where alert rabbits were rotated for 12 hr with continuous visual stimulation. With the slit light at a fixed position, the eye movement was gradually augmented as measured either in temporary darkness or with the slit light illuminated. At 12 hr after starting the rotation, the eye movement, particularly that with the slit light presented, attained much improved compensation of the head rotation as shown in Fig. 2C. Likewise, continuous rotation with the moving slit light caused gradual reduction of the eye movement, as shown in Fig. 2D. At 12 hr, there was virtually no rotation of the eye. These effects would improve the constancy of retinal images of the slit light, either stationary or moving. The progressive effects of visual stimulation on the horizontal vestibular-ocular reflex were totally absent when the flocculus had been extirpated on the side of the stimulated eye. Conversely, in those rabbits whose cerebral visual cortex or cerebellar visual area (lobules VI and VII) had been destroyed chronically, the effects were the same or even more prominent than in normal rabbits. Thus, the progressive effects appear to support the "learning" capability postulated for the cerebellar flocculus.

SIMPLE SPIKE DISCHARGES FROM FLOCCULUS PURKINJE CELLS

With extracellular microelectrodes, two kinds of spikes can be recorded from Purkinje cells, i.e., *simple* and *complex* spikes (Fig. 3B). Complex spikes represent the activity induced via synapses from climbing fibers; simple spikes reflect activities at other synapses (4,25). Linsberger and Fuchs (13) demonstrated in alert monkey that simple spike responses of flocculus Purkinje cells to horizontal head rotation were modified very effectively during visual fixation. Simple spike discharges from flocculus Purkinje cells of alert rabbits also exhibited marked effects when the vestibulo-ocular reflex is performed in the presence of visual stimuli (6).

Simple spike discharges from flocculus Purkinje cells of alert rabbits occurred at 10 to 60 per second in the absence of both vestibular and visual stimuli. When the animal was rotated sinusoidally, this activity was modulated sinusoidally at the frequency of the head rotation. As surveyed during rotation in darkness, there are two major response types; one is with the modulation occurring in phase with the instantaneous head velocity and the other with the outphase modulation as shown in Fig. 3D and E. Intermediate response patterns were seen only in a relatively small number of cells examined.

As pointed out by Linsberger and Fuchs (13), inphase responses of flocculus Purkinje cells would have the effect of cancelling the excitatory action of primary vestibular signals on second-order vestibular neurons (see Fig. 1), since the primary vestibular afferents discharge impulses in phase with head velocity. In contrast, outphase responses of the flocculus Purkinje cells would facilitate the excitatory action of primary vestibular afferents, as the

inhibition waxes and wanes in opposition to the excitation. Hence, the flocculus should have a dual action to enhance or depress the horizontal vestibulo-ocular reflex, depending on whether Purkinje cells there discharge predominantly with the outphase or the inphase pattern. The above-described results in rabbits that chronic destruction of the flocculus causes a gain decrease of the horizontal vestibulo-ocular reflex therefore does not contradict the postulate that cerebellar Purkinje cells have solely inhibitory action.

When the slit light alone was moved sinusoidally around a stationary rabbit, there was little modulation of simple spike discharges. However, it was very effective in modifying the amplitude and phase angle of simple spike modulation provoked by simultaneous head rotation. With the fixed slit light presented, it frequently occurred that an outphase response was augmented, that an inphase response was depressed, or that an inphase response was converted to another response type. Even though the effect was opposite in a minority of examined cells or neutral in another minority, the fixed slit light caused a shift of the dominance to the outphase response type. Conversely, the moving slit light simulating vision reversal caused a shift of the dominance to the inphase response type; in the majority of examined cells, the observed changes were augmentation of an inphase response, reduction of an outphase response or conversion from an outphase to another response. For the reason discussed above, the dominance of outphase responses during presentation of the fixed slit light should have the effect to enhance the horizontal vestibulo-ocular reflex, while the dominance of inphase responses produced by the moving slit light should cause the opposite effect to depress the reflex. Thus, the immediate effects of the slit light upon the horizontal vestibulo-ocular reflex can satisfactorily be accounted for by the population shift seen in flocculus Purkinje cells between the outphase and inphase response types.

Two questions arise. First, how are the two major Purkinje cell response types, inphase and outphase, generated? Second, how does vision affect the simple spike activity? As to the first question, it is pointed out that the primary vestibular afferents from the vestibular organ ipsilateral to the flocculus concerned convey inphase signals and those from the contralateral vestibular organ outphase ones. Both of these signals converge onto the flocculus (20). Also, the phase of signals in primary vestibular afferents can be shifted by 180° through inhibitory relay by cerebellar cortical cells. Concerning the second question, it is natural to assume that the visual mossy fiber pathway (Fig. 1) is responsible. In fact, chronic lesion placed in the climbing fiber visual pathway does not impair the immediate effects of the slit light on the rabbit horizontal vestibulo-ocular reflex and the underlying modulation of simple spike discharges in flocculus Purkinje cells (Ito and Miyashita, *to be published*).

COMPLEX SPIKE DISCHARGES FROM FLOCCULUS PURKINJE CELLS

In the absence of both vestibular and visual stimuli, complex spikes of flocculus Purkinje cells discharge at 1 to 2 per second. By presenting pattern light stimuli to stationary rabbits, receptive areas have been defined in the visual field from which both facilitation and inhibition are elicited in complex spike discharges (16). Complex spike discharges of flocculus Purkinje cells have also been shown to have a direction sensitivity for moving light targets (23). The sinusoidally moving slit light affected complex spike discharges frequently, mostly in phase with the forward movement of the slit light (6). Complex spike discharges were also affected by head rotation even in the absence of visual stimuli (6). This is in accord with the previous report that caloric and galvanic stimulation of the labyrinth causes modulation of not only simple but also complex spikes in the cerebellum (5).

Just as for simple spikes, visual stimulation with the slit light effectively modified the modulation of complex spikes provoked by vestibular stimulation. Response patterns of complex spikes varied from cell to cell, but there was a certain tendency for the inphase pattern to prevail under the fixed slit light and the outphase pattern to prevail under the moving slit light. This is in contrast to the effects on simple spikes described above. Further, when both simple and complex spikes were tested under the same series of alternated rotation with and without the slit light presented, opposite effects for simple and complex spikes were consistently observed (6).

The above-described observations raise questions about the following two kinds of neuronal mechanisms. First, how do vestibular signals influence the complex spike discharges of flocculus Purkinje cells? There must be a pathway through which vestibular signals impinge on the climbing fiber visual pathway somewhere in its course through the midbrain to the inferior olive. Second, what do the complex spike discharges serve? As mentioned above, the activity of simple spikes, behaving oppositely to complex spikes, satisfactorily explains the effect of visual stimulation on the vestibulo-ocular reflex. Further, complex spike discharges occur at a considerably lower rate than do the simple spikes; even though one complex spike may be equivalent to several simple spikes as propagating signals, simple spikes would predominate over complex spikes in their effect on the second-order vestibular neurons. It is unlikely that the complex spikes are responsible for any immediate modification by visual stimulus of the vestibulo-ocular reflex.

Positive meanings for the complex spike activity may be searched for in the long-term learning process of the cerebellum. One may imagine that complex spikes serve a process intrinsic to the cerebellar cortex, such as controlling the plastic modifiability of synaptic transmission from granule cells onto Purkinje cells (18). Indeed, chronic destruction of the climbing fiber visual pathway resulted in loss of the progressive modification of the rabbit horizontal vestibulo-ocular reflex (Ito and Miyashita, *to be published*) that normally occurred during sustained application of combined vestibular and visual stimulation (Fig. 2C and D). Neuronal activities in the flocculus underlying this plasticity are now under study.

COMMENT

Studies of a neuronal system require new techniques and strategies in addition to those that have been utilized for analyses at cellular levels. Close association of different disciplines would indeed be useful in bringing together as many available lines of approach as possible, with a carefully chosen focus. Although there is still much to be done, it is hoped that the flocculo-vestibulo-ocular system can be one such focus that may lead to knowledge of essential mechanisms of cerebellar function.

REFERENCES

1. Baarsma, E. A., and Collewijn, H. (1974): Vestibulo-ocular and optokinetic reactions to rotation and their interaction in the rabbit. *J. Physiol.,* 238:603–625.
2. Carpenter, R. H. S. (1972): Cerebellectomy and the transfer function of the vestibulo-ocular reflex in the decerebrate cat. *Pro. R. Soc. Lond.* [Biol.], 181:353–374.
3. Dow, R. S., and Moruzzi, G. (1958): *The Physiology and Pathology of the Cerebellum.* University of Minnesota Press, Minneapolis.
4. Eccles, J. C., Ito, M., and Szentágothai, J. (1967): *The Cerebellum as a Neuronal Machine.* Springer, New York.
5. Ferin, M., Grigorian, R. A., and Strata, P. (1971): Mossy and climbing fibre activation in the cat cerebellum by stimulation of the labyrinth. *Exp. Brain Res.,* 12:1–17.
6. Ghelarducci, B., Ito, M., and Yagi, N. (1975): Impulse discharges from flocculus Purkinje cells of alert rabbits during visual stimulation combined with horizontal head rotation. *Brain Res.,* 87:66–72.
7. Gonshor, A., and Melvill-Jones, G. (1973): Changes of human vestibulo-ocular response induced by vision-reversal during head rotation. *J. Physiol. (Lond.),* 234:102–103.
8. Ito, M. (1972): Neural design of the cerebellar motor control system. *Brain Res.,* 40:81–84.
9. Ito, M., Nishimaru, N., and Yamamoto, M. (1973): Specific neural connections for the cerebellar control of vestibulo-ocular reflexes. *Brain Res.,* 60:238–243.
10. Ito, M., Shiida, T., Yagi, N., and Yamamoto, M. (1974): Visual influence on rabbit horizontal vestibulo-ocular reflex presumably effected via the cerebellar flocculus. *Brain Res.,* 60:238–243.
11. Ito, M., Shiida, T., Yagi, N., and Yamamoto, M. (1974): The cerebellar modification of rabbit's horizontal vestibulo-ocular reflex induced by sustained head rotation combined with visual stimulation. *Proc. Japan Acad.,* 50:85–89.
12. Kornhuber, H. H. (1971): Motor functions of the cerebellum and basal ganglia, the cerebello-cortical saccadic (ballistic) clock, the cerebellonuclear hold regulator, and the basal ganglia ramp (voluntary speed smooth movement) generator. *Kybernetik,* 8:157–162.
13. Linsberger, S. G., and Fuchs, A. F. (1974): Response of flocculus Purkinje cells to adequate vestibular stimulation in the alert monkey: Fixation vs. compensatory eye movements. *Brain Res.,* 69:347–353.
14. Lorente de Nó, R. (1931): Ausgewalte Kapitel aus der vergleichenden Physiologie des Labyrinthes. Die Augenmuskelreflexe beim Kaninchen und ihre Grundlagen. *Ergeb. Physiol.,* 32:73–242.
15. Maekawa, K., and Simpson, J. I. (1973): Climbing fiber responses evoked in the vestibulo-cerebellum of rabbit from visual system. *J. Neurophysiol.,* 36:649–666.
16. Maekawa, K., and Kimura, K. (1974): Inhibition of climbing fiber responses of rabbit's flocculus Purkinje cells induced by light stimulation of the retina. *Brain Res.,* 65:347–350.
17. Manni, D. E. (1950): Localizzazioni cerebellari corticali della cavia nota 29, Effetti di lesioni delle "parti vestibolari" del cervelletto. *Arch. Fisiol.,* 50:110–123.
18. Marr, D. (1969): A theory of cerebellar cortex. *J. Physiol. (Lond.),* 202:437–470.
19. Miles, F. A., and Fuller, J. H. (1974): Adaptive plasticity in the vestibulo-ocular responses of the Rhesus monkey. *Brain Res.,* 80:512–516.
20. Precht, W., and Llinás, R. (1969): Functional organization of the vestibular afferents to the cerebellar cortex of frog and cat. *Exp. Brain Res.,* 9:30–52.
21. Robinson, D. A. (1974): The effect of cerebellectomy on the cat's vestibulo-ocular integrator. *Brain Res.,* 71:195–207.
22. Robinson, D. A. (1975): Oculomotor control signals. In: *Basic Mechanisms of Ocular Motility and Their Clinical Implications,* edited by P. Bach-y-Rita and G. Lennerstrand. Pergamon Press, Oxford. (*In press.*)
23. Simpson, J. I., and Alley, K. I. (1974): Visual climbing fiber input to rabbit vestibulo-cerebellum: A source of direction-specific information. *Brain Res.,* 82:302–308.
24. Takemori, S., and Cohen, B. (1974): Loss of visual suppression of vestibular nystagmus after flocculus lesions. *Brain Res.,* 72:213–224.
25. Thach, W. T. (1968): Discharge of Purkinje and cerebellar nuclear neurons during rapidly alternating arm movements in the monkey. *J. Neurophysiol.,* 26:785–797.

The Nervous System, Donald B. Tower, Editor-in-Chief. *Vol. 1: The Basic Neurosciences.* Raven Press, New York, 1975.

Control of Spinal Mechanisms From The Brain

A. Lundberg

The spinal cord has a central role in the history of neurophysiology. From Sherrington's work on spinal reflexes emerged principles of utmost importance for the advancement of research on the function of the central nervous system — above all, the principle of central inhibition as an active process and of reciprocal innervation. The explosive development that resulted from the application of modern electrophysiological technique to the study of the central nervous system started with the spinal cord. As a result we now possess extensive information regarding neuronal properties, synaptic mechanism, and pathways in the spinal cord.

Motoneurons are controlled by pathways descending from the brain, by propriospinal pathways, and by reflex pathways from primary afferents. Five pathways descending from the brain have monosynaptic connections with motoneurons (for references see ref. 2). Four of them are excitatory: the corticospinal, rubrospinal and vestibulospinal tracts, and a reticulospinal tract. The monosynaptic connections from the two former pathways presumably have evolved to serve manipulatory movements requiring a high degree of precision; phylogenetically they are late, being found in primates but not in the cat. Monosynaptic excitation from the pathways originating in the lower brainstem, which is found also in lower vertebrates, and is matched by monosynaptic inhibition of motoneurons to neck and trunk muscles from the medial vestibular nucleus, probably has special importance in fast postural adjustments. Nonetheless, most of the effects from the brain to motoneurons seem to be mediated by propriospinal neurons and spinal interneurons.

For many years descending and reflex effects were treated as separate entities, but there is now strong evidence that they are not apart from each other. It all started with Merton's hypothesis of servo control via the γ-operated stretch reflex. Also in its modern version with Granit's α-γ-linkage and servo assistance from the stretch reflex (8,35), the essential element remains — higher centers are using a spinal reflex to control movements. In this special case the control depends on the remarkable arrangement of γ-operated muscle spindles from which the motoneurons are excited monosynaptically. For the major part of reflexes which are not mediated monosynaptically there is another possibility — the control may be exerted at the interneuronal level. There is now extensive evidence showing convergence of descending pathways and primary afferents on common interneurons projecting to motoneurons. In this chapter I discuss the integrative significance of this convergence in relation to segmental mechanisms governing transmission in some reflex pathways. I also briefly consider some new findings regarding propriospinal pathways.

THE DESCENDING CONTROL OF INTERNEURONAL PATHWAYS FROM PRIMARY AFFERENTS TO MOTONEURONS

Most of the information regarding convergence on interneurons has been obtained with the indirect technique of recording synaptic potentials in motoneurons. This simple technique is illustrated diagrammatically in Fig. 1. In the cases represented by A, separate stimulation of either I or II is without effect on the motoneuron while combined stimulation of I and II gives a postsynaptic potential (PSP). The explanation must be subliminal excitatory convergence on common interneurons from I and II and summation of their effects on combined stimulation which gives discharge in a number of interneurons and results in a PSP in the motoneuron. In most cases it is more convenient to use stimuli which separately applied do excite some interneurons; excitatory

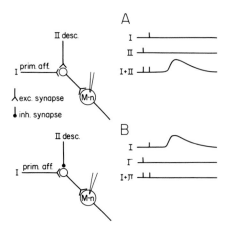

FIG. 1. Diagram showing indirect technique used to investigate convergence in interneurons in reflex pathways to motoneurons. See text for explanation. The example refers to convergence from descending fibers and primary afferents but the technique can be used for convergence from any source.

convergence is then inferred when the PSP on combined stimulation is larger than the algebraic sum of the PSPs evoked by separate stimuli.

The variant of the technique, used to establish convergence of excitation and inhibition on interneurons, is shown in Fig. 1B. Stimulus I evokes a test PSP while the conditioning stimulus II is without effect on the motoneurons. A decrease or abolishment of the test PSP on combined stimulation shows that the conditioning volley II has inhibitory effect on the interneurons, provided that it neither changes the membrane conductance in the motoneurons nor gives presynaptic inhibition of transmission from I. In Fig. 1 inhibition is indicated as postsynaptic on the soma of the interneurons, in which case the decrease of the PSP in the motoneurons is due to a corresponding decrease in the number of excited interneurons. Alternatively the decrease in the test PSP may be due to presynaptic inhibition of transmission from the terminals of interneurons which would give a decreased PSP in the motoneurons without change in number of discharging interneurons. There is one example of an inhibitory action of the latter type (29) but in most cases inhibition is probably postsynaptic on the cell body of the interneurons. By varying the conditioning-test interval it is possible to deduce the latency and time course of the PSP evoked in interneurons by conditioning stimuli.

When investigating the effect of descending conditioning volleys on a disynaptic test PSP from primary afferents, the results are easy to interpret because there is only one interneuron in the tested pathway. However, when the test PSP is mediated by a chain of interneurons it is usually not possible to decide at which level the descending action is exerted. In such cases it is sometimes an advantage to reverse the technique and use a disynaptic descending PSP as test. Effects produced on it by conditioning volleys in polysynaptic reflex pathways then give a measure of convergence on last order interneurons projecting directly to motoneurons (1).

Descending Inhibition

Intracellular recordings from interneurons have revealed that stimulation of virtually any motor center in the brain can produce inhibitory PSPs (IPSPs) in interneurons. These IPSPs may be evoked in two different ways. Descending fibers excite many inhibitory interneurons belonging to pathways from primary afferents. These interneurons may in turn inhibit other interneurons from which IPSPs are recorded although the primary descending effect is a facilitation of a pathway from primary afferents (13,29). Such inhibitory effects are thus a consequence of the commonly occurring inhibitory interaction between interneuronal pathways in the spinal cord. In other cases there is no evidence for facilitation of transmission from primary afferents and inhibition seems to be the *primary* event. It may then be mediated either monosynaptically as indicated in Fig. 1B or else by excitation of a "private" inhibitory interneuron.

All the four known pathways giving primary inhibition of interneuronal transmission in reflex pathways originate in the lower brainstem (28,29). Two of them are monoaminergic and their existence has been inferred from experiments in which the precursors DOPA or 5-HTP were administered intravenously in acute spinal cats. Of the two nonmonoaminergic pathways, only the dorsal reticulospinal system has been subject to a detailed analysis. Activity in this system is responsible for the tonic inhibition of the segmental reflex pathways found in the decerebrate cat. It suppresses a variety of reflexes but is without effect on reciprocal Ia inhibition. The other pathway is also activated by electrical stimulation in the reticular formation but its axons descend in the ventral half of the spinal cord. It has been shown that activation of this pathway inhibits transmission in some reflex paths to motoneurons but a systematic analysis has been difficult because of the concomitant activation of fibers giving postsynaptic inhibition in motoneurons. It is of interest that this pathway very effectively inhibits the transmission in the reflex pathways that mediate depolarization to primary afferent terminals, including those of Ia afferents.

Since I last reviewed this field (29) there has been very little advance in knowledge regarding these descending inhibitory pathways. It would be particularly important to learn how these inhibitory systems interact with the descending tracts which have excitatory action on interneurons in the same reflex pathways and how they are governed from other centers in the brain. Within the last domain there is some new information: Stimulation of the mesencephalic locomotor center activates the noradrenergic reticulospinal pathway thereby releasing the spinal locomotor center for action (9,11).

Descending Excitation

The corticospinal, rubrospinal, and vestibulospinal tracts all have excitatory action on interneurons of segmental reflex paths to motoneurons (10,28,29,35), and similar effects are produced by long propriospinal fibers that originate in forelimb segments and descend to the lumbosacral segments (24). Important effects are exerted on the reflex pathways from the flexor reflex afferents (FRA) but the following discussion is restricted to the excitatory actions on interneurons of reflex pathways from Ia, Ib and cutaneous afferents.

Ia afferents

Impulses in the large Ia muscle spindle afferents evoke monosynaptic excitation in motoneurons to homonymous and synergic muscles

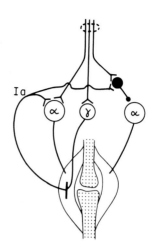

FIG. 2. Schematic representation of connections assumed to give "α-γ-linked reciprocal inhibition" showing that any neuronal system which mediates excitation to agonist α- and γ-motoneurons also evokes excitation in Ia inhibitory interneurons (*black*) projecting to antagonist motoneurons.

and reciprocal inhibition in motoneurons to antagonists. It is firmly established that Ia inhibition is mediated by a disynaptic pathway (3,23). Although not in all cases limited to antagonists at the same joint, the pattern of reciprocal Ia inhibition is a relatively simple one. It operates between flexors and extensors and there is no indication of alternative Ia inhibitory reflex pathways (12). The convergence on the interneuron of the reciprocal Ia inhibitory pathway—the Ia inhibitory interneuron—has been thoroughly investigated. The diagram of convergence on them given by Lindström (27) in his Fig. 1 includes eight excitatory paths, but three additional connections have been revealed since then, most notably monosynaptic excitation from corticospinal fibers in the primate (26). Figure 2 illustrates the principle organization that all neuronal systems with excitatory action on α- and γ-motoneurons to a certain group of muscles give parallel excitation to the interneurons of the reciprocal Ia inhibitory pathway. The physiological significance of these connections appears from a consideration of the functional role of reciprocal inhibition. In order to provide relaxation of the antagonist during agonist contraction, inhibition should be coupled, not to the synaptic depolarization of agonist motoneurons but to

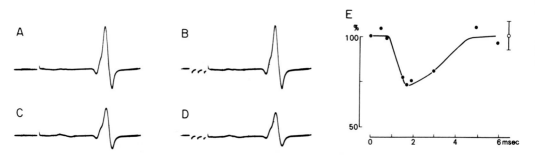

FIG. 3. Reciprocal Ia inhibition during voluntary ankle dorsiflexion in man. **A–D:** H-reflexes in triceps surae. Left records are controls and right records (**B, D**) show the effect of triple conditioning weak group-I volleys in the peroneal nerve. **A** and **B** were obtained at rest, **C** and **D** during a weak voluntary dorsiflexion of the foot. The inhibition in **D** was evoked by the third conditioning volley and abscissa in curve **E** is the interval between the third conditioning shock and the test shock (38).

their *activation.* In movements depending on α-γ-linkage, the activation of motoneurons depends on convergent excitation from the direct α-route and from Ia afferents as part of the indirect γ-route. Accordingly the same type of convergence would be required in the inhibitory pathway in order to achieve a coupling of reciprocal inhibition (=activation of the Ia inhibitory interneurons) to activation of agonist motoneurons. Hence the concept of "α-γ-linked reciprocal inhibition" (12) which has been discussed in more detail elsewhere (15,30).

Recent experiments by Tanaka (38) suggest that "α-γ-linked reciprocal inhibition" operates in man. At rest, conditioning volleys in low-threshold group-I afferents from pretibial flexors failed to inhibit the H-reflex to an antagonist ankle extensor (Fig. 3A,B). During a voluntary dorsiflexion of the foot, on the other hand, the same conditioning volleys evoked a clear inhibition (C,D) with the expected latency and time course of reciprocal Ia inhibition (E). Clearly these findings are well explained by the hypothesis that the voluntary command for a dorsiflexion of the foot also provides facilitation of the interneurons mediating Ia inhibition to antagonists.

I will now turn to one of the most intriguing developments in spinal cord physiology—the recurrent inhibition of Ia inhibitory interneurons from motor axon collaterals. For some time it has been known that impulses in motor axon collaterals not only evoke recurrent IPSPs in motoneurons but also inhibit inhibitory interneurons projecting directly to motoneurons (3).

Efforts to analyze the pathway to which these inhibitory interneurons belong soon revealed that the recurrent inhibition is exerted on the Ia inhibitory interneurons (16). This effect was demonstrated with the indirect technique of investigating the depression of the Ia IPSP by conditioning volleys in motor axon collaterals. The segmental latency and the time course of this depression was the same as that of the recurrent IPSP in motoneurons suggesting similar postsynaptic inhibition of Ia inhibitory interneurons. Careful studies of the distribution of recurrent effects revealed that the Ia inhibitory interneurons receive their recurrent inhibition from the efferents to the same muscle from which they are monosynaptically excited (Fig. 4). In other words, α-motoneurons and inhibitory interneurons with the same Ia input appear to be acted upon together, probably by the same Renshaw cells (15,18,27).

These findings led to the identification of the Ia inhibitory interneurons. Hultborn et al. (17) searched for interneurons monosynaptically

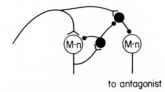

FIG. 4. Diagram showing that motoneurons and inhibitory interneurons with the same monosynaptic Ia input receive recurrent inhibition from the same efferents. Thus Ia activity may excite the interneurons directly and inhibit them indirectly via activation of motoneurons and Renshaw cells (16,18).

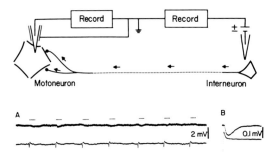

FIG. 5. The experiment proving projection of Ia inhibitory interneuron to its target motoneuron. The interneuron was functionally identified since it received monosynaptic Ia excitation and recurrent inhibition. Simultaneous recording was made extracellularly from the interneuron and intracellularly from its target motoneuron (*diagram*). **A:** Parallel records of spikes in the interneuron (*lower traces*) and small unitary IPSPs (*dashed lines*) in the motoneuron (*upper traces*). **B:** As in **A** but averaged records triggered by the spikes in the interneuron (25).

excited from Ia afferents and disynaptically inhibited from motor axon collaterals. They found them in the ventral horn in a region just dorsal and dorso-medial to the motor nucleus. Subsequently, Jankowska and Roberts (25) were able to prove that the axons of these interneurons have monosynaptic inhibitory connections with motoneurons. Their elegant technique with simultaneous recording of impulses in single interneurons and of unitary IPSPs in their target motoneurons is illustrated in Fig. 5. [For other physiological and anatomical aspects on the Ia inhibitory interneurons, see Jankowska (23) and Burke and Rudomin (2).]

Since the Ia interneurons are identified, it is possible to investigate convergence onto them also by direct recording. Hultborn, Illert, and Santini (*unpublished*) have now confirmed many of the conclusions drawn from experiments with the indirect technique and also obtained additional new information. They showed, for example, mutual inhibitory connections between Ia inhibitory interneurons projecting to antagonist motor nuclei as shown in Fig. 6; the activity in either reciprocal inhibitory pathway may thus depress the activity in the opposite one. It is noteworthy that the parallelism in convergence to agonist motoneurons and Ia inhibitory interneurons (Fig. 2) is not restricted to their excitatory input but also extends to inhibitory inputs like Renshaw

inhibition (Fig. 4) and Ia inhibition (Fig. 6).

Feldman and Orlovsky (5) have succeeded in recording from Ia inhibitory interneurons during locomotion in mesencephalic cats – a remarkable technical achievement. During stepping the interneurons became active with the muscle supplying their Ia afferent input. From ingenious experiments on cats with de-efferented hindlimbs they were able to prove that the activity was evoked by convergent excitation from Ia afferents and from the central program generating the stepping movements. Thus these authors have shown not only that reciprocal Ia inhibition functions during stepping but also that "there is α-γ-linked reciprocal inhibition," indeed the first demonstration that it operates in cats.

The recurrent control of the Ia inhibitory interneurons provides an interesting segmental mechanism for regulation of reciprocal inhibition in movements depending on α-γ-linkage. The essence of the Ia servo-assistance hypothesis is that a load on a contracting muscle gives an acceleration in the Ia discharge which increases the motoneuronal firing. The increased Ia discharge will also reach the Ia inhibitory interneurons and tend to accelerate their firing rate and thereby augment the depth of the reciprocal inhibition. This may be a disadvantage since the role of inhibition is to prevent excita-

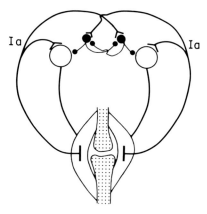

FIG. 6. The mutual inhibitory connection between Ia inhibitory interneurons projecting to antagonist muscles was revealed with intracellular recording from Ia inhibitory interneurons. The collateral connection to the "opposite" interneuron is evidenced by recurrent depression from motor axon collaterals also of the Ia IPSP in the interneuron (Hultborn, Illert, and Santini, *unpublished findings*).

tion, and inhibition beyond this level may compromise the readiness for activation should the need arise. However, the existence of the recurrent control might counteract the excess excitatory action in the Ia inhibitory interneurons by inhibition produced by the increased motoneuronal firing. It has been suggested that the recurrent control may keep the depth of reciprocal inhibition constant during different degrees of agonist activity in Ia servo-assisted movements (19).

In order to test this hypothesis, inhibition of the monosynaptic test reflex to knee flexors was investigated during static stretch of the knee extensor in decerebrate cats with effective tonic inhibition of transmission in reflex pathways from the FRA and Ib afferents. A diagrammatic representation of the results is given in Fig. 7. In exceptional cats without stretch reflexes there was a linear relationship between muscle length, Ia impulse frequency, and inhibition of the test reflex (B). When a stretch reflex was evoked (C, EMG indicated in lower graph), a break appeared and with further stretch, increasing the EMG activity, the inhibitory curve remained level. However, in many experiments the plateau was not maintained but with further extension inhibition again increased as shown in D. The further

analysis indicates that the latter finding does not invalidate the hypothesis because the increment in inhibition at high degrees of extension is not due to an increased activity in the Ia inhibitory pathway but to another mechanism. Excitability measurements revealed that corresponding to the increment in inhibition a depolarization was evoked in terminals of the Ia afferents mediating the test reflex. Furthermore, the degree of depolarization measured with the excitability technique was shown to give presynaptic inhibition of test reflex transmission of roughly the same order of magnitude as the increment in inhibition (Fu, Hultborn, Larsson, and Lundberg, *unpublished*). The observations made so far thus indicate that there is a reasonable balance between the two opposing systems controlling the excitability of the Ia inhibitory interneurons when an excess of Ia excitation produces an increased motoneuronal firing.

Accordingly it seems that subsidiary to the "α-γ-linkage in reciprocal inhibition," there is an autoregulatory segmental mechanism keeping the depth of the reciprocal inhibition constant during different degrees of agonist activity. The sensitivity of this autoregulatory mechanism can in all likelihood be "set" by different neuronal systems controlling transmission from motor axon collaterals to Renshaw cells (15).

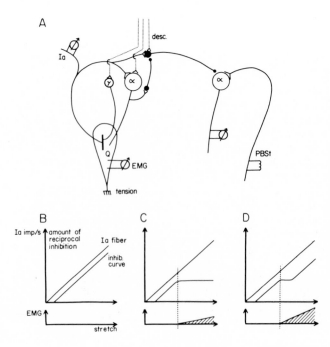

FIG. 7. Reciprocal inhibition during the decerebrate stretch reflex (schematic representation). **A:** Experimental arrangement with simultaneous recording of EMG and tension in the knee extensor (Q), activity in a single Ia afferent from Q and of the monosynaptic test reflex from the knee flexors (PBSt posterior biceps semitendinosus). The test reflex was recorded in the severed S1 ventral root. For explanation of **B–D** see text. Observe that **C** and **D** refer to experiments in which there is a continuous increase in the EMG throughout the extension. In some experiments the EMG activity saturated at less than full extension, even so an increment in inhibition occurred with further extension; in this case probably caused largely by excess Ia excitation not matched by recurrent inhibition (refs. 15 and 19 and Fu, Hultborn, Larsson, and Lundberg, *unpublished findings*).

In view of all the care taken by the central nervous system to regulate reciprocal Ia inhibition it is now desirable to test its role in motor regulation, for example in rapid reversal of antagonist movements. Is there a difference in this respect between flexion-extension and movements not subserved by Ia inhibition like abduction-adduction? Is the disability for rapid reversal after cerebellar inflictions at least in part due to a defect regulation of reciprocal Ia inhibition? In this connection it is relevant that the ventral spinocerebellar tract may give information regarding transmission in the Ia inhibitory pathway (27).

Ib Afferents

These afferents originate from Golgi tendon organs and are effectively activated by increased muscular tension. It is generally believed that Ib afferents have both disynaptic and trisynaptic reflex pathways to motoneurones but so far there is no information suggesting unlike functions of Ib reflex pathways with these different linkages. Starting out from the "lengthening reaction" in decerebrate cats the interest has been focused on autogenetic Ib inhibition as a feedback mechanism regulating tension—force feedback (35). The analysis by Houk et al. (14) of the stretch reflex indicates a rather small gain of the force feedback in decerebrate cats, which is not surprising in view of the effective tonic descending inhibition of interneurons belonging to Ib reflex pathways to motoneurons in this preparation (28). There is convergent excitation to these interneurons (Fig. 8) from the corticospinal and rubrospinal tracts (12,33) and the setting of the gain of the force feedback through interneuronal facilitation may be a very important mechanism for the brain to command muscular force. Houk et al. (14) have postulated that the Ib force loop may serve to reduce the sensitivity to muscular fatigue and also indicated the possibility that during certain motor tasks, e.g., exploratory movements, length feedback may be inhibited and force feedback facilitated "so far to provide a system controlling muscular force rather than length."

It should be emphasized that Ib reflex regulation is not predominantly autogenetic. To any given motor nucleus the effect is drawn from many muscles, which suggests Ib regulation

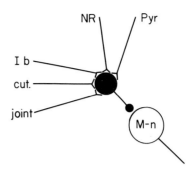

FIG. 8. These excitatory connections to interneurons in the Ib inhibitory pathway to motoneurons were revealed with the use of the indirect technique. Rubrospinal (NR) and probably also corticospinal (Pyr) connections are monosynaptic. Excitation from cutaneous (Cut) and joint afferents is mediated by oligosynaptic pathways but they may not be monosynaptic (12,32,33).

between co-contracting muscles. Spinal cats have rather stereotyped Ib patterns but rubrospinal facilitation has revealed more complex patterns including Ib inhibition of extensor motoneurons from flexors as well as of flexor motoneurons from extensors (12). These findings indicate the existence of alternative Ib reflex patterns which in turn suggests that a command for a complex movement, perhaps with co-contraction of some flexors and extensors, may be accompanied by a mobilization of an appropriate Ib reflex pattern.

A recent investigation has revealed the existence of segmental mechanisms which may contribute to regulation of Ib transmission (32). With the aid of the spatial facilitation technique it was shown that the interneurons of Ib reflex pathways receive convergent short-latency excitation from low threshold cutaneous afferents and from joint afferents (Fig. 8). These findings may have interesting functional implications. Consider that an exploratory limb movement commanded by the brain meets an obstacle. The resulting exteroceptive activity may facilitate the Ib inhibitory transmission with the result that the muscular tension is decreased not to force the obstacle. Postsynaptic inhibition of α-motoneurons from private reflex pathways from cutaneous afferents might also contribute, but a control of Ib inhibitory transmission increasing the gain in the Ib force loop would provide an elegant type of regulation since otherwise this feedback mechanism would tend to maintain constant force. The facilitation from low threshold joint afferents might have a similar function. The receptor origin of these afferents is not known. However, should they turn out to be those activated at the end of flexion and extension (see ref. 35), the facilitation of Ib inhibition might provide a mechanism to give decreased force when a movement approaches the limit given by the range over which the joints operate.

It would be of interest to use the method by Houk et al. (14) to investigate if the force feedback gain in decerebrate cats can be influenced by adequate stimulation of skin and joint receptors. Perhaps it is also of some interest to keep these convergent effects on the Ib inhibitory pathway in mind with respect to the "lengthening reaction." Although autogenetic Ib inhibition is believed to contribute, the mechanism of the "lengthening reaction" essentially remains obscure (35). Hongo (personal communication) has found that "lengthening" in an extensor evoked with intact muscle insertion by flexion of the joint is not observed when the isolated tendon is stretched in the same preparation.

The excitatory pathways from Ib afferents have received little attention. They are subject to the same facilitatory influences from the corticospinal and rubrospinal tracts as the Ib inhibitory pathways. It is not known if the more complex Ib excitatory patterns brought out during rubrospinal facilitation are reciprocal to the Ib inhibitory patterns. I have discussed the possibility that Ib excitation from synergically active muscles may give a reinforcing positive feedback which should have a powerful load-compensating effect (31). However, in view of the complete parallelism in facilitatory effects from low threshold cutaneous and low threshold joint afferents on Ib inhibitory and Ib excitatory pathways, I now prefer to view Ib excitation as a mechanism subsidiary to Ib inhibition. Let us assume that Ib excitation is reciprocal to Ib inhibition also in the more complex Ib pattern. When transmission in the Ib inhibitory pathway is facilitated from cutaneous afferents or joint afferents under the conditions described above, then the parallel facilitation of Ib excitatory pathways may give excitation of antagonist motoneurons. This would clearly be a purposeful brake of a movement when there is an obstacle or when it becomes extreme. It should

not necessarily be assumed that the Ib excitatory pathways are continuously active in parallel with the Ib inhibitory ones. They may have lower transmittability and come into operation only under special conditions such as those just referred to.

Reciprocal Ib excitation has also been discussed as a mechanism that might contribute to regulation of reciprocal inhibition (31).

Cutaneous Afferents

Generally, our knowledge about reflex pathways from cutaneous afferents is limited. It is known that cutaneous afferents contribute to a variety of reflex pathways to motoneurons. As part of the FRA, they can mediate excitation or inhibition to motoneurons via a large number of alternative reflex pathways (31). Cutaneous afferents may also act on motoneurons via the Ia inhibitory pathway (15) and results referred to in the preceding section suggest a corresponding action via the Ib reflex paths. Nevertheless, it seems likely that there are also "private" reflex pathways from cutaneous afferents.

It has long been believed that the minimal linkage in reflex pathways from cutaneous afferents is trisynaptic. The minimal central latency for cutaneous PSP in hindlimb motoneurons is about 1.8 msec (12). Since Ib PSPs or group II PSPs with the same central latency are considered as disynaptically mediated, why should the cutaneous PSP be trisynaptic? The reason is that activation of dorsal horn interneurons from cutaneous afferents occurs with very short latency, about 0.5 msec. Accordingly if these interneurons are part of the reflex pathway there is ample time for transmission via second-order interneurons. However, should it turn out that the first-order interneurons of pathways from cutaneous afferents to motoneurons are more ventrally located and that there is an appreciable intraspinal slowing of the conduction velocity in cutaneous afferents, then the assumption of a trisynaptic linkage must be reconsidered.

Volleys in the corticospinal and rubrospinal tracts give effective excitation to interneurons of reflex pathways from cutaneous afferents (4,12,33). It has been shown that rubrospinal fibers have monosynaptic connection with last-order interneurons in cutaneous reflex pathways while more indirect evidence suggests that corticospinal fibers act monosynaptically on first-order interneurons (13). Facilitation of a trisynaptic reflex pathway at two stations by two different descending systems would indicate a high degree of selectivity in the control of transmission.

The only clear example of a specialized cutaneous reflex in acute spinal cats is given by the reflex activation of toe extensors from pressure receptors of the central plantar cushion (4). This reflex may have its main significance in relation to descending activation of its interneurons from rubrospinal and corticospinal fibers. Assume that a brain command for plantar flexion of the toes is mediated by activation of these interneurons. During contact with the ground activation will be effectively reinforced by the convergent excitation from the plantar cushion to the same interneurons. It is tempting to extend this idea of a positive feedback reinforcement from cutaneous receptors to the control of the grip of the hand in primates. Intuitively it seems clear that the muscular force of the grip should increase when an object is seized. Marsden et al. (34) showed that a load compensating servo-control of thumb flexion in man was abolished when the skin of the thumb was made anesthetic. The authors assume that the servo is due to a transcortical reflex from Ia afferents, which is gated at a cortical level by impulses from the skin. I believe it is important to consider the possibility that such a servo may be spinal; impulses from pressure receptors in the skin might reinforce thumb flexion through convergence on interneurons, which also receive descending excitatory action as part of the voluntary command for thumb flexion.

The examples given above emphasized the conjoint activation of interneurons from descending fibers and cutaneous afferents. In some cases the main function may be the reflex action and the descending action may then more suitably be described as facilitation of a reflex. Progress in the study of spinal reflexes from exteroceptors has been slow; effects evoked by electrical stimulation of cutaneous nerves are difficult to interpret and, except for the toe extensor reflex mentioned above, light adequate stimuli are largely ineffective after anesthesia or in unanesthetized spinal cats. Recently, investigations of tactile reflexes have been made

in kittens that were spinalized a few weeks after birth and kept for some months. These animals have tactile placing reactions which are virtually indistinguishable from those found in the intact cat (17). The authors postulate that tactile placing also in the intact cats is dependent on a true spinal circuit which is normally under supraspinal control. Thus, the well-known disappearance of tactile placing after cortical lesion may indicate that the interneurons of its spinal reflex pathway require descending facilitatory support—a possibility that has been referred to previously (31,33).

In further investigations on chronic spinal cats Forssberg et al. (6) have analyzed tactile reflexes evoked during locomotion. They found a phase-dependent reflex reversal. During the swing phase there is additional activation of flexors but in the stance phase an increased rapid extension. These reflexes appear functionally meaningful in allowing the animal to overcome an obstacle impeding the movement of the limb. As one of three possible explanations the authors suggest that the spinal generator of locomotion "could phasically switch between reflex pathways." If so, a descending command may give a switching of reflexes from cutaneous afferents secondary to its activation of the spinal generator for locomotion.

INTEGRATION IN A PROPRIOSPINAL PATHWAY

In the previous section it was tacitly assumed that interaction in transmission to motoneurons from primary afferents and descending tracts took place in interneurons. However, in some cases (13,29) the experimental conditions did not allow a differentiation between interneurons and short propriospinal neurons. It may turn out to be important to differentiate between effects at these two levels.

Stewart et al. (37) first showed that in cats corticospinal volleys act on hindlimb motor nuclei through activation of propriospinal neurons. They investigated effects which remained after transection of the corticospinal tract in L3 but were abolished by a corresponding lesion in C3, thus being mediated by neurons originating between these levels. Using the same technique with lesions of the corticospinal tract at different segmental levels it has now been shown that disynaptic corticospinal excitation to forelimb motoneurons is mediated by propriospinal neurons originating in the C3 and C4 segments (see ref. 21). With the spatial facilitation technique it was shown that these neurons also receive monosynaptic excitation from rubrospinal fibers and from fibers activated in the contralateral subtectal region, presumably belonging to the tectospinal tract (Fig. 9), as well as short-latency excitation from low threshold cutaneous forelimb afferents ascending in the dorsal column (22).

Intracellular recording was then made from propriospinal neurons in C3 (20). They were identified by antidromic stimulation of their axons at different spinal cord levels; the axons of some of them terminate in the lower cervical segments where the forelimb motor nuclei are located. These cells received convergent monosynaptic EPSPs from corticospinal, rubrospinal, and presumed tectospinal fibers, as required for the system defined with the indirect technique. The somata of these cells were found at a depth of 2.5 to 3.5 mm from the cord dorsum, mainly in the lateral part of Rexed's laminae VI and VII. Furthermore, horseradish peroxidase was injected into certain forelimb motor nuclei. Subsequent histological exploration of the C3 and C4 segments revealed cells to which the enzyme was transported from terminals in the motor nuclei (Grant, Illert, and Tanaka, *unpublished findings*). Since these cells had a similar location as those recorded from, there is strong evidence that the propriospinal neurons investigated with the direct and indirect technique are identical. Accordingly Fig. 9 includes the connections found also with direct recording from propriospinal cells. Fibers in the dorsal column (DC) with monosynaptic excitatory connections to these cells presumably mediate the short-latency excitation revealed with the use of the indirect technique. Figure 9 shows that the monosynaptic EPSPs evoked in the propriospinal neurons from the corticospinal and rubrospinal traces are mediated by collaterals from fibers proceeding caudally. This was established with the collision technique. Since these fibers project to forelimb segments there is presumably "a built-in coordination at a spinal level in the activation of propriospinal and segmental mechanism" (20). Observe in Fig. 9 that three of the pathways with monosynaptic connections to

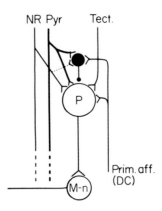

FIG. 9. Connections to propriospinal neurons (P) with somata in C3 and monosynaptic excitatory projection to forelimb motoneurons (Mn). See text for explanation. The convergence from corticospinal fibers and primary forelimb afferents interneuron to P was established with the indirect spatial facilitation technique using intracellular recording from somata of propriospinal neurons (20,21,22).

the propriospinal neurons also have disynaptic inhibitory connections. The inhibition, which seems to be of feed-forward type, may provide for a high degree of selectivity in activation of these propriospinal neurons. Another inhibitory connection to the propriospinal neurons is not shown in Fig. 9. Stimulation of ventrally located fibers in C5 evoked monosynaptic IPSPs in many of the propriospinal neurons recorded. If these fibers are descending this inhibition may provide a mechanism for switching-off the propriospinal system, for example during urgent postural adjustments.

Integration in this propriospinal system should be considered in relation to the general problem of how activity in a variety of motor pathways is coordinated. There can be little doubt that such a coordination occurs between the motor centers in the brain as well as in the spinal cord, both at a propriospinal and a segmental level. As regards coordination between the motor centers in the brain, it seems likely that the cerebellar loops allow commands in different motor centers to be shaped with due consideration to the activity in other motor centers. However, information transfer via the cerebellar loop implies a time lag which is undesirable in fast movements. Integration in the propriospinal neurons may have a time-saving function by allowing a command from a motor center, e.g., the motor cortex, to be influenced from other centers at time intervals too brief to permit an influence on the original command. The influence from tectum and from cutaneous afferents on corticomotoneuronal transmission is of particular interest in this connection, suggesting that a command from the motor cortex for a forelimb movement can be influenced *en route* by on-going visual activity and exteroceptive activity from the forelimb. Thus, a command for a ballistic movement may not have to be entirely preprogrammed in the brain. Studies of connections to other propriospinal systems are highly desirable.

COMMENTS

I have not aimed at giving a complete survey but chosen to exemplify in more detail how some spinal mechanisms are controlled.

Among the segmental mechanisms not dealt with, the reflex pathways from the FRA must at least be mentioned here because important principles have come out from the investigations of these pathways. Thus, the concept of alternative reflex pathways from the same afferents, with inhibitory interactive connections between them, first emerged for the pathways from the FRA (28). The role of the descending pathways inhibiting interneuronal transmission, a field in which knowledge is scant, is also best illustrated with regard to transmission from the FRA. For example, activity in the noradrenergic reticulospinal tract inhibits transmission in some pathways from the FRA, thereby releasing transmission in alternative reflex pathways. This release in fact represents a complete switch in spinal cord function bringing out locomotor mechanisms (9,28,29). The many different actions evoked from the FRA in the spinal cord are bewildering and there is need for some unifying concept. I have outlined a working hypothesis (31), its essence being that the active movement evokes activity in the FRA which gives reinforcing activation of interneurons already activated by the brain command for the movement. The descending activation of any particular excitatory pathway is assumed to give interactive inhibition of the alternative pathways from the FRA with the result that the reinforcing feedback is channeled back to the inter-

neuronal pathway already activated. The FRA are viewed as a segmental activating system subserving descending activation of a variety of interneuronal pathways to motoneurons.

A reference must also be made to problems related to the reflex pathways from secondary spindle afferents. Matthews (35) has provided powerful stimuli for further research in this field. Whether or not the secondaries contribute excitation in the decerebrate stretch reflex and whether or not they are part of the FRA, there is experimental evidence suggesting that they have alternative excitatory and inhibitory paths to both flexor and extensor motoneurons. Interneuronal switching may give a wide range of operational possibilities to the γ-operated secondaries.

It is also important not to neglect presynaptic inhibition—the general interest in this field seems to be on the wane. Transmission in reflex pathways to primary afferent terminals is subject to the same intricate descending control as the reflex pathways to motoneurons (28). The ideas regarding the functional role of presynaptic inhibition are largely based on the available information regarding connections to primary afferent terminals. In many cases the giving and receiving fibers are the same, thus proving a segmental negative feedback circuit. It is often stated that its function may be to give spatial sharpening by eliminating stray excitation (36, see however 2). Somehow this hypothesis tends to obscure its potential role as a general mechanism for regulation of transmission to first-order interneurons. If, as has been discussed in this chapter, descending activation of interneurons is subserved by a positive reinforcing feedback from peripheral receptors, then there seems to be a need for a mechanism regulating the positive feedback—presynaptic inhibition of transmission from primary afferent terminals seems suited for such a purpose.

Feedback control of movements is one of the most intensely discussed topics in neurophysiology. While there can be no doubt about the existence of a feedback control at all levels in the central nervous system the recent tendency has been to emphasize that occurring in higher centers perhaps at the expense of the spinal cord. My own plea is for the spinal cord because time is essential in motor regulation. It would surprise me if relatively simple tasks like servo regulation of length and tension were carried out through circuits involving higher brain centers. Although higher centers certainly have to order suitable segmental mechanisms into operation and to control that they function, they have the much more difficult task of giving shape to the motor command. The manyfold intricate ways of regulation of spinal cord mechanisms are indicative of the importance of these mechanisms in motor regulation, but it is regrettable that current ideas regarding feedback control of movements to such a large extent depends merely on knowledge of neuronal connections. Such knowledge, however, must precede functional tests and we may have to learn much more in order to devise appropriate tests during function. The spinal cord may have many feedback mechanisms at its disposal and for any given movement it may be crucial to test the appropriate one.

A review dealing with components of the spinal cord machinery tends to give a simplistic picture of how the spinal cord functions. The spinal cord has the ability to generate rhythmic alternating movements and Grillner (9) has reviewed the extensive literature regarding locomotion in intact, mesencephalic, and spinal animals. Although locomotion essentially is generated by intrinsic spinal mechanisms it is clearly subject to a very intricate control from higher centers (for references, see 9). Nonetheless it is worth noting the surprisingly well-integrated motor behavior in chronic spinal animals both in locomotion, in posture, and in response to tactile stimuli (9).

ACKNOWLEDGMENT

The author is indebted to H. Hultborn and E. Jankowska for valuable comments on the manuscript.

REFERENCES

1. Bruggencate, G. ten, and Lundberg, A. (1974): Facilitatory interaction in transmission to motoneurones from vestibulospinal fibres and contralateral primary afferents. *Exp. Brain Res.*, 19: 248–270.
2. Burke, R. E., and Rudomin, P. (1975): Spinal neurons and synapses. In: *Handbook of Physiology.* Am. Physiol. Soc. (*in press*).
3. Eccles, J. C. (1964): *The Physiology of Synapses.* Springer-Verlag, Berlin.
4. Engberg, I. (1964): Reflexes to foot muscles in the cat. *Acta Physiol. Scand.*, 62:Suppl. 235.
5. Feldman, A. G., and Orlovsky, G. N. (1975): Activity of interneurones mediating reciprocal Ia inhibition during locomotion. *Brain Res.*, 84:181–194.
6. Forssberg, H., Grillner, S., and Rossignol, S. (1975): Phase dependent reflex reversal during walking in chronic spinal cats. *Brain Res.*, 85: 103–107.
7. Forssberg, H., Grillner, S., and Sjöström, A. (1974): Tactile placing reactions in chronic spinal kittens. *Acta Physiol. Scand.*, 92:114–120.
8. Granit, R. (1970): *The Basis of Motor Control.* Academic Press, London and New York.
9. Grillner, S. (1975): Locomotion in vertebrates — Central mechanisms and reflex interaction. *Physiol. Rev.*, 55:247–304.
10. Grillner, S., and Hongo, T. (1972): Vestibulospinal effects on motoneurones and interneurones in the lumbosacral cord. In: *Basic Aspects of Central Vestibular Mechanisms*, edited by A. Brodal and O. Pompeiano. *Progr. Brain Res.*, 37:244–262.
11. Grillner, S., and Shik, M. L. (1973): On the descending control of the lumbosacral spinal cord from the "mesencephalic locomotor region." *Acta Physiol. Scand.*, 87:320–333.
12. Hongo, T., Jankowska, E., and Lundberg, A. (1969): The rubrospinal tract. II. Facilitation of interneuronal transmission in reflex paths to motoneurones. *Exp. Brain Res.*, 7:365–391.
13. Hongo, T., Jankowska, E., and Lundberg, A. (1972): The rubrospinal tract. IV. Effects on interneurones. *Exp. Brain Res.*, 15:54–78.
14. Houk, J. C., Singer, J. J., and Goldman, M. R. (1970): An evaluation of length and force feedback to soleus muscles of decerebrate cats. *J. Neurophysiol.*, 33:784–811.
15. Hultborn, H. (1972): Convergence on interneurones in the reciprocal Ia inhibitory pathway to motoneurones. *Acta Physiol. Scand.*, 85:Suppl. 375.
16. Hultborn, H., Jankowska, E., and Lindström, S. (1971): Recurrent inhibition from motor axon collaterals of transmission in the Ia inhibitory pathway to motoneurones. *J. Physiol. (Lond.),* 215:591–612.
17. Hultborn, H., Jankowska, E., and Lindström, S. (1971): Recurrent inhibition of interneurones monosynaptically activated from group Ia afferents. *J. Physiol. (Lond.)*, 215:613–636.
18. Hultborn, H., Jankowska, E., and Lindström, S. (1971): Relative contribution from different nerves to recurrent depression of Ia IPSPs in motoneurones. *J. Physiol. (Lond.)*, 215:637–664.
19. Hultborn, H., and Lundberg, A. (1971): Reciprocal inhibition during the stretch reflex. *Acta Physiol. Scand.*, 85:136–138.
20. Illert, M., Lundberg, A., Padel, Y., and Tanaka, R. (1975): Convergence on propriospinal neurones which may mediate disynaptic corticospinal excitation to forelimb motoneurones. *Brain Res.*, 93:530–534.

21. Illert, M., Lundberg, A., and Tanaka, R. (1974): Disynaptic corticospinal effects in forelimb motoneurones in the cat. *Brain Res.*, 75:312–315.

22. Illert, M., Lundberg, A., and Tanaka, R. (1975): Integration in a disynaptic cortico-motoneuronal pathway to the forelimb. *Brain Res.*, 93:525–529.

23. Jankowska, E. (1975): Identification of interneurones interposed in different spinal reflex pathways. In: *Golgi Centennial Symposium Proceedings*, edited by M. Santini, pp. 235–246. Raven Press, New York.

24. Jankowska, E., Lundberg, A., and Stuart, D. (1973): Propriospinal control of last order interneurones of spinal reflex pathways in the cat. *Brain Res.*, 53:227–231.

25. Jankowska, E., and Roberts, W. J. (1972): Synaptic actions of single interneurones mediating reciprocal Ia inhibition of motoneurones. *J. Physiol. (Lond.)*, 222:623–642.

26. Jankowska, E., and Tanaka, R. (1974): Neural mechanism of the disynaptic inhibition evoked in primate spinal motoneurones from the corticospinal tract. *Brain Res.*, 75:163–166.

27. Lindström, S. (1973): Recurrent control from motor axon collaterals of Ia inhibitory pathways in the spinal cord of the cat. *Acta Physiol. Scand.*, Suppl. 392.

28. Lundberg, A. (1966): Integration in the reflex pathway. In: *Muscular Afferents and Motor Control*, Nobel Symposium 1, edited by R. Granit, pp. 275–305. Almqvist & Wiksell, Stockholm.

29. Lundberg, A. (1969): Convergence of excitatory and inhibitory action on interneurones in the spinal cord. In: *The Interneuron*, edited by M. A. B. Brazier, UCLA Forum Med. Sci., No. 11, pp. 231–265. University of California Press, Los Angeles.

30. Lundberg, A. (1970): The excitatory control of the Ia inhibitory pathway. In: *Excitatory Synaptic Mechanisms*, edited by P. Andersen and J. K. S. Jansen, pp. 333–340. Universitetsforlaget, Oslo.

31. Lundberg, A. (1972): The significance of segmental spinal mechanisms in motor control. *Fourth International Biophysics Congress*, Moscow.

32. Lundberg, A., Malmgren, K., and Schomburg, E. D. (1975): Convergence from Ib, cutaneous and joint afferents in reflex pathways to motoneurones. *Brain Res.*, 87:81–84.

33. Lundberg, A., and Voorhoeve, P. (1962): Effects from the pyramidal tract on spinal reflex arcs. *Acta Physiol. Scand.*, 56:201–219.

34. Marsden, C. D., Merton, P. A., and Morton, H. B. (1972): Servo action in human voluntary movement. *Nature*, 238:140–143.

35. Matthews, P. B. C. (1972): *Mammalian Muscle Receptors and Their Central Actions*. Edward Arnold Ltd., London.

36. Schmidt, R. F. (1971): Presynaptic inhibition in the vertebrate central nervous system. *Ergebn. Physiol.*, 63:19–101.

37. Stewart, D. H., Preston, J. B., and Whitlock, D. G. (1968): Spinal pathways mediating motor cortex evoked excitability changes in segmental motoneurons in pyramidal cats. *J. Neurophysiol.*, 31:928–937.

38. Tanaka, R. (1974): Reciprocal Ia inhibition during voluntary movements in man. *Exp. Brain Res.*, 21:529–540.

The Nervous System, Donald B. Tower, Editor-in-Chief. *Vol. 1: The Basic Neurosciences*. Raven Press, New York, 1975.

Membrane Specializations of Ependymal Cells and Astrocytes

M. W. Brightman and T. S. Reese

The venerable inference that glial and ependymal cells influence the exchange of substances between blood, cerebrospinal fluid (CSF), and neurons was initially derived from the spatial position of these nonneuronal cells. Astrocytes, interposed between blood vessels and neurons, were regarded as intermediaries that could deliver substances from blood to nerve cell and vice versa (10). This very relationship was later interpreted as a means of restricting exchanges of certain substances. Dyes and other colloids were supposed to be prevented from reaching the neuron by the perivascular astrocytic sheath (7). The notion that the astrocyte acts as a barrier to smaller substances between blood and neuron persists but remains unproven.

Like the blood space, the CSF compartments are separated from neurons by either astrocytes alone or, as long recognized, by glial cells together with an additional epithelial barrier, the ependyma (25). However, an intercellular flow of proteins, e.g., ferritin (4) and horseradish peroxidase (HRP) (5), can take place between adjacent ependymal cells except in certain regions where contiguous ependymal cells are fastened by tight junctions (21). A similar but limited passage can also take place from the subarachnoid CSF across the subpial or marginal astrocytes that cover neuronal processes at the outer surface of the brain (5). The following discussion concerns the membrane specializations of glial cells. We examine the possibility that these specializations are not merely attachment devices, but may be involved in both the uptake and the cell-to-cell transfer of substances exchanged between the brain and its surrounding fluids.

EPENDYMAL JUNCTIONS

The ventricles of the vertebrate brain are lined by a continuous, simple epithelium, the ependyma. Adjacent ependymal cells are connected by junctions limited in extent (3) and can, therefore, be circumvented by proteins migrating along the lateral extracellular clefts between the cells (4,5). In such experiments, approximately 0.5 ml of a 0.5% solution of HRP is infused at approximately 0.02 ml/min through one lateral ventricle of an anesthetized mouse and allowed to flow out of the cisterna magna through a hole in the atlantooccipital membrane. After 5 to 90 min of perfusion, the HRP is replaced by aldehyde fixative. The fixed brains are then processed for peroxidatic activity (20).

Even after a few minutes of perfusion with peroxidase, the electron-dense reaction product of HRP activity coats not only the membrane of cilia and microvilli belonging to the ependymal cells but also the intercellular clefts (Fig. 1). The extracellular space is abruptly narrowed to a width of approximately 20 to 40 Å where it becomes the median slit of gap junctions (Fig. 1). These discontinuous junctions are bypassed so that protein fills the cleft on either side of them and readily flows into the extracellular clefts of the subependymal neural parenchyma.

The discrete, discoid nature of the gap junctions is best appreciated in replicas of freeze-fractured membranes. The technique includes fixation in aldehydes, cryoprotection in 20% glycerol, and freezing in liquid Freon near liquid nitrogen temperatures. Under vacuum, the specimen is cleaved and a thin film of platinum and carbon is then deposited onto the fractured surface. The underlying brain tissue is digested in Clorox bleach and the freed replica is washed and dried onto electron-microscope grids. Within the cell membrane, the fracture plane is through the hydrophobic midportion; two membrane halves are so revealed. The inner or cytoplasmic half is viewed from its outer aspect toward the cytoplasm and is usually studded with particles (about 70 to 100 Å

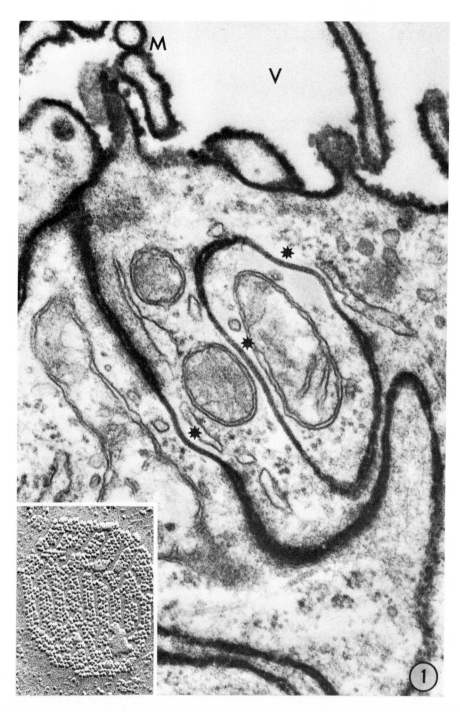

FIG. 1. Horseradish peroxidase crosses the ependyma by moving extracellularly between adjacent cells and around discontinuous gap junctions (asterisks). Peroxidase reaction product coats the lateral and luminal cell membrane including that of the microvilli (M) projecting into the ventricle (V). Free peroxidase has been flushed from the lumen (V) during ventricular perfusion of fixative. Mouse, × 80,000. **Inset:** Freeze-fracture replica of an ependymal gap junction. On the inner half of the cleaved cell membrane, particles about 90 Å wide are frequently aligned in orderly rows. The whole aggregate is discoid and sharply delimited from surrounding particles that are small and randomly dispersed. × 75,000. (From ref. 5.)

wide) thought to be protein (2). The outer half is viewed from its inside toward the extracellular space and usually has fewer particles than the inner half of the plasma membrane.

As in other epithelia, the ependymal gap junctions viewed *en face* appear as discoid aggregates of large particles on the inner half of the cell membrane (Fig. 1, inset). The particles (about 90 Å wide) are often regularly arranged in linear rows with particle-free strips, uniformly wide, between the rows. Complementary pits, into which the particles fit, occur on the outer half of the cell membrane belonging to the contiguous ependymal cell.

The elongated ependymal cells over the median eminence and those over the area postrema are linked by both tight and gap junctions (21). At the tight junction, the outer leaflet of contiguous cell membranes are fused to occlude the extracellular space. When these tight junctions form continuous belts around the perimeter of endothelial cells of cerebral capillaries, choroid plexus epithelial cells, and the special ependyma just mentioned, protein is prevented from moving between blood and extracellular fluid or CSF (5,20).

When the tight and gap junctions are sufficiently large, they are easily recognized as members of a junctional complex in thin, plastic sections. Either junction may be so small, however, that it can only be distinguished unequivocally in freeze-fracture replicas. Thus, between ependymal cells near the median eminence, the usual discoid aggregates of large particles characteristic of gap junctions becomes interlaced with simple ridges that belong to "rudimentary" tight junctions. Directly over the median eminence, these ridges become branched, extensive, and actually touch the border of gap junctions in the junctional complexes of this region. It has been proposed that this regional increase in the complexity of tight junctions imparts the properties of a graded sieve to the wall of the third ventricle; as a result, progressively smaller molecules, as they approach the floor of the third ventricle over the median eminence proper, are impeded from passing between cells (6). Gap and tight junctions, fully formed, are closely interwoven in other epithelia (8).

Cell processes containing small profiles resembling synaptic vesicles lie free within the cerebral ventricles (3). These neuronal-like processes are unmyelinated and make desmosome-like contacts with the luminal surface of ependymal cells (13,17,26). The granular and agranular vesicles within these "endings" do not abut directly against the cell membrane; and the cytoplasmic fuzz at the point of contact is symmetric as at a desmosome rather than asymmetric as at a synaptic contact. The supraependymal neuronal processes may be receptors (17,26) and probably do not transmit impulses to the ependymal cells with which they form contacts. The predominant junction between ependymal cells differs markedly from the desmosome-like contacts. This principal contiguity, the gap junction, unites all ependymal cells throughout the ventricular system and is structurally very similar to the gap junctions between astrocytes.

ASTROCYTIC JUNCTIONS

Astrocytes at the subpial border, around blood vessels, and throughout the neural parenchyma are united by gap junctions; as far as we have been able to ascertain, such cells are never linked by tight junctions in the mammalian brain. The gap junctions, like those between ependymal cells, have a regular curvilinear contour and a median slit (approximately 20–40 Å wide) continuous with the extracellular space (Fig. 2). In the brain of the goldfish *Cassius auratus* the narrowing of the wide extracellular space where it becomes confluent with the junctional gap is extremely abrupt (Fig. 2). These astrocytic junctions are numerous in the synaptic bed of Mauthner's cell within the medulla oblongata of the goldfish (5), in the spinal cord of the cat, and presumably throughout the rest of the brain.

The astrocytic gap junctions of the goldfish medulla are very similar to those of the contacts, presumably electrotonic, between the club endings of VIII nerve axons and the lateral dendrite of the Mauthner cell. The external leaflets of the cell membrane at neuronal gap junctions, however, have periodic indentations more pronounced than those of neighboring astroglial gap junctions. In both neuronal and ependymal gap junctions tangentially cut after being stained by permanganate fixative (23), a polygonal subunit of these junctions is outlined. This unit is similar to that of gap junctions, first recognized by Revel and Karnovsky (22), between liver cells.

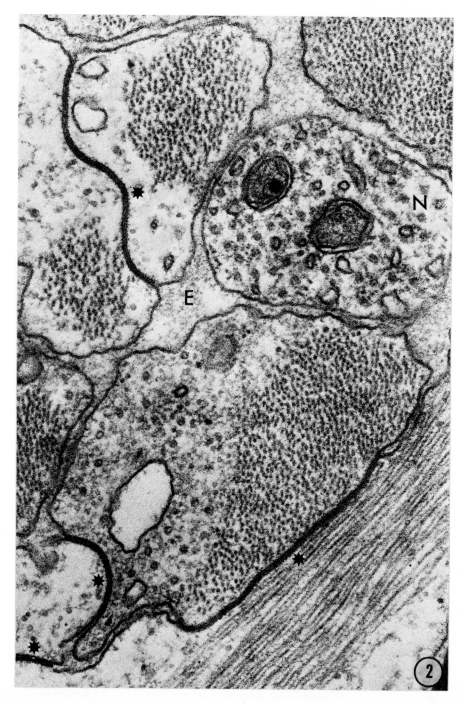

FIG. 2. Contiguous astrocytes containing bundles of 100 Å-thick filaments are interconnected by extensive gap junctions (asterisks). The cytoplasmic fuzz subjacent to the cytoplasmic leaflets of these particular junctions is barely perceptible at this magnification. The wide extracellular spaces (E) between astrocytes and a neuronal process (N) contain a fluffy substance and are abruptly narrowed at every gap junction. Synaptic bed of Mauthner's cell in the medulla oblongata of the goldfish. (From ref. 5.)

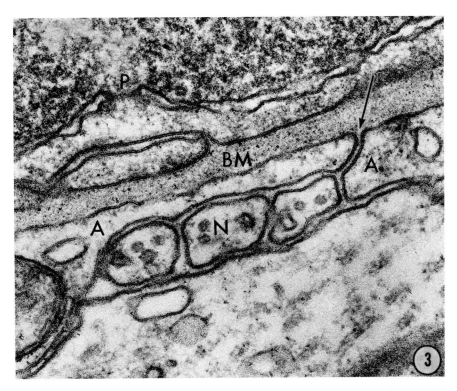

FIG. 3. Thin perivascular astrocytes (A) are separated by a cleft (arrow), the walls of which bear no apparent specialization but which are somewhat more regular in contour and slightly denser than the rest of the astrocytic plasmalemma. The cleft opens into a periendothelial basement membrane (BM) at one end and into a space enclosing small neurites (N) at the other end. *Upper left:* An endothelial cell nucleus with its nuclear membrane perforated by a pore (P). *Lower right:* A broad process, presumably neuronal. Mouse brain, × 107,000. (From ref. 5a.)

In freeze-fracture replicas, astroglial junctions have a subunit comparable to that of ependymal contacts (24).

A second kind of junction is that between extracellular substance and both perivascular and subpial astrocytes. This type of contact, the hemidesmosome, usually consists of a dense, amorphous fuzz extending from the cytoplasmic leaflet of the junctional membrane well into the cytoplasm. Hemidesmosomes are especially well developed in astrocytes bordering vessels larger than capillaries. Whether they face a vessel wall or the pia, astrocytic hemidesmosomes, like those of the arachnoid membrane (16), are always covered by an external basement membrane (Fig. 4).

A third type of contiguity recently recognized appears to be confined to those astrocytes fronting the CSF of the subarachnoid space and, perhaps the cerebral blood (Fig. 3). The evidence for special appositions between perivascular astrocytes is, in part, only suggestive. They are recognized where, despite the absence of cytoplasmic fuzz subjacent to the junction membrane, the leaflets at the apposition are somewhat less undulating than the remainder of the cell membrane. Because of this regular contour, the leaflets of the apposition are usually not grazed but, instead, are more readily sectioned traversely so that the leaflets appear crisper and slightly denser than those in the rest of the cell membrane (3). It is questionable if this apposition forms an actual junction.

The junctional nature of the appositions between marginal astrocytes beneath the pia is more certain (16). Here, although the junctional membranes undulate slightly with respect to each other, there may be focal constrictions of the extracellular cleft. Perhaps more significantly, a fuzzy material abuts the cytoplasmic

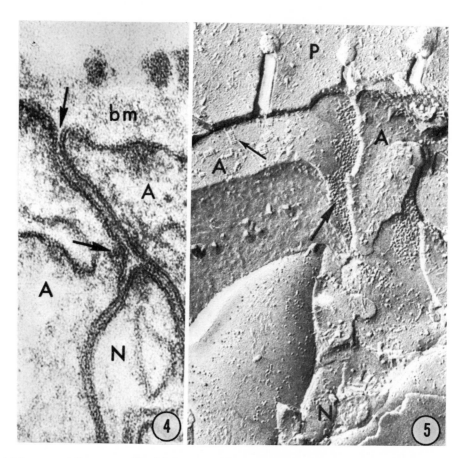

FIG. 4. Mouse cerebellar cortex. Subpial, marginal astrocytes (A) may be connected by junctions where the interglial cleft is narrowed at one end (upper arrow) and bordered by cytoplasmic fuzz at the lower end (lower arrow). The cleft bifurcates to enclose a process (N) that is probably neuronal. Just above the upper letter "A" is cytoplasmic fuzz that may be part of a hemidesmosome. Three collagen fibrils lie in the subarachnoid space above the basement membrane (BM). Specimen tilted about 35°. × 200,000. (From ref. 16.)

FIG. 5. Mouse cerebellar cortex. Freeze-fracture replica of two marginal astrocytes (A) that face each other with neuropil (N) below. The cytoplasmic half of the cell membrane belonging to the left astrocyte contains an aggregate of particles (large arrow) that are smaller than the particles of gap junctions and that occur in the same region as the fuzzy material shown in Fig. 4. The same membrane surface fronting the pia (P) is studded with assemblies consisting of rectangular aggregates of small particles (small arrow). × 90,000. (From ref. 16.)

leaflet bilaterally (Fig. 4). The most convincing evidence that the apposition is junctional, is afforded by freeze-fracture replicas. The inner half of the cleaved, lateral cell membrane at the apposition has an aggregation of particles (Fig. 5). The particles are about as big as those randomly distributed over the cell membrane and smaller than those of gap junctions. However, a distinctive attribute of a junction is, in addition to the size of the constituent particles, the packing of these particles into a well-defined aggregate. The clustering is not as orderly as that of ependymal gap junctions. Like the gap junc-

tion, the subunits of the border junction extend through both halves of the cleaved membrane; regions of the outer half are indented by small, closely packed indentations that are probably complementary to the aggregated particles on the opposite half of the junction membrane (Fig. 7).

ASSEMBLIES

A specialization of both astrocytic (12) and ependymal (6) cell membranes consists of small, particles assembled into tightly packed ortho-

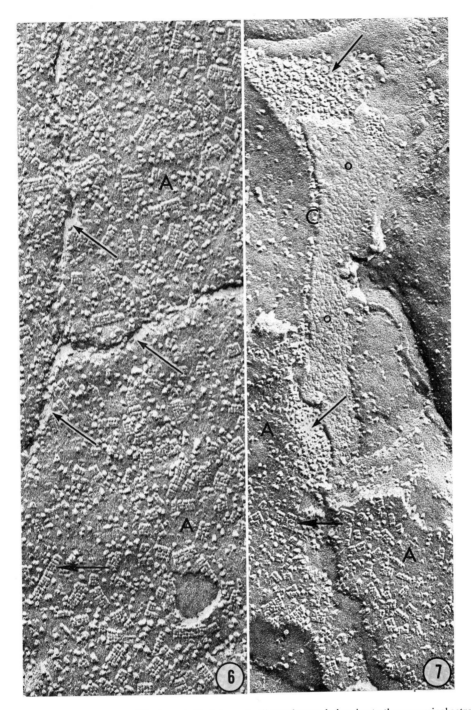

FIG. 6. Mouse cerebellar cortex. The inner half of cleaved cell membranes belonging to three marginal astrocytic end-feet (A) that face the pia is festooned by numerous assemblies (horizontal arrow). At the entrances to three extracellular clefts (diagonal arrow), the cell membranes turn in to form their walls. × 100,000. (From ref. 16.)

FIG. 7. The inner half of the left fractured subpial astrocyte (A), bears aggregates of particles (diagonal arrows) that are smaller than those belonging to gap junctions. The external half of the adjacent astrocyte on the right (A) is covered with minute pits (open circles) which appear to fit over the particles of the left cell. The packing of particles and their symmetrical arrangement on either side of the intercellular cleft (C) suggest that they comprise an astrocytic border junction. The fracture face of the left cell also bears assemblies (horizontal arrow). × 100,000. (From ref. 16.)

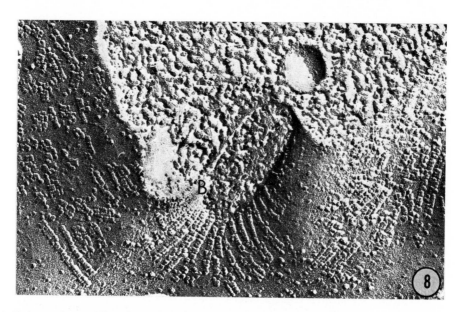

FIG. 8. Orthogonal assemblies of small particles on the inner half of the ependymal cell membrane resemble the assemblies of astrocytes; the ependymal ones form trains near cell branches (B). Mouse ependyma, × 119,000. (From ref. 6.)

gons within the membranes (Figs. 5–8). Invisible in thin plastic sections, the assemblies are readily discernible on the inner half of cleaved cell membranes. Each assembly is rectangular with very closely packed particles or subunits that are approximately 60 to 70 Å wide (Figs. 6 and 7). The counterpart of each assembly pattern on the outer half of the membrane is a rectangular reticule of closely matching grooves on the inner half. Although some assemblies occur in the abluminal part of the cell membrane that does not face the CSF or blood spaces, they are not as numerous there as in the luminal part of the plasma membrane where it fronts the spaces (12). In astrocytes that are satellites of neurons, the number of assemblies is also considerably less than in astrocytes facing fluid compartments (12).

In the ependyma, assemblies that appear to be identical to those in astrocytes also cover parts of the inner half of the plasma membrane (6). There is a tendency for the assemblies to form parallel trains, especially near a branch of the ependymal cell (Fig. 8). Even in these localities, however, the ependymal assemblies are not as numerous or as closely packed as in some regions of the perivascular astrocytes. The assemblies in astrocytes and ependymal

cells may be close to or at some distance from gap or border junctions and do not bear any consistent spatial relationship to junctions.

SOME IMPLICATIONS OF MEMBRANE SPECIALIZATIONS

Gap Junctions

The median slit of gap junctions can be penetrated by lanthanum hydroxide, perfused along with aldehyde fixative and the larger molecule HRP (MW, 40,000), that has been infused into the peripheral blood of the living animal. The greater amount of either colloid, nevertheless, is able to bypass the discontinuous gap junctions. This type of junction may thus impede but does not prevent molecules as large as protein from migrating between the CSF and extracellular fluid of the cerebral parenchyma (4,5).

A major function attributable to the gap junction is electrical and metabolic coupling between both excitable and nonexcitable cells. Recently, the evidence concerning this function was thoroughly reviewed by Bennett (1). A number of substances, when injected either iontophoretically or pneumatically into the cytoplasm of one cell, move into their electrically coupled neighbor. Fluorescein (MW, 330) when injected into one septate axon of crayfish, crosses into a second intact axon that is electrically coupled to the first (18), although larger molecular weight peroxidases cannot (1a). The supposition that the gap junction is the pathway for this cell-to-cell transfer of current and molecules in a variety of cells has been based on coincidence: gap junctions, although possibly only one member of a junctional complex, always unite cells that are electrically coupled. The other types of junction in the complex may vary but the gap junction is consistently present (1,6).

Nevertheless, the role of the gap junction as the electrotonic contact would be more convincing if this type of junction were the only one that joined electrically coupled cells. Conversely, to rule out the participation of tight junctions in electric coupling, we thought at one time that the choroid plexus epithelial cells might provide a good test. According to their fine structure visible in thin plastic sections, only tight junctions appear to link these cells. However, freeze-fracturing has exposed small gap junctions sequestered among the tight junctions (14).

A similar circumstance makes it uncertain whether or not gap junctions are solely responsible for the transfer of metabolites between cultured cells exhibiting metabolic and ionic coupling. Certain genetic strains of fibroblasts are able to incorporate a tritiated purine into their nucleic acids; others cannot. In culture, the metabolically competent cells can pass the labeled purine along to other competent (but not to incompetent) fibroblasts after making physical contact with them. The metabolically coupled cells are, however, connected not only by gap junctions but also by focal tight junctions (9). It is unclear, therefore, whether or not the gap junction provides the exclusive path for cell-to-cell passage of this metabolite.

The structure of the gap junction would be appropriate for such transfer. The sometimes shadowy outlines of the subunits in gap junctions have been visualized with lanthanum tracer in heart, liver (22), and, subsequently, in a variety of excitable and nonexcitable cells (6). Lanthanum hydroxide is small enough to trickle into narrow (10 to 20 Å wide) crevices that are continuous with the rest of the extra-

cellular space. The crevices outline each subunit bridging the median split of the gap junction. When viewed *en face* in thin plastic sections, the outlined subunits appear as a tightly packed honeycomb of hexagons (22), although the irregularity of their shape likens them more to polygons (6).

A comparable pattern had been demonstrated at junctions connecting the electrically coupled club endings and Mauthner's cell dendrite in goldfish brains fixed, and simultaneously stained, by permanganate (23). In the spinal cord of Mormyrid electric fish, electrically interacting dendrites are linked by closely apposed junctions. Originally regarded as tight, these extensive junctions when cut tangentially, appear to have a 90 Å periodicity similar to that of Mauthner's cell junctions (19).

In lanthanum-treated gap junctions, the electron-lucent subunits surrounded by lanthanum-filled crevices contain a faintly dense central core [10 Å or less in width (22)] that is somewhat more prominent in permanganate-fixed neuronal tissue (23). This core has come to be regarded as representing a channel which leads from the cytoplasm of one cell to that of its adjoined neighbor and which is isolated by the wall of the subunit from the extracellular space (1,6). The subunit wall is thus assumed to prevent the leakage of substances within the cytoplasm to the outside and to prevent the entry of extracellular substances, such as lanthanum, into the cell. In frozen-cleaved gap junctions, the 10 Å channels surrounded by each subunit wall, would be well below the resolution of about 30 Å in the replication procedure, but would be expected to course through either the large particles or their equivalent pits. Although the channels figure prominently in schematic representations of gap junctions (14,19), they have yet to be clearly demonstrated in either thin plastic sections or replicas of fractured junctions.

If it is still assumed that, despite the shortcomings discussed above, gap junctions provide a low-resistance pathway for electric current, then we might adduce that some astrocytes are electrically coupled to certain oligodendroglial cells, since such cells have been reported to be united by gap junctions (15). Such an inference has been made for astrocyte-to-astrocyte coupling. It has been suggested that in the optic nerve of the amphibian *Necturus,* electrical interaction between astrocytes may be mediated by gap junctions between these cells (11). In the cat spinal cord, gap junctions have been described between astrocytes and oligodendroglial cells (15). A similar junction between an astrocyte and a dendrite is also illustrated (15). Before accepting the induction that electrotonic coupling occurs between these cell types *in situ,* it would be important to establish whether or not the contacts have a 90 Å periodicity. However, it seems likely that astrocytes throughout the brain are electrically coupled.

Astrocytic Junctions at the Pial Border

The function of the newly recognized contacts between astrocytes that form the subpial marginal border of the brain is unknown. These junctions do not resemble gap junctions in either thin sections or in freeze-fracture replicas. Furthermore, there are no tight junction ridges in the vicinity of the border junctions. If the border junctions are responsible only for the adhesion of contiguous astrocytes, it would be expected from their configuration that the adhesion would not be an occlusive one that would prevent the extracellular flow of small substances. Alternatively, the strategic positioning of these membrane specializations at the sides of clefts would obligate substances crossing the actrocytic border to run a gauntlet between the specializations where the substances could be taken up by the astrocytic membranes at these points.

Assemblies

A purported function of the assemblies on the inner half of cell membranes belonging to astrocytes has been inferred from the position of these cells. Although assemblies lie within the plasma membranes of parenchymal astrocytes that are satellites of neurons, they are considerably more numerous within astrocytic membranes that front the CSF and blood compartments of the brain (12). It has been suggested that, in other organs (e.g., liver and intestine), the cells facing a fluid space also contain assemblies, which, like those of astrocytes, may in some way be implicated in the transport of material (12). The trains of assemblies that oc-

cupy the plasma membranes of ependymal cells would also be expected to be involved in the exchange of substances in and out of the ependymal cells and thus, across the ependyma. However, the epithelial cells of the choroid plexus which actively take up organic anions and other substances contain few, if any, assemblies (6). If the assemblies are involved in the uptake of material from extracellular fluid, this activity may thus be confined to only certain substances or may be associated with different transport systems within the membrane. Alternatively, the presence or absence of assemblies may depend on the functional state of cells since astrocytic assemblies rapidly disappear during circulatory arrest (12a).

Conclusion

We may now restate Golgi's general inference in terms of the recent, but still fragmentary, evidence outlined herein. Perivascular and subpial astrocytes, as well as ependymal cells, have morphological specializations in the form of intercellular junctions and assemblies of membrane particles. Certain substances could be actively incorporated into glial cells through the activity of the assemblies or other specializations. Such substances or their metabolic products could then be transferred from cell to cell across the very gap junctions that are circumvented by other substances moving passively and extracellularly between the cells.

REFERENCES

1. Bennett, M. V. L. (1973): Permeability and structure of electrotonic junctions and intercellular movements of tracers. In: *Intracellular Staining in Neurobiology,* edited by S. D. Kater and C. Nicholson, pp. 115–133. Elsevier, New York.
1a. Bennett, M. V. L., Feder, N., Reese, T. S., and Stewart, W. (1973): Movement during fixation of peridoxases injected into the crayfish septate axon. *J. Gen. Physiol.,* 61:254.
2. Branton, D. (1969): Membrane structure. *Annu. Rev. Plant Physiol.,* 20:209–238.
3. Brightman, M. W., and Palay, S. L. (1963): The fine structure of ependyma in the brain of the rat. *J. Cell Biol.,* 19:415–439.
4. Brightman, M. W. (1965): The distribution within the brain of ferritin injected into cerebrospinal fluid compartments. I. Ependymal distribution. *J. Cell Biol.,* 26:99–123.
5. Brightman, M. W., and Reese, T. S. (1969): Junc-

tions between intimately apposed cell membranes in the vertebrate brain. *J. Cell Biol.,* 40:648–677.

5a. Brightman, M. W. et al. (1970): *J. Neurol. Sci.,* 10:215–239.

6. Brightman, M. W., Prescott, L., and Reese, T. S. (1975): Intercellular junctions in specialized ependyma. In: *Second Conference on Brain-Endocrine Interaction,* S. Karger AG, Switzerland. (*In press.*)

7. Dempsey, E. W., and Wislocki, G. B. (1955): An electron microscopic study of the blood-brain barrier in the rat, employing silver nitrate as a vital stain. *J. Biophys. Biochem. Cytol.,* 1:245–256.

8. Friend, D. S., and Gilula, N. B. (1973): Variations in tight and gap junctions in mammalian tissues. *J. Cell Biol.,* 53:758–776.

9. Gilula, N. B., Reeves, O. R., and Steinbach, A. (1972): Metabolic coupling, ionic coupling and cell contacts. *Nature,* 235:262–265.

10. Golgi, C. (1903): *Opera Omnia,* Vol. 1, p. 40. U. Hoepli, Milano.

11. Kuffler, S. W., and Nicholls, J. G. (1966): The physiology of neuroglial cells. *Ergeb. Physiol.,* 57:1–90.

12. Landis, D. M. D., and Reese, T. S. (1974): Arrays of particles in freeze-fractured astrocytic membranes. *J. Cell Biol.,* 60:316–320.

12a. Landis, D. M. D., and Reese, T. S. (1974): Membrane structure in rapidly frozen freeze-fractured cerebellar cortex. *J. Cell Biol.,* 63:184a.

13. Leonhardt, H., and Backus-Roth, A. (1969): Synapsenartige Kontakte zwischen intraventrikulären Axonendigungen und freien Oberflächen von Eoendymzellen des Kaninchengehirns. *Z. Zellforsch.,* 97:369–376.

14. McNutt, N. S., and Weinstein, R. S. (1972): Membrane ultrastructure at mammalian intercellular junctions. *Prog. Biophys. Mol. Biol.,* 26:45–101.

15. Morales, R., and Duncan, D. (1975): Specialized contacts of astrocytes with astrocytes and with other cell types in the spinal cord of the cat. *Anat. Rec.,* 182:255–265.

16. Nabeshima, S., Reese, T. S., Landis, D. M. D., and Brightman, M. W. (1975): Junctions in the meninges and marginal glia. *J. Comp. Neurol.* (*In press*).

17. Noack, W., and Wolff, J. R. (1971): Axon-like processes within the lateral ventricle of cat (corpus callosum and nucleus caudatus). *Experientia,* 27:172.

18. Pappas, G. D., and Bennett, M. V. L. (1966): Specialized junctions involved in electrical transmission between neurons. *Ann. NY Acad. Sci.,* 137:495–508.

19. Pappas, G. D., Asada, Y., and Bennett, M. V. L. (1971): Morphological correlates of increased coupling resistance at an electrotonic synapse. *J. Cell Biol.,* 49:173–188.

20. Reese, T. S., and Karnovsky, M. J. (1967): Fine structural localization of a blood-brain barrier to exogenous peroxidase. *J. Cell Biol.,* 34:207–217.

21. Reese, T. S., and Brightman, M. W. (1968): Similarity in structure and permeability to peroxidase of epithelia overlying fenestrated cerebral capillaries. *Anat. Rec.,* 160:414.

22. Revel, J. P., and Karnovsky, M. J. (1967): Hexagonal array of subunits in intercellular junctions of the mouse heart and liver. *J. Cell Biol.,* 33:C7–C12.

23. Robertson, J. D. (1963): The occurrence of a subunit pattern in the unit membranes of club endings in Mauthner cell synapses in goldfish brains. *J. Cell Biol.,* 19:201–221.

24. Tani, E., Nishiura, M., and Higashi, N. (1973): Freeze-fracture studies of gap junctions of normal and neoplastic astrocytes. *Acta Neuropathol.,* 26:127–138.

25. Virchow, R. (1863): *Cellular Pathology.* Translated from the second edition by F. Chance, pp. 310–320. J. B. Lippincott and Co., Philadelphia.

26. Westergaard, E. (1972): The fine structure of nerve fibers and endings in the lateral cerebral ventricles of the rat. *J. Comp. Neurol.,* 144:345–354.

The Nervous System, Donald B. Tower, Editor-in-Chief. *Vol. 1: The Basic Neurosciences*. Raven Press, New York, 1975.

Permeability of the Blood-Brain Barrier

William H. Oldendorf

After they are introduced into blood, foreign small molecules distribute throughout the extracellular fluid (ECF) of all tissues within a few seconds. For the past century, it has been recognized that many such foreign molecules do not distribute to the ECF of brain. This easily demonstrated observation has perpetuated the concept of a blood-brain barrier (BBB). During the past decade the anatomical basis of this barrier has been established, and, almost certainly, it is an effect of several unique structural characteristics of brain capillaries (1).

Although the term BBB implies an impermeable barrier between blood and brain, it could be deduced from our fund of general information that the barrier must be permeable to some solutes in blood because some drugs (such as barbiturates) have an instantaneous effect on brain function and because the brain is metabolically active and must receive its substrates from blood. It is clear that the BBB is more correctly thought of as selectively permeable rather than impermeable. The molecular basis of this selectivity is the relative affinity of the plasma solute for the several substances present at the interface at which entry from plasma into brain takes place. These molecular criteria have partially been established and seem to follow a reasonably predictable pattern.

The entire central nervous system (CNS) parenchyma has a BBB except for a few small regions in the floor of the third ventricle surrounding the stalk of the pituitary, an area in the preoptic recess, and the area postrema beneath the floor of the fourth ventricle near the obex. In these regions capillary permeability resembles that found in nonneural tissues.

Although the anatomical location of the BBB and many of its transfer characteristics are known, the teleology of this unique capillary bed is not all clear. Certain advantages to brain suggest themselves, but their relative importance is quite unknown.

An attempt will be made here to define certain of the unique structural features of the BBB, to establish the apparent molecular correlates of its selective permeability and, finally, to speculate upon its teleology and its possible role in brain disease.

STRUCTURE AND FUNCTION OF CAPILLARIES

Multicellular organisms, such as mammals, have each of their cells immersed in an ECF common to them all. One of the apparent objectives of evolution has been to reduce the volume of this fluid (presumably to improve portability) while maintaining its composition optimal for maintaining cell viability. The individual cells seem to have adapted relatively little to a changing environment, but rather they have generated complex communities of specialized cells, each class of which is devoted to optimizing some parameter, or a related group of parameters, of their common ECF. The spectacular success of this evolution is demonstrated in mammals and other vertebrates in which only about 20% of the organism's volume is ECF.

Each of the cells is brought functionally into close apposition to all other cells by virtue of the mixing of the ECF. Since it would require an enormous amount of energy to pump all of the ECF past all of the cells, only about 20% of the ECF (blood plasma) is actually pumped about the body. It is broken up into narrow vessels (capillaries) so numerous that they are within about 100 μm of most extracellular fluid. Since the time of diffusional equilibrium between two points in a liquid diminishes with the inverse square of their separation, diffusional exchange is very rapid between blood plasma in the capillaries and the adjacent more stationary interstitial ECF.

This exchange is possible because of the permeability of the capillary walls to plasma solutes (1,2). For general (nonneural) capillaries, this permeability is based solely upon molecular

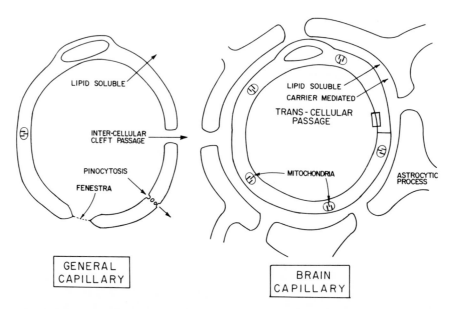

FIG. 1. Diagram of the major differences between a general (nonneural) and a brain capillary. Small molecules can equilibrate between the moving extracellular fluid (plasma) in the general capillary and the stationary extracellular fluid outside by diffusion through the intercellular cleft. The role of fenestrae in exchange is unclear but they are especially prominent in capillary walls passing considerable quantities of fluid such as in renal glomerules and choroid plexus. Pinocytosis is a relatively inefficient mechanism of permeability but probably is independent of molecular size and can pass even very large macromolecules.

In the brain capillary, these nonspecific routes of exchange are missing; the intercellular clefts are sealed shut by tight junctions, there is markedly reduced pinocytosis and no fenestrae. Transcapillary exchange must, accordingly, take place through the cells of the capillary wall, the major barrier of which is the plasma membranes (inner and outer) of the capillary endothelial cells. This transcapillary exchange is selective and is based upon the likelihood of a solute molecule leaving the plasma water and entering the membrane lipid. The small rectangle is the domain shown in Fig. 2. The rat capillary endothelial cell in brain has about five times as many mitochondria as in skeletal muscle, suggesting that this is an energetic cell perhaps carrying out energy-dependent transport of ions.

size. Molecules smaller than about 20,000 to 40,000 MW equilibrate between plasma and the interstitial ECF with half-times of 10 to 30 sec following intravenous injection into small animals (3). Larger molecules, such as albumin (60,000 MW), remain relatively confined to the plasma and are lost from blood with half-times of several hours.

Whereas general capillary permeability is based upon molecular size, BBB permeability is based upon quite different criteria. Figure 1 diagrammatically shows the paths of exchange between general and brain capillaries and their surrounding ECF. General capillaries appear to allow all small molecules to diffuse through clefts between endothelial cells and through fenestrae across which is suspended a rather ill-defined membrane. In addition to these pathways for small molecules, the capillary cell

cytoplasm contains numerous pinocytotic vesicles presumably containing plasma. The role of these vesicles in capillary transport is not well defined, but they probably are the major mechanism by which large molecules traverse the capillary wall. Capillary cell pinocytosis appears to be a mechanism that is inefficient but is independent of molecular size. The electron microscopy of capillary structure has been reviewed by Karnovsky (4).

In brain capillaries these routes of nonspecific exchange are not present. The endothelial cells are fused to each other by tight junctions, no fenestrae are seen, and pinocytosis is virtually absent. To traverse the brain capillary wall a molecule must pass directly through the cells. It must escape from plasma proteins and water, enter the cell membrane, escape into and traverse the cytoplasm, and similarly penetrate the outer

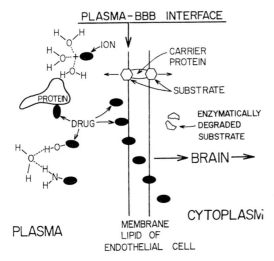

PLASMA-BBB INTERFACE

CARRIER PROTEIN

SUBSTRATE

PROTEIN

DRUG

ENZYMATICALLY DEGRADED SUBSTRATE

⟶ **BRAIN** ⟶

CYTOPLASM

PLASMA

MEMBRANE LIPID OF ENDOTHELIAL CELL

FIG. 2. A diagrammatic representation of the plasma-capillary cell membrane interface located at the small rectangle in Fig. 1. Whether or not a molecule in solution in plasma will penetrate the capillary cell wall (the BBB) depends on the likelihood of its entering the lipid of the cell membrane. This, in turn, will be determined by the relative affinity of the solute molecule for the four major molecular species present at the interface (plasma water, plasma proteins, membrane lipid, and membrane carrier proteins). The black ovals represent drug molecules and the hexagons represent metabolic substrate molecules (such as glucose). If a drug molecule is not attached to plasma protein and has a relative affinity for the membrane lipid and plasma water such that it can leave the water and enter the membrane, then it will diffuse through the BBB.

Affinity for the polar water molecules is high if the drug is ionized or if the nonionized molecule has a considerable hydrogen bond-forming capability. Such molecules remain anchored in the water. Substrate molecules generally are quite polar and enter the membrane by virtue of carrier proteins in the membrane that have high affinities for specific substrate molecular configurations, whereas lipid-mediated entry into the membrane can take place at an essentially infinite number of sites and penetration is accordingly not saturable. Carrier-mediated entry can occur at a finite number of carrier protein receptor sites and is saturable. The water-lipid membrane interface can be simulated *in vitro* by a simple lipid-water two-phase system in which relative lipid versus water affinities can be measured. The separation of drug and substrate molecules here is arbitrary and some drugs may have carrier affinities allowing transport that would not be predicted by relative lipid-water affinity.

By forcing plasma solutes to pass through the endothelial cells, they are brought into contact with cytoplasmic enzymes which may degrade them before they ever actually enter the brain ECF.

membrane. This transcellular passage probably occurs in general capillaries, but is overshadowed by the efficient nonspecific exchange routes.

By virtue of the BBB, the brain ECF does not exchange all small molecules with the general ECF. In addition to a possible site of such exchange at the brain capillary wall, exchange also could take place at the ependymal cell layer of the choroid plexus and at the arachnoid membrane. At all of these sites, nonselective exchange is prevented by formation of tight junctions between adjacent cells. The CNS ECF is, accordingly, in a selective relationship with the general ECF and achieves a greater degree of homeostasis than the remainder of the organism. The arachnoid membrane is probably properly considered the outer boundary of the CNS, because the ECF of the dura immediately outside the arachnoid, having no BBB, freely exchanges with the general ECF.

The ability of a solute in free solution in plasma to penetrate the BBB is based upon the relative affinity for plasma water and the endothelial cell plasma membrane (Fig. 2). Sufficiently lipid-soluble materials penetrate BBB and these presumably can enter the membrane at a nearly infinite number of sites. Certain lipid insoluble substances, such as glucose, also penetrate the BBB, and it is presumed that these enter the membrane because of the presence in the membrane of specialized proteins having high-affinity sites specific for the transported substances. In effect these carrier proteins create a high solubility in the membrane for these substances, much as hemoglobin in red cells greatly increases the solubility of oxygen in blood. Hemoglobin can be thought of as a prototype for the many carrier transport proteins greatly increasing the capacity for their transported substances in the anatomic compartment in which these proteins are present. In the case of membrane transport proteins, this compartment is the cellular membrane.

BBB penetration can thus be lipid-mediated or carrier-mediated. Lipid mediation is of great importance in pharmacology since this apparently is the mechanism by which certain drugs penetrate the BBB (5). Carrier mediation is of particular importance in neurochemistry because metabolic substrates are polar molecules and thus insoluble in lipids. Their BBB penetration is largely dependent on carrier transport. Many substances show penetration caused by slight lipid solubility (a diffusible component) and a superimposed carrier-mediated transport, which increases BBB flux of the solute much beyond that due to simple diffusion.

LIPID MEDIATED PENETRATION

The plasma-endothelial cell membrane interface can be simulated *in vitro* by an oil-water (nonpolar versus polar) two-phase system. If a radiolabeled substance is placed in a bottle, some buffered water and oil (such as olive oil) is added, shaken violently, and allowed to separate to oil and water, the concentration in the oil divided by the concentration in the water is the oil/water partition coefficient (PC). It can be used to estimate the readiness with which the labeled molecule will enter the membrane lipid from water. This relative affinity is crucial rather than the absolute solubility of the labeled molecule in either lipid or water.

The PC of a particular molecule can be predicted by noting the polar characteristics of the molecule (6). If the molecule is ionized, the charge site is anchored to surrounding water molecules because of strong charge-dipole interactions. Nonionized molecules have more or less polar side groups such as —OH- and —NH$_2$-forming hydrogen bonds to water. Other substituted groups form weaker hydrogen bonds. In terms of attachment to water, one ionic site is equivalent to several —OH groups (Fig. 2).

We have measured BBB permeability to over 150 test substances using a rat model in which we rapidly inject a ^{14}C-labeled test substance and ^{3}H-water into the common carotid artery (7,8). The ratio of ^{14}C to ^{3}H in the brain is measured 15 sec later and compared with the same ratio in the injected solution. The ^{3}H-water serves as a highly diffusible reference which nearly completely remains in brain. This test measures the percentage clearance of the test substance during a single brain passage. This percent clearance relative to water has been expressed as a brain uptake index (BUI).

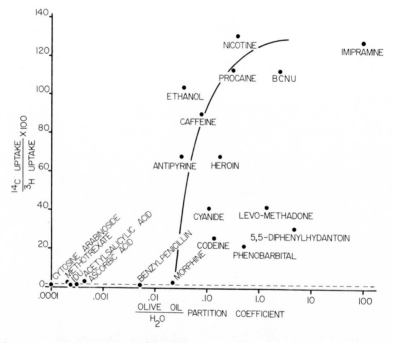

FIG. 3. Showing the relationship between olive oil/water partition coefficient of certain drugs and their percentage clearance by brain during the first circulatory passage after rapid arterial injection. The clearance rises above the 2% method background when the partition coefficient exceeds 0.02 to 0.04. The relatively low uptakes of some drugs may represent immediate plasma protein binding.

We have correlated the olive oil/water PC and BUI of a number of drugs (9). Above a PC of 0.03 to 0.04 substantially all of a drug is cleared by brain during a single microcirculatory passage (Fig. 3). Since the BBB is in effect a continuous biological membrane, this simple procedure, studied in more than 10,000 rats, may have produced more experimental data about this membrane than any other living membrane system.

CARRIER-MEDIATED PENETRATION

Seven independent carrier transport systems have been demonstrated in the BBB. They are for glucose (and certain other hexoses), short-chain monocarboxylic acids, certain neutral amino acids, basic amino acids, certain purines, and certain nucleosides. By injecting unlabeled substances mixed with the labeled water reference and test substance, saturation kinetics can be established, and it can be shown that each of these carriers (except those for amino acids) is approximately half-saturated in the presence of normal blood concentrations of their transported substances (10). The neutral and basic amino acid carriers are considerably more than half-saturated and show affinities for most of the alpha-amino acids in their class (Table 1).

TABLE 1. *Affinity constants and stereospecificity of BBB carriers[a]*

Carrier systems and metabolites	Usual rat plasma conc. (mM)[b]	$K_m(L)$ (mM)	$K_m(D)$ (mM)	$\dfrac{K_m(D)}{K_m(L)}$
Neutral amino acid carrier				
Methionine	0.07	0.19	0.66	3.5
Leucine	0.17	0.15	0.42	2.8
Phenylalanine	0.08	0.12	0.73	6
Tyrosine	0.07	0.16	2.5	16
Histidine	0.08	0.28	9	32
Tryptophan	0.07	0.19	25	>100
DOPA	–	0.44	>25	>100
Isoleucine	0.10	0.33	>25	>100
Valine	0.20	0.63	>25	>100
Threonine	0.30	0.73	>25	>100
Basic amino acid carrier				
Arginine	0.20	0.09	1.8	20
Ornithine	0.09	0.23	–	–
Lysine	0.40	0.10	>25	>100
Carboxylic acid carrier				
Pyruvic	0.14	0.38[c]	–	–
Lactic	1.1	1.9	Immeasurably high	>100
Hexose carrier				
Glucose	6.3	Immeasurably high	9.0	0
Mannose	–	–	21	–
Galactose	–	–	40	–
Fructose	0.4	–	Immeasurably high	–

[a] Affinity constants of some of the BBB carriers as determined by the carotid-diffusible reference method. Half-saturation (K_m) was determined by including serially increasing concentrations of unlabeled substance in the injectate and noting the inhibitory effect on the brain uptake of the radiolabeled species. Using this method the amino acid carriers appear to be substantially more than half-saturated in the presence of normal plasma amino acid concentrations.

[b] This refers to the concentrations of the L-form.

[c] Pyruvate is listed here although it does not have an asymmetric center.

The ratio of affinities for the L and D enantiomers is an index of stereospecificity. In the case of amino acids a high ratio indicates high stereospecificity whereas for glucose the low number indicates high stereospecificity.

These transport carriers are stereospecific. In the case of the amino acids, this is variable and, although some D-amino acid affinities can be measured, the L-form is always preferred (11).

ACTIVE TRANSPORT BY BBB

Carrier-mediated BBB permeability to glucose and other metabolic substrates probably is bidirectional (in and out of brain). If the brain is utilizing them, a concentration gradient will be maintained between plasma and brain and no energy-dependent mechanism would be needed to pump them since simple diffusion would tend to abolish this gradient if the BBB were permeable. There are substantial ionic gradients across the BBB, which are not due to brain utilization. Potassium, for example, is about 40% lower in brain ECF than in plasma. This gradient probably is maintained by energy-dependent transport out of CNS. Although the regulation of CNS ECF potassium probably is an interaction of choroid plexus, glia, and BBB, the BBB participation must be active in this regulation because of the large concentration gradient existing across it. That the brain capillary carries out some substantial energy-dependent transport is suggested by our unpublished observation that rat cerebellar capillary endothelial cells contain five times as many mitochondria as similar cells in skeletal muscle (Fig. 1). The greater work capacity of the brain capillary suggested by this observation could be directed to unidirectional ion transport. It is also possible that it is related to the maintenance of the unique brain capillary structural features creating the BBB.

Certain of the acidic end products of brain monoamines may also be transported out of brain since probenecid (which competes with organic anion transport) results in an elevation of their concentration in cerebrospinal fluid (CSF) and brain. Although this excretion from brain has been suggested to be a function of choroid plexus, it is unlikely that choroidal excretion is important in humans since the organic anions would have to be brought from all parts of brain to the choroid plexus by circulating CSF. Cisternography has shown that cortical subarachnoid CSF does not circulate back into the ventricles. It would be more reasonable to suggest this excretion is a function of each brain region's capillaries (12).

TELEOLOGY OF BBB

There undoubtedly are many reasons for the BBB, but the most widely held belief is that it protects the brain from potentially neurotoxic substances in blood. It undoubtedly performs this function, but a more inclusive generalization would be to state that the BBB facilitates the optimization of the fluid environment of the brain cells by providing a second order of stabilization beyond the homeostatic mechanisms stabilizing the general ECF. Protection from toxic polar substances in blood probably is only a part of this more general function.

Serum bilirubin is an example of a blood-borne substance kept out of brain. Although bilirubin is itself lipid-soluble and thus readily enters brain, it is held out of free solution in plasma by being bound to plasma protein (13). The protein-bilirubin complex is polar and does not penetrate the BBB. Even severely icteric patients show very little staining of the brain or CSF. Bilirubin is neurotoxic when it does get into brain in appreciable quantities, and presumably it is the cause of kernicterus, the neurological disease of early infancy in which visible brain staining occurs, particularly in certain of the extrapyramidal nuclei, in the presence of neonatal jaundice. This staining most likely is due to inadequate plasma protein complexing of bilirubin in the newborn.

In a natural setting, very few significantly lipid-soluble substances appear in blood. Ethanol from intestinal fermentation can make some animals intoxicated but the lack of a BBB for lipid-soluble solutes probably has not significantly affected survival. The common drugs taken for their mental effects (ethanol, caffeine, amphetamine, nicotine, marijuana, and heroin) all have sufficient lipid affinity that they immediately penetrate the BBB (Fig. 3). Ideally, a drug taken for a brief mental effect should have a PC high enough to allow rapid BBB penetration but low enough to prevent significant depot fat accumulation. Ethanol has this ideal PC of about 0.04. This correlates with the ease with which even obese people can become heavily intoxicated with ethanol and yet sober up quickly.

In the design of drugs for transient mental effects, extreme lipid solubility is undesirable. The extreme PC of tetrahydrocannabinol (> 5,000) probably correlates with its unfortunately prolonged minor effects. A drug with such an extremely high affinity for lipid could exhibit significant sequestration in lung lipid, perhaps in lung surfactant, particularly when inhaled. An optimum PC for a short-acting psychotropic drug probably is between about 0.1 and 1.0.

Many drugs (such as most antibiotics) are kept out of the brain by the BBB. It is sometimes possible to make such molecules reversibly nonpolar thereby allowing passage into brain. If the brain has the enzymatic mechanism for restoring the polarity of the molecule to its original form, the drug has been made to penetrate the BBB. This process of latentiation is utilized in making heroin by acetylating the two hydroxyl groups of morphine. Heroin, being much more lipid soluble by virtue of the shielding of these two polar sites, readily penetrates the BBB, whereas morphine does not (14). Once in brain the heroin is deacetylated back to the relatively polar morphine, which cannot readily leak back out of brain. It probably is in the form of morphine that heroin is pharmacologically active (15). By making morphine transiently lipid soluble a considerable increase in therapeutic efficacy can be realized and heroin is about five times more effective, on a molar basis, than is morphine. Antibiotics and other therapeutic agents probably can similarly be made to penetrate the BBB by this mechanism (16).

The rapid entry of heroin into brain following intravenous injection may be correlated with its apparently greater addictive properties relative to morphine. The immediacy of brain entry may more strongly reinforce the association between the act of administration and the drug's central effects.

Once a lipid-soluble molecule is introduced into the body, the usual effect of metabolism is to render the molecule more polar. This increasing polarity can be thought of as a protective mechanism on the part of the body since the organism has no ability to confine or otherwise transport lipid-soluble substances that readily diffuse through all cell membranes and tissue compartments. Only when rendered polar can biological membranes efficiently transport these substances.

The ability of BBB to obstruct passage of some substances is enhanced by enzymatic mechanisms in the cytoplasm of the brain capillary endothelial cells. These cells contain monoamine oxidase (MAO) (17), which probably serves to restrict the passage of biogenic amines in or out of brain. This MAO activity may be located on the surface of the mitochondria in brain capillary cells. One could readily imagine a burst of systemic norepinephrine upon jumping into cold water. Entrance of this norepinephrine into brain could substantially alter its function and isolation of brain from such systemic perturbations probably is a significant effect of the BBB. This enzymatic barrier probably enhances simple physical exclusion of the BBB. DOPA-decarboxylase, and other enzymes are also present in these cells.

TELEOLOGY OF CARRIER-MEDIATED TRANSPORT

The BBB behaves as though all substances in plasma are prevented from entering brain but specific classes of molecules are, in effect, issued passes to allow entry. The advantages to brain are not entirely evident, but such an arrangement could provide considerable stabilization of the flux into brain of metabolic substrates such as glucose. To be most effective as a control mechanism, such a carrier transport system should be about half-saturated in the presence of the usual concentration of substrate to which the carrier protein is exposed. This is the case with several of the BBB carriers, including the glucose carrier. The flux of glucose into brain is rendered relatively constant in the event of hyper- or hypoglycemia. With hyperglycemia, the carrier is oversaturated and efficiency of transport is diminished. With hypoglycemia the carrier is undersaturated and transport efficiency is increased.

A similar situation probably occurs when there are bursts of systemic lactate from muscle cells in response to intense muscular exertion. The short-chain monocarboxylic acid carrier is ordinarily about half-saturated, and oversaturation in the presence of high blood lactate would prevent an excessive flux into brain where acid-base balance could be disturbed, as a result.

The precursors of the recognized central neurotransmitters (glucose, DOPA, histidine, tryptophan) readily penetrate the BBB by virtue of various carrier systems. The transmitters themselves are polar substances without affinity for any of the carriers. As a result, they are trapped in the brain by the BBB. In searching for new transmitter substances, this inability to penetrate the BBB might be used as a criterion since ready flux of a central transmitter agent out of the brain would be uneconomical, requiring large amounts of transmitter to be formed. The brain presumably seeks to keep its transmitters to some degree localized to the region in which they are released. Any transmitters lost to blood plasma through a permeable capillary bed would reappear in all regions of brain upon recirculation. It therefore seems prudent for the brain to use as transmitters those substances it can make from accessible precursors and which will not quickly be lost from brain to plasma. The plasma would act as a sink for those substances that were in higher concentration in brain ECF and to which the BBB was permeable. In pathological lesions in which the BBB has failed, and the capillaries are nonspecifically permeable, the plasma could become an effective regional sink for ECF transmitters thereby changing local neural responsivity.

POSSIBLE ROLE OF BBB IN BRAIN DISEASE

The role of BBB in human disease is unclear because so little is known about it. It seems reasonable to suggest, however, that this unique capillary bed, with its dependence on specific carrier systems, does become disarranged and plays a part in some CNS pathophysiology.

The BBB is lost in virtually all lesions in which normal histology is significantly altered (18). The brain capillary bed functionally comes to resemble nonneural capillaries. The BBB behaves as though it is maintained as a function of normal brain and any serious pathophysiology results in a loss of this function; the brain no longer keeps its capillaries shut off.

The radioisotope brain scan atraumatically maps the distribution of large human brain lesions having an abnormally permeable BBB. The technique is designed to show regional hot spots and does not measure overall BBB permeability. Despite its limitations, the brain scan is very useful clinically and constitutes about $\frac{1}{3}$ of the work load of most nuclear medicine departments. If the technique were more absolutely quantitative, general abnormalities of BBB might be demonstrated in many brain

and systemic diseases. As long as the technique aims solely at detecting focal pathology, we may be discarding much clinically useful information. Radioisotope brain scanning is handicapped by an inherently poor spatial resolution that seems likely to remain above about 10 mm because of several physical factors. When nonradioactive water-soluble iodinated contrast media are used with the newer computerized transmission section radiography (the EMI-scan), BBB defects are defined with a spatial resolution of 2 to 3 mm. In this case the contrast medium leaks through the abnormally permeable BBB in a manner similar to the radionuclide in the isotope scan but provides a substantially sharper picture and correspondingly more information about specific lesions.

The brain is dependent on the BBB carrier systems to exchange its metabolites with plasma. If we were somehow to inactivate the BBB glucose carrier, for example, within a few minutes the brain would show signs of glucose deprivation and become irreversibly damaged. Because this carrier makes the BBB freely permeable to glucose, the CSF glucose is about $\frac{2}{3}$ of plasma glucose and presumably would equal plasma if the brain were not so actively consuming it. It has been suggested that one of the factors responsible for the reduction of CSF glucose in meningitis is the failure of the BBB glucose carrier (19). The glucose carrier can be denatured *in vivo* by carotid injection of $HgCl_2$ (20), and it would be interesting to assess the long-term effect on brain function of such an induced isolated lesion.

In some pathological lesions it is conceivable that the BBB glucose carrier is regionally inactivated, thereby creating what would be, in effect, a regional hypoglycemia. This could be quite localized since the diffusion of glucose into a lesion from surrounding healthy brain would be inadequate because of the limited diffusional flux which can take place between two points separated by even a few millimeters.

The two major BBB amino acid transport systems (for neutral and for basic amino acids) each show affinities for most of the alpha amino acids within their category. The individual affinities are such that, in the presence of the normal complement of plasma free amino acids, the carriers are substantially more than half-saturated. As a result the flux of some amino acids into brain is probably rate limited by the BBB. This may not be a major problem in the mature brain where the flux required is small. In the infant human brain, with its higher rate of protein synthesis, this limitation of amino acid influx may be important. In phenylketonuria, in which there is a very high blood phenylalanine level, this amino acid (which has the highest affinity for the neutral amino acid carrier) may so fully occupy the carrier transport sites that the flux of other neutral amino acids into brain is impaired and the developing brain is, in effect, subjected to an amino acid deficiency comparable to that found with a diet inadequate in protein (21). It can be demonstrated that the brain uptake of ^{75}Se-selenomethionine (a neutral amino acid) is measurably impaired in humans suffering from phenylketonuria (22). In animals this impaired uptake caused by high blood phenylalanine can be shown to effect only the neutral amino acids and to spare the basic amino acids (23). If this transport mechanism saturation is indeed an important cause of the mental retardation in phenylketonuria, the excessive occupation of the neutral amino acid carrier by phenylalanine would be somewhat analogous to the occupation by carbon monoxide of hemoglobin sites normally carrying oxygen.

It is interesting to speculate on how much of a limitation on brain development is imposed by the heavily saturated BBB amino acid carriers in the normal infant and what interactions take place in disease between various amino acids using the same carrier system. There is evidence that the rate of production of brain serotonin is limited by the flux of tryptophan through the BBB (24). Tryptophan is a neutral alpha amino acid that enters brain by virtue of the neutral amino acid carrier system. Since this carrier is so heavily saturated, the flux of tryptophan is sensitive not only to changes in serum tryptophan but to the other neutral amino acids (25). Changes in dietary intake may, through this mechanism, result in changes in brain serotonin content offering a mechanism for the mood changes commonly seen after eating.

There is an independent BBB transport system for short-chain monocarboxylic acids which increases BBB permeability to lactate, pyruvate, *b*-hydroxybutyrate, and several related acids (26). Since jugular venous lactate is about 5% higher than arterial lactate, it is reasonable to suggest that this carrier normally functions to facilitate loss of lactate from brain where its production exceeds the capacity of the brain's enzymatic mechanism for metabolizing it. Lactate can diffuse measurably through the BBB without its carrier mechanism, but at ordinary blood lactate levels the rate of exchange is some three to five times greater by virtue of the carrier. This carrier appears to be about half-saturated in the presence of normal blood and brain levels of pyruvate and lactate. When brain becomes acutely hypoperfused, the brain lactate rises within 3 to 5 min from its normal 2 mM to about 15 mM. This parallels an accumulation of CO_2, and these two factors are largely responsible for the drop in brain pH in hypoperfusion. The mechanisms involved have been well-studied (27), but its precise pathophysiology remains unknown. Looking at the problem teleologically, the cardinal importance of a stable pH to brain is suggested by the observation that it is apparently the regional extracellular pH that is the major parameter used by the brain to adjust regional blood flow (28).

Based upon the normal brain scan seen during the first few days after cortical infarction, the BBB seems quite resistant to acute ischemia. The scan commonly becomes positive after about 1 week. During this first week, the capillary bed in the lesion does not become nonspecifically leaky and blood-brain metabolic exchange must depend on the BBB carrier system. The BBB lactate carrier, which seems to have adapted to normal brain lactate concentration, probably becomes oversaturated in the presence of the high ischemic brain lactate and can no longer effectively transport this lactate out of brain. If this sequence of speculations is shown to be real, the brain's exceptional vulnerability to ischemia may, in part, be a price we pay for the BBB.

Included in Fig. 1 is the indication that there are about five times as many mitochondria in the brain capillary endothelial cells as in corresponding nonneural cells. This is based upon unpublished electron microscopic mitochondrial counts in rat cerebellar capillaries versus skeletal muscle capillaries. This observation suggests that the metabolic work capacity of the brain capillary endothelial cell is several times greater than in general capillaries. We can only speculate about what work is being carried out by the BBB that is not being performed by the general capillary. There are considerable ionic concentration gradients between brain ECF and plasma (29). Potassium, for example, is considerably lower in brain ECF as judged by its concentration in CSF. This lower neuronal environmental potassium must result in a hyperpolarization and stabilization of the neuronal membrane. These gradients are present across the wall of the brain capillary. To maintain such gradients must consume energy, and it may be this work that correlates with the BBB's greater number of mitochondria.

If it is of great importance for the BBB to be able to actively pump ions up concentration gradients, then this may constitute an important clue in unraveling the teleology of the BBB. It would be impossible to maintain a concentration gradient between one side and the other of a sheet of cells if the junctions between the cells leaked freely. Such nonspecific leakage paths would abolish any local concentration gradients by diffusional flux. If uphill transport were to take place with any degree of efficiency, nonspecific leakage paths must be sealed. This could well be a major reason for having a unique brain capillary bed, which is fundamentally impermeable to all water-soluble substances. Carrier-mediated BBB transport could be looked upon as a way of living with this impermeability in the face of the brain's considerable requirements for metabolite exchange with blood.

ACKNOWLEDGMENTS

Many helpful suggestions were provided by Mrs. Stella Z. Oldendorf. Technical assistance was provided by Mrs. Shigeyo Hyman and Mr. Leon Braun. Support was in part provided by U.S. Public Health Service Grant NS8711 from the National Institute of Neurological Diseases and Stroke and the Veterans Administration Los Angeles.

REFERENCES

1. Crone, C., and Lassen, N. (1970): *Capillary Permeability*. Academic Press, New York.
2. Landis, E. M., and Pappenheimer, J. R. (1963): Exchange of substances through the capillary walls. In: *Handbook of Physiology, Circulation, Vol. II,* edited by W. F. Hamilton, pp. 961–1074. American Physiology Society, Washington, D.C.
3. Oldendorf, W. H., and Kitano, M. (1972): The early disappearance of extracellular tracers from plasma after intravenous injection. *Proc. Soc. Exp. Biol. Med.,* 141:940–943.
4. Karnovsky, M. J. (1967): The ultrastructural basis of capillary permeability studied with peroxidase as a tracer. *J. Cell. Biol.,* 35:213–236.
5. Stein, W. D. (1967): *The Movement of Molecules Across Cell Membranes.* Academic Press, New York.
6. Oldendorf, W. H. (1974): Blood-brain barrier permeability to drugs. *Ann. Rev. Pharmacol.,* 14:239–248.
7. Oldendorf, W. H. (1970): Measurement of brain uptake of radiolabeled substances using a tritiated water internal standard. *Brain Res.,* 24:372–376.
8. Oldendorf, W. H. (1971): Brain uptake of radiolabeled and amino acids, amines, and hexoses after arterial injection. *Am. J. Physiol.,* 221:1629–1639.
9. Oldendorf, W. H. (1974): Lipid solubility and drug penetration of the blood-brain barrier. *Proc. Soc. Exp. Med. Biol.,* 147:813–816.
10. Pappenheimer, J. R., and Setchell, B. P. (1973): Cerebral glucose transport and oxygen consumption in sheep and rabbits. *J. Physiol. (Lond.),* 233:529–551.
11. Oldendorf, W. H. (1973): Stereospecificity of blood-brain barrier permeability to amino acids. *Am. J. Physiol.,* 224:967–969.
12. Wolfson, L. I., Katzman, R., and Escriva, A. (1974): Clearance of amine metabolites from the cerebrospinal fluid: The brain as a "sink." *Neurology,* 24:772–779.
13. Diamond, I. (1969): Bilirubin binding and kernicterus. *Adv. Pediatr.,* 16:99–119.
14. Oldendorf, W. H., Hyman, S., Braun, L., and Oldendorf, S. Z. (1972): Blood-brain barrier: Penetration of morphine, codeine, heroin, and methadone after arterial injection. *Science,* 178:984–988.
15. Way, E. L. (1968): Distribution and metabolism of morphine and its surrogates. In: *Addictive States,* edited by A. Wickler, pp. 13–31. Williams and Wilkins, Baltimore.
16. Oldendorf, W. H. (1974): Blood-brain permeability to drugs. *Ann. Rev. Pharmacol.,* 14:239–248.
17. Bertler, A., Falck, B., Owman, C. H., and Rosengren, E. (1966): The localization of monoaminergic blood-brain barrier mechanisms. *Pharmacol. Rev.,* 18:369–385.
18. Broman, T. (1949): *The Permeability of the Cerebrospinal Vessels in Normal and Pathological Conditions.* Munksgaard, Copenhagen.
19. Prockop, L. D., and Fishman, R. A. (1968): Experimental pneumococcal meningitis. Permeability changes influencing the concentration of sugars and macromolecules in cerebrospinal fluid. *Arch Neurol.,* 19:449–463.
20. Steinwall, O., and Klatzo, I. (1966): Selective

vulnerability of the blood-brain barrier in chemically induced lesions. *J. Neuropathol. Exp. Neurol.*, 25:542–559.

21. Udenfriend, S. (1961): Phenylketonuria. *Am. J. Clin. Nutr.*, 9:691–694.

22. Oldendorf, W. H. (1973): Saturation of blood-brain barrier transport of amino acids in phenylketonuris. *Arch. Neurol.*, 28:45–48.

23. Oldendorf, W. H., Sisson, W. B., Mehta, A., and Treciokas, L. (1971): Brain uptake of Selenomethionine Se-75: I. Effects of elevated blood levels of methionine and phenylalanine. *Arch. Neurol.*, 24:423–430.

24. Fernstrom, J. D., and Wurtman, R. J. (1971): Brain serotonin content: Physiological dependence on plasma tryptophan levels. *Science*, 173:149–151.

25. Fernstrom, J. D., and Wurtman, R. J. (1972): Brain serotonin content: Physiological regulation by plasma neutral amino acids. *Science*, 178: 414–416.

26. Oldendorf, W. H. (1973): Carrier-mediated blood-brain barrier transport of short-chain monocarboxylic organic acids. *Am.J. Physiol.*, 1450–1453.

27. MacMillan, V., and Siesjo, B. K. (1972): Cerebral energy metabolism. In: *Scientific Foundations of Neurology*, pp. 21–32. F. A. Davis Co., Philadelphia.

28. Siesjo, B. K., and Sorensen, S. C. (1971): *Ion Homeostasis of the Brain*. Academic Press, New York.

29. Katzman, R., and Pappius, H. M. (1973): *Brain Electrolytes and Fluid Metabolism*. Williams and Wilkins, Baltimore.

The Nervous System, Donald B. Tower, Editor-in-Chief. *Vol. 1: The Basic Neurosciences.* Raven Press, New York, 1975.

Cerebrospinal Fluid Physiology: Role of Secretory and Mediated Transport Systems

Robert Katzman

Neurologists and neurosurgeons have long been aware of the importance of the cerebrospinal fluid (CSF) both in diagnostic neuroradiology and as a source of accessible fluid for the diagnosis of neurological disorders. During the past twenty years, physiologists and biochemists have become aware of the importance of the CSF as a counterpart of the brain extracellular fluid, the internal environment of the brain.

The CSF is a unique internal body fluid with a concentration of proteins and other organic molecules dramatically lower than in other internal body fluids. In fact, the CSF is primarily, but not exclusively, a mixed electrolyte solution which differs in its electrolyte composition from the serum from which it is derived, but probably closely reflects the electrolyte composition of the brain extracellular fluid. It has become apparent that the blood-CSF barrier, secretory processes at the choroid plexus, and mediated transport systems important in clearing the CSF of unwanted metabolites are responsible for the unique chemical composition of CSF.

CSF PHYSIOLOGY *IN VIVO*

A major advance in the understanding of CSF physiology was provided by the elegant application of methods used in renal and other areas of physiology by Pappenheimer and his associates (1–3). Their technique involved the steady-state perfusion of the ventriculocisternal system using an artificial CSF perfused into a lateral ventricle at a constant infusion rate and under constant pressure conditions with the effluent removed at the cisterna magna. To measure the rate of CSF formation, a tracer molecule, such as inulin, which does not readily diffuse into the adjacent brain parenchyma, is added to the perfusate. Then, the rate of CSF

formation can be calculated by determining the dilution of the tracer by newly formed CSF, once a steady-state condition is obtained. Similarly, by adding radioactively labeled molecules of interest to the perfusate, the removal or clearance of molecules from CSF can be determined by the degree to which such molecules are removed in excess of the clearance of the nondiffusible inert tracer itself, the latter clearance reflecting the rate of absorption of CSF as a bulk fluid. Also, such techniques can be used to note the rate of appearance of substances in CSF when radioactive tracers are injected intravenously. This method has been extended to perfusions of other portions of the CSF spaces, including the spinal and cerebral subarachnoid spaces. A detailed review of these various applications is contained in the monographs of Davson (4) and Katzman and Pappius (5).

Physiological measurements made with the steady-state perfusion techniques must be carried out with care. The method is deceptively easy, and misinterpretations can easily arise. It is essential that a true steady state be obtained. The CSF spaces are large compared, for example, to the volume of fluid directly involved in the ventriculocisternal perfusions. If one is measuring CSF formation or absorption utilizing a ventriculocisternal perfusion, the tracer must have distributed throughout the entire volume of CSF, as shown by Pappenheimer et al. (3). Moreover, the tracer must be an inert substance of sufficient molecular weight to minimize diffusion and sufficiently lipophobic that it will not readily cross membranes adjacent to the CSF spaces. The most commonly used tracer is inulin, which, if used as a purified molecule, fits the criteria very well. However, inulin, a polymer of fructose with a molecular weight of about 5,600, is sometimes unstable and may be partially degraded with some release of fructose which can be metabolized. Moreover, radioactively labeled inulin, either as a ^{14}C-carboxy or as tritiated inulin, is sometimes degraded during storage; therefore, its purity must be established prior to use. Other molecules, such as the high molecular weight, blue dextran, and radioactively labeled serum albumin, have been used as tracers.

Although the steady-state ventriculocisternal perfusion technique provided the methodology underlying several specific findings which we will discuss below, certain general features of the system were immediately identified by Pappenheimer and his associates. These investigators varied the pressure of the system by raising or lowering the cisternal outflow cannula and demonstrated that the rate of CSF formation was largely independent of CSF pressure, although there was a very slight decrease in the rate of formation at high pressures. This independence of formation rate and CSF pressure strongly supports the concept that CSF is secreted and not a simple dialysate of serum. In contrast, the rate of CSF absorption is directly proportional to the pressure and appears to represent a physical process. Whereas the secretion of CSF is believed to take place at the choroid plexus and at other extrachoroidal sites, the absorption of CSF occurs at arachnoid villi present near sagittal and other sinuses, along nerve roots, and along nerve root sheaths. Some questions have been recently raised as to the possibility of CSF absorption in the Virchow–Robin spaces over the cerebral cortex, but these have not yet been resolved. The fact that CSF absorption is pressure dependent, however, suggests the existence of a one-way valvular system. If, as proposed, the arachnoid villi serve as such valves (6), the morphological basis of this action is not yet well understood. It should be noted that in experimental animals such as the dog, a major route of CSF egress may occur via the olfactory and optic nerves.

FORMATION OF CSF: SECRETION BY CHOROID PLEXUS

That the richly vascular choroid plexus may act as a secretory organ was postulated in the 1850s by pioneer anatomists describing the ventricular and subarachnoid systems, including Faivre and Luschka. Although subsequent histological studies suggested that the choroidal epithelium contained secretory cells, and several neurosurgeons observed the formation of fluid droplets on the surface of the exposed choroid plexus in man, it remained for deRougemont et al. (7) in 1960 to demonstrate conclusively that CSF was secreted by the choroid plexus. Their demonstration depended upon the ability to carry out an accurate electrolyte analysis in droplets of fluid removed from the surface of the choroid plexus in animals in which the lateral ventricle had been unroofed and filled with a light oil. The fluid droplets which formed on the surface of the choroid plexus were removed by a micropipette and found to have the ionic constitution of CSF rather than that of an ultrafiltrate of plasma. Subsequently, Welch (8) confirmed the production of CSF by choroid plexus by demonstrating that the change in hematocrit in the blood flowing through the choroid plexus in experimental animals could be accounted for by the rate of secretion of CSF.

In every mammalian species studied, acetazolamide, a drug that inhibits the enzyme carbonic anhydrase, has been found to reduce the rate of CSF formation by about 40% as measured by the ventriculocisternal perfusion technique. This effect of acetazolamide has been utilized in the treatment of hydrocephalus in certain patients, although the drug has not been found to be as effective in such conditions as had been hoped. Of significance in terms of the physiology, however, was the fact that acetazolamide not only reduced the rate of total CSF formation as measured by the ventriculocisternal perfusion technique, but also reduced production of choroid plexus fluid as measured by the use of choroid plexus hematocrit (8) or as measured by the micropuncture technique (9). It should be noted that for acetazolamide to be effective, it must be given in doses sufficient to reduce the activity of carbonic anhydrase by over 99.5%. Cerebrospinal fluid production is also reduced by the drug, ouabain, a cardiac glycoside that inhibits Na-K dependent ATPase. In the case of this drug, however, there is variation in both its effectiveness and required dosage between species. Recently, a potent diuretic, furosemide, has been demonstrated to be capable of reducing CSF production, being slightly more effective than acetazolamide (10). Furosemide is a powerful diuretic known to act on the kidney tubule by a mechanism which is believed to be different from the action of this drug on carbonic anhydrase, an enzyme which it also inhibits. The extent to which the action of furosemide on CSF production is a reflection of its inhibition of carbonic anhydrase or whether in this situation it acts via a different, as yet undescribed, mechanism has not been finally established.

CSF FORMATION, OSMOLALITY, AND WATER FLOW

An interesting observation of Heisey et al. (1) was that the formation of CSF continued, even when the ventriculocisternal system was perfused with a hypo-osmotic solution. Again, this observation is in accord with the role of secretion in the formation of CSF. However, the net rate of formation was linearly related to total osmotic pressure differences between plasma and CSF. Recently, Hochwald et al. (11) studied the effect of changes in serum osmolality upon the change in CSF formation, and demonstrated that as serum osmolality was increased, CSF formation decreased; the converse occurring with infusion of hypo-osmolar solutions. Experiments such as those of Hochwald et al. require a redefinition of the term "CSF formation."

Water is known to exchange with CSF as it does with every body fluid. Years ago, Bering (12) demonstrated that the rate of exchange of D_2O with CSF was much slower than in brain tissue, in the order of about 7 min as compared to 12 to 25 sec for brain parenchyma. This, however, reflected the large volume and distance from capillaries in CSF. In fact, Heisey et al. (1) estimated the osmotic permeability of the ependyma, TOH, and found it comparable to that of other body membranes and greater than the diffusional permeability of the same membrane. Pape and Katzman (13) demonstrated that the CSF osmolality will reflect serum osmolality due to water shifts, but with a delay in the cat of about 45 min. Under these circumstances, it would appear that when there is a change in serum osmolality, water will shift in or out of the CSF in a passive but somewhat slow process. This will, of course, result in an apparent change in CSF formation if measured by the dilution of the tracer. Should such water movement be considered to be equivalent to bulk formation or absorption of CSF? Or, would it be preferable to define bulk fluid as the sum of the solute and solvents moving together. If the latter is accepted as a definition, the present evidence must be interpreted to indicate that some bulk formation of CSF can occur by secretion when CSF osmolality is lowered. At present, there is no evidence that either bulk formation of CSF or bulk absorption is altered by changes in serum osmolality, and, in fact, the latter influences only the water component of the CSF.

CONSTANCY OF THE IONIC CONSTITUENTS OF THE CSF

As long ago as 1931, it had been discovered that the CSF cation, calcium, was present in a concentration significantly different from that in serum and remained unaltered as serum concentrations were altered by changes in the activity of parathyroid hormone (14). Subsequently, it has been shown that the concentration of K and Mg are different in CSF than in serum and remain relatively constant in CSF despite changes in serum concentrations. Utilizing the ventriculocisternal perfusion techniques together with appropriate isotopes of these cations, it has been possible to demonstrate that a twofold system operates to maintain this constancy. On the one hand, the entry of cations into CSF via the process of CSF secretion is carefully controlled. Ames et al. (15) demonstrated that newly formed choroidal plexus CSF is markedly constant at about 3 mM once the plasma K exceeds a level of about 3.5 mM. Even with a plasma K of 1.5 mM, the choroid plexus K is over 2 mM. Thus, there appears to be a saturable mediated transport system involved in the secretion of choroid plexus K. In addition to the control of CSF ion concentrations by carrier-mediated transport between blood and CSF, mediated transport mechanisms seem to be involved in clearance of ions from CSF, when their concentration exceeds the usual concentration. This can easily be demonstrated by bypassing the formation process with a ventriculocisternal perfusion at a rate of 5 to 10 times that of the rate of formation of CSF. Under such conditions, it has been demonstrated that the K in the cisternal effluent tends towards a value of 3 mM, although the K perfused might be much lower or higher in concentration (16). This exchange of K occurs both with the adjacent brain tissue and with blood. Bradbury and Stulcova (17) have reported that the clearance of K from CSF to blood is predominantly controlled by Na-K ATPase. Both this movement and the exchange with brain are altered by administration of the ATPase inhibitor, ouabain. The enzymatic basis of clearance mechanisms for Ca and Mg, which parallel those for K, has not yet been defined. In contrast to the concentrations of K, Ca, and Mg, which are maintained at very stable levels in all species, the concentrations of Na and Cl in CSF vary somewhat with alterations in serum osmolality and Na and Cl content. However, the movement of both ^{24}Na and ^{36}Cl into CSF occurs via mediated transport systems. In the case of ^{24}Na, the rate of transport into CSF is altered by acetazolamide to the same extent that CSF formation is altered. The existence of a chloride pump was demonstrated by Bourke et al. (18) who have shown that the movement of tracer amounts of Cl into CSF continued even though body Cl was replaced by isethionate. On the other hand, the bicarbonate present in CSF may reflect brain metabolism and varies, depending upon metabolic conditions.

The fact that CSF K is maintained at a level of about 3 mM in all mammalian species; the fact that the K concentration from CSF obtained from different sites is always between the range of 2.5 and 3 mM whatever the serum level (serum K is usually greater than 4 mM), and the fact that ^{42}K perfused through the ventriculocisternal system exchanges rapidly with adjacent brain K had led to the postulate that the CSF K reflected the extracellular K of the brain. To test this hypothesis, recently developed highly selective ion exchanger electrodes have been used to measure the extracellular K concentration in brain tissue. Extensive work with these electrodes have now demonstrated that, in fact, brain extracellular K is maintained at a level just under 3 mM as had been predicted. Thus, the probability that brain extracellular K and CSF K are identical lends further credence to the hypothesis that the CSF reflects the extracellular fluid of the brain and, perhaps, serves as a reservoir of such extracellular fluid.

ACTIVE CLEARANCE OF ANIONS AND ORGANIC ACIDS FROM THE CSF

It had been known for many years that halide anions, particularly bromide, appeared in the CSF in concentrations lower than those in plasma. This had been ascribed to the blood-CSF barrier to these anions. However, in 1961, Becker (19) postulated that the low concentration of these anions in CSF was due to their active transport out of CSF. He found that the choroid plexus of rabbits could accumulate ^{131}I in vitro at a concentration 30 times that of the medium. This accumulation was blocked by metabolic inhibitors and was temperature dependent. It was competitively inhibited by perchlorate or thiocyanate and self-saturation could be demonstrated. In 1964, Coben et al. (20) reported that when ^{131}I was injected into the lateral ventricle of the dog, its removal was so rapid that less than 10% of the initial injectant was present at the end of 20 min, but that this clearance could be blocked by the intraperitoneal administration of perchlorate. Thus, a single carrier-mediated transport system capable of removing these inorganic anions from the CSF and characterized as a group by the ability of perchlorate to block their removal was ascribed to choroid plexus transport. Recently, however, Davson and Hollingsworth (21) have shown that an identical clearance mechanism for iodide exists at the level of the brain capillary. Hence, the relative importance of the choroid plexus for the clearance of iodide versus the capillaries near ependymal or subarachnoid surfaces is now uncertain, but the evidence available from the work of Davson would tend to suggest that the cerebral capillaries may play as important a role as the choroid plexus.

A second transport system operating via a clearance mechanism present both in the choroid plexus and in other structures is capable of removing weak organic acids. This phenomenon was first discovered by Dandy and Blackfan in 1913 (22), who found that if phenolsulfonaphthalein (PSP) was injected into the lateral ventricle, it would normally quickly appear in urine, but if there were an aqueductal block, its clearance from the ventricle was greatly slowed. Subsequently, Pappenheimer et al. (2) demonstrated that the removal of both diodrast and

PSP was by an active process, that is, the clearance from CSF to bloodstream occurred when the levels of these substances in the bloodstream were greater than those in CSF. Pappenheimer et al. adduced evidence that the clearance occurred in or near the choroid plexus of the fourth ventricle in the goat. Probenecid is a molecule originally developed to block specifically the excretion of penicillin into the urine. Fishman (23) demonstrated that the low concentration of penicillin found in normal CSF was due to a clearance mechanism that could be blocked by probenecid which would also block the clearance of PSP and related compounds. In recent years, because of the great interest in the metabolites of dopamine and serotonin, the presence of the organic acid end products, homovanillic acid (HVA) and 5-hydroxyindoleacetic acid (5-HIAA), in CSF has been studied. It has been found that these substances are present in the lateral ventricle in concentrations much greater than those in the cisterna magna and greater in the cisterna magna than in the lumbar subarachnoid fluid. For both compounds, the administration of probenecid will reduce their clearance from CSF and reduce the size of the ventricular lumbar gradient. Since choroid plexus *in vitro* will accumulate these substances, an accumulation that depends upon active metabolism by the choroid plexus which can be blocked by probenecid, it has been assumed that the choroid plexus of the fourth ventricle again is involved in the removal of these metabolites. Recent work by Wolfson et al. (24), however, has shown that the rate of removal from the subarachnoid space is much greater than from the ventriculocisternal system. This clearance of 5-HIAA from the subarachnoid space is a probenecid-sensitive clearance mechanism. The removal of 5-HIAA from the subarachnoid space shows typical saturation kinetics and, hence, appears to be removed by a mediated transport system. It is interesting to note that Dandy and Blackfan (22) initially assumed that PSP was removed diffusely throughout the subarachnoid space, a conclusion that now appears to have been correct. Thus, the role of the choroid plexus may now have to be redefined; although it is capable of concentrating these substances *in vitro,* it may not play as important a part in their removal from CSF *in vivo* as do

other vascular elements. However, which vascular elements are involved in the weak organic acid transport mechanism has not been clearly delineated. Although one would, *a priori,* suppose that capillaries near the subarachnoid surface would be most important, there is the possibility that the pial vasculature itself (25) may also be involved. Thus, two clear-cut but distinct clearance mechanisms, one for the inorganic halide anions and the other for the weak organic acids including many metabolites, have been identified. For the inorganic anion transport mechanism, perchlorate serves as a useful competitive inhibitor; for the weak organic acid system, probenecid serves the same function. In the latter instance, probenecid has been used clinically in an attempt to determine the "true" levels of HVA and 5-HIAA in spinal fluid in the hope of monitoring the state and activity of brain aminergic systems.

Similarly, amino acids are transported from CSF to blood against a concentration gradient (26). The removal of the amino acid, leucine, from the subarachnoid and ventricular spaces has been clearly shown to be via a carrier-mediated transport system with usual saturation kinetics. Lorenzo (27) has suggested that this system may be located in the choroid plexus on the basis that the kinetic coefficients of CSF clearance and those of choroid plexus uptake *in vitro* are similar. However, the problem remains that the removal from subarachnoid spaces is more rapid than with ventriculocisternal perfusion. Again, the localization of the clearance mechanism in the subarachnoid space is not known.

COMMON PROPERTIES OF CHOROIDAL EPITHELIUM AND CEREBRAL CAPILLARY ENDOTHELIUM

In the studies that we have reviewed, it is apparent that there is a startling similarity between the function of the choroidal epithelium and the cerebral capillary endothelium. The extracellular fluid of the brain, presumably formed at the capillary endothelium, is identical with CSF in at least two instances—its low protein content and specific K concentration. Whether the clearance of halides, weak organic acids, and amino acids occurs primarily via the choroid plexus or via capillary endothelium is uncertain. It is clear that both have similar transport properties and the *capability* of appropriate mediated transport. These transport processes are not unique for the central nervous system; certainly, they are shared by the kidney tubule (as in the case of the probenecid system) or by other tissues (iodide transport into the thyroid by a perchlorate-inhibited system; amino acid and K transport by ubiquitous carrier mechanisms). Yet, not all epithelial tissues nor all capillary endothelium are involved in such transport activities. The "set" of the transport systems, at least in regard to K, is obviously different in the central nervous system where the extracellular K is maintained at 3 mM as compared to the remainder of the body where the extracellular K tends to a value between 4 to 5.5 mM. Morphologically, as described by Brightman (*this volume*), the capillary endothelium and the choroidal epithelium share the presence of tight junctions, but otherwise there are many morphological differences (for example, the multiple invaginations and processes that characterize the choroidal epithelium). The choroidal epithelium which represents specialized ependymal cells and the cerebral capillary endothelium which is of mesenchymal origin have arisen from diverse embryological cell lines, yet have expressed the same phenotypic transport processes. Both the choroidal epithelium and the capillary endothelium have particularly high gamma glutamyl transpeptidase activities, an enzyme implicated in amino acid transport. This is, indeed, an extraordinary evolutionary event which occurs in species higher than Elasmobranchs and lower than mammals. (Klatzo has demonstrated that the blood-brain barrier in the shark occurs at the level of the glial cell membranes investing the capillary rather than at the capillary endothelium.) Much remains to be learned about these systems in intermediary species.

SUMMARY

We have reviewed several mediated transport systems involved in the elaboration and clearance of the cerebrospinal fluid. The similarity, perhaps identity, of the CSF and the brain extracellular fluid has been stressed. The remarkable coincidence of similar transport mechanisms in choroid plexus epithelium and brain capillary endothelium has been emphasized.

The consequence of these transport mechanisms is important for the function of the nervous system both in health and in disease. In normal health, the maintenance of a constant internal environment in the brain extracellular fluid and in the CSF helps to provide an extraordinary degree of stability for the functioning of the nervous system. The rapidity with which metabolites are removed serves a similar function. In disease states, understanding of the existence of these transport systems can be of clinical importance. Levels of penicillin in the brain can, if needed, be elevated by the administration of probenecid to block the clearance of this molecule. Evaluation of the dopaminergic systems as in Parkinson's disease can be made more precise by determining the HVA level after the administration of probenecid. In a similar manner, the effects of many neuroleptic drugs upon these systems may be studied by what has become known as the "probenecid test." We do not know if any disease states are characterized by abnormalities in transport systems. We do know, however, that the transport of individual neutral amino acids into brain can be controlled by manipulating the plasma levels of other neutral amino acids competing for the same transport site. This phenomenon is most striking in the case of tryptophan, the essential amino acid present in the blood in the lowest concentration. Variations in diet change the amount of tryptophan entering the brain and as a consequence alter the level of its neurotransmitter metabolite, serotonin (28). But as yet, the transport molecules themselves have not been isolated and identified. If it will ever be possible to modify or control these molecules remains a question for the future.

ACKNOWLEDGMENTS

This work was supported by USPHS grants NS 03356, NS 09649, NS 01450, and a Career Development Award, NB 17044.

REFERENCES

1. Heisey, S. R., Held, D., and Pappenheimer, J. R. (1962): Bulk flow and diffusion in the cerebrospinal fluid system of the goat. *Am. J. Physiol.*, 203:775–781.

2. Pappenheimer, J. R., Heisey, S. R., and Jordon, E. F. (1961): Active transport of Diodrast and phenolsulfonphthalein from cerebrospinal fluid to blood. *Am. J. Physiol.,* 200:1–10.

3. Pappenheimer, J. R., Heisey, S. R., Jordon, E. F., and Downer, J. deC. (1962): Perfusion of the cerebral ventricular system in unanesthetized goats. *Am. J. Physiol.,* 203:763–774.

4. Davson, H. (1967): *Physiology of the Cerebrospinal Fluid.* Little, Brown, Boston.

5. Katzman, R., and Pappius, H. M. (1973): *Brain Electrolytes and Fluid Metabolism.* Williams & Wilkins, Baltimore.

6. Welch, K., and Friedman, V. (1960): The cerebrospinal fluid valves. *Brain,* 83:454–469.

7. deRougemont, J., Ames, A., III, Nesbett, F. D., and Hofmann, H. F. (1960): Fluid formed by choroid plexus. A technique for its collection and a comparison of its electrolyte composition with serum and cisternal fluids. *J. Neurophysiol.,* 23:485–495.

8. Welch, K. (1963): Secretion of cerebrospinal fluid by choroid plexus of the rabbit. *Am. J. Physiol.,* 205:617–624.

9. Ames, A., III, Higashi, K., and Nesbett, F. B. (1965): Effects of pCO_2, acetazolamide and ouabain on volume and composition of choroid-plexus fluid. *J. Physiol. (Lond.),* 181:516–524.

10. McCarthy, K. D., and Reed, D. J. (1974): The effect of acetazolamide and furosemide on cerebrospinal fluid production and choroid plexus carbonic anhydrase activity. *J. Pharmacol. Exp. Ther.* 189:194–201.

11. Hochwald, G. M., Mald, A., DiMattio, J., and Malhan, C. (1974): The effects of serum osmolarity on cerebrospinal fluid volume flow. *Life Sci.,* 15:1309–1316.

12. Bering, E. A. (1952): Water exchange of central nervous system and cerebrospinal fluid. *J. Neurosurg.,* 9:275–287.

13. Pape, L., and Katzman, R. (1970): Effects of hydration on blood and cerebrospinal fluid osmolalities. *Proc. Soc. Exp. Biol. Med.,* 134:430–433.

14. Merritt, H. H., and Bauer, W. (1931): The equilibrium between cerebrospinal fluid and blood plasma. III. The distribution of calcium and phosphorus between cerebrospinal fluid and blood serum. *J. Biol. Chem.,* 90:215–232.

15. Ames, A., III., Higashi, K., and Nesbett, F. B. (1965): Relation of potassium concentration in choroid-plexus fluid to that in plasma. *J. Physiol. (Lond.),* 181:506–515.

16. Katzman, R., Graziani, L., Kaplan, R., and Escriva, A. (1965): Exchange of cerebrospinal fluid potassium with blood and brain. *Arch. Neurol.,* 13:513–524.

17. Bradbury, M. W. B., and Stulcova, B. (1970): Efflux mechanism contributing to the stability of the potassium concentration in cerebrospinal fluid. *J. Physiol. (Lond.),* 208:415–430.

18. Bourke, R. S., Gabelnick, H. L., and Young, O. (1970): Mediated transport of chloride from blood into cerebrospinal fluid. *Exp. Brain Res.,* 10:17–38.

19. Becker, B. (1961): Cerebrospinal fluid iodide. *Am. J. Physiol.,* 201:1149–1151.

20. Coben, L. A., Loeffler, J. D., and Elsasser, J. C. (1964): Spinal fluid iodide transport in the dog. *Am. J. Physiol.,* 206:1373–1378.

21. Davson, H., and Hollingsworth, J. R. (1973): Active transport of ^{131}I across the blood-brain barrier. *J. Physiol. (Lond.),* 233:327–347.

22. Dandy, W. E., and Blackfan, K. D. (1913): An experimental and clinical study of internal hydrocephalus. *JAMA,* 61:2216–2217.

23. Fishman, R. A. (1966): Blood-brain and CSF barriers to penicillin and related organic acids. *Arch. Neurol.,* 15:113–124.

24. Wolfson, L. I., Katzman, R., and Escriva, A. (1974): Clearance of amine metabolites from the cerebrospinal fluid: The brain as a "sink." *Neurology,* 24:772–779.

25. Levin, E., Sepulveda, F. V., and Yudilevich, D. L. (1974): Pial vessels transport of substances from cerebrospinal fluid to blood. *Nature,* 249:266–268.

26. Lajtha, A., and Toth, J. (1961): The brain barrier system. II. Uptake and transport of amino acids by the brain. *J. Neurochem.,* 8:216–225.

27. Lorenzo, A. V. (1974): Amino acid transport mechanisms of the cerebrospinal fluid. *Fed. Proc.,* 33:2079–2085.

28. Fernstrom, J. D., and Wurtman, R. J. (1971): Brain serotonin content: Physiological dependence on plasma tryptophan levels. *Science,* 173:149–152.

The Nervous System, Donald B. Tower, Editor-in-Chief. *Vol. 1: The Basic Neurosciences*. Raven Press, New York, 1975.

Mechanisms of Ion Distribution Between Blood and Brain

Joseph D. Fenstermacher

Systems for the precise regulation of the internal environment of the brain, the extracellular fluid (ECF), are very highly developed and exceedingly effective in most vertebrate species. Ionic homeostasis in the ECF of the brain is a function of transport mechanisms which are located not only at the blood-brain barrier (the capillary endothelium and surrounding structures) but also at the blood-cerebrospinal fluid (CSF) barrier (the choroid plexus and, possibly, the pial vessels) and the CSF-brain interfaces (the ependymal and pial-glial membranes). In addition a certain degree of local electrolytic control may be facilitated by some of the glial cells within the brain parenchyma. Because the movements of ions between blood and brain are clearly dependent upon these various constituents of the system, all of them will be considered in this presentation. Studies of transport across these membranes or barriers, with the exception of direct blood-CSF exchange at the choroid plexuses, are complicated by the uncertainty of the ionic concentrations in the several—extracellular, glial, and neuronal—brain fluid compartments. Despite this limitation, a significant body of useful observations which suggest the nature of the transfer processes at the principal transport interfaces has accumulated. The results from the more pertinent papers will be presented and discussed herein. In addition, theoretical calculations of material flow in this system which indicate the role of the blood-brain barrier in the regulation of the electrolytic composition of the brain ECF are given.

MECHANISMS OF MEMBRANE PERMEATION

General Mechanisms

The movements of ions across membranes occur, in general, by one or more of the following mechanisms—simple passive diffusion, facilitated diffusion, and active transport. In addition, if fluid formation or secretion takes place across a membrane, the flux of electrolytes may be coupled to or affected by this process and, depending on the arrangement, either be actively or passively transported.

Simple Diffusion

The passive diffusion of an ion across a membrane separating two different fluids, e.g., plasma and CSF, is defined as the spontaneous movement of that substance from the fluid of higher electrochemical potential to the one of lower potential. The flow is driven by the electrochemical forces, proceeds in the direction opposite to the electrochemical gradient, and continues until the gradient is dissipated. When the latter condition is reached, no net transport of the electrolyte occurs since the electrical and chemical forces become equal and opposite, and an ionic equilibrium, which is mathematically stated by the Nernst equation,[1] is achieved. The source of the electrical component of the potential is the separation of charges which takes place because of the presence, for example, of both permeable and impermeable ions on either side of the membrane or an electrogenic pump in the membrane.

Facilitated Diffusion

The movements of many substances across membranes occur by a process called facili-

---

[1] The Nernst equation is

$$E = (RT/ZF) \ln (C_1/C_2)$$

where E is the electrical potential, R is the gas constant, T is the absolute temperature, Z is the valence, F is Faraday's constant, and C_1 and C_2 are the ionic concentrations (or more correctly, activities) in the two solutions which are separated by the membrane.

tated diffusion. Generally this mechanism is envisioned as the combination of the transported material, the substrate, with a membrane "carrier" which then transfers the substrate across the membrane and releases it on the other side. Facilitated diffusion proceeds down the electrochemical gradient, utilizes no energy, and leads to a condition of electrochemical equilibrium. Such a transport set-up selectively carries only those materials of appropriate physicochemical properties (stereospecificity) and possess a finite transfer capacity (saturability). If two different substrates share the same carrier system, they will compete for the available transport sites and mutually inhibit or reduce their rates of movement across the membrane (competition). The term, exchange diffusion, is applied to a facilitated diffusion arrangement when all of the carrier molecules are combined with substrate, i.e., completely saturated, as they shuttle back and forth across the membrane. The transport of ions by exchange diffusion is quite common in membrane biology; part of the transfer of tracer sodium across red cell membranes takes place by this mechanism.

Active Transport

Active transport shares many of the features ·saturation, competition, inhibition, and stereospecificity – of a facilitated diffusion system; however, it differs from the latter because an energy input is required and the substrate is moved from a solution of lower electrochemical potential to one of higher potential ("uphill" transfer). Demonstration of the energy dependency of active transport is usually made by observing the effects of various metabolic inhibitors upon the exchange process. The test for uphill transfer or pumping is made by comparing data on steady-state distribution ratios with the Nernst equation and/or undirectional fluxes with the Ussing flux ratio equation[2]; if the experimental and calculated results are significantly different, the second criteria of active

transport is satisfied. Sodium movement across frog skin is an example of active transport.

Fluid Secretion

One of the principal functions of the choroid plexus is the production of cerebrospinal fluid. The available evidence suggests that this process occurs by the development of an osmotic gradient across the choroidal epithelium – probably by the active transport of Na^+ from the choroidal ECF to the CSF – which then osmotically draws water across the epithelium (for reviews of this see refs. 1 and 2). Because the pumping of an ionic species leads to a charge separation and the movement of water causes concentration and, perhaps, pressure changes on both sides of the membrane, localized electrochemical potential gradients are induced by the process of CSF formation at the choroid plexus. The movements of ions in this situation become a complex function of the characteristics of the specific ions which are actively transported, the rate of fluid production and flow, the passive permeability of the choroidal epithelium to the various electrolytes, and the geometrical arrangement of the cellular membranes and the ion pump(s).

Experimental Indicators of Mechanisms

In a system such as the frog skin or toad bladder, studies of ion movements are simpler than in the blood-brain-CSF system since the transmembrane chemical and electrical gradients can be easily controlled and samples of the two opposing fluids readily obtained. Exchange between blood and CSF at the choroid plexus is the exception since techniques of *in situ* and *in vivo* isolation have been developed over the last decade. For blood-ECF or CSF-ECF transport, only the blood and CSF can be changed or sampled with assurance, the concentration in the brain's ECF remaining unknown or uncertain for both cases.

The most general way of studying electrolyte movements in this system involves the raising or lowering of the ionic concentrations in either blood or CSF and measuring the changes in the exchange of a radioactive isotope of that electrolyte (saturation or self-inhibition) or of another related ion (competition). If the transfer mecha-

---

[2] The Ussing flux ratio equation is

$$J_{12}/J_{21} = (C_2/C_1)\ e^{-zFE/RT},$$

where J_{12} and J_{21} are the undirectional fluxes from solution 1 to solution 2 and solution 2 to solution 1, respectively.

nism is passive diffusion, the undirectional flux should be linearly related to the concentration of the electrolyte in the blood or CSF and the time course of net exchange should be the same in control and experimental animals provided that the membrane itself or the electrical gradient is not altered by the procedure. Measurements of these two transport parameters, undirectional flux and net exchange, and evaluation of the transfer process have also been studied in situations where the electrical gradient, and not the chemical gradient, has been varied. Attempts to modify the ECF concentrations of ions have been made by osmotically withdrawing or adding water to the brain and by CSF perfusion with solutions of differing ionic compositions; however, these techniques generate uncertain or imprecise changes in ECF concentrations of electrolytes and make the data analysis very difficult and hazardous.

If competition and saturation can be demonstrated, a differentiation between active transport and facilitated diffusion—the two processes that display these characteristics—can be made by using various transport and metabolism inhibitors. Sensitivity to known inhibitors of active ion transport in other membrane systems implies that a similar transfer mechanism is involved at the site or sites being studied.

The production of CSF at the choroid plexus, however, confuses the application of the above criteria to electrolytic transport across this structure. For example, the bulk flow of the forming CSF across the choroidal epithelium could well carry along various ions by solvent drag, and, based on the electrochemical gradient, the distribution ratio might indicate active transport. Yet, if the movement of the ions was driven by the water flow, the transfer would be considered passive. Bulk flow of fluid across the brain capillaries and the ependymal and pial-glial membranes apparently is so small, if it exists at all, that it does not appreciably affect ion fluxes at these sites.

ION TRANSPORT AT THE CHOROID PLEXUS

Direct studies of ion transport across the choroid plexus have been conducted by four different research groups. Ames and collaborators (3–5) and Miner and Reed (6) have collected freshly formed choroid plexus fluid (CSF) under oil, analyzed the fluid plus the plasma or serum for electrolytes, and determined distribution ratios. A technique of isolating and perfusing the *in situ* sheep choroid plexus was developed and used for ion flux experiments by Pollay and co-workers (7,8). Wright (9) placed the fourth ventricle choroid plexus of the bullfrog in a chamber and studied undirectional fluxes of labeled ions across this membrane. Ideally, the measured distribution ratios and undirectional fluxes should be compared to those calculated by the Nernst and Ussing flux ratio equations, respectively. Experimentally, however, all of the driving forces were not measured or controlled in most of these studies; therefore, the authors assumed that a passive distribution across the choroid plexus would lead to CSF concentrations which are identical to those of a plasma or serum ultrafiltrate. Such an assumption may be questioned, however, since the various filtration membranes used have differing properties—fixed charges, aqueous channel sizes, etc.—and the ultrafiltration process itself develops electrical and osmotic gradients which may be unrelated to the *in vivo* situation.

Sodium

Ames et al. (3) and Miner and Reed (6) compared the Na^+ concentration in the choroidal CSF to that of a plasma or serum ultrafiltrate. Their results were identical and yielded CSF:ultrafiltrate ratios of 1.05, a value which agreed with that reported by Pollay et al. (7) for the *in situ* perfused sheep choroid plexus. A significant electrical potential, 5 to 14 mV (CSF positive), exists between blood and CSF (10,11); whether or not such potentials would be found for those studies in which the plexus was surrounded by oil is uncertain. Assuming, nevertheless, that the transmembrane potential was as low as 5 mV and inserting this value into the Nernst equation, a CSF:plasma water distribution ratio of 0.83 is calculated; the experimentally determined ratio was 0.97. Since both of these analyses indicate that the Na^+ concentration in the CSF produced by the choroid plexus is higher than the chemical and electrical forces would passively generate, the exchange of this cation seems to involve an uphill transport process or pump. The work of Wright (9) with the isolated choroid plexus of the bull frog supports this conclusion. The flux of ^{22}Na from blood to CSF was about 40% greater than the flux in the opposite direction, the likely result of an active transport mechanism since the transchoroidal potential in this preparation was less than 1 mV.

Considerations of two other characteristics of such transfer systems, drug inhibition and self-saturation, also tend to support this conclusion. Although the plasma concentration range was fairly limited (153–169 mEq/liter H_2O), Ames et al. (4) found no significant change in the Na$^+$ concentration of choroid plexus fluid. Wright (9) reported that the active component of Na$^+$ transport in the frog choroid plexus was blocked by ouabain, a potent inhibitor of Na-K activated ATP-ase, and was directly dependent upon the bicarbonate concentration of the surrounding medium. Similar sensitivities of the transchoroidal Na$^+$ flux upon ouabain and bicarbonate were indicated by the observations of Ames et al. (5) on the *in situ* cat choroid plexus. Surprisingly, Wright found no effects of the carbonic anhydrase inhibitor, acetazolamide, on ^{22}Na transport in his study, whereas Ames et al. discovered that this drug diminished both CSF secretion and net Na$^+$ transfer.

In summary, the body of extant evidence indicates that Na$^+$ transport from blood to CSF at the choroid plexus is mediated, in part, by an active transport mechanism.

Potassium

In the work of Ames et al. (3) and Miner and Reed (6), the reported plasma ultrafiltrate to plasma ratios for K$^+$ were around 0.80; the calculated ratio, based on a blood-CSF electrical gradient of 5 mV (CSF positive) and the Nernst equation, was 0.83. Both studies yielded CSF: plasma or serum water ratios of about 0.75 for K$^+$. Although the agreement between these ratios is relatively close and suggests that the electrochemical forces of the system could virtually account for the observed K$^+$ distribution, other studies indicate that an active process may be involved.

Ames et al. (4) changed the plasma concentration of K$^+$ and measured the K$^+$ concentra-

TABLE 1. *Potassium concentrations in plasma and CSF (mEq/liter) from rabbits after 3 weeks of special diets*[a]

	Control	Low K$^+$	High K$^+$
Plasma	4.15 ± 0.27	1.58 ± 0.09	7.09 ± 0.59
CSF	2.83 ± 0.08	2.72 ± 0.06	3.02 ± 0.12

[a] Data from Bradbury and Kleeman (1967); values are means $\pm$ SE.

tion in the choroidal fluid (CSF) during the next hour. Over a plasma concentration range of 2.1 to 7.9 mEq/kg water, the CSF concentration of K$^+$ varied from 2.5 to 3.4 mEq/kg water. As has been mentioned by various authors (e.g., 1,2), the relative constancy of the choroidal fluid K$^+$ implies that the transfer of this cation from blood to CSF is mediated by a process which is saturated or nearly saturated at plasma concentration of 2.5 mEq/kg water or greater. Support for the constancy of the K$^+$ concentration in CSF was obtained by the chronic studies of Bradbury and Kleeman (12) given in Table 1. In view of the nearly fivefold differences in plasma K$^+$, the concentration of this cation in CSF remained strikingly constant.

Studies of the undirectional flux of K$^+$ across the choroid plexus of the bullfrog and sheep by Wright (9) and Pollay et al. (7,8), respectively, gave somewhat conflicting results. For the bullfrog choroid plexus *in vitro*, the fluxes appeared to be very small (about $\frac{1}{50}$ of the Na$^+$ flux) and passive; however, the CSF to blood transport of K$^+$ was slightly greater than the flux in the opposite direction at low fluid concentrations (2 mEq/liter) and became clearly greater at high concentrations (10 mEq/liter). For the vascularly perfused sheep choroid plexus, the CSF to blood transfer of K$^+$ was linearly related to the CSF concentration of K$^+$, whereas the blood-to-CSF flux seemed to be a complex function of the serum K$^+$, a relationship which resembled that found by Ames et al. (4) for the cat choroid plexus. At low to normal ventricular fluid (CSF) concentrations, 1 to 5 mEq/kg water, the K$^+$ flow from blood to CSF was equal to or greater than the CSF to blood flux, but at higher concentrations the relationship was reversed, CSF to blood transfer being the greater.

The transport of K$^+$ across the plexus also seemed to be affected by other experimental conditions which inhibit or accelerate active ion translocation processes in other cellular systems. The results of Ames et al. (5) indicate that the inhalation of 10% CO_2, which caused a rise in both arterial H^+ and HCO_3^- concentrations, increased CSF secretion and the blood to CSF flux of K^+; on the other hand the topical application of 10^{-3} M acetazolamide decreased both secretion and K^+ flux. In a study by Pollay et al. (8), ouabain in either blood or CSF decreased the blood to CSF transfer of K^+, yet did not affect the transfer of this cation in the other direction. Ames et al. (5) found, likewise, that topical ouabain (10^{-4} M) decreased K^+ transfer from blood to CSF and CSF formation. As Wright (9) has pointed out, studies of ouabain effects on K^+ flux across multicellular membranes are fraught with difficulty since the cells themselves, in addition to the fluids on both sides, can be a source of K^+. In a non-steady-state condition such as ouabain might cause, a significant portion of the apparent transependymal fluxes may arise from the leakage of ions from the cellular K^+ pool. Also if significant amounts of tracer K^+ accumulate in the choroidal cells during the earlier portion of an experiment, flux studies performed thereafter with ouabain could be distorted by the loss of ^{42}K from the cells.

The preceding findings do not easily lend themselves to the development of a simple, satisfactory model for K^+ exchange at the choroid plexus; nevertheless these observations—low levels of K^+ in CSF, virtual constancy of the K^+ concentration of the CSF, apparent differences in the undirectional fluxes, and effects of various transport stimulators and inhibitors—indicate that diffusion is not the only transport mechanism involved. Some combination of passive diffusion, facilitated diffusion, and active transport—possibly from CSF to blood—must be responsible for the regulation of K^+ flow across the choroid plexus.

Calcium and Magnesium

In the previously cited studies of Ames et al. (3) and Miner and Reed (6) Ca^{2+} and Mg^{2+} concentrations were also determined. For Mg^{2+} the results of these studies clearly indicate that an active transport system which moves this cation from blood to CSF is involved. The concentration of Mg^{2+} in the CSF is around 60% higher than would be expected in an appropriate ultrafiltrate. In addition, if the distribution of Mg^{2+} between CSF and blood were in accord with the electrical gradient, the concentration of this electrolyte in CSF would be much less than in the plasma. The findings with Ca^{2+} are more conflicting, mainly because of the discrepancies in the degree of plasma protein binding. Ames et al. (3) found a CSF:plasma ultrafiltrate ratio of 0.91 for Ca^{2+}; Miner and Reed (6) obtained a CSF:serum ultrafiltrate ratio of about 1.90. In the latter study nearly twice as much Ca^{2+} was found to be protein "bound" as in the former one. Based on an electrical potential of 5 mV (CSF positive), the ratio that would be found if the free Ca^{2+} ions distributed passively across the choroid plexus is 0.69, a value significantly less than those reported by Ames et al. and Miner and Reed.

Wright (9), in his work on the bullfrog choroid plexus *in vitro*, determined that the fluxes of Ca^{2+} across this tissue were very small (about one-third of the K^+ flux) and that the undirectional transfer from blood to CSF was somewhat larger than the flux in the opposite direction. In the unpublished observations of Ames and Nesbett which are cited by Cserr in her review (1), the effects of increasing plasma Ca^{2+} and Mg^{2+} on the ionic composition of the fluid which formed on the surface of the choroid plexus gave further indications that some degree of blood-CSF exchange regulation of these divalent cations takes place. When the Mg^{2+} concentration in the plasma was elevated to five times the normal level, the choroidal fluid concentration only increased by 33%; when the plasma Ca^{2+} concentration was raised fivefold, the CSF concentration was nearly tripled. These results imply that Mg^{2+} exchange across the choroid plexus is fairly tightly controlled, whereas the flow of Ca^{2+} is regulated to a lesser degree.

Additional support for this suggestion comes from the ventriculocisternal perfusion studies of Graziani et al. (13) and Ginzburg (*unpublished observations* cited by Katzman and Pappius, ref. 2). These data, although not a direct examination of transchoroidal exchange as the preceding ones are, indicate that Ca^{2+} enters the CSF both by a diffusional leak and a pump and that Mg^{2+} is transferred from blood to CSF almost entirely by a pump. Since the net movements of these two divalent cations apparently are against their respective electrochemical gradients, the transport systems for both of them seem to be active.

Chloride

The concentration of Cl⁻ in the CSF which is secreted by the choroid plexus is fairly similar to that of a plasma (3) or serum (6) ultrafiltrate. Since the CSF is electrically positive relative to blood, the concentration of Cl⁻ in the choroidal fluid would be expected to be somewhat higher (theoretical ratio of 1.20 for a potential of 5 mV) than in plasma or serum water.

In studies with the *in vitro* frog choroid plexus, Wright (9) found that the undirectional fluxes across the plexus were equal and agreed with the Ussing flux ratio equation for passive ionic distribution; furthermore these fluxes were similar in magnitude, but not identical, to the Na⁺ fluxes in this system. By a technique of hemodialysis, Gabelnick et al. (14) and Bourke et al. (15) partially replaced blood and tissue Cl⁻ with isethionate and lowered the plasma Cl⁻ from 120 to 60 mM/liter plasma. Over this concentration range the uptake of ³⁶Cl by CSF from blood continued at a constant rate, indicating some sort of linkage with cationic (e.g., Na⁺) transport or CSF secretion or the operation of a special chloride transporting mechanism. Measurements of the electrical potential between blood and CSF during a similar chloride-isethionate replacement procedure indicated little or no change in this driving force during a comparable experimental period (16). Although the latter experiment suggests an active mechanism for Cl⁻ transport between blood and CSF, the ability of the isethionate ion, a negatively charged particle of larger size (MW = 125) and lower membrane permeability than chloride, to follow transported cations into the forming CSF may have been much less than that of Cl⁻, and thus the Cl⁻ may have been preferentially driven as the most permeable anion in the system down a locally developed electrical gradient which was generated by a cation pump.

The existing experimental evidence does not clearly establish the presence of an active transport mechanism for all or part of the translocation of Cl⁻ across the choroid plexus. Passive processes – diffusion and/or linkage to CSF secretion – seem to explain the movements of this anion between blood and CSF adequately.

ION TRANSPORT AT THE CSF-BRAIN INTERFACE

Many solutes, ranging in size from albumin to urea, have been found to move from ventricular and subarachnoid fluid (CSF or CSF + perfusate) into brain tissue. The ependymal and pial-glial membranes, therefore, do not seem to be significant barriers to molecular and ionic exchange. Material transport across these membranes and, subsequently, through the extracellular fluid (ECF) of the brain mainly occurs by diffusion. The rates of diffusion through the brain extracellular space (ECS) range from about 20% (white matter) to 40 to 50% (gray matter) of their respective diffusion rates in water at the same temperature; the size of the brain ECS is around 13 to 18%, the space of white matter being somewhat smaller than that of gray matter (all of the preceding information is more completely discussed in a review by Fenstermacher and Patlak, 17). In addition the diffusional transport of a particular ion or molecule through the ECS can be modified by cellular uptake and capillary exchange (18).

Sodium

Very little direct information on the movement of Na⁺ between CSF and brain exists. The work of Ames et al. (3) and Miner and Reed (6) indicate that the concentration Na⁺ in the CSF changes little as it passes from the lateral ventricles to the cistern magna. This could be the result of either ependymal impermeability to Na⁺ or a condition of diffusional equilibrium between CSF and brain ECF for this electrolyte. Subsequently, the ventriculocisternal perfusion studies of Patlak and Fenstermacher (19) indicate that ²⁴Na passes across the ependyma and through the ECF of the dog caudate nucleus by diffusion and that its apparent rate of diffusion in brain ECF is equal to or higher than that of many other substances.

Potassium

Reports from many different laboratories (3,6,20,21) show that the concentration of K$^+$ in CSF decreases as CSF flows through the ventricular system. Direct evidence that this change in CSF K$^+$ resulted from a loss to brain tissue (and, subsequently, to blood) was obtained by ventriculocisternal perfusion studies with ^{42}K. Cserr (22) found that the flux of ^{42}K across the ependyma was 4 to 5 times that of tracer Na$^+$ and 6 to 10 times that of ^{36}Cl; likewise, Katzman et al. (23) reported that ^{42}K clearance from CSF by brain was 5 to 6 times that of ^{28}Mg and ^{45}Ca. The preceding works all indicate that the transfer of K$^+$ across the ependyma is quite rapid. In a later study Pape and Katzman (24) found that the K$^+$ permeability of the ependyma is about twice as high as that of the pial-glial membrane.

Various studies (21,22,25) have shown that the transfer of ^{42}K from ventricular perfusate (CSF) to brain tissue is directly proportional to the concentration of K$^+$ in the perfusate, an observation which suggests that this exchange is diffusional; furthermore the ^{42}K tissue profiles found by Pape and Katzman (24) after ventricular and subarachnoid perfusions were consistent with those predicted for a system in which the ion diffused into and through the brain ECF and was taken up by brain cells. All of these observations indicate that K$^+$ moves readily between CSF and brain ECF, that this exchange occurs by diffusion, that the K$^+$ concentration of the CSF approaches that of the adjacent brain ECF, and that a continual net flux of this electrolyte from CSF to brain ECF to plasma takes place.

Calcium and Magnesium

As the CSF flows from the lateral ventricles to the subarachnoid space, Ca^{2+} and Mg^{2+} concentrations decrease — a likely reflection, in the steady state, of a net loss of these electrolytes to brain tissue and, ultimately, to blood (3,6, 20,26). Katzman and his co-workers (23,27) have demonstrated that significant amounts of ^{45}Ca enter the surrounding brain during ventriculocisternal perfusions with this radioisotope and that the flux of ^{45}Ca into the brain is proportional to the Ca^{2+} concentration in the perfusate. Similar observations with Mg^{2+} and ^{28}Mg were made by Katzman et al. (23). The CSF to brain flux coefficients reported for Ca^{2+} and Mg^{2+} in this study were much smaller than that of K$^+$ as would be expected from their differences in diffusability and tissue distribution. In brief, all of the available evidence indicates that these two divalent cations diffuse between CSF and brain ECF and that there is a continual net flow of Ca^{2+} and Mg^{2+} from CSF to blood via the brain ECF.

Chloride

As for most of the cations, only limited evidence concerning the CSF-brain exchange of Cl$^-$ exists. The differences between the Cl$^-$ concentrations of ventricular and cisternal CSF are small and do not indicate any net flux of this anion between CSF and brain ECF (3,6). The only other study on the transependymal movement of Cl$^-$ indicated that ^{36}Cl moved rapidly from CSF to brain parenchyma and that its subsequent distribution within the brain ECS was compatible with diffusional kinetics (18).

ION TRANSPORT BETWEEN BLOOD AND BRAIN EXTRACELLULAR FLUID

In comparison to the rates of transcapillary exchange in most other organs, the movements of many molecules and ions across the capillary complex of the brain are surprisingly slow; nevertheless, the transport of certain substances, e.g., glucose and phenylalanine (28), from blood to brain is very fast. The older notion of a simple capillary wall which restricts the transfer of materials or reduces their rates of flux, the so-called blood-brain barrier phenomena, has developed into a more dynamic concept of blood-brain exchange, one which combines limited permeability to materials in general with special transport systems for certain specific molecules and ions.

Sodium

The movement of Na$^+$ between blood and brain has been repeatedly demonstrated to be slow. For example, Davson and Welch (29) reported an exchange half-time for ^{24}Na of about 2.5 hr and a permeability coefficient which was one-tenth that of ^{42}K.

Although the transport of Na$^+$ under the circumstances of markedly elevated or lowered plasma concentrations have not been reported, attempts to study Na$^+$ uptake by brain from blood with conditions which apparently altered the electrochemical driving forces of the system have been made. Held et al. (10) varied the blood-CSF and, presumably, the blood-ECF electrical potential by 15 to 20 mV and found no detectable difference in the net rate of ^{24}Na uptake in the rat brain, whereas Davson and Segal (30) observed that the brain uptake of ^{22}Na in the rabbit was lowered when extracellular Na$^+$ was partially replaced by choline via ventriculo-cisternal perfusion of a choline-containing solution. The results imply that some mechanism other than passive diffusion mediates the transfer of this cation; however studies with various inhibitors and accelerators of Na$^+$ transport only gave partial support to this suggestion. Drugs such as ouabain, acetazolamide, and amiloride, had no effects on the blood-brain exchange of ^{22}Na; only two agents, vasopressin which increased the turnover rate (30) and furosemide which decreased the net uptake (31), caused any change in the distribution pattern of this radioisotope. On the basis of the various findings cited, none of the possible mechanisms of Na$^+$ transport—passive diffusion, exchange diffusion, or active transport—can be ruled out. Perhaps, as in the red cell, all three processes are involved in Na$^+$ transfer at the blood-brain barrier.

Potassium

The net uptake of ^{42}K by brain from blood appears to be quite slow, having a brain exchange half-time of about 24 hr (2); this rate of transfer, however, is not only a function of brain-capillary permeability but also of brain cellular exchange since most (95% or more of the total) of the brain's K$^+$ is intracellular. This large cellular pool of K$^+$ complicates the analysis of transcapillary exchange studies with this cation and its isotopes. By means of a detailed mathematical model which took transport processes across both capillary and cellular

membranes into account and data from published ^{42}K uptake studies, Davson and Welch (29) estimated that the blood to brain ECF flux of this isotope was ten times larger than that of ^{22}Na and had a transfer half-time of less than 30 min.

Experiments in which the plasma K$^+$ concentration was markedly altered for either 24 hr (21) or 3 weeks (12) have shown that the K$^+$ content of the brain is amazingly stable. The plasma concentrations of K$^+$ ranged from 1.6 to 9.4 mEq/liter-plasma; yet the brain levels did not change in either the short or long term groups. In these same studies, the distribution of ^{42}K between blood and brain was also observed and the rates of K$^+$ influx calculated. In most regions of the brain, there was a linear relationship between influx rate and plasma K$^+$ concentration. Analysis of graphs of the experimental data suggested that K$^+$ exchange between blood and brain occurred by both a diffusion-like process and a constant or saturated influx mechanism which could be either exchange diffusion or active transport. Bradbury and co-workers (32,33) have also modified the K$^+$ concentration of brain ECF by ventriculo-cisternal and subarachnoid perfusion of low and high K$^+$ solutions and observed brain uptake of ^{42}K from either blood or CSF (perfusate). When the tracer was introduced into the blood, the most rapid influx across brain capillaries occurred with the low perfusate (and ECF?) concentrations of K$^+$; on the other hand, when the tracer was contained in the perfusate, the brain uptake was fairly constant, but the loss to blood via the capillaries of the choroid plexus or brain, or both, was greatest with the high perfusate (and ECF?) concentrations of K$^+$. Although other alternatives were offered, the authors proposed that an active transport mechanism which is sensitive to the concentration of K$^+$ in the ECF and moves K$^+$ from ECF to blood was the most likely explanation of their experimental findings and those of others (12,21).

Ready acceptance of Bradbury and co-workers' intriguing hypothesis must be cautioned, however, since K$^+$ transport between brain ECF and cells confuses the interpretation of these data and the understanding of this cation's blood-brain transfer processes. Nevertheless, regulation of brain capillary exchange of K^+ by a special process does seem likely, but further evidence is needed before an accurate description of the mechanism or mechanisms can be made.

Calcium and Magnesium

Very little information about the transport of Ca^{2+} and Mg^{2+} from blood to brain exists. The equilibrium half-times for these two cations have been reported to be quite different, 8 hr for Ca^{2+} and about 24 hr for Mg^{2+} (Katzman and Pappius, ref. 2, citing unpublished observations of Graziani and Escriva and of Ginzburg, respectively). No conclusions about transport mechanisms can be made from these data.

Chloride

Davson and Welch (29) reported that the time of ^{36}Cl exchange between blood and brain ECF is similar to that of ^{22}Na. Gabelnick et al. (14) found that Cl^- uptake by brain was directly proportional to the plasma concentration of Cl^- when the latter was varied from 60 to 120 mEq/liter-plasma; on the other hand Held et al. (10) found no variation in brain exchange of ^{36}Cl when the blood-CSF electrical potential was altered. The former finding suggests that Cl^- movement across brain capillaries is passive and diffusional, whereas the latter hints that other mechanisms may be involved. In view of the paucity of data on Cl^- transport between blood and brain ECF, any further comments on this anion's mechanism of movement seem unwarranted.

GLIAL CELL REGULATION OF EXTRACELLULAR FLUID

A role for the glial cells in the regulation of ECF electrolytes, especially K^+, has been postulated for a number of years. These cells have high resting potentials which are very sensitive to the ECF concentration of K^+ and a sizable amount of Na-K-activated ATPase, which is much more sensitive to the external concentration of K^+ than is the neuronal enzyme (34). Furthermore, glial cells are linked morphologically and electrically to each other, but not to neurons, by gap junctions.

Orkand et al. (35) suggested that these cells might serve as "spatial buffers" for the brain ECF by conducting K^+ ions away from local areas in which extracellular K^+ increased due to neuronal activity. Such an arrangement could serve to regulate the immediate fluid environment and maintain a spatially and temporally limited homeostasis but would be incapable of handling or controlling the K^+ concentration of the ECF in the face of a significant leakage of K^+ from blood into brain ECF. Also, the relative importance of this transport process in even very transient circumstances is uncertain since the diffusion of K^+ through the ECS and reuptake of this ion by the neurons would also help dissipate localized changes in the ECF composition. Nevertheless, the peculiar electrical and membrane properties of glial cells are intriguing and, no doubt, important in some aspect or aspects of brain function.

CONCLUDING ANALYSIS AND DISCUSSION

Although many of the specific details for the various ions and transport sites are lacking, certain general conclusions about the transport mechanisms involved in the movements of electrolytes across three of the possible regulatory membranes—the choroid plexus, the pia-glia, and the ependyma—can be made from the results presented in the preceding sections. At the choroid plexuses, both active and passive processes operate to maintain a fairly constant composition in the newly formed CSF. As this fluid flows through the ventricular and subarachnoid spaces, free exchange of ions between the CSF and the adjacent brain ECF occurs. This transfer across the ependymal and pial-glial membranes and the subsequent distribution through the ECF to deeper tissue sites seem to happen by simple diffusion. These transport steps certainly would contribute to ionic homeostasis within the brain, but are they adequate to control the ECF concentration throughout the entire brain? Most investigators in the field of blood-brain-CSF transport physiology would guess that these processes in themselves are not enough to maintain the constancy of the brain's internal environment unless the blood-brain barrier is virtually impermeable to electrolytes, a situation which tracer studies have shown is not true.

Despite the general agreement that the brain capillary complex must be more than a passive barrier to ion transport, only limited experimental proof of this has been generated; nevertheless by combining these observations with the general properties of blood-CSF and CSF-brain exchange and a mathematical treatment of the system, certain conclusions about the nature of the transport processes at the blood-brain barrier can be made. The approach to the problem and the equations for the CSF-brain-blood transport system are similar to those published by Pape and Katzman (24) and Patlak and Fenstermacher (19). For the present treatment, the following assumptions are used: the CSF-brain interfaces (ependyma and pia-glia) are highly permeable; the only mechanism of ionic movement through the ECF is diffusion; the concentrations in the ECF at the ependymal and pial-glial surfaces are equal; the concentrations of electrolytes in the CSF, ECF, and intracellular fluid are constant with reference to time (steady-state assumption); and the geometry of the system is effectively rectangular. The differential equation for this situation is equation (2) of Patlak and Fenstermacher (19). Applying the appropriate boundary conditions yields the following solution which relates the concentration in the ECF, C_x, at a distance, x, from the brain surface to the variables of the system:

$$C_x = 2(C_f - C_a k_{po}/k_{pi}) \frac{\sinh(\lambda L/2)}{\sinh(\lambda L)}$$

$$\left\{ \cosh[\lambda(x - L/2] \right\} + C_a k_{po}/k_p \quad (1)$$

In this equation, C_f and C_a are the effective concentrations of the electrolyte in the CSF and arterial plasma, respectively; k_{pi} and k_{po} are the transfer coefficients of the brain capillary complex for the movement of the ion from brain ECF to plasma and plasma to ECF, respectively (for this treatment the k_p's are assumed to be constant with respect to distance and concentration); λ equals $(k_{pi}/D)^{1/2}$; D is the effective diffusion coefficient of the electrolyte through the brain ECF; and L equals the thickness of the brain. In the following tables and discussion, the capillary exchange half-time ($t_{1/2}$) will be used instead of the transfer coefficient; the relationship between these two constants is: $t_{1/2} = (1/k_p)\ln 2$. In addition, the capillary exchange process for the model system is considered to be diffusion, and thus k_{po} and k_{pi} are equal.

For the analysis, typical values for the several variables of the system will be substituted into Eq.(1) and the ECF concentration profiles generated in attempt to demonstrate that the transfer of electrolyte across the blood-brain barrier cannot occur only by diffusion if the brain ECF is to be regulated. Because the system is symmetrical around the midpoint, $x = L/2$, the C_x's only need to be calculated up to $L/2$. As previously presented, the apparent rates of material diffusion through the brain ECF vary from 20 to 50% of their comparable diffusion rates in water. On the basis of this, reasonable estimates for the D of Na+, K+, and Cl− in brain at 37°C range from 5 to 10×10^{-6} cm²/sec; for all calculation an intermediate value of 8×10^{-6} cm²/sec was used.

The effects of decreasing diffusional capillary exchange (increasing $t_{1/2}$) are shown in Table 2. In all cases a constant concentration of the ion

TABLE 2. *The effects of various capillary exchange rates on the relative ECF concentrations of a model ion at various points in the brain[a]*

Capillary $t_{1/2}$ (min)	Distance from CSF-brain interface (cm)					
	0.0	0.1	0.2	0.3	0.4	0.5
15	0.75	0.91	0.96	0.99	0.99	1.00
30[b]	0.75	0.88	0.94	0.97	0.98	0.98
90	0.75	0.83	0.88	0.91	0.93	0.93
300	0.75	0.79	0.82	0.84	0.85	0.85

[a] The following values for the variables were used: $D = 8 \times 10^{-6}$ cm²/sec; relative CSF concentration = 0.75; relative plasma concentration = 1.00; and brain thickness = 1.00.

[b] This capillary $t_{1/2}$ corresponds to the one for ⁴²K calculated by Davson and Welch (29).

TABLE 3. *The effects of brain thickness on the relative ECF concentrations of a model ion at various points in the brain*[a]

Brain thickness (cm)	Distance from CSF-brain interface (cm)					
	0.0	0.05	0.10	0.2	0.4	0.8
0.4	0.75	0.81	0.85	0.88	—	—
1.0	0.75	0.82	0.88	0.94	0.98	—
2.0	0.75	0.82	0.88	0.94	0.98	1.00

[a] The following values of the variables were used: $D = 8 \times 10^{-6}$ cm^2/sec; capillary $t_{1/2} = 30$ min; relative CSF concentration = 0.75; and relative plasma concentration = 1.00.

in the ECF has been established within 3 mm of the surface. The value of this steady-state concentration approaches the plasma level (1.0) for the shorter transfer times, 15 and 30 min; whereas a figure between the CSF (0.75) and plasma concentrations was found for the case of low capillary permeability ($t_{1/2} = 300$ min).

The brain thicknesses that were chosen and the animals which correspond to those dimensions are: 0.4 (rabbit), 1.0 (dog), and 2.0 (human) cm. The results are presented in Table 3. For the smallest sized brain, the ECF concentrations throughout the tissue remain significantly below the plasma levels. For the larger sized ones, a plateau which approached the plasma concentration was reached around 0.3 cm as noted in the previous paragraph. This distance seems to define the upper limit of the CSF's diffusional effectiveness for the regulation of ECF electrolyte composition for ions with D's and k_p's in the range considered to be realistic for Na$^+$ and K$^+$. Lower values of the capillary transfer coefficient ($t_{1/2} = 6$ hr), however, yielded ECF concentrations which were relatively close to the CSF values.

Table 4 shows the changes in the ECF profiles caused by plasma concentration perturbations. Lowering the plasma concentration to one-half the normal caused an appreciable lowering of the profile compared to the "control," whereas raising it produced a marked elevation of the profile. If ionic exchange between plasma and brain ECF occurs only by diffusion (the situation which was mathematically modelled), one would expect to see detectable changes in the brain levels of an electrolyte when its blood concentration is markedly altered. Such changes were not found for K$^+$ (12) but were suggested for Cl$^-$ (15).

In view of the evidence that tracers of Na$^+$, K$^+$, and other ions exchange at slow but reasonable rates between blood and brain, the results of the above calculations indicate that significant concentration gradients of electrolyte would exist in the brain ECF if the control of this fluid's ionic content was dependent only on diffusional exchange between a highly regulated CSF and the ECF. It, therefore, appears likely that the degree of ionic homeostasis which is known to occur in the brain during various experimental and pathological conditions could

TABLE 4. *The effects of plasma concentration on the relative ECF concentrations of a model ion at various points in the brain*[a]

Relative plasma concentration	Distance from CSF-brain interface (cm)					
	0.0	0.1	0.2	0.3	0.4	0.5
0.5	0.75	0.62	0.56	0.53	0.52	0.52
1.0	0.75	0.88	0.94	0.97	0.98	0.98
2.0	0.75	1.37	1.68	1.83	1.90	1.92

[a] The following values of the variables were used: $D = 8 \times 10^{-6}$ cm^2/sec; capillary $t_{1/2} = 30$ min; relative CSF concentration = 0.75; and brain thickness = 1.0 cm.

only be produced by a brain capillary system which serves as something more than a "tight" membrane or passive barrier to electrolytic transfer. Although the existing experimental evidence and the preceding computations provide a reasonable foundation for making such a statement, much work remains to be done before the precise mechanisms, the interrelationships with the flows of other ions and water, the energy sources, and the specific enzymes are established for the blood-brain exchange of the major ions.

ACKNOWLEDGMENTS

The author thanks Dr. Clifford S. Patlak for his generous assistance with the mathematical analysis and his critical review of the manuscript and Mrs. Josephine Clem for her excellent secretarial support.

REFERENCES

1. Cserr, H. F. (1971): Physiology of the choroid plexus. *Physiol. Rev.*, 51:273–311.
2. Katzman, R., and Pappius, H. (1973): *Brain Electrolytes and Fluid Metabolism.* Williams & Wilkins, Baltimore.
3. Ames, A., Sakanoue, M., and Endo, S. (1964): Na, K, Ca, Mg, and Cl concentrations in choroid plexus fluid and cisternal fluid compared with plasma ultrafiltrate. *J. Neurophysiol.*, 27:672–681.
4. Ames, A., Higashi, K., and Nesbett, F. B. (1965): Relation of potassium concentration in choroid-plexus fluid to that in plasma. *J. Physiol.*, 181:506–515.
5. Ames, A., Higashi, K., and Nesbett, F. B. (1965): Effects of P_{CO_2}, acetazolamide and ouabain on volume and composition of choroid-plexus fluid. *J. Physiol. (Lond.)*, 181:516–524.
6. Miner, L. C. and Reed, D. J. (1972): Composition of fluid obtained from choroid plexus tissue isolated in a chamber *in situ. J. Physiol.*, 227:127–139.
7. Pollay, M., Stevens, A., Estrada, E., and Kaplan, R. (1972): Extracorporeal perfusion of choroid plexus. *J. Appl. Physiol.*, 32:612–617.
8. Pollay, M., Kaplan, R., and Nelson, K. M. (1973): Potassium transport across the choroidal ependyma. *Life Sci.* II, 12:479–487.
9. Wright, E. M. (1972): Mechanisms of ion transport across the choroid plexus. *J. Physiol. (Lond.)*, 226:545–571.
10. Held, D., Fencl, V., and Pappenheimer, J. R. (1964): Electrical potential of cerebrospinal fluid. *J. Neurophysiol.*, 27:942–959.
11. Welch, K. and Sadler, K. (1965): Electrical potentials of choroid plexus of the rabbit. *J. Neurosurg.*, 22:344–351.
12. Bradbury, M. W. B., and Kleeman, R. (1967): Stability of the potassium content of cerebrospinal fluid and brain. *Am. J. Physiol.*, 213(2):519–528.
13. Graziani, L., Kaplan, R., Escriva, A., and Katzman, R. (1967): Calcium flux into CSF during ventricular and ventriculocisternal perfusion. *Am. J. Physiol.*, 213:629–636.
14. Gabelnick, H. L., Dedrick, R. L., and Bourke, R. S. (1970): *In vivo* mass transfer of chloride during exchange hemodialysis. *J. Appl. Physiol.* 28:636–641.
15. Bourke, R. S., Gabelnick, H. L., and Young, O. (1970): Mediated transport of chloride from blood into cerebrospinal fluid. *Exp. Brain Res.*, 10:17–38.
16. Abbott, J., Davson, H., Glen, I., and Grant, N. (1971): Chloride transport and potential across the blood-CSF barrier. *Brain Res.*, 29:185–193.
17. Fenstermacher, J., and Patlak, C. (1975): The exchange of material between cerebrospinal fluid and brain. In: *The Fluid Environment of the Brain,* edited by H. Cserr, J. Fenstermacher, and V. Fencl. New York, Academic Press (*in press*).
18. Fenstermacher, J. D., Patlak, C. S., and Blasberg, R. G. (1974): Transport of material between brain extracellular fluid, brain cells and blood. *Fed. Proc.*, 33:2070–2074.
19. Patlak, C., and Fenstermacher, J. (1975): Measurements of dog blood-brain transfer constants by ventriculocisternal perfusion. *Am. J. Physiol.* (*in press*).
20. Bito, L. Z. (1969): Blood-brain barrier: evidence for active cation transport between blood and the extracellular fluid of brain. *Science*, 165:81–83.
21. Bradbury, M. W. B. and Davson, H. (1965): The transport of potassium between blood, cerebrospinal fluid and brain. *J. Physiol. (Lond.)*, 181:151–174.
22. Cserr, H. (1965): Potassium exchange between cerebrospinal fluid, plasma, and brain. *Am. J. Physiol.*, 209(6):1219–1226.
23. Katzman, R., Graziani, L., and Ginsburg, S. (1968): Cation exchange in blood, brain and CSF. In: *Progress in Brain Research,* edited by A. Lajtha and D. H. Ford, pp. 283–294. American Elsevier, New York.
24. Pape, L. G. and Katzman, R. (1972): K^{42} distribution in brain during simultaneous ventriculocisternal and subarachnoid perfusion. *Brain Res.*, 38:49–69.
25. Katzman, R., Graziani, L., Kaplan, R., and Escriva, A. (1965): Exchange of cerebrospinal fluid potassium with blood and brain. *Arch. Neurol.*, 13:513–524.
26. Bradbury, M. W. B. (1965): Magnesium and calcium in cerebrospinal fluid and in the extracellular fluid of brain. *J. Physiol. (Lond.)*, 179:67–68P.

27. Graziani, L., Escriva, A., and Katzman, R. (1965): Exchange of calcium between blood, brain, and cerebrospinal fluid. *Am. J. Physiol.*, 208(6):1058–1064.

28. Oldendorf, W. (1971): Brain uptake of radiolabeled amino acids, amines, and hexoses after arterial injection. *Am. J. Physiol.*, 221:1629–1637.

29. Davson, H. and Welch, K. (1971): The permeation of several materials into the fluids of the rabbit's brain. *J. Physiol. (Lond.)*, 218:337–351.

30. Davson, H. and Segal, M. B. (1970): The effects of some inhibitors and accelerators of sodium transport on the turnover of ^{22}Na in the cerebrospinal fluid and the brain. *J. Physiol. (Lond.)*, 209:131–153.

31. Buhrley, L. E. and Reed, D. J. (1972): The effect of furosemide on sodium-22 uptake into cerebrospinal fluid and brain. *Exp. Brain Res.*, 14:503–510.

32. Bradbury, M. W. B. and Stulcova, B. (1970): Efflux mechanism contributing to the stability of the potassium concentration in cerebrospinal fluid. *J. Physiol. (Lond.)*, 208:415–430.

33. Bradbury, M., Segal, M., and Wilson, J. (1972): Transport of potassium at the blood-brain barrier. *J. Physiol. (Lond.)*, 221:617–632.

34. Henn, F., Haljamae, H., and Hamberger, A. (1972): Glial cell function: active control of extracellular K^+ concentration. *Brain Res.*, 43:437–443.

35. Orkand, R., Nicholls, J., and Kuffler, S. (1966): Effects of nerve impulses on the membrane potential of glial cells in the central nervous system of amphibia. *J. Neurophysiol.*, 29:788–806.

The Nervous System, Donald B. Tower, Editor-in-Chief. *Vol. 1: The Basic Neurosciences*. Raven Press, New York, 1975.

Pathophysiologic Aspects of Cerebral Ischemia

Igor Klatzo

Cerebral ischemia can be divided into two types: (1) *total or global* and (2) *regional or partial.* In the former the blood circulation is affected in a generalized fashion, such as occurs in cardiac arrest or shock; in the latter there is a regional interference with blood supply to particular regions of the brain. The regional ischemia, being the basic pathologic component of the stroke, constitutes the main subject of this article. In spite of its paramount clinical importance the understanding of cerebral ischemia with regard to its pathophysiologic effects on the brain tissue has been rather poor. One of the difficulties in this respect has been that, due to the great efficiency of the circulus of Willis, experimental models based on interruption of arterial blood supply have necessitated lengthy operations—a circumstance which has not been conducive to collecting adequate groups of animals for meaningful interpretation of the findings. The other difficulty has been related to the complexity of pathophysiologic conditions present in some experimental models. Criticism of this kind may apply, e.g., to a popular Levine's model (1) where hypoxia and ischemia (admittedly different in their effects upon brain tissue) are used in a combined way and the findings sometimes are indiscriminately interpreted in reference to the one or the other condition. For similar reasons embolism or acute hypotonia when used as experimental models to study cerebral ischemia should be recognized as different conditions from "pure" ischemia where the main pathophysiologic event constitutes the interference with the arterial blood supply.

Since the beginning of modern neuropathology of all elements of brain parenchyma the neurons have been considered as especially sensitive to both anoxia and ischemia. The "ischemic cell change" described by Spielmeyer (2) remains in the textbooks of neuropathology as the most characteristic neuronal alteration in ischemia. In further histopathologic studies, however, it became apparent that some changes ascribed to ischemia can be produced also by delayed or faulty fixation of the brain tissue. In this respect the occurrence of so-called "dark neurons" became particularly controversial (3). The advent of electron microscopy has brought another area of confusion in differentiation between anoxic, ischemic and fixation artifact changes since swelling of cellular organelles, such as mitochondria, and, especially, of the perivascular astrocytic processes was recognized as the common finding in all these three conditions. It is only recently with marked improvement in brain tissue processing for electron microscopy (EM) and with application of strictly controlled experimental conditions that the specific effect of ischemia upon brain tissue can be evaluated on the ultrastructural level; and it has been established that the above mentioned hydrophilic alterations within various cellular compartments represent true *in vivo* changes produced by ischemia, and not merely fixation artifacts.

The Mongolian gerbils (*Meriones unguiculatus*) which are characterized by frequent anomalies of the circulus of Willis offer special advantages, and the interpretations of cerebral ischemia proposed in this chapter are based primarily on the study of these animals. Although the unilateral occlusion of the common carotid artery in the neck results in ischemic infarction of the corresponding hemisphere in 30% of gerbils only, the simplicity of the experimental procedure allows for an easy and quick processing of a larger number of animals and for collecting statistically meaningful data based on many parameters of experimentation.

For obtaining an overall dynamic profile of morphological changes and their relationship to the duration of ischemic and postischemic periods, light microscopy, although inferior to EM in providing cytologic detail, presents obvious advantages and it was extensively used in the studies on Mongolian gerbils (4). Our observations revealed that the lesions develop during the ischemic period, as well as *after reestablishment of the circulation,* and this presents one facet of a *"maturation" phenomenon* which seems to be a general principle applicable to various parameters of ischemic injury. The rate of "maturation" of ischemic lesions in gerbils was directly related to the intensity (duration) of an ischemic insult, a lesser intensity resulting in slower development of the lesions. Thus, it took 1 week for a selective disintegration of the H2 sector of the hippocampus in carotid occlusions of short (8 to 15 min) duration, whereas similarly severe damage of this sector was observed in a few days following more prolonged occlusions. In another example, animals sacrificed almost immediately after 30 min occlusion showed practically no recognizable ischemic changes in the basal ganglia, whereas extensive, severe ischemic injury was observed in these structures in gerbils sacrificed after 20 hr release following occlusion of the same duration. The phenomenon of "maturation" was also recognizable in other parameters of ischemic injury. Thus, with regard to the behavior of the blood-brain barrier (BBB), in shorter unilateral carotid occlusion (e.g., 15 min), the gerbils previously injected with Evans Blue tracer never disclosed BBB damage. With 1 hr occlusion it took 20 hr for animals to show BBB changes, whereas with 6 hr occlusion all gerbils revealed Evans Blue discoloration of the brain within 1 hr after release of the clip (5). Another instance of the "maturation" phenomenon can be deduced from carbohydrate and biogenic amine assays in ischemic gerbils (6,7). Data for glycogen, serotonin, dopamine, and norepinephrine determinations revealed in animals with shorter occlusion periods peaks that were delayed but of similar magnitude to those that were reached in a relatively short time after more severe ischemic insults. In sensitive (symptom-positive) animals the lowest level glycogen (250 μmoles/kg) was recorded in the ipsilateral hemisphere at a 1 hr period of carotid occlusion; with longer occlusion the glycogen levels climbed steadily, reaching higher than starting point values at 9 hr. In nonsensitive (symptom-negative) animals, obviously much less affected by ischemia, the glycogen in the occluded hemisphere dropped to a similarly low level, but this oc-

curred after 3 hr of ischemic occlusion. With regard to biogenic amines, serotonin was considerably elevated in the affected hemisphere when the gerbils were sacrificed after 6 hr of carotid occlusion. However, when the occlusion lasted only 15 min and then the clip was released, it took 20 hr for the serotonin to reach almost the same level as in animals sacrificed immediately after 6 hr of carotid occlusion (7). Determinations for dopamine and norepinephrine showed that the lowest levels occurred much sooner after 1 hr than after 15 min of occlusion (7). Observations which could be interpreted as revealing similar "maturation" phenomenon were made by Van Harreveld and Marmont (8) in studies of asphyxia of the lumbosacral region in cats, the asphyxia being produced by raising the intradural pressure. In these experiments there was a secondary disappearance of tendon reflexes and tone after a certain time related to the duration of asphyxia. In similar, later experiments Van Harreveld and Trubatch (9) suggested that the delay in the final disappearance of the reflexes could be due to the fact that although the neurons are irreversibly damaged during the period of asphyxia, they retain enough of the enzymatic apparatus for their temporary repolarization and functioning, until it is exhausted.

As is evident from the foregoing observations, the intensity of injury in regional ischemia is primarily determined by degree of interference with blood supply and by duration of the period following release of occlusion, i.e., a period which allows for "maturation" of the lesions. It may be assumed, however, that even when the release of occlusion and reestablishment of circulation does not occur, there can be regional, zonal gradients in the intensity of injury around the foci with maximally impaired blood circulation. Thus, it is possible that a certain degree of "maturation" may follow definitive arterial occlusions, resulting in "growth" of ischemically damaged brain territories. It is intriguing to speculate whether deterioration in clinical condition or emergence of positive isotope scanning, not infrequently observed after a certain period of latency, may be related to the described "maturation" phenomenon.

Another finding brought out by our light microscopic observations on gerbils was the feature of *selective vulnerability* to ischemia

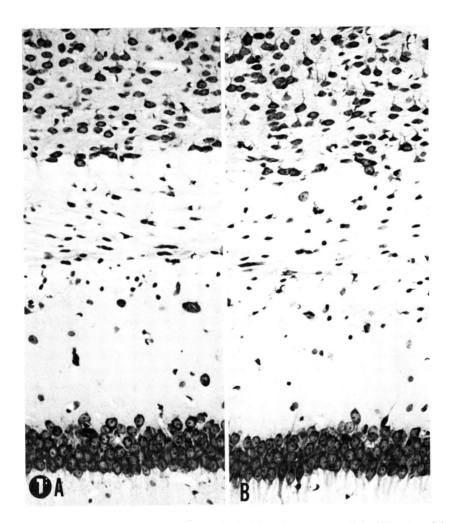

FIG. 1. A: Control gerbil perfused with paraformaldehyde. Normal appearance of the H2 sector of the hippocampus and the cerebral cortex. B: Corresponding area from the gerbil occluded for 4 min bilaterally and sacrificed 1 hr later showing accentuated staining of neuronal processes in the H2 sector and in the cerebral cortex. Both preparations stained with cresyl violet; × 150.

displayed by certain topistic units and most clearly observed in the hippocampus (4). There, the earliest recognizable effect of ischemia was expressed by the accentuated Nissl staining of the neuronal processes, confined strictly to H2 sector in the gerbils sacrificed shortly after 4 min occlusion of the common carotid arteries bilaterally. In the animals which were allowed to live 1 hr after 4 min of bilateral occlusion this change became much more prominent and it appeared to involve also the cortical neurons (Fig. 1). The most striking topistic lesion was the *"reactive change"* that was confined to the

H3 sector of the hippocampus. This change occurred only in those animals subjected to relatively slight ischemic insult (7 min bilateral or 15 min unilateral occlusion) and it was fully developed only after 20 hr of maturation. At this stage it was characterized by a peripheral shift of the nucleus whereas the voluminous cytoplasm showed a central chromatolysis (Figs. 2 and 3), the overall picture resembling that of *primäre Reizung* described by Nissl (10). The electron microscopic study on the reactive change revealed this region of the perikaryon filled with a dense accumulation of various

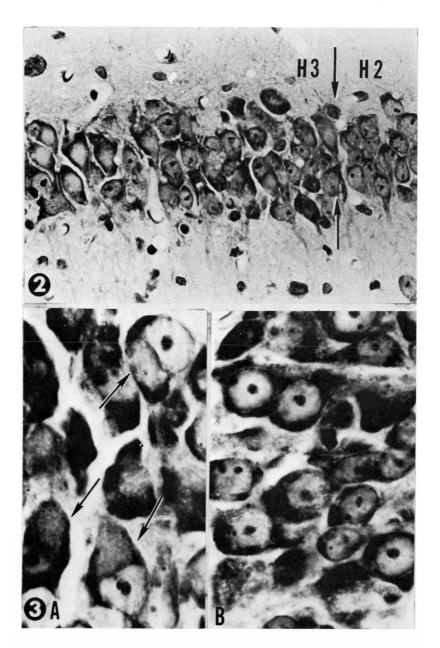

FIG. 2. Left common carotid artery occlusion for 15 min and 20 hr release. Arrows indicate the border between H2 and H3 sectors of the left hippocampus. The neurons of the H3 sector reveal the "reactive change." Cresyl violet stain; × 300.

FIG. 3. A: Area of H3 sector of the left hippocampus in a gerbil subjected 15 min occlusion of the left common carotid artery and 20 hr release. Arrows indicate neurons showing the "reactive change." **B:** Similar area from H3 of a normal gerbil. Cresyl violet stain; × 900 (both photographs).

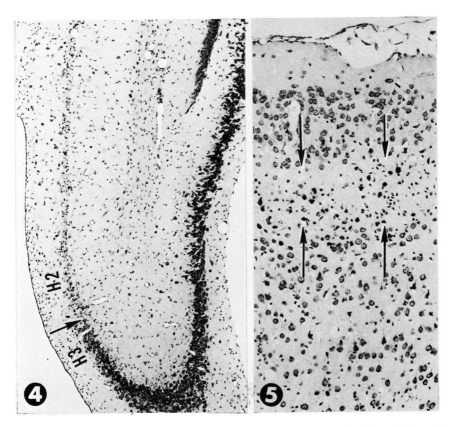

FIG. 4. Left hippocampus of the gerbil with 15 min of left carotid occlusion sacrificed 1 week later. There is almost complete neuronal disintegration of the H2 sector, whereas H3 sector appears to be well preserved. Cresyl violet stain; × 90.

FIG. 5. Left cerebral cortex of the gerbil with 1 hr left carotid occlusion and 20 hr release. Intense damage of the third layer (arrows). Cresyl violet stain; × 110.

organelles (11). Conspicuous among those were bizarrely shaped mitochondria, membrane-bound lysosomal structures, and unidentifiable, nonmembrane bound particles. Histochemical observations on the reactive change showed intense activity within the cytoplasm of affected neurons with regard to such enzymes as various dehydrogenases and acid phosphatase (12). The animals subjected to the duration of ischemia which produces reactive change at 20 hr, when sacrificed 1 week later, showed mostly excellent preservation of the H3 sector whereas the H2 sector revealed widespread disintegration of neurons (Fig. 4). It is thus evident that the reactive change represents a cellular reaction to ischemia in which the neurons are capable of full recovery from an ischemic injury. Our studies on gerbils showed that

selective vulnerability was also discernible in a laminar injury of cortical neurons with special predilection for the third layer. This finding was conspicuous 20 hr after release of the clip in the gerbils subjected to 1 hr unilateral occlusion (Fig. 5).

The feature of selective vulnerability is one of the tenets of Vogt and Vogt's (13) theory of pathoclisis which postulates a different affinity of different structural CNS units to different noxious agents. The basic assumptions of this theory were strongly supported by histochemical observations (14) demonstrating different enzymatic compositions of various neuronal units, e.g., individual layers of the cerebral cortex. More recently Folbergrova et al. (15) showed a differential behavior of metabolites of energy reserves in individual layers of the cortex in animals subjected to ischemia and anesthesia. Brierley (16) described a laminar pattern of ischemic cell damage in the cerebral cortex as a result of cardiac arrest. Is selective vulnerability dependent on regional differences in blood supply? It can be argued that regional differences in cerebral blood flow, demonstrated in various neuronal topistic units (17), reflect primarily metabolic requirements of particular types of neurons and thus are of secondary significance in the selective vulnerability phenomenon.

The acceptance of a pathoclisis role would support an assumption that the basic pathomechanism of ischemia is related to the *metabolic energy disturbance* and therefore the sensitivity of various CNS cellular units to ischemia is influenced by their metabolic state. Additional support for this assumption could be found by relating the histopathologic finding of considerable differences in the degree of ischemic damage frequently displayed by adjacent individual neurons in an ischemically affected region with Hydén's (18) cytochemical analysis indicating marked differences in metabolic and functional state of individual neurons within an anatomic unit.

It is possible that in cerebral ischemia two modalities of ischemic injury are operative. (a) The *fast* modality—related to an acute energy crisis as expressed in precipitous drops in levels of glucose, glycogen and energy phosphates, associated with a concomitant rise in lactate and pyruvate. Simultaneously affected may be energy-dependent osmotic regulation resulting in increased water uptake by various cellular compartments. (b) The *slow* modality—related to depletion of enzymic and structural protein reserves combined with inability to replenish them by nuclear or cytoplasmic synthesis. The latter type of ischemic injury may account for the described "maturation" phenomenon.

Unquestionably, one of the most serious complications of ischemia is the *brain edema* and its sequelae. The abnormal accumulation of fluid, which is the basic definition of edema, begins promptly following an ischemic injury. The fluid accumulates predominantly in neurons and astrocytes—neuronal mitochondria, astrocytic vascular processes, and dendrites being especially susceptible to swelling. In light

microscopic observations the initial cellular water uptake can be recognized as a vacuolization of the neuropil. The water distention affecting most of the cellular elements is very conspicuous in the later stages of ischemic injury (Fig. 6). It is a matter of definition when such microscopically evident cellular water uptake reaches an extent to be called brain edema. Clearly the water uptake and grossly recognizable brain edema greatly increase with the advent of a necrotic disintegration of the tissue, which considerably changes osmotic balances in the affected area. According to the proposed classification of brain edemas (19), the edema occurring as a complication of cerebral ischemia should be classified as basically of a *cytotoxic* type. This assumption is supported by observations on the BBB which indicate that only in the later stages of ischemia, associated with rather severe tissue injury, is there a breakdown of the BBB which introduces a *vasogenic* component into the existing cytotoxic edema developed by intracellular imbibition of fluid (5). The edema of brain tissue as a complication of ischemia introduces an important factor into the subsequent dynamic development of ischemic injury. Intracellular water uptake produces an increased tissue pressure that may have several consequences, the most serious of which derives from the compression of arteries caught between bony confines of the skull or rigid tentorium and edematous brain tissue (Fig. 7). The resulting secondary ischemia of this origin may start a *circulus vitiosus,* edema-ischemia-edema, and this is presumably the mechanism which operates in the clinical cases of uncal and cerebellar herniations. Increased tissue pressure also might be responsible for the frontal advancement of ischemic territory by compression of adjacent cellular structures, their swelling and further advancement by involvement of new marginal zones. In support of such an assumption are our observations in gerbils showing areas of the cerebral cortex affected by ischemia being demarcated from unaffected regions by narrow zones of dark, compressed neurons and the observations of Garcia and Kamijyo (20) demonstrating progressive extension in time of ischemic lesions in monkeys subjected to middle cerebral artery occlusion.

Cerebral ischemia being a cerebrovascular

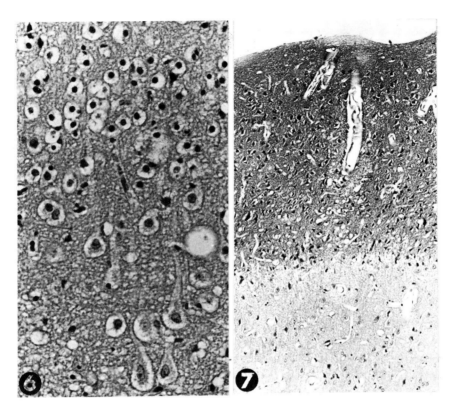

FIG. 6. Cerebral cortex of the gerbil occluded for 6 hr and sacrificed following one hour release. All cellular elements show intense cytoplasmic vacuolization which is also prominent in the neuropil. H. & E. stain; × 300.

FIG. 7. Gerbil occluded for 1 hr and sacrificed 20 hr later. There is a sharp demarcation between the severely damaged upper layers and the lower layers of the cerebral cortex. The animal showed an extensive necrotic focus in the underlying basal ganglia. H. & E. stain; × 90.

disturbance is greatly influenced by the systemic *blood pressure.* An *acute hypotension* has been used to produce ischemic lesions (21), and recently Dodson et al. (22) demonstrated in an ultrastructural study that the compound effects of hypotension plus ischemia result in more widespread and complex morphologic response than either hypotension or ischemia alone. In our studies on gerbils an acute hypotension, which was found to follow immediately the release of arterial occlusion, was closely associated with the appearance of a "no-reflow" phenomenon (23). The no-reflow phenomenon was evaluated by intravascular injections of carbon particle suspensions before the termination of experiments at different time intervals after carotid clip release. The appearance of a no-reflow phenomenon was of a transitory nature and its incidence was correlated closely

with a drop in the levels of systemic blood pressure. It could not be demonstrated after periods longer than 15 min following release of occlusion during which time there was full recovery from the drop in blood pressure. Also indicating a close relationship between systemic blood pressure and the no-reflow phenomenon was the fact that the latter could be abolished by administration of pharmacological agents such as epinephrine, which prevented a drop in blood pressure following release of an occlusion. It is then likely that acute hypotension in areas with presumably compromised vascular autoregulation may cause sludging, stasis, and circulatory standstill which would have deleterious effects propagating further ischemic injury.

Our studies on gerbils revealed similarly damaging effects of *hypertension* on the brain tissue subjected to ischemia (5). The animals

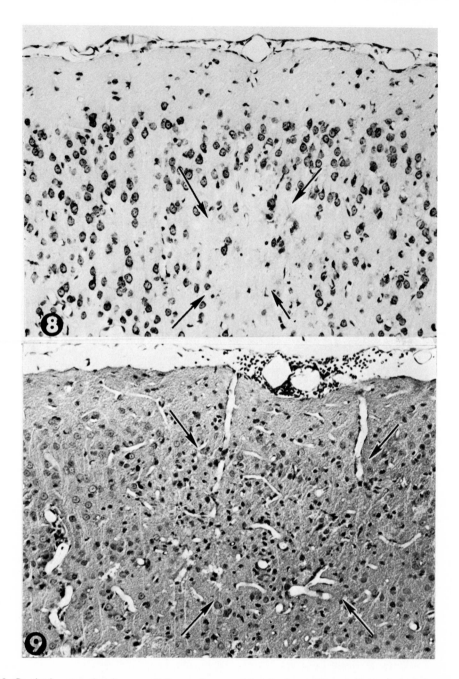

FIG. 8. Cerebral cortex showing a small focus of neuronal loss in the gerbil occluded unilaterally for 1 hr and sacrificed 1 week later. The adjacent neurons appear to be well preserved. Cresyl violet stain; × 140.

FIG. 9. Other area in the cortex of the same animal. The ischemic injury is recognizable by the presence of inflammatory cells in the subarachnoid space overlying small focus of condensation of glial cells and capillaries (arrows). H. & E. stain; × 140.

made hypertensive during the period of release of occlusion revealed consequently much more severe and earlier occurring damage to the BBB. Comparison between two groups of gerbils, which were all subjected to identical durations of occlusion and release but differed in one group with elevated blood pressure, showed that the histopathologic picture of ischemic injury was conspicuously more severe in the hypertensive group. The biochemical assays on these two groups revealed that in the hypertensive animals the lactate levels following release of occlusion kept rising, in contrast to the control normotensive group. It appears then that for brain tissue subjected to ischemia both systemic hypotension and hypertension may have very harmful effects and this should be of significance for the clinical management of stroke patients.

The clinically important question of *neuronal recovery* has been a controversial one, primarily because of the difficulty in ascertaining the functional state of neurons from static morphologic pictures. Nonetheless, the light microscopic observations on gerbils (4) indicated that a considerable neuronal recovery from ischemia is possible. For example, the comparison between groups of animals all occluded for 1 hr but sacrificed at different intervals after release of the clip revealed the following: In all animals sacrificed 20 hr after release the cerebral cortex showed extensive neuronal changes. On the other hand, the majority of gerbils sacrificed 1 week later showed remarkably well-preserved cortical neurons. Only occasional foci of cell disappearance (Fig. 8), glial modules, or capillary proliferations (Fig. 9) testified that such areas had been affected by ischemia. Thus, this comparison suggests that many of the neurons which showed marked ischemic changes at 20 hr have by now completely recovered. Another instance of apparent neuronal recovery has been described above as a reactive change in the H3 neurons in gerbils occluded for short periods of time and sacrificed 20 hr later. An indication of neuronal ability to recover from ischemia is also provided by histochemical observations in gerbils (12), demonstrating a strong enzymatic activity in neurons with pronounced ischemic changes such as chromatolysis, cytoplasmic vacuolization, or intense hyperchromasia. The intense enzymatic activity in these neurons clearly indicates their viability at the time of the termination of the experiment. Finally, a remarkable reversibility of ischemic brain damage after 1 hr of total ischemia has been reported by Hossmann and Kleihues (24).

These brief pathophysiologic considerations of cerebral ischemia are thus concluded on an optimistic note that a considerable recovery of brain from ischemic injury can be achieved. This should provide encouragement for further elucidation of the pathomechanisms involved, with the hope of developing new approaches for successful clinical management of many stroke patients.

REFERENCES

1. Levine, S. (1960): Anoxic-ischemic encephalopathy in rats. *Am. J. Pathol.*, 36:1–17.
2. Spielmeyer, W. (1922): *Histopathologie des Nervensystems*, pp. 74–79. Springer, Berlin.
3. Cammermeyer, J. (1961): The importance of avoiding dark neurons in experimental neuropathology. *Acta Neuropathol.* (Berlin), 1:245–270.
4. Ito, U., Spatz, M., Walker, J. T., Jr., and Klatzo, I.: Experimental cerebral ischemia in Mongolian gerbils. I. Light microscopic observations. *Acta Neuropathol.* (*in press*).
5. Ito, U., Spatz, M., and Klatzo, I.: Experimental cerebral ischemia in Mongolian gerbils. III. Behaviour of the blood-brain barrier. *Acta Neuropathol.* (in press).
6. Mrsulja, B. B., Mrsulja, B. J., Ito, U., Spatz, M., and Klatzo, I.: Experimental cerebral ischemia in Mongolian gerbils. II. Carbohydrate changes. *Acta Neuropathol.* (*in press*).
7. Mrsulja, B. B., Mrsulja, B. J., Ito, U., Spatz, M., and Klatzo, I.: Experimental cerebral ischemia in Mongolian gerbils. V. Behaviour of biogenic amines. *In preparation.*
8. Van Harreveld, A., and Marmont, G. (1939): The course of recovery of the spinal cord from asphyxia. *J. Neurophysiol.*, 11:101–111.
9. Van Harreveld, A., and Trubatch, J. (1974): Reflex figures during asphyxial rigidity. *Exp. Neurol.*, 45:161–173.
10. Nissl, F. (1892): Über die Veränderungen der Ganglienzellen am Facialiskern des Kaninchens nach Ansreissung der Nerven. *Allg. Z. Psychiatr.*, 48:197–206.
11. Bubis, J., Mrsulja, B. J., Ito, U., Spatz, M., and Klatzo, I.: Experimental cerebral ischemia in Mongolian gerbils. VII. Ultrastructural observations on the "reactive change" in the hippocampus. *In preparation.*
12. Mrsulja, B. J., Bubis, J., Ito, U., Spatz, M., and

Klatzo, I.: Experimental cerebral ischemia in Mongolian gerbils. VI. Histochemical observations on the reactive change in the hippocampus. *In preparation.*

13. Vogt, C., and Vogt, O. (1922): Erkrankungen der Grosshirnrinde in Lichte der Topistik, Pathoklise und Pathoarchitektonik. *J. Psychol. Neurol.,* 28:9–68.

14. Friede, R. L. (1968): Mappings of oxidative enzymes in the brain. In: *Pathology of the Nervous System,* edited by J. Minckler, pp. 306–320. McGraw-Hill, New York.

15. Folbergrova, J., Lowry, O. H., and Passonneau, J. V. (1970): Changes in metabolites of the energy reserves in individual layers of mouse cerebral cortex and subjacent white matter during ischemia and anesthesia. *J. Neurochem.,* 17:1155–1162.

16. Brierley, J. B. (1972): Pathology of cerebral ischemia. In: *Cerebral Vascular Diseases, VIII Conference,* edited by F. H. McDowell and R. W. Brennan, pp. 59–75. Grune and Stratton, New York and London.

17. Reivich, M. (1972): Regional cerebral blood flow in physiologic and pathophysiologic states. In: *Cerebral Blood Flow,* edited by J. S. Meyer and J. P. Schade, *Progress in Brain Research,* Vol. 35, pp. 191–228. Elsevier, Amsterdam.

18. Hydén, H. (1943): Die Funktion des Kernkör-penchens bei der Eiweissbildung in Nervenzellen. *Zeit. Mikr.-anat. Forschung,* 54:96–129.

19. Klatzo, I. (1967): Presidential Address: Neuropathological aspects of brain edema. *J. Neuropathol. Exp. Neurol.,* 26:1–13.

20. Garcia, J. H., and Kamijyo, Y. (1974): Cerebral infarction. Evolution of histopathologic changes after occlusion of a middle cerebral artery in primates. *J. Neuropathol. Exp. Neurol.,* 33:408–421.

21. Brierley, J. B., Brown, A. W., Excell, B. J., and Meldrum, B. S. (1969): Brain damage in the Rhesus monkey resulting from profound arterial hypotension. I. Its nature, distribution and general physiological correlates. *Brain Res.,* 13:68–100.

22. Dodson, R. F., Aoyagi, M., Hartmann, A., and Tagashira, Y. (1974): Acute cerebral infarction and hypotension: An ultrastructural study. *J. Neuropathol. Neurol.,* 33:400–407.

23. Klatzo, I., Ito, U., Go, K. G., and Spatz, M. (1974): Observations on experimental cerebral ischemia in Mongolian gerbils. In: *Pathology of Cerebral Microcirculation,* edited by J. Cervós-Navarro, pp. 338–341. Walter de Gruyter Publ., New York and Berlin.

24. Hossmann, K.-A., and Kleihues, P. (1973): Reversibility of ischemic brain damage. *Arch. Neurol.,* 29:375–384.

The Nervous System, Donald B. Tower, Editor-in-Chief. *Vol. 1: The Basic Neurosciences.* Raven Press, New York, 1975.

Introduction to Section on Neuropharmacology

Neuropharmacology since 1950 has developed from the concept of chemical neurotransmission and the concept that drug receptors are specific molecular entities. Both of these ideas were strongly disputed and ill defined in 1950. Evidence for the role of acetylcholine at neuroeffector and ganglionic junctions had accumulated slowly with the help of specific blocking agents. Otherwise, neuropharmacology was empirical and the availability of drugs as tools to study the nervous system was limited.

Then, within about 5 years a rapid evolution of ideas and methods for their investigation took place. The roles of norepinephrine and epinephrine as neurotransmitter and as hormone, respectively, began to be defined. Sensitive methods for chemical and histochemical detection of enzymes and neurotransmitters became available. The biosynthetic and degradative pathways of these agents were analyzed. This led to the classification and discovery of drugs that influenced the synthesis, release, metabolism, and reuptake of neurotransmitters. Neuroendocrinology grew from the discoveries of the anatomical relation between the pituitary and the hypothalamus, the concept of feed-back control, and the discovery of release mechanisms of hormones and of pineal function and its control. The idea of narcotic analgesic receptors slowly emerged from the discovery of narcotic antagonists. The availability of membranes rich in nicotinic receptors (the *Electrophorus* and *Torpedo* electroplax), of sensitive and specific methods for measuring ligand-receptor binding, and of site-specific blocking agents led to the development of the concept that drug receptors are specific molecular entities and to criteria for their isolation and identification.

The papers included in this Section on Neuropharmacology represent many of the accomplishments that have come out of the background I have briefly described. They also indicate that by the time of the 50th anniversary of the National Institute of Neurological and Communicative Disorders and Stroke there will be more significant advances in neuropharmacology. These will have great impact on knowledge of the etiology, pathogenesis, and treatment of diseases of the nervous systems and on understanding of the differentiation and function of neural pathways. Examples of the kinds of problems we can expect to be solved include: identification of the endogenous ligand for narcotic analgesic receptors and the molecular basis of addiction and tolerance; the reconstitution of some functional neuronal systems *in vitro;* the mechanisms of the coupling of receptor activation to postsynaptic permeability changes; the role of cyclic AMP as an intracellular postsynaptic messenger; and the mechanism of transsynaptic enzyme synthesis and hormone release.

The NINCDS has been a source of financial support and its staff has been a source of inspiration and guidance for neuropharmacological research. The contributions to this section leave no doubt about the value of this support. The Institute will have no difficulty in attracting skilled and imaginative investigators who will continue to help it to fulfill its missions.

Steven E. Mayer
La Jolla, California
July 1, 1975

The Nervous System, Donald B. Tower, Editor-in-Chief. *Vol. 1: The Basic Neurosciences*. Raven Press, New York, 1975.

The Acetylcholine Receptor: Isolation and Characterization

Arthur Karlin

The acetylcholine receptor (AChR) transduces the binding of acetylcholine (ACh) into an increase in the permeability of the postsynaptic membrane. One goal of current research is a molecular description of this phenomenon, namely of the interactions of the AChR with ACh and its congeners, with permeating cations, and with near-neighbors in the membrane, all in terms of the chemical and physical properties of the AChR. Another goal is the determination of the mechanisms controlling the synthesis, localization, and degradation of the AChR. Significant progress toward these goals has been made in the last few years as means have been developed for identifying the AChR, other than by the physiological response to ACh.

In order to achieve a complete molecular description it is necessary to return to a study of the physiological response (i.e., of the permeability changes), not only in cells but also in membrane systems reconstituted from purified AChR and other characterized membrane components. The description of the physiological response in intact cells has been much refined recently with the introduction of the analysis of "noise" (1,2), and thus the demands on a molecular description are more rigorous. This review encompasses work on the nicotinic, excitatory type of AChR found in vertebrate skeletal muscle and in the homologous electrogenic cells (electroplax) of the fish, *Electrophorus electricus* and *Torpedo sp.* (For a more detailed review, see ref. 3.)

REVERSIBLE BINDING OF ACh AND ITS CONGENERS

All approaches to the AChR begin with the response of cells to ACh and the modification of this response. The binding properties of the AChR are inferred from the variation of the response as a function of the concentration of ACh and of its congeners. The occupation of binding sites is usually taken to be determined by the Langmuir adsorption isotherm, formally equivalent to the Michaelis–Menten equation. The response to agonists (or activators) is assumed to increase with increasing occupation. If the response were linearly proportional to occupation, then the equilibrium dissociation constant for an activator-AChR complex would be equal to the concentration of activator eliciting a half-maximal response. The latter quantity is taken as the apparent dissociation constant (K_{app}) even though the relationship between the measured response and the extent of occupation is not likely to be a simple proportionality. This difficulty can be circumvented in the case of competitive inhibitors, the K_I for which can be determined independently of the type of response measured (4).

The electric tissue of the electric eel (*Electrophorus electricus*) has proved to be a most valuable source for AChR. The pharmacological characterization of the AChR in intact cells (electroplax) dissected from this tissue has been carried out largely in the laboratory of David Nachmansohn (e.g., 5). The results are in fact similar to those obtained previously with skeletal muscle by similar methods (6). The archetype competitive inhibitor, (+)-tubocurarine, for example, has a K_I of about 2×10^{-7} M.

One approach, the first one tried, to the direct assay of AChR is to test for the binding of ligands such as (+)-tubocurarine. It is to be remembered that such ligands dissociate from the receptor very rapidly so that a ligand-receptor complex cannot be isolated free of unbound ligand. Early attempts to isolate AChR from electric tissue and to assay it by the binding of (+)-tubocurarine (7) or gallamine (8) were unsuccessful. Aqueous extracts were retained, and particulate fractions were discarded; the latter are now known to contain all of the AChR. Binding data were incomplete and not comparable to dose-response data. Waser (9), however, was able to demonstrate by autoradiography localized, saturable binding of ^{14}C-toxiferine at the end-plate regions of mouse diaphragm, though, of course, this was not useful in the isolation of AChR.

The first successful use of reversible binding to identify AChR in a subcellular fraction was that of O'Brien and Gilmour (10) who looked at the binding of ^{3}H-muscarone (both a nicotinic and muscarinic agonist) to particulate fractions of electric tissue of the rays *Torpedo marmorata* and *T. oscellata*. The binding was found to saturate at 2 nmoles/g of original tissue with a dissociation constant of 7×10^{-6} M. In addition, ACh and other nicotinic agents competed with this binding in a manner consistent with dose-response data for these agents (obtained with other tissues). Despite this early success, reversible binding did not prove practical as a primary assay in the isolation of AChR. Nevertheless, the determination of the binding of ACh and other nicotinic agents competed with of characterizing the AChR, once isolated.

BINDING OF α-NEUROTOXINS

The venoms of elapid and hydrophid snakes contain highly toxic polypeptides (11). A class of these, the α-neurotoxins (MW of 7,000 to 8,000), act specifically on the AChR in the postsynaptic membrane of vertebrate muscle and electroplax. They produce a nondepolarizing block similar to that produced by (+)-tubocurarine, and this block is reversed only very slowly if at all by washing. Lee and his associates (11) demonstrated in the 1960s that ^{131}I-labeled α-neurotoxins bind specifically to neuromuscular junctions and that this binding is inhibited by (+)-tubocurarine.

Changeux, Kasai, and Lee (12) demonstrated that α-bungarotoxin acts on the electroplax of *Electrophorus* as it does on vertebrate muscle and that, in addition, it displaced the binding of ^{14}C-decamethonium to subcellular membrane vesicles prepared from *Electrophorus* electric tissue. Miledi, Molinoff, and Potter (13), also proceeding on the basis of the work of Lee and his associates, demonstrated

the binding of ^{131}I-α-bungarotoxin to a crude membrane fraction of *Torpedo marmorata*. They showed that the toxin-binding component is solubilized from the membranes by a solution containing the nonionic detergent Triton X-100. The rate of binding of α-bungarotoxin to the membranes was shown to be decreased in the presence of high concentrations of carbamylcholine and of (+)-tubocurarine. Raftery et al. (14), Meunier et al. (15), and Fulpius et al. (16) described the binding of various radioactively tagged α-toxins to membrane fragments from *Electrophorus* electric tissue and to detergent extracts of the membrane fractions. It was confirmed that toxin binding is retarded in the presence of reversible AChR ligands.

Further evidence for the specificity of the binding of the α-toxins for the AChR is that the extent of binding of radioactively tagged toxin correlates with the extent of physiological inhibition, although the latter lags behind the former initially (17,18). Both by dissection and by autoradiography, toxin at low concentrations binds predominantly at the end-plate of normal muscle, and this binding is decreased by about 50% in the presence of a high concentration of (+)-tubocurarine (19–21). That portion of the binding to the end-plate which can be blocked with (+)-tubocararine is that relevant to the response to ACh (22). Correlated with increased sensitivity to ACh, non-end-plate binding of toxin increases by an order of magnitude following denervation (19,20,23). During differentiation of myogenic cells in culture, binding of toxin correlates with the development of a depolarizing response to ACh (17,24).

AFFINITY LABELING

The successful affinity labeling of the AChR depends on the fortuitous presence of an easily reducible disulfide bond in the close vicinity of the ACh binding site (25). Reduction of this disulfide group with dithiothreitol alters the pharmacological specificity of the AChR in *Electrophorus* electroplax: the response to monoquaternary activators (ACh, carbamylcholine, butyltrimethylammonium) is decreased; the response to the bis-quaternary activator decamethonium is increased; and hexamethonium, normally an inhibitor, is an activator of the reduced receptor. All effects of reduction are fully reversed by oxidizing agents. This reversal is blocked if the oxidizing agent is preceded by an alkylating agent such as *N*-ethylmaleimide (NEM). Similar effects have been observed in muscle of other vertebrate species (3).

Maleimide derivatives bearing a quaternary ammonium group act similarly to NEM in preventing the reversal of the effects of dithiothreitol by oxidizing agents, but at apparent rates three orders of magnitude greater than NEM. An optimal enhancement in the apparent rate of alkylation of 1,100-fold is obtained with 4-(*N*-maleimido)benzyltrimethylammonium ion (MBTA), one of a series of quaternary ammonium derivatives (25). The reaction with the quaternary ammonium derivatives but not that with the uncharged maleimides is retarded by reversible AChR ligands. In the absence of prior reduction of the AChR, the quaternary ammonium maleimides act as completely reversible, competitive inhibitors. These maleimides are affinity labels (26) of the reduced receptor. The distance from the quaternary ammonium group of MBTA to the reactive maleimide double bond is about 1 nm, suggesting a similar distance in the ACh binding site from the negative subsite binding the ammonium group to at least one of the SH groups formed by reduction (25).

The quantity of AChR was determined for the first time in intact electroplax (*Electrophorus*) using the tritiated affinity label, 4-(*N*-maleimido)benzyltri(^{3}H)methylammonium ion (^{3}H-MBTA). Following the procedures used in the physiological experiments, cells were reduced with dithiothreitol and then alkylated with ^{3}H-MBTA, labeling the AChR and also some of the more slowly reacting, but more numerous, nonreceptor SH groups. Other cells were labeled similarly except that the addition of an AChR ligand or of an affinity oxidizing agent was interposed between reduction and alkylation, protecting the AChR but not the nonreceptor sites from alkylation. The difference between the extents of labeling of unprotected and of the protected group of cells was taken as the specific labeling. Quantitatively it approaches an asymptotic limit as the concentration of ^{3}H-MBTA increases. This limit, an estimate of the quantity of AChR, is about 10 pmoles labeled sites per gram wet weight of

cell (27), in fair agreement with subsequent estimates by α-toxin binding.

The affinity labeled AChR can be dissociated in sodium dodecyl sulfate (SDS) solutions and the covalently labeled polypeptide separated and characterized by SDS-polyacrylamide gel electrophoresis (28). This is not possible with the α-toxin-labeled AChR, since the α-toxins dissociate from the AChR in SDS (e.g., 20). The specifically affinity labeled component of intact electroplax was shown to be a polypeptide of about 40,000 daltons (28). Thus, a subunit of the AChR was identified that bears all or part of the ACh binding site.

PURIFICATION OF THE AChR

The various types of assays described above are based on properties of the ACh binding site(s), and it is the quantity and/or reactivity of these sites which are determined and for which direct evidence of purification is obtained. It is conveniently assumed that when the binding sites are present, the complete AChR is also present. The first step in purification has been in all cases to prepare a more or less crude membrane fraction of electric tissue from *Electrophorus* or *Torpedo*. This fraction is in some cases extracted with 1 M NaCl to remove a large part of the acetylcholinesterase (29). In all cases, the AChR is extracted from the membrane by a 1 to 3% solution of a nonionic detergent (usually Triton X-100). The AChR in the extract is then adsorbed to an affinity gel consisting of either an α-toxin or a small AChR ligand attached covalently to beads of agarose (Table 1). After the "nonspecifically" adsorbed proteins are eluted with media of elevated ionic strength, the AChR is eluted with media containing high concentrations of small AChR ligands (e.g., carbamylcholine, benzoquinonium, hexamethonium). The eluted AChR is subjected to dialysis and/or in some cases additional procedures such as sedimentation in a sucrose-density gradient to remove the eluting ligand and to purify further. The reported overall purifications have been 2,000- to 4,000-fold from *Electrophorus* and 100- to 300-fold from *Torpedo*. (*Torpedo* tissue contains about 15-fold as much AChR per gram as *Electrophorus* tissue.)

There are obvious differences in the specific

TABLE 1. *Purification of AChR*

Gel ligand[a]	Specific activity[b] (μmoles sites/g protein)	MW SDS-PGE[c] (10³ daltons)	Ref.
Electrophorus			
N. naja toxin	7.5	42, 54	(30)
N. N. siam. toxin	11	160[d]	(31)
—HNφ(—OCH₂CHṄEt₃)₂	6	43, 48	(32)
—HNφṄMe₃	4.5	44, 50	(33)
—OCφṄMe₃	4.5[e]	40, 47, 53	(34)
Torpedo			
—HN(CH₂)₃ṄMe₃	10	40, 50, 65	(35)
N. n. siam. toxin	2	45, 50	(36)
N. n. siam. toxin	2.8, 8[f]	46, —, —[g]	(37,38)
—OCφṄMe₃	4[e]	39, 48, 58, 64	(39)

[a] Toxin is linked directly to agarose. The small ligands are linked to agarose by an arm 7 to 22 atoms long.

[b] Assay is by toxin binding, except e and f.

[c] These are the apparent molecular weights of major staining bands on polyacrylamide gel electrophoresis of reduced AChR preparation in SDS, except that [d] is unreduced.

[e] Assay is by affinity labeling with ³H-MBTA. Toxin binding gives about twice the specific activity.

[f] This value is the sum of two classes of ACh binding sites which are only 50% blocked by high concentrations of (+)-tubocurarine.

[g] Molecular weights of additional components not given.

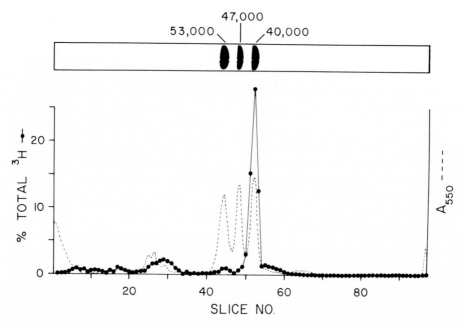

FIG. 1. Acrylamide gel electrophoresis in SDS of purified receptor from *Electrophorus electricus* affinity labeled with ³H-MBTA. **Top:** Photograph of gel stained with Coomassie Brilliant Blue. **Bottom:** ³H activity (45,000 cpm total) in 1 mm slices of the same gel superimposed on the densitometer trace obtained before slicing.

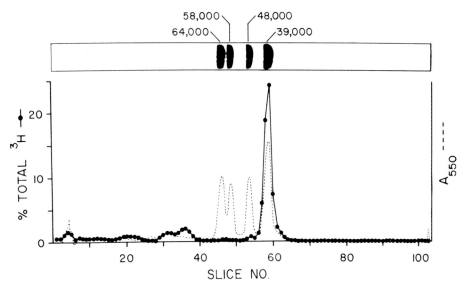

FIG. 2. Acrylamide gel electrophoresis in SDS of purified receptor from *Torpedo californica* affinity labeled with ³H-MBTA. Details are as in Fig. 1.

activities reported for purified AChR (Table 1). Some of these differences depend on the assays used. In the assay by reduction and affinity alkylation with ³H-MBTA, all of the labeling of purified AChR is blocked by pretreatment of the AChR with the α-toxin of *Naja naja siamensis* (34,39,40). Conversely, less than half of the binding of ³H-α-toxin is blocked by prealkylation of the AChR with MBTA (40). In fact, there appear to be twofold as many α-toxin binding sites as ³H-MBTA reactive sites on the AChR purified either from *Electrophorus* (40) or *Torpedo* (39). These results are consistent with the reports that twice the number of moles of α-toxin are bound compared to ACh to *Torpedo* (41) and *Electrophorus* (32) AChR. The reason for the greater binding of α-toxin is not known. It is possible, however, that even in purified AChR there are at least two classes of α-toxin binding sites.

SUBUNITS

All purified AChR preparations, with the possible exception of one (31), contain two or more molecular weight classes of polypeptides as determined by SDS-polyacrylamide gel electrophoresis (Table 1). There is the ubiquitous presence of a polypeptide component

of about 40,000 daltons. In addition, there are higher molecular weight components. In comparing *Electrophorus* and *Torpedo* AChR, it is apparent that components of about 40,000 and 48,000 daltons are present in both. An even more striking similarity is that reduction and affinity labeling with ³H-MBTA of purified AChR from either species results in the incorporation of radioactivity exclusively into the approximately 40,000 dalton components (34,39; Figs. 1 and 2). These components are in fact the only ones for which a function has been defined, namely the bearing of all or part of the ACh binding site, and which have certain status as subunits of the AChR. The functions of the other components remain to be determined. There is little evidence as to the stoichiometry of the putative subunits in the complete AChR.

HYDRODYNAMIC PROPERTIES

The α-toxin binding component of *Electrophorus* membrane extracted in nonionic detergent (14,15,31) and purified (33), or extracted in bile salt solution (15), has an apparent Stokes radius by gel filtration on agarose of about 7 nm. This is approximately equivalent to the Stokes radius of β-galactosidase, of molecular weight

540,000. The affinity-labeled component in *Electrophorus* membrane is obtained in an aggregate of similar size to the toxin-binding component after extraction in nonionic detergent (42). The nonionic detergent extract of *Torpedo* membrane contains two components with different Stokes radii binding toxin with differing affinities: the higher affinity component has a greater Stokes radius and the lower affinity component has the same Stokes radius as β-galactosidase (43).

The sedimentation coefficients of the toxin binding component from *Electrophorus* (15,30), from rat muscle (20), and the smaller of the two from *Torpedo* (43) are close to that of catalase, of molecular weight 240,000. This difference from the results of gel filtration is due partially to bound detergent, which increases the effective Stokes radius and decreases the density of the complex, and partially to shape factors (44). The molecular weight of the toxin-AChR complex, corrected for bound detergent, was estimated to be 360,000. The complex of toxin and purified AChR from *Electrophorus* was cross-linked with glutaraldehyde in nonionic detergent; a broad peak centered at an apparent molecular weight of 260,000 was obtained by SDS-polyacrylamide gel electrophoresis (33). It may be concluded that in uncharged detergents or in bile salts the AChR is an aggregate of a molecular weight of about 3×10^5. The specific activities obtained for purified AChR are consistent with 1 to 2×10^5 daltons per ACh binding site. There is as yet little information as to the state of aggregation of the AChR in the membrane.

CHEMICAL COMPOSITION

Amino acid analyses have been reported (e.g., 32,35,51) which are of course composites of all the components present. They show no unusual features. Only the similarity of *Electrophorus* and *Torpedo* receptors is remarkable (51). There is some direct evidence for the presence of sugar residues. In addition, plant lectins bind to the AChR. There is no information on specific associations of the AChR with lipids. Such interactions are likely to be disrupted in detergent solutions.

BINDING SITE PROPERTIES

It is obvious from the success of the assay procedures that the ACh binding site is not radically altered by the extraction of the AChR from its native environment with nonionic detergents or bile salts. The rate of affinity alkylation of the AChR in intact electroplax and of AChR purified in detergent solution are nearly the same. Also unchanged is the enhancement in the rate of reaction of ^{3}H-MBTA compared with ^{14}C-NEM (34). The geometry of the site is thus not appreciably altered. Nevertheless, some differences in the binding of agonists to AChR in membrane and in solution have been found. The affinities of *Electrophorus* AChR for agonists appear to increase 20-fold upon its extraction with detergent from membrane (32). The affinities for antagonists are unchanged. In contrast, solubilization of AChR from *Torpedo* membrane results in a decrease in the affinities for agonists (45). The relevance of these results to the functional properties of the AChR remains uncertain. It is reassuring that the affinities for antagonists are comparable to those obtained from dose-response data. No cooperativity has been observed in the binding of either agonists or antagonists to solubilized AChR.

ANTIBODIES TO AChR

Purified AChR from *Electrophorus* has been injected into rabbits, producing in them a flaccid paralysis similar in some aspects to that seen in myasthenia gravis. The rabbit serum precipitates AChR and inhibits the response of the intact electroplax to carbamylcholine (46,47). Rabbit anti-*toxin* serum also precipitates purified AChR, presumably because AChR is eluted from the toxin-agarose column on which it is purified by these workers with a considerable amount of toxin bound to it (47). Similar results have been obtained by others who reported that anti-*Electrophorus* AChR precipitates all toxin binding activity in crude extracts of *Torpedo* membrane and of embryonic chick muscle (48). The cross-reaction of the two species of AChR has been demonstrated directly (51). The production of specific antisera may permit correlation of separate antigenic sites with separable functions of the AChR, as for example, the binding of ACh and ion permeation.

REINCORPORATION OF AChR INTO MEMBRANE

Strong proof that a purified preparation of AChR is both complete and functional would be provided by the incorporation of purified AChR into a characterized lipid membrane with reconstitution of the control of Na^+ and K^+ permeability characteristic of the AChR in intact cells. Such a result has not yet been convincingly achieved, but some preliminary results have been reported. Hazelbauer and Changeux (49) were able to dissolve a *Torpedo* membrane preparation rich in AChR in cholate and by dialyzing away the cholate reconstitute vesicles which in some cases showed increased Na^+ permeability in the presence of carbamylcholine. This suggested that solubilization *per se* does not necessarily inactivate the permeability control function of the AChR. Kemp et al. (50) added a detergent extract of muscle to a thin lipid film which spontaneously showed increasing permeability with time. The rate of increase was greater in the presence of carbamylcholine.

Purified AChR from *Electrophorus* and that from *Torpedo* have been incorporated into phospholipid vesicles. The AChR-containing vesicles appear to be denser than phospholipid vesicles without AChR (40). The Na^+ permeability of these vesicles, however, has not been significantly sensitive to carbamylcholine. Michaelson et al. (35) have reported that vesicles reconstituted from AChR and lipids, both purified from *Torpedo*, occasionally show increased permeability to Na^+ in the presence of carbamylcholine and that this effect is blocked by α-toxin. Conditions for consistent reconstitution of membrane containing functional AChR have yet to be described.

CONCLUSION

Much progress has been made toward the molecular characterization of the AChRs from the electric tissues of *Electrophorus electricus* and species of *Torpedo*. Less is known about

the less plentiful AChR in vertebrate muscle. Similar binding specificities and subunits and immunological cross-reactivity suggest that the physiological and pharmacological similarities among these AChRs are based on similar molecular structures. Undoubtedly many features of the AChR have been conserved during evolution, and the mechanism of permeability control by the AChR is probably very general. It appears that we are on the verge of discovering this mechanism.

ACKNOWLEDGMENTS

Support by the National Institute of Neurological and Communicative Disorders and Stroke, the National Science Foundation, and the New York Heart Association, Inc. is gratefully acknowledged.

REFERENCES

1. Katz, B., and Miledi, R. (1972): The statistical nature of the acetylcholine potential and its molecular components. *J. Physiol.*, 224:665–699.
2. Anderson, C. R., and Stevens, C. F. (1973): Voltage clamp analysis of acetylcholine produced end-plate current fluctuations at frog neuromuscular junction. *J. Physiol.*, 235:655–691.
3. Karlin, A. (1974): The acetylcholine receptor: progress report. *Life Sci.*, 14:1385–1415.
4. Rang, H. P. (1971): Drug receptors and their function. *Nature*, 231:91–96.
5. Higman, H. B., Podleski, T. R., and Bartels, E. (1963): Apparent dissociation constants between carbamylcholine *d*-tubocurarine, and the receptor. *Biochim. Biophys. Acta*, 75:187–193.
6. Jenkinson, D. H. (1960): The antagonism between tubocurarine and substances which depolarize the motor end-plate. *J. Physiol.*, 152:309–324.
7. Ehrenpreis, S. (1960): Isolation and identification of the acetylcholine receptor protein of electric tissue. *Biochim. Biophys. Acta*, 44:561–577.
8. Chagas, C. (1959): Curare fixation by cells. In: *Curare and Curare-Like Agents*, edited by D. Bovet, F. Bovet-Nitti, and G. B. Marini-Bettolo, pp. 327–345. Elsevier, New York.
9. Waser, P. G. (1970): On receptors in the postsynaptic membrane of the motor endplate. In: *Molecular Properties of Drug Receptors*, edited by R. Porter and M. O'Connor, pp. 59–69. Churchill, London.
10. O'Brien, R. D., and Gilmour, L. P. (1969): A muscarone-binding material in electroplax and its relation to the acetylcholine receptor I. Centrifugal assay. *Proc. Natl. Acad. Sci. USA*, 63:496–503.

11. Lee, C. Y. (1972): Chemistry and pharmacology of polypeptide toxins in snake venoms. *Ann. Rev. Pharmacol.*, 12:265–286.
12. Changeux, J.-P., Kasai, M., and Lee, C. Y. (1970): Use of a snake venom toxin to characterize the cholinergic receptor protein. *Proc. Natl. Acad. Sci. USA*, 67:1241–1247.
13. Miledi, R., Molinoff, P., and Potter, L. T. (1971): Isolation of the cholinergic receptor protein of *Torpedo* electric tissue. *Nature*, 229:554–557.
14. Raftery, M. A., Schmidt, J., Clark, D. G., and Wolcott, R. G. (1971): Demonstration of a specific α-bungarotoxin binding component in *Electrophorus electricus* electroplax membranes. *Biochem. Biophys. Res. Commun.*, 45:1622–1629.
15. Meunier, J.-C., Olsen, R. W., Menez, A., Fromageot, P., Boquet, P., and Changeux, J.-P. (1972): Some physical properties of the cholinergic receptor protein from *Electrophorus electricus* revealed by a tritiated α-toxin from *Naja nigricollis* venom. *Biochemistry*, 11:1200–1210.
16. Fulpius, B., Cha, S., Klett, R., and Reich, E. (1972): Properties of the nicotinic acetylcholine receptor macromolecule of *Electrophorus electricus*. *Febs. Lett.*, 24:323–326.
17. Patrick, J., Heineman, S. F., Lindstrom, J., Schubert, D., and Steinbach, J. H. (1972): Appearance of acetylcholine receptors during differentiation of a myogenic cell line. *Proc. Natl. Acad. Sci. USA*, 69:2762–2766.
18. Albuquerque, E. X., Barnard, E. A., Jansson, S. E., and Wieckowski, J. (1973): Occupancy of the cholinergic receptors in relation to changes in the end-plate potential. *Life Sci.*, 12:545–552.
19. Miledi, R., and Potter, L. T. (1971): Acetylcholine receptors in muscle fibers. *Nature*, 233:599–603.
20. Berg, D. K., Kelly, R. B., Sargent, P. B., Williamson, P., and Hall, Z. W. (1972): Binding of α-bungarotoxin to acetylcholine receptors in mammalian muscle. *Proc. Natl. Acad. Sci. USA*, 69:147–151.
21. Porter, C. W., Chiu, T. H., Wieckowski, J., and Barnard, E. A. (1973): Types and locations of cholinergic receptor-like molecules in muscle fibers. *Nature New Biol.*, 241:3–7.
22. Albuquerque, E. X., Barnard, E. A., Chiu, T. H., Lapa, A. J., Dolly, J. O., Jansson, S. E., Daly, J., and Witkop, B. (1973): Acetylcholine receptor and ion conductance modulator sites at the murine neuromuscular junction: Evidence from specific toxin reactions. *Proc. Natl. Acad. Sci. USA*, 70:949–953.
23. Hartzell, H. C., and Fambrough, D. M. (1972): Acetylcholine receptors: distribution and extra-junctional density in rat diaphragm after denervation correlated with acetylcholine sensitivity. *J. Gen. Physiol.*, 60:248–262.
24. Paterson, B., and Prives, J. (1973): Appearance of acetylcholine receptor in differentiating cultures of embryonic chick breast muscle. *J. Cell Biol.*, 59:241–245.
25. Karlin, A. (1969): Chemical modification of the active site of the acetylcholine receptor. *J. Gen. Physiol.*, 54:245s–264s.
26. Singer, S. J. (1970): Affinity labelling of protein active sites. In: *Molecular Properties of Drug Receptors*, edited by R. Porter and M. O'Connor, pp. 229–242. Churchill, London.
27. Karlin, A., Prives, J., Deal, W., and Winnik, M. (1970): Counting acetylcholine receptors in the electroplax. In: *Molecular Properties of Drug Receptors*, edited by R. Porter and M. O'Connor, pp. 247–259. Churchill, London.
28. Reiter, M., Cowburn, D. A., Prives, J. M., and Karlin, A. (1972): Affinity labeling of the acetylcholine receptor in the electroplax: Electrophoretic separation in sodium dodecyl sulfate. *Proc. Natl. Acad. Sci. USA*, 69:1168–1172.
29. Silman, H. I. and Karlin, A. (1967): Effect of local pH changes caused by substrate hydrolysis on the activity of membrane-bound acetyl-cholinesterase. *Proc. Natl. Acad. Sci. USA*, 58:1664–1668.
30. Lindstrom, J. and Patrick, J. (1974): Purification of the acetylcholine receptor by affinity chromatography. In: *Synaptic Transmission and Neuronal Interaction*, edited by M. V. L. Bennett, pp. 191–216. Raven Press, New York.
31. Klett, R. P., Fulpius, B. W., Cooper, D., Smith, M., Reich, E., and Possani, L. D. (1973): The acetylcholine receptor 1. Purification and characterization of a macromolecule isolated from *Electrophorus electricus*. *J. Biol. Chem.*, 248:6841–6853.
32. Meunier, J.-C., Sealock, R., Olsen, R., and Changeux, J.-P. (1974): Purification and properties of the cholinergic receptor protein from *Electrophorus electricus* electric tissue. *Eur. J. Biochem.*, 45:371–394.
33. Biesecker, G. (1973): Molecular properties of the cholinergic receptor purified from *Electrophorus electricus*. *Biochemistry*, 12:4403–4409.
34. Karlin, A., and Cowburn, D. A. (1973): The affinity-labeling of partially purified acetylcholine receptor from electric tissue of *Electrophorus*. *Proc. Natl. Acad. Sci. USA*, 70:3636–3640.
35. Michaelson, D., Vandlen, R., Bode, J., Moody, T., Schmidt, J., and Raftery, M. A. (1974): Some molecular properties of an isolated acetylcholine receptor ion-translocation protein. *Arch. Biochem. Biophys.*, 165:796–804.
36. Heilbronn, E., and Mattson, C. (1974): The nicotinic cholinergic receptor protein: improved purification method, preliminary amino acid composition and observed autoimmuno response. *J. Neurochem.*, 22:315–316.
37. Eldefrawi, M. E., and Eldefrawi, A. T. (1973): Purification and molecular properties of the acetylcholine receptor from *Torpedo* electroplax. *Arch. Biochem. Biophys.*, 159:362–373.
38. Carroll, R. C., Eldefrawi, M. E., and Edelstein, S. J. (1973): Studies on the structure of the acetylcholine receptor from *Torpedo marmorata*. *Biochem. Biophys. Res. Commun.*, 55:864–872.

39. Weill, C. L., McNamee, M. G., and Karlin, A. (1974): Affinity-labeling of purified acetylcholine receptor from *Torpedo californica. Biochem. Biophys. Res. Commun.,* 61:997–1003.

40. McNamee, M. G., Weill, C. L., and Karlin, A. (1975): Further characterization of purified acetylcholine receptor and its incorporation into phospholipid vesicles. In: *Protein-Ligand Interactions,* edited by H. Sund and G. Blauer, pp. 316–327. Verlag Walter de Gruyter, Berlin.

41. Raftery, M. A., Schmidt, J., Vandlen, R., and Moody, T. (1974): Large-scale isolation and characterization of an acetylcholine receptor. In: *Neurochemistry of Cholinergic Receptors,* edited by E. DeRobertis and J. Schacht, pp. 5–18. Raven Press, New York.

42. Karlin, A., and Cowburn, D. A. (1974): Molecular properties of membrane-bound and of solubilized and purified acetylcholine receptor identified by affinity labeling. In: *Neurochemistry of Cholinergic Receptors,* edited by E. DeRobertis and J. Schacht, pp. 37–48. Raven Press, New York.

43. Raftery, M. A., Schmidt, J., and Clark, D. G. (1972): Specificity of α-bungarotoxin binding to *Torpedo californica* electroplax. *Arch. Biochem. Biophys.,* 152:882–886.

44. Meunier, J.-C., Olsen, R. W., and Changeux, J.-P. (1972): Studies on the cholinergic receptor protein from *Electrophorus electricus. FEBS Lett.,* 24:63–68.

45. Franklin, G. I., and Potter, L. T. (1972): Studies of the binding of α-bungarotoxin to membrane-bound and detergent-dispersed acetylcholine receptors from *Torpedo* electric tissue. *FEBS Lett.,* 28:101–106.

46. Patrick, J., and Lindstrom, J. (1973): Autoimmune response to acetylcholine receptor. *Science,* 180:871–872.

47. Patrick, J., Lindstrom, J., Culp, B., and McMillen, J. (1973): Studies in purified eel acetylcholine receptor and anti-acetylcholine receptor antibody. *Proc. Natl. Acad. Sci. USA,* 70:3334–3338.

48. Sugiyama, H., Benda, P., Meunier, J.-C., and Changeux, J.-P. (1973): Immunological characterization of the cholinergic receptor protein from *Electrophorus electricus. FEBS Lett.,* 35:124–128.

49. Hazelbauer, G. L., and Changeux, J.-P. (1974): Reconstitution of a chemically excitable membrane. *Proc. Nat. Acad. Sci. USA,* 71:1479–1483.

50. Kemp, G., Dolly, J. O., Barnard, E. A., and Werner, C. E. (1973): Reconstitution of a partially purified endplate acetylcholine receptor. *Biochem. Biophys. Res. Commun.,* 54:607–613.

51. Karlin, A., Weill, C. L., McNamee, M. G., and Valderrama, R. (*in press*): Facets of the structures of acetylcholine receptors from *Electrophorus* and *Torpedo, Cold Spr. Harb. Symp. Quant. Biol.,* 40.

The Nervous System, Donald B. Tower, Editor-in-Chief. *Vol. 1: The Basic Neurosciences.* Raven Press, New York, 1975.

Isolation of the Opiate Receptor: A Progress Report

Avram Goldstein

In 1971, my co-workers and I proposed, in detail, a method for identifying opiate receptors (1), which took advantage of the pharmacologic stereospecificity of the D(−) opiates related to morphine. We pointed out that since L(+) isomers in this series were quite inert, having neither agonist nor antagonist properties, it could be surmised that they were incapable of entering the receptor sites. If the L(+) isomers entered the sites but failed to trigger an effect there because of the wrong positioning of essential groups, they would at least act as competitive antagonists, since at appropriate concentration they would exclude the active isomers. The minimum conclusion, therefore, was that mole for mole, the L(+) isomers were far less likely to occupy receptor sites. On this basis we concluded that the necessary (though not suffi-cient) condition for identifying an opiate receptor was that it must bind any active opiate stereospecifically, i.e., despite the simultaneous presence of its inactive enantiomer.

We also discussed the problem of nonspecific nonsaturable binding. To determine the binding of a radioactive D(−) isomer in the presence of excess nonradioactive L(+) isomer would not be an accurate measure of receptor binding in most cases, since an unknown part of the observed radioactivity would represent simple solution in membranes or ligand trapped in the aqueous interior of cells or synaptosomes. It was essential, we pointed out, to include an incubation of the radioactive ligand with an excess of nonradioactive D(−) pharmacologically active isomer. In this incubation condition, virtually all the radioactive ligand would be ex-

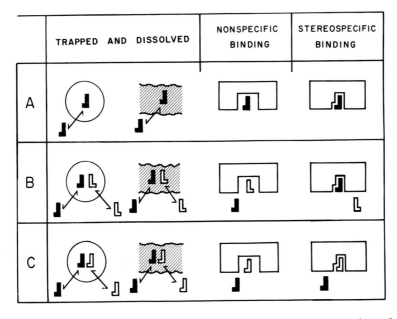

FIG. 1. Methodology for measuring opiate receptor binding in tissue homogenates or membrane fractions. *Solid symbols* represent a radioactive opiate ligand; *open symbols* indicate a large excess of nonradioactive dextrorphan [an inert L(+) isomer] in **B**, or the same excess of nonradioactive levorphanol [an active D(−) isomer] in **C**. Stereospecific binding, considered equivalent to opiate receptor binding, is given by the difference between the incubations with dextrorphan (**B**) and with levorphanol (**C**). From Goldstein et al. (1).

cluded from receptor sites, leaving the nonspecific nonsaturable binding undiminished. Thus, the only suitable measure of receptor binding is a difference between the binding of radioactive ligand under the two incubation conditions, e.g., in the presence of nonradioactive dextrorphan [L(+)] on the one hand, and nonradioactive levorphanol [D(−)] on the other. Figure 1, p. 333, taken from our 1971 publication, illustrates the conceptual basis of the procedure. Using this technique we showed that about 2% of the total binding of radioactive levorphanol in mouse brain homogenate met the criterion of stereospecificity. This binding was confined to membrane fractions. Its subcellular distribution depended upon the ligand concentration; at low concentration most of the binding was in a fraction containing synaptosomal membranes. We found also that calcium ion reduced the binding and that EDTA increased it.

Unfortunately, at that time, a radioactive opiate ligand of sufficiently high specific activity was not available to us, so we were unable to carry out the procedure with low enough ligand concentration to maximize the stereospecific binding relative to the nonspecific binding. This important step forward was taken by two other groups, nearly simultaneously, using our conceptual approach and our methodology (2,3). They succeeded in raising the fraction stereospecifically bound to as high as 80% with the antagonist naloxone or the highly potent agonist etorphine. Dramatic progress followed from this significant technical success. A convincing correlation was found between receptor binding and pharmacologic potency for a large series of opiates. Opiate receptors were localized at high density in the limbic system of brain, and at lower density in other parts of the nervous system. And opiate receptors were discovered to be restricted to the vertebrates, in agreement with the phylogenetic distribution of pharmaco-

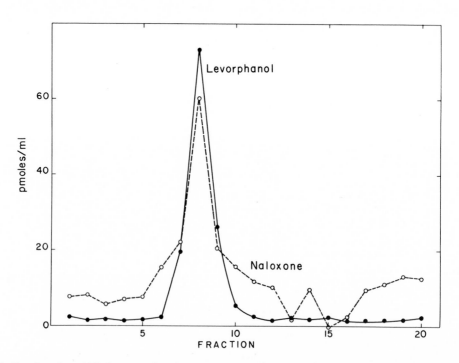

FIG. 2. Fractionation of binding capacity for levorphanol and for naloxone in the chloroform-methanol (C-M) 1:1 eluate. An ether precipitate of C-M extract from two pooled mouse brains was fractionated on Sephadex LH-20, with the following elution sequence: C, 25 ml; C-M 4:1, 80 ml; C-M 1:1, 100 ml. Fractions of the C-M 1:1 eluate were collected, as shown (4 ml each), after discarding the first 20 ml (void volume). Duplicate 0.2 ml aliquots from each fraction were dried under N_2, redissolved in heptane, and assayed for binding capacity by phase partition. Aqueous phase = 0.1 M Tris, pH 7.4, 1 ml, containing 4×10^{-7} M ^{14}C-levorphanol or ^{14}C-naloxone. *Solid lines,* levorphanol; *broken lines,* naloxone.

logic activity. These and other important findings are amply described in recent reviews (4–6).

FRACTIONATION IN CHLOROFORM-METHANOL

It was soon evident that opiate receptors belong to the class of membrane receptors that is very difficult to extract into aqueous solution. This posed a major problem for purification—a problem not yet really solved. Detergents, both ionic and nonionic, either failed to extract the receptor or extracted it but simultaneously destroyed its unique ability to bind opiates. This presented the classical problem of receptor pharmacology: Once removed from its natural environment, where it has a characteristic functional activity, how do we know that a specific binding material is really a receptor? Sooner or later the receptor function has to be demonstrated. And if the extraction procedure destroys even the specific binding capacity,

how can we ever accomplish a complete purification? We explored two approaches to this problem. One, about which some progress has already been reported (7–10), employed organic solvents to solubilize the specific binding material and purify it, using procedures introduced in the laboratory of E. DeRobertis. Chloroform-methanol extracts were found to retain the stereospecific binding capacity. Ether precipitated the binding material, and most of the nonspecifically interacting lipids could thus be removed in the ether supernatant. The precipitate was redissolved and then fractionated with increasing methanol concentration on a Sephadex LH-20 column. This yielded a single peak of levorphanol-binding material, of variable stereospecificity, up to 100% in some experiments, as low as 10% in others. The causes of this variability are still not well understood. Typical results with two opiate ligands—an agonist and an antagonist—are illustrated in Fig. 2.

The results shown in Fig. 2 suggested strongly

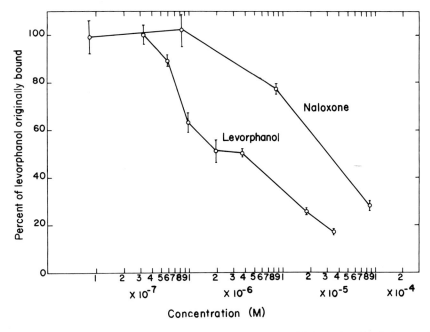

FIG. 3. Reduction of radioactive levorphanol binding by preincubation with levorphanol or naloxone. Fractions 7, 8, and 9 of the C-M 1:1 eluate (Fig. 2), which had the capacity to bind levorphanol and naloxone, were pooled and diluted to 20 ml (50 mg tissue equivalent/ml) with C-M 1:1. 0.3 ml aliquots were used in the phase partition procedure, as previously described. Nonradioactive levorphanol or naloxone was added to the buffer phase at the indicated concentrations, and mixed for 5 min at room temperature prior to adding 4×10^{-7} M ^{14}C-levorphanol. In the absence of a competing ligand, the total levorphanol originally bound (=100%) was $2,600 \pm 110$ pmoles/g tissue. Mean and SEM are shown for the triplicate determinations at each concentration in the aqueous phase.

that levorphanol and naloxone were binding to the same sites. To ascertain if there was a competition between the two ligands for these sites, the phase distribution assay was conducted with ^{14}C-levorphanol as ligand, in the simultaneous presence of either nonradioactive levorphanol or nonradioactive naloxone at various concentrations. The results, shown in Fig. 3, indicate the competitive relationship between the two ligands.

Several methodologic problems with the Sephadex LH-20 procedures have slowed further progress. The measurement of binding, fraction by fraction, employs an equilibrium phase distribution method; the radioactive ligand partitions between a buffer phase and the organic phase. An apparent increase of ligand solubility in the organic phase indicates the presence of binding material there. This method is very efficient with ligands such as levorphanol, where the partition strongly favors the buffer phase, but it has proved to be impractical for ligands of high lipophilicity like etorphine (Table 1), since the increase in partition coefficient resulting from the binding interaction is then too small, relatively, to measure accurately. Another problem involving this method is that

TABLE 1. *Some partition coefficients of opiates in different solvents[a]*

Drug	Organic solvent	Partition coefficient (org./aq.)
MAPL	Chloroform	0.28
MAPL	*n*-Heptane	<0.005
Morphine	*n*-Heptane	<0.005
Levorphanol	Chloroform	0.83
Levorphanol	Chloroform:methanol (2:1; v/v)	0.67[b]
Levorphanol	*n*-Heptane	0.007
Naloxone	*n*-Heptane	0.054
Etorphine	*n*-Heptane	0.41
APL	*n*-Heptane	3.3

[a] All compounds were tested at concentrations within the range 10^{-8} to 4×10^{-7} M, by equilibrium at 23°C between 0.1 M Tris buffer (pH 7.4) and the indicated solvent. MAPL and APL were protected from light during equilibration. Radioactive drugs were used and both phases were assayed by liquid scintillation counting. APL = *p*-azidophenylethylnorlevorphanol HCl; MAPL = *p*-azidophenylethyl-N-methylnorlevorphanol HCl.
[b] The presence of methanol alters the composition of the aqueous phase.

under some conditions, treatment of an organic solution of binding material with aqueous buffer may cause the formation of a fine insoluble precipitate at the interface which contains some or all of the binding capacity and is very difficult to work with. Finally, we have found that the Sephadex LH-20 column preferentially retains methanol, introducing a complication into the desired regularity of the stepwise changes of chloroform:methanol ratio in the effluent solution.

The most significant finding with Sephadex LH-20 columns was the altered behavior of the binding material after complexing with an opiate ligand. This provided a means for efficient purification, since the complex could be separated from adventitious impurities by recycling through the column. We concluded, from analysis of the complex, that the material was probably proteolipid in nature, but Loh et al. (11) later claimed it was largely or entirely cerebroside sulfate. This issue is not yet settled. If the binding substance is indeed cerebroside sulfate without protein, the number of amine groups released on hydrolysis indicates that each binding site must represent a considerable array of glycolipid residues in some sort of micellar aggregate. Our finding that the opiate ligand can be removed by dialysis, while the binding capacity is nondialysable, can be reconciled with either interpretation.

PHOTOAFFINITY LABELING

Our second approach to the problem has been to attempt affinity labeling of the opiate receptors. Once the receptor material is attached covalently to an appropriate opiate ligand, vigorous purification can be carried out without regard to the loss of binding capacity, since the ligand is already bound irreversibly. A photoaffinity label seemed especially desirable, because the reversible interaction with the receptor sites could be studied in the dark, the permanent attachment being carried out at will by exposure to ultraviolet light. Our first attempts along these lines were encouraging but not adequate. We knew from the structure-activity relationships in the opiate series that bulky substituents are permissible on the lone N atom, which usually carries only a methyl group. Indeed, groups like phenethyl in place of methyl greatly increase the agonist potency. The reagent we developed was the ^{3}H-labeled p-azido phenylethyl analogue of levorphanol (12), which we now call APL (Fig. 4).

Phenyl azides are stable in the dark but upon exposure to ultraviolet light cleave off N_2, leaving a reactive nitrene capable of forming a covalent bond to any of several chemical groups. We showed that this compound was indeed a typical opiate agonist. It produced analgesia, locomotor activity, and Straub tail reaction in mice, and it inhibited electrically stimulated muscle twitches in the guinea pig ileum preparation. It acted stereospecifically, and its effects were blocked and reversed by naloxone. It became firmly attached to tissues upon irradiation, but, unfortunately, there was so much nonspecific attachment that any stereospecific attachment was masked.

Assuming that the very high lipophilicity of APL was responsible for the nonspecific attachment, probably because most of it was dissolved in membranes at the time of irradiation, we synthesized MAPL, the N-methyl quaternary derivative of APL (13). As expected, MAPL has a much lower organic/aqueous partition coefficient. (Table 1). It remains an effective agonist (although of lower potency) in the guinea pig ileum myenteric plexus-longitudinal muscle preparation, where the sites of opiate action on the plexus neurons are readily accessible from the ambient solution. Results with MAPL are encouraging. Most interesting has been the finding that irreversible attachment of MAPL to the receptor sites yields a permanent agonist effect (14). The measurement of this effect was the decrease in acetylcholine (ACh) output due to electrical stimulation, a well-established opiate action in this tissue (15–18). In the dark, MAPL reduces ACh output, and this effect is completely reversible after sufficient washing out of the drug. After irradiation in the presence of MAPL, the reduction of ACh output is irreversible. This result was by no means a foregone conclusion. It might have been expected that permanent attachment of an opiate agonist at its receptor sites would block those sites and thus prevent other agonists from exerting their effects, i.e., that the agonist would become an antagonist. The actual result is decisive in refuting—at least for this system—the concept (19) that agonistic effects require repetitive association and dissociation at the receptor.

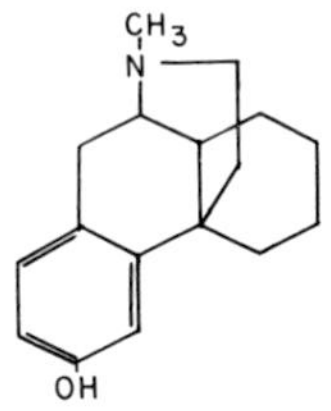

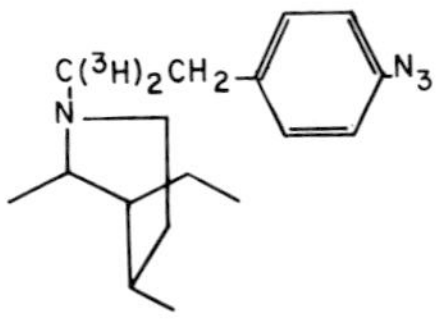

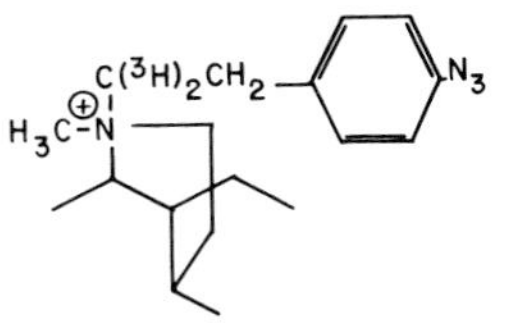

Another interesting outcome of these experiments concerns the effects of the antagonist naloxone. Even when long-lasting agonists like etorphine or APL (in the dark) are used, which cannot be reversed by prolonged exhaustive washing, naloxone nevertheless causes an immediate reversal. After MAPL has been attached irreversibly, however, naloxone is unable to reverse its effect. On the other hand, if naloxone is present before and during the irradiation of MAPL, the irreversible effect does not occur, i.e., naloxone protects the receptor sites against photoaffinity labeling with MAPL. We interpret these results to indicate that naloxone reacts with the same receptor sites as does MAPL, in agreement with pharmacologic (20–24) and binding (3,6) data.

We have argued elsewhere (25) in favor of an allosteric model of the receptor, in which agonists produce a conformation change, and antagonists prevent and reverse such change. The conformation of the agonist complex is incompatible with normal function. Thus, for example, if the receptor extends through a neu-

FIG. 4. Structures of two photoaffinity labels. Both compounds are derived from norlevorphanol. APL is the p-azidophenylethyl analogue of levorphanol. MAPL is the N-methyl quaternary derivative of APL. The azide group liberates N_2 and forms a reactive nitrene on exposure to ultraviolet light, but it is stable in the dark. All three compounds shown here are active opiates in the guinea pig myenteric plexus-longitudinal muscle preparation.

ronal membrane, with an opiate recognition unit on the external surface coupled to an enzyme unit on the internal surface, the conformation associated with the agonist complex would inactivate the enzyme function. According to Collier (26), the enzyme thus incorporated into the receptor complex might be a prostaglandin-stimulated adenylate cyclase. After covalent attachment of MAPL, the enzyme inactivation would be persistent, and naloxone could no longer revert it to normal. Operationally identical would be a model, such as proposed by Changeux (27) for other receptors, in which naloxone stabilizes the receptor in its functional conformation, whereas agonists stabilize it in the nonfunctional conformation. This model does not require separate sites; the interaction of agonist or antagonist with the receptor shifts the equilibrium toward the nonfunctional or functional conformation, respectively.

Consistent with the effects of MAPL on function in the myenteric plexus are the results on binding of radioactive MAPL. In the dark, stereospecific reversible binding can be demonstrated in the intact myenteric plexus preparation, using the filtration technique (3). In the intact myenteric plexus preparation, stereospecific attachment (i.e., irreversible binding) is produced by irradiation. In homogenates, however, there is a very large increase in nonspecific attachment due to irradiation, and the small amount of stereospecific attachment (on the order of 10 pmole/g tissue) is masked. This finding suggests strongly that the opiate receptor sites are located on external membrane surfaces. Further evidence is provided by the fact that MAPL, which is a quaternary charged compound, is pharmacologically active although it would not be expected to penetrate membranes.

Autoradiographic studies are in progress with myenteric plexus (13). It is already clear the MAPL localizes stereospecifically in the ganglia, but details of the localization at higher resolution are not yet available. Extraction and fractionation of the covalent MAPL-receptor complex are also in progress, both with SDS-polyacrylamide gel electrophoresis and with chloroform-methanol fractionation on Sephadex LH-20.

Despite the exciting progress of the last few years in several laboratories, advances in the purification and characterization of the opiate receptor have been slow. Deeper understanding of opiate action and of the pathophysiology of the addictive process requires that we elucidate how the combination of an opiate molecule with its receptor site initiates the chain of events leading to the typical pharmacologic effect. It appears that this goal may be nearing achievement soon.

ACKNOWLEDGMENTS

Work summarized in this paper was supported by National Institute on Drug Abuse grants DA-972 and DA-249 and by the Drug Abuse Council. I thank Louise Lowney, Brian M. Cox, and Kent Opheim for reviewing the manuscript.

REFERENCES

1. Goldstein, A., Lowney, L. I., and Pal, B. K. (1971): Stereospecific and nonspecific interactions of the morphine congener levorphanol in subcellular fractions of mouse brain. *Proc. Natl. Acad. Sci. USA*, 68:1742–1747.
2. Simon, E. J., Hiller, J. M., and Edelman, I. (1973): Stereospecific binding of the potent narcotic analgesic (^{3}H)etorphine to rat brain homogenate. *Proc. Natl. Acad. Sci. USA*, 70:1947–1949.
3. Pert, C. B., and Synder, S. H. (1973): Opiate receptor: Demonstration in nervous tissue. *Science*, 179:1011–1014.
4. Goldstein, A. (1974): Opiate receptors. *Life Sci.*, 14:615–623.
5. Simon, E. J. (1973): In search of the opiate receptor. *Am. J. Med. Sci.*, 226:160–168.
6. Snyder, S. H., Pert, C. B., and Pasternak, G. W. (1974): The opiate receptor. *Ann. Int. Med.*, 81: 534–540.
7. Pal, B. K., Lowney, L. I., and Goldstein, A. (1971): Further studies on the stereospecific binding of levorphanol by a membrane fraction from mouse brain. In: *Agonist and Antagonist Actions of Narcotic Analgesic Drugs*, edited by H. W. Kosterlitz, H. O. J. Collier, and J. E. Villarreal, pp. 62–69. Macmillan, London.
8. Goldstein, A. (1973): The search for the opiate receptor. In: *Pharmacology and the Future of Man*. Proc. 5th Int. Congr. Pharmacol., San Francisco, July 24–29, 1972, pp. 140–150, Karger, Basel.
9. Goldstein, A. (1973): Recent studies on the binding of opiate narcotics to possible receptor sites. In: *New Concepts in Neurotransmitter Regulation*, edited by A. J. Mandell, pp. 297–309. Plenum Press, New York.
10. Lowney, L. I., Schulz, K., Lowery, P. J., and Goldstein, A. (1974): Partial purification of an opiate receptor from mouse brain. Identification

of a membrane proteolipid that binds opiate narcotics stereospecifically. *Science,* 183:749–753.

11. Loh, H. H., Cho, T. M., Wu, Y., and Way, E. L. (1974): Stereospecific binding of narcotics to brain cerebrosides. *Life Sci.,* 14:2231–2245.

12. Winter, B. A., and Goldstein, A. (1972): A photochemical affinity-labelling reagent for the opiate receptor(s). *Mol. Pharmacol.,* 6:601–611.

13. Cox, B. M., Opheim, K. E., and Goldstein, A. (1975): *Photoaffinity Labelling of Opiate Receptors.* Marcel Dekker, New York.

14. Schulz, R., and Goldstein, A. (1975): Irreversible alteration of opiate receptor function by a photoaffinity labelling reagent. *Life Sci.,* 16:1843–1848.

15. Schaumann, W. (1957): Inhibition by morphine of the release of acetylcholine from the intestine of the guinea-pig. *Brit. J. Pharmacol.,* 12:115–118.

16. Paton, W. D. M. (1957): The action of morphine and related substances on contraction and on acetylcholine output of coaxially stimulated guinea-pig ileum. *Brit. J. Pharmacol.,* 12:119–127.

17. Cowie, A. L., Kosterlitz, H. W., and Watt, A. J. (1968): Mode of action of morphine-like drugs on autonomic neuro-effectors. *Nature,* 220:1040–1042.

18. Cox, B. M., and Weinstock, M. (1966): The effect of analgesic drugs on the release of acetylcholine from electrically stimulated guinea-pig ileum. *Brit. J. Pharmacol.,* 27:81–92.

19. Paton, W. D. M. (1961): A theory of drug action based on the rate of drug-receptor combination. *Proc. Roy. Soc. Ser. B.,* 154:21–69.

20. Beckett, A. M., Casy, A. F., and Harper, N. J. (1956): Analgesics and their antagonists: Some steric and chemical considerations. *J. Pharm. Pharmacol.,* 8:874–884.

21. Cox, B. M., and Weinstock, M. (1964): Quantitative studies of the antagonism by nalorphine of some of the actions of morphine-like analgesic drugs. *Brit. J. Pharmacol.,* 22:289–300.

22. Archer, S., and Harris, L. S. (1965): Narcotic antagonists. In: *Progress in Drug Research,* edited by E. Jucker, pp. 262–320. Birkhäuser, Verlag, Basel und Stuttgart.

23. Takemori, A. E. Kupferberg, H. J., and Miller, J. W. (1969): Quantitative studies of the antagonism of morphine by nalorphine and naloxone. *J. Pharmacol. Exp. Ther.,* 169:39–45.

24. Portoghese, P. S. (1966): Stereochemical factors and receptor interactions associated with narcotic analgesics. *J. Pharm. Sci.,* 55:865–887.

25. Goldstein, A. (1974): Interactions of narcotic antagonists with receptor sites. *Advan. Biochem. Psychopharmacol.,* 8:471–481.

26. Collier, H. O. J., and Roy, A. C. (1974): Hypothesis: Inhibition of E prostaglandinsensitive adenyl cyclase as the mechanism of morphine analgesia. *Prostaglandins* 7:361–376.

27. Changeux, J. (1966): Responses of acetylcholinesterase from *Torpedo marmorata* to salts and curarizing drugs. *Mol. Pharmacol.,* 2:369–392.

The Nervous System, Donald B. Tower, Editor-in-Chief. *Vol. 1: The Basic Neurosciences*. Raven Press, New York, 1975.

Factors Regulating Catecholamine Biosynthesis in Peripheral and Central Catecholaminergic Neurons

Norman Weiner

In the past two decades, biochemical, pharmacological, and morphological studies have contributed immensely to our knowledge of the complex structure and function of the adrenergic neuronal unit. These investigations have demonstrated that, in addition to releasing norepinephrine consequent to nerve stimulation, the adrenergic neuron is able to store the transmitter in specific intracellular particles, whether the norepinephrine is formed endogenously or taken up from the circulation. These vesicles, when appropriately fixed with osmium tetroxide and examined by electron microscopy, exhibit characteristic dense osmiophilic cores. The vesicles are analogous to the chromaffin granules of the adrenal medulla.

Studies of these isolated vesicles have revealed that the storage of catecholamines involves an active uptake process from the cytoplasm. This process is temperature dependent and requires ATP and magnesium. Depleting agents, notably of the reserpine class, selectively block this uptake mechanism. In addition to the uptake process into the isolated vesicles, there is an active, sodium-dependent amine pump in the axonal membrane. Axonal membrane uptake of amines is not blocked by reserpine but appears to be selectively blocked by another group of agents, among which are cocaine, imipramine, desmethylimipramine, and protriptyline. Tyramine and other sympathomimetic amines also are substrates for the axonal uptake mechanism, and their uptake is blocked in a similar fashion by cocaine and by imipramine. There is general agreement that this uptake process is responsible for the termination of the biological effects of released catecholamines. In contrast, when enzymatic degradation of the amine is blocked by appropriate inhibitors, potentiation of the actions of catecholamines generally does not result.

Monoamine oxidase, an enzyme localized in mitochondria, is also present in the adrenergic neuron. This enzyme is responsible for the degradation of free intraneuronal norepinephrine. If uptake into the vesicles is blocked, for example by reserpine, the free amine is rapidly degraded by monoamine oxidase, largely in the intraneuronal site. Catechol-*o*-methyl transferase, a second major enzyme responsible for the ultimate degradation of catecholamines, although present in small amounts in the adrenergic neuron, is apparently not significantly involved in metabolizing intraneuronal norepinephrine. The enzyme, located principally in the liver and kidney, is more important in the metabolism of circulating catecholamines.

BIOSYNTHESIS OF CATECHOLAMINES

In addition to the ability of this structure to release, recapture, store, and catabolize norepinephrine, the adrenergic neuronal unit is capable of synthesizing norepinephrine from precursor amino acids. After postganglionic denervation of an organ, there is a progressive loss of the ability of that tissue to synthesize dihydroxyphenylalanine (DOPA) from tyrosine or to synthesize norepinephrine from dopamine. When the nerve is completely degenerated, these attributes of the tissue are totally absent. It thus appears that the enzymes which catalyze these two reactions, tyrosine 3-monooxygenase (tyrosine hydroxylase) and dopamine-β-hydroxylase, are exclusively localized within the adrenergic neuron.

Tyrosine hydroxylase is able to catalyze the aromatic hydroxylation of both phenylalanine and tyrosine (1–3). The enzyme is present in the adrenal medulla, in adrenergic neurons, and in brain. Although there is some controversy over the intracellular localization of the enzyme, the bulk of the evidence supports the view that tyrosine hydroxylase is a soluble enzyme present in the axoplasm of the adrenergic nerve. Petrack and co-workers have demonstrated that a large fraction of the tyrosine hydroxylase activity in bovine adrenal medulla may be recovered in the particulate fraction of sucrose homogenates and the enzyme can be solubilized by treatment of the tissue with proteolytic enzymes (4). Wurzburger and Musacchio have accumulated considerable evidence that suggests that the particulate localization of the bovine adrenal medulla enzyme is an artifact resulting from both the self-aggregation of tyrosine hydroxylase in homogenates and the ability of the enzyme to adsorb irreversibly to particulate structures (5). Studies in our laboratory support the results of Musacchio. We have demonstrated that soluble bovine adrenal medulla enzyme will rapidly aggregate and may easily be sedimented by centrifugation. Furthermore, when soluble bovine adrenal medulla enzyme is mixed with membranes from a variety of tissues and the membranes are sedimented by centrifugation, the bulk of the enzyme is found in the sediment. This is in contrast to soluble adrenal enzyme from a variety of other species, including man, guinea pig, rat, and rabbit. Tyrosine hydroxylase from the adrenals of these species is found mostly or entirely in the cytosol and the enzyme exhibits little tendency to aggregate or to adsorb to membranes in a nonspecific fashion (6). In homogenates of sympathetic ganglia and of bovine splenic nerves, tyrosine hydroxylase appears to be largely in the soluble supernatant fraction. Some of the brain tyrosine hydroxylase, notably in the striatum, is associated with particles (7). Although much of the enzyme present in the particulate fraction of brain tissue may actually be present in solution in the axoplasm that is trapped within synaptosomes, a significant fraction does appear to be membrane bound (8). Two types of tyrosine hydroxylase may exist that exhibit different kinetic properties and may be localized in different cell fractions (8).

Tyrosine hydroxylase requires oxygen and a reduced pterin cofactor for activity (9–11). A pterin cofactor has been isolated from bovine adrenal medulla and the cofactor appears to be similar to or identical with tetrahydrobiopterin, the cofactor that is also required for activity of liver phenylalanine hydroxylase (12). Iron also enhances the enzymatic hydroxylation of tyrosine to DOPA (9). Shiman and co-workers (2) suggest that iron may be involved largely in the degradation of hydrogen peroxide, which accumulates during the enzymatic reaction and adversely affects enzyme activity. We have confirmed that iron is required for optimal activity in the tyrosine hydroxylation reaction and have demonstrated complete loss of activity in the presence of iron chelators, such as α,α-dipyridyl. Although catalase does increase the activity of tyrosine hydroxylase to some degree, it is unable to replace completely iron in the system. Our results (6) are in agreement with those of Udenfriend and co-workers who claim that iron may be an essential cofactor in the tyrosine hydroxylase reaction.

Kinetic studies on the mechanism of the tyrosine hydroxylation reaction indicate that, during the conversion of tyrosine to DOPA, the enzyme itself is oxidized to an inactive form. The reduced pterin combines with the inactive oxidized form of the enzyme, converting the hydroxylase to the active reduced form. Tetrahydropterin is simultaneously converted to the dihydro form and must be enzymatically reduced before it may function again to regenerate reduced tyrosine hydroxylase (9). Pteridine reductase catalyzes the latter reaction. Pteridine reductase has been demonstrated in adrenal glands and brain and appears to be distinct from dihydrofolate reductase (13). Studies in our laboratory (14) and in the laboratory of Musacchio indicate that methotrexate, a potent inhibitor of dihydrofolate reductase, does not inhibit pteridine reductase (13).

L-Aromatic amino acid decarboxylase (DOPA decarboxylase), the enzyme that catalyzes the formation of dopamine from dihydroxyphenylalanine, is also located within the adrenergic neuron, although it is not present exclusively in this structure. When tissues containing a dense adrenergic innervation are denervated, a significant reduction in the DOPA decarboxylase activity of the tissue can be demonstrated. DOPA decarboxylase is a typical amino acid decarboxylase that requires pyridoxal phosphate for activity. In adrenergic nervous tissue and adrenal chromaffin cells, the enzyme appears to be restricted to the cytosol. Suggestions that a portion of DOPA decarboxylase in brain is particulate may be explained by the presence of the enzyme in the cytosol that is trapped within synaptosomes (15). Recent studies have suggested that enzymes that decarboxylate DOPA and 5-hydroxytryptophan are distinct and possess different kinetic characteristics (16).

Dopamine-β-hydroxylase, the enzyme that catalyzes the synthesis of norepinephrine from dopamine, is a copper-containing enzyme that requires oxygen and a reducing agent as cosubstrates in the reaction (17). Thus, like tyrosine hydroxylase, this enzyme may be classified as a mixed-function oxidase. The natural reducing substance is probably ascorbic acid. The enzyme is present in the storage vesicle, and, therefore, the site of storage of norepinephrine is also the site at which norepinephrine is finally synthesized. The enzyme is to some extent located within, or attached to, the membrane of the granule and a portion of the enzyme is present in soluble form within the storage particle. Uptake of dopamine into the storage vesicle is a necessary prerequisite to the hydroxylation of this substrate (18). The demonstration of dopamine-β-hydroxylase activity in intact storage particles requires the presence of adenosine triphosphate (ATP) and magnesium in the system. However, when the enzyme is solubilized, the necessity for ATP and magnesium disappears, suggesting that the ATP and magnesium are actually required for the uptake process rather than for the catalytic transformation (19).

The mechanism by which dopamine-β-hydroxylase catalyzes the hydroxylation of dopamine and related phenylethylamines has been studied extensively. Two copper (Cu^{2+})ions in the active site region of the enzyme are reduced by ascorbate to cuprous ion, which in turn complexes with molecular O_2. The cuprous ions transfer two electrons to the oxygen molecule in the complex. The activated oxygen then reacts with dopamine, which is bound at the active site of the enzyme, to yield the hydroxylated product, norepinephrine. The second atom of oxygen reacts with two protons to form water. The oxidized (Cu^{2+}) form of the enzyme must again be reduced to the active (Cu^+) form by ascorbic acid in order to continue the

enzymatic process. The enzyme is activated by fumarate and other dicarboxylic acids and is inhibited by disulfiram and related sulfhydryl reagents (20,21).

Thus norepinephrine formation from tyrosine involves three enzyme-catalyzed reactions. In addition tyrosine must be taken up from the extracellular fluid into the adrenergic neuron prior to aromatic hydroxylation to DOPA. This apparently involves an active transport process, since uptake is concentrative, stereospecific, is inhibited by oxygen deprivation and metabolic inhibitors, and is competitively antagonized by other aromatic amino acids. Because adrenergic nervous tissue comprises only a small fraction of most adrenergically innervated organs, the nature and kinetics of tyrosine uptake into neurons are virtually unknown. Preliminary studies in our laboratory on tyrosine uptake and retention indicate that the rate of uptake and retention of tyrosine in chronically denervated nictitating membranes cannot be distinguished from these processes in innervated membranes (R. A. Bjur and N. Weiner, *unpublished observations*).

Conversion of tyrosine to DOPA and, in turn, conversion of the latter substrate to dopamine appear to occur in the axoplasm of the adrenergic neuron. Dopamine must then be taken up into the storage vesicle before it can be converted to norepinephrine by the enzyme dopamine-β-hydroxylase. The norepinephrine may then be incorporated into the storage complex, the biochemical nature of which is unknown, although it presumably involves some noncovalent interaction with ATP and perhaps with soluble chromogranins and divalent cations in the vesicle (22). Newly synthesized norepinephrine either may be discharged from the nerve terminal consequent to nerve stimulation by an exocytotic process or may leak spontaneously from the storage vesicle into the axoplasm. The amine is either again taken up into the vesicle from the cytosol or it is metabolized, primarily by oxidative deamination. Thus the synthesis and turnover of norepinephrine is dependent not only on the amounts and activities of the biosynthetic enzymes but also on the kinetics of the processes that mediate tyrosine uptake into the neuron and catecholamine uptake into the storage vesicles, on the ability of the storage vesicles to retain catecholamines, on the rate of oxidative deamination of free norepinephrine within the axoplasm, and on neuronal release and reuptake of both norepinephrine and dopamine. Many studies, including several in our laboratory, indicate that the rate of norepinephrine synthesis is critically dependent on many or all of these factors and the relative importance of each may vary to a considerable degree, depending on the physiological and pharmacological stresses applied to the system (23).

REGULATION OF NOREPINEPHRINE SYNTHESIS

Although it is generally agreed that reuptake mechanisms are of major importance in the termination of the action of that norepinephrine that is released from adrenergic neurons by physiological stimuli, much of the amine which is taken back into the neuron appears to be metabolized by intraneuronal monoamine oxidase (24). There is a preponderance of evidence that suggests that norepinephrine synthesis must play a critical role in the maintenance of the stores of this amine and that synthesis is responsive to, and proportional to, the intensity of adrenergic neuronal activity. For example, in spite of varying intensities and durations of adrenergic nerve stimulation and norepinephrine release, the tissue levels of this amine either do not change significantly or are reduced only briefly. Several workers have shown that, in man and animals, stress and adrenergic nerve stimulation lead to increased urinary excretion of norepinephrine and norepinephrine metabolites (23). If the adrenergic nerve stores are maintained, increased synthesis must have taken place. Increased synthesis associated with sympathetic nerve stimulation was first clearly demonstrated in the adrenal gland. The stimulation of one gland leads to an outpouring of catecholamines, and, after a considerable period of stimulation, the total catecholamine content of the stimulated gland plus the amount in the perfusate exceeds that present in the contralateral unstimulated gland and its perfusate. More recently, studies with inhibitors of norepinephrine synthesis and turnover studies have shown that the turnover of norepinephrine in

tissues is rapid and, in the presence of such synthesis inhibitors as α-methyl-p-tyrosine, tissue norepinephrine is rapidly depleted. This is particularly true if the animal is simultaneously stressed.

END-PRODUCT FEEDBACK REGULATION OF TYROSINE HYDROXYLASE ACTIVITY

In investigations of the tyrosine hydroxylase enzyme of beef adrenal medulla, Nagatsu and co-workers demonstrated that catecholamines and other catechols were able to inhibit the activity of the enzyme (11). Ikeda and co-workers presented evidence that this inhibition represents competition between the catecholamine and the pterin cofactor for the oxidized form of the enzyme (9). Employing a synthetic pterin cofactor at a concentration of 1 mM, Udenfriend et al. (25) demonstrated that approximately 50% inhibition of tyrosine hydroxylase activity is obtained with a similar concentration of norepinephrine. It is quite likely that considerably smaller concentrations of catecholamines in the axoplasm of the neuron may severely inhibit tyrosine hydroxylase activity *in situ,* since the concentration of the cofactor within the neuron may be considerably less than 1 mM (12). Since the tyrosine hydroxylase reaction appears to be the rate-limiting step in the biosynthesis of norepinephrine (11), end-product feedback inhibition of tyrosine hydroxylase may be an extremely critical regulatory mechanism for the biosynthesis of catecholamines.

Numerous pharmacological studies indicate that the *in situ* activity of tyrosine hydroxylase may be profoundly affected by intraneuronal catecholamines. Alousi and Weiner (26) demonstrated that tyrosine hydroxylase activity is markedly reduced in intact vasa deferentia 2 hr after administration of reserpine. In addition, tyramine inhibited the activity of tyrosine hydroxylase in intact tissue. Neither of these agents affected the activity of partially purified tyrosine hydroxylase (27,28). It was concluded from these studies that a small pool of free intraneuronal norepinephrine regulates the activity of tyrosine hydroxylase by end-product feedback inhibition. Drugs that release norepinephrine from storage sites, such as reserpine and tyramine, increase the concentration of the catecholamine in the axoplasm. Since tyrosine hydroxylase is present in the cytosol (*vide supra*), the catecholamine would be expected to inhibit the activity of the enzyme in proportion to its concentration in the same intracellular compartment. Similar results were obtained for other amines such as α-methyl-phenylethylamines (29).

Intraneuronal monoamine oxidase would be expected to deaminate cytosol catecholamines rapidly and might therefore function to sustain a high level of tyrosine hydroxylase activity by minimizing end-product feedback inhibition. Conversely it might be anticipated that monoamine oxidase inhibitors would tend to preserve free intraneuronal catecholamines and, indirectly, inhibit tyrosine hydroxylase activity. Alousi and Weiner (26) demonstrated that pheniprazine inhibited tyrosine hydroxylase activity and, subsequently, Bjur and Weiner (30) and Weiner et al. (28) showed that other monoamine oxidase inhibitors, such as pargyline and tranylcypromine, were also able to reduce tyrosine hydroxylase activity in intact tissue. Furthermore, when the vesicle amine uptake system was blocked by reserpine, the inhibitory effect of norepinephrine or pargyline on tyrosine hydroxylase activity in intact mouse vasa deferentia was potentiated. All these studies support the contention that the level of free intraneuronal norepinephrine is a significant factor in the regulation of the activity of tyrosine hydroxylase.

The importance of this regulatory mechanism was demonstrated further by the observation that a synthetic pterin cofactor, 2-amino-4-hydroxy-6,7-dimethyltetrahydropteridine (DMPH₄), could enhance the activity of tyrosine hydroxylase in intact vasa deferentia. Furthermore, the inhibitory effects of reserpine, tranylcypromine (28,30), and norepinephrine (31) on the *in situ* enzyme could be reversed in a competitive fashion by addition of the pterin cofactor to the medium.

In these studies (30) it was observed that the apparent K_m for the synthetic pterin cofactor, DMPH₄, was not significantly different, whether this kinetic constant was determined in intact mouse vasa deferentia or in a partially purified enzyme preparation of the same tissue. A similar apparent K_m for norepinephrine synthesis was obtained in intact vasa deferentia and in

homogenates of this tissue when the putative natural cofactor, tetrahydrobiopterin, was examined. Since norepinephrine would be expected to increase the apparent K_m of pterin cofactor for the enzyme, these results suggest that, under normal circumstances, the enzyme is minimally inhibited by catecholamines *in situ*.

ENHANCED NOREPINEPHRINE SYNTHESIS DURING NERVE STIMULATION

In the past decade a considerable amount of evidence has accumulated to support the concept that increased adrenergic nervous activity is associated with enhanced synthesis of norepinephrine from tyrosine both *in vivo* and *in vitro* (23,26,32). We have examined this phenomenon utilizing the isolated hypogastric nerve-vas deferens preparation of the guinea pig. In this organ, nerve stimulation is associated with an approximate doubling of the synthesis of norepinephrine from tyrosine (33). This enhanced synthesis can be partially or completely prevented by the addition of norepinephrine to the bath (32,33). When DOPA is used as precursor, synthesis of norepinephrine is not enhanced by nerve stimulation, suggesting that the effect of nerve stimulation is at the tyrosine hydroxylase step. Since the total amount of norepinephrine in the stimulated preparation is not different from that in the contralateral sham-stimulated organ, it is presumed that a small, chemically indetectable pool of norepinephrine is critical for the regulation of norepinephrine synthesis. This small compartment, which we presume to be free intraneuronal norepinephrine, may be depleted during nerve stimulation (26,32).

If reduced end-product feedback inhibition of tyrosine hydroxylase is responsible for the enhanced synthesis of norepinephrine associated with nerve stimulation, elimination of end-product feedback inhibition with excess added cofactor would be expected to erase any differences in tyrosine hydroxylase activity between stimulated and unstimulated vas deferens preparations. Although added pterin cofactor did increase norepinephrine synthesis in unstimulated guinea-pig vas deferens preparations, the cofactor increased the rate of catecholamine synthesis to an even greater degree in preparations subjected to hypogastric nerve stimulation. Kinetic analysis of the effect of pterin cofactor on norepinephrine synthesis in stimulated and unstimulated preparations revealed that nerve stimulation was associated with an approximate doubling of the V_{max} for synthesis. However, no significant change in the apparent K_m for pterin cofactor was demonstrable. This is in contrast to the interaction between added norepinephrine and pterin cofactor in the same intact preparation. Addition of norepinephrine to the medium is associated with a significant increase of the apparent K_m of the pterin cofactor for norepinephrine synthesis, whereas the V_{max} of the synthesis of catecholamines is not affected (28,31). Although these results suggest that the reduction in the level of free intraneuronal norepinephrine is responsible for the enhanced tyrosine hydroxylase activity associated with nerve stimulation, the mechanism does not appear to involve reduced end-product feedback inhibition of the enzyme, which is competitive with the pterin cofactor.

In addition to the increase in norepinephrine synthesis, which occurs during nerve stimulation, there is a considerable increase in norepinephrine synthesis in the vas deferens, which occurs for several hours following stimulation of the hypogastric nerve (34). In contrast to the enhancement of norepinephrine synthesis, which occurs during nerve stimulation, this poststimulation increase in norepinephrine synthesis is blocked if puromycin is present in the incubation medium during the stimulation period but is not inhibited by addition of norepinephrine to the incubation medium during stimulation (34). Puromycin does not affect the poststimulation increase in norepinephrine synthesis, if it is added only in the period following nerve stimulation, at the time that norepinephrine synthesis in the intact tissue is assessed. However, the effect does not appear to be mediated by synthesis either of enzyme protein or a protein activator, since cycloheximide, at a concentration that virtually completely inhibits the incorporation of amino acids into protein, fails to block the poststimulation activation of tyrosine hydroxylase (14). No increase in enzyme activity is apparent in homogenates of vasa deferentia assayed under optimal conditions for tyrosine hydroxylase after an hour of stimulation, suggesting that there is no increase in enzyme protein.

POSSIBLE ALLOSTERIC FACTORS MODULATING THE ACTIVITY OF TYROSINE HYDROXYLASE

Studies in several laboratories suggest that a number of factors may modify the activity of tyrosine hydroxylase by an allosteric effect. Kuczenski and Mandell (35) observed that the activity of soluble tyrosine hydroxylase from the rat caudate nucleus increases with increasing ionic strength. In particular, sulfate ion appears to stimulate the activity of the enzyme. The K_m for $DMPH_4$ is unaffected by sulfate ion, but the V_{max} is approximately doubled. Even greater effects on the enzyme were demonstrable when the sulfated polysaccharide, heparin, was employed. In the presence of heparin, the K_m of $DMPH_4$ was reduced from 0.7 mM to 0.15 mM and the V_{max} of the enzymatic reaction was increased approximately two-fold (8). Furthermore these workers observed that the K_i of the soluble enzyme for dopamine increased in the presence of heparin. In these studies addition of heparin seemed to alter the kinetic properties of soluble tyrosine hydroxylase so that the enzyme resembled the particulate enzyme more closely. These workers postulated that physiological stimuli (? nerve stimulation) may modify the soluble enzyme in some manner that converts it to a particulate form (membrane bound), and this alteration is responsible for the changes in the kinetic properties of the enzyme. The enzyme becomes more active in the presence of either optimal or suboptimal concentrations of cofactor and becomes more resistant to inhibition by dopamine.

These provocative studies are difficult to assess because there is no evidence that a sulfated polysaccharide, such as heparin, is present in catecholaminergic neurons. Furthermore, although the effects observed by Kuczenski and Mandell (8,35) are quite striking in the presence of Tris acetate buffer, they are not duplicated if sodium acetate buffer is employed in place of Tris acetate (3). The reasons for the special role of Tris in this phenomenon are unclear, as is the physiological relevance of the observation.

In what appear to be a related series of observations, Lloyd and Kaufman (36) have shown that phosphatidyl-L-serine stimulates partially purified tyrosine hydroxylase obtained from bovine caudate nucleus. This phospholipid lowers the K_m of the enzyme for tetrahydrobiopterin, DMPH$_4$, and 6-methyltetrahydropterin approximately fourfold. No effect of the phospholipid on the tyrosine K_m was apparent. In addition phosphatidyl-L-serine increased the pH optimum of the enzyme from 6.0–6.1 to 6.6–6.8. Polyglutamic acid was also observed to decrease the K_m for pterin cofactor. This polyanionic macromolecule also increased the V_{max} of the enzyme, similar to the effect of heparin. It may be that anions or salts facilitate the interaction of soluble tyrosine hydroxylase with other macromolecular tissue components and that this interaction is associated with a conversion of the enzyme to a more active form.

Recent studies suggest that the activity of tyrosine hydroxylase may also be modulated by cations. Gutman and Segal (37) reported that increased concentrations of sodium ion and decreased concentrations of potassium ion enhanced the activity of soluble adrenal tyrosine hydroxylase. This is a particularly intriguing observation, since analogous changes in cation concentration in the nerve terminal would be associated with nerve terminal depolarization. However, using homogenates of guinea-pig vas deferens preparations, we were unable to demonstrate any significant effects of variations in sodium or potassium ions on tyrosine hydroxylase activity (33). Similar negative results were obtained by Ikeda et al. (9), using an enzyme preparation from bovine adrenal medulla.

Another cation that is presumably taken up into the neuron during stimulation is calcium. Gutman and Segal (37) reported that 0.1 mM calcium chloride slightly activated bovine adrenal tyrosine hydroxylase whereas 0.2 mM calcium chloride reduced the activity of the enzyme modestly.

Morgenroth et al. (38) recently reported that tyrosine hydroxylase activity in homogenates of guinea pig vasa deferentia is activated by calcium ions and this activation is blocked by ethylene glycol bis-(β-aminoethylether)-N,N'-tetraacetic acid (EGTA). The activation of the enzyme appears to be a consequence of an increase in the affinity of the enzyme for both

tyrosine and DMPH$_4$ and a decrease in its affinity for norepinephrine. For these studies, suboptimal concentrations of substrate and cofactor were employed.

Of particular interest was the observation of Morgenroth et al. (38) that similar changes in the kinetic properties of a soluble preparation of tyrosine hydroxylase could be elicited either by prior electrical stimulation of the intact vas deferens preparation or by incubating the intact preparation in the presence of depolarizing concentrations of potassium. These changes in the enzyme could be prevented by deletion of Ca^{2+} from the incubation medium. Morgenroth et al. (38) propose that the activation of tyrosine hydroxylase as a consequence of nerve stimulation may be the result of an influx of calcium caused by nerve terminal depolarization and consequent activation of the enzyme by the cation. Analogous results have been observed with a tyrosine hydroxylase preparation obtained from adrenergic neurons in the central nervous system subsequent to stimulation of the locus coeruleus (39).

Thoa et al. (14) studied the activity of tyrosine hydroxylase in homogenates prepared from guinea-pig vasa deferentia 1 hr following nerve stimulation. In contrast to the results of Morgenroth et al. (38), they were unable to demonstrate a change in tyrosine hydroxylase activity in these preparations either in the presence of suboptimal or optimal concentrations of tyrosine, although considerable increases in tyrosine hydroxylase activity in the intact stimulated preparations were still apparent.

In contrast to the reported effects of calcium ion on the guinea pig vas deferens enzyme and the enzyme in adrenergic neurons in the central nervous system, Goldstein et al. (40) observed that, when rat brain striatal slices were incubated with different concentrations of calcium ion, synthesis of [^{14}C]-dopamine from [^{14}C]-tyrosine was reduced as the calcium ion concentration was raised. Similarly Roth et al. have observed that calcium ion inhibits the activity of a high-speed supernatant preparation of rat striatal tyrosine hydroxylase (41). Conversely EGTA activates this enzyme by increasing its affinity for substrate and cofactor and reducing its affinity for the catecholamine endproduct. Reducing impulse flow in the nigrostriatal dopaminergic pathway, either by placing lesions in the nigrostriatal tract or administering γ-hydroxybutyrolactone, is associated with increased tyrosine hydroxylase activity in the neostriatum (41). These surprising observations have been explained by assuming that dopamine presynaptic receptors in some way serve as negative-feedback modulators of tyrosine hydroxylase in dopamine-containing neurons. The absence of dopamine in the synaptic space or the blockade of these dopamine receptors by haloperidol, phenothiazines, or related drugs is associated with a diminution in this negative feedback system and an activation of tyrosine hydroxylase in the dopamine nerve terminals (41). Support for this speculation is not available nor is an explanation for the quite paradoxical effects observed in adrenergic neuronal systems. Furthermore the effects of cessation of impulse flow and EGTA on the activity of striatal tyrosine hydroxylase are difficult to reconcile with more recent observations from the same laboratory that stimulation of the nigrostriatal tract is associated with an enhanced affinity of substrate and cofactor for the striatal tyrosine hydroxylase and a reduced affinity of the enzyme for dopamine (42). Thus, both increased and decreased impulse flow appear to be associated with similar changes in the kinetics of striatal tyrosine hydroxylase. These results would suggest that the enzyme should normally be found in the activated state.

POSTULATED ROLES FOR CYCLIC AMP AND CYCLIC AMP-DEPENDENT PROTEIN KINASE IN MODULATING TYROSINE HYDROXYLASE ACTIVITY

Anagnoste et al. (43) demonstrated that addition of dibutyryl cyclic AMP (cAMP) to incubating slices of rat striatum is associated with a considerable increase in the rate of formation of $[^{14}C]$-dopamine from $[^{14}C]$-tyrosine. They suggested that cAMP, which is elevated in brain tissue subjected to high potassium or electrical stimulation (44), may be responsible for the increased tyrosine hydroxylase activity associated with nerve stimulation. Dibutyryl cAMP appears to increase the V_{max} of the enzyme in striatal slices but does not influence the K_m for tyrosine. Unfortunately, since pterin

cofactor either is not taken up into synaptosomes or does not stimulate tyrosine hydroxylase in these particles, kinetic studies with pterin cofactor are not possible in this preparation.

Harris et al. (45) have recently claimed that dibutyryl cAMP is able to stimulate tyrosine hydroxylase when the cyclic nucleotide is added to rat striatal homogenates. cAMP was reported to produce a similar effect on soluble striatal tyrosine hydroxylase. The stimulation of the enzyme by 10 μM cAMP is associated with a reduction in the K_m for $DMPH_4$ (from 0.62 to 0.08 mM) and an increase in the K_i for dopamine (from 0.09 to 0.64 mM). The K_m for tyrosine was also reduced from 54 to 23 μM. The V_{max} of the enzyme was not altered (45).

In contrast to these results, Lovenberg et al. (46) were unable to demonstrate an effect of cAMP on the kinetic properties of rat striatal tyrosine hydroxylase solubilized by addition of 0.2% Triton X-100. On the other hand, these workers demonstrated a severalfold reduction in the K_m for pterin cofactor when the soluble enzyme was incubated in a system optimal for protein kinase activity (added constituents were ATP, cAMP, Mg^{2+}, EGTA, NaF, and theophylline).

Morgenroth et al. (47) found that cAMP alone is able to activate tyrosine hydroxylase present in a crude high speed supernatant from rat striatum. [This discrepancy with the results of Lovenberg et al. (46) may be explained by the use of Triton X-100 in the studies of the latter workers. In the absence of detergent, the brain supernatant may contain sufficient quantities of ATP and protein kinase (and Mg^{2+}) to produce some degree of enzyme activation without further additions.] When the enzyme was further purified on a Sephadex G-25 column, cAMP was no longer able to activate the enzyme. However, activation could be produced by addition of ATP, Mg^{2+}, and cAMP and further activation could be obtained by addition of protein kinase. Both Lovenberg et al. (46) and Morgenroth et al. (47) conclude that activation of tyrosine hydroxylase may be mediated by a cAMP-dependent protein kinase. Whether tyrosine hydroxylase or an activator of the enzyme is phosphorylated remains to be elucidated.

Brostrom et al. (48) have recently demonstrated the presence of a calcium-binding protein in pig cerebral cortex that activates adenylate cyclase in this system. The activation of adenylate cyclase is Ca^{2+} dependent and is prevented by addition of excess EGTA. The calcium-binding protein appears to be identical to a previously recognized phosphodiesterase-activating factor, which is also Ca^{2+} dependent. Brostrom et al. speculate that the activation of this system leads to enhanced synthesis of cAMP and preferential enhanced hydrolysis of cyclic guanosine monophosphate (cGMP). If these events occur in catecholaminergic nerve terminals, they may be responsible for the initiation of the reactions that ultimately lead to tyrosine hydroxylase activation and induction of the enzyme (*vide infra*).

Although the above studies suggest that the activation of tyrosine hydroxylase may be mediated by nerve terminal depolarization, uptake of Ca^{2+}, activation of adenylate cyclase, production of cAMP and activation of a cAMP-dependent protein kinase, there remain major unanswered questions that should temper an enthusiastic acceptance of this regulatory model.

The similar activation of rat brain striatal tyrosine hydroxylase by reduced and increased impulse flow in the nigrostriatal system remains unexplained. It is possible that the enzyme in this region is different from that in peripheral and central noradrenergic neurons, and that the enzyme in dopamine neurons exhibits special regulatory properties, such as polyanion sensitivity. Joh and Reis (49) have presented preliminary evidence that suggests that the striatal enzyme(s) is (are) of different molecular weight(s) from that in adrenergic neurons and may be immunochemically different. Whether there are different enzymes or interchangeable forms of the same enzyme complexes is not yet certain. Lloyd and Kaufman (50) demonstrated cross-reactivity between antibody to bovine adrenal tyrosine hydroxylase and other tyrosine hydroxylases, including that from the striatum. Recently Numata and Nagatsu (51) were unable to demonstrate changes in the kinetic properties of bovine mandibular nerve tyrosine hydroxylase in the presence of either heparin or lysolecithin, suggesting the adrenergic and dopaminergic isoenzymes may be different.

A major problem, yet unresolved, relates to the changes in tyrosine hydroxylase activity *in situ* during nerve stimulation, reported by Weiner et al. (33) and Cloutier and Weiner (31). As noted above, these studies suggest that the change in tyrosine hydroxylase after nerve stimulation is largely a V_{max} effect. No significant change in the apparent K_m for either tyrosine or $DMPH_4$ was demonstrated in these studies, although a change in the apparent K_m for $DMPH_4$ could be produced by addition of norepinephrine to the intact tissue. Furthermore the enzyme activated by nerve stimulation appeared to be at least as sensitive to inhibition by catecholamines as is the enzyme present in the contralateral, unstimulated vas deferens preparation. These *in situ* analyses of the enzyme are in sharp distinction to the behavior of the enzyme when it is examined in disrupted cell systems after similar treatments of the intact tissue.

The physiological relevance of the cAMP and Ca^{2+}-mediated changes in the enzyme described above remains a matter of conjecture. Changes in tyrosine hydroxylase activity during nerve stimulation do not appear to be mediated by norepinephrine-sensitive activation of adenylate cyclase, since these effects are not prevented by either propranolol or phenoxybenzamine (F.-L. Lee, and N. Weiner, *unpublished observations*). It is possible that the cAMP-protein kinase mediated changes in tyrosine hydroxylase are not responsible for the increased activity of the enzyme during nerve stimulation, but may be the mediators of the poststimulation increase in tyrosine hydroxylase, which is prevented by puromycin, but not by norepinephrine.

Finally the possibility that the changes in the kinetic properties of the enzyme associated with activation of neural systems are an artifact has not been totally excluded. Activation of adenylate cyclase appears to occur in many brain cells as well as in smooth muscle and other tissues. There is no unequivocal evidence that this enzyme system exists in catecholaminergic nerve terminals. It is conceivable that, during the tissue homogenization and enzyme assay procedures, activated adenylate cyclase and protein kinase from other cells could come into contact with the tyrosine hydroxylase and produce the kinetic changes that have been observed. Studies in which this type of posthomogenization artifact has been excluded must be carried out before the physiological significance of this mechanism for the activation of this enzyme is established.

THE INDUCTION OF NOREPINEPHRINE BIOSYNTHETIC ENZYMES FOLLOWING PROLONGED STIMULATION

In addition to the enhanced activity of tyrosine hydroxylase that occurs during and shortly following nerve stimulation, other mechanisms for the regulation of the biosynthesis of this transmitter exist. Increased sympathetic activity for many hours or days is associated with an increase in the content of tyrosine hydroxylase in the adrenal gland, in sympathetic nervous tissue, and in the central nervous system (23). Immunochemical studies with specific antibody indicate that the amount of enzyme protein increases both in the central nervous system after reserpine treatment (52) and in the adrenal gland after either immobilization stress, cold exposure, or 6-hydroxydopamine administration (53).

A large number of pharmacological agents that affect adrenergic nervous function either directly or indirectly can influence the level of tyrosine hydroxylase in peripheral or central adrenergic neurons. Insulin administration and the consequent hypoglycemia is associated with reflex increases in adrenergic stimulation and elevated levels of tyrosine hydroxylase and dopamine-β-hydroxylase in the adrenal medulla. The administration of either reserpine, which impairs sympathetic function by depletion of catecholamine stores, or phenoxybenzamine, which produces blockade of sympathetic function at the postsynaptic receptor site, presumably leads to a reflex increase in adrenergic nervous activity as a compensatory mechanism and consequent increases in the levels of the biosynthetic enzymes. These effects can be inhibited at least in part by administration of inhibitors of protein synthesis or actinomycin D (54,55). Conversely, after chronic denervation of the adrenal gland, the level of tyrosine hydroxylase is significantly less than that in the contralateral, innervated gland.

The mechanism by which tyrosine hydroxylase is induced in adrenergic nervous tissue with chronic nervous stimulation has been examined in a variety of systems. Waymire et al. (56) demonstrated that the addition of dibutyryl cAMP, cAMP analogues, or phosphodiesterase inhibitors to growing neuroblastoma C-1300 cells in culture was associated with arrest of cell division, cell differentiation, and increased levels of tyrosine hydroxylase after 48–72 hr. Immunotitration studies revealed that the level of enzyme protein in the neuroblastoma cells was increased (N. Weiner and M. Posiviata, *unpublished observation*). The kinetic properties of the induced enzyme were not different from those of the enzyme present in control cell cultures (56). Mackay and Iversen (57) noted a similar increase in tyrosine hydroxylase in sympathetic ganglia which were cultured in the presence of dibutyryl cAMP.

Guidotti and Costa (58) demonstrated a rapid and transient increase in adrenal medulla cAMP after administration of carbachol or reserpine to rats. This increase was followed by an elevation in adrenal tyrosine hydroxylase 24 hr later. In contrast Paul et al. (59) demonstrated a rise in rat adrenal cortex cAMP after immobilization stress, but these workers were unable to show an elevation of the cyclic nucleotide in the adrenal medulla. Immobilization stress is associated with elevated levels of tyrosine hydroxylase after one or more days (60). Otten et al. (61) administered reserpine to rats or subjected groups of these animals either to intermittent swimming or cold stress and measured cAMP and tyrosine hydroxylase levels in the adrenal medulla and superior cervical ganglia at intervals thereafter. Early increases in adrenal cAMP and later elevations in tyrosine hydroxylase were detectable after each of these procedures. However, a good correlation between the extent of the rise in adrenal medulla cAMP and the subsequent induction of tyrosine hydroxylase was not apparent. Furthermore no elevation in cAMP was demonstrable in the superior cervical ganglion after swimming stress although a subsequent elevation in tyrosine hydroxylase was noted. Further studies by Otten et al. (62) also suggest that there may not be a causal relationship between elevations of cAMP and induction of tyrosine hydroxylase. These workers showed that isoproterenol administration, which results in considerable increases in cAMP levels in the superior cervical ganglion, is not associated with elevated tyrosine hydroxylase levels subsequently. Furthermore, propranolol administration to rats markedly diminishes the rise in adrenal medulla cAMP after reserpine treatment but does not modify the subsequent rise in tyrosine hydroxylase. Clearly more information is required before the precise role of cyclic nucleotides in the induction of tyrosine hydroxylase *in vivo* is ascertained.

Cyclic nucleotides also may be involved in the release of catecholamines by nerve stimulation (63,64). Both cAMP and cGMP analogues and phosphodiesterase inhibitors enhance release of norepinephrine and dopamine-β-hydroxylase during nerve stimulation of the isolated, perfused cat spleen. In this preparation these substances do not appear to initiate the release process, since they do not affect the release of neurotransmitter in the absence of nerve stimulation (64). It remains to be determined whether the cyclic nucleotide mediated release of neurotransmitter during nerve stimulation either is responsible for, or is intimately linked to, the concomitant or subsequent changes in biosynthetic enzyme activities or levels.

Dopamine-β-hydroxylase levels in adrenergic nervous tissue and in the adrenal medulla are also increased following prolonged sympathetic activity (65). It has been proposed that cAMP may be involved in the induction of this enzyme (66). Adrenal cortical hormonal factors also appear to play significant roles in the determination of the synthesis and levels of norepinephrine biosynthetic enzymes, especially in the adrenal gland (67).

In addition to the effects of nerve stimulation and hormones on dopamine-β-hydroxylase levels in adrenergic nervous tissue and in the adrenal gland, other factors may regulate the activity of this enzyme *in situ*. Potent endogenous inhibitors of dopamine-β-hydroxylase have been demonstrated in tissues (68–70), and some of these inhibitory substances may be present in the storage vesicles where dopamine-β-hydroxylase is localized (68–70). The physiological significance of these inhibitors in the regulation of norepinephrine synthesis remains to be assessed.

CONCLUSION

The sympathetic nervous system is an important component of the complex homeostatic systems involved in regulation of blood pressure, cardiac output, blood glucose, carbohydrate, and lipid metabolism and other peripheral functions. Central catecholaminergic neurons are vitally involved in the adjustments of complex functions mediating motor function, affect, perception, arousal, and other types of behaviors. These peripheral and central functions must be modulated according to the physiological inputs and stresses to which the normal organism is subjected. Furthermore these processes are modified in response to cardiovascular, metabolic, psychiatric, and other disease processes, and many of the useful therapeutic agents in the management of these diseases are presumed to produce their effects by altering the function of these peripheral and central neural systems. It is obvious that the biosynthesis of catecholamine neurotransmitters is in turn modified in response to the needs of the organism and in response to pathological and pharmacological stresses that impinge upon the individual. It is also apparent that primary disturbances in these catecholamine-containing neural systems are responsible for some pathological processes. Obvious examples of this are Parkinson's disease and pheochromocytoma. Others in which a primary role of the catecholamine systems is suspected include disorders of affect, schizophrenia, and hypertension. Our knowledge of adrenergic function and the regulation of neurotransmitter synthesis and metabolism has been developed enormously in the past 25 years, and insights into the role of these systems in disease processes and in treatment have advanced accordingly. Nevertheless in view of the many questions that remain unanswered, our knowledge may still be considered rudimentary. It is to be expected that, as additional information about this complex system is accumulated in the years ahead, our understanding of, and our ability to deal effectively with, diseases in which these neural systems play a role will be correspondingly advanced.

ACKNOWLEDGMENTS

The research work of the author summarized in this report was supported by U.S. Public Health Service Grants NS 07642, NS 07927, and NS 09199 from the National Institute of Neurological Diseases and Stroke.

REFERENCES

1. Ikeda, M., Levitt, M., and Udenfriend, S. (1967): Phenylalanine as substrate and inhibitor of tyrosine hydroxylase. *Arch. Biochem. Biophys.*, 120: 420–427.
2. Shiman, R., Akino, M., and Kaufman, S. (1971): Solubilization and partial purification of tyrosine hydroxylase from bovine adrenal medulla. *J. Biol. Chem.*, 246:1330–1340.
3. Weiner, N., Lee, F. L., Waymire, J. C., and Posiviata, M. (1974): The regulation of tyrosine hydroxylase activity in adrenergic nervous tissue. In: *Ciba Foundation Symposium 22, Aromatic Amino Acids in the Brain*, edited by R. J. Wurtman, pp. 135–147. Elsevier, Amsterdam.
4. Petrack, B., Sheppy, F., and Fetzer, V. (1968): Studies on tyrosine hydroxylase from bovine adrenal medulla. *J. Biol. Chem.*, 243:743–748.
5. Wurzburger, R. J., and Musacchio, J. M. (1971): Subcellular distribution and aggregation of bovine adrenal tyrosine hydroxylase. *J. Pharmacol. Exp. Ther.*, 177:155–167.
6. Waymire, J. C., Weiner, N., Schneider, F. H., Goldstein, M., and Freedman, L. S. (1972): Tyrosine hydroxylase in human adrenal and pheochromocytoma: Localization, kinetics, and catecholamine inhibition. *J. Clin. Invest.*, 51:1798–1804.
7. McGeer, P. L., Bagchi, S. P., and McGeer, E. G. (1956): Subcellular localization of tyrosine hydroxylase in beef caudate nucleus. *Life Sci.*, 4:1859–1867.
8. Kuczenski, R. T., and Mandell, A. J. (1972): Regulatory properties of soluble and particulate rat brain tyrosine hydroxylase. *J. Biol. Chem.*, 247:3114–3122.
9. Ikeda, M., Fahien, L. A., and Udenfriend, S. (1966): A kinetic study of bovine adrenal tyrosine hydroxylase. *J. Biol. Chem.*, 241:4452–4456.
10. Brenneman, A. R., and Kaufman, S. (1964): The role of tetrahydropteridines in the enzymatic conversion of tyrosine to 3,4-dihydroxyphenylalanine. *Biochem. Biophys. Res. Comm.*, 17:177–183.
11. Nagatsu, T., Levitt, B. G., and Udenfriend, S. (1964): Tyrosine hydroxylase: The initial step in norepinephrine biosynthesis. *J. Biol. Chem.*, 238:2910–2917.
12. Lloyd, T., and Weiner, N. (1971): Isolation and characterization of a tyrosine hydroxylase cofactor from bovine adrenal medulla. *Mol. Pharmacol.*, 7:569–580.
13. Musacchio, J. M., D'Angelo, G. L., and McQueen, C. A. (1971): Dihydropteridine reductase: Implication on the regulation of catecholamine biosynthesis. *Proc. Natl. Acad. Sci. USA*, 68:2087–2091.
14. Thoa, N. B., Johnson, D. G., Kopin, I. J., and Weiner, N. (1971): Acceleration of catecholamine formation in the guinea-pig vas deferens following hypogastric nerve stimulation: Roles of tyrosine

hydroxylase and new protein synthesis. *J. Pharmacol. Exp. Ther.*, 178:442–449.
15. Laduron, P., and Belpaire, F. (1968): Tissue fractionation and catecholamine. II. Intracellular distribution patterns of tyrosine hydroxylase, dopa decarboxylase, dopamine-β-hydroxylase, phenylethanolamine-*N*-methyltransferase and monoamine oxidase in adrenal medulla. *Biochem. Pharmacol.*, 17:1127–1140.
16. Sims, K. L., Davis, G. A., and Bloom, F. E. (1973): Activities of 3,4-dihydroxy-L-phenylalanine and 5-hydroxy-L-tryptophan decarboxylases in rat brain: Assay characteristics and distribution. *J. Neurochem.*, 20:449–464.
17. Kaufman, S., and Friedman, S. (1965): Dopamine-β-hydroxylase. *Pharmacol. Rev.*, 17:71–100.
18. Kirshner, N., Rorie, M., and Kamin, D. L. (1965): Inhibition of dopamine uptake *in vitro* by reserpine administered *in vivo*. *J. Pharmacol. Exp. Ther.*, 141:285–289.
19. Levin, E. Y., and Kaufman, S. (1961): Studies on the enzyme catalyzing the conversion of 3,4-dihydroxyphenylethylamine to norepinephrine. *J. Biol. Chem.*, 236:2043–2049.
20. Goldstein, M., Joh, T. H., and Garvey, T. G., III (1968): Kinetic studies of the enzymatic dopamine β-hydroxylation reaction. *Biochemistry*, 7:2724–2730.
21. Craine, J. E., Daniels, G. H., and Kaufman, S. (1973): Dopamine-β-hydroxylase: The subunit structure and anion activation of the bovine adrenal enzyme. *J. Biol. Chem.*, 248:7838–7844.
22. Weiner, N. (1964): The catecholamines; biosynthesis, storage and release, metabolism and metabolic effects. In: *The Hormones, Vol. 4*, edited by G. Pincus, K. V. Thimann, and E. B. Astwood, pp. 403–479. Academic Press, New York.
23. Weiner, N. (1970): Regulation of norepinephrine biosynthesis. *Ann. Rev. Pharmacol.*, 10:273–290.
24. Cubeddu, L. X., Barnes, E., Langer, S. Z., and Weiner, N. (1974): Release of norepinephrine and dopamine-beta-hydroxylase by nerve stimulation. I. Role of neuronal and extraneuronal uptake and of alpha-presynaptic receptors. *J. Pharmacol. Exp. Ther.*, 190:431–450.
25. Udenfriend, S., Zaltzman-Nirenberg, P., and Nagatsu, T. (1965): Inhibitors of purified beef adrenal tyrosine hydroxylase. *Biochem. Pharmacol.*, 14:837–845.
26. Alousi, A., and Weiner, N. (1966): The regulation of norepinephrine synthesis in sympathetic nerves. Effect of nerve stimulation, cocaine and catecholamine releasing agents. *Proc. Natl. Acad. Sci. USA*, 56:1491–1496.
27. Weiner, N., and Selvaratnam, I. (1968): The effect of tyramine on the synthesis of norepinephrine. *J. Pharmacol. Exp. Ther.*, 161:21–33.
28. Weiner, N., Cloutier, G., Bjur, R., and Pfeffer, R. I. (1972): Modification of norepinephrine synthesis in intact tissue by drugs and during short-term adrenergic nerve stimulation. *Pharmacol. Rev.*, 24:203–221.

29. Kopin, I. J., Weise, V. K., and Sedvall, G. C. (1969): Effect of false transmitters on norepinephrine synthesis. *J. Pharmacol. Exp. Ther.,* 170:246–252.

30. Bjur, R. A., and Weiner, N. (1975): The activity of tyrosine hydroxylase in intact adrenergic neurons of the mouse vas deferens. *J. Pharmacol. Exp. Ther.,* 194:9–26.

31. Cloutier, G., and Weiner, N. (1973): Further studies on the increased synthesis of norepinephrine during nerve stimulation of guinea-pig vas deferens preparation: Effect of tyrosine and 6,7-dimethyltetrahydropterin. *J. Pharmacol. Exp. Ther.,* 186:75–85.

32. Weiner, N., and Rabadjija, M. (1968): The effect of nerve stimulation on the synthesis and metabolism of norepinephrine in the isolated guinea-pig hypogastric nerve-vas deferens preparation. *J. Pharmacol. Exp. Ther.,* 160:61–71.

33. Weiner, N., Bjur, R., Lee, F. L., Becker, G., and Mosimann, W. F. (1973): Studies on the mechanism of regulation of tyrosine hydroxylase activity during nerve stimulation. In: *Frontiers in Catecholamine Research,* edited by E. Usdin and S. H. Snyder, pp. 211–221. Pergamon Press, New York.

34. Weiner, N., and Rabadjija, M. (1968): The regulation of norepinephrine synthesis. Effect of puromycin on the accelerated synthesis of norepinephrine associated with nerve stimulation. *J. Pharmacol. Exp. Ther.,* 164:103–114.

35. Kuczenski, R. T., and Mandell, A. J. (1972): Allosteric activation of hypothalamic tyrosine hydroxylase by ions and sulphated mucopolysaccharides. *J. Neurochem.,* 19:131–137.

36. Lloyd, T., and Kaufman, S. (1974): The stimulation of partially purified bovine caudate tyrosine hydroxylase by phosphatidyl-L-serine. *Biochem. Biophys. Res. Comm.,* 59:1262–1269.

37. Gutman, Y., and Segal, J. (1972): Effect of calcium, sodium and potassium on adrenal tyrosine hydroxylase activity *in vitro. Biochem. Pharmacol.,* 21:2664–2666.

38. Morgenroth, V. H., III, Boadle-Bider, M., and Roth, R. H. (1974): Tyrosine hydroxylase: Activation by nerve stimulation. *Proc. Natl. Acad. Sci. USA,* 71:4283–4287.

39. Roth, R. H., Salzman, P. M., and Morgenroth, V. H., III (1974): Noradrenergic neurons: Allosteric activation of hippocampal tyrosine hydroxylase by stimulation of the locus coeruleus. *Biochem. Pharmacol.,* 23:2779–2784.

40. Goldstein, M., Backstrom, T., Ohi, Y., and Frenkel, R. (1970): The effects of Ca^{++} ions on the C^{14} catecholamine biosynthesis from C^{14}-tyrosine in slices from the striatum of rats. *Life Sci.,* 9:919–924.

41. Roth, R. H., Walters, J. R., and Morgenroth, V. H., III (1974): Effects of alterations in impulse flow on transmitter metabolism in central dopaminergic neurons. In: *Neuropsychopharmacology of Monoamines and Their Regulatory Enzymes,* edited by E. Usdin, pp. 369–384. Raven Press, New York.

42. Murrin, L. C., Morgenroth, V. H., III, and Roth, R. H. (1974): Activation of striatal tyrosine hydroxylase by increase in impulse flow. *Pharmacologist,* 16:213.

43. Anagnoste, B., Shirron, C., Friedman, E., and Goldstein, M. (1974): Effect of dibutyryl cyclic adenosine monophosphate on ^{14}C-dopamine biosynthesis in rat brain striatal slices. *J. Pharmacol. Exp. Ther.,* 191:370–376.

44. Kakiuchi, S., Rall, T. W., and McIlwain, H. (1969): The effect of electrical stimulation upon the accumulation of adenosine 3′,5′-phosphate in isolated cerebral tissue. *J. Neurochem.,* 16:485–491.

45. Harris, J. E., Morgenroth, V. H., III, Roth, R. H., and Baldessarini, R. J. (1974): Regulation of catecholamine synthesis in rat brain *in vitro* by cyclic AMP. *Nature,* 252:156–158.

46. Lovenberg, W., Bruckwick, E. A., and Hanbauer, I. (1975): The effect of phosphorylating conditions on rat striatal tyrosine hydroxylase (TH). *Fed. Proc.,* 34:624.

47. Morgenroth, V. H., III, Hegstrand, L. R., Roth, R. H., and Greengard, P. (1975): Evidence for involvement of protein kinase in the activation by cAMP of brain tyrosine 3-monooxygenase. *J. Biol. Chem.,* 250:1946–1948.

48. Brostrom, C. O., Huang, Y. C., Breckenridge, B. McL., and Wolff, D. J. (1975): Identification of a calcium-binding protein as a calcium-dependent regulator of brain adenylate cyclase. *Proc. Natl. Acad. Sci. USA,* 72:64–68.

49. Joh, T. H., and Reis, D. J. (1975): Different forms of tyrosine hydroxylase in central dopaminergic and noradrenergic neurons and sympathetic ganglia. *Brain Res.,* 85:146–151.

50. Lloyd, T., and Kaufman, S. (1973): Production of antibodies to bovine adrenal tyrosine hydroxylase: Cross-reactivity studies with other pterin-dependent hydroxylases. *Mol. Pharmacol.,* 9:438–444.

51. Namata (Sudo), Y., and Nagatsu, T. (1975): Properties of tyrosine hydroxylase in peripheral nerves. *J. Neurochem.,* 24:317–322.

52. Joh, T. H., Gregham, C., and Reis, D. (1973): Immunochemical demonstration of increased accumulation of tyrosine hydroxylase protein in sympathetic ganglia and adrenal medulla elicited by reserpine. *Proc. Natl. Acad. Sci. USA,* 70:2667–2771.

53. Hoeldtke, R., Lloyd, T., and Kaufman, S. (1974): An immunochemical study of the induction of tyrosine hydroxylase in rat adrenal glands. *Biochem. Biophys. Res. Comm.,* 57:1045–1053.

54. Weiner, N., and Mosimann, W. F. (1970): The effect of insulin on the catecholamine content of cat adrenal glands. *Biochem. Pharmacol.,* 19:1189–1199.

55. Thoenen, H., Mueller, R. A., and Axelrod, J. (1969): Trans-synaptic induction of adrenal tyrosine hydroxylase. *J. Pharmacol. Exp. Ther.,* 169:249–254.

56. Waymire, J. C., Weiner, N., and Prasad, K. N.

(1972): Regulation of tyrosine hydroxylase activity in cultured mouse neuroblastoma cells: Elevation by analogs of cAMP. *Proc. Natl. Acad. Sci. USA,* 69:2241–2245.

57. Mackay, A. V. P., and Iversen, L. L. (1972): Increased tyrosine hydroxylase activity of sympathetic ganglia cultured in the presence of dibutyryl cyclic AMP. *Brain Res.,* 48:424–426.

58. Guidotti, A., and Costa, E. (1973): Involvement of adenosine 3′,5′-monophosphate in the activation of tyrosine hydroxylase elicited by drugs. *Science,* 179:902–904.

59. Paul, M. I., Kvetňanský, R., Cramer, R., Silbergeld, S., and Kopin, I. J. (1971): Immobilization stress induced changes in adrenocortical and medullary cyclic AMP content in the rat. *Endocrinology,* 88:338–344.

60. Kvetňanský, R., Weise, V. K., and Kopin, I. J. (1970): Elevation of adrenal tyrosine hydroxylase and phenylethanolamine-*N*-methyl transferase by repeated immobilization of rats. *Endocrinology,* 87:744–749.

61. Otten, U., Oesch, F., and Thoenen, H. (1973): Dissociation between changes in cyclic AMP and subsequent induction of TH in the rat superior cervical ganglion and adrenal medulla. *Naunyn-Schmiedeberg's Arch. Pharmacol.,* 280:129–140.

62. Otten, U., Mueller, R. A., Oesch, F., and Thoenen, H. (1974): Location of an isoproterenol-responsive cyclic AMP pool in adrenergic nerve cell bodies and its relationship to tyrosine 3-monooxygenase induction. *Proc. Natl. Acad. Sci. USA,* 71:2217–2221.

63. Wooten, F. G., Thoa, N. B., Kopin, I. J., and Axelrod, J. (1973): Enhanced release of dopamine-β-hydroxylase and norepinephrine from sympathetic nerves by dibutyryl cyclic adenosine 3′,5′-monophosphate and theophylline. *Mol. Pharmacol.,* 9:178–183.

64. Cubeddu, L. X., Barnes, E., and Weiner, N. (1975): Release of norepinephrine and dopamine-β-hydroxylase by nerve stimulation. IV. An evaluation of a role for cyclic adenosine monophosphate. *J. Pharmacol. Exp. Ther.,* 193:105–127.

65. Molinoff, P. B., Brimijoin, S., and Axelrod, J. (1972): Induction of dopamine-β-hydroxylase in rat hearts and sympathetic ganglia. *J. Pharmacol. Exp. Ther.,* 182:116–129.

66. Gewirtz, G. P., Kvetňanský, R., Weise, V. K., and Kopin, I. J. (1971): Effect of ACTH and dibutyryl cyclic AMP on catecholamine synthesizing enzymes in the adrenals of hypophysectomized rats. *Nature,* 230:462–464.

67. Weiner, N. (1975): Control of the biosynthesis of adrenal catecholamines by the adrenal cortex. In: *Handbook of Physiology. Section 7: Endocrinology. Vol. VI. Adrenal Gland,* edited by H. Blaschko, G. Sayers, and A. D. Smith, pp. 357–366. American Physiological Society, Washington, D.C.

68. Duch, D. S., Viveros, O. H., and Kirshner, N. (1968): Endogenous inhibitor(s) in adrenal medulla of dopamine-β-hydroxylase. *Biochem. Pharmacol.,* 17:255–264.

69. Chubb, I. W., Preston, B. N., and Austin, L. (1969): Partial characterization of a naturally occurring inhibitor of dopamine-β-hydroxylase. *Biochem. J.,* 111:245–246.

70. Molinoff, P. B., Nelson, D. L., and Orcutt, J. C. (1974): Dopamine-β-hydroxylase and the regulation of the noradrenergic neuron. In: *Neuropsychopharmacology of Monoamines and Their Regulatory Enzymes,* edited by E. Usdin, pp. 95–104. Raven Press, New York.

The Nervous System, Donald B. Tower, Editor-in-Chief. *Vol. 1: The Basic Neurosciences*. Raven Press, New York, 1975.

Amino Acid Neurotransmitters: Biochemical Pharmacology

Solomon H. Snyder

The study of amino acids as neurotransmitters is a most exciting area of neurobiology, because it appears likely that quantitatively these compounds may be the major neurotransmitters in the brain. Research in this area, however, is still in its infancy as is evident by the considerable efforts still being devoted simply to establishing conclusively that one or another amino acid is in fact a neurotransmitter. For several amino acids, this evidence is sufficiently advanced that research is now directed toward an analysis of synaptic mechanisms and identifying the actions of certain psychotropic drug via amino acid neurotransmitters.

The major criteria for a neurotransmitter include the occurence of the compound localized predominantly to nerve terminals and, ideally, within synaptic vesicles in nerve terminals. A neurotransmitter should be released selectively upon nerve stimulation. Since many chemicals are released when nervous tissue is depolarized, the word "selective" is particularly crucial in deciding if a given chemical satisfies this criterion. There should be a mechanism to terminate the synaptic action of the putative transmitter substance. Perhaps the most important consideration is that the compound in question should mimic the synaptic effects of the natural transmitter. Studies of the detailed ionic alterations induced by natural neurotransmission and various amino neurotransmitters have not been particularly fruitful, since several compounds share similar actions. Thus both glycine and γ-aminobutyric acid (GABA) increase chloride conductance with similar reversal potentials. One of the most valuable tools in determining whether a compound mimics the natural transmitter has been the use of drug antagonists which should block effects of the natural transmitter and the test compound in a similar fashion.

Clearly, the above criteria include neuro-chemical and neurophysiological considerations. The most conclusive evidence for amino acids as neurotransmitters has derived from neurophysiologic studies with some neurochemical support. Recently, advanced neurochemical techniques, such as the ability to label the "transmitter pool" of an amino acid with a radioactive isotope and the ability to assay the postsynaptic receptor biochemically have accelerated neurochemical research to the point where in coming decades they may provide a major source of information about synaptic actions of amino acid transmitters.

GLYCINE

It is now reasonably well established that glycine is a major inhibitory neurotransmitter particularly in the spinal cord and brainstem. Within the spinal cord it is the transmitter of interneurons which synapse upon motor cells to elicit "postsynaptic inhibition." Its exact function in the brain is unclear. However, it is reasonable to suppose that glycine is the transmitter of interneurons in the brainstem which are analogous to those in which it is contained in the spinal cord.

The notion that glycine can be a potent inhibitor of motor cells in the spinal cord derives from classic studies in which the synaptic influences of all known amino acids were carefully screened and glycine appeared to be a reasonable transmitter candidate (1). Subsequently, neurochemical studies of endogenous levels of glycine suggested that it might be the transmitter mediating postsynaptic inhibition in the spinal cord (2). Thus glycine levels are two to three times higher in the brainstem and spinal cord than in higher brain centers. Within the spinal cord, glycine levels are higher in the ventral than the dorsal gray. Asphyxiation of the spinal cord by occluding the thoracic aorta of cats results in the selective death of interneurons and a well-correlated lowering of glycine levels. This suggestive but inconclusive neurochemical data prompted detailed neurophysiological studies which demonstrated that glycine mimics all the synaptic properties of the natural transmitter of postsynaptic inhibition in the spinal cord. The most convincing evidence made use of strychnine, which is a potent antagonist of postsynaptic inhibition. While both GABA and glycine hyperpolarize motor cells in the spinal cord, only the actions of glycine can be antagonized by strychnine at low doses (3).

LABELING GLYCINE NEUROTRANSMITTER POOLS BY SPECIFIC NERVE TERMINAL UPTAKE

Biochemical studies of glycine as a neurotransmitter were greatly hampered by the fact that glycine participates in numerous metabolic schemes in addition to its role as a neurotransmitter. How might one label selectively the neurotransmitter pool? Considerable advance in neurochemical studies of glycine and other amino acid neurotransmitters derived from the concept that the synaptic actions of amino acid neurotransmitters might be terminated by reuptake into the nerve endings which had released them as had been shown by Axelrod and other workers to occur for norepinephrine. Synaptosome preparations (pinched off nerve terminals which can be isolated from the brain by a combination of appropriate homogenization plus differential and sucrose gradient centrifugation) from the spinal cord accumulate radiolabeled glycine by a high affinity uptake process which is absolutely sodium dependent (4). By contrast, although other amino acids can be accumulated into synaptosomes by high affinity uptake processes, these are not sodium dependent, except in the case of transmitter candates. The high affinity, sodium-dependent glycine uptake occurs also in the brainstem but is not readily demonstrable in the cerebral cortex. In this way high affinity glycine uptake parallels the distribution of presumed glycine neurons. Since the glycine nerve terminals must be only a subpopulation of spinal cord nerve terminals, it might conceivably be possible to separate them from the general population of nerve terminals in the

spinal cord. If radioactive glycine is accumulated selectively by glycine nerve terminals in synaptosomes preparations while other nontransmitter amino acids are accumulated homogeneously by all synaptosomes, then physical properties of glycine synaptosomes may differ from those of the general population of spinal cord synaptosomes. Indeed, when the spinal cord is labeled with a large number of radioactive amino acids, one can separate by sucrose density gradient centrifugation glycine accumulating synaptosomes from those which accumulate other amino acids. The unique glycine synaptosomes occur in the spinal cord and brainstem but not in the cerebral cortex (5). The unique glycine synaptosomes can be labeled only by the high affinity sodium-dependent uptake process and not by low affinity uptake.

Biochemical studies of amino acid neurotransmitters involving uptake have been rendered more complex by the realization that glia as well as nerve terminals may possess high-affinity, sodium-requiring uptake systems (6,7). This appears to be only a relatively minor component for glycine, but assumes greater importance with GABA and glutamic acid uptake, as will be discussed below.

By taking advantage of the high affinity uptake system, autoradiographic studies have provided an estimate of the proportion of synapses in the spinal cord which utilize glycine as a neurotransmitter. Tracer amounts of ^{3}H-glycine label about 25% of nerve terminals in the spinal cord. Regardless of variations in the concentrations of ^{3}H-glycine or prolonged exposure periods, the proportion of synapses labeled with glycine appears constant (8). By contrast, nontransmitter amino acids such as leucine label all nerve terminals homogeneously and to a very limited extent. The amount of labeling with leucine increases with the duration of exposure until all nerve terminals are labeled.

Transmitter release from a given synapse biochemically is not so readily demonstrated in the brain as in the peripheral nervous system. A relatively crude but technically feasible procedure is to study the release of compounds from superfused brain slices or synaptosomes and evaluate the influence of electrical or potassium induced polarization. Only low levels of endogenous transmitter candidates are released from these preparations. Accordingly most studies have made use of radiolabeled amino acids. To demonstrate specificity, one must show that an amino acid transmitter candidate is released by relatively physiological depolarization while nontransmitter amino acids are not released. While there have been some conflicting results with different techniques, several studies have shown a selective release of radiolabeled glycine from brain slices (9,10). In confirmation of the notion that the neurotransmitter pool is labeled by high affinity sodium dependent uptake processes, some studies have shown that glycine and other amino acid transmitter candidates are released only if the slices have been labeled by the high affinity sodium dependent process (4).

BIOCHEMICAL IDENTIFICATION OF THE GLYCINE RECEPTOR

The ability to identify glycine receptor binding biochemically has facilitated study of its synaptic mechanisms (11–13). In synaptic membrane preparations of the spinal cord and brainstem, the glycine receptor can be labeled by binding with radioactive strychnine. Strychnine possesses high affinity for the glycine receptor with a dissociation constant of only about 2 to 4 nM. Glycine has much less affinity itself, requiring about 10,000 nM concentration to inhibit strychnine binding 50%. Because most chemicals will bind to most biological membranes, one must be cautious in receptor binding studies to ensure that the binding involves the physiologically relevant receptor. Strychnine binding can be shown to label the glycine receptor selectively, because the relative affinities of a series of amino acids for strychnine binding sites closely parallel their ability to mimic glycine neurophysiologically. Moreover, the regional distribution of strychnine binding in the central nervous system closely parallels the distribution of endogenous glycine, high affinity glycine uptake into unique accumulating synaptosomes and the ability of glycine to mimic natural inhibition. Strychnine binding is highest in the spinal cord and brainstem with lower levels as one ascends the neuraxis.

Studies of strychnine binding to the glycine receptor have provided considerable insight into the nature of synaptic transmission at this synapse. Shortly after the development of the allosteric model of enzymes, Changeux (14) postulated that neurotransmitters may also satisfy an allosteric model. In its simplest formulation, one assumes that there are two interconvertible receptor conformations, one which has a selective high affinity for the antagonist, and one which prefers the agonist. Antagonists exert their pharmacological activity by shifting the equilibrium between the free forms of agonist and antagonist receptor making fewer agonist receptors available for the action of the neurotransmitter. In this model recognition of the neurotransmitter is translated into an alteration in ionic conductance, because the appropriate ion binds with preferential affinity to one or the other of the two receptor conformations. Neurotransmitter binding to the receptor changes the equilibrium between receptor conformations, altering the affinity of the ion and triggering its passage through the synaptic membrane. Experiments using protein modifying reagents have indicated that the binding of glycine and its antagonist strychnine to the receptor occur to different states of the glycine receptor, which interact in a cooperative fashion (12,13). The binding of strychnine appears to be associated with the ion conductance mechanism for the glycine receptor, because chloride and other anions in physiological concentrations inhibit strychnine binding in close accordance with their ability to mimic the neurophysiologic synaptic actions of chloride at glycine synapses. Thus, ions whose hydrated radius is similar to that of chloride or smaller can pass through the "chloride pore" and reverse postsynaptic inhibitory potentials when injected into motor cells, while larger anions are ineffective. Strychnine binding can be inhibited only by those anions which also reverse the inhibitory postsynaptic potential.

DRUG EFFECTS

Very few psychotropic drugs are known to exert their actions via amino acid neurotransmitters. Of a large series of psychotropic drugs screened for their influence on the glycine receptor, most have no influence even at high concentrations. However, the benzodiazepine tranquilizers such as diazepam (Valium®) do compete for glycine receptor binding at concentrations similar to those which occur in the brain after pharmacologic doses of the drugs. Diazepam has about the same affinity as glycine itself for the glycine receptor. To test whether the effects of benzodiazepines on the glycine receptor might be related to their therapeutic actions, a series of 21 benzodiazepines with known pharmacologic potencies in animals and man were examined for their influence on glycine receptor binding. There was an extremely close correlation between pharmacologic potency and affinity for the glycine receptor (15). One might argue that both receptor binding and pharmacologic potency are related simply to solubility in the lipid membranes of the brain. If this were the case, then pharmacologic potency of benzodiazepines should also correlate with receptor binding for other neurotransmitters in the same brain membranes. However, there is no correlation between affinity of benzodiazepines for the opiate and muscarinic cholinergic receptors and their pharmacologic potency. Moreover much higher concentrations of benzodiazepines are required to compete for muscarinic and opiate receptor binding than are required to compete for the glycine receptor. The benzodiazepines have muscle relaxant, antianxiety, and sedative actions. A compound can compete for receptor binding if it is either an agonist or an antagonist. Since the known glycine antagonist strychnine causes muscular tenseness and convulsions, one would assume that benzodiazepines mimic glycine at its receptor sites. The sedative actions of benzodiazepines exhibit cross tolerance with barbiturates and numerous other sedatives. However, barbiturates have negligible affinity for the glycine receptor. Thus the sedative actions of drugs probably do not involve the glycine receptor. Perhaps the muscle relaxant and antianxiety actions of benzodiazepines involve mimicking of glycine at its receptor sites in the spinal cord and brainstem. The possibility that sedative actions of benzodiazepines are related to GABA mechanisms in presynaptic inhibition will be described below.

GABA

Biochemical studies of GABA as a neurotransmitter are much easier than investigations of other amino acid transmitters, because GABA probably does not have any general role in intermediary metabolism and protein synthesis. Indeed, the fact that GABA is localized almost exclusively to the central nervous system provided the initial impetus for believing that GABA might be a neurotransmitter. Upon subcellular fractionation, endogenous GABA is confined to synaptosomes, though when these are lyzed, GABA is not recovered from synaptic vesicles. As with glycine, GABA is accumulated by nerve terminals by a high-affinity, sodium-dependent uptake system. Depolarization of brain tissue results in a selective release of GABA.

As with glycine, the proportion of synapses in various brain areas which contain GABA can also be estimated by autoradiography. In numerous brain regions, the density of GABA synapses varies between 25 and 40% (8). Glial uptake of GABA seems to be more prominent than with glycine. Depending on the method of tissue preparation, autoradiography can show accumulated GABA to label exclusively the Muller glial cells in the retina or the amacrine neuronal cells (16). In sensory ganglia, exogenous GABA selectively labels glia (6). It is assumed that there are no GABA neurons in sensory ganglia. Accordingly, it is striking that these ganglia do possess endogenous GABA as well as its synthetic enzyme glutamic acid decarboxylase.

Direct evidence that GABA is a neurotransmitter at particular synapses in the central nervous system has made extensive use of specific GABA antagonists (17). Picrotoxin is a GABA antagonist, although it may act more at the ion conductance site than at the GABA recognition site itself. Moreover, picrotoxin does not appear to be extraordinarily potent or selective. Bicuculline has been the most effective GABA antagonist. At many inhibitory synapses throughout the central nervous system bicuculline antagonizes natural synaptic inhibition as well as the actions of GABA but not those of glycine. Postsynaptic inhibition in the spinal cord, however, is not antagonized by bicuculline, consistent with the notion that glycine is the transmitter at this synapse. The neurophysiologic evidence suggests that in areas rostral to the spinal cord and brainstem, GABA is the principal if not sole inhibitory neurotransmitter.

Within the spinal cord GABA appears to be involved in presynaptic inhibition, a unique neuronal mechanism which modulates sensory input and also occurs in the brainstem. It is thought that presynaptic inhibition is mediated via the effects of an interneuron which possesses axoaxonal synapses upon nerve terminals of primary sensory afferent fibers. The transmitter is thought to be excitatory and therefore to depolarize partially the nerve terminals of the sensory afferent fibers resulting in less transmitter release from them. Because presynaptic inhibition is antagonized by bicuculline and picrotoxin, it is thought to be GABA mediated, although in this case GABA must act as an excitatory transmitter.

Some psychotropic drugs may act clinically by altering GABA transmission in presynaptic inhibition. Extremely low doses of barbiturates and other sedatives as well as benzodiazepines facilitate presynaptic inhibition (18). It seems reasonable to postulate that this action accounts for the sedative effects of these drugs. Perhaps benzodiazepines exert their sedative effects by facilitating GABA-mediated presynaptic inhibition while the muscle relaxant actions of benzodiazepines, not shared by barbiturates, involve glycine mimicry.

As with the glycine receptor, the GABA receptor can be labeled biochemically. In this case, the effective ligand has been GABA itself. GABA binds to synaptic membrane preparations of the central nervous system in the absence of sodium with an affinity of about 0.1 μM (19). The close similarity between the relative affinities of amino acids for the GABA binding sites and their ability to mimic GABA neurophysiologically ensures that the binding involves the postsynaptic receptor sites for GABA. With fresh tissue in the presence of sodium, GABA binds to brain membranes by a process unrelated to the postsynaptic receptor and which probably involves uptake sites. The substrate specificity for the sodium dependent GABA binding process suggests that it involves glial rather than neuronal uptake sites for GABA (20). A wide range of psychotropic drugs examined, including barbiturates and benzodiazepines, have negligible affinity for the GABA receptor binding sites. Thus, if barbiturates do act at GABA synapses to facilitate presynaptic inhibition, the mechanism involved is probably not a mimicry of GABA.

GLUTAMIC AND ASPARTIC ACIDS

As with glycine, glutamic and aspartic acids have many "jobs" in the central nervous system besides being possible neurotransmitters. These two compounds present an additional problem. Because of their structural similarity, if both of them exert a particular type of action, one cannot determine which is normally involved. There are very few neurochemical events which have been shown to discriminate these two amino acids.

Both glutamic and aspartic acids are powerful excitants of almost all neurons in the brain. Studies of endogenous levels of glutamic acid provided some weak suggestions that it might be the primary sensory afferent transmitter in the spinal cord, because its levels are slightly higher in the dorsal than the ventral gray. However, one should expect the levels of the sensory afferent transmitter to fall after lesions of the dorsal root. Glutamic acid levels in the spinal cord are unchanged after this procedure. It is more likely that the peptide Substance P is the primary afferent neurotransmitter. Its levels are up to 50 times greater in the dorsal than in the ventral gray. Moreover, Substance P is almost completely depleted from the dorsal gray after section of the dorsal root. In addition, Substance P is about 250 times more potent than glutamic acid in exciting single cells in the dorsal gray of the spinal cord (21).

As with glycine and GABA there exist high affinity sodium dependent uptake systems into synaptosomes for glutamic and aspartic acids (4). The two acidic amino acids compete in a mutual fashion so that it is difficult to ascertain whether the uptake system is specific for one or the other compound. As discussed above for glycine, if glutamic acid is accumulated by unique nerve terminals which use it or aspartic acid as their neurotransmitter, it might be possible to discriminate the physical properties of these nerve endings from the general population of nerve terminals. Accordingly, it is of interest that unique glutamic and aspartic acid accumulating synaptosomes can be separated from those which accumulate all other amino acids in sucrose gradient centrifugation of brain slices (4). However, the recent evidence that, like GABA, glutamic and aspartic acids can be accumulated by glia (6,7) raises the possibility that the apparent glutamic acids synaptosomes are in fact glial particles or "gliosomes."

The one neuron for which there is impressive evidence that glutamic acid is the neurotransmitter is the granule cell of the cerebellum.

Quantitatively, cerebellar granule cells are more prominent than any other neurons in the brain. One can selectively deplete the hamster cerebellum of its granule cells by innoculating newborn brain with a unique virus which destroys granule cell precursors at a time that other neuronal and glial elements in the cerebellum have already developed and are resistant to destruction. In the cerebellum of adult hamsters in which granule cells were destroyed by virus treatment, synaptosomal uptake of all neurotransmitters and amino acids is normal with the exception of glutamic and aspartic acids. Uptake of these two amino acids is reduced by 70 to 80% (22). From these data one could not determine whether glutamic or aspartic acid is the transmitter of granule cells. Measurement of endogenous levels of all amino acids shows that only glutamic acid is depleted by about 40%, while aspartic acid levels as well as all other amino acids are normal. Thus glutamic acid is apparently the neurotransmitter of the granule cells. This is consistent with the neurophysiologic evidence that the transmitter of granule cells is excitatory. Interestingly, these findings indicate that at least 40% of all the glutamic acid in the cerebellum is in a neurotransmitter pool in granule cells.

Additional evidence that glutamic and/or aspartic acids are central nervous transmitters is obtained from release studies. Potassium depolarization of brain slices labeled with a variety of radioactive amino acids results in a selective release of glutamic and aspartic acids as well as GABA and glycine (from spinal cord) (4,9). Numerous other amino acids are not released.

There is some recent neurophysiologic evidence that may differentiate glutamic from aspartic acid synapses. Some synapses in the spinal cord are more sensitive to glutamic acid than aspartic acid. Kainic acid, a rigid analogue which can be superimposed upon the conformation of glutamic but not aspartic acid, is highly active at the apparent glutamic acid preferring synapses but not those where aspartic acid is most active (23). This suggests that there are indeed separate glutamic and aspartic acid nerve terminals and synapses. Moreover, the glutamic acid receptor may be highly selective. Biochemical evidence supports these suggestions. Radiolabeled kainic acid binds to synaptic membranes of brain tissue with an affinity constant of about 25 nM (24). Of numerous amino acids examined, only L-glutamic acid is a potent competitor with half maximal inhibition at 1000 nM, while the D-isomer is inactive. Dramatically, aspartic acid possesses negligible affinity for kainic acid sites and numerous other amino acids are inactive. Saturable high affinity kainic acid binding cannot be detected in tissues other than brain, further supporting its selectivity. Glutamic acid binds to brain membranes but binds just as well to the liver and does not display nearly so great a structural specificity.

Despite the strongly suggestive neurophysiologic and biochemical evidence for glutamic and aspartic acids as neurotransmitters, it is difficult to develop an overwhelming case for these compounds in the absence of highly selective and potent antagonists. Compounds such as glutamic acid diethyl ester have been suggested as receptor blockers for glutamic acid, but none are particularly potent in neurophysiologic studies. Because of the difficulty in establishing glutamic and aspartic acids definitively as neurotransmitters, it is not surprising that no psychotropic drugs are known to exert their actions by modulating synaptic effects of these amino acids.

In summary, neurophysiologic and neurochemical studies have provided substantial evidence that amino acids such as glutamic and aspartic acids, GABA and glycine, are quantitatively prominent neurotransmitters in the central nervous sytem. There is already evidence that important psychotropic agents such as sedatives, antianxiety drugs, and muscle relaxants may exert their actions via certain of these amino acid neurotransmitters.

ACKNOWLEDGMENTS

Supported by USPHS grant MH-18051 and RSDA Award MH-33128.

REFERENCES

1. Curtis, D. R., and Crawford, J. M. (1969): Central synaptic transmission-microelectrophoretic studies. *Ann. Rev. Pharmacol.,* 9:209–240.
2. Aprison, M. H., Davidoff, R. A., and Werman, R. (1970): Glycine: its metabolic and possible transmitter roles in nervous tissue. In: *Handbook of Neurochemistry,* edited by A. Lajtha, pp. 381–397. Plenum, New York.

3. Curtis, D. R., Duggan, A. W., and Johnston, G. A. R. (1971): The specificity of strychnine as a glycine antagonist in the mammalian spinal cord. *Exp. Brain Res.*, 12:547–565.
4. Snyder, S. H., Young, A. B., Bennett, J. P., and Mulder, A. H. (1973): Synaptic Biochemistry of amino acids. *Fed. Proc.*, 32:2039–2047.
5. Arregui, A., Logan, W. J., Bennett, J. P., and Snyder, S. H. (1972): Specific glycine-accumulating synaptosomes in the spinal cord of rats. *Proc. Natl. Acad. Sci., U.S.A.*, 69:3485–3489.
6. Schon, F. E., and Kelly, J. S. (1974): The characterization of ^{3}H-GABA uptake into the satellite glial cells of rat sensory ganglia. *Brain Res.*, 66: 289–300.
7. Henn, F. A., and Hamberger, A. (1971): Glial cell functions: uptake of transmitter substances. *Proc. Natl. Acad. Sci. U.S.A.*, 68:2686–2690.
8. Iversen, L. L., and Bloom, F. E. (1972): Studies of the uptake of ^{3}H-GABA and [^{3}H]glycine in slices and homogenates of rat brain and spinal cord by electron microscopic autoradiography. *Brain Res.*, 41:131–143.
9. Hammerstad, J. P., and Cutler, R. W. P. (1972): Sodium ion movements and the spontaneous and electrically stimulated release of [^{3}H]GABA and [^{14}C]glutamic acid from rat cortical slices. *Brain Res.*, 47:401–413.
10. Hopkin, J., and Neal, M. J. (1971): Effect of electrical stimulation and high potassium concentrations on the efflux of [^{14}C]glycine from slices of spinal cord. *Brit. J. Pharmacol.*, 42: 215–223.
11. Young, A. B., and Snyder, S. H. (1973): Strychnine binding associated with glycine receptors of the central nervous system. *Proc. Natl. Acad. Sci. U.S.A.*, 70:2832–2836.
12. Young, A. B., and Snyder, S. H. (1974): Strychnine binding in rat spinal cord membranes associated with the synaptic glycine receptor: cooperativity of glycine interactions. *Mol. Pharmacol.*, 10:790–809.
13. Young, A. B., and Snyder, S. H. (1974): The glycine synaptic receptor: evidence that strych-

nine binding is associated with the ionic conductance mechanism. *Proc. Natl. Acad. Sci. U.S.A.*, 71:4002–4005.
14. Changeux, J. P. (1966): Responses of Acetylcholinesterase from Torpedo marmorata to salts and curarizing drugs. *Mol. Pharmacol.*, 2:369–392.
15. Young, A. B., Zukin, S. R., and Snyder, S. H. (1974): Interaction of benzodiazepines with central nervous glycine receptors: possible mechanism of action. *Proc. Natl. Acad. Sci. U.S.A.*, 71:2246–2250.
16. Neal, M. J., and Iversen, L. L. (1972): Autoradiographic localization of ^{3}H-GABA in rat retina. *Nature New Biol.*, 235:217–218.
17. Krnjević, K. (1974): Chemical nature of synaptic transmission in vertebrates. *Physiol. Rev.*, 54: 418–540.
18. Schmidt, R. F. (1963): Pharmacological studies on the primary afferent depolarization of the toad spinal cord. *Arch. Gen. Physiol.*, 277: 325–346.
19. Zukin, S. R., Young, A. B., and Snyder, S. H. (1974): Gamma-aminobutyric acid binding to receptor sites in the rat central nervous system. *Proc. Natl. Acad. Sci. U.S.A.*, 71:4802–4807.
20. Enna, S. J., and Snyder, S. H. (1975): Properties of γ-aminobutyric acid (GABA) receptor binding in rat brain synaptic membrane fraction. *Brain Res. (in press)*.
21. Konishi, S., and Otsuka, M. (1974): The effects of Substance P and other peptides on spinal neurons of the frog. *Brain Res.*, 65:397–410.
22. Young, A. B., Oster-Granite, M. L., Herndon, R. M., and Snyder, S. H. (1974): Glutamic acid: selective depletion by viral induced granule cell loss in hamster cerebellum. *Brain Res.*, 73:1–13.
23. Johnston, G. A. R., Curtis, D. R., Davies, J., and McCulloch, R. M. (1974): Spinal interneuron excitation by conformationally restricted analogues of L-glutamic acid. *Nature*, 248:804–805.
24. Simon, J. R., and Kuhar, M. J. (1975): Specific [^{3}H]-kainic acid binding to brain membranes: evidence for association with the L-glutamate receptor. *J. Neurochem. (in press)*.

The Nervous System, Donald B. Tower, Editor-in-Chief. *Vol. 1: The Basic Neurosciences.* Raven Press, New York, 1975.

Microanatomy and Pharmacology of Cholinergic Synapses

George B. Koelle

In the evolution of the nervous system, a strange turn was taken by the cholinergic component. Evidence of neurohumoral transmission is doubtful among the coelenterates and their evolutionary predecessors. Above this level, where acetylcholine (ACh) and other transmitters appear, the animal kingdom apparently divided along two distinct lines: the deuterostomes, which include the echinoderms and all the vertebrates; and the protostomes, among which are the various worms, mollusks, crustaceans, and insects (1). In the former group, ACh is the major or sole neurohumoral transmitter of primary efferent fibers from the central nervous system (CNS) to the periphery (i.e., preganglionic sympathetic and parasympathetic, and somatic motor fibers) (Fig. 1). Among the protostomes, ACh generally trans-

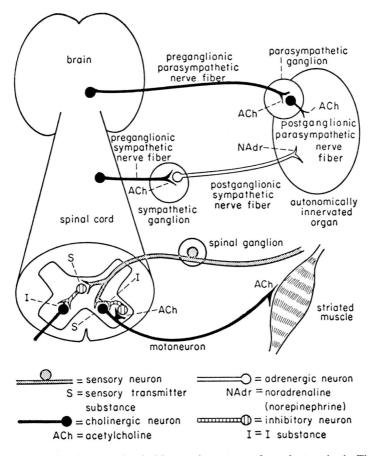

FIG. 1. Diagram representing the neurochemical innervation pattern of vertebrate animals. The sensory transmitter (S) is now believed to be glutamic acid, and the inhibitory transmitters (I) glycine and gamma-aminobutyric acid (GABA). (From Florey, ref. 2. Courtesy of W. B. Saunders Co., Division of C.B.S., Inc.)

mits impulses only in the reverse direction from the primary afferent fibers to the CNS; certain annelids utilize ACh as the transmitter of both afferent and efferent peripheral fibers (2–5). In both major divisions of the animal kingdom, it is likely that glutamic acid (GA) is the chief complementary peripheral transmitter, i.e., for primary afferent fibers in vertebrates and for excitatory efferent fibers in insects and crustaceans (6,7). ACh and GA probably function as neurohumoral transmitters within the CNS of both divisions. The transmitter actions of ACh no doubt are confined to specific synaptic sites, in contrast to the monoamines which apparently function both in this manner and diffusely through release by neurosecretory cells into the cerebrospinal fluid (8).

The two-dimensional structural formulas of ACh and GA bear a certain resemblance to each other:

$$\text{ACh}$$

$$\begin{array}{ccc} H_3C & & O \\ \diagdown & + & \parallel \\ H_3C\!-\!NCH_2CH_2OC\!-\!CH_3 \\ \diagup \\ H_3C \end{array}$$

$$\text{GA}$$

$$\begin{array}{ccc} H & & O \\ \diagdown & +\,H & \parallel \\ H\!-\!NCCH_2CH_2C\!-\!OH \\ \diagup & | \\ H & {}^-OC\!=\!O \end{array}$$

However, there are marked differences in the extent of distribution and manner of disposition of the two compounds. ACh and the enzyme involved immediately in its synthesis, choline acetyltransferase (ChAc), are restricted in their localization almost entirely to cholinergic neurons; the specific enzyme which brings about the extremely rapid hydrolysis of ACh, acetylcholinesterase (AChE), is present both there and at immediate postjunctional sites. In contrast, GA is distributed extensively throughout the CNS and peripheral tissues. Its transmitter action is probably terminated not by enzymatic destruction, but by reuptake into the axonal terminals and adjacent glial cells (9). In view of these differences, it is remarkable that the two compounds should have evolved as neurohumoral transmitters along distinct lines but otherwise practically interchangeably

at sites such as the motor endplate (MEP) of striated muscle, where extremely narrow temporal and spatial limitations of transmitter action are required.

MICROANATOMY OF CHOLINERGIC JUNCTIONS

The MEP of vertebrate skeletal muscle has served as the prototype of cholinergic junctions from which much of our detailed knowledge of structure, function, and mechanisms of drug action at such sites has been derived. This is due to certain unique features of the MEP in comparison with most other cholinergic synapses; they include its positive identification as a cholinergic junction, its ready accessibility for both intracellular recording and the microiontophoretic application of drugs at selected pre- and postjunctional sites, and the relatively wide cleft (approximately 500 Å) between the pre- and postjunctional membranes. For biochemical studies of the specific enzymes and receptors involved in cholinergic transmission, homologous structures (the electric organs of certain fish) have been of particular value, providing a source of large quantities of these components in highly concentrated form. The electroplaques of the electric eel, *Electrophorus electricus,* represent MEPs in association with a minimal amount of the homologue of the conducting membrane of the muscle fiber; those of electric rays (*Torpedo* and *Raia*) consist of the homologue of the ACh-excitable postjunctional membrane only.

Modern studies of the anatomy of the MEP date from the light microscopic description in 1947 by Couteaux (10) which focused attention on the palisade-like postjunctional structures that can be stained selectively by Janus green B. Subsequent light microscopic histochemical staining for AChE (11,12) and early electron microscopic observations (13) confirmed that the palisades represented the extensive invaginations of the postjunctional membrane into the sarcoplasm. Further details of the structure of the MEP, including the dense concentration of synaptic vesicles of the motor nerve terminal and the transverse tubular system and sarcoplasmic reticulum of the muscle fiber, were described by Andersson-Cedergren (14) and others.

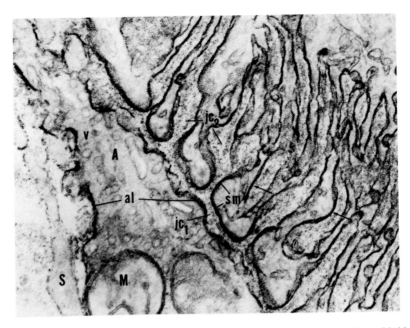

FIG. 2. Localization of AChE and ChE at the MEP of mouse intercostal muscle by the gold-thiolacetic acid method. The entire terminal axolemmal membrane (al) and postjunctional sarcolemmal membrane (sm) at both the primary (jc_1) and secondary (jc_2) clefts are coated with a fine deposit of aurous sulfide, indicating the sites of enzymatic activity. A: axonal terminal; M: mitochondria; S: Schwann sheath cell; v: synaptic vesicles. Magnification × 63,000. (From ref. 21. Courtesy of *J. Cell Biol.*)

Much progress has been made during the past decade toward elucidating the structures, localizations, and dynamic functional aspects of the specific proteins that participate in cholinergic transmission, as reviewed both by Michelson and Zeimal (5) and in recent symposia (15, 16). AChE has been crystallized from the electric organs of both *Electrophorus* (17) and *Torpedo* (18). The enzyme has a unit molecular weight of approximately 80,000 and occurs in tetramers which in turn form larger aggregates. At each active center, there are two critical sites: the anionic site, to which the quaternary N^+ atom of ACh is attracted by coulombic forces, and the esteratic site, where the electrophilic carbonyl C atom of the substrate combines by dipole-dipole interaction with a serine-hydroxyl group, the nucleophilicity of which is enhanced by hydrogen binding with an adjacent histidine-imidazole group. The subsequent steps leading to the hydrolysis of ACh take place at an extremely high velocity with a turnover number of approximately 80 μsec (19,20).

Refinement of electron-microscopic histochemical techniques for AChE has provided direct evidence that the enzyme is present in high concentration at the entire surfaces of the pre- and postjunctional membranes (Fig. 2), along with a considerably lower concentration of pseudocholinesterase, the function of which is unknown (21). Equivalent localization of AChE has been demonstrated more recently at cholinergic synapses of the superior cervical ganglion (22).

Studies on the isolation and characterization of the nicotinic cholinergic receptor from electric organs are reviewed elsewhere in this volume (see also refs. 5,15,16). The receptor and AChE share several features in common: both probably combine with ACh at anionic and esteratic sites, have approximately the same unit size, and are grouped in tetramers. In addition, both have been estimated to be present at the postjunctional membrane of the mouse MEP in equal numbers (23,24). Whereas now there is no doubt that the receptor and AChE comprise separate and distinct active sites, it has generally been assumed that they are located in close apposition in a mosaic-like pattern, and may even be bound to a common macromolecule along with the still hypothetical ionophore that presumably regulates the ionic permeability of the postjunctional membrane (25). On the other hand, electron-microscopic observations (discussed below) have suggested that, in contrast to AChE which is distributed throughout the infoldings of the postjunctional membrane, the receptors are confined to its immediate juxtaneural portions.

To date, histochemical attempts to localize ChAc have been based on the relatively non-specific procedure of trapping coenzyme A (CoA) released enzymatically from acetyl-CoA, which serves as the acetyl donor for the enzyme (26,27). More specific immunofluorescence methods will probably become available in the near future as a result of the high degrees of purification of the enzyme which have now been achieved (28). From fractionation studies by sucrose density-gradient centrifugation, it seems likely that, in most species, ChAc is present chiefly within the cytoplasm of the cholinergic terminal. Following the active uptake of choline from the extracellular fluid, it is probably acetylated in the cytoplasm and then incorporated into the synaptic vesicles along with ATP and a specific protein, vesiculin (29).

Calcium ion is essential for coupling the arrival of the nerve action potential with the synchronous discharge of the contents of approximately 100 vesicles into the subsynaptic space. At present, the most satisfactory model to account for the electrophysiological, biochemical, and electron miscroscopic observations concerning the formation, storage, and release of ACh is the membrane recycling sequence proposed for the frog MEP by Heuser and Reese (30). In this scheme (Fig. 3), the vesicles fuse with the plasma membrane at specific sites adjacent to the postjunctional membrane and discharge their contents into the cleft by exocytosis. The vesicular membranes are incorporated into the plasma membrane; then, in the vicinity of the Schwann sheath or teloglial cells, equivalent amounts of membrane are retrieved into the cytoplasm as coated vesicles. The latter lose their coats and coalesce to form cisternae from which the new vesicles, charged with ACh, are formed. A modified version of this sequence probably takes place in electric organs and at cholinergic synapses in the peripheral and central nervous systems (29).

In conventional thin-section electron micrographs of MEPs, areas of increased density have been noted at both the pre- and postjunctional membranes near the regions bordering the invaginations of the latter; within the nerve terminal, synaptic vesicles tend to be concentrated in the vicinity of the electron-dense bars

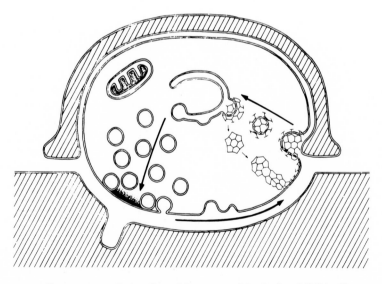

FIG. 3. Membrane recycling sequence of synaptic vesicles proposed for the frog MEP by Heuser and Reese (30). See text for description. (Courtesy of *J. Cell Biol.*)

running transversely to its long axis, suggesting that both the discharge and the action of ACh may be confined to restricted sites at the two membranes (31–33). These relationships have been visualized more clearly in freeze-fracture preparations in which membranes are split along the plane of their internal hydrophobic lamella, shadowed with platinum, then viewed toward either the cytoplasmic (A face) or external (B face) surface (34). In such preparations, the transverse dense bars of the prejunctional membrane are represented by parallel narrow ridges facing the openings of the postjunctional invaginations. Both the prejunctional ridges and the corresponding postjunctional sites are bordered by rows of particles which have been postulated to represent the active zones of transmitter release and the specific sites of the receptors, respectively. In keeping with the former proposal, it has been found that, whereas the synaptic vesicles are distributed randomly during the resting stage, following brief periods of stimulation, considerable numbers align themselves along the prejunctional ridges (35). The identification of the particles along the juxtaneural portions of

the postjunctional membrane with the receptors has been strengthened by autoradiographic demonstrations that, in sections treated with ^{125}I-labeled-α-bungarotoxin which binds tightly to the receptor with high selectivity, the peptide is localized only at the top of the junctional folds (36,37). These relationships are illustrated in Fig. 4. Structures equivalent to those described above have also been identified at synapses in the CNS where the presynaptic active zones and the corresponding postsynaptic specific sites are much more tightly packed in hexagonal patterns (38).

PHARMACOLOGY

The actions of most drugs at the neuromuscular junction and at other cholinergic synapses can at present be described to varying degrees of precision in terms of the structures and processes discussed above (for references, see ref. 39). Representative examples are briefly summarized here in the sequence shown in Fig. 5.

Local anesthetics block conduction by a still undefined mechanism which suppresses the increase in ion conductance of the axonal

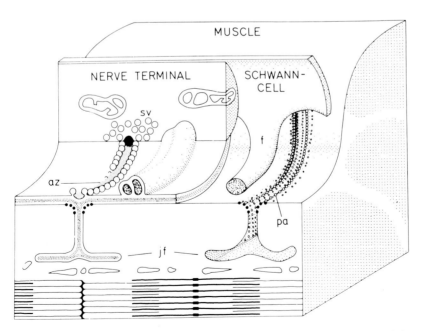

FIG. 4. Schema of the main structural features in the frog motor endplate. Active zones (az) of the presynaptic membrane and particle aggregations (pa) representing the specific sites at the postsynaptic membrane are facing each other. This striking arrangement may represent the structural correlate of secretion-excitation coupling. sv = Synaptic vesicles, jf = junctional folds, f = Schwann cell finger. (From ref. 38. Courtesy of Raven Press.)

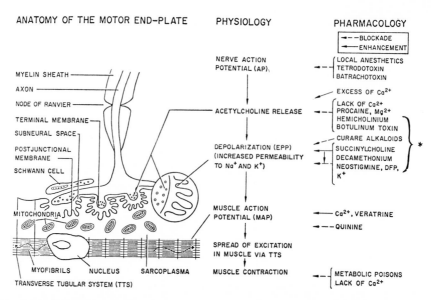

FIG. 5. Sites of action of drugs at the neuromuscular junction and adjacent structures. The anatomy of the MEP is shown at the left, and the sequence of events from liberation of ACh by the nerve action potential (AP) to contraction of the muscle fiber are indicated in the middle column. The modification of these processes by various agents is shown on the right. Dashed arrows, inhibition or block; solid arrows, enhancement or activation. Circled insert, enlargement of indicated structures. Drugs included in the bracket (*) modify specifically some stage of cholinergic transmission; those above and below act on conduction of the nerve or muscle AP or on muscle contraction. (Modified from Waser, ref. 40.)

membrane associated with the action potential. *Tetrodotoxin*, a complex molecule isolated from the puffer fish and terrestrial newts, produces the same effect by selectively blocking the inflow of sodium ions which is the basis of the upsweep of the spike of the nerve action potential. Batrachotoxin, obtained from the skin of a South American frog, has the opposite action, causing depolarization block by maintaining enhanced permeability of the sodium channels.

Calcium ion, as mentioned earlier, is probably essential for coupling the nerve action potential with the release of all neurohumoral transmitters from the presynaptic terminals. Accordingly, ACh release is enhanced at high, and reduced at low, levels of Ca^{2+} in the extracellular fluid. Either the action of Ca^{2+} or its lack is complicated by its effects at other sites, which include stabilization of the postjunctional membrane and coupling of the muscle action potential with the contractile process. Magnesium ion has the opposite effect on transmitter release, competing here with Ca^{2+}; in an investigation by Heuser et al. (35), Mg^{2+} was found to prevent the mobilization of synaptic vesicles at the active zone of the prejunctional membrane in response to repetitive nerve stimulation. Procaine and other local anesthetics also block transmitter release, usually at concentrations lower than those required to produce axonal conduction block.

Hemicholinium and botulinus toxin interfere with transmitter release selectively at cholinergic junctions. Hemicholinium blocks the active transport of choline across the prejunctional membrane and thus shuts off the supply for replenishment of the store of ACh. The exact site and mechanism of action of botulinus toxin are not known. Black widow spider venom has the opposite effect, causing massive discharge and subsequent depletion of synaptic vesicles.

The short-acting (e.g., physostigmine, neostigmine) and long-acting (e.g., DFP and other organophosphates) anti-ChE agents initially cause enhancement of cholinergic transmission which is succeeded by blockade. At the MEP, the former effect is due to moderate prolongation of the endplate potential (EPP) through persistence of ACh, which results in repetitive firing of the muscle action potential in response to single nerve impulses. However, when depolarization of the postjunctional membrane is extended beyond a limited time, transmission block ensues. This is probably not directly attributable to the depolarization itself but to a poorly understood process that has been described, for want of a more precise term, as densitization of the receptors.

There are two categories of classic neuromuscular blocking drugs: the competitive and the depolarizing agents. The competitive agents (e.g., *d*-tubocurarine and related natural alkaloids and synthetic compounds) combine with the cholinergic receptors and produce no direct effect but block the depolarizing action of endogenous or applied ACh. The depolarizing agents (e.g., succinylcholine, decamethonium) act as relatively stable cholinomimetic agents thus producing the same sequence of effects as the anti-ChE agents: brief excitation manifested by twitching and fasciculation followed by paralysis. It is probable that, whereas drugs of both classes combine with the same anionic sites of the ACh-receptors, the rigid molecular structures of the competitive agents prevent the conformational changes induced by ACh and the flexible depolarizing agents that result in the increased cation permeability of the postjunctional membrane recorded as the EPP (41).

The receptors at the MEP are exclusively of the nicotinic type, whereas only muscarinic receptors, which are blocked selectively by atropine, are present on smooth muscle and other autonomic effector cells; autonomic ganglion cells contain predominantly nicotinic but a complement of muscarinic receptors, and most cholinoceptive neurons of the CNS probably contain both types also, with one or the other predominating. These distinctions have permitted varying degrees of selectivity of drug action at peripheral sites. For example, the neuromuscular blocking agents mentioned above are virtually devoid of direct effects on either smooth muscle or gland cells. Although at present there is no direct information concerning structural differences between nicotinic and muscarinic receptors, pharmacological studies of structure-activity relationship within series of drugs, along with the measurement of critical molecular parameters of the drugs by X-ray diffraction analysis and the construction of rigid molecular models, have permitted some rational

speculation in this regard. Thus it has been shown that numerous muscarinic-activating and -blocking agents possess the combination of a quaternary-N^+ atom and an atom capable of H-bonding, separated by approximately 4.3 Å; this is equivalent to the distance between the N^+ atom and the ester-O atom of ACh. In many nicotinic drugs, the corresponding distance is 5.9 Å, similar to that between the N^+ atom and the carbonyl-O atom of the transmitter. Drugs of both classes may show enhanced activity with the attachment of hydrophobic groups to the N^+ atom. From these data, it has been deduced that both types of receptor resemble AChE in possessing anionic and nucleophilic sites with adjacent hydrophobic areas, and that the major difference between muscarinic and nicotinic receptors is the distance between the two critical sites (42). Alternative but similar interpretations of these relationships have been offered (43).

The remaining drugs listed in Fig. 5 act predominantly beyond the loci of the cholinergic receptor. Potassium ion produces depolarization at both the subsynaptic membrane and sarcolemna, leading to activation succeeded by block. Veratrine and related alkaloids cause repetitive firing following single stimuli in all excitable cells, probably by increasing the sodium conductance of the membrane. Whereas quinine appears to possess competitive nicotinic-blocking activity, the total response is complicated by other depressant effects, including an increase in the refractory period of the sarcoplasmic membrane.

As a final cautionary note in any discussion of this type, the first adage of pharmacology should be mentioned: no drug has a single action. This is important to both the clinician who must be aware of possible side effects in his patients, and the investigator who uses drugs as tools to elucidate physiological mechanisms. Although many drugs produce relatively selective effects, a multiplicity of actions at the MEP has been demonstrated with essentially all that have been studied sufficiently thoroughly (44).

REFERENCES

1. Ivanov, A. V., Khozatsky, L. I., Takhtadjan, A. L., and Polyansky, V. I. (1956): Phylogenesis. *Great Soviet Encylopedia (Moscow)*, 45:109–119.

2. Florey, E. (1966): *An Introduction to General and Comparative Animal Physiology*, p. 495. W. B. Saunders Co., Philadelphia.
3. Florey, E. (1967): Neurotransmitters and modulators in the animal kingdom. *Fed. Proc. Am. Soc. Exp. Biol.*, 26:1164–1178.
4. Barker, D. L., Herbert, E., Hildebrand, J. G., and Kravitz, E. A. (1972): Acetylcholine and lobster sensory neurones. *J. Physiol. (Lond.)*, 226:205–229.
5. Michelson, M. J. and Zeimal, E. V. (1973): *Acetylcholine. An Approach to the Molecular Mechanism of Action*. Pergamon Press, New York.
6. Kravitz, E. A., Slater, C. R., Takahashi, K., Bownds, M. D., and Grossfeld, R. M. (1970): Excitatory transmission in invertebrates—glutamate as a potential neuromuscular transmitter compound. In: *Excitatory Synaptic Mechanisms*, edited by P. Andersen and J. K. S. Jansen, pp. 85–93. Universitetsforlaget, Oslo.
7. Hammerschlag, R., and Weinreich, D. (1972): Glutamic acid and primary afferent transmission. In: *Studies of Neurotransmitters at the Synaptic Level*, edited by E. Costa, L. L. Iversen, and R. Paoletti, pp. 165–180. Raven Press, New York.
8. Konstantinova, M. (1973): Monoamines in the liquor-contacting nerve cells in the hypothalamus of the lamprey, *Lampetra fluviatilis L. Z. Zellforsch.*, 144:549–557.
9. Iversen, L. L. (1970): Neuronal uptake processes for amines and amino acids. In: *Advances in Biochemical Psychopharmacology, Vol. 2*, edited by E. Costa and E. Giacobini, pp. 109–132. Raven Press, New York.
10. Couteaux, R. (1947): Contribution à l'étude de la synapse myoneurale; buisson de kühne et plaque motrice. *Rev. Can. Biol.*, 6:563–711.
11. Koelle, G. B., and Friedenwald, J. S. (1949): A histochemical method for localizing cholinesterase activity. *Proc. Soc. Exp. Biol. Med.*, 70:617–622.
12. Couteaux, R., and Taxi, J. (1952): Recherches histochimiques sur la distribution des activités cholinestérasiques au niveau de la synapse myoneurale. *Arch. Anat. Microsc. Morphol. Exp.*, 41:352–392.
13. Robertson, J. D. (1956): Some features of the ultrastructure of reptilian skeletal muscle. *J. Biophys. Biochem. Cytol.*, 2:369–392.
14. Andersson-Cedergren, E. (1959): Ultrastructure of motor end plate and sarcoplasmic components of mouse skeletal muscle fiber. *J. Ultrastructr. Res. (Suppl.)*, 1:1–191.
15. De Robertis, E. and Schacht, J. (Eds.) (1974): *Neurochemistry of Cholinergic Receptors*. Raven Press, New York.
16. Waser, P. G. (Ed.) (1975): *Cholinergic Mechanisms*. Raven Press, New York.
17. Leuzinger, W., Baker, A. L., and Cauvin, E. (1968): Acetylcholinesterase. II. Crystallization, absorption spectra, isoionic point. *Proc. Natl. Acad. Sci. USA*, 59:620–623.
18. Hopff, W. H., Riggio, G., and Waser, P. G. (1975): Progress in isolation of acetylcholinesterase. In: *Cholinergic Mechanisms*, edited by P. G. Waser, pp. 293–298. Raven Press, New York.
19. Froede, H. C., and Wilson, I. B. (1971): Acetylcholinesterase. In: *The Enzymes, Vol. 5*, edited by P. D. Boyer, pp. 87–114. Academic Press, New York.
20. Kitz, R. J. (1973): Molecular pharmacology of acetylcholinesterase. In: *Modern Pharmacology. Part I, A Guide to Molecular Pharmacology-Toxicology*, edited by R. M. Featherstone, pp. 333–374. Marcel Dekker, Inc., New York.
21. Davis, R., and Koelle, G. B. (1967): Electron microscopic localization of acetylcholinesterase and nonspecific cholinesterase at the neuromuscular junction by the gold-thiocholine and gold-thiolacetic acid methods. *J. Cell Biol.*, 34:157–171.
22. Koelle, G. B., Davis, R., Smyrl, E. G., and Fine, A. V. (1974): Refinement of the bis-(thioacetoxy) aurate (1) method for the electron microscope localization of acetylcholinesterase and nonspecific cholinesterase. *J. Histochem. Cytochem.* 22:252–259.
23. Waser, P. G. (1970): On receptors in the postsynaptic membrane of the motor endplate. In: *Molecular Properties of Drug Receptors*, edited by R. Porter and M. O'Connor, pp. 59–75. J. & A. Churchill, Ltd., London.
24. Hubbard, J. I. (1973): Microphysiology of vertebrate neuromuscular transmission. *Physiol. Rev.*, 53:674–723.
25. Csillik, B. (1965): *Functional Structure of the Postsynaptic Membrane in the Myoneural Junction*. Akadémiai Kiadó Publishing House of the Hungarian Academy of Sciences, Budapest.
26. Burt, A. M., and Silver, A. (1973): Histochemistry of choline acetyltransferase: A critical analysis. *Brain Res.*, 62:509–516.
27. Kaśa, P. (1975): Histochemistry of choline acetyltransferase. In: *Cholinergic Mechanisms*, edited by P. G. Waser, pp. 271–281. Raven Press, New York.
28. Rossier, J., Bauman, A., Rieger, F., and Benda, P. (1975): Immunological studies on the enzymes of the cholinergic system. In: *Cholinergic Mechanisms*, edited by P. G. Waser, pp. 283–292. Raven Press, New York.
29. Whittaker, V. P., and Dowdall, M. J. (1975): Current state of research on cholinergic synapses. In: *Cholinergic Mechanisms*, edited by P. G. Waser, pp. 23–42. Raven Press, New York.
30. Heuser, J. E., and Reese, T. S. (1973): Evidence for recycling of synaptic vesicle membrane during transmitter release at the frog neuromuscular junction. *J. Cell Biol.*, 57:315–344.
31. Birks, R., Huxley, H. E., and Katz, B. (1960): The fine structure of the neuromuscular junction of the frog. *J. Physiol. (Lond.)*, 150:134–144.
32. Couteaux, R., and Pécot-Dechavassine, M. (1970): Vésicules synaptiques et poches au niveau des zones actives de la jonction neuro-

musculaire. *C. r. hebd. Seanc. Acad. Sci., Paris,* 271:2346–2349.

33. Rash, J. E., and Ellisman, M. H. (1974): Studies of excitable membranes. I. Macromolecular specializations of the neuromuscular junction and the nonjunctional sarcolemma. *J. Cell Biol.,* 63:567–586.

34. Moor, H. (1971): Recent progress in the freeze-etching technique. *Philos. Trans. R. Soc. Long. (Biol. Sci.),* 261:121–131.

35. Heuser, J. E., Reese, T. S., and Landis, D. M. D. (1974): Functional changes in frog neuromuscular junctions studied with freeze fracture. *J. Neurocytol.,* 3:109–131.

36. Fertuck, H. C., and Salpeter, M. M. (1974): Localization of acetylcholine receptor by ^{125}I-labeled α-bungarotoxin binding at mouse motor endplates. *Proc. Natl. Acad. Sci. USA,* 71:1376–1378.

37. Albuquerque, E. X., Barnard, E. A., Porter, C. W., and Warnick, J. E. (1974): The density of acetylcholine receptors and their sensitivity in the postsynaptic membrane of muscle endplates. *Proc. Natl. Acad. Sci. USA,* 71:2818–2822.

38. Akert, K., Peper, K., and Sandri, C. (1975): Structural organization of motor end plate and central synapses. In: *Cholinergic Mechanisms,* edited by P. G. Waser, pp. 43–57. Raven Press, New York.

39. Koelle, G. B. (1975): Neurohumoral transmission and the autonomic nervous system. In: *The Pharmacological Basis of Therapeutics,* 5th Edition, edited by L. S. Goodman and A. Gilman, pp. 404–444. Macmillan, New York.

40. Waser, P. (1958): Pharmakologie der Muskelendplatten. *Schweiz. Arch. Neurol. Psychiatr.* 82: 298–319.

41. Pauling, P., and Petcher, T. J. (1973): Neuromuscular blocking agents: Structure and activity. *Chem. Biol. Interact.,* 6:351–365.

42. Beers, W. H., and Reich, E. (1970): Structure and activity of acetylcholine. *Nature (Lond.),* 228:917–922.

43. Chothia, C. (1970): Interaction of acetylcholine with different cholinergic nerve receptors. *Nature (Lond.),* 225:36–38.

44. Karczmar, A. G., Nishi, S., and Blaber, L. C. (1972): Synaptic modulations. In: *Brain and Human Behavior,* edited by A. G. Karczmar and J. C. Eccles, pp. 63–92. Springer-Verlag, New York.

The Nervous System, Donald B. Tower, Editor-in-Chief. *Vol. 1: The Basic Neurosciences*. Raven Press, New York, 1975.

Central Noradrenergic Synaptic Mechanisms

Floyd E. Bloom

There are several ways to subdivide classes of central neurons. They can be distinguished morphologically on the basis of the number of dendrites, or of their size, shape, or location. Neurons may also be characterized physiologically on the basis of their input connections or output projections or be considered as excitatory or inhibitory in function. In this chapter we consider the distribution and functional characteristics of a class of central neuron characterized by its neurotransmitter substance, norepinephrine. The biochemistry and pharmacology of norepinephrine (NE) have already been extensively resolved. As a result of the application of this knowledge, the cytological and functional analysis of norepinephrine-containing neurons in the brain has advanced steadily since the earliest reports (see 1,2) that the iontophoretic administration of NE could in fact alter the discharge rates and patterns of brain cells.

Early microiontophoretic studies assumed that such responses were meaningful and that quantitative assessment of the proportion of neurons which would or would not respond to NE in a given brain region implied "importance" of noradrenergic transmission there. There are only two possible general types of positive responses which neurons can manifest to microiontophoretic administration of NE: the cell can fire either faster or slower. Thus, depending on the cell type tested, NE can either depress discharge rates, as it does in several cortical areas (see below), or facilitate discharge rates as with certain groups of hindbrain and spinal neurons (1–5).

However, some conceptual problems of interpretation arise when apparently similar neurons under apparently identical conditions respond to NE by qualitatively opposite changes. For example, in earlier reports, only a few relatively unimpressive and generally depressant effects of NE were observed in cerebral cortex (1,2), while others observed excitatory responses of cortical neurons. More recent studies (6) of cerebral cortex indicate that the major actions of NE are depressant.

By proper regard for each of the necessary experimental controls peculiar to microiontophoresis (2), it has been possible to observe reproducible effects of NE on neuronal discharge. However, such data do not necessarily indicate that the responses reflect underlying NE-mediated input to the cells being tested. To corroborate this inference requires the demonstration that selective stimulation of the afferent NE axons will reproduce the effects produced by microiontophoresis of NE. Since the cells of origin for the cortical NE projections have only recently been established (2), the next best evidence has been to establish cytochemically that the cells being tested receive NE-containing synapses. In the absence of such corroborative data, iontophoretic responses simply cannot be interpreted functionally.

LOCALIZING NE-CONTAINING SYNAPSES

The varicosities of the axons demonstrated by fluorescence histochemistry indicate presumed sites of transmitter release. However, because of the limited resolution of the optical microscope relative to the very fine nature of the complexly interrelated cellular processes of the neuropil, electron microscopic methods are needed to determine precisely which neurons in a given region receive synaptic contact from NE-containing axons.

No single electron microscopic histochemical method has yet achieved the consistency and selectivity of localization desired for analysis of NE-transmitting synapses. Permanganate fixation methods (see ref. 7) offer the most direct approach to the successful visualization of small granular synaptic vesicles, which seem identical morphologically and pharmacologically to the storage vesicles of NE in peripheral sympathetic nerve terminals. However, technical problems (such as poor penetration, yielding small usable tissue samples) generally limit this method to regions with a high density of NE axons (e.g., pons, hypothalamus). Recently it has been possible to observe permanganate-positive terminals within the cerebellar cortex of certain mouse mutant strains (8).

We have found most useful for our purposes a combination of two methods (see 7): autoradiographic localization of processes which accumulate tracer amounts of ^{3}H-NE *in vivo* or *in vitro:* and the acute degeneration which occurs in NE terminals within 8 to 48 hr after injection of 6-hydroxydopamine (6-OHDA) into the cerebrospinal fluid.

For these reasons we have attempted to apply as many of the available methods as are possible when seeking to localize NE-containing synaptic terminals, and find the most satisfactory localizations to be based upon complementary results from multiple approaches (7). A promising auxiliary line of investigation is based upon the exploitation of axoplasmic transport. The distribution of a specific NE axonal pathway can now be revealed by autoradiographic localization of labeled macromolecules which are synthesized exclusively in a few perikarya after a restricted microinjection of labeled precursor, directly to the NE-containing neurons.

By application of the combination of fluorescence histochemistry, autoradiography of ^{3}H-NE and acute degeneration after 6-OHDA, NE-containing synapses have been identified as projecting to olfactory mitral cells, to hypothalamic neurons of the supraoptic nucleus (9,10), to a portion of the neurons of the rat and cat raphe nuclei, as well as to particular neurons in certain cortical regions described below.

EFFECTS OF NE ON CENTRAL NEURONS

A number of different procedures have been employed to study the effects of NE on central neurons. For example, injection of precursors parenterally (see ref. 11) has been reported to alter both cortical slow waves and unit potentials. The most useful technique, however, for evaluating the effects of NE on central neurons utilizes microiontophoretic application from multibarrel micropipettes, thus circumventing

many of the temporal, chemical, and structural restrictions suffered with other drug testing procedures (see refs. 1,2,11).

Overview of Microiontophoretic Studies

In contrast to earlier studies which indicated negligible NE effects on cortical (12) and spinal (1,2) neurons, recent experiments have indicated that NE can affect nerve cells at virtually all levels of the neuraxis (see Table 1). The critical parameters underlying the presence or absence, and qualitative nature of responses to NE have been clarified by a number of recent studies. Thus, in the cerebral cortex, the response to iontophoresis of NE depends partially on the type of anesthesia: excitatory responses are more prevalent with halothane or in certain unanesthetized preparations (13,14). The pH of the drug solution also may be critical: unidentified cortical neurons are reported to be excited by NE ejected from solutions with pH less than 4.0 and inhibited by NE from solutions greater than 4.0 (6). However, we have not observed a strict pH dependency for NE responses in other brain areas including the unanesthetized squirrel monkey cortex (15,16); in fact, with pH 4.5 NE, tests by Weight and Salmoiraghi (11), on spinal interneurons revealed both excitatory and inhibitory responses to NE on the same cell. These responses were antagonized selectively by alpha adrenergic antagonists, so that they could not have been due to "proton" receptors.

Identification of Test Neurons

When attempting to evaluate the results of iontophoretic tests in any brain region, the primary concern is the identity of the cells tested. Such identifications can be made during the test on the basis of characteristic discharge patterns or from the response of the test cells to stimulation of specific antidromic or orthodromic projections, or by marking recording sites with any of several methods and examining the recording sites cytologically after the experiment.

Such identifications offer several interpretative advantages. First, the cells tested can then be categorized into homogeneous functional or cytological groupings for cleaner interpre-

TABLE 1. *Studies on the pharmacological characterization of NE receptors through-out the mammalian CNS as studied by microiontophoresis on various regions and cell types*

Brain region	Receptor studies	Ref.
Cortex		
1. Cerebral (general)	Excitations blocked by α and β blockers, depressions not blocked by either	13
	Depressions blocked with "calcium antagonists"	27
2. Polysensory cells	Depressions potentiated by desmethylimipramine	16a
3. Pyramidal cells	Depressions blocked with MJ-1999 and potentiated with monoamine oxidase inhibitors	28
Limbic system		
1. Hippocampus pyramidal cells	Depressions blocked by MJ-1999, prostaglandins E_1 and E_2; potentiated with phosphodiesterase inhibitors and desmethylimipramine	23,24
2. Olfactory bulb mitral cells	Depressions blocked with dibenamine and LSD	(see 1)
Diencephalon		
1. Medial geniculate	Depressions blocked with strychnine	16b
2. Hypothalamus, supraoptic	Depressions blocked with MJ-1999; potentiated with DMI	9
Brainstem		
1. Paramedian reticular nucleus	Excitations blocked with chlorpromazine	29,4
2. Unidentified cells	Amphetamine sensitivity correlated with NE response	3
	Excitation blocked by alpha methyl NE	
Spinal cord		
1. Interneuron	Depressions and excitations blocked with phenoxybenzamine	30 (see 11)
Cerebellum		
1. Purkinje	Depressions blocked by MJ-1999, prostaglandin E_1, nicotinate; potentiated by DMI, methylxanthines, papaverine	17,19 21,23

See also refs. 10,13.

tation of heterogeneous responses. The differences in responsiveness to NE between "all-cells-in-a-region" and specific identifiable cell types within a region have been described for olfactory bulb, hypothalamus, cerebral cortex, cerebellum, thalamus, limbic system, pons, and spinal cord (see ref. 2). In all of these cases, the response to NE of identified cells is inhibitory, with the exception of border cells in the ventromedial nucleus of the hypothalamus (2), the cells of the paramedian reticular nucleus (4), and some cells in the pontine raphe nucleus (5), which respond to NE with excitatory responses. In no cases do identified cells exhibit significant instances of mixed responses (i.e., some cells faster, some cells slower) as seen when "all-cells-in-a-region" are artificially lumped together.

Second, identification of tested cells is even more important when drug responses are to be compared to a specific synaptic input to a test cell, or in attempts to determine the molecular basis of the synaptic or drug response. Here, the cells must be identified so that it can be established cytologically (7) that the pathway under examination does, indeed, synapse with the cells to be tested. However, in the case of catecholaminergic synaptic projections, precise source neurons to specific postsynaptic cells can be stimulated only for a very few synaptic targets. Nevertheless, a synaptic inference to iontophoretic responses requires that the cells tested be shown to receive this chemical class of synaptic inputs whether or not their nucleus of origin can at present be stimulated.

Third, identification of the test cells can define which of the iontophoretic responses observed may never be utilized by normal synaptic connections (e.g., the excitatory beta receptors of neurons in the deep cerebellar nuclei of the cat where no evidence for catecholaminergic synapses exists; see refs. 1,2). Finally, identification of test cells is required so that data may be accumulated on homogenous cell populations for evaluation of the antagonists or potentiators of the test synapses or test substances.

ACTION OF NE ON DEFINED POSTSYNAPTIC NEURONS

NE-containing synapses have been demonstrated by a combination of fluorescence histochemistry, autoradiography after ^{3}H-NE, and acute degeneration after 6-OHDA in a number of structures where neurons have also been tested with NE by iontophoresis. Supraoptic (9) and olfactory bulb (1) neurons are reproducibly inhibited by NE, but alpha receptor blockade did not completely eliminate the recurrent type of synaptic inhibition in either case. Cells of the medial geniculate body are also inhibited by NE (16b), as are cat motoneurons (11). In neither of these cases, however, has it been possible to activate the noradrenergic pathway selectively.

Cytochemical studies have shown that polysensory cortex of the squirrel monkey contains an extensive network of fine NE-containing axons that establish both axosomatic and axodendritic synapses on these neurons (16a). Moreover, NE, administered by microiontophoresis, depresses spontaneous or induced discharge in well over 90% of these neurons.

The NE responses were usually of short latency and had very low thresholds. Only a few excitatory responses were seen, and these could readily be reversed to inhibition by concurrent iontophoresis of desmethylimipramine.

The most serious obstacle to physiologic analysis of these implied central noradrenergic physiological receptors has been the inability to activate the pathway selectively. The noradrenergic projections to rat cerebellar Purkinje cells and hippocampal pyramidal cells have, however, been recently studied by both electrophysiological and cytochemical methods.

The Noradrenergic Projection to Rat Cerebellar Purkinje Cells

Localization

The NE-containing axons of the cerebellar cortex can be localized, at the light microscopic level, using either formaldehyde-induced fluorescence in normal animals or *in vitro* incubation with catecholamine analogues. These techniques may be combined with 6-OHDA pretreatment to ensure that NE- rather than serotonin-containing fibers are being visualized (7). The thin fluorescent fibers branch extensively and manifest multiple varicosities in the molecular layer of the cerebellar cortex, giving off branches which run in both frontal and sagittal planes.

NE-containing synapses in the cerebellum can be localized at the electron microscopic level by degeneration after 6-OHDA exposure or autoradiography of sites taking up ^{3}H-NE. These ultrastructural studies indicate that NE-containing fibers synapse on the Purkinje cell dendritic tree, in the mid-to-outer molecular layer. Recent techniques for facilitating visualization of these fibers suggest that they are of sufficient density to permit contact with each Purkinje cell.

Characterization of the Purkinje Cell Adrenergic Receptor

When NE is applied to Purkinje cells from micropipettes by iontophoresis, there is a uniform and powerful depression of spontaneous discharge (17). Interspike interval histograms show that NE produces no effects on climbing fiber bursts or on the most probable single spike interval, but rather, that NE specifically augments the population of long pauses seen during normal Purkinje cell firing.

Several lines of evidence suggest that a beta receptor is involved in the Purkinje cell response. For example, epinephrine and isoproterenol produce changes in mean rate and in the interspike interval histogram analogous to those of NE (17). Moreover, iontophoretic administration of MJ-1999, a specific beta-adrenergic blocking agent (17), antagonizes NE responses. Yet, iontophoresis of NE slows Purkinje cell discharge even when adrenergic synaptic terminals are selectively destroyed by prior injection of 6-OHDA (see 2), and before significant numbers of synapses have been formed (18).

Mechanism of the Noradrenergic Receptor on Central Neurons

It has also been possible to record intracellularly from Purkinje cells during extracellular application of NE (19). The result is hyperpolarization with either no change or an increase in membrane resistance. Similar transmembrane changes after iontophoresis of NE have recently been described in cat motoneurons by Engberg and Marshall (20).

The hyperpolarization with increased resistance seen with NE is in direct contrast to changes seen with classical inhibitory postsynaptic potentials (IPSPs) or during iontophoresis of gamma-aminobutyric acid (GABA) (19). The classical inhibitory pathways and amino acids are thought to operate exclusively through mechanisms which increase conductance to ionic species whose equilibrium potentials are more negative than the resting membrane potential. In such cases, the hyperpolarization is associated with decreased membrane resistance. Hyperpolarization produced by NE, on the other hand, may be due to a decrease in conductance to some ion such as sodium or calcium, or activation of an electrogenic pump.

Activation of the Adrenergic Pathway to Cerebellum

Experiments utilizing changes in formaldehyde-induced fluorescence of neurons and axons, in animals with lesions of the ascending NE bundles, or cerebellar peduncles, or auto-

radiography after microinjections into NE nuclei have shown that the cerebellar adrenergic projection arises from the nucleus locus coeruleus (21,22), a bilateral group of NE-containing neurons in the dorsal pontine reticular formation.

Purkinje cells showed remarkably uniform inhibitory responses to stimulation of locus coeruleus (LC) with trains of pulses: 94 of 102 cells (20 animals) recorded extracellularly displayed depression of spontaneous discharge rate (21). Complete cessation of discharge outlasting the stimulation period by 4 to 65 sec (mean, 21 sec) could be obtained with 20 to 100 pulses at 10 Hz.

Mechanism of the NE Receptor Activated by NE Pathway Stimulation

Intracellular recording of some Purkinje cells during stimulation of LC with single shocks revealed late hyperpolarizations (not directly related to climbing fiber responses) which were usually quite small. With trains of pulses, large hyperpolarizations extending well beyond the stimulation period and averaging 14 mV (range, 2 to 39 mV) were recorded. An index of membrane resistance was obtained by measuring the size of climbing fiber excitatory postsynaptic potentials (EPSPs), and by measuring the potential deflexions produced by hyperpolarizing currents (0.5 to 1 nA, 40 msec duration) passed through the recording micropipette in conjunction with a Wheatstone bridge circuit. In all cases, input resistance, as measured by these two parameters, either increased (10 cells) or did not change (two cells) during the LC evoked hyperpolarizations. Thus, LC stimulation exactly mimicked the action of exogenous NE: both produce hyperpolarization without a decrease in membrane resistance (21,23).

Pharmacological Studies on the Response to NE Pathway Stimulation

Although the effects of LC stimulation produce the same qualitative effect on Purkinje cells as the iontophoretic administration of NE, additional studies were undertaken to confirm the noradrenergic nature of the LC effects. When catecholamine-containing pathways were selectively and chronically destroyed by intracisternally injected 6-OHDA, only 5 of 60 cells were inhibited when the LC was stimulated directly. Furthermore, when animals are acutely pretreated with reserpine (1.5 mg/kg, i.v.) and alpha-methyl-tyrosine (100 to 200 mg/kg, i.p.), the loss of the LC inhibitory effects, whether to single or multiple shocks, correlates well with the loss and subsequent recovery of NE content.

The Noradrenergic Projection to Rat Hippocampal Pyramidal Cells

Recently, the hippocampal cortex, a brain region known to receive an extensive input of NE-containing fibers has been examined (23, 24). We have confirmed the presence of NE terminals by both fluorescence histochemistry, 6-OHDA induced degeneration (Bloom and Segal, *in prep.*) and by autoradiography after microinjection of labeled precursors into the locus coeruleus. These studies also indicate that the hippocampal NE projections onto pyramidal cells function in a fashion quite similar to the effects of the locus coeruleus on cerebellar Purkinje cells: LC and NE slow pyramidal cell discharge with long-latency and long-duration actions; the receptor is blocked with MJ-1999 and by prostaglandins of the E series, and the action of the pathway is totally blocked by chronic pretreatment with 6-OHDA or acute pretreatment with reserpine and alpha-methyl-tyrosine (23,24). Preliminary evidence suggests that in the hippocampus, as in the cerebellum (see below), the NE inhibitory actions may be mediated postsynaptically by formation of cyclic AMP.

Other LC-NE Synaptic Sites

Inhibitions of neurons in other brainstem areas have also been found with LC stimulation. Thus, cells in the spinal trigeminal nucleus and lateral geniculate nucleus (25) show a decreased probability of discharge following LC activation. However, no pharmacological characterizations here have yet been reported.

CYCLIC 3'5'-ADENOSINE MONOPHOSPHATE AS A MEDIATOR OF NE ACTION IN THE CNS

When the combined cytological and iontophoretic studies above demonstrated that rat cerebellar Purkinje and hippocampal pyramidal

neurons received NE-containing synapses and that these neurons gave uniform inhibitory response to NE, subsequent studies could proceed to investigate the mechanism of the inhibitory response. In both test systems, cyclic 3'5'-adenosine monophosphate (cyclic AMP) was observed to mimic the ability of NE to depress spontaneous activity, and the NE receptor could be blocked by the beta sympatholytic MJ-1999.

In order to pursue the possibility that this action of cyclic AMP in the CNS might indicate a "second messenger" hypothesis for central NE synapses, many other experiments have been conducted. Biochemical evidence suggested that NE could elevate cerebellar cyclic AMP levels (2). Furthermore, parenteral administration of phosphodiesterase inhibitors such as aminophylline or theophylline potentiated NE depressions of Purkinje cells, while iontophoretic administration of these methylxanthines and of papaverine converted weak excitant actions of iontophoretic cyclic AMP into pronounced depressions (19). These observations led us to propose that the actions of NE (19), and later those of the NE-mediated locus coeruleus synaptic projection to Purkinje cells (23), could be mediated by cyclic AMP (21). Subsequently, the proposal has been strengthened by observations that the actions of NE of the NE pathway, and of cyclic nucleotides all hyperpolarize Purkinje cells through an unexplained membrane action in which membrane conductance to passive ion flow is not increased (as it is with most other known synaptic chemicals) (21). The cyclic AMP mediation of the NE actions also finds support from the observations that prostaglandins E_1 and E_2 and nicotinate will selectively block NE effects on Purkinje cells and pyramidal cells (24) as they do on the cyclic AMP-mediated adrenergic responses of adipocytes. Even more direct confirmation of the hypothesis stems from the observation that NE and the NE pathway will selectively increase the immunocytochemical assay of Purkinje cell cyclic AMP content (2). These studies have been recently reviewed exhaustively (1,2,21).

CONCLUSIONS

At the present time, characterization of central noradrenergic synaptic function requires a combination of cytochemical and electro-physiological experiments. These combinations are required in order to specify the nature of homogeneous test cells bearing what are assumed to be examples of the natural synaptic receptor. For the only two cellular test systems in which the required fundamental observations have been gathered, the cerebellar Purkinje cell and the hippocampal pyramidal cell, the central noradrenergic receptor is characterized as a beta type, inhibitory in function. The inhibitory response to NE may be mediated intracellularly by activation of cyclic AMP synthesis through a membrane-related receptor stimulating adenylate cyclase. Some aspect of this receptor site can also be antagonized by prostaglandins of the E series and by nicotinate, and the overall effects across such receptors can be potentiated by phosphodiesterase inhibitors. Whether or not such enzyme-activated central receptors are typical of all central noradrenergic receptors remains to be determined. Of further interest through the next decade of research will be studies designed to determine whether the participation of NE neurons in such functions as sleep (26) and their intimate association with the powerful biological consequences of activating cyclic AMP synthesis (2) can provide a better understanding of the more general neurobiological roles played by these important neurons.

REFERENCES

1. Bloom, F. E. (1968): Electrophysiological pharmacology of single nerve cells. In: "Psychopharmacology—A Ten Year Progress Report" edited by D. H. Efron, pp. 355–373, U.S. Govt. Printing Office, Washington, D.C.
2. Bloom, F. E. (1974): To spritz or not to spritz: The doubtful value of aimless iontophoresis. *Life Sci.,* 14:1819–1834.
3. Boakes, R. J., Bradley, P. B., Brookes, N., Candy, J. M., and Wolstencroft, J. H. (1971): Actions of noradrenaline, other sympathomimetic amines and antagonists on neurones in the brainstem of the cat. *Brit. J. Pharmacol.,* 41:262–271.
4. Bradley, P. B., Wolstencroft, J. H., Hosli, L., and Avanzino, G. L. (1966): Neuronal basis for the central action of chlorpromazine. *Nature,* 212:1425–1427.
5. Couch, J. (1970): Responses of neurons in the raphe nuclei to serotonin, norepinephrine and acetylcholine and their correlation with an excitatory synaptic input. *Brain Res.,* 19:137–150.
6. Frederickson, R., Jordan, L., and Phillis, J. W.

(1972): The action of noradrenalin on cortical neurons. *Brain Res.,* 35:556–560.
7. Bloom, F. E. (1973): Ultrastructural identification of catecholamine-containing central synaptic terminals. *J. Histochem. Cytochem.,* 21: 333–348.
8. Landis, S. C., and Bloom, F. E. (1974): Fluorescence and electron microscopic analysis of catecholamine-containing fibers in mutant mouse cerebellum. *Anat. Rec.,* 178:398.
9. Barker, J. L., Crayton, J. C., and Nicoll, R. A. (1971): Supraoptic neurosecretory cells: Adrenergic and cholinergic sensitivity. *Science,* 171: 208–210.
10. Nicoll, R. A., and Barker, J. L. (1971): The pharmacology of recurrent inhibition in the supraoptic neurosecretory system. *Brain Res.,* 35:501–516.
11. Salmoiraghi, G. C., and Stefanis, C. (1971): Central synapses and suspected transmitters. *Int. Rev. Neurobiol.,* 10:1–30.
12. Krnjevic, K., and Phillis, J. W. (1963a): Iontophoretic studies of neurons in mammalian cerebral cortex. *J. Physiol.,* 165:274–304.
13. Johnson, E. S., Roberts, M. H. T., Sobieszek, A., and Straughan, D. W. (1969a): Noradrenaline sensitive cells in cat cerebral cortex. *Int. J. Neuropharmacol.,* 8:549–557.
14. Johnson, E. S., Roberts, M. H. T., and Straughan, D. W. (1969b): The responses of cortical neurones to monoamines under differing anesthetic conditions. *J. Physiol.,* 203:261–275.
15. Foote, S. L., Freedman, R., and Oliver, A. P. (1975): Effects of putative neurotransmitters on neuronal activity in monkey auditory cortex. *Brain Res.,* 86:229–242.
16a. Nelson, C. N., Hoffer, B. J., Chu, N-s., and Bloom, F. E. (1973): Cytochemical and pharmacological studies on polysensory neurons in the primate frontal cortex. *Brain Res.,* 62:115–133.
16b. Tebecis, A., (1970): Effects of monoamines and amino acids on medial geniculate neurons of the cat. *Neuropharmacology,* 9:381–390.
17. Hoffer, B. J., Siggins, G. R., and Bloom, F. E. (1971): Studies on norepinephrine-containing afferents to Purkinje cells of rat cerebellum: II. Sensitivity of Purkinje cells to norepinephrine and related substances administered by microiontophoresis. *Brain Res.,* 25:523–534.
18. Woodward, D. J., Hoffer, B. J., Siggins, G. R., and Bloom, F. E. (1971): The ontogenetic development of synaptic junctions, synaptic activation and responsiveness to neurotransmitter substances in rat cerebellar Purkinje cells. *Brain Res.,* 34:73–79.
19. Siggins, G. R., Hoffer, B. J., and Bloom, F. E. (1971): Studies on norepinephrine-containing afferents to Purkinje cells of rat cerebellum: III. Evidence for mediation of norepinephrine effects by cyclic 3',5'-adenosine monophosphate. *Brain Res.,* 25:535–553.
20. Engberg, I., and Marshall, K. C. (1971): Mechanism of noradrenaline hyperpolarization in spinal cord motoneurons of the cat. *Acta Physiol. Scand.,* 83:142–144.

21. Hoffer, B. J., Siggins, G. R., Oliver, A. P., and Bloom, F. E. (1973): Activation of the pathway from locus coeruleus to rat cerebellar Purkinje neurons: pharmacological evidence of noradrenergic central inhibition. *J. Pharmacol. Exp. Ther.*, 184:553–569.

22. Segal, M., and Bloom, F. E. (1974): The action of norepinephrine in the rat hippocampus: II. Activation of the input pathway. *Brain Res.*, 72:99–114.

23. Siggins, G. R., Hoffer, B. J., Oliver, A. P., and Bloom, F. E. (1971): Activation of a central noradrenergic projection to cerebellum. *Nature*, 233:481–483.

24. Segal, M., and Bloom, F. E. (1974): The action of norepinephrine in the rat hippocampus: I. Iontophoretic studies. *Brain Res.*, 72:79–97.

25. Sasa, M., Muneyiko, K., Ikeda, H., and Takaori, S. (1974): Noradrenaline-mediated inhibition by locus coeruleus of spinal trigeminal neurons. *Brain Res.*, 80:443–460.

26. Chu, N-s., and Bloom, F. E. (1974): Activity patterns of catecholamine-containing pontine neurons in the dorso-lateral tegmentum of unrestrained cats. *J. Neurobiol.*, 5:527–544.

27. Phillis, J. W., Lake, N., and Yarborough, G. G. (1973): Calcium mediation of the inhibitory effects of biogenic amines on cerebral cortical neurons. *Brain Res.*, 53:465–469.

28. Stone, T. W. (1973): Pharmacology of pyramidal tract cells in the cerebral cortex. *Naunyn Schmiederbergs Arch.Pharmacol.,*278:333–346.

29. Avanzino, G. L., Bradley, P. B., and Wolstencroft, J. H. (1966): Pharmacological properties of neurones of the paramedian reticular nucleus. *Experientia*, 22:410.

30. Biscoe, T. J., and Curtis, D. R. (1966): Noradrenaline and inhibition of Renshaw cells. *Science*, 151:1231–1232.

The Nervous System, Donald B. Tower, Editor-in-Chief. *Vol. 1: The Basic Neurosciences.* Raven Press, New York, 1975.

Regulation of Adenylate Cyclase Activity by Neurotransmitters and Its Relation to Neural Function

John P. Perkins

Adenosine 3',5'-monophosphate (cAMP) is now established as the intracellular mediator of the actions of a variety of substances that affect cell function upon interaction with extracellular receptors (1). In each effector-target cell system studied, the circumstances that led to the demonstration of an involvement of cAMP have been similar. Namely, an identifiable substance, usually a hormone, was known to cause a measurable alteration in a specific biochemical or physiological function of a cell or tissue. In this setting the now familiar experimental criteria proposed by Robison et al. (1) (Table 1) were demonstrated. It should be noted that these criteria are stated in terms of

TABLE 1. *Criteria for establishing a mediatory role for cAMP in the action of hormones and neurohumors*

1. The hormone should be capable of stimulating adenyl cyclase in broken cell preparations from the appropriate cells, whereas hormones that do not produce the response should not stimulate adenyl cyclase.
2. The hormone should be capable of increasing the intracellular level of cyclic AMP in intact cells, whereas inactive hormones should not increase cyclic AMP levels. It should be demonstrated that the effect on the level of cyclic AMP occurs at dose levels of the hormone that are at least as small as the smallest levels capable of producing a physiological response. The increase in the level of cyclic AMP should precede or at least not follow the physiological response.
3. It should be possible to potentiate the hormone (i.e., increase the magnitude of the physiological response) by administering the hormone together with theophylline or other phosphodiesterase inhibitors. The hormone and the phosphodiesterase inhibitor should act synergistically.
4. It should be possible to mimic the physiological effect of the hormone by the addition of exogenous cyclic AMP.

(Taken from Robison et al., ref. 1, p. 36.)

a prior knowledge of an effector-induced alteration of cell function. Unfortunately, with regard to establishing a role for cyclic nucleotides in the function of the nervous system, one is quite limited in terms of measurable neuronal or glial cell functions. The functions of neurons are characteristically described in terms of electrophysiological parameters rather than biochemical parameters, e.g., chemically or electrically evoked changes in resting membrane potentials or changes in the frequency of propagated action potentials. The physiologically relevant functions of glial cells are not known at all with assurance. Thus, for sometime after it had been shown that adenylate cyclase was present at high levels in nervous tissue (2), any effect of cyclic nucleotides on a specific function remained obscure.

If one assumed that cAMP played the same role in the nervous system that it did in the target cells of hormones, i.e., an intracellular mediator of the actions of extracellular effectors, then a possible role in nervous system function was apparent on theoretical grounds. In many instances, especially in the peripheral nervous system, the identities of specific synaptic transmitters were known. In fact the neurotransmitter of postganglionic sympathetic neurons, norepinephrine (NE), was known to cause alterations in metabolic functions of innervated organs by a mechanism that involved the stimulation of adenylate cyclase and the subsequent activation by cAMP of specific phosphorylation reactions. Thus it was a short extrapolation to imagine that cAMP might also mediate the electrophysiological effects of NE on postsynaptic neurons. However, only recently has convincing evidence in support of such a role for cAMP been obtained.

Attempts to satisfy the four basic criteria of Sutherland for implication of a mediatory role for cAMP in the action of NE or any other neurotransmitter have been confronted with special problems.

Criterion 1. Two characteristics of nervous tissue prevent the ready demonstration of neurotransmitter-specific stimulation of adenylate cyclase activity. First, it has commonly been observed that although high levels of this enzyme activity are present in homogenates of nervous tissue, no significant stimulation of activity is elicited in the presence of added neurotransmitter (3,4). Second, the extreme cellular heterogeneity of nervous system tissue, especially the central nervous system (CNS), makes it quite difficult to obtain a homogenate of only the "appropriate" cells. Not only will such homogenates contain fragments of glial cells but also fragments of a variety of functionally different neurons, each of which may respond selectively to different neurotransmitters.

Criterion 2. Fortunately, intact cell preparations of nervous tissue, such as slices and minces, have been found to respond to a variety of putative neurotransmitters with a rise in cAMP content. However, the investigator is still plagued by the problem of cellular heterogeneity when attempting to demonstrate neurotransmitter-specific changes in cAMP that correlate with neurotransmitter-specific changes in physiologic function. Furthermore establishing the quantitative relationship between an electrophysiological response and the "dose" of neurotransmitter is quite difficult, even if the problem of heterogeneity is overcome by studying the response of single cells upon iontophoretic application of effectors (5). Finally, the electrophysiological events to be measured occur very rapidly, within milliseconds, and it is impossible with current technology to make a biochemical determination of changes in cAMP content within such time limitations.

Criterion 3. Synergistic interactions of neurotransmitters and inhibitors of cyclic nucleotide–phosphodiesterase (PDE) activity have been observed in experiments with nervous tissue preparations (6–9). However, anomalous effects of methylxanthines also have been reported (10,11). Methylxanthine inhibitors of PDE have little or no effect on the accumulation of cAMP elicited in guinea pig brain slices by catecholamines or histamine (10).

Criterion 4. In certain experimental situations, in which the electrophysiological effects of catecholamines have been defined, appropriate application of cAMP or analogues of cAMP can be shown to mimic the effects of the catecholamine (6–8,11,12). The relative ease with which cAMP or its analogues can be shown to accurately mimic these effects of catecholamines has made this criterion the one most readily satisfied.

In spite of the inherent technical difficulties just alluded to, a reasonably coherent picture of the role of cAMP as a mediator of at least certain of the effects of catecholamine neurotransmitters on neuronal function is beginning to appear. In the following sections, I briefly review the three basic experimental approaches that have contributed most to our current level of understanding. Many of the early studies were oriented toward demonstrating the existence in nervous tissues of the enzymic components of the cAMP second messenger system and characterizing their properties. There also have been numerous studies designed to characterize the factors that influence cyclic nucleotide levels in slices or cultured cell preparations of nervous system tissues. Finally, there have been some very elegant studies designed to correlate the effects of neurotransmitters on cyclic nucleotide levels with their effects on electrophysiological function.

DEMONSTRATION OF THE ENZYMIC COMPONENTS OF THE CYCLIC NUCLEOTIDE SECOND MESSENGER SYSTEMS IN NERVOUS TISSUE

In 1962 Klainer et al. (2) reported the presence of adenylate cyclase activity in homogenates and subcellular membrane fractions of certain nervous system tissues. Such preparations exhibited little or no increased activity in the presence of catecholamines. Many subsequent studies have documented the presence of adenylate cyclase activity in every portion of the nervous system examined to date. However, with rare exceptions, adenylate cyclase activities in broken cell preparations of CNS tissues do not respond to neurotransmitters with increased activity (3,4). Dopamine- and catecholamine-sensitive adenylate cyclases have been demonstrated in homogenates of rat brain caudate nucleus (13). Maximally effective concentrations of either catecholamine increase enzyme activity about twofold. The lack of effector sensitivity of CNS-derived adenylate cyclases has been attributed to a unique degree of lability of the association between regulatory and catalytic components of the enzyme system. Such a conclusion seems reasonable, since a number of different neuroactive substances can increase the rate of synthesis of cAMP in intact cell preparations of nervous system tissues.

Chasin et al. (14) and Shimizu et al. (15) have demonstrated that homogenates of guinea pig cerebral cortex prepared in Krebs-Ringer buffer exhibit the same effector sensitivity as do slices of the same tissue. However, these preparations appear to be composed of intact vesicles and cannot utilize exogenous adenosine triphosphate (ATP) as substrate for adenylate cyclase activity. When the vesicles are suspended in Tris buffer, basal activity increases and exogenous ATP can be utilized as substrate. However, effector sensitivity is lost and the vesicles become swollen and the membranes thinned and distorted. The subcellular origins of the vesicles are not known. Such preparations may offer certain technical advantages over slice or mince preparations, but at their present stage of characterization they would not appear to be any more suitable for the direct measurement of adenylate cyclase activity than whole cell preparations. The magnitude of the rise in cAMP in the vesicles should be the net result of synthesis and degradation since the vesicles surely contain PDE activity. Thus, one is faced with the same complex kinetic situation that exists in intact cells exposed to activators of adenylate cyclase.

Brostrom et al. (16) have recently identified a calcium-binding protein from porcine cerebral cortex that acts as a calcium-dependent regulator of adenylate cyclase activity. This protein appears to be identical to the calcium-binding protein that regulates brain PDE activity (17). Detergent-dispersed (Lubrol-PX) adenylate cyclase activity was completely inhibited by 50 μM EGTA and stimulated 50% by 30 μM Ca^{2+}. Inhibition by EGTA was overcome by Ca^{2+}. Chromatography of the detergent-dispersed preparation on ECTEOLA-cellulose resulted in a marked reduction in adenylate cyclase activity even in the presence of optimal Ca^{2+} concentrations. However, adenylate cyclase activity was increased about ninefold upon addition of the calcium-binding protein. Brostrom et al. (16) propose a physiological role for Ca^{2+} and the binding protein in the regulation of adenylate cyclase activity as a function of the intracellular Ca^{2+} concentration. Still to be determined is the effect of such Ca^{2+}-binding proteins on the activity of adenylate cyclases from other tissues, especially those that do not appear to be stimulated by Ca^{2+} or inhibited by EGTA (see ref. 18).

To date, the only unique properties of the adenylate cyclases of nervous tissue are the aforementioned lability of responsiveness to effectors and the recent observation by Brostrom et al. (16) just referred to. The variations in the anatomical localization of adenylate cyclase throughout the nervous system and its subcellular distribution have been analyzed in previous reviews (19–21).

Guanylate cyclase activity has been demonstrated in broken cell preparations of most CNS tissues examined to date (see ref. 22), but a stimulatory effect of an appropriate neurotransmitter on enzyme activity has not been convincingly demonstrated. However, guanylate cyclase activity from most tissues is not stimulated by those agents that cause increases in intracellular levels of guanosine 3′,5′-monophosphate (cGMP). No properties of guanylate cyclase, unique to the enzyme from nervous system tissues have been reported.

Phosphodiesterase activity selective for cAMP and cGMP have been demonstrated in a variety of preparations from the nervous system (23–25). Kakiuchi (17) has proposed, based on kinetic evidence, that the Ca^{2+}-dependent PDE activity of brain preferentially hydrolyzes cGMP rather than cAMP at substrate concentrations in the physiologically significant range. There is a marked variation of PDE activity throughout different regions of the brain and a marked variation in the ratio of adenylate cyclase:PDE activities. No functional significance has, as yet, been ascribed to this observation, however.

Protein kinase activities specifically stimulated by either cGMP or cAMP have been demonstrated in nervous tissue (26,27). Phosphorylation of endogenous protein substrates by endogenous cAMP-dependent kinases can be readily demonstrated in synaptic membrane-containing subcellular fractions of cerebral cortex (see 28). These same membrane fractions contain phosphoprotein phosphatase activity capable of removing phosphate from substrate protein after it has been phosphorylated by cAMP-dependent protein kinase (29).

Thus it appears that nervous system tissues possess all the known components of the cAMP second messenger system and that, in general, the enzymes involved are not obviously unique in their properties. That is not to suggest that no unique features will be found, but it may well be that, as in other tissues, specificity of action of extracellular effectors is primarily related to the cell-specific expression of receptor molecules linked to adenylate cyclase and to cell-specific expression of substrates for cAMP-dependent protein kinases. However, there also is some indication that the enzymic components of the second messenger system exhibit a degree of tissue-specific subcellular localization, which may be involved in ordering their function.

EFFECTS OF NEUROACTIVE SUBSTANCES ON THE CYCLIC NUCLEOTIDE CONTENT OF INTACT CELL PREPARATIONS OF BRAIN

In 1968 Kakiuchi and Rall (30,31) reported their initial studies on the actions of catecholamines and histamine on the cAMP content of slices of rabbit cerebellum and cerebral cortex. Since that time, numerous workers have established that a variety of neuroactive substances can increase the cAMP and cGMP content of slices from a number of different anatomical areas of brain (for reviews see 10,20,22,32–35). The specificity of action of the various agents is marked, and variations in effect are observed in different anatomical areas of the brain in the same species and in the same brain area in different species. In fact quantitative differences in responsiveness have been observed in the same brain area of different strains of the same species (mentioned in 34). I will not attempt to summarize all of the studies in this area, but will focus on specific aspects of current interest.

The studies of Kakiuchi and Rall (30,31) indicated that the effect of catecholamines on

cAMP formation in cerebellar slices of rabbit brain was mediated by β-adrenergic receptors. Subsequent studies with slices from a number of brain areas and from different species suggest that catecholamines can, in fact, interact with a variety of different "receptors" to increase cAMP content. Such receptors are, of course, defined only in operational terms of agonist and antagonists specificity. Variation in the expression of these receptors is observed in the same anatomical region of different species and in different anatomical areas in the same species (36).

Chasin et al. (37) were first to focus attention on the α-like nature of the receptors mediating the effects of catecholamines on the cAMP content of guinea pig cerebral cortex slices. These early observations have been confirmed and extended by Schultz and Daly (reviewed in 34) and extended and discussed in detail by Sattin et al. (36). In rat cerebral cortex, catecholamines increase the accumulation of cAMP levels by interacting with both α- and β-receptors (34,35). Finally, in rat and rabbit cerebellum, only β-adrenergic receptors appear to be involved (10).

In those brain regions that exhibit α-receptor-mediated responses, catecholamines and adenosine produce a synergistic effect on cAMP content. This interaction is most obvious in slices of guinea pig cerebral cortex, since the effects of catecholamines alone are quite small (see 36). In rat cerebral cortex, it appears that the synergistic effects of catecholamines and adenosine also are primarily mediated by the α-like receptors (35; however, see discussion in 34).

In an attempt to provide a mechanism to explain the synergism of effect that has been observed when two or more effectors of cAMP formation are added together to brain slices, Sattin et al. (36) have proposed a new concept of *dependent* and *independent* receptors. In essence they propose the existence of a class of receptors linked to adenylate cyclase that cause activation of the enzyme only when two different agonist molecules are bound concomitantly. If, in fact, such a class of receptors exists, the regulation of adenylate cyclase activity in brain is a complicated affair indeed. Adenylate cyclases linked to independent α-receptors, β-receptors, adenosine receptors, and histamine receptors must exist as well as dependent receptors for adenosine-catecholamine, adenosine-histamine, histamine-catecholamine, and perhaps dependent α-β-receptors (see discussion in 36). The hypothesis is of some interest, since it does provide a plausible mechanism to account for synergistic interactions; however, it is too early to assess its validity. It will be difficult to obtain direct evidence for the existence of specific cells with dependent receptors in view of the cellular heterogeneity of brain. To date, brain slices are the only experimental preparations in which such synergistic interactions have been noted. In clonal cell lines that respond to adenosine and/or catecholamines, no evidence for a synergistic interaction of combinations of the two effectors has been reported. However, if it is assumed that cells that contain dependent receptors would not have independent receptors for the same effectors, then the existence of dependent receptors could have gone undetected during the screening of potential effectors added singly to clonal cell lines.

The actions of adenosine and analogues of adenosine on cAMP formation in brain slices and in cultured cells of neural origin have been thoroughly investigated since the initial demonstration of their effect (4). Although adenosine is readily taken up into cells and can serve as a precursor of cAMP, it does not raise cAMP levels in this manner. There is now strong support for the idea that adenosine increases cAMP levels in brain slices and in certain cultured cells by interacting with extracellular receptors linked to adenylate cyclase (reviewed in 10,34–36).

Although the evidence cannot be presented here, the effects on cAMP formation in brain slices of electrical stimulation, increased extracellular K^+, ouabain, veratridine, and batrachotoxin appear to be mediated, at least in part, by the release of adenosine from the slices and its subsequent direct action on adenylate cyclase. However, other factors also have been implicated as mediators of the effects of these agents especially of the actions of K^+ and ouabain (reviewed in 10,21,32).

The evidence supporting a role for adenosine and adenosine analogues as neurotransmitters in the peripheral nervous system has been reviewed by Burnstock (38). The effects of adenosine on cAMP formation and the observation

that adenosine is released from brain slices by field stimulation implicate it as a transmitter in the CNS as well. The examination of this hypothesis and the investigation of the mechanism of synergism between adenosine and biogenic amines provide interesting directions for future research.

Finally I would like to mention that Shimizu et al. (15,39) have demonstrated that another class of neuroactive agents, acidic amino acids, can cause marked increases in the formation of cAMP in slices and homogenates of guinea pig cerebral cortex. The authors suggest that release of acidic amino acids (aspartate, glutamate) and their subsequent effects on cAMP formation may be involved in the stimulatory action of depolarizing stimuli on cAMP accumulation.

EFFECTS OF NEUROACTIVE SUBSTANCES ON THE CYCLIC AMP CONTENT OF CULTURED CELLS OF NERVOUS SYSTEM ORIGIN

General Comments

As mentioned previously the cellular heterogeneity of CNS tissue presents a formidable problem in attempts to correlate the effects of neuroactive agents on cyclic nucleotide content with effects on function. One possible solution to this problem would be to separate the two basic cellular components of nervous tissue, neurons, and glia, and to conduct such correlative studies in the purified cell populations. However, attempts to separate the neurons and glia of brain by physical techniques have been plagued by poor yields, insufficient resolution, and damaged cells. Rather than intact neurons, neuronal cell bodies are most often the product of such procedures. To date, little information concerning cyclic nucleotides and brain function has come from such studies.

Primary cultures of nervous system tissue can be manipulated to provide populations of cells enriched in neurons or glia. However, since differentiated neurons lose the capacity to proliferate, cultures of neurons of sufficient purity or sufficient density to allow biochemical analyses are difficult to obtain. Furthermore, the probability is high that such cultures of neurons, derived from even very circumscribed areas of brain, will contain a variety of neuronal "species" that will be sensitive to different effector agents. Primary cultures of glia can be freed of neurons with relative ease but such cultures are usually heavily contaminated with fibroblasts. Clonal lines of transformed cells of nervous system origins have been extensively studied but have the inherent problem of not fully expressing all differentiated functions.

Primary culture systems and clonal cell lines of neural origins also have been used to seek answers to the simpler question of which type of cell, neuron or glia, responds to a given neuroactive substance with a rise in cAMP content. Unfortunately, results of such studies also have not been very illuminating; for example, both neuroblastoma and glioma cell lines respond to catecholamines, adenosine, and prostaglandins under appropriate conditions.

Primary Cultures of Dispersed Brain Cells

Gilman and Schrier (40) have examined the effects of a number of neuroactive substances on cAMP formation in dispersed-cell cultures of whole fetal rat brain. Although they did not conduct a strict comparison of the responsiveness of normal brain slices and the cultured cells, it is clear from their results that there are marked differences as well as similarities in the responses of the two preparations. No synergism of action between catecholamines and adenosine was observed in the cultured-cell preparation. Prostaglandin E_1 had a marked effect on the cAMP content of the cultured cells but has little or no effect on cAMP content in whole rat brain slices. In the cultures the effects of catecholamines appeared to be mediated entirely by β-receptors. Adenosine also increased cAMP formation, and its effect was blocked by theophylline, as is also the case in brain slices. The authors concluded that catecholamines increased cAMP formation primarily in glia, since the magnitude of the effect increased with increasing cell proliferation.

One potential disadvantage of this type of culture is that the normal three-dimensional relationships of cells is lost. In reaggregated brain cell cultures, little cell division occurs and the proportion of cell types and their orientation to one another are, to a degree, similar to those of normal brain (41). In reaggregated cultures of mouse brain cells, the responsiveness to catecholamines develops more slowly in culture, and the magnitude of the increase in cAMP content is much smaller than in cultures of dispersed cells (42).

Explant Cultures of Rat Cerebral Cortex

We have conducted a comparison of the development and characteristics of responsiveness

TABLE 2. *Comparison of the effects of certain neuroactive agents on cAMP formation in slices of rat cerebral cortex and explant cultures of cerebral cortex*

	Relative cAMP content			
	Rat cerebral cortex slice		Rat cerebral cortex explant	
Effector	rat age: 8 days	rat age: 40 days	6 days in culture	12 days in culture
None	100	100	100	100
Norepinephrine (NE)	100–150	800	1,000	600
Isoproterenol (ISO)	100–150	400	2,000	1,200
NE + Propranolol	100	200	100	100
ISO + Propranolol	100	100	100	100
NE + Phentolamine	100	400	2,000	1,200
ISO + Phentolamine	100	400	2,000	1,200
Adenosine (Ads)	600	800	100–150	100–150
NE + Ads	1,300	2,000	700	450
Prostaglandin E_1	100–150	100–150	300	600

Maximally effective concentrations of the effectors were used in each case NE, 100 μM; ISO, 30 μM; phentolamine, 10 μM; propranolol, 10 μM; adenosine, 100 μM; prostaglandin E_1, 10 μM.

to catecholamines, adenosine, and prostaglandins in normal rat cerebral cortex and in explant cultures of newborn rat cortex. Explant cultures were used in an attempt to maintain normal cell proportions and orientation. Briefly, cerebral cortex was removed sterilely from newborn Spraque-Dawley rats, cut into $0.3 \times 0.3 \times 0.5$ mm sections and placed into culture in collagen-coated plastic petri dishes. The cultures were viable for at least 30 days but unfortunately did not maintain their three-dimensional integrity for more than 4 days in culture. All attempts to prevent cell migration, which was the prelude to cellular proliferation, also affected either cell viability or morphology.

A comparison of certain properties of the explant cultures and cerebral cortex slices is shown in Table 2. The overall impression from the comparison is that the culture system is not a predictive model of the responsiveness of cortex slices. The observation of an apparent α-receptor-mediated inhibitory effect on cAMP formation is of interest and has not been observed in other experimental CNS preparations. The responsiveness to prostaglandins develops late in culture (8 to 16 days) and may be a reflection of the increased proportion of fibroblasts in cultures of this age.

If specific cell-cell interactions form the basis for the complex effects of neuroactive substances on cAMP formation in brain slices, e.g., synergistic interactions of effectors, then it is to be expected that such functions will be lost in culture systems that fail to maintain or reconstitute these interactions.

Clonal Cell Lines of Neural Origins

Clonal lines of neuroblastoma and glioma cells have received much attention recently as potential model systems for the study of neuronal and glial function. A detailed appraisal of the usefulness of this general approach would be premature at this time and review of the many published studies in this field is outside the scope of this article. My comments will be limited to a brief survey of the effects of neuroactive agents on cyclic nucleotide content in these cell lines.

Neuroblastoma C1300

Early studies suggested that C1300 cells were remarkably insensitive to most of the effectors that increase cyclic nucleotide content in brain slices or brain cultures (42). However, when such agents were tested in the presence of inhibitors of PDE activity, their capacity to increase the synthesis of cAMP could be readily detected (43,44). This observation coupled with the fact that inhibitors of PDE alone can increase cAMP levels in certain clones of C1300 cells (45), indicated that the PDE activity in these cells is quite high and that under basal conditions there is a rapid turnover of cAMP. To date it has been shown that β-catecholamines (46), prostaglandins of the E-series (42), and adenosine and adenosine analogues (43,44) all cause marked increases in certain clones of C1300 neuroblastoma. The report (47) that cholinergic agents increase adenylate cyclase activity in certain clones of C1300 cells goes somewhat against the dogma of this field and awaits confirmation by other workers in the field. However, in intact cells of this same clone, cholinergic agents inhibited the accumulation of cAMP in response to stimulation by prostaglandins (48). The recent observation that morphine acts as an antagonist of the catecholamine-sensitive adenylate cyclase of a neuroblastoma-glial cell hybrid line may provide some much welcomed insight into the mechanism of action of this important class of drugs (49).

Glioma and Astrocytoma Cell Lines

Both the C-6 rat glioma cell lines and the human astrocytoma lines were derived from brain tumors and thus are probably transformed cell lines. Their similarity to normal glial cells is difficult to assess, since so little is known of glial cell-specific functions. DeVellis and co-workers (50) have demonstrated some biochemical similarities between the C-6 line and supposed glial cell functions; namely, C-6 contains the S-100 protein and responds to cortisol with induction of glycerol-phosphate dehydrogenase activity. The C-6 lines respond to β-catecholamines with a rise in intracellular cAMP, but do not respond to any other known neuroactive agents.

The human astrocytoma line 1321N1 responds to β-catecholamines, prostaglandins of the E-series, and adenosine and adenosine analogues (51). We have not been able to demonstrate a synergistic interaction of any two of these three effectors. To the contrary, combinations of the agents usually elicit a rise in cAMP that is less than the sum of the effect induced by each agent separately. The adenylate cyclase of membrane preparations of both C-6 and 1321N1 cell lines can be activated by the appropriate effectors.

The observation that normal and transformed glial cells in culture respond to catecholamines provides the basis for an often-proposed hypothesis that neuronally released NE could influence the metabolism of glial cells located near the synaptic cleft to the end of providing some support function for the neuron. This hypothesis remains an unverified speculation worthy of further examination.

The characteristics of the regulation of cAMP formation in clonal cell lines of neural origin do not firmly establish such preparations as predictive models of normal neurons and glia. However, such studies are important preliminaries to the study of mixed cultures of homogeneous populations of neurally derived cells. One obvious goal of the study of neural cells in culture is to be able to reconstitute a synaptically linked neuronal system of two or more homogeneous populations of cells with defined neural function. Such a goal does not appear to be attainable within the near future.

RELATION OF CHANGES IN CYCLIC NUCLEOTIDE CONTENT TO CHANGES IN FUNCTION

Over the past 4 years, Greengard and his collaborators have carried out an impressive series of experiments relating the effects of dopamine and acetylcholine on cAMP and cGMP content to changes in synaptic potentials in the superior cervical ganglion. This work has been summarized in detail by Greengard (28) and Greengard and Kebabian (52) recently and will be addressed here only briefly.

Based on the results of biochemical, pharmacological, morphological, and electrophysiological studies, a model of the superior cervical ganglion has been proposed (Fig. 1) (52). It is suggested that the predominant cell type of the ganglion, the postganglionic sympathetic neuron, receives at least three types of innervation. The primary innervation is through preganglionic, cholinergic fibers, which release acetyl-

choline onto nicotinic cholinergic receptors. It is this synaptic event that generates the fast excitatory postsynaptic potential (f-EPSP). The postsynaptic ganglion cell also is thought to receive innervation through two modulatory pathways. The available evidence indicates the existence of an interneuron that releases dopamine onto dopamine receptors that are linked to adenylate cyclase in the postganglionic cell. The activation of adenylate cyclase leads to increased levels of cAMP, which causes a hyperpolarization of the postganglionic neuron. This event is detected as a slow inhibitory postsynaptic potential (s-IPSP). The dopaminergic interneuron receives cholinergic innervation through muscarinic receptors. An excitatory modulatory pathway is proposed to be composed of preganglionic cholinergic innervation of the postganglionic cell through muscarinic receptors. Activation of these receptors results in the formation of cGMP and depolarization of the postganglionic neuron. This event is detected as a slow excitatory postsynaptic potential (s-EPSP). The evidence in support of this model of the superior cervical ganglion is listed below:

1. Dopamine causes an increase in the cAMP content of slices of ganglia. This effect is potentiated by inhibitors of PDE activity and antagonized by α-adrenergic antagonists. Dopamine also causes a hyperpolarization of postganglionic neurons which is potentiated by PDE inhibitors and blocked by α-adrenergic antagonists.

2. Stimulation of preganglionic fibers leads to an increase in the cAMP content of the ganglia. This effect is potentiated by PDE inhibitors and antagonized by α-adrenergic antagonists as well as by muscarinic cholinergic antagonists. Nicotinic receptor antagonists do not prevent the rise in cAMP.

3. Stimulation of preganglionic fibers causes the three changes in synaptic potential shown in Fig. 1. Nicotinic antagonists prevent the f-EPSP but not the s-EPSP or the s-IPSP. Muscarinic inhibitors prevent the s-EPSP and s-IPSP but not the f-EPSP. Alpha-receptor inhibitors prevent only the s-IPSP. The effects of stimulation on the s-IPSP and s-EPSP are potentiated by PDE inhibitors.

4. Application of cholinomimetic drugs (carbachol, bethanechol) cause an increase in cAMP and cGMP in ganglia slices. This effect

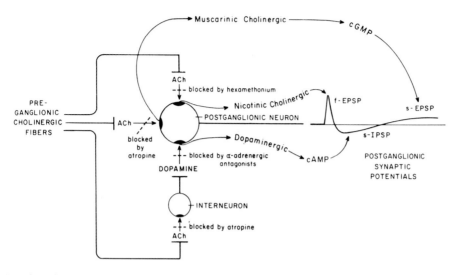

FIG. 1. A simplified schematic diagram of the principal synaptic connections in the mammalian superior cervical ganglion, and the postulated role of these connections in the genesis of the postganglionic synaptic potentials. The diagram shows the relationship between the various neuronal elements; the neurotransmitters released at the various synapses; the sensitivity of the synaptic receptors to different classes of specific antagonists; the electrical signs that accompany activation of the various postganglionic receptors following preganglionic stimulation; and the postulated involvement of cyclic nucleotides in the production of the electrophysiological responses. ACh, acetylcholine; cAMP, cyclic AMP; cGMP, cyclic GMP; f-EPSP, fast excitatory postsynaptic potential; s-IPSP, slow inhibitory postsynaptic potential; s-EPSP, slow excitatory postsynaptic potential. (Taken from Greengard, ref. 28.)

is blocked by muscarinic — but not by nicotinic-receptor antagonists.

5. Application of cAMP to ganglia causes a prolonged hyperpolarization characteristic of the s-IPSP while application of cGMP causes a prolonged depolarization characteristic of the s-EPSP. These effects are potentiated by PDE inhibitors.

6. Immunohistochemical methods demonstrate that dopamine causes an accumulation of cAMP selectively in postganglionic neurons.

Thus, building on previous knowledge of the anatomy and electrophysiological properties of the mammalian superior cervical ganglion, Greengard and his co-workers have utilized a variety of complementary experimental techniques to demonstrate the probable role of cyclic nucleotides in synaptic function. The ganglion is composed of a heterogeneous cell population and their experimental approach has necessarily been indirect. However, the good correlation between effects of a variety of probes on function and cyclic nucleotide content make alternate interpretations of these results unlikely.

Recent studies of the properties of the adenylate cyclase-linked dopamine receptor of cells in the caudate nucleus (13,28) coupled with the observations of Siggins et al. (53) that iontophoretic application of dopamine or cAMP depresses the spontaneous or drug-evoked discharges of neurons in the caudate nucleus indicate a similar function of cAMP in both peripheral and central neurons, i.e., inhibitory modulation of excitatory events. In fact, in each of the four neural systems studied to date, superior cervical ganglion (8,28,52), caudate nucleus (53,54), cerebellar Purkinje cells (7,54), and pyramidal tract neurons of the cerebral cortex (53,54,55) cAMP appears to subserve an inhibitory role. On the other hand, cGMP may serve an excitatory modulatory role in the superior cervical ganglion as well as in the cerebral cortex pyramidal tract cells (53). Bloom (54) presents a detailed discussion of work from his laboratory elsewhere in this volume.

MECHANISM BY WHICH CYCLIC NUCLEOTIDES ALTER NEURONAL FUNCTION

In mammalian systems the only thoroughly documented direct action of cyclic nucleotides is the activation of a class of protein kinases. Thus it is reasonable to assume that cyclic nucleotides may elicit their electrophysiological effects on neurons by activation of protein kinases. Greengard (28,52) has proposed a model of the mechanism by which cAMP acts as the mediator of dopaminergic transmission and thus as a modulator of cholinergic transmission in the superior sympathetic ganglion. Cyclic AMP is thought to activate a protein kinase located in the postsynaptic membrane. The activated kinase is then presumed to phosphorylate a specific protein component of the membrane leading to a change in the ion permeability of the membrane resulting in hyperpolarization (s-IPSP). Reversal of the process is thought to involve removal of the phosphate moiety by a specific phosphoprotein phosphatase. No evidence has been presented in support of the existence in the superior cervical ganglion of an appropriately located kinase or phosphatase, nor any evidence that membrane phosphorylation occurs in the presence of dopamine. However, Greengard and his colleagues (see 28,52) have accumulated some indirect evidence in other experimental preparations (cerebral cortex synaptic membranes, caudate nucleus membranes, frog bladder, and avian erythrocyte) for which there is evidence that cyclic nucleotides alter membrane permeability. Basically the evidence is of two kinds: (a) a demonstration in membrane fractions of the existence of cAMP or cGMP-dependent phosphorylation and dephosphorylation of a limited number of endogenous proteins by endogenous kinase(s) and phosphatase(s), respectively; (b) demonstration of phosphorylation of specific proteins upon addition to intact cell preparation of agents that specifically alter ion permeability. The results to date are consistent with the hypothesis that cAMP may alter neuronal function by altering the phosphorylation state of membrane proteins. However, basically what has been shown is that in homogenates, membrane preparations, or intact cells, when cAMP content rises, certain proteins become phosphorylated. In the nonneural systems phosphorylation occurs over the same time course as does the change in ion permeability; but, in the neural preparations, the changes in ion permeability occur much too rapidly to carry out the appropriate biochemical analysis of changes in phosphorylation.

There is currently no indication of the function of the phosphorylated proteins that have been observed. In the two neural preparations studied by Greengard and his co-workers to date, neurotransmitter-induced phosphorylation of specific membrane proteins has not been demonstrated. In fact the cell of origin of the cAMP-induced phosphorylated protein is not known with any assurance. Perhaps some support for the functional relevance of the phosphorylation can be gleaned from the fact that, in studies with caudate nucleus, the endogenous protein that underwent cAMP-dependent phosphorylation was localized in the same subcellular fraction that contained the dopamine-sensitive adenylate cyclase.

Thus, although significant progress has been made in establishing a role for cAMP as the mediator of the inhibitory effects of NE and dopamine in a number of neural systems, we are still quite naive in our understanding of the molecular events initiated by cAMP which result in altered ion permeability of postsynaptic membranes.

INVOLVEMENT OF CYCLIC NUCLEOTIDE IN PRESYNAPTIC PHENOMENA

Early observations by Breckenridge et al. (56) and Singer and Goldberg (6) suggested that cyclic nucleotides might also play a role in the regulation of release of acetylcholine by nerve endings at the neuromuscular junction. Singer and Goldberg (6) presented electrophysiological evidence that epinephrine, theophylline, and dibutyryl cAMP all increased the compound EPP elicited by nerve stimulation and increase the frequency of MEPPs and the quantal content of the EPP. Their preliminary results indicated that the selective β-receptor agonist isoproterenol did not have such effects on neuromuscular transmission. However, the use of specific receptor antagonists to further delineate the class of adrenergic receptor involved was not reported.

More recent studies by Miyamoto and Breckenridge (12) and by Wilson (11) indicate that cAMP is not a required factor in transmitter release but a regulatory factor whose actions are seen more prominently in fatigued nerve preparations. Although these workers agree that cAMP is not required for neuromuscular transmission, they do not agree on the mechanism of regulation. Miyamoto and Breckenridge analyzed MEPP frequency in unstimulated and KCl-treated nerve-muscle preparations and suggested that both catecholamines and dibutyryl cAMP increased MEPP frequency by accelerating the influx of calcium. On the other hand, Wilson analyzed various properties of EPPs evoked by nerve stimulation and concluded that neither theophylline nor dibutyryl cAMP affected calcium influx but acted to increase the releasable store of acetylcholine. He suggests that cAMP regulates metabolic activity in the nerve terminal that is associated with synthesis, mobilization, and storage of acetylcholine. Thus the precise role of cAMP in the catecholamine-induced increase in acetylcholine release is yet to be determined, as is the nature of the adrenergic receptor mediating the effect.

There is now substantial support for the theory that NE released at adrenergic nerve terminals regulates its own further release by interacting with α-receptors apparently located on the surface of the presynaptic membrane (57). An involvement of cAMP in potentiating the nerve stimulation-induced release of NE has recently been established (9,58). Wooten et al. (58) demonstrated an enhancement of the nerve stimulation-mediated release of NE and dopamine-β-hydroxylase (DBH) activity in the isolated guinea pig vas deferens preparation by dibutyryl cAMP or theophylline. Cubeddu et al. (9) have extended these studies in an examination of the role of cyclic nucleotides in the release of NE and DBH from the perfused cat spleen upon nerve stimulation. Analogues of cAMP (monobutyryl cAMP and 8-methylthio cAMP) as well as potent inhibitors of PDE activity (isobutylmethylxanthine and Ro-20–1724) enhanced nerve stimulation-induced release of NE and DBH. Of significance was the observation that synergistic effects on NE and DBH release were obtained with a combination of monobutyryl cAMP and RO-20–1724 at low concentrations; concentrations that did not have an effect when either drug was added alone. No significant effect of any of these agents was observed on spontaneous release of NE or DBH.

The α-blocker phentolamine was shown to potentiate markedly the release of NE and DBH, but the combination of phentolamine and either monobutyryl cAMP or a PDE inhibitor had no greater effect on release than phentolamine alone. Of some surprise was the observation that 8-bromo-cGMP had the same effect on release (potentiation) as did the cAMP analogues. Unfortunately, 8-bromo-cGMP apparently was tested only at concentrations of 10 and 100 μM. Goldberg et al. (22) have demonstrated that high concentrations of cGMP or cGMP analogues can mimic effects of cAMP. Thus, in Yin-Yang, bidirectional control systems where the effects of cAMP are dominant, high concentrations of cGMP may produce the same effect as cAMP, but low concentrations may produce the opposite effect, i.e., act as a true mimic of endogenous cGMP. It would be of interest to examine the effect of low concentrations of cGMP on the release of NE and DBH in the presence of phentolamine. Under this condition, one should see the greatest sensitivity to cGMP if in fact cGMP mediates the inhibition of release caused by NE acting on presynaptic α-receptors. It is interesting to note that in both adrenergic nerves and cholinergic nerves cyclic nucleotides do not seem to be required for release of the neurotransmitter. They appear to be involved in the regulation of release by yet to be determined mechanisms.

CONCLUSIONS

To the extent that it is now apparent, cyclic nucleotides play the same fundamental role in the nervous system as in other organ systems, as intracellular mediators of the actions of extracellular effectors. In specific neurons of the superior cervical ganglion, cerebellum, cerebral cortex, and caudate nucleus, cAMP has been shown to mediate inhibitory influences of catecholamines. Although less extensively studied, cGMP appears to mediate excitatory influences; and in the postganglionic adrenergic neuron and in the pyramidal tract cells of the cerebral cortex, cAMP and cGMP have demonstrable opposing actions on neuronal function. It will be of interest to determine if all the various substances that have been shown to elicit a rise in cAMP content in brain slices also have inhibitory influences on neuronal activity. In that regard Phillis et al. (55) have recently demonstrated that adenosine has potent inhibitory effects on the spontaneous electrical activity of certain pyramidal tract cells (Betz cells) in the cerebral cortex.

It is clear from their effects on the electrical properties of neurons that cyclic nucleotides mediate changes in ion permeability. However, there is only a limited amount of indirect evidence that indicates the molecular events leading to such changes. As is the case for most types of cells, that sequence of events initiated by stimulators of adenylate cyclase that occurs after the activation of the cyclic nucleotide-dependent protein kinase remains essentially unknown.

With regard to future directions for research it seems apparent that the combination of pharmacological, biochemical, and electrophysiological techniques should continue to provide the most fruitful approach to the analysis of a mediatory role for cyclic nucleotides in neuronal function. Unfortunately, to date, such an approach has been undertaken on a large scale by only a few laboratories.

The extreme cellular heterogeneity of the CNS remains as a problem that markedly limits progress. Although immunofluorescence techniques have been used to advantage for the demonstration of the cellular location of cyclic nucleotides in heterogeneous tissues, the resolving power of this procedure is limited. The availability of a histochemical method for the demonstration of cAMP and cGMP at the electronmicroscopic level would be a significant advance.

Finally, the long-range goal of reconstituting a functioning neural system from its fully characterized component parts seems a long way off. A great deal of progress has been made in the culturing of nervous system tissue, but homogeneous populations of functioning neurons are not yet available in sufficient quantity to allow biochemical analyses. The fundamental limitation remains unresolved—primary cultures of nervous tissue are usually composed of mixed populations of functional neurons, whereas transformed neuroblasts can be obtained as clonal lines but they do not retain sufficient differentiated function.

ACKNOWLEDGMENT

Studies from the author's laboratory mentioned in this article were supported by U.S. Public Health Service Grant NS10233 from the National Institute of Neurological Diseases and Stroke and were conducted in collaboration with R. B. Clark, A. Kalisker, R. Ortmann, Y. F. Su, G. L. Johnson, and M. M. Moore.

REFERENCES

1. Robison, G. A., Butcher, R. W., and Sutherland, E. W. (1971): *Cyclic AMP*. Academic Press, New York.
2. Klainer, L. M., Chi, Y.- M., Friedberg, S. L., Rall, T. W., and Sutherland, E. W. (1962): Adenyl Cyclase IV. The effects of neurohormones on the formation of adenosine 3':5'-phosphate by preparations from brain and other tissues. *J. Biol. Chem.*, 237:1239–1243.
3. Forn, J., and Krishna, G. (1971): Effect of norepinephrine; histamine and other drugs on cyclic 3':5'-AMP formation in brain slices of various animals species. *Pharmacology*, 5:193–204.
4. Sattin, A., and Rall, T. W. (1970): The effect of adenosine and adenine nucleotides on the cyclic adenosine 3':5'-phosphate content of guinea pig cerebral cortex slices. *Mol. Pharmacol.*, 6:13–23.
5. Shoemaker, W. J., Balentine, L. T., Siggins, G. R., Hoffer, B. J., Henriksen, S. J., and Bloom, F. E. (1975): Characteristics of the release of adenosine 3':5'-monophosphate from micropipets by microiontophoresis. *J. Cyc. Nucl. Res.*, 1:97–106.
6. Singer, J. J., and Goldberg, A. L. (1970): Cyclic AMP and transmission at the neuromuscular junction. In: *Advances in Biochemical Psychopharmacology, Vol. 3*, edited by E. Costa and P. Greengard, pp. 335–348. Raven Press, New York.
7. Hoffer, B. J., Siggins, G. R., Oliver, A. P., and Bloom, F. E. (1971): Cyclic AMP mediation of norepinephrine inhibition in rat cerebellar cortex: A unique class of synaptic responses. *Ann. N.Y. Acad. Sci.*, 185:531–549.
8. McAfee, D. A., and Greengard, P. (1972): Adenosine 3':5'-monophosphate: Electrophysiological evidence for a role in synaptic transmission. *Science*, 178:310–312.
9. Cubeddu, L. X., Barnes, E., and Weiner, N. (1975): Release of norepinephrine and dopamine-β-hydroxylase by nerve stimulation IV. An evaluation of a role for cyclic adenosine monophosphate. *J. Pharmacol. Exp. Ther.*, 193:105–127.
10. Rall, T. W., and Sattin, A. (1970): Factors influencing the accumulation of cyclic AMP in brain tissue. In: *Advances in Biochemical Psychopharmacology, Vol. 3*, edited by E. Costa and P. Greengard, pp. 113–133. Raven Press, New York.
11. Wilson, D. F. (1974): The effects of dibutyryl cyclic adenosine 3':5'-monophosphate, theophylline and aminophylline on neuromuscular transmission in the rat. *J. Pharmacol. Exp. Ther.*, 188: 447–452.
12. Miyamoto, M. D., and Breckenridge, B. (1974): A cyclic adenosine monophosphate link in the catecholamine enhancement of transmitter re-

lease at the neuromuscular junction. *J. Gen. Physiol.*, 63:609–624.

13. Kebabian, J. W., Petzold, G., and Greengard, P. (1972): Dopamine-sensitive adenylate cyclase in the caudate nucleus of the rat brain and its similarity to the "dopamine-receptor." *Proc. Natl. Acad. Sci. USA*, 69:2145–2149.

14. Chasin, M., Mamrak, F., and Samaniego, S. G. (1974): Preparation and properties of a cell-free, hormonally responsive adenylate cyclase from guinea pig brain. *J. Neurochem.*, 22:1031–1038.

15. Shimizu, H., Ichishita, H., and Mizokami, Y. (1975): Stimulation of the cell-free adenylate cyclase from guinea pig cerebral cortex by acidic amino acids and veratridine. *J. Cyc. Nucl. Res.*, 1:61–67.

16. Brostrom, C. O., Huang, Y.-C., Breckenridge, B., and Wolff, D. J. (1975): Identification of a calcium-binding protein as a calcium-dependent regulator of brain adenylate cyclase. *Proc. Natl. Acad. Sci. USA*, 72:64–68.

17. Kakiuchi, S. (1975): Ca^{2+} plus Mg^{2+}-dependent phosphodiesterase and its modulator from various rat tissues. In: *Advances in Cyclic Nucleotide Research, Vol. 5*, edited by G. I. Drummond, P. Greengard, and G. A. Robison. Raven Press, New York.

18. Perkins, J. P. (1973): Adenyl cyclase. In: *Advances in Cyclic Nucleotide Research, Vol. 3*, edited by P. Greengard and G. A. Robison, pp. 1–64. Raven Press, New York.

19. Weiss, B., and Kidman, A. D. (1969): Neurobiological significance of cyclic 3':5'-adenosine monophosphate. In: *Advances in Biochemical Psychopharmacology, Vol. 1*, edited by E. Costa and P. Greengard, pp. 131–164. Raven Press, New York.

20. Rall, T. W., and Gilman, A. G. (1971): The role of cyclic AMP in the nervous system. In: *Neurosciences Research Symposium Summaries, Vol. 5*, edited by F. O. Schmitt, G. Adelman, T. Melnechuk, and F. G. Worden, pp. 215–311. MIT Press, Cambridge, Mass.

21. Daly, J. W., Huang, M., and Shimizu, H. (1972): Regulation of cyclic AMP levels in brain tissue. In: *Advances in Cyclic Nucleotide Research, Vol. 1*, edited by P. Greengard, R. Paoletti, and G. A. Robison, pp. 375–388. Raven Press, New York.

22. Goldberg, N. D., O'Dea, R. F., and Haddox, M. K. (1973): Cyclic GMP. In: *Advances in Cyclic Nucleotide Research, Vol. 3*, edited by P. Greengard and G. A. Robison, pp. 155–224. Raven Press, New York.

23. Breckenridge, B., and Johnson, R. E. (1969): Cyclic 3':5'-nucleotide phosphodiesterase in brain. *J. Histochem. Cytochem.*, 17:505–511.

24. Weiss, B., and Costa, E. (1968): Regional and subcellular distribution of adenyl cyclase and 3':5'-cyclic nucleotide phosphodiesterase in brain and pineal gland. *Biochem. Pharmacol.*, 17: 2107–2116.

25. Appleman, M. M., Thompson, W. J., and Russell, T. R. (1973): Cyclic nucleotide phosphodiester-

ase In: *Advances in Cyclic Nucleotide Research, Vol. 3*, edited by P. Greengard and G. A. Robison, pp. 65–98. Raven Press, New York.

26. Maeno, H., Johnson, E. M., and Greengard, P. (1971): Subcellular distribution of adenosine 3':5'-monophosphate-dependent protein kinase in rat brain. *J. Biol. Chem.*, 246:134–142.

27. Kuo, J. F. (1974): Guanosine 3':5'-monophosphate-dependent protein kinases in mammalian tissues. *Proc. Natl. Acad. Sci. USA*, 71:4037–4041.

28. Greengard, P. (1975): Cyclic nucleotides, protein phosphorylation, and neuronal function. In: *Advances in Cyclic Nucleotide Research, Vol. 5*, edited by G. I. Drummond, P. Greengard, and G. A. Robison. Raven Press, New York.

29. Maeno, H., and Greengard, P. (1972): Phosphoprotein phosphatase from rat cerebral cortex: Subcellular distribution and characterization. *J. Biol. Chem.*, 247:3269–3277.

30. Kakiuchi, S., and Rall, T. W. (1968): The influence of chemical agents on the accumulation of adenosine 3':5'-phosphate in slices of rabbit cerebellum. *Mol. Pharmacol.*, 4:367–378.

31. Kakiuchi, S., and Rall, T. W. (1968): Studies on adenosine 3':5'-phosphate in rabbit cerebral cortex. *Mol. Pharmacol.*, 4:379–388.

32. Shimizu, H., Creveling, C. R., and Daly, J. W. (1970): Effect of membrane depolarization and biogenic amines on the formation of cyclic AMP in incubated brain slices. In: *Advances in Biochemical Psychopharmacology, Vol. 3*, edited by E. Costa and P. Greengard, pp. 135–154. Raven Press, New York.

33. Krishna, G., Forn, J., Voigt, K., Paul, M., and Gessa, G. L. (1970): Dynamic aspects of neurohormonal control of cyclic 3':5'-AMP synthesis in brain. In: *Advances in Biochemical Psychopharmacology, Vol. 3*, edited by E. Costa and P. Greengard, pp. 155–172. Raven Press, New York.

34. Daly, J. W. (1973): Regulation of cyclic AMP levels in brain. In: *Frontiers in Catecholamine Research*, edited by E. Usdin and S. Snyder, pp. 301–306. Pergamon Press, New York.

35. Perkins, J. P., Moore, M. M., Kalisker, A., and Su, Y. F. (1975): Regulation of cyclic AMP content in normal and malignant brain cells. In: *Advances in Cyclic Nucleotide Research, Vol. 5*, edited by G. I. Drummond, P. Greengard, and G. A. Robison. Raven Press, New York.

36. Sattin, A., Rall, T. W., and Zanella, J. (1975): Regulation of cyclic adenosine 3':5'-monophosphate levels in guinea pig cerebral cortex by interaction of alpha adrenergic and adenosine receptor activity. *J. Pharmacol. Exp. Ther.*, 192:22–32.

37. Chasin, M., Rivkin, I., Mamrak, F., Samaniego, S. G., and Hess, S. M. (1971): α and β-adrenergic receptors as mediators of accumulation of cyclic adenosine 3':5'-monophosphate in specific areas of guinea pig brain. *J. Biol. Chem.*, 246:3037–3041.

38. Burnstock, G. (1972): Purinergic nerves. *Pharmacol. Rev.*, 24:509–581.

39. Shimizu, H., Ichishita, H., and Odagiri, H. (1974): Stimulated formation of cyclic adenosine 3':5'-monophosphate by aspartate and glutamate in cerebral cortical slices of guinea pig. *J. Biol. Chem.,* 249:5955–5962.

40. Gilman, A. G., and Schrier, B. K. (1972): Adenosine cyclic 3':5'-monophosphate in fetal rat brain cell cultures. I. Effect of catecholamines. *Mol. Pharmacol.,* 8:410–416.

41. Sidman, R. L. (1970): Cell proliferation, migration and interaction in the developing mammalian central nervous system. In: *Neurosciences Second Study Program,* edited by F. O. Schmitt. Rockefeller University Press, New York.

42. Gilman, A. G. (1972): Regulation of cyclic AMP metabolism in cultured cells of the nervous system. In: *Advances in Cyclic Nucleotide Research, Vol. 1,* edited by P. Greengard, R. Paoletti, and G. A. Robison, pp. 389–410. Raven Press, New York.

43. Hamprecht, B., and Schultz, J. (1973): Stimulation by prostaglandin E_1 of adenosine 3':5'-cyclic monophosphate formation in neuroblastoma cells in the presence of phosphodiesterase inhibitors. *FEBS Lett.,* 34:85–89.

44. Blume, A. J., Dalton, C., and Sheppard, H. (1973): Adenosine-mediated elevation of cyclic 3':5'-adenosine monophosphate concentrations in cultured mouse neuroblastoma cells. *Proc. Natl. Acad. Sci. USA,* 70:3099–3102.

45. Prasad, K. N., Gilmer, K., and Kumar, S. (1973): Morphologically "differentiated" mouse neuroblastoma cells induced by non-cyclic AMP agents: Levels of cyclic AMP, nucleic acid and protein *Proc. Soc. Exp. Biol. Med.,* 143:1168–1171.

46. Prasad, K. N., Sahu, S. K., and Kumar, S. (1975): Relationship between cyclic AMP and differentiation of neuroblastoma cells in culture. In: *Differentiation and Control of Malignancy of Tumor Cells,* pp. 287–309. Gann Monograph on Cancer Research, Tokyo.

47. Prasad, K. N., Gilmer, K., and Sahu, S. K. (1974): Demonstration of acetylcholine-sensitive adenyl cyclase in malignant neuroblastoma cells in culture. *Nature,* 249:765–767.

48. Sahu, S. K., and Prasad, K. N. (1975): Effect of neurotransmitters and prostaglandin E_1 on cyclic AMP levels in various clones of neuroblastoma cells in culture. *J. Neurochem., in press.*

49. Sharma, S. K., Nirenberg, M., and Klee, W. A. (1975): Morphine receptors as regulators of adenylate cyclase activity. *Proc. Natl. Acad. Sci. USA,* 72:590–594.

50. De Vellis, J., and Brooker, G. (1973): Induction of enzymes by glucocorticoids and catecholamines in a rat glial cell line. In: *Tissue Culture of the Nervous System,* edited by G. Sato, pp. 231–245. Plenum Press, New York.

51. Clark, R. B., Su, Y. F., Ortmann, R., Cubeddu, L. X., Johnson, G. L., and Perkins, J. P. (1975): Factors influencing the effect of hormones on the accumulation of cyclic AMP in cultured human astrocytoma cells. *Metabolism,* 24:343–358.

52. Siggins, G. R., Hoffer, B. J., and Ungerstedt, U. (1974): Electrophysiological evidence for involvement of cyclic adenosine monophosphate in dopamine responses of caudate nucleus. *Life Sci.,* 15:779–792.

53. Stone, T. W., Taylor, D. A., and Bloom, F. E. (1975): Cyclic AMP and Cyclic GMP may mediate opposite neuronal responses in the rat cerebral cortex. *Science,* 187:845–847.

54. Bloom, F. E. (1975): In: *This Volume.*

55. Phillis, J. W., Kostopoulas, G. K., and Limacher, J. J. (1975): A potent depressant action of adenine derivatives on cerebral cortical neurons. *Eur. J. Pharmacol.,* 30:125–129.

56. Breckenridge, B. M., Burn, J. H., and Matschinsky, F. M. (1967): Theophylline, epinephrine, and neostigmine facilitation of neuromuscular transmission. *Proc. Natl. Acad. Sci. USA.,* 57:1893–1897.

57. Langer, S. Z. (1973): The regulation of transmitter release elicited by nerve stimulation through a presynaptic feedback mechanism. In: *Frontiers in Catecholamines Research,* edited by E. Usdin and S. Snyder, pp. 543–549. Pergamon Press, New York.

58. Wooten, F. G., Thoa, N. B., Kopin, I. J., and Axelrod, J. (1973): Enhanced release of dopamine-β-hydroxylase and norepinephrine from sympathetic nerves by dibutyryl cyclic adenosine 3':5'-monophosphate and theophylline. *Mol. Pharmacol.,* 9:178–183.

The Nervous System, Donald B. Tower, Editor-in-Chief. *Vol. 1: The Basic Neurosciences.* Raven Press, New York, 1975.

The Pineal Gland: A Model to Study the Regulation of the β-Adrenergic Receptor

Julius Axelrod

After a long period of neglect the pineal gland has become a subject of considerable interest to neurobiologists. Over the past decade this tissue has proved to be a productive experimental model for the study of biological rhythms and the interaction between neurotransmitters and excitable cells. The pineal gland has been shown to be involved in the pigmentation of fish and amphibians, gonadal function, and light reception (1). The ability of extracts of pineal glands to blanch the skin of tadpoles led Lerner and his co-workers (2) to isolate the skin-lightening principle. With use of a variety of separation techniques, the skin-lightening principle of the pineal was separated and identified as 5-methoxy-N-acetyltryptamine (melatonin). The isolation and characterization of melatonin initiated a new era in pineal gland research.

The availability of melatonin made it possible to examine its physiological activities. Melatonin is the most potent agent for causing contractions of melanophores in frog and fish skin (1). This indole exerts inhibitory effects on gonads; it delays vaginal opening and reduces ovarian weight in young rats (1). When implanted in the median eminence of the rat it lowers the luteinizing hormone (LH) concentration in plasma and blocks the rise of LH in the pituitary (3). During proestrus, melatonin inhibits ovulation by preventing the release of LH. The early-morning surge in plasma prolactin is mediated by an increased release of a still unidentified pineal hormone (4). Blinding male hamsters causes a fall in testes weight, but when pineals are removed or when sympathetic nerves to the pineal are cut, the fall in testes weight is prevented (5). The pineal can serve as a time-measuring device in birds (6).

β-ADRENERGIC RECEPTORS AND REGULATION OF INDOLE METABOLISM IN THE PINEAL

The mammalian pineal gland is heavily innervated by sympathetic nerves arising from the superior cervical ganglia (7) and contains high levels of norepinephrine, serotonin, and histamine (8). Our interest in the pineal was stimulated by high levels of serotonin and the presence of the methoxyindole melatonin. We soon found the two enzymes involved in the biosynthesis of melatonin in the pineal: serotonin N-acetyltransferase (9) and hydroxyindole-O-methyltransferase (HIOMT) (10). The N-acetyltransferase was found to be the critical enzyme that was regulated by sympathetic nerves as will be shown later. HIOMT, the enzyme involved in the final step in melatonin synthesis, is highly localized in the pineal cell of animals. The biosynthesis of melatonin in the pineal cell is shown to proceed as follows: tryptophan → 5-hydroxytryptophan → serotonin → N-acetylserotonin → melatonin. The initial step is catalyzed by tryptophan hydroxylase, the second by l-aromatic amino acid decarboxylase, the third by N-acetyltransferase, and the final step by HIOMT.

The role of sympathetic nerves in the regulation of melatonin synthesis was first examined by studying the effects of light and darkness on pineal HIOMT activity. It had been observed that continuous light causes an increase in the incidence of estrus in rats. This effect of light is abolished by an injection of melatonin (1). Thus, it appeared that the increased incidence of estrus in rats kept in light might be due to a decreased formation of the inhibitory hormone (melatonin). There was a marked reduction in pineal HIOMT activity when rats were left in constant light, as compared to those left in constant darkness (11). This indicated that continuous light reduces the activity of HIOMT which then leads to less melatonin synthesis. A decrease in the synthesis of the inhibitory hormone melatonin would result in the increased incidence of estrus.

The pineal gland lies deep between the two cerebral hemispheres of the rat, and it appeared that information about environmental lighting might reach the pineal via a neural route. Neural impulses reaching the pineal can be readily abolished by the bilateral removal of the superior cervical ganglia. When rats were ganglionectomized, the difference in HIOMT activity in rats exposed to continuous light and darkness was abolished (11). Blinding of rats also had the same effects as denervation. All of these experiments implicated the retina and the norepinephrine-containing sympathetic nerves in the regulation of melatonin synthesis.

These experiments raised a number of questions. If norepinephrine released from sympathetic nerves regulates melatonin formation, does it do it by stimulating α- or β-adrenergic receptors? Is adenylate cyclase involved, and what is the critical step that is regulated in the synthesis of melatonin from tryptophan? To answer these questions, a pineal organ culture system was developed that was able to carry out all of the steps in the synthesis of melatonin from tryptophan (12). The addition of radioactive tryptophan to the pineal culture medium resulted in the formation of serotonin, N-acetylserotonin, and melatonin. The protein synthesis inhibitor cyclohexamide blocked the synthesis of melatonin as well as of the intermediate steps, indicating that new enzyme protein is necessary for the formation of melatonin in organ culture. The rat pineal cultured in vitro made it possible to elucidate the mechanisms of regulation of the synthesis of a hormone by a neurotransmitter. The addition of l-norepinephrine to the pineal organ culture caused a marked stimulation of melatonin synthesis from tryptophan (13). The increased formation of melatonin by norepinephrine was prevented by propranolol, a β-adrenergic blocking agent, but not by α-adrenergic blocking agents. Many biological actions are initiated by the action of norepinephrine on the β-adrenergic receptor which in turn stimu-

lates the synthesis of cyclic AMP by adenylate cyclase. It was not surprising that dibutyryl cyclic AMP was found to markedly stimulate the formation of ^{14}C-melatonin from ^{14}C-tryptophan. These results indicate that norepinephrine released from sympathetic nerves stimulates a β-adrenergic receptor on the pineal cell membrane. This then caused an activation of adenylate cyclase inside the cell to form cyclic AMP from ATP (Fig. 1).

The specific enzyme regulated by the β-adrenergic receptor was found to be N-acetyltransferase, the enzyme that converts serotonin to N-acetylserotonin. This latter compound serves as the substrate for HIOMT, that forms melatonin. Dibutyryl cyclic AMP, norepinephrine, and isoproterenol stimulated the formation of N-acetyltransferase in pineal organ culture (14). The elevation of N-acetyltransferase by cyclic nucleotides or catecholamines was blocked by protein synthesis inhibition.

The temporal relationship between stimulation of the β-adrenergic receptor, cyclic AMP, and the induction of N-acetyltransferase in the rat pineal was examined in vivo (15). Injection of l-isoproterenol during the daytime (when the enzyme levels are low), resulted in a 15-fold increase in pineal cyclic AMP levels within 2 min, reached a maximum in 10 min, and returned to baseline level 30 min after the administration of the catecholamine. One hour following the injection of isoproterenol and 30 min after cyclic AMP returned to its low baseline level, N-acetyltransferase showed its initial rise. The enzyme

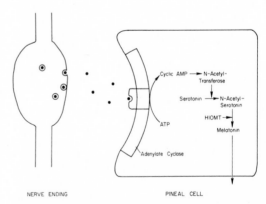

FIG. 1. Stimulation of the β-adrenergic receptor in pineal cell by the neurotransmitter norepinephrine and the subsequent synthesis of the hormone melatonin.

reached a peak 2 hr later and then returned to its low daytime level 2 hr later. Propranolol injected before isoproterenol prevented the elevation of both cyclic AMP and N-acetyltransferase activity. When the β-adrenergic blocking agent was given 1 hr after isoproterenol – at a time when cyclic AMP had risen and fallen to its low baseline level – the elevation in N-acetyltransferase was still prevented. The injection of a protein synthesis inhibitor, cyclohexamide, before the administration of the catecholamine, blocked the induction of N-acetyltransferase but allowed the rise and fall of cyclic AMP to proceed in a normal manner. When cyclohexamide was administered 1 hr after isoproterenol and after the rise and fall of cyclic AMP, the formation of N-acetyltransferase was still blocked. These experiments demonstrated that isoproterenol (and presumably norepinephrine released from nerve terminals) stimulates a β-adrenergic receptor (Fig. 1). The binding of the catecholamine to the β-adrenergic receptor on the outside of the pineal cell membrane then activates the adenylate cyclase on the inner membrane. This in turn converts ATP to cyclic AMP. The cyclic AMP induces the synthesis of new N-acetyltransferase (Fig. 1). Recent studies in our laboratory have demonstrated that cyclic AMP acts at both transcriptional and translational sites in N-acetyltransferase synthesis.

SUPERSENSITIVITY AND SUBSENSITIVITY OF THE β-ADRENERGIC RECEPTOR OF THE PINEAL

Changes in the responsiveness of excitable membranes are still poorly understood. After denervation or administration of drugs that deplete biogenic amines, there is a marked increase in the responsiveness of postsynaptic membranes. Administration of cocaine causes an increase in response to norepinephrine. This supersensitivity is due to the ability of cocaine to block reuptake of the catecholamines by sympathetic nerves, an important mechanism for the inactivation of neurotransmitters (16). Thus, supersensitivity can result from presynaptic and postsynaptic events. Recent work with the pineal gland has uncovered ways in which postsynaptic β-adrenergic receptors can be modified.

During daytime the activity of N-acetyltrans-

ferase in the pineal is low (14). After the injection of catecholamines such as norepinephrine or isoproterenol, a 20- to 30-fold increase in enzyme activity results (17). When the pineal is denervated surgically by the unilateral removal of the superior cervical ganglion or chemically by the injection of 6-hydroxydopamine, the administration of catecholamines caused a 100-fold increase in N-acetyltransferase. This enhanced induction of the enzyme after denervation is blocked by propranolol. This finding demonstrates that denervation causes a supersensitivity of the pineal β-adrenergic receptor in inducing N-acetyltransferase activity.

The supersensitivity of the pineal β-adrenergic receptor after sympathetic nerve denervation might be due to the absence of the nerve or to the depletion of its neurotransmitter norepinephrine. To test this possibility, sympathetic nerves were depleted of their norepinephrine by an injection of reserpine. The administration of isoproterenol caused a increased induction of N-acetyltransferase in these reserpine-treated rats. Supersensitivity resulting from reserpine treatment developed very rapidly, in less than 1 day. Light reduces the release of neurotransmitter. Prolonged exposure of rats to light resulted in a supersensitive response of the pineal. Thus, the reduced firing of nerves can cause a supersensitive response in the induction of N-acetyltransferase by isoproterenol. Supersensitivity of the pineal β-adrenergic receptor after the rat was subject to denervation, reserpine treatment, or light exposure was also shown in pineal culture in vitro as well as in vivo.

The observation that reduced exposure of b-adrenergic receptor to the neurotransmitter norepinephrine causes supersensitivity suggested that this hyperresponsiveness could be overcome by the administration of a catecholamine (17). The repeated administration of isoproterenol to denervated or reserpine-treated rats not only suppressed the superinduction of N-acetyltransferase but also profoundly reduced the induction of the enzyme when the pineal was later removed and stimulated with catecholamines in organ culture. These observations indicated that a reduced exposure of the postjunctional β-adrenergic receptor to catecholamines results in an increased responsiveness while increased exposure results in subsensitivity. Thus, super- and subsensitivity of responsive cells are opposite poles of the same phenomenon.

Depletion of catecholamine neurotransmitter by treatment with reserpine or denervation also causes a greater increase in cyclic AMP as compared to the intact pineal. Experiments using dibutyryl cyclic AMP instead of isoproterenol to induce N-acetyltransferase showed that super- and subsensitivity occurs at two sites in the pineal cell, one in the cell membrane β-adrenergic receptor and another in an intracellular site.

CIRCADIAN RHYTHMS IN THE PINEAL GLAND

The pineal gland has high levels of serotonin, which is about equally divided between the parenchymal cell and sympathetic nerve terminals. Soon after the discovery of serotonin in the pineal, Quay (18) observed a circadian rhythm of this biogenic amine in the rat pineal gland. Under normal lighting conditions, serotonin levels are highest about midday and fall rapidly soon after the onset of darkness. To determine the driving mechanism for the 24-hr rhythm in pineal serotonin, we kept rats in continuous darkness or light. When rats were left in continuous darkness, the serotonin rhythm persisted with about a 24-hr cycle (19). These findings indicated that the serotonin rhythm in the pineal was circadian and driven by an internal clock. The rhythm was abolished when rats were left in constant light. The circadian rhythm of serotonin can be turned around about 180° by placing the rats in an artifically reversed lighting environment. This indicated that even though the serotonin rhythm is endogenous, environmental lighting can serve as a synchronizer.

In a series of experiments it was established that the pineal serotonin rhythm is controlled by a nervous pathway (19). Denervation of the pineal by removal of the superior cervical ganglia abolished the pineal serotonin rhythm. Decentralization of the superior cervical ganglia or depletion of brain biogenic amine by reserpine also repressed this pineal circadian rhythm. These observations suggested that biogenic amine-containing nerve tracts in the brain control the serotonin rhythm.

There are also circadian rhythms in pineal N-acetylserotonin, melatonin, N-acetyltransferase, and hydroxyindole-O-methyltransferase which are approximately 180° out of phase with that of serotonin. One hour after the onset of darkness there is about a 30-fold increase in N-acetyltransferase activity in the pineal followed by a smaller elevation of N-acetylserotonin and melatonin. The rhythm in pineal N-acetyltransferase persists in continuous darkness and is suppressed in continuous light (14). The enzyme rhythm is abolished by denervation of the sympathetic nerve to the pineal or by interrupting nerve impulses from the brain. Recent work has shown that lesions that destroy the suprachiasmatic nucleus will eliminate the circadian rhythm of pineal N-acetyltransferase (20). Cutting the nerve tracts leaving suprachiasmatic nucleus will also abolish this rhythm but interrupting tracts entering this nucleus does not.

These observations suggest that the biological clock in the brain that generates circadian rhythm in the pineal is located in or near the suprachiasmatic nucleus.

The observation that circadian rhythms in pineal serotonin and N-acetyltransferase are prevented by cutting sympathetic nerves to the pineal suggested that these rhythms might be driven by diurnal changes in the release of the neurotransmitter norepinephrine. A 24-hr rhythm in the turnover of norepinephrine in sympathetic nerves in the pineal was demonstrated (21). This rhythm in turnover of norepinephrine persisted in blinded rats and was suppressed in continuous light. This suggested that the circadian rhythm of N-acetyltransferase in the pineal cell is generated by day and night changes in the turnover and presumably the release of norepinephrine. The role of the catecholamine neurotransmitter in driving the circadian rhythms in the pineal was established by a series of experiments *in vivo* (22). Exposing animals to light (reducing the release of norepinephrine) or interrupting sympathetic nerve impulses by ganglionectomy or decentralization prevented the night-time elevation of N-acetyltransferase. The administration of the β-adrenergic blocking agent propranolol or the biogenic amine depletor reserpine also suppressed the circadian rhythm of N-acetyltransferase. The protein synthesis inhibitor cyclohexamide, when injected immediately before darkness, abolished the rise of N-acetyltransferase. These experiments demonstrate that the increased release of norepinephrine at the onset of darkness stimulated the β-adrenergic receptor in the pineal cell. This in turn initiates events that lead to the synthesis of new N-acetyltransferase molecules. The rise in N-acetyltransferase during the night results in a fall in the substrate for this enzyme, serotonin, and an elevation of its product N-acetylserotonin (23). The rise in N-acetylserotonin at night causes an increased formation of melatonin by HIOMT. These events are reversed during the daytime. Thus the driving mechanism for the circadian rhythms of indole in the pineal are the changes in N-acetyltransferase which in turn are controlled by the β-adrenergic receptor. Exposure of rats to a few minutes of light during the night or the administration of propranolol results in a precipitous fall in N-acetyltransferase activity. Injection of isoproterenol prevents the fall of the enzyme. Thus, maintenance of N-acetyltransferase activity requires the continuous occupation of the β-adrenergic receptor on the cell surface.

A diurnal rhythm in the responsiveness of pinealocytes to β-adrenergic stimulation was also observed (24). Pineals were removed from rats housed in diurnal lighting in various times of the day. The pineals were then cultured *in vitro* in the presence of isoproterenol and the increase in N-acetyltransferase measured. The longer the rat was exposed to daylight and decreased sympathetic activity, the more responsive the pineal became to isoproterenol in its induction of N-acetyltransferase. Thus a 30-to-40-fold rise in enzyme activity after the onset of darkness can be caused by a small increase in the concentration of the neurotransmitter onto a supersensitive β-adrenergic receptor. The fall in enzyme activity late at night could result from a decreased sensitivity of the receptor and decreased nerve firing. Changes in the same direction in signal intensity and receptor sensitivity could serve as an effective amplification and dampening system.

REFERENCES

1. Wurtman, R. J., Axelrod, J., and Kelly, D. (1968): *The Pineal.* Academic Press, New York.
2. Lerner, A. B., Case, J. C., Takahashi, Y., Lee, T. H., and Mori, W. (1958): Isolation of mela-

tonin, the pineal gland factor that lightens melanocytes. *J. Am. Chem. Soc.,* 80:2587.
3. Fraschini, F., Collu, R., and Martini, L. (1971): Mechanisms of inhibitory action of pineal principles on gonadotropin secretion. In: *Ciba Foundation Symposium on the Pineal Gland,* edited by G. E. W. Wolstenholme and J. Knight, pp. 259–273. Churchill Livingstone, London.
4. Ronnekleiv, O. K., Krulich, L., and McCann, S. M. (1973): An early morning surge of prolactin in the male rat and its abolition by pinealectomy. *Endocrinology,* 92:1339–1342.
5. Reiter, R. J., and Sorrentino, S., Jr. (1971): Factors influential in determining the gonad-inhibiting activity of the pineal gland. In: *Ciba Foundation Symposium on the Pineal Gland,* edited by G. E. W. Wolstenholme and J. Knight, pp. 329–340. Churchill Livingstone, London.
6. Gaston, S., and Menaker, M. (1968): Pineal function: The biological clock in the sparrow? *Science,* 160:1125–1127.
7. Kappers, J. A. (1960): The development, topographical relations and innervation of the epiphysis cerebri in the albino rat. *Z. Zellforsch. Mikrosk. Anat.,* 52:163–215.
8. Giarman, N. J., and Day, N. (1959): Presence of biogenic amines in the bovine pineal body. *Biochem. Pharmacol.,* 1:235.
9. Weissbach, H., Redfield, B. G., and Axelrod, J. (1960): Biosynthesis of melatonin: Enzymic conversion of serotonin to N-acetylserotonin. *Biochim. Biophys Acta,* 43:352–353.
10. Axelrod, J., and Weissbach, H. (1961): Purification and properties of hydroxyindole-O-methyltransferase *J. Biol. Chem.,* 236:211–213.
11. Axelrod, J., Wurtman, R. J., and Snyder, S. H. (1965): Control of hydroxyindole O-methyltransferase activity in the rat pineal gland by environmental lighting. *J. Biol. Chem.,* 240:949–954.
12. Wurtman, R. J., Larin, F., Axelrod, J., Shein, H. M., and Rosasco, K. (1968): Formation of melatonin and 5-hydroxyindoleacetic acid from ^{14}C-tryptophan by rat pineal glands in organ culture. *Nature,* 217:953–954.
13. Axelrod, J., Shein, H. M., and Wurtman, R. J. (1969): Stimulation of C^{14}-melatonin synthesis from C^{14}-tryptophan by noradrenaline in rat pineal in organ culture. *Proc. Natl. Acad. Sci. USA,* 62:544–549.
14. Klein, D. C. (1974): Circadian rhythms in indole metabolism in the rat pineal glands. In: *The Neurosciences, Third Study Program,* edited by F. O. Schmitt and F. G. Worden, pp. 509–515. MIT Press, Cambridge, Mass.
15. Deguchi, T. (1973): Role of the *beta*-adrenergic receptor in the elevation of adenosine cyclic 3′,5′-monophosphate and induction of serotonin N-acetyltransferase in rat pineal glands. *Molec. Pharmacol.,* 9:184–190.
16. Whitby, L. G., Hertting, G., and Axelrod, J. (1960): Effect of cocaine on the disposition of noradrenaline labelled with tritium. *Nature,* 187: 604–605.

17. Deguchi, T., and Axelrod, J. (1973): Supersensitivity and subsensitivity of the β-adrenergic receptor in pineal gland regulated by catecholamine transmitter. *Proc. Natl. Acad. Sci. USA,* 70: 2411–2414.

18. Quay, W. B. (1963): Circadian system in rat pineal serotonin and its modification by estrous cycle and photo periods. *Gen. Comp. Endocrinol.,* 3:473–479.

19. Snyder, S. H., Zweig, M., Axelrod, J., and Fischer, J. E. (1965): Control of the circadian rhythm in serotonin content of the rat pineal gland. *Proc. Natl. Acad. Sci. USA,* 53:301–305.

20. Moore, R. Y., and Klein, D. C. (1974): Visual pathways and the central neural control of a circadian rhythm in pineal serotonin *N*-acetyltransferase activity. *Brain Res.,* 71:17–33.

21. Brownstein, M. J., and Axelrod, J. (1974): Pineal gland: 24-hour rhythm in norepinephrine turnover. *Science,* 184:163–165.

22. Deguchi, T., and Axelrod, J. (1972): Control of circadian change of serotonin *N*-acetyltransferase activity in the pineal organ by the β-adrenergic receptor. *Proc. Natl. Acad. Sci. USA,* 69:2547–2550.

23. Axelrod, J. (1974): The pineal gland: A neurochemical transducer. *Science,* 184:1341–1348.

24. Romero, J. A., and Axelrod, J. (1974): Pineal β-adrenergic receptor: Diurnal variation in sensitivity. *Science,* 184:1091–1092.

The Nervous System, Donald B. Tower, Editor-in-Chief. *Vol. 1: The Basic Neurosciences*. Raven Press, New York, 1975.

Neuroendocrine Control of Ovulation

Charles H. Sawyer

Until the late 1940s the control of ovulation —the shedding of mature ova from the ovary— was considered largely a nonnervous, pituitary–ovarian interaction except in a relatively small group of "reflex" ovulators. In that group, which included the cat and rabbit, the release of pituitary ovulating hormone was triggered by sensory or psychic stimuli related to coitus. The discovery by Sawyer et al. (1) that reflex ovulation in the rabbit could be blocked with antiadrenergic and anticholinergic drugs provided a tool with which to test the brain's involvement in "spontaneous" ovulation in the rat (2,3). With the use of dibenamine, atropine, or barbiturates, Everett and Sawyer (4) found that, under controlled lighting conditions in the proestrous rat, the central nervous system activates the release of an ovulatory quantum of pituitary gonadotropin between 2 and 4 p.m., an interval which came to be known as the "critical period" (5,6).

NEUROVASCULAR CONCEPT AND LUTEINIZING HORMONE-RELEASING HORMONE

The late 1940s and early 1950s were also the period during which neurohumoral control of the adenohypophysis was demonstrated by experiments involving pituitary stalk section, transplantation of the gland to sites distant from the hypothalamus, and finding it inexcitable *in situ* to direct electrical stimulation [see Markee et al. (7) and Harris (8,9)]. According to the neurovascular concept humoral mediators, later known as "releasing factors" and finally as "releasing hormones" (9,10), are poured into the proximal capillary plexus of the hypophysial portal system from nerve endings in the median eminence. These factors or hormones are then transported by the portal veins to the anterior pituitary gland where they activate or inhibit release of adenohypophysial hormones. The first demonstrations of a gonadotropic releasing factor in hypothalamic extracts were made in-

dependently in 1960 by McCann et al. (11) and by Harris and Nikitovitch-Winer (12). Ten more years of intensive research disclosed the structure of luteinizing hormone-releasing hormone (LRH) as a decapeptide (10), and its synthesis made it readily available for experiments to be described later.

EFFECT OF BRAIN LESIONS AND DEAFFERENTATION

Meanwhile, also in the 1940s and 1950s, it was noted that localized electrolytic lesions discretely placed by stereotaxic methods in the basal hypothalamus resulted in ovarian atrophy and anestrus, whereas lesions further rostral induced a condition of persistent vaginal cornification ("constant estrus") with large anovulatory ovarian follicles [see Sawyer (13) for review]. Median eminence lesions often destroyed the proximal capillary plexus of the portal system, and were tantamount to pituitary stalk section. In 1964, Halasz (14) introduced a new method of isolating the hypothalamus with a stereotaxic knife which could partially or totally "deafferent" the basal "hypophysiotrophic" area, but leave intact its efferent connections with the pituitary gland by the portal system. Halasz, Gorski, and others (14) showed that anterior deafferentation of the hypothalamus interrupted cyclic ovulation and induced "constant estrus" by permitting a "tonic" secretion of gonadotropin like that which followed the placement of preoptic lesions. On the other hand, deafferentation rostral and superior to the medial preoptic area permitted ovulation, suggesting that the timing mechanism for "phasic" release of luteinizing hormone (LH) in the rat lay in the preoptic area (Fig. 1).

Like the rat, the rhesus monkey ovulates in a cyclic pattern and in response to administration of exogenous estrogen. According to Knobil (15), this continues after complete deafferentation of the basal hypothalamus (Fig. 1), and he

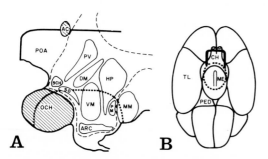

FIG. 1. A: Schematic sagittal drawing of the brain showing anterior deafferentation of the preoptic area (solid line) as projected by Halasz (1969) in the rat and total deafferentation of the basal hypothalamus (broken line) as reported by Knobil (1974) in the monkey. **B:** Base of the brain showing locations of the cuts. Redrawn with permission.

proposes that in the monkey the "Zeitgeber" lies in the ovary itself rather than in the brain. However, Spies et al. (16) questioned these findings by blocking cyclic release of LH in the monkey with lesions over the optic chiasm; more research is needed to resolve the conflicting claims.

STEROID FEEDBACK EFFECTS

The work of Everett and Sawyer (4) suggested that a cyclic neural stimulus for LH release might be transmitted to the pituitary gland during the critical period daily but be effective in triggering LH release only if hormonal conditions were right, as they are during proestrus. A surge of estrogen secretion precedes the LH surge on proestrus (17), and treatment with antibodies to estrogen blocks LH release and ovulation (18). Figure 2 shows in a semidiagrammatic manner the relationships of secretion of estrogen, LH, and progesterone prior to ovulation in the rat estrous cycle (19).

The sites of stimulatory and inhibitory feedback actions of ovarian steroids relative to ovulation have remained a subject of continuous research (20). Kawakami and Sawyer (21) suggested that the steroids might control gonadotropic secretion by acting exclusively on the brain via changes in thresholds of rhinencephalic-hypothalamic nervous transmission. Later findings (22) revealed that the steroids could also alter pituitary thresholds to the direct application of exogenous LRH. Considerable

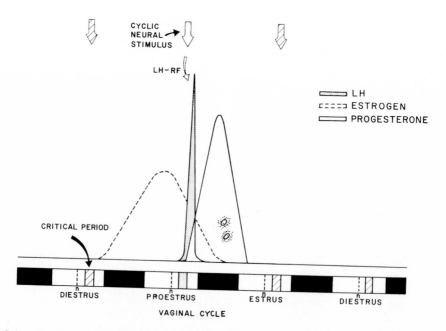

FIG. 2. Schematic diagram of cyclic changes in plasma LH, estrogen, and progesterone during the rat estrous cycle. The proestrous discharge of LH which results in follicular rupture (at ova) is triggered by a cyclic neural stimulus which activates release of LRH (here abbreviated LH-RF) during the critical period which begins about 2 hr after noon (n). (Adapted, with permission, from a figure by R. A. Gorski.)

evidence from the laboratories of Davidson (23) and McCann (24) indicates that the median eminence is a major focus for the inhibitory feedback action of estrogen, and that the anterior pituitary itself is a primary size of stimulatory feedback effects. Estrogen can also exert inhibitory effects at the pituitary level (25). On the other hand, stimulatory feedback actions of estrogen have also been reported far from the median eminence–pituitary complex, i.e., in the preoptic region under the anterior commissure (20) and more recently in the medial amygdala or bed nucleus of the stria terminalis (26). These are areas of marked estrogen uptake by the brain as demonstrated by radioautographic methods (27,28).

SITES OF LRH PRODUCTION

Where in the brain is LRH produced? The availability of pure synthetic LRH has shed new light on this subject by enabling immunologists to produce antibodies to LRH–protein complexes and to use them in visualizing sites of LRH localization in thin sections of brain tissue by immunohistochemical methods (see 29 for review). LRH is seen as a brown precipitate in the immunoperoxidase system and as fluorescent granules in the immunofluorescence preparation. High concentrations of the hormone have been seen repeatedly in the external zone of the median eminence, especially at its lateral angle (Fig. 3). A few authors have described LRH fluorescence in the perikarya of neurons in and around the preoptic area as well as the arcuate nucleus, but others have attributed such localization to nonspecific staining. High concentrations of the hormone have been localized in the arcuate nucleus and median eminence by another technique in which tiny cylinders are punched out of frozen sections of the brain and pooled for radioimmunoassay (RIA) of LRH (30). Knigge et al. (31) have suggested that LRH might be secreted by nerve endings into the

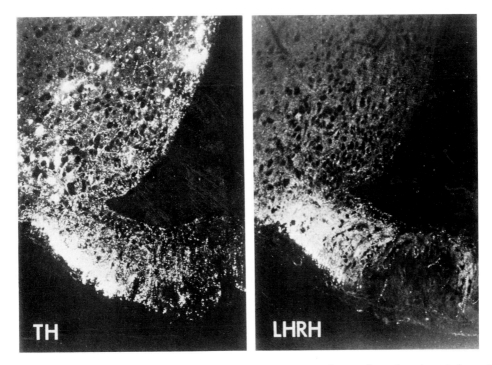

FIG. 3. Fluorescence immunohistochemical preparations of successive microscopic sections through the median eminence-arcuate nucleus region of the rat hypothalamus showing comparative localizations of tyrosine hydroxylase (TH) (*left*) and LHRH (*right*). The enzyme, which converts tyrosine to DOPA, and hormone, LRH, show overlapping distributions in the lateral external zone of the median eminence. (Figure from T. Hökfelt and K. Fuxe.)

third ventricle and carried by cerebrospinal fluid to the median eminence, where it is absorbed and transported by tanycytes of the ependymal epithelium to the proximal capillary plexus of the portal system. This concept is discussed and its physiological significance questioned by Sawyer (29).

ELECTRICAL STIMULATION AND RECORDING EXPERIMENTS

Information on brain areas and pathways involved in control of ovulation has also been obtained from electrical stimulation and recording experiments. Earlier findings in the rat with the application of electrical or electrochemical (anodal DC with stainless-steel electrodes) stimulation have been reviewed by Everett (32) and by Taleisnik and Carrer (33). Stimulation of the medial amygdala, septum, preoptic area, or dorsal tegmentum of the midbrain as well as the median eminence-arcuate zone induces ovulation, whereas stimulation of the hippocampus or midbrain raphe nuclei inhibits cyclic ovulation. The effects of stimulation of various areas of the brain on LH release as measured by RIA have been studied by many investigators and reviewed by Barraclough (34). In some of these studies the electrical stimuli have been applied following deafferentation cuts to trace pathways to the median eminence.

In our laboratory Terasawa recorded elevated multiunit activity (MUA) in the arcuate nuclei following ovulation-inducing electrochemical stimulation of the preoptic area and ovulation-advancing treatment with progesterone on the morning of proestrus [see Sawyer (29) for references]. That review (29) also describes the findings of Gallo et al. that electrochemical stimulation of the hippocampus which blocked ovulation in proestrous rats and lowered plasma LH levels in ovariectomized animals induced a rise in MUA in the ventromedial hypothalamus, and the observation of Carrer that ovulation-inhibiting electrochemical stimulation of the midbrain raphe nuclei elevates MUA in the preoptic area.

In Kawakami's laboratory in Yokohama, Terasawa et al. (26) have employed unit and MUA recording methods in a wide variety of experiments. They have shown (Fig. 4) that ovulation-inducing electrical stimulation of the medial amygdala elevates MUA in the medial

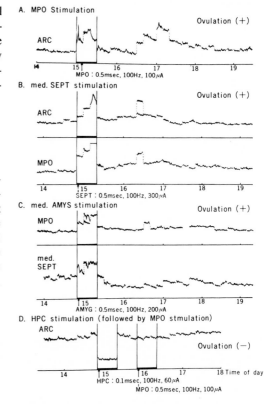

FIG. 4. Correlated changes in multiunit activity in the arcuate nucleus (ARC), medial preoptic area (MPO), and medial septum (med SEPT) following ovulation-inducing electrical stimulation of a more distant site in the brain. Hippocampal (HPC) stimulation which blocks the ovulatory effect of MPO stimulation prevents the rise in MUA in ARC. (From Kawakami and Terasawa, 26.)

septum, medial preoptic area (MPO), and arcuate nuclei, whereas inhibitory stimulation from the hippocampus lowers the MUA level in the arcuate nucleus and prevents the rise following MPO stimulation. In female rats spontaneous elevations of the MUA in septum, preoptic area, and arcuate nuclei were recorded on the afternoon of proestrus (26). Similar findings by Moss, Dyer, Wuttke, and their colleagues were reviewed by Sawyer (29), which contains the references to their papers. The 1975 review (29) also cites the findings of Faure, Vincent, Dufy, Bensch, and their colleagues in Bordeaux that ovulation-inducing vaginal stimulation in the rabbit elevates single and multiple unit activity in the basal premammillary area.

ADRENERGIC CONTROL OF LRH RELEASE

Catecholamine involvement in brain-pituitary-ovarian function was suggested more than 25 years ago when we found that ovulation could be induced in the rabbit by intrapituitary or intraventricular infusions of epinephrine, and that coitally induced ovulation could be prevented with adrenergic blocking agents (1,7). Donovan and Harris (8) made very slow infusions of epinephrine into the rabbit pituitary with negative results, and concluded correctly that the catecholamine was not acting at the pituitary level as a gonadotropin releasing factor. Our results with intraventricular infusions, combined with electrical recording methods, were interpreted as a central stimulatory effect of the norepinephrine (6). Meanwhile, high concentrations of norepinephrine had been demonstrated in the hypothalamus by Vogt and dopamine in the brainstem by Carlsson, and Swedish investigators had developed an elegant formaldehyde-fluorescence method of histochemically localizing catecholamines in the brain [see Fuxe and Hökfelt, (35) for earlier references]. Note also tyrosine hydroxylase (TH) immunohistochemistry (Fig. 3).

About 5 years ago renewed interest developed in hypothalamic adrenergic mechanisms controlling gonadotropin secretion. On the basis of experiments on rats, it was proposed by Schneider, McCann, Kamberi, and Porter [see McCann (24) for references] that dopamine was more effective than norepinephrine in stimulating LH release. Fuxe and Hökfelt (35), however, had maintained that dopamine was inhibitory in this regard. With Rubinstein and Weiner [see Weiner et al. (36) for references] we found in the rat that intraventricular infusions of epinephrine and norepinephrine stimulated multiunit activity in the median eminence (Fig. 5) and induced ovulation, whereas dopamine gave negative results. More recently in the rabbit we have observed (37) that intraventricular dopamine not only fails to stimulate LH release or ovulation, but it can actually inhibit the LH-releasing effect of a subsequent infusion of norepinephrine. Recent work by the Kalras in McCann's laboratory (24) confirms the stimulatory action of norepinephrine on LH release in the rat.

IONTOPHORESIS OF CATECHOLAMINES TO ANTIDROMICALLY IDENTIFIED NEURONS

During the past few years neurons have been antidromically "dissected" projecting from medial preoptic nuclei to the ventromedial-arcuate region and from the basal hypothalamus to the median eminence (38,39). Stimulating electrodes on axons or their endings can fire antidromic action potentials which are identified by their firing characteristics and recorded with a microelectrode at the nerve cell body. If the microelectrode is a multibarreled micropipette, one can then apply drugs or hormones to the neuron by microiontophoresis. With

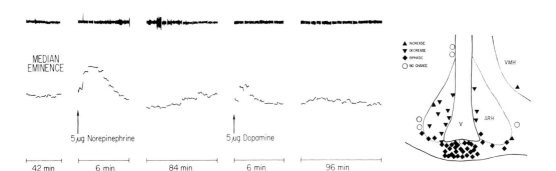

FIG. 5. Changes in multiple unit activity (MUA) in the rat median eminence induced by infusing norepinephrine and dopamine into the third ventricle. Epinephrine and norepinephrine induced biphasic effects on MUA in the median eminence and depressed activity in the arcuate nucleus (ARH), summarized in drawing at right. Dopamine exerted very little, if any, effect. [From Weiner et al. (1971): *Science.*]

such a system Moss (40) has recently tested the effects of applying norepinephrine (NE) and dopamine iontophoretically to antidromically identified tuberoinfundibular neurons in female rats. He reports on 23 such neurons which were excited by NE but either inhibited or unaffected by dopamine; conversely, 14 units excited by dopamine were unresponsive to or inhibited by NE. However, among 70 unidentified neurons, some were excited by both catecholamines, some inhibited by both, and others excited by one and inhibited or unaffected by the other, i.e., the overall sensitivity of unidentified neurons was nonspecific. Moss concludes that both NE and dopamine may play functional roles in modulating activity of hypophysiotropic neurons.

"SHORT-LOOP" AND "ULTRA-SHORT-LOOP" FEEDBACK EFFECTS

Kawakami and Sakuma (41) have recently employed the microiontophoretic technique to apply LRH, LH, and follicle stimulating hormone (FSH) to antidromically identified tuberoinfundibular neurons in the arcuate nucleus and to MPO neurons projecting to the medial basal hypothalamus. Of 74 antidromically identified neurons in the arcuate nucleus, LRH was excitatory to 33 and inhibitory to 11. Similarly, LH excited 28 and inhibited 5 of 58 units tested among the identified neurons. Follicle stimulating hormone was excitatory to only 12 and inhibitory to 4 of 41 units tested. When applied to MPO units, LH excited 12 of 14 units, whereas FSH was stimulatory to 5 and inhibitory to 1; on the other hand, LRH was excitatory to only 2 of 45 units in the MPO. An autoregulatory role is thus suggested for LRH in its tuberoinfundibular secretion, and more widespread feedback roles are indicated for LH and FSH at both basal hypothalamic and MPO sites.

SUMMARY

Figure 6 summarizes many of the brain-pituitary-ovarian relationships discussed above. Luteinizing hormone-releasing hormone is produced by neurons in the arcuate nucleus of the hypophysiotropic area and secreted into the proximal capillary plexus of the pituitary

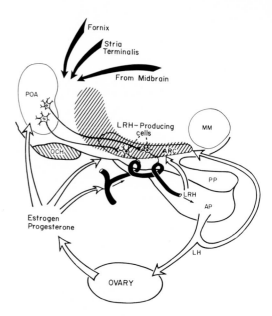

FIG. 6. Diagram of some brain-pituitary-ovary interrelationships. For explanation see text of summary. (From Sawyer, 29.)

portal system in the median eminence. LRH production is modulated in the rat and possibly also in the monkey by direct input from the preoptic region and less directly by facilitatory and inhibitory projections from the amygdala, hippocampus, and midbrain. Ovarian steroids are shown feeding back directly to the pituitary and to several sites in the brain where they influence both pituitary–ovarian function and sexual behavior. Electrophysiological evidence has been presented for "ultrashort" feedback action of LRH on arcuate neurons as well as the "short" feedback loop of LH. Evidence has been presented that adrenergic mechanisms influence LRH release with norepinephrine facilitatory and dopamine inhibitory to the process. Rapid strides are now being made in these areas of research with the use of immunological methods such as radioimmunoassay and immunohistochemistry.

ACKNOWLEDGMENT

This research was supported by grants from NINDS (NS 01162) and from the Ford Foundation.

REFERENCES

1. Sawyer, C. H., Markee, J. E., Townsend, B. F. (1949): Cholinergic and adrenergic components in the neurohumoral control of the release of LH in the rabbit. *Endocrinology*, 44:18–37.

2. Sawyer, C. H., Everett, J. W., and Markee, J. E. (1949): A neural factor in the mechanism by which estrogen induces the release of luteinizing hormone in the rat. *Endocrinology*, 44:218–233.

3. Everett, J. W., Sawyer, C. H., and Markee, J. E. (1949): A neurogenic timing factor in control of the ovulatory discharge of luteinizing hormone in the cyclic rat. *Endocrinology*, 44:234–250.

4. Everett, J. W., and Sawyer, C. H. (1950): A 24-hour periodicity in the "LH-Release Apparatus" of female rats, disclosed by barbiturate sedation. *Endocrinology*, 47:198–218.

5. Everett, J. W. (1961): The mammalian female reproductive cycle and its controlling mechanisms. In: *Sex and Internal Secretions*, 3rd ed., edited by W. C. Young, pp. 497–555. Williams and Wilkins, Baltimore.

6. Sawyer, C. H. (1963): Mechanisms by which drugs and hormones activate and block release of pituitary gonadotropins. *Proceedings of the First International Pharmacological Meeting*, Vol. 1, edited by R. Guillemin, pp. 27–46. Pergamon Press, New York.

7. Markee, J. E., Everett, J. W., and Sawyer, C. H. (1952): The relationship of the nervous system to the release of gonadotrophin and the regulation of the sex cycle. *Rec. Progr. Hormone Res.*, 7: 139–163.

8. Harris, G. W. (1955): *Neural Control of the Pituitary Gland*. Edward Arnold, London.

9. Harris, G. W. (1972): Humours and hormones. *J. Endocrinol.*, 53:ii–xxiii.

10. Schally, A. V., Arimura, A., Kastin, A. J., Matsuo, H., Baba, R., Redding, T. W., Nair, R. M. G., and Debeljuk, L. (1971): Gonadotropin-releasing hormone: one polypeptide regulates secretion of luteinizing and follicle stimulating hormones. *Science*, 173:1036–1038.

11. McCann, S. M., Taleisnik, S., and Friedman, H. M. (1960): LH-releasing activity in hypothalamic extracts. *Proc. Soc. Exp. Biol. Med.*, 104:432–434.

12. Harris, G. W. (1961): The pituitary stalk and ovulation. In: *Control of Ovulation*, edited by C. Villee, pp. 56–74. Pergamon Press, London.

13. Sawyer, C. H. (1969): Regulatory mechanisms of secretion of gonadotrophin hormones. In: *The Hypothalamus*, edited by E. Anderson, W. Haymaker, and W. J. H. Nauta, pp. 389–422. Charles C Thomas, Springfield, Illinois.

14. Halasz, B. (1969): The endocrine effects of isolation of the hypothalamus from the rest of the brain. In: *Frontiers in Neuroendocrinology*, edited by W. Ganong and L. Martini, pp. 307–342. Oxford University Press, New York.

15. Knobil, E. (1974): On the control of gonadotropin secretion in the rhesus monkey. *Rec. Progr. Hormone Res.*, 30:1–46.

16. Spies, H. G., Resko, J. A., and Norman, R. L. (1974): Evidence of preoptic hypothalamic influence on ovulation in the Rhesus monkey. *Fed. Proc.*, 33:222. Abstract.

17. Brown-Grant, K. (1971): The role of steroid hormones in the control of gonadotropin secretion in adult female mammals. In: *Steroid Hormones and Brain Function*, edited by C. H. Sawyer and R. A. Gorski, pp. 269–288. University of California Press, Los Angeles.

18. Ferin, M., Tempone, A., Zimmerling, P. E., and VandeWiele, R. L. (1969): Effect of antibodies to 17 β-estradiol and progesterone on the estrous cycle of the rat. *Endocrinology*, 85:1070–1078.

19. Gorski, R. A. (1971): Steroid hormones and brain function: Progress, principles and problems. In: *Steroid Hormones and Brain Function*, edited by C. H. Sawyer and R. A. Gorski, pp. 1–26. University of California Press, Los Angeles.

20. Davidson, J. M. (1969): Feedback control of gonadotropin in secretion. In: *Frontiers in Neuroendocrinology 1969*, edited by W. Ganong and L. Martini, pp. 343–388. Oxford University Press, New York.

21. Kawakami, M., and Sawyer, C. H. (1959): Neuroendocrine correlates of changes in brain activity thresholds by sex steroids and pituitary hormones. *Endocrinology*, 65:652–668.

22. Sawyer, C. H. and Hilliard, J. (1971): Sites of feedback action of estrogen and progesterone. 3rd Int. Congr. Horm. Ster. *Excerpta Med. Int. Congr. Ser. No. 219*, 716–721.

23. Davidson, J. M., Chiung, C., Smith, E. R., Damossa, D., and Johnston, P. (1973): Feedback mechanisms in relation to reproduction. *Excerpta Med. Int. Congr. Ser. No. 273*, 191–196.

24. McCann, S. M., Krulich, L., Cooper, K. J., Kalra, P. S., Kalra, S. P., Libertun, C., Negro-Vilar, A., Orias, R., Rønnekleiv, O., and Fawcett, C. P. (1973): Hypothalamic control of gonadotrophin and prolactin secretion, implications for fertility control. *J. Reprod. Fertil.*, Suppl. 20: 43–59.

25. Blake, C. A., Norman, R. L., and Sawyer, C. H. (1974): Localization of inhibitory actions of estrogen and nicotine on release of luteinizing hormone in rats. *Neuroendocrinology*, 16:22–35.

26. Kawakami, M., and Terasawa, E. (1974): Role of limbic structures on reproductive cycles: In: *Biological Rhythms in Neuroendocrine Activity*, edited by M. Kawakami, pp. 197–219. Igaku Shoin Ltd., Tokyo.

27. Stumpf, W. E. (1971): Hypophysiotropic neurons in the periventricular brain: topography of estradiol concentrating neurons. In: *Steroid Hormones and Brain Function*, edited by C. H. Sawyer and R. A. Gorski, pp. 215–227. University of California Press, Los Angeles.

28. Pfaff, D., and Keiner, M. (1973): Atlas of estradiol-concentrating cells in the central nervous system of the female rat. *J. Comp. Neurol.*, 151: 121–157.

29. Sawyer, C. H. (1975): Some recent developments in brain-pituitary-ovarian physiology. First

Geoffrey Harris Memorial Lecture (International Society of Neuroendocrinology, sponsors), XXVI International Physiological Congress, New Delhi, 1974. *Neuroendocrinology,* 17:97–124.

30. Palkovits, M., Arimura, A., Brownstein, M., Schally, A. V., and Saavedra, J. M. (1974): Luteinizing hormone-releasing hormone (LH-RH) content of hypothalamic nuclei in rat. *Endocrinology,* 95:554–558.

31. Knigge, K. M., Joseph, S. A., Silverman, A. J., and Vaala, S. (1973): Further observations on the structure and function of the median eminence, with reference to the organization of RF-producing elements in the endocrine hypothalamus. In: *Drug Effects on Neuroendocrine Regulation,* edited by E. Zimmerman, B. H. Marks, W. H. Gispen, and D. DeWied, *Prog. Brain Res.,* 39:7–20.

32. Everett, J. W. (1972): Brain, pituitary gland, and the ovarian cycle. *Biol. Reprod.,* 6:3–12.

33. Taleisnik, S., and Carrer, H. F. (1973): Facilitatory and inhibitory mesencephalic influence on gonadotropin release. In: *Hormones and Brain Function,* edited by K. Lissak, pp. 335–345. Plenum Press, New York.

34. Barraclough, C. A., Turgeon, J., Mann, D. R., and Cramer, O. M. (1973): Further analysis of the CNS regulation of adenohypophysial LH release: Facilitation of the ovulatory LH surge by oestrogen and progesterone. *J. Reprod. Fertil.,* Suppl. 20.

35. Fuxe, K., and Hökfelt, T. (1969): Catecholamines in the hypothalamus and the pituitary gland. In: *Frontiers in Neuroendocrinology 1969,* edited by W. Ganong and L. Martini, pp. 47–96. Oxford University Press, New York.

36. Weiner, R. I., Gorski, R. A., and Sawyer, C. H. (1972): Hypothalamic catecholamines and pituitary gonadotrophic function. In: *Brain-Endocrine Interaction, Median Eminence: Structure and Function,* edited by K. M. Knigge, D. E. Scott and A. Weindl, pp. 236–244. S. Karger, Basel.

37. Sawyer, C. H., Hilliard, J., Kanematsu, S., Scaramuzzi, R., and Blake, C. A. (1974): Effects of intraventricular infusions of norepinephrine and dopamine on LH release and ovulation in the rabbit. *Neuroendocrinology,* 15:328–337.

38. Cross, B. A. (1973): Unit responses in the hypothalamus. In: *Frontiers in Endocrinology 1973,* edited by W. Ganong and L. Martini, pp. 133–171. Oxford University Press, New York.

39. Cross, B. A. (1973): Toward a neurophysiological basis for ovulation. *J. Reprod. Fertil.,* Suppl. 20: 97–117.

40. Moss, R. L., Kelly, M., and Riskind, P. (1975): Tuberoinfundibular neurons: dopaminergic and norepinephrinergic sensitivity. *Brain Res.* 89: 265–277.

41. Kawakami, M., and Sakuma, Y. (1974): Responses of hypothalamic neurons to the microiontophoresis of LH-RH, LH and FSH under various levels of circulating ovarian hormones. *Neuroendocrinology,* 15:290–307.

The Nervous System, Donald B. Tower, Editor-in-Chief. *Vol. 1: The Basic Neurosciences*. Raven Press, New York, 1975.

Central Monoaminergic Function

Alfred Heller

The isolation and identification of pharmacologically active compounds from nerve tissue has been essential to the evolution of current concepts regarding the mechanisms by which information is transmitted from cell to cell within the nervous system and from nerve cells to peripheral effectors. Investigation of the pharmacology of compounds such as acetylcholine, norepinephrine, dopamine, serotonin, and γ-aminobutyric acid (GABA) was stimulated by the realization that such substances could have physiological functions in the nervous system. The experimental evidence supporting the role of acetylcholine and norepinephrine as neurotransmitters in peripheral nerve is well known, and these studies remain the model for investigations of the function of such compounds at central synapses. For this reason, it is important that concepts underlying our understanding of the physiological role of established neurotransmitters in the periphery be considered before discussing their possible central functions. In particular, attention should be directed to the modulatory influences that such neurotransmitters exert on peripheral effectors. Norepinephrine at postganglionic adrenergic junctions acts as a modulator of endogenous activity inherent to the tissue. Regulation of cardiac rate and contractility, regulation of the tonicity of smooth muscle of blood vessels and viscera, as well as glandular secretion, are examples of this type of modulatory influence. Removal of the adrenergic innervation leading to a loss of tissue norepinephrine in structures such as the heart or the vascular bed has important consequences, but does not abolish the inherent endogenous activity of the structure. On the other hand, denervation of striated skeletal muscle by removal of the cholinergic motor nerves results in a flaccid paralysis and atrophy.

Neurotransmitters not only regulate the endogenous activity of visceral musculature, but at least at some junctions in the periphery

the release of norepinephrine has modulatory effects on a variety of ongoing intracellular metabolic processes. These effects are believed to be mediated by stimulation of the enzyme adenylate cyclase, resulting in an elevation of intracellular cyclic 3'5'-adenosine monophosphate (cyclic AMP), which as a "second messenger" (1) regulates a variety of metabolic processes including glycogenolysis and glycogen synthesis. Stimulation of sympathetic innervation to the liver produces an increase in the activities of hepatic phosphorylase and glucose 6-phosphatase, leading to a reduction in the level of glycogen in this organ and an increase in blood glucose. Parasympathetic stimulation with release of acetylcholine raises glycogen synthetase levels, an effect which is blocked by simultaneous sympathetic stimulation (2). It is clear from these studies that stimulation of the autonomic innervation to the liver can cause coordinated and rapid changes in the activities of enzymes regulating liver glycogen levels. The loss of such regulation is seen with chronic sympathetic denervation of the heart which produces a rise in cardiac glycogen as would be predicted if norepinephrine released from such nerve endings functions to elevate cyclic AMP synthesis in cardiac cells. Loss of the transmitter and presumably a decrease in the "second messenger" should result in an appropriate change in the activities of phosphorylase and glycogen synthetase so as to result in elevated glycogen levels. However, despite the rise in cardiac glycogen these effects at the enzymatic level have not been observed when activity is assayed *in vitro* (3). Although the mechanisms are clearly complex, tissue glycogen levels as well as those of other metabolic substrates appear to be regulated by the activity of autonomic nerves in an antagonistic but reciprocal manner, as is characteristic of autonomic regulation of many peripheral functions.

A useful system for studying the modulatory

role of peripheral adrenergic neurons on biosynthetic processes within an effector tissue has been developed from studies of the effects of environmental lighting on melatonin biosynthesis in the pineal. The biosynthesis of melatonin, the active principle of the pineal, requires *N*-acetylation of serotonin by the enzyme serotonin *N*-acetyltransferase with subsequent *O*-methylation to form melatonin. The last step requires an enzyme, hydroxyindole-*O*-methyltransferase found in mammals only in pineal, retina, and the Harderian gland. Melatonin itself, as well as the activities of the enzymes *N*-acetyltransferase and hydroxyindole-*O*-methyltransferase in the pineal, exhibit diurnal rhythms which can be modified by environmental lighting. Complex polyneuronal pathways originating in the retina are involved in the transmission of lighting information to the pineal. The final common pathway for all such information involves the sympathetic adrenergic outflow to the pineal arising from the superior cervical ganglia. Decentralization of the ganglia by cutting of the preganglionic fibers or denervation of the pineal by ganglionectomy abolishes the rhythmicity in both enzyme activities (for review, see 4,5).

The active participation of postganglionic sympathetic fibers in mediating afferent input to the pineal and thus regulating enzyme activity has been shown by nerve stimulation experiments. The activities of both *N*-acetyltransferase and hydroxyindole-*O*-methyltransferase can by "fixed" by appropriate manipulation. Hydroxyindole-*O*-methyltransferase activity can be elevated by blinding or bilateral lesions of the inferior accessory optic tract, the central pathway mediating information on environmental lighting for this enzyme. *N*-acetyltransferase activity can be suppressed by exposure of rats to continuous light. Changes in afferent input to the pineal can be produced by stimulation of the preganglionic sympathetic trunk. Such nerve stimulation has been shown to produce a time-dependent linear *reduction* in pineal hydroxyindole-*O*-methyltransferase activity in rats in which this enzyme has been fixed at high levels. In animals where pineal *N*-acetyltransferase activity has been suppressed by constant light, 2 hr of nerve stimulation will *increase* enzyme activity threefold. There is good reason from both *in vitro* and *in*

vivo studies, to believe that the rise in *N*-acetyltransferase activity induced by such sympathetic stimulation is mediated by norepinephrine through an adenylate cyclase-cyclic AMP mechanism. Isolated pineals incubated in norepinephrine or dibutyryl-cyclic AMP show an increase in *N*-acetyltransferase activity. This increase in enzyme activity is partially blocked by cycloheximide, an inhibitor of protein synthesis. Norepinephrine will also elevate pineal adenylate cyclase activity *in vitro* and will raise light-suppressed levels of *N*-acetyltransferase in the intact animal. The nerve stimulation-induced increase in *N*-acetyltransferase appears to involve a similar mechanism since the effect is completely abolished by either propranolol, a beta-adrenergic blocking agent or cycloheximide. Thus, afferent input mediated by sympathetic fibers appears capable of regulating the synthesis of specific pineal proteins (for review, see 5,6).

The participation of the nervous system and norepinephrine in pineal function has characteristics common to autonomic regulation in general. Neuronal input plays a modulatory role on ongoing enzyme activity. Denervation or decentralization of the gland does not result in an absence of appropriate biosynthetic enzyme activity, but rather in a loss of diurnal variations. These coordinated diurnal variations are an example of the modulatory role of norepinephrine on ongoing "tonic" activity. One puzzling aspect of the effects of sympathetic regulation is related to the finding that increased afferent input is capable of *lowering* hydroxyindole-*O*-methyltransferase activity when it is elevated and *raising* *N*-acetyltransferase activity when it is suppressed. This paradox may represent an analogue of the general characteristic of autonomic regulation that response to nerve stimulation depends on the tone of the tissue stimulated. The possibility should be considered that in this system a change in afferent input *per se* signals the pineal to alter its enzyme activities appropriately depending on the level of enzyme present at the time of change in afferent input.

The central nervous system contains the established peripheral neurotransmitters, acetylcholine and norepinephrine, as well as a series of other pharmacologically active compounds including dopamine, serotonin, and

GABA. These compounds are distributed in a nonuniform pattern and have been the subject of considerable speculation and research as to their neuronal function, particularly in relation to central drug action. It is clear from a variety of studies that many centrally active pharmacologic agents have effects on acetylcholine, catecholamine and indolealkylamine levels, metabolism, biosynthesis, and storage, and that reasonable models of drug action can be derived from such considerations. Since drugs can produce important changes in behavioral states, pharmacologic studies at various levels of organization provide an important approach to elucidation of the role of these substances in physiological function. Such studies, however, require a neuroanatomic-neurochemical basis if meaningful interpretations are to be drawn. Direct information is necessary as to the association of particular transmitter candidates with specific neuronal elements; information which was, of course, essential to formulation of our current understanding of transmitter function in peripheral systems. Such neuroanatomic-neurochemical correlations are more difficult to obtain in the central nervous system in part due to the relative inaccessibility of the tissue. The most serious problem, however, is the complexity of central neuronal connections and interrelations. Despite the inherent difficulties, the last 10 to 15 years have yielded a wealth of such information and newer analytical techniques, both biochemical and microscopic, promise that the relation of biologically active compounds to specific neuronal elements will be understood in considerable anatomic and neurochemical detail.

Transection of peripheral nerve to produce denervation of specific tissues has been applied with great success in the periphery to establish the presence of a particular transmitter in specific neurons, e.g., acetylcholine in preganglionic and norepinephrine in postganglionic fibers within the sympathetic division of the autonomic nervous system. Similarly in brain, central lesions can be used to destroy identifiable neuronal elements and to then study the neurochemical consequences of the resultant neuronal degeneration. By this approach, it was possible to identify the medial forebrain bundle, a complex tract interconnecting the hypothalamus, the basal telencephalon, and the

midbrain as being essential for the maintenance of brain serotonin and norepinephrine. Destruction of this fiber system at various levels in the brain leads to a marked and permanent loss in the biosynthesis and storage of these monoamines over widespread areas of brain. Both norepinephrine and serotonin are affected by transection of this fiber system at the diencephalic level while selective reductions can be produced by lateral (norepinephrine) versus medial (serotonin) ablation in the mesencephalon (for review, see 7,8).

During the last decade, the application of a variety of histochemical, pharmacological, and biochemical techniques frequently in conjunction with central lesions, has provided additional information on the association of monoamines with specific central neurons. These techniques, and in particular the fluorescence method of Falck and Hillarp, which allows visualization of the monoamines at the cellular level, has permitted an extensive mapping of cell bodies and fiber pathways containing these putative transmitters.

Norepinephrine-containing cell groups in the brainstem give rise to both descending and ascending fibers. The ascending norepinephrine fibers form distinct fiber systems. The more dorsal of these, the dorsal or dorsal tegmental bundle, receives fibers primarily from the locus coeruleus. These fibers ascend via the medial forebrain bundle to innervate diencephalic and telencephalic structures. Ascending fibers from more caudally placed nuclei as well as from the locus coeruleus ascend via a more ventrally placed system of fibers supplying innervation to brainstem structures including the medulla, the pons, and the mesencephalon as well as entering the medial forebrain bundle to innervate diencephalic structures and possibly telencephalic areas. Another prominent and complex catecholamine-containing fiber system has been described within the periventricular and periaqueductal gray of the medulla, pons, mesencephalon, and diencephalon. Ascending dopamine neurons arise from the substantia nigra and ventral tegmentum and project cranially via the internal capsule and medial forebrain bundle to supply the striatum. Mesencephalic dopamine-containing cell bodies also send fibers to the nucleus accumbens, the olfactory bulb, and the interstitial nucleus of the stria terminalis (the so-called mesolimbic dopamine system). A dopamine projection from the mesencephalon to the septum, the amygdala, and the cortex has also been described. Serotonin-containing cell bodies occupy a medial position extending through the medulla, pons, and mesencephalon in the raphe nuclei with fibers passing cranially via the medial forebrain bundle. Extensive anatomic descriptions of these systems are available (9,10).

The functional role of monoamines in brain has been approached at various levels of organization from the synaptic to the behavioral. Central monoamines have been implicated in the mediation of a variety of physiological and behavioral states including regulation of body temperature, sleep, eating behavior, central drug action, regulation of release of pituitary hormones, motoneuron activity, and extrapyramidal motor function (11).

Information on neurochemical-neuroanatomic correlations is necessary for the interpretation of functional studies and provides an essential basis for the use of lesions, stimulation, or pharmacological manipulation. With selectively placed central lesions, either electrolytic or chemical, it is possible to produce specific depletions of brain monoamines as an approach to the study of function. It should be noted, however, that at least in some cases the mechanisms underlying lesion effects on putative neurotransmitter content may be more complex than such losses in peripheral tissues following transection of autonomic nerves. There is reason to believe on the basis of anatomic and neurochemical data, that at least in some areas of telencephalon, the loss of norepinephrine and serotonin following lesions is not entirely attributable to direct denervation, but rather is secondary to a disruption of neuronal control of monoamine biosynthesis mediated across polyneuronal systems, not unlike the situation described above for regulation of enzyme activity in the pineal (8,12).

Another interesting complexity of the mapping of monoaminergic innervation in brain arises from studies utilizing sensitive isotopic assays for the monoamines permitting analysis of these compounds in individual nuclei. These studies show that essentially all hypothalamic nuclei contain norepinephrine, dopamine, and serotonin in varying proportions and that there

is even a nonuniform distribution of norepinephrine within some nuclei (13). These results suggest that the "real" maps of innervation to specific nuclei by monoamine pathways may be more complex than can be appreciated at present.

Considering the widespread distribution of monoamine-containing neurons in brain and the physiological functions in which they have been postulated to participate, it is indeed surprising as Vogt has noted, "that extensive damage to this system of neurones is not lethal and does not even cause very conspicuous signs" (11). This is analogous to the well-known fact that peripheral sympathectomy is likewise nonlethal if stress is avoided. Nevertheless, the loss of monoamines from brain induced by either lesions or chemical methods is not without consequences. For example, it can be shown that medial forebrain bundle lesions which reduce telencephalic monoamines produce an increased sensitivity to electric foot-shock and this increase in sensitivity can be reversed by administration of 5-hydroxytryptophan, the precursor of serotonin, but not by L-DOPA, the precursor of dopamine and norepinephrine (14). Rotational and postural abnormalities have been reported with unilateral 6-hydroxy-dopamine-induced destruction of the substantia nigra, the origin of the dopamine-containing nigrostriatal system. There is a decrement in this rotational behavior with time, but it can then be elicited by tail pinching. Dopamine-releasing drugs such as amphetamine cause rotation toward the lesion side while dopamine "receptor" stimulating drugs such as apomorphine cause rotation toward the intact side (9).

The interpretation of behavioral or drug effects observed following loss of central monoamines is far from simple. No lesion technique results in destruction specific to a single neuronal system. Damage to other systems is invariably a consequence of the destructive technique. While "chemical" lesioning is thought to be more selective such as when 6-hydroxydopamine is injected intracerebrally, there is good reason to believe that neurons other than those of the monoaminergic system are destroyed due to the mechanical trauma associated with the injection (15). Transection of a fiber system at various brain levels can be helpful in determining if a functional effect is specific to a particular neuronal group. For example, both septal (telencephalic) and dorsomedial tegmental lesions (mesencephalic) reduce brain serotonin and produce marked potentiation of thiopental-induced "sleep" in the rat. This effect is, however, probably not related to destruction of serotonin neurons since medial forebrain bundle lesions in the diencephalon which also reduce serotonin by transection of the monoamine pathway interconnecting these areas, is without effect on thiopental action (16).

Since drug- or lesion-induced monoamine depletions are rarely complete, it is of importance to consider the functional status of the remaining monoamines in relation to alterations in central physiology. Consideration must also be given to the effects of the loss of one transmitter on the utilization of other transmitter candidates innervating similar anatomic loci. The analysis of monoamine "turnover" in the lesioned animal, despite the technical problems involved, undoubtedly would more accurately reflect ongoing monoaminergic function than the levels of the transmitters *per se*. The importance of assessing monoamine "turnover" is emphasized by recent findings demonstrating that ongoing behavior, itself, can modify catecholamine metabolism in the central nervous system (CNS). When rats are treated with α-methyl-*p*-tyrosine, there is a greater decrease in brain norepinephrine and dopamine if the animals are performing in an operant situation, than in controls (17). The concept that operant behavioral performance affects norepinephrine "turnover" is supported by isotopic tracer experiments. Two hours after intraventricular injection of ^{3}H-norepinephrine the specific activity of brainstem-diencephalic norepinephrine is 25% lower in rats lever-pressing for water as compared to the specific activity found in untrained control animals with free access to water or to that found in an untrained water-deprived group. These findings are important in the interpretation of drug effects on behavior, since behavior, itself, is apparently capable of "changing the chemical substrate on which the drugs act" (18).

In general, most investigators have taken the reasonable point of view, that central monoamines function as synaptic transmitters in the CNS. The most direct experimental evidence has come from microiontophoretic studies of the responsiveness of individual central neurons to putative transmitters and drugs (for a comprehensive and critical review of this subject, see 19). This approach was initially used to identify the cholinoceptive inhibitory spinal Renshaw cells which are innervated by recurrent branches of motor fibers. It has been subsequently applied to almost all other regions of the CNS. There is now abundant evidence from such microiontophoretic studies that many central neurons have monoaminergic receptors, inhibitory or excitatory, depending on the area of brain. In some cases, such receptors may be utilized for physiological function. Yet it is fair to say that there is no central synapse for which it can be stated with certainty that any given monoamine functions as a synaptic transmitter in the classical sense. Nevertheless, considering the diffuse and widespread distribution of monoamine-containing neurons in the CNS, it is difficult to believe that this is not the case at least for some of the synaptic contacts made by these cells.

In order to illustrate the problems involved in assessing the role of monoamines in the CNS, it is helpful to consider a single case in some detail. The postulated role for dopamine as an inhibitory transmitter in the mammalian basal ganglia has been extensively studied. The basal ganglia are a particularly useful subdivision of the telencephalon for the study of the interrelationship of monoamines to CNS function. This area of brain has high levels of almost all of the neurotransmitter candidates including acetylcholine, serotonin, and GABA, as well as containing norepinephrine. Most striking, however, is the fact that the basal ganglia contain the highest level of dopamine of any major subdivision of brain. The presence of dopamine in the caudate was first reported by Bertler and Rosengren and its relation to extrapyramidal function suggested by Hornykiewicz's description of reduced levels of this monoamine in the basal ganglia of patients suffering from Parkinson's disease. This finding led to the introduction of L-DOPA as a form of replacement therapy in this disease. In addition, the finding spurred a lively and productive interest in the participation of this catecholamine in extrapyramidal function (20).

Just as with the other monoamines, it is useful to examine the pharmacology of dopamine in the periphery which is complex and distinct from that of either norepinephrine or epinephrine. Dopamine, like norepinephrine, has stimulatory effects on cardiac contractility and rate due to its action on β-adrenergic receptors. It produces vascular constriction by an α-adrenergic mechanism, but is also capable of producing dilation in specific vascular beds. The vasodilation of the renal and mesenteric beds are of considerable interest since they indicate the existence of a specific dopamine "receptor" despite the fact that peripheral "dopaminergic" nerves to these vascular beds have never been demonstrated. The vasodilation produced by dopamine is not antagonized by propranolol, a β-receptor blocker, and a potency series, dopamine = epinine > 6-propylnoraporphine-10-11-diol > apomorphine has been described. Specific partial antagonism to dopamine-induced vasodilation has been obtained with haloperidol and other butyrophenones. Such pharmacological characterization in peripheral systems has been useful in studying α- and β-adrenergic receptors in the CNS. The characteristics of the peripheral dopamine "receptor" are similarly important (21).

In the superior cervical ganglion, the role of dopamine contained within small interneurons in mediating the inhibitory effects of preganglionic stimulation has been extensively investigated. Preganglionic nerve stimulation produces an initial fast excitatory postsynaptic potential (EPSP) followed by a slow inhibitory postsynaptic potential (IPSP) and a slow EPSP. Such stimulation also results in an increase in ganglionic cyclic AMP. The ganglion contains an adenylate cyclase more sensitive to dopamine than norepinephrine. It has been suggested that the slow IPSP is mediated by dopamine release from the small intensely fluorescent cells of the ganglion which contain this catecholamine. Stimulation of the adenylate cyclase of postsynaptic elements results in a rise in cyclic AMP and this "secondary messenger" acting via its ability to regulate membrane protein kinases is thought to produce changes in membrane properties involved in ion movements required for the generation of potentials (22).

One aspect of dopamine action on the ganglion is its facilitatory effect on the slow EPSP. Dopamine release appears to be a necessary condition for generation of this potential. It is striking that the facilitatory effect of dopamine persists for long periods of time (2 hr or more) and that this persistence is not dependent on the initial dopamine–receptor interaction since phenoxybenzamine which blocks the initial facilitatory effect will not reverse the facilitation once it has been elicited by dopamine. It has been suggested that this dopamine action consists of "a long-lasting metabolic or structural change in the post-synaptic neuron induced by the initial action of the modulating transmitter dopamine" and may be a mechanism for "coupling synaptic action to long-lasting changes in neuronal metabolism and molecular structure" (23).

In the basal ganglia, the presence of dopamine is a function of a dopamine-containing nigrostriatal projection whose cell bodies lie within the pars compacta of the substantia nigra and the adjacent ventral tegmentum. Axons pass through the ventral tegmentum and ascend via the internal capsule and medial forebrain bundle to innervate the putamen and caudate nucleus. Lesions placed along the course of this projection lead to marked reductions in striatal dopamine and the enzyme activities essential for its biosynthesis, i.e., tyrosine hydroxylase and DOPA decarboxylase (24). The cells receiving innervation from the dopamine-containing pathway to the striatum have been the subject of considerable investigation. In the adult animal, the caudate exhibits an intense diffuse fluorescence probably due to the fact that the nerve fibers seem to be very small. The precise striatal cells innervated by the dopamine system are as yet unclear. The neuronal population within the caudate consists mainly of interneurons and electrophysiological studies indicate that only 5% of the cells are output neurons. Electron microscopic studies of "false-transmitter tagged" boutons indicate the presence of both axodendritic and axosomatic monoamine junctions in the striatum. These studies suggest that at least part of the prejunctional vesicular monoamine may be "apposed to lakes of extracellular space" and "that the vesicle content may be released either by exocytosis or through narrow pits directly into the extracellular space" allowing for diffusion of the transmitter away from the immediate vicinity of release; a situation not unlike that suggested for release of norepinephrine from sympathetic nerves at peripheral junctions with smooth muscle (25).

Many workers have suggested an interaction between dopaminergic and cholinergic neurons in the striatum. Dopamine from the nigrostriatal projection is thought to have an inhibitory effect on interneurons which may be cholinergic. Although studies of acetylcholine in the striatum do indicate that dopamine antagonists accelerate acetylcholine metabolism and apomorphine, a dopamine-like agonist, reduces utilization, the physiological significance of these drugs effects is much less clear (26).

As discussed above, there is considerable evidence that catecholamines function, in part, as modulators of intracellular metabolism in peripheral systems. A variety of studies suggest that dopamine may have a similar function in the caudate. Transection of the nigrostriatal system represents a central analogue to peripheral studies of the metabolic consequences for postsynaptic elements of monoamine depletion secondary to denervation. The destruction of the nigrostriatal dopamine input does indeed produce a long-standing increase in glycogen in the caudate ipsilateral to the lesion. This increase in glycogen may represent a central metabolic response to denervation-induced loss of monoamines similar to the elevation of cardiac glycogen following surgical sympathectomy. The rise in glycogen occurs only in the caudate despite the fact that the lesions employed routinely destroy other fibers resulting in losses of norepinephrine and serotonin over widespread areas of the telencephalon (27). Since this effect is restricted to the caudate, it is reasonable to focus on participation of dopamine in caudate metabolic function despite the fact that the lesions also reduce norepinephrine and serotonin in this structure. Dopamine may, indeed, have a unique metabolic regulatory role in the caudate. Homogenates of rat caudate contain an adenylate cyclase which is activated twofold by dopamine at relatively low concentrations while being less sensitive to norepinephrine (28). Homogenates from other areas of brain in general have different potency patterns. For example, cerebellar adenylate cyclase has a high basal activity which is increased by norepinephrine and relatively unaffected by dopamine. Following administration to rats of L-DOPA, the precursor of dopamine, there is a rise in caudate cyclic AMP, but no effect on cerebellar cyclic AMP (29). In addition, recent studies have shown that following unilateral ablation of the nigrostriatal pathway and a loss of dopamine from the caudate, there is an enhancement of the dopamine-stimulated adenylate cyclase activity in caudate suggesting a denervation supersensitivity related to this enzymatic function (30). Taken together, these results (i.e., the presence of a dopamine-sensitive adenylate cyclase in the caudate, enhancement of its sensitivity to dopamine by denervation, and the rise in glycogen seen following chronic denervation) are consistent with the notion that the dopamine-containing nigrostriatal pathway plays a role in the regulation of metabolic events in the caudate.

Whether or not such regulation is related to cell activity *per se* is difficult to answer. Cyclic nucleotides applied by microiontophoresis can effect neuronal activity. For example, pyramidal tract cells in the rat cerebral cortex are inhibited by norepinephrine and cyclic AMP, but excited by acetylcholine and cyclic GMP. These opposing responses to the cyclic nucleotides are in accord with the hypothesis that cyclic AMP and cyclic GMP act in opposing fashion as intracellular mediators of specific hormonal responses (31). Such a function for dopamine and the cyclic nucleotides in regulating caudate cell firing rates has not yet been fully elucidated. Most investigators have taken the view that dopamine functions as an inhibitory neurotransmitter in the caudate. The effects of dopamine applied iontophoretically onto caudate neurons are generally inhibitory although some reports of excitatory responses exist. These inhibitory actions on cell firing rates are similar to effects obtained with dopamine in other portions of the CNS. It has been noted, however, that dopamine is seldom as effective as the inhibitory amino acids, GABA or glycine, on caudate cells (19). Dopamine acting as a caudate inhibitory transmitter fits well with the frequently expressed concept that Parkinson's disease is the result of an unimpeded activity of cholinergic caudate neurons whose activities are normally damped by the dopamine nigrostriatal projection. This concept is, of course, supported by the clinical efficacy of cholinergic antagonists and L-DOPA in parkinsonism. Although this model is attractive, a careful examination of the electrophysiological literature is difficult to reconcile with the concept that the nigrostriatal input is purely inhibitory in the caudate. First, when *intracellular* potentials are recorded from caudate neurons in response to nigral stimulation in the cat, they are most frequently characterized by initial excitation rather than by inhibition (see 32 for references). In addition, the long-latency monosynaptic excitation triggered in cells of the caudate by stimulation of the substantia nigra persists even when striatal dopamine is removed by various manipulations including 6-hydroxydopamine, reserpine, or α-methyl-*p*-tyrosine. In normal cats, nigral stimulation suppresses glutamate-induced firing in the striatum. This response persists in animals subjected to the dopamine-depleting treatments mentioned above. Considering the sensitivity of caudate neurons to GABA, it has been suggested that at least part of the inhibition may be mediated by GABA-releasing interneurons rather than by dopaminergic inputs (33).

In an attempt to assess the role of the dopamine-containing nigrostriatal system in regulation of the firing rates of caudate cells, unilateral hypothalamic lesions were placed in the cat destroying the nigrostriatal projection. Spontaneous firing rates and patterns in both the ipsilateral and contralateral caudates were simultaneously recorded. This design avoids problems related to spontaneous changes in the arousal state of the animals. In nonlesioned control cats, cells in the right and left caudates fire at approximately equal rates. In lesioned animals, there was some tendency for the firing rates to increase in the caudate ipsilateral to the lesion, but this increase was not statistically significant. However, quite surprisingly, in the caudate contralateral to the lesion the spontaneous firing rate decreased threefold. Similar effects were seen with lesions which destroyed portions of the red nucleus and surrounding tegmentum, but did not damage the substantia nigra and produced no effects on dopamine levels in the caudate nuclei. Studies in the monkey with chronic recording from the caudate following unilateral "supranigral" lesions,

produced results in general agreement with those obtained in the acute cat experiments (32). Subsequent work has provided evidence that the contralateral slowing is the result of the simultaneous destruction of striatofugal fiber systems by the lesions employed to interrupt the nigrostriatal dopaminergic system (34). The results of these lesion studies illustrate the general principle discussed above, that the assignment of particular functions to a given neuronal system requires its interruption at more than one anatomic level.

The failure to observe marked statistically significant increases in the firing rates of caudate cells ipsilateral to the lesion is surprising if dopamine functions solely as an inhibitory transmitter in the caudate. Any interpretation of the effects of ablation, however, must take into account the complex neurochemical milieu remaining following lesions of the nigrostriatal bundle. A more complete appreciation of the participation of caudate acetylcholine, GABA, and serotonin in the regulation of cell firing rates will be necessary to interpret the observed effects.

In light of evidence that dopamine does participate in regulation of metabolic functions in the caudate, presumably via the adenylate cyclase system and considering evidence for its role in both inhibitory and excitatory processes in autonomic ganglia, it is reasonable to postulate similar functions for dopamine in the caudate via the adenylate cyclase system. Monoamines in general may function in the CNS in a manner quite different than that ascribed to classical transmitters in peripheral systems. Indeed, some transmitter candidates may function in part to modulate events which have considerably longer time courses than processes such as initiation of action potentials. Bloom has suggested that "sequential intracellular mediation of synaptic messages by cyclic nucleotides offers at least the possibility for longer term changes in neuronal membrane, and in carbohydrate and protein metabolism by the intermediary role of cyclic nucleotide-dependent protein kinases. It should at least be considered that some synapses whose actions are translated into intracellular nucleotides or other forms of second messenger molecules may thus carry out trophic effects which far outweigh the more transient electrophysiological actions generated immediately at the cell surface membrane" (35).

Such long-term trophic effects for central monoamines may be best examined by a careful study of the role that monoamines may play in the ontogenesis of CNS function at the biochemical, cellular, and behavioral level. There is little doubt that afferent input plays a role, presumably via some chemical mediator(s), in neuronal development. In the periphery, preganglionic fibers and probably the transmitter–tissue interaction appear to exert a general regulatory effect on the growth and biochemical maturation of the postganglionic adrenergic neurons (36). In the case of the central monoamine systems, there is now a considerable body of information on their pre- and postnatal development. Although the monoamine pathways make their appearance early in life and fibers are laid down at least in part at birth, levels of the monoamines and their biosynthetic enzymes increase markedly during the postnatal period. This postnatal development is complex and varies in different regions of brain. In the rat, telencephalic levels of catecholamines are only 70% of adult values even by 6 weeks of age (37). There is, therefore, an extended period of time for manipulation of these systems prior to their full neurochemical expression. Examination of the role of monoamines in neuronal development, particularly as a means of assessing their function can be approached by early neuronal disruption. For example, unilateral diencephalic lesions transecting the medial forebrain bundle and medial internal capsule in the 3- to 4-day-old rat prevents the subsequent increases with development of telencephalic norepinephrine and dopamine and the animals grow to adulthood without experiencing throughout their life span normal monoaminergic systems (38). A variety of pharmacological, electrophysiological, neurochemical, and behavioral evaluations of CNS function in such animals during their postnatal development in the absence of specific monoamine systems should be of considerable value in assessing whether or not the presence of monoamines affects the long-term processes of neuronal growth and development necessary for the full expression of potential central nervous system function.

The study of monoamine function in the central nervous system is an important but difficult problem. It appears clear, for example, that despite considerable experimental effort, our understanding of the role of dopamine in the striatum is far from complete. Models derived from studies on the peripheral nervous system, while essential, cannot be applied to the CNS without critical appreciation of their limitations within the context of the complexity of the CNS. Elucidation of the physiological role of monoamines in the CNS presents a fascinating but challenging problem, the complexity of which we may not as yet fully appreciate.

ACKNOWLEDGMENTS

The author wishes to express his appreciation to his colleague, Dr. Philip C. Hoffmann, for his help in the planning and preparation of this manuscript.

REFERENCES

1. Sutherland, E. W., Øye, I., and Butcher, R. W. (1965): The action of epinephrine and the role of the adenyl cyclase system in hormone action. Rec. Prog. Hormone Res., 21:623–642.
2. Shimazu, T. (1967): Glycogen synthetase activity in liver: Regulation by the autonomic nerves. Science, 156:1256–1257.
3. Daw, J. C., and Berne, R. M. (1967): Effect of sympathectomy on cardiac UDPG-glycogen transferase activity in the cat. Am. J. Physiol., 213:1480–1484.
4. Wurtman, R. J., Axelrod, J., and Kelly, D. E. (1968): The Pineal. Academic Press, New York.
5. Klein, V. C., Weller, J. L., and Moore, R. Y. (1971): Melatonin metabolism: Neural regulation of pineal serotonin: Acetyl coenzyme A N-acetyltransferase activity. Proc. Natl. Acad. Sci. USA, 12:3107–3110.
6. Heller, A., Volkman, P., and Browning, R. (1973): Neuronal control of monoamines in brain and melatonin-forming systems in the pineal. Progr. Brain Res., 39:237–250.
7. Heller, A. (1972): Neuronal regulation of brain serotonin levels. Fed. Proc., 31:81–90.
8. Heller, A., and Moore, R. Y. (1968): Control of brain serotonin and norepinephrine by specific neural systems. Advan. Pharmacol., 6A:191–206.
9. Ungerstedt, U. (1973): Selective lesions of central catecholamine pathways: Application in functional studies. In: Neurosciences Research, Vol. 5: Chemical Approaches to Brain Function, edited by S. Ehrenpreis and I. J. Kopin, pp. 73–96. Academic Press, New York.
10. Lindvall, O., and Björklund, A. (1974): The

organization of the ascending catecholamine neuron systems in the rat brain as revealed by the glyoxylic acid fluorescence method. *Acta Physiol. Scand.*, Suppl. 412:1–48.

11. Vogt, M. (1973): Functional aspects of the role of catecholamines in the central nervous system. *Brit. Med. Bull.*, 29:2,168–171.

12. Moore, R. Y. (1970): Brain lesions and amine metabolism. *Int. Rev. Neurobiol.*, 13:67–91.

13. Palkovits, M., Brownstein, M., Saavedra, J. M., and Axelrod, J. (1974): Norepinephrine and dopamine content of hypothalamic nuclei of the rat. *Brain Res.*, 77:137–149.

14. Lints, C. E., and Harvey, J. A. (1969): Drug induced reversal of brain damage in the rat. *Physiol. Behav.*, 4:29–31.

15. Sotelo, C., Javoy, F., Agid, Y., and Glowinski, J. (1973): Injection of 6-hydroxydopamine in the substantia nigra of the rat. I. Morphological study. *Brain Res.*, 58:269–290.

16. Harvey, J. A., Heller, A., Moore, R. Y., Hunt, H. F., and Roth, L. J. (1964): Effect of central nervous system lesions on barbiturate sleeping time in the rat. *J. Pharmacol. Exp. Therap.* 144:24–36.

17. Schoenfeld, R. I., and Seiden, L. S. (1969): Effect of α-methyltyrosine on operant behavior and brain catecholamine levels. *J. Pharmacol. Exp. Therap.*, 167:319–327.

18. Lewy, A. J., and Seiden, L. S. (1972): Operant behavior changes norepinephrine metabolism in rat brain. *Science*, 175:454–456.

19. Krnjevic, K. (1974): Chemical nature of synaptic transmission in vertebrates. *Physiol. Rev.*, 54:418–540.

20. Hornykiewicz, O. (1973): Dopamine in the basal ganglia. Its role and therapeutic implications (including the clinical use of L-DOPA). *Brit. Med. Bull.*, 29:2,172–178.

21. Goldberg, L. I. (1974): Commentary: The dopamine vascular receptor. *Biochem. Pharmacol.*, 23:1–3.

22. Greengard, P., and Kebabian, J. W. (1974): Role of cyclic AMP in synaptic transmission in the mammalian peripheral nervous system. *Fed. Proc.*, 33:4,1059–1067.

23. Libet, B., and Tasaka, T. (1970): Dopamine as a synaptic transmitter and modulator in sympathetic ganglia: A different mode of synaptic action. *Proc. Natl. Acad. Sci. USA*, 67:2,667–673.

24. Moore, R. Y., Bhatnagar, R. K., and Heller, A. (1971): Anatomical and chemical studies of a nigro-neostriatal projection in the cat. *Brain Res.*, 30:119–135.

25. Tennyson, V. M., Heikkila, R., Mytilneou, C., Coté, L., and Cohen, G. (1974): 5-Hydroxydopamine "tagged" neuronal boutons in rabbit neostriatum: Interrelationship between vesicles and axonal membrane. *Brain Res.*, 82:341–348.

26. Guyenet, P. G., Javoy, F., Agid, Y., Beaujouan,

J. C. and Glowinski, J. (1975): Dopamine receptors and cholinergic neurons in the rat neostriatum. In: *Advances in Neurology, Vol. 9: Dopaminergic Mechanisms*, edited by D. B. Calne, T. N. Chase, and A. Barbeau, pp. 43–51. Raven Press, New York.

27. Hoffmann, P. C., Toon, R., Kleinman, J., and Heller, A. (1973): The association of lesion-induced reductions in brain monoamines with alterations in striatal carbohydrate metabolism. *J. Neurochem.*, 20:69–80.

28. Kebabian, J. W., Petzold, G. L., and Greengard, P. (1972): Dopamine-sensitive adenylate cyclase in caudate nucleus of rat brain, and its similarity to the "dopamine receptor." *Proc. Natl. Acad. Sci. USA*, 69:2145–2149.

29. Garelis, E., and Neff, N. H. (1974): Cyclic adenosine monophosphate: Selective increase in caudate nucleus after administration of L-DOPA. *Science*, 183:532–533.

30. Mishra, R. K., Gardner, E. L., Katzman, R., and Makman, M. H. (1974): Enhancement of dopamine-stimulated adenylate cyclase activity in rat caudate after lesions in substantia nigra: Evidence for denervation supersensitivity. *Proc. Natl. Acad. Sci. USA*, 71:3883–3887.

31. Stone, T. W., Taylor, D. A., and Bloom, F. E. (1975): Cyclic AMP and cyclic GMP may mediate opposite neuronal responses in the rat cerebral cortex. *Science*, 187:845–847.

32. Hull, C. D., Levine, M. S., Buchwald, N. A., Heller, A., and Browning, R. A. (1974): The spontaneous firing pattern of forebrain neurons. I. The effects of dopamine and non-dopamine depleting lesions on caudate unit firing patterns. *Brain Res.*, 73:241–262.

33. Feltz, P., and De Champlain, J. (1972): Persistence of caudate unitary responses to nigral stimulation after destruction and functional impairment of the striatal dopaminergic terminals. *Brain Res.*, 43:595–600.

34. Levine, M. S., Hull, C. D., Buchwald, N. A., and Villablanca, J. (1974): The spontaneous firing patterns of forebrain neurons. II. Effects of unilateral caudate nuclear ablation. *Brain Res.*, 78:411–424.

35. Bloom, F. E. (1973): Dynamic synaptic communication: Finding the vocabulary. *Brain Res.*, 62:299–305.

36. Black, I. B., and Geen, S. C. (1974): Inhibition of the biochemical and morphological maturation of adrenergic neurons by nicotinic receptor blockade. *J. Neurochem.*, 22:301–306.

37. Porcher, W., and Heller, A. (1972): Norepinephrine, dopamine and their associated biosynthetic and degradative enzymes in developing rat brain. *J. Neurochem.*, 19:1917–1930.

38. Erinoff, L., and Heller, A. (1973): Failure of catecholamine development following unilateral diencephalic lesions in the neonatal rat. *Brain Res.*, 58:489–493.

The Nervous System, Donald B. Tower, Editor-in-Chief. *Vol. 1: The Basic Neurosciences.* Raven Press, New York, 1975.

The Coming of Age of Neurochemistry and Related Disciplines

One of the obvious landmarks of the silver anniversary of the NINCDS is the ascension of neurochemistry from the efforts of a small number of pioneers at the end of the last century and through the early days of the NINCDS in the 1950's to the present complement of the American and International Neurochemistry Societies of nearly 1,000 members. Except for a few investigators such as Thudicum, Klenk, Blix, and a handful of others working in relative isolation, neurochemistry was looked on by biochemists as a horrible area in which to conduct experiments. Interest in this field began to accelerate when top-flight investigators such as Herbert Carter, Jordi Folch-Pi, Heinrich Waelsch, and Eugene Roberts turned their principal efforts toward studying the chemistry of the brain. These early investigations were primarily of an analytical nature. Biochemists examining metabolic events tended, usually, to eschew experiments with neural tissue. The classic metabolic approach was to devise a procedure to assay the reaction under investigation, then carry out a survey to see which tissue contained the highest activity. Brain was often excluded from such surveys! Examination of the details of the process was then pursued with the tissue selected.

An experience of my own in the late 1950's is an example of how some potential advantages of experimentation with brain may have been overlooked. We wished to determine the stoichiometry of long-chain fatty acid synthesis. We knew that acetyl coenzyme A (CoA) and malonyl CoA were the sources of carbon atoms for fatty acids and that the highest level of fatty acid synthesis occurred in the liver of animals recently fed a carbohydrate-rich meal. However, the presence of a high level of malonyl CoA decarboxylase activity prevented the determination of the stoichiometry of the reaction in extracts and partially purified enzyme preparations from liver and other tissues. One day I was discussing this problem with R. Wayne Albers, who is still a member of the intramural research staff of the NINCDS, and he suggested that I look at fatty acid synthesis in neonatal brain tissue since lipid deposition in that organ occurs at a rapid rate during that period of development. Following Albers' suggestion, after a few conventional enzyme purification steps, I obtained a fatty acid-synthesizing preparation from young rat brain tissue where the requirements and stoichiometry of long-chain fatty acid synthesis were readily demonstrated (1). Thus, the brain enzyme system provided a much needed bit of essential information which otherwise might have taken years to obtain. Since that time, Albers had devoted much of his efforts to the isolation and characterization of Na^+,K^+-activated adenosine triphosphatase, a critical enzyme for nerve impulse generation and propagation(2).

At the present moment, the situation in neurochemistry is vastly changed. A large number of scientists have committed their talents and resources almost exclusively to investigations in this field, and a journal devoted strictly to this topic has met with great success. Thus, as the quantity and the quality of neurochemical publications rapidly increase with each passing year, one might expect similar advances and expansion in allied disciplines. In particular, neuroimmunology and neurovirology seem likely candidates for important developments in both basic and applied areas. Somewhat more difficult to foresee at this moment is the certain amplification of our concepts of learning and behavior. Since the exploitation of the discovery of Flexner and his associates that antibiotics impair memory consolidation, comparatively few conceptual advances have been made in this area (see Agranoff, *this volume*). One asks whether investigations of minute neural nets perhaps established *in vitro* should be expanded or whether we should try to approach this problem by devising larger computer-analyzed data collection systems with noise-reduction devices to examine cerebral activity *in situ*.

Probably the approach undertaken by Benzer (3) and others of a detailed anatomical and physiological analysis of simple central nervous systems in lower orders will provide a practical system for these critical studies.

These considerations ultimately lead to thoughts of physiological, biophysical, and biochemical correlates of behavior. The editors are pleased to present some of Eric Kandel's views in this area. Clearly, here, too, one expects major advances by the NINCDS' golden anniversary. I, for one, look with eager anticipation to the elaboration and execution of novel concepts that are certain to occur in this important aspect of neuroscience. I trust the reader shares my optimism for the fruition of these "inner space" explorations.

References

1. Brady, R. O. (1960): Biosynthesis of fatty acids. II. Studies with enzymes from rat brain. *J. Biol. Chem.*, 235:302–309.
2. Siegel, G. J., and Albers, R. W. (1970): Nucleoside triphosphate phosphohydrolases. In: *Handbook of Neurochemistry, Vol. 4*, edited by A. Lajtha, pp. 13–44. Plenum Press, New York.
3. Benzer, S. (1973): Genetic dissection of behavior. *Scientific American* 229, No. 6: 24–37.

Roscoe O. Brady
Bethesda, Maryland
July 1975

The Nervous System, Donald B. Tower, Editor-in-Chief. *Vol. 1: The Basic Neurosciences.* Raven Press, New York, 1975.

Permeable Junctions: Permeability, Formation, and Genetic Aspects

Werner R. Loewenstein

In formulating one of the basic tenets of Cell Theory, Schleiden (1) wrote in 1838: "Every higher organism is an aggregate of fully individual and independent units, the cells." He used the precise German wording, *"in sich selbst abgeschlossene Einzelwesen,"* circumscribed, self-contained unit beings. This tenet has been extraordinarily fruitful and influential in biology and medicine; in particular, in the neurosciences, where it took the special form of the Neuron Doctrine, its influence continues unabated. We have now become aware, to be sure, that the self-containment is not absolute. Over the past 15 years, cells in a wide variety of excitable and inexcitable tissues have been found to be coupled by channels built into the plasma membrane where the cells are joined (2,3). Small molecules pass freely from one cell to another through these channels, which implies that the coupled cell system rather than the single cell is the unit in many functional respects, although in respect to macromolecules, which do not pass through the channels, the cell individuality is maintained. This form of direct intercellular communication is nearly a universal feature of cells in organized tissues. The only known exceptions are skeletal muscle and much of the nervous system, in which the cells seem to have undergone a special evolution insuring that the membrane surface barrier is continuous, as is required for private-line communication. However, in the embryo, even these cells make junctional channels; in fact, very early the entire embryo appears interconnected.

I deal here with the permeability of the channels, with their formation, and with some aspects of their genetics. In my own work, I have used epithelial tissues, which offer the advantage of large cell size, abundant channels, and ohmic membrane behavior. As it turns out, the channel properties in these cells are quite similar, if not identical, to those in excitable tissues, and so, I hope, the electrically silent epithelial cell may serve as a model.

THE MEMBRANE CHANNELS

Channel Permeability

Small Ion Permeability

The concept of the cell-to-cell channel, which Gilula deals with from the morphological point of view elsewhere in this volume, was originally formulated on the basis of purely electrical measurements of high spatial resolution and fluorescent and colorant tracer diffusion in epithelial cells (2). These measurements described the channel as consisting of two highly permeable membrane elements, one on each membrane of the junction (junctional membrane), and an element of insulation, a diffusion barrier sealing the interior of the connected cell system from the exterior (junctional insulation) (Fig. 1). The electrical specific resistance of the junctional membrane is much smaller than that of the nonjunctional membrane (2–7). A low resistance in the region of the junction has, in fact, been implicit ever since the discovery of electric synaptic transmission by Furshpan and Potter (8). In giant newt embryo cells, where measurements were recently done on single cell pairs, the upper limit of specific junctional membrane resistance is estimated at $10^{-2}\Omega/cm^2$, six orders of magnitude lower than that of nonjunctional membrane (9,10). Given this limit and assuming a channel spacing (d) of 100 Å and a packing of $1/2(\sqrt{3}d^2)$ channels per unit area, an upper limit of resistance for the single channel is obtained of the order of 10^{10} Ω.[1]

This value fits reasonably well with the re-

---

[1] The channel spacing in this computation is based on the spacing between the membrane particles seen in the freeze-fractured gap junction, assumed to contain the channels (see refs. 11–14). Although the particle packing is not strictly hexagonal, the error introduced by this assumption does not change the order of magnitude of the calculated resistance.

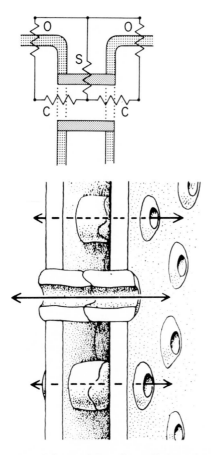

Then the resistance of the single channel is given by

$$\frac{l\tau}{\pi a^2} + \tau df(2a/d),$$

where the first term is the resistance of the isolated channel and the second term the additional resistance resulting from the electrostatic interaction between channels: a is the channel radius; l the channel length; τ the resistivity of the channel core; d the channel spacing; and $f(2a/d)$, the ratio of the resistance of the channel system to that of a single isolated channel (see 15). Computations for a channel of 10 Å radius, 200 Å length (two membrane thicknesses), and a core resistivity of 50 Ωcm (cytoplasm) give a resistance of the order of 10^{10} Ω.

Permeability to Larger Molecules

The junctional membrane elements are also quite permeable to molecules larger than the inorganic ions. This was first shown for the junctions in salivary gland, using the strongly fluorescent fluorescein (330 MW) as a tracer (16) and confirmed for a variety of cells, including an electrical synapse (3,17–21). A number of dyes that do not significantly permeate nonjunctional membranes have since been shown to pass through junctions: several colorant molecules ranging from 300 to 990 MW (22,23), the 550 MW fluorescent Procion yellow (18,24,25), and the fluorescent 370 MW dansyl-DL-aspartate and the 380 MW dansyl-L-glutamate (25).

The range of junctional permeability probes has recently been enlarged by the *ad hoc* synthesis of fluorescent polymers of glucose and glycine, and the use of fluorescent polypeptides (I. N. Simpson, B. Rose, H. Wiegandt, and W. R. Loewenstein, *unpublished*). Our results with these probes spanning a broad range of molecular sizes suggest an upper limit between 1,000 and 2,000 MW for permeation of the junctional channels in *Chironomus* salivary gland cells (Table 1).[2]

FIG. 1. **Top:** Scheme of the cell-to-cell channel as defined by electrical measurements and by intracellular tracer diffusion. O, nonjunctional membrane, 10^4 Ωcm²; C, junctional membrane, 10^{-2} Ωcm²; S, junctional insulation. The cell-to-cell channel resistance, $2r_c \leq 10^{10}$ Ω. (From Loewenstein, ref. 2.) **Bottom:** A schematic representation of a model of membrane junction in which the cell-to-cell channels are pictured as two abutting protein channels traversing the membranes. The junctional insulation is assumed to be given by the hydrophobic regions of the protein particles and their abutment. (Reproduced with permission from Loewenstein, ref. 75.)

sistance expected *a priori* for a channel with a 10 Å radius, the radius suggested by the studies with fluorescent probes described below. The channel may be treated, in a first approximation, as a cylindrical volume conductor. The effect of the interaction between the potential fields of the neighboring channels can be estimated on the assumption that the potential field is similar to that of a boundary tube of a diameter equal to the channel spacing with the channel on axis.

---

[2] An earlier estimate of a limit of the order of 10^4 MW, based on experiments with fluorescent serum albumin as a tracer in *Drosophila* salivary cells (22), is now shown to be wrong. The protein was probably degraded inside the cells and a fluorescent-labeled peptide fragment had crossed the junction.

TABLE 1. *Tracer molecules used for probing junctional permeability*

Molecule	Mol. weight	Cell junction	Cell-cell passage	Reference
Fluorescent dyes				
Fluorescein	332	salivary gland[a]	+	Loewenstein and Kanno, 1964 (16)
		electrical synapse	+	Pappas and Bennett, 1966 (17)
		cultured fibroblasts	+	Furshpan and Potter, 1968 (3)
		cult. epithelial cells	+	Azarnia and Loewenstein, 1971 (20)
		isolated embryo cells	+	Sheridan, 1971 (19)
Procion yellow	550	electrical synapse	+	Payton et al., 1969 (24)
		salivary gland[a]	+	Rose, 1971 (18)
		fibroblasts	+	Johnson and Sheridan, 1971 (25)
Colorants				
Azur B	305	salivary gland[a]	+	Kanno and Loewenstein, 1966 (22)
Orange G	452	salivary gland[a]	+	Kanno and Loewenstein, 1966 (22)
Solantine turquoise[b]	700	salivary gland[a]	+	Kanno and Loewenstein, 1966 (22)
Tripan blue[b]	960	salivary gland[a]	+	Kanno and Loewenstein, 1966 (22)
Evans blue[b]	961	salivary gland[a]	+	Kanno and Loewenstein, 1966 (22)
Chicago blue	993	embryo	+[c]	Potter et al., 1966 (23)
Fluorescent amino acids				
Dansyl-DL-aspartate	366	cultured fibroblasts	+	Johnson and Sheridan, 1971 (25)
Dansyl-L-glutamate	380	cultured fibroblasts	+	Johnson and Sheridan, 1971 (25)
Rhodamine glutamate	688	salivary gland[a]	+	Simpson et al., 1975[d]
Fluorescent polymers				
Dansyl-glycine	308	salivary gland[a]	+	Simpson et al., 1975[d]
Dansyl-hexaglycine	594	salivary gland[a]	+	Simpson et al., 1975[d]
FITC-hexaglycine	794	salivary gland[a]	+	Simpson et al., 1975[d]
FITC[e]-glucose	565	salivary gland[a]	+	Simpson et al., 1975[d]
FITC-maltose	725	salivary gland[a]	+	Simpson et al., 1975[d]
FITC-maltotriose	899	salivary gland[a]	+	Simpson et al., 1975[d]
FITC-maltotetraose	1,058	salivary gland[a]	+	Simpson et al., 1975[d]
Fluorescent peptides				
Dansyl insulin, A chain	3,200	salivary gland	−	Simpson et al., 1975[d]
FITC insulin, A chain	2,900	salivary gland	−	Simpson et al., 1975[d]
FITC insulin, B chain	4,300	salivary gland	−	Simpson et al., 1975[d]
FITC microperoxidase	2,800	salivary gland	−	Simpson et al., 1975[d]
FITC polylysine	127,000	salivary gland	−	Kanno and Loewenstein, 1966 (22)
Nucleic acid				
RNA bacteriophage F-2	10^6	salivary gland	−	Loewenstein, 1967[f]

[a] Tests were made showing that passage is blocked by rise in cytoplasmic Ca^{2+} concentration.
[b] Relatively poor tracer that binds to cytoplasm.
[c] Variable results.
[d] I. Simpson, B. Rose, H. Wiegandt, and W. R. Loewenstein, *unpublished results*.
[e] FITC = fluoresceinisothiocyanide.
[f] *Unpublished data.*

Table 1 lists the tracer substances that so far have been employed. The general method here was to microinject the fluorescent or colorant molecules into a cell and to observe under a microscope their passage to adjacent cells. In the case of the nucleic acid, active RNA-phage was microinjected into a cell, and the content of cell neighbors was seeded and assayed with the usual agar plaque method.

Another method makes use of certain enzyme-deficient mutant cells that are rendered metabolically competent when grown in contact with wild-type cells (26). Low–molecular weight molecules appear to be transferred from the wild-type cell to the mutant cell (27,28), a transfer shown to be related to the presence of permeable junctions (21,29). In this method the mutant cell is simply cocultured with the wild-type cell, and the incorporation of the radioactive material into the corresponding metabolic pathways of the mutant is determined by autoradiography. With the aid of this method, nucleotides, sugar phosphate, choline phosphate, and the cofactor tetrahydrofolate, but not large proteins or nucleic acids, were found to be exchanged by junction-forming cells (30).

Channel Insulation

The channel insulation is a diffusion barrier for all molecules including the small inorganic ions; the lower limit of the electrical resistance of this barrier in *Drosophila* gland cell junction, expressed as surface resistance, is shown to be greater than 10^4 Ωm^2, the resistance of nonjunctional membrane (16). In newt embryo cells, where the absolute resistance could be determined, the total resistance of all channel insulations in one junction containing $> 10^4$ channels is of the order of 10^8 Ω (10); i.e., the insulation for the single channel amounts to $> 10^{12}$ Ω.

At the time I postulated the cell-cell channel unit at the Membrane Conference of 1966 (2), there was little information on the nature of the channel insulation. The nature, to be sure, is still unknown, but the general physical and chemical knowledge of cell membranes has since much increased and, for membrane junctions, freeze-fracture electron microscopy has now provided at least a basis for reasonable guessing. Thus, for instance, if the membrane particles seen in the freeze-fractured gap junction (11–14) contain the channels and the channels are made of protein (31,32), then, in the light of present membrane concepts (see 33), it is plausible that the cell-cell channel is given by two abutting protein channels and that the insulation, by the hydrophobic regions of the proteins, and by their abutment (Fig. 1). Be this as it may, the insulation is an essential channel feature permitting rather leak-proof exchange of molecules between cells.

Channel Formation

The channels are not patent while the cells, that can make them, are separate. They become functional when the cells are joined. The development of a fully coupled system takes on the order of minutes in many kinds of cells (19,34–39). The channels are blocked or disappear rapidly when the cells are separated. This is shown conveniently in macroblastomeres isolated from newt embryo (morula) (9). Junction formation is readily induced in these giant cells (0.5 mm diameter) by manipulating them into contact, and it is feasible to keep the electrodes inside them throughout the development of coupling (Fig. 2). When the cells are pushed together, they make permeable channels within 4 to 20 min. When the cells are pulled apart, the channels seal. New channels form when the cells are joined at different spots; and so on. Thus, a large part of the surface membrane of these cells, perhaps all of it, is capable of channel formation (9). A similar conclusion followed from a study of junction formation in sponge cells in which channel formation was induced by random cell contact (34).

Figure 2 illustrates a continuous electrical measurement during the formation of a junction between two newt embryo cells. Current (i) is pulsed between interior and exterior of cell 1, and the resulting changes in membrane potential (V) are measured in cells 1 and 2. Coupling develops progressively, as reflected in the gradual rise of V_2 and the gradual fall in V_1.

Such a simple two-cell system reduces to a

$\longrightarrow$

FIG. 2. Channel formation. Evolving resistances of junctional membrane and junctional insulation during junction formation *in vitro* between two newt embryo cells. The two cells were isolated from the embryo and micromanipulated into contact. **A:** Record of a continuous electrical measurement during development of coupling. Current ($i = 0.9 \times 10^{-8}$ A) is passed between the interior of cell 1 and the exterior, and the resulting steady-state changes (V) in membrane potential (E) are continuously measured in cells 1 and 2. The V_2 electrode was inside cell 2 since the establishment of cell contact (time = 0); the V_1 electrode was inserted when V_2 became detectable (c mark). **B:** Coupling coefficient V_2/V_1. **C:** V_1 (●) and V_2 (▲). **D:** Computed total junctional membrane resistance ($2 r_c$; ●); junctional insulation resistance (r_s; ▲); logarithmic scale. The time scale is common for the record and the plotted curves.

Top inset: *right,* circuit diagram; *left* **a,** photomicrograph of a developing junction between two cells; **b,** two coupling cells; the three measuring electrodes are visible; **c,** breaking of the junction; the cells were micromanipulated apart (the last connecting strand is seen breaking). Calibration 160 μm for a; 100 μm for b and c. (Reproduced with permission from Ito et al., ref. 10.)

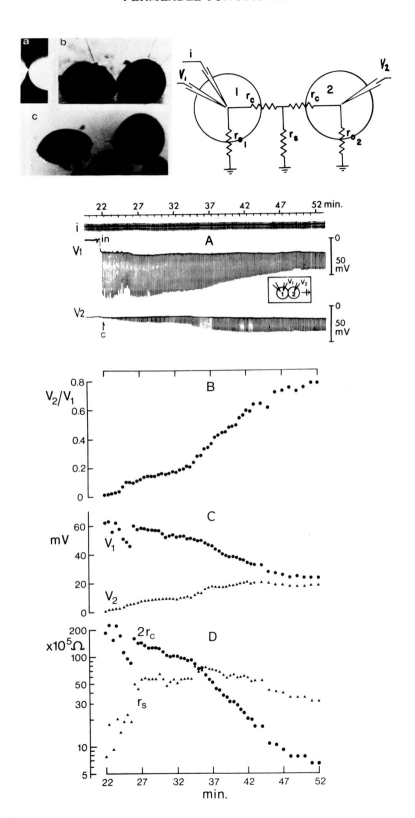

manageable number the continuous electrical measurements needed for determining the conductance of the evolving junctional membrane and junctional insulation. We determine first the cell membrane resistances, r_{o1}, r_{o2}, while the cells are separate; we measure next V_1 and V_2 (and i) while the cells are coupling; and again r_{o1} and r_{o2} after separating the cells. Then, with the aid of Kirchoff's laws, the total junctional membrane resistance, $2r_c$ and the total junctional resistance, r_s, are given by

$$r_c = \frac{V_1 - V_2}{i - \left(\dfrac{V_1}{r_{o1}} - \dfrac{V_2}{r_{o2}}\right)},$$

$$r_s = \frac{V_1}{i - \left(\dfrac{V_1}{r_{o1}} + \dfrac{V_2}{r_{o2}}\right)} - \frac{i - \dfrac{V_1}{r_{o1}}}{i - \left(\dfrac{V_1}{r_{o1}} + \dfrac{V_2}{r_{o2}}\right)} \; r_c$$

The general result of such a measurement, as exemplified by Fig. 2D, is that r_c falls two orders of magnitude over an average period of 20 min, while r_s rises one to three orders of magnitude and then settles somewhat below peak. A plausible and simple interpretation of this result is that *junctional coupling develops by progressive addition of channel units* and that the channel insulation, the unit r_s, initially improves and/or that the resistance of the extracellular leakage pathway in between the channels increases during channel accretion.[3]

We have as yet no electron microscopic information on the newt embryo cell junction to ponder the notion of coupling development by accretion of channel units. However, for junctions of Novikoff's hepatoma fibroblasts, there is freeze-fracture evidence that the first clusters of gap-junction particles appear within 5 min of

---

[3] In the case of an improvement of channel insulation, the rising phase of total r_s would reflect the dominance of the increasing unit r_s over the effect of parallel leak contribution of the growing number of channels, and the falling phase, the shift in dominance. The increase in resistance of the extracellular leakage pathway in between channels is conceivable, for instance, if a significant r_s component is associated with the convolution and restriction of leakage of this pathway, constraints which would multiply as more and more channels are formed; the rise of (total) r_s would then represent dominance of the increasing constraints over increasing leakage contributions.

cell aggregation, at about the time coupling between these cells becomes detectable; and that the number of particles increases with time (40).

Action of Ca^{2+}

Uncoupling by Ca^{2+}

The permeability of the junctional channels depends on Ca^{2+}. In an established junction, where the channels sealed off from the exterior by the junctional insulation face the low Ca^{2+} concentration of the cytoplasm ($<10^{-6}$ M), the permeability is high. The permeability dependence on Ca is shown by two classes of experiments. In one, the interior of the coupled cell system is allowed to equilibrate with known concentrations of Ca^{2+} in the external medium through a hole in the nonjunctional cell membrane. The channel conductance and permeability for molecules of the size of fluorescein fall drastically at Ca^{2+} concentrations above 5 to 8×10^{-5} M (Fig. 3) (41).

In another class of experiments, performed on the closed cell system, aequorin is used as an indicator of cytoplasmic Ca^{2+} while uncoupling is produced by microinjection of Ca^{2+} into a cell or by treatment with agents that inhibit the energized sequestering and extrusion of cytoplasmic Ca^{2+}. The aequorin (30,000 MW) is injected into a pair of coupled *Chironomus* salivary gland cells and its light emission (which increases as a function of Ca^{2+} concentration; 42) is viewed through a microscope with the aid of an image intensifier coupled to a television camera (Fig. 4) (43). This novel aspect of the aequorin technique allows one to see where inside the cell the Ca^{2+} concentration is changing and by how much. The method has a spatial resolution of 1 μm and a sensitivity for 10^{-6} M Ca^{2+} concentration over a 2- μm diameter cytoplasmic volume in the steady state.

Figure 5 gives an example in which Ca^{2+} (buffered with EGTA) is injected into a cell. Short puffs of 5 to 10×10^{-5} M free Ca^{2+} are seen as aequorin glows that are confined to the immediate vicinity of the injection pipette (Fig. 5). As described below, the confinement is mainly caused by rapid energized Ca^{2+} sequestering. Such a local Ca^{2+} puff into cell center does not affect the junctional channels. The channel conductance, however, is promptly reduced (un-

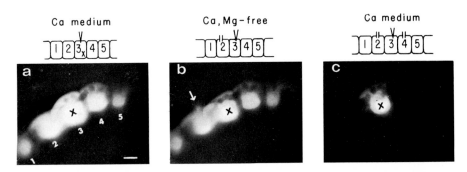

FIG. 3. Channel block by Ca^{2+}. Junctional permeability in a chain of *Chironomus* salivary gland cells is probed by fluorescein (300 MW). The darkfield photomicrographs show the spread of this fluorescent dye injected into cell 3: **a,** in the intact cell system; **b,** after making a hole into cell 2 in Ca,Mg-free medium (fluorescein leaks visibly through the hole; arrow); **c,** in Ca-containing (12 mM) medium (a hole was made here also in cell 4, bracketing the injected cell). Calibration 50 μm. (From Oliveira-Castro and Loewenstein, ref. 41.)

coupling) when the puff is fast and long enough to saturate the local sequestering capacity and the aequorin reaches the junction. The channels open again after the cells have rid themselves of the excess Ca^{2+} by pumping it out (Fig. 5B).

In a variant of this experiment, the Ca^{2+} puff is delivered close to one of the junctions (junction 1/2) of a cell with two junctions. Here the rise in cytoplasmic Ca^{2+} concentration encompasses junction 1/2 but not the other junction (1/3), 100 μm away; significant electrical uncoupling is shown to occur at the former junction alone (Fig. 6) (47).

In another set of experiments, the cells are treated with ionophores A23187 (2×10^{-6} M) or X537A (1×10^{-5} M). This leads, within 1 min, to a diffuse rise in cytoplasmic Ca^{2+} concentration, detectable as a diffuse aequorin glow that reaches all junctions of the cell. The rise in cytoplasmic Ca^{2+} is then invariably associated with uncoupling (Fig. 7). Similar results and an equally good correlation between rising cytoplasmic Ca^{2+} and uncoupling are obtained in experiments in which the cells are poisoned with cyanide (5×10^{-3} M)(Fig. 8) (43).

In all these conditions, the rise in cytoplasmic Ca^{2+} concentration is accompanied by depolarization (the Na conductance of nonjunctional membrane increases). Hence, the question needed to be resolved of whether the cytoplasmic Ca^{2+} or the depolarization is the primary cause of the uncoupling: Ca^{2+} was injected while the cell membrane potential was clamped near resting level with a feedback system. Uncoupling ensued nonetheless when-

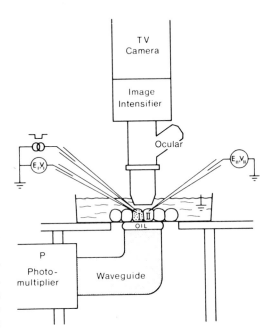

FIG. 4. Set-up for visualizing free cytoplasmic Ca^{2+}. One or two cells contain aequorin, and the $[Ca^{2+}]$-dependent aequorin luminescence is scanned by an image intensifier-television system and integrated separatedly by a photomultiplier. Electrical coupling is measured as in Fig. 2. Photomultiplier current P, and the coupling parameters i, E_1, E_2, V_1, and V_2 are displayed on a chart recorder and a storage oscilloscope onto which a second TV camera is focused. The two camera outputs are displayed simultaneously on a monitor and videotaped. (Reproduced with permission from Rose and Loewenstein, ref. 43.)

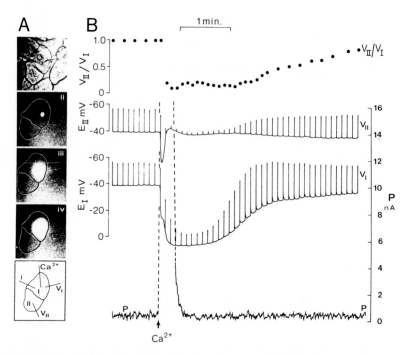

FIG. 5. Junctional uncoupling by intracellular injection of Ca^{2+}. **A:** Darkfield TV pictures (ii–iv) of aequorin luminescence, produced by three puffs of 5×10^{-5} M free Ca^{2+} (buffered with EGTA) of increasing magnitude, delivered to about the center of the basal region of a *Chironomus* salivary gland cell. The pictures are each taken at the time of maximum luminescence spread. Cell diameter ca. 100 μm. Puffs *ii* and *iii* do not reach the junction of the cell and do not affect coupling. Puff *iv* reaches one junction causing transient uncoupling, as shown by electrical measurements in **B:** chart records of P, E_I, E_{II}, V_I, V_{II} (i = 4×10^{-8} A) and plot of coupling coefficient V_{II}/V_I. Note the rapid recoupling after restoration of normal Ca^{2+} activity. *i*, brightfield TV picture of the cells. *Bottom*, cell diagram showing location of microelectrodes and of Ca injection pipette (hydraulic); dotted cell preinjected with aequorin. (Reproduced with permission from Rose and Loewenstein, ref. 43.)

ever the aequorin glow produced by the injection reached the junction (Fig. 9). Uncoupling was even observed when the membrane potential was raised above the original level. Depolarization is thus clearly not necessary for uncoupling.

In a complementing series of experiments, the cells were exposed to high K (90 mM) medium. Within 2 to 5 min, the membrane potentials fell to near zero or overshot zero by 5 to 10 mV. The depolarized cells nevertheless stayed well coupled much longer, often for several hours. Eventually and rather abruptly, they uncoupled, and this was invariably associated with an abrupt rise in cytoplasmic Ca^{2+} concentration (43). Depolarization is thus also not sufficient for uncoupling.

In sum, *the cytoplasmic Ca^{2+} concentration in the domain of the junction seems to determine the permeability of the channels.* We do not know the mechanism by which the calcium

ion alters the permeability. Conceivably Ca^{2+} binds to junctional membrane changing the conformation of the channels (44). We favor this simple notion, because the permeability change is readily reversed when the normal cytoplasmic Ca^{2+} concentration is restored in cells with normal Ca-sequestering and Ca-pumping activity.[4]

Selective Uncoupling by Ca^{2+}

The decrease in junctional conductance in the foregoing experiments occurs when the

---

[4] The permeability reversal typically lags behind the fall of the cytoplasmic Ca^{2+} concentration (Fig. 5B). We don't know the lag in respect to restoration of the original Ca^{2+} level. However, such a lag may be expected if the affinity for Ca^{2+} binding to junctional membrane is high. A variety of physiological Ca^{2+} binding reactions to cellular proteins are known to exhibit this behavior.

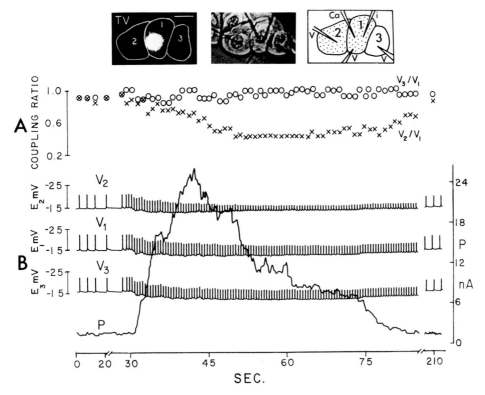

FIG. 6. Local uncoupling. Ca^{2+} is iontophoresed close to cell junction 1/2. The resulting aequorin glow encompasses this junction, but not junction 1/3 of the same cell; only junction 1/2 uncouples significantly. Test current ($i = 4 \times 10^{-8}$ A) is pulsed into cell 1, and V is measured in cell 2 and 3. **Top:** Darkfield TV picture at time of maximum luminescence spread (peak on P record). Calibration, 100 μm. To the right, brightfield TV picture of the cells and diagram of the electrode arrangement. Cells 1 and 2 contain aequorin. **B:** Chart record of E_1, E_2, E_3, V_1, V_2, V_3, and P. **A:** Coupling coefficients V_2/V_1 and V_3/V_1. (From Rose and Loewenstein, ref. 47.)

cytoplasmic Ca^{2+} concentration in the junctional region is above 5×10^{-5} M. This decrease in junctional permeability to the small inorganic ions goes hand in hand with a decrease in permeability to the larger fluorescein anion; the cell-to-cell passage of this molecule is blocked or the rate of passage is slowed by more than one order of magnitude (41,45). However, at Ca^{2+} concentrations somewhat lower than 5×10^{-5} M, the junctional change appears more selective: fluorescein passage is blocked or markedly slowed, whereas little or no change in electrical coupling is detectable (Fig. 10) (46). Possible interpretations of this result are the following. (a) The effective channel bore is reduced even at the lower Ca^{2+} concentration (although less than at the higher ones) and this reduction is more limiting for the 300-MW fluorescein anion than for the smaller inorganic

ions. (b) The effect of Ca^{2+} is an all-or-none channel closure, but relatively few channels are closed at the low Ca^{2+} concentration. This seems possible, because the resolution for detecting closure of a small channel fraction may be greater in the fluorescein method than in the measurement of electrical coupling. The coupling coefficient is a very sensitive indicator in the low range but relatively insensitive in the high range.

Another possibility—that the fluorescein and inorganic ions take altogether different routes— seems unlikely for the following reasons. (a) Most of the tracer molecules listed in Table 1 do not permeate nonjunctional membrane, but since, like fluorescein, they all pass from cell to cell in fractions of a second, they must clearly take the junctional route. (b) In developing junctions between reaggregated *Xenopus* em-

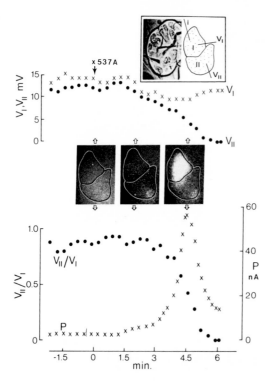

FIG. 7. Uncoupling produced by Ca^{2+} transporting ionophore X537A. Exposure to 1×10^{-5} M X537A starts at black arrow and continues throughout the remainder of the experiment. **Top:** V_I, V_{II} ($i = 4 \times 10^{-8}$ A); **center:** darkfield TV pictures of luminescence (open arrows indicate their time correspondence); **bottom:** coupling coefficient V_{II}/V_I; photocurrent P. Peak of luminescence in cell II (not shown) occurred 5 min after peak in I. **Top inset:** Brightfield TV picture and cell diagram; cells I and II contain aequorin. (Reproduced with permission from Rose and Loewenstein, ref. 43.)

bryo cells, fluorescein passes only between the cells that are electrically coupled; mere adhesive contact between these cells is not sufficient for fluorescein passage (19). (c) Cell-to-cell passage of fluorescein in *Chironomus* and *Drosophila* salivary glands and in mammalian liver cells is blocked whenever these cells are electrically uncoupled by elevation of cytoplasmic Ca^{2+} concentration (2,22,41,44,45,47). This, and not the converse, is, of course, the condition for the small and large molecules sharing the same channel, a condition fulfilled by all tracer substances in Table 1 so tested (marked by ^{a}). (c) Certain cell strains, which by genetic defect are incapable of transferring inorganic ions through junctions are also in-

capable of transferring fluorescein; the correction of the latter defect by genetic manipulation goes hand in hand with correction of the former defect (see below). For all these reasons, I have tacitly assumed in this chapter that there is only one kind of junctional channel in a given cell junction type.

Possible Functional Roles of Uncoupling by Ca^{2+}

Among the possible functional adaptations of junctional uncoupling by Ca^{2+}, the most obvious one is the capacity of the connected cell ensemble to uncouple from an unhealthy member. Thus, for example, if Ca^{2+} pumping in (nonjunctional) cell membrane is abnormally slow or the cell membrane is injured, the ensuing unbalanced or excessive Ca^{2+} influx will lead to the sealing of the junctions of the abnormal cell.

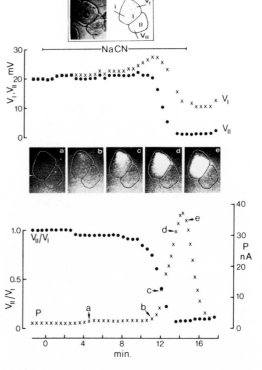

FIG. 8. Uncoupling by cyanide. Exposure to 5 mM sodium cyanide (*top signal*); Ca-free medium. Time correspondence of TV pictures marked on P curve. $i = 4 \times 10^{-8}$ A. (Reproduced with permission from Rose and Loewenstein, ref. 43.)

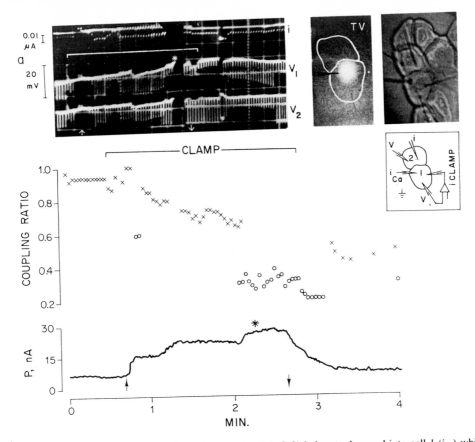

FIG. 9. Uncoupling by Ca^{2+} at clamped membrane potential. Ca^{2+} is ionotophoresed into cell I (i_{Ca}) while the membrane potential is held near resting value by a feed-back controlled inward current (i clamp) for the period marked "clamp." Coupling is measured in both directions across the junction with test current pulse into cell I (x) or cell 2 (o). Electrode i_{Ca} is filled with Ca-EGTA and serves to inject Ca^{2+} (outward current) and to pass the (inward) test current pulses (EGTA$^-$), 200 msec duration, 0.4/sec. The feedback gain used allows passage of attenuated V pulses, but, as coupling between the two cells diminishes, V_1 is more attenuated than V_2, as reflected in the discrepancy of the coupling ratios x and o; the true ratios lie then somewhere between the observed values. P, photomultiplier current indicating the cytoplasmic Ca^{2+} concentration; arrows mark "on" and "off" of Ca^{2+} iontophoresis. **a:** Storage oscilloscope records of i_{Ca}, i_1, i_2 (*top trace*), E_1, E_2, V_1, V_2; *white bar*, clamp period, *arrows*, the period of iontophoresis. *TV*, sample of darkfield pictures of aequorin luminescence showing the spatial intracellular distribution of Ca^{2+} at the time marked by asterisk on the P curve and oscilloscope record. Calibration, 100 μm. To the right, the brightfield TV picture of the cells and the microelectrodes. Both cells contain aequorin. (From Rose and Loewenstein, ref. 63.)

The elements of the sealing reaction are built into the normal cell system and are critically poised: the Ca^{2+} concentration profile falls off steeply across the cell membrane in the inward direction and the junctional channels are capable of rapid closure in the presence of a sufficiently high Ca^{2+} concentration. All that is required to set the reaction into motion is a sufficient depression of the cellular energy metabolism on which the Ca^{2+} pump depends, or a discontinuity in the cell membrane. The experiments of Figs. 3 and 8, in fact, are good micromodels of what one expects to happen during, respectively, ordinary tissue wounds

and abnormalities in cell energy metabolism. If it were not for this fast mechanism of channel closure, a tissue-like skin, with widely interconnected cells, would not survive an injury; or a liver, in which most cells are interconnected (48), could not survive the death of even a single cell. Indeed, in skin wounds, junctional uncoupling is one of the first reactions to injury; the junctional channels of the intact cells at the wound border seal themselves off from the injured ones (49).

Another interesting, although a more speculative possibility is that uncoupling plays a role in embryonic development, namely in the fixa-

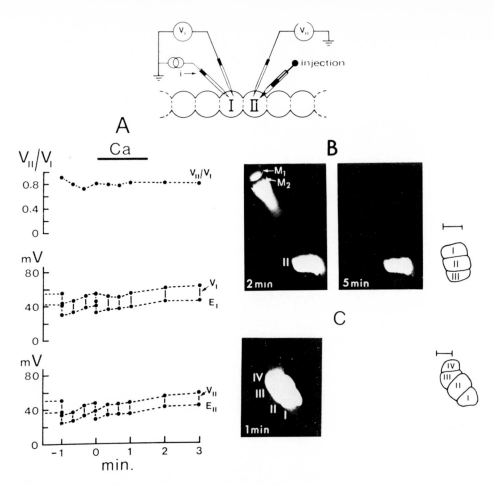

FIG. 10. "Selective" uncoupling. Injection of 5 pmole of Ca (unbuffered) into a *Chironomus* salivary gland cell causes block of cell-to-cell flow of fluorescein (**B**), without significant changes in electrical coupling (**A**). Ca and fluorescein (isotonic solution) are injected together (hydraulically) into cell II for the period signaled by the bar in *A*. V_I and V_{II} are plotted here as displacements of E_I. **B**: Darkfield photomicrographs of the fluorescence, 2 and 5 min after injection, which is seen confined to the injected cell II at the lower right corner of the photograph. Superposed (*top left*) are photographs of the fluorescent solution in the micropipette, showing the meniscus M_1, M_2 before and after the injection; the injected volume was calculated from the difference in meniscus height. **C**: A control experiment, in another preparation, in which an isotonic fluorescein–KCl solution is injected into a cell (III). *Calibrations,* 100 μm. No aequorin is used in these experiments. (From Délèze and Loewenstein, ref. 46.)

tion of cellular differentiations. I have discussed this in detail elsewhere for both total and selective uncoupling (50,51). Here I mention only that selective uncoupling, which seemed then remote, emerges now as a serious, although experimentally no less dreaded, possibility in the light of the experiments illustrated in Fig. 10. In the same direction point also the results obtained with some embryos in which, following a general embryo characteristic (23,52–56), the cells are electrically coupled; yet they show no fluorescein transfer within the limits of the methods (57–59; but see also 19).

THE DOMAIN OF CYTOPLASMIC Ca^{2+} DIFFUSION AND INTERCELLULAR COMMUNICATION

There are various tissues with permeable junctions, such as heart muscle, smooth muscle, endocrine and exocrine glands in which the intracellular Ca^{2+} concentration rises during physiological activity. However, this is not necessarily incompatible with a high junctional permeability, because the domain of free Ca^{2+} diffusion in the aqueous phase of the cytoplasm (cytosol), unlike that of all other

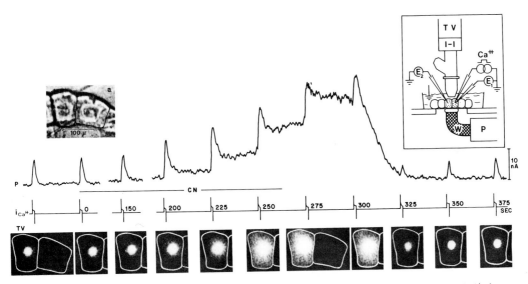

FIG. 11. Energy-dependent Ca^{2+} diffusion restriction in the cytosol. Standard Ca^{2+} test pulses, 2.4/min, are iontophoresed into the basal region of a salivary gland cell. *TV*, darkfield TV pictures giving the spatial distribution of the resulting aequorin luminescence at the time of maximum spread of each luminescence pulse. *P*, chart records of photomultiplier current giving the time course of the corresponding luminescent pulses. Iontophoretic current pulses $i_{Ca} = 1.5 \times 10^{-8}$ A; 1 sec duration. For the period indicated by the bar (CN), the preparation is superfused with 2 mM cyanide; the numbers indicate the time (sec) after the beginning of superfusion (time for half maximal concentration change in the bath is of the order of 0.5 min). The Ca^{2+}-injected cell and the adjacent one contain aequorin. Note that there is no detectable intracellular release of Ca^{2+} at this cyanide concentration. Cells in Ca-free medium. **a:** Brightfield TV pictures of the two aequorin loaded cells. (Reproduced with permission from Rose and Loewenstein, ref. 63.)

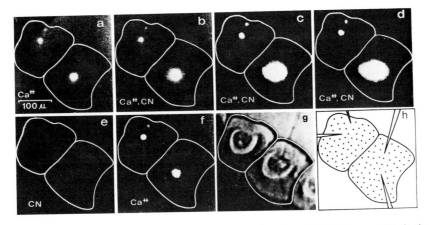

FIG. 12. Cytoplasmic Ca^{2+} diffusion restriction at membrane leak points. Ca^{2+} leaks are visible in the darkfield TV pictures a–f as three luminescent dots. The two dots on the left cell are the Ca^{2+} leaks at the points of insertion of two microelectrodes of <0.2 μm tip diameter. The larger leak in the right cell was produced by vibrating such a microelectrode for a few sec before **a**. **a:** Leaks in medium containing 4 mM Ca; **b–d:** 1, 2, 3 min after application of medium containing 4 mM Ca and 2 mM cyanide. **e:** Ca-free medium containing 2 mM cyanide. **f:** 2 min after return to medium of **a**. **g:** Brightfield TV pictures of the two aequorin-loaded cells. **h:** Cell diagram showing electrode location. There was no detectable leak at the upper electrode insertion in the right cell (Reproduced with permission from Rose and Loewenstein, ref. 63.)

cellular inorganic ions, is severely restricted (60–62). Figure 11 illustrates this for the case of a Ca^{2+} injection into a *Chironomus* salivary gland cell, where the Ca^{2+} distribution is displayed by the glow of aequorin. The immediately striking feature here is that the rise in Ca^{2+} concentration is confined to the vicinity of the micropipette tip: the Ca^{2+} concentration, which is $>10^{-4}$ M within a radius of 16 μm of the glow sphere around the tip, falls precipitously within the next 1 to 2 μm to below 10^{-6} M, the limit of the method. This remarkable restriction of Ca^{2+} diffusion is primarily due to sequestering by mitochondria or other intracellular energized Ca^{2+} sinks: when the cell is injected with ruthenium red (0.1 mM), a blocker of mitochondrial Ca^{2+} uptake, or when it is treated with cyanide (2 mM), the injected Ca^{2+} spreads throughout the cytoplasm. The Ca^{2+} concentration then falls off more gradually with distance, approaching the pattern of a more freely diffusing molecule[5] (Fig. 11) (63).

A further illustration of the restriction for Ca^{2+} diffusion is given in Fig. 12 for the case of Ca^{2+} entry through cell membrane. Here Ca^{2+} is seen to leak in at the points of insertion of three microelectrodes. Again, the increase in cytoplasmic Ca^{2+} concentration is highly localized. In the example of the smallest of the three leaks (around an ordinary microelectrode where the Ca^{2+} flux is probably not more than five times the flux through intact membrane), the rise in Ca^{2+} is confined to within 1 to 2 μm from the membrane leak points so long as intracellular Ca^{2+} sequestering is unimpaired (Fig. 12c,d).

The limiting factors in the restriction of Ca^{2+} spread in both kinds of experiments are thus clearly the metabolically driven Ca^{2+} sinks (mitochondria, etc., see 64) inside the cells. Ca^{2+}, of course, binds also to the aequorin, and to cytoplasmic protein (in fact, Ca^{2+} binds strongly to axoplasmic protein; P. F. Baker and W. Schlaepfer, *personal communication*) but, these bindings are not predominant factors here, as shown by the experiments with cyanide and ruthenium red. (Aequorin light emission itself is not affected by cyanide).

---

[5] At this cyanide concentration, there is no detectable intracellular Ca^{2+} release, as determined between the earlier pulses (0 to 200 sec, Fig. 11) in the test cell and throughout the experiment in the adjacent cell.

The restriction for Ca^{2+} spread in the cytosol explains why in the experimental situations of Figs. 5 (ii, iii) and 6, the channels stay open even though a substantial rise in Ca^{2+} concentration occurs only short distances away. Thus, to return to the above question, it seems quite possible that junctional permeability in gland, heart, and smooth muscle cells may not be perturbed during physiological activities involving local elevations of cytoplasmic Ca^{2+} concentration. In the following, I shall attempt to state this in a wider sense, as it might apply to intracellular communication by Ca^{2+} signals in general.

THE DOMAIN OF CYTOPLASMIC Ca^{2+} DIFFUSION AND INTRACELLULAR COMMUNICATION

Hypothesis of Private-Line Intracellular Communication

In a variety of physiological processes, Ca^{2+} seems to be a messenger between events in the cell surface membrane and in the cell interior. Examples are the processes of muscle contraction (65), synaptic transmitter release (66, 67), gland secretion (68,69), and visual cell

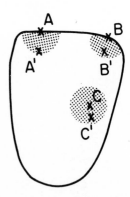

FIG. 13. Hypothesis of intracellular private-line communication by Ca^{2+}. Membrane processes A and B (transducer sites for transmembrane Ca^{2+} flux) and intracellular process C (a Ca^{2+} release site) are connected by the Ca^{2+} flux (the communication line) respectively to Ca-sensitive intracellular processes A', B', C'. The domains over which Ca^{2+} concentration is significant for messenger function are represented in gray. Where these domains are small, because of sufficiently dense and fast Ca^{2+} sequestering elements, there is no cross-talk between communication lines.

excitation (70,71). Thus, from the result that the domain of Ca^{2+} diffusion in the cytosol is so uniquely restricted, emerges the interesting possibility that in some of these intracellular messenger functions, Ca^{2+} may operate within such restricted domains, that is, several such domains may coexist in a cell, without message interference; or, to state this in different terms, in cells equipped with sufficient Ca^{2+} sinks, cellular processes may be connected by discrete Ca^{2+} lines of communication.

Consider, for example, the case of two re-

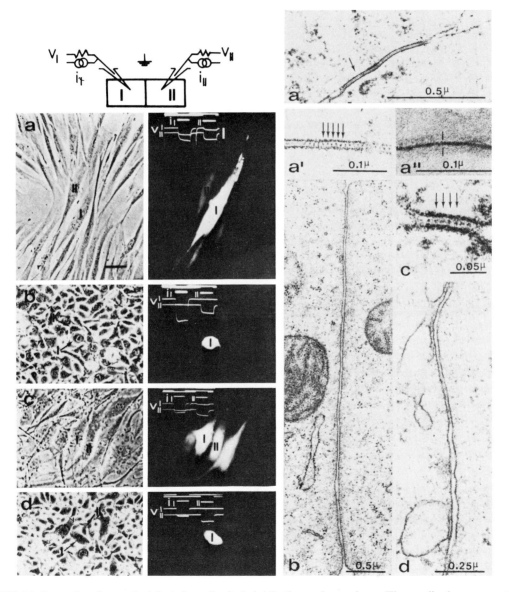

FIG. 14. Correction of a genetic defect of coupling by hybridization, and reversion. **a:** The coupling human parent cell. **b:** The noncoupling mouse parent cell. **c:** Early hybrid cell. **d:** A segregant cell, after loss of certain human chromosomes a few generations later. **Left:** Photomicrographs of the cells (electrode locations for coupling measurements are marked; electrode i_I contained fluorescein); **center:** oscilloscope record of i_I, i_{II}, V_I, V_{II} (input and transfer resistances are measured in both I and II); **right:** electron micrographs of the corresponding cell junctions (**a″**, after lanthanum infiltration. (From Azarnia et al., ref. 74.)

ceptor processes *A* and *B* on the cell membrane, which, in an extension of the experiments in Fig. 12, transduce Ca^{2+} flux through the membrane. The flux may now connect *A* with a sensitive intracellular process *A'* without significant crosstalk with a similar connection between *B* and *B'*, or between intracellular processes *C* and *C'* (Fig. 13). The number of such private lines will depend on the local density of the sequestering elements and on the rate and the capacity for sequestering. In the case of the basal region of the salivary gland cell (where the Ca^{2+} spread of the experiments of Figs. 11 and 12 was determined), which is crammed full with mitochondria (18), one may suspect that the number of such possible lines is high.

GENETIC ASPECTS OF JUNCTION FORMATION

The capacity of junctional channel formation seems to be a nearly universal feature of cells. The only exceptions among normal tissues seem to be skeletal muscle and most nerve fibers, which interestingly also do not divide. In normally dividing cells, the capacity is so basic that permeable junctions are made even between cultured cells from different organs and different species. For instance, a lens cell from the rabbit eye makes perfectly viable channels with a liver cell from mouse or a fibroblast from man (72).

We have been searching for some time for the rare exceptions among dividing cells that are unable to make permeable junctions. We have found so far seven cell strains that do not couple with each other or with normal cells: they show no detectable transfer of small ions, of fluorescein or of radioactive-labeled nucleotide derivatives, and, in the two strains thus tested, there are no detectable gap-junctions (20,29,73,74). We have used these strains to look into some genetic aspects of channel formation, by fusing the cells with normally coupling ones and by examining the coupling characteristics of the hybrids. In the hybrid systems so far examined, the capacity of channel formation behaves like a dominant character: the hybrids between the coupling and noncoupling cells are coupling.

I shall briefly describe the results obtained with one hybrid system, a cross between a human cell and a mouse cell. The human cell is

a skin fibroblast and the mouse cell, a derivative (Cl-1D) of an L-cell. This system is unusually suited for genetic analysis: the parent cells are genetically marked by enzyme defects permitting easy hybrid selection (the human cell is deficient in inosine pyrophosphorylase and the mouse cell in thymidine kinase), the karyotypes are readily distinguishable, and the hybrids lose chromosomes at a rate appropriate for segregant analysis. To summarize the junctional properties of the parent cells, the human cell is coupling and has gap junctions; the mouse cell is noncoupling and lacks gap junctions.

The hybrids between these cells took in all these respects after the human parent, while they contained the nearly complete chromosome complement of the two parent cells (Fig. 14). As the hybrid cells lost some of the human chromosomes after some generations, clones appeared which had reverted to the non-coupling trait of the mouse parent. In all instances, this reversion went hand in hand with reversion to the gap-junction deficient trait (as shown by both transmission- and freeze-fracture electron microscopy), although the noncoupling trait had segregated from a number of other phenotypic traits which originally went together in the mouse parent cell (74). The results thus show a genetic correlation between gap junction and coupling: the coupling cell contributes a factor to the hybrids, presumably linked to one or more of the human chromosomes, that corrects the junctional deficiency of the noncoupling cell.

REFERENCES

1. Schleiden, M. J. (1838): Beiträge zur Phytogenesis. *Müller's Arch. Anat. Physiol. Wiss. Medic.*, 1838:137–176.
2. Loewenstein, W. R. (1966): Permeability of membrane junctions. *Ann. N.Y. Acad. Sci.*, 137:441–472.
3. Furshpan, E. J., and Potter, D. D. (1968): Low resistance junctions between cells in embryos and tissue culture. *Curr. Top. Dev. Biol.*, 3:95–127.
4. Weidmann, S. (1966): The diffusion of radiopotassium across intercalated discs of mammalian cardiac muscle. *J. Physiol. (Lond.)*, 187:323–342.
5. Bennett, M. V. L. (1966): Physiology of electrotonic junctions. *Ann. N.Y. Acad. Sci.*, 137:509–539.
6. Woodbury, J. W., and Crill, W. E. (1970): The potential in the gap between two abutting cardiac muscle cells. A closed solution. *Biophys. J.*, 10:1076–1083.

7. Spira, A. W. (1971): The nexus in the intercalated disc of the canine heart: Quantitative data for estimation of its resistance. *Ultrastr. Res.*, 34: 409–425.

8. Furshpan, E. J., and Potter, D. D. (1959): Transmission at the giant motor synapse of the crayfish. *J. Physiol. (Lond.)*, 145:289–325.

9. Ito, S., and Loewenstein, W. R. (1969): Ionic communication between early embryonic cells. *Dev. Biol.*, 19:228–243.

10. Ito, S., Sato, E., and Loewenstein, W. R. (1974): Studies on the formation of a permeable membrane junction. II. Evolving junctional conductance and junctional insulation. *J. Membr. Biol.*, 19:339–355.

11. Goodenough, D. A., and Revel, J. P. (1970): A fine structural analysis of intercellular junctions in the mouse liver. *J. Cell Biol.*, 45:272–290.

12. Chalcroft, J. P., and Bullivant, S. (1970): An interpretation of liver cell membrane and junction structure based on observations of freeze-fracture replicas of both sides of the fracture. *J. Cell Biol.*, 47:49–60.

13. Pinto da Silva, P., and Gilula, N. B. (1972): Gap junctions in normal and transformed fibroblasts in culture. *Exp. Cell Res.*, 71:393–401.

14. McNutt, N., and Weinstein, R. S. (1973): Membrane ultrastructure at mammalian intercellular junction. *Progr. Biophys. Mol. Biol.*, 26: 45–101.

15. Kanno, Y., and Loewenstein, W. R. (1963): A study of the nucleus and cell membrane of oocytes with an intracellular electrode. *Exp. Cell Res.*, 31:149–166.

16. Loewenstein, W. R., and Kanno, Y. (1964): Studies on an epithelial (gland) cell junction. I. Modifications of surface membrane permeability. *J. Cell Biol.*, 22:565–586.

17. Pappas, G. D., and Bennett, M. V. L. (1966): Specialized junctions involved in electrical transmission between neurons. *Ann. N.Y. Acad. Sci.*, 137:495–508.

18. Rose, B. (1971): Intercellular communication and some structural aspects of cell junction in a simple cell system. *J. Membr. Biol.*, 5:1–19.

19. Sheridan, J. (1971): Dye movement and low resistance junctions between reaggregated embryonic cells. *Dev. Biol.*, 26:627–636.

20. Azarnia, R., and Loewenstein, W. R. (1971): Intercellular communication and tissue growth. V. A cancer cell strain that fails to make permeable junctions with normal cells. *J. Membr. Biol.*, 6:368–385.

21. Azarnia, R., Michalke, R. W., and Loewenstein, W. R. (1972): Intercellular communication and tissue growth. VI. Failure of exchange of endogenous molecules between cancer cells with defective junctions and noncancerous cells. *J. Membr. Biol.*, 10:247–258.

22. Kanno, Y., and Loewenstein, W. R. (1966): Cell-to-cell passage of large molecules. *Nature*, 212: 629.

23. Potter, D. D., Furshpan, E. J. and Lennox, E. S. (1966): Connections between cells of the developing squid as revealed by electrophysiological methods. *Proc. Natl. Acad. Sci. USA*, 55:328–335.

24. Payton, B. W., Bennett, M. V. L., and Pappas, G. D. (1969): Permeability and structure of junctional membranes at an electrotonic synapse. *Science*, 166:1641–1643.

25. Johnson, R., and Sheridan, J. D. (1971): Junctions between cancer cells in culture: ultrastructure and permeability. *Science*, 174:717–719.

26. Subak-Sharpe, H., Bürk, R. R., and Pitts, J. D. (1969): Metabolic cooperation between biochemically marked mammalian cells in culture. *J. Cell Sci.*, 4:353–367.

27. Cox, R. P., Kraus, M. R., Balis, M. E., and Dancis, J. (1970): Evidence of transfer of enzyme product as the basis of metabolic cooperation between tissue culture fibroblasts of Lesch-Nyhan Disease and normal cells. *Proc. Natl. Acad. Sci. USA*, 67:1573–1579.

28. Pitts, J. D. (1971): In: *Growth Control in Cell Culture, a Ciba Foundation Symposium*, edited by G. Wolstenholme and J. Knight, p. 89. Churchill and Livingstone, London.

29. Gilula, N. B., Reeves, O. R., and Steinbach, A. (1972): Metabolic coupling, ionic coupling and cell contacts. *Nature*, 235:262–265.

30. Pitts, J. D. (1975): How do animal cells communicate? *Nature*, 255:371–372.

31. Gilula, N. (1975): Biochemical and morphological characterizations of the gap junction. In: *Cellular Membranes and Tumor Cell Behavior, 28th Annual Symposium on Fundamental Cancer Research*. Williams and Wilkins. Baltimore.

32. Goodenough, D. (1975): The structure and permeability of isolated hepatocyte gap junctions. *Cold Spr. Harbor Symp. Quant. Biol.*, in press.

33. Singer, S. J. (1975): Architecture and topography of biological membranes. In: *Cell Membranes: Biochemistry, Cell Biology, and Pathology*, edited by G. Weisman and R. Clayborne. H. P. Publishing Co., New York.

34. Loewenstein, W. R. (1967): On the genesis of cellular communication. *Dev. Biol.*, 15:503–520.

35. Hülser, D. R., and Peters, J. H. (1972): Contact cooperation in stimulated lymphocytes. II. Electro-physiological investigations on intercellular communication. *Exp. Cell Res.*, 74:319–326.

36. DeHaan, R. L. and Hirakow, R. (1972): Synchronization of pulsation rates in isolated cardiac myocytes. *Exp. Cell Res.*, 70:214–220.

37. Oliveira-Castro, G. M., Barcinski, M. A., and Cukierman, J. (1973): Intercellular communication in stimulated human lymphocytes. *J. Immunol.*, 111:1616–1619.

38. Hammer, M., Epstein, E., and Sheridan, J. (1973): Gap junction formation in reaggregating systems. *J. Cell Biol.*, 59:130a.

39. Ito, S., Sato, E., and Loewenstein, W. R. (1974): Studies on the formation of a permeable membrane junction. I. Coupling under various conditions of membrane contact. Colchicine, Cytochalasin B., Dinitrophenol. *J. Membr. Biol.*, 19:305–337.

40. Johnson, R., Hammer, M., Sheridan, J., and Revel, J. P. (1974): Gap junction formation be-

tween reaggregated Novikoff hepatoma cells. *Proc. Natl. Acad. Sci. USA*, 71:4536–4540.

41. Oliveira-Castro, G. M., and Loewenstein, W. R. (1971): Junctional membrane permeability: effects of divalent cations. *J. Membr. Biol.*, 5:51–77.

42. Shimomura, O., and Johnson, F. H. (1969): Properties of the bioluminescent protein aequorin. *Biochemistry*, 8:3991–3997.

43. Rose, B., and Loewenstein, W. R. (1975): Permeability of cell junction depends on local cytoplasmic calcium activity. *Nature*, 254:250–252.

44. Loewenstein, W. R. (1967): Cell surface membranes in close contact. Role of calcium and magnesium ions. *J. Colloid Interface Sci.*, 25:34–46.

45. Rose, B., and Loewenstein, W. R. (1971): Junctional membrane permeability. Depression by substitution of Li for extracellular Na, and by long-term lack of Ca and Mg; restoration by cell repolarization. *J. Membr. Biol.*, 5:20–50.

46. Délèze, J., and Loewenstein, W. R. (1975): Permeability of a cell junction during intracellular injection of divalent cations. *J. Membr. Biol.*, in press.

47. Rose, B., and Loewenstein, W. R. (1975): Junctional membrane permeability and its dependence on cytoplasmic ionic calcium concentration. A study with aequorin. *J. Membr. Biol.*, in press.

48. Penn, R. D. (1966): Ionic communication between liver cells. *J. Cell Biol.*, 29:171–173.

49. Loewenstein, W. R., and Penn, R. D. (1967): Intercellular communication and tissue growth. II. Tissue regeneration. *J. Cell Biol.*, 33:235–242.

50. Loewenstein, W. R. (1968): Some reflections on growth and differentiation. *Persp. Biol. Med.*, 11:260–272.

51. Loewenstein, W. R. (1968): Communication through cell junctions. Implications in growth control and differentiation. *Dev. Biol.*, 19(Suppl. 2):151–183.

52. Ito, S., and Hori, N. (1966): Electrical characteristics of *Triturus* egg cells during cleavage. *J. Gen. Physiol.*, 49:1019–1027.

53. Sheridan, J. (1968): Electrophysiological evidence for low-resistance intercellular junctions in the early chick embryo. *J. Cell Biol.*, 37:650–659.

54. Bennett, M. V. L., and Trinkaus, J. P. (1970): Electrical coupling between embryo cells by way of extracellular space and specialized junctions. *J. Cell Biol.*, 44:592–607.

55. DiCaprio, R. A., French, A. S., and Saunders, E. J. (1974): Dynamic properties of electrotonic coupling between cells of early Xenopus embryos. *Biophys. J.*, 14:387–411.

56. Warner, A. E. (1970): Electrical connexions between cells at neural stages of the axolotl. *J. Physiol. (Lond.)*, 210:150P.

57. Slack, C., and Palmer, J. P. (1969): The permeability of intercellular junctions in the early embryo of *Xenopus laevis*, studies with fluorescent tracer. *Exp. Cell Res.*, 55:416–419.

58. Tupper, J., and Saunders, J. W. (1972): Intercellular permeability in the early Asterias embryo. *Dev. Biol.*, 27:546–554.

59. Bennett, M. V. L., Pappas, G. D., and Spira, M. E. (1972): Properties of electrotonic junctions between embryonic cells of *Fundulus*. *Dev. Biol.*, 29:419–435.

60. Hodgkin, A. L., and Keynes, R. D. (1957): Movements of labeled calcium in squid giant axons. *J. Physiol. (Lond.)*, 138:253–281.

61. Baker, P. F., and Crawford, A. C. (1972): Mobility and transport of magnesium in squid giant axons. *J. Physiol. (Lond.)*, 227:835–875.

62. Baker, P. F. (1972): Transport and metabolism of calcium ions in nerve. *Prog. Biophys. Biophys. Chem.*, 24:177–223.

63. Rose, B., and Loewenstein, W. R. (1975): Calcium distribution in cytoplasm visualized by aequorin: distribution in the cytosol is restricted due to energized sequestering. *Science, in press.*

64. Lehninger, A. L., Carafoli, E., and Rossi, C. J. (1967): Energy-linked ion movements in mitochondrial systems. *Adv. Enzymol.*, 29:259–322.

65. Ebashi, S., and Endo, M. (1968): Calcium ion and muscle contraction. *Prog. Biophys. Mol. Biol.*, 18:123–183.

66. Katz, B., and Miledi, R. (1967): A study of synaptic transmission in the absence of nerve impulse. *J. Physiol. (Lond.)*, 192:407–436.

67. Llinás, R., Blinks, J. R., and Nicholson, C. (1973): Calcium transient in presynaptic terminal of squid giant synapse: detection with aequorin. *Science*, 176:1127–1129.

68. Douglas, W. W. (1968): Stimulus-secretion coupling: the concept and clues from chromaffin and other cells. *Br. J. Pharmacol. Chemother.*, 34:451–474.

69. Rasmussen, H. (1970): Cell communication, calcium ion, and cyclic AMP. *Science*, 170:404–412.

70. Hagins, W. A. (1972): The visual process: excitatory mechanisms in the primary receptor cells. *Ann Rev. Biophys. Bioeng.*, 1:131–158.

71. Brown, J. E., and Blinks, J. R. (1974): Changes in intracellular free calcium concentrations during illumination of invertebrate photoreceptors. *J. Gen. Physiol.*, 64:643–665.

72. Michalke, W., and Loewenstein, W. R. (1971): Communication between cells of different types. *Nature*, 232:121–122.

73. Borek, C., Higashino, S. and Loewenstein, W. R. (1969): Intercellular communication and tissue growth. IV. Conductance of membrane junctions of normal and cancerous cells in culture. *J. Membr. Biol.*, 1:274–293.

74. Azarnia, R., Larsen, W., and Loewenstein, W. R. (1974): The membrane junctions in communicating and non-communicating cells, their hybrids and segregants. *Proc. Natl. Acad. Sci. USA*, 71:880–884.

75. Loewenstein, W. R. (1974): Cellular communication by permeable membrane junctions. *Hosp. Prac. (Membrane Series)*, 9:113–122; also (1975): In: *Cell Membranes: Biochemistry, Cell Biology and Pathology*, edited by G. Weismann and R. Clayborne, H. P. Publishing Co., N.Y.

The Nervous System, Donald B. Tower, Editor-in-Chief. *Vol. 1: The Basic Neurosciences*. Raven Press, New York, 1975.

The Isolation of Specific Cell Types from Mammalian Brain

Shirley E. Poduslo and Guy M. McKhann

The understanding of the brain at a cellular level has occurred, in recent years, through the techniques of neurophysiology and neuroanatomy. In addition these two disciplines have now gone a step further and are providing information about interconnecting groups of cells or systems. In contrast neurochemists have been limited to talking about brain as a whole, regions of brain, which may be enriched in a particular cell type, or to the examination of subcellular fractions. In a sense this is a denominator problem; instead of the denominator for neurochemical studies being individual neurons or groups of neurons, it is a relatively large mass of tissue.

There have been two approaches to changing this denominator for neurochemical studies. One is the dissection of single neurons and their subsequent chemical analysis. The other is the bulk isolation of specific cell types. In this chapter, we present some observations about the techniques for the separation of individual cell types, comment on the present status of these studies, and discuss their potential use for the study of normal and abnormal brain.

A number of different investigators have developed techniques for isolation of individual cell types from mammalian brain (1–6). We will emphasize the technique described by Poduslo and Norton (1), as we are most familiar with this technique.

The separation of cells involves the following steps.

1. *Dissection and prior treatment of tissue.* The tissue is dissected and chopped into a fine mince. Then it is incubated with an exogenous histolytic enzyme, trypsin, or collagenase, to soften or loosen the extracellular attachments.

2. *Dissociation of tissue.* The treated tissue is separated into a single cell suspension by passing it through a series of nylon and stainless steel screens of known pore sizes.

3. *Separation of cell types.* At present, neuronal perikarya and highly branched astrocytes can be separated from each other and from myelin and cell fragments by sucrose density gradient centrifugation. Using white matter, oligodendroglia perikarya can be separated from myelinated processes and debris by a similar technique.

The existing techniques can yield fractions that are markedly enriched in neurons, astrocytes, or oligodendroglia (Fig. 1). These enriched fractions have been used for studies of cellular composition, localization of enzymes, and preparation of subcellular fractions, including a plasma membrane fraction from oligodendroglia.

STUDIES OF COMPOSITION

The comparison of different cell types are indicated in Table 1, taken from the work of Poduslo and Norton (8).

The most striking findings in these studies are the enrichment of myelin components (galactolipids and 2′,3′-cyclic nucleotide 3′-phosphohydrolase) in oligodendroglia and the presence of gangliosides, possibly components of plasma membranes, in all three cell types.

Enzyme Localization

The determination of the enzyme content or enrichment of specific enzymes in individual cell types has turned out to be more difficult than one might expect. Figure 2 shows some studies from our laboratory (9) that indicate some of the problems.

These problems, more specifically, are the following:

1. The separation procedure damages cells by shearing off cell processes, thereby exposing

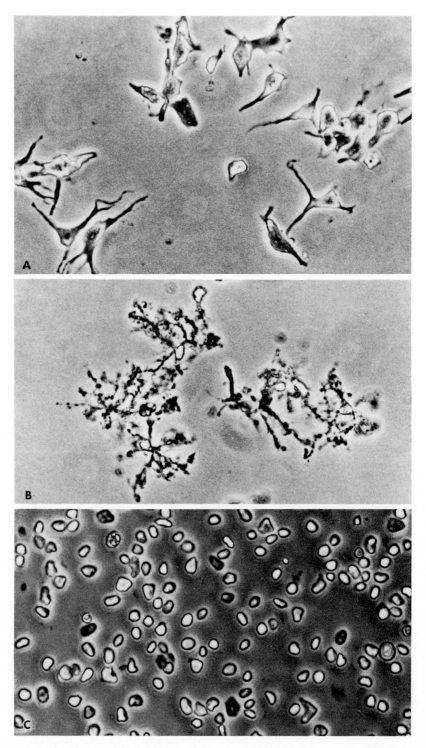

FIG. 1. Phase-contrast micrographs. × 740. **A:** Rat brain neurons; **B:** Rat brain astrocytes; **C:** Calf brain oligo-dendroglia.

TABLE 1. *Comparison of three isolated cell types and myelin*

Species preparation	Rat		Beef	
	Neurons	Astrocytes	Oligodendroglia	Myelin
Yield, 10^6 cells/g fresh tissue	17	3.5	11.4	–
Dry wt, pg/cell	178	590	25^a	–
RNA, pg/cell	24.2	29.1	1.95 ± 0.43^b	–
DNA, pg/cell	8.18	11.2	5.14 ± 0.75^b	–
DNA/RNA ratio	0.34	0.38	2.6	–
2',3'-cAMPase, μmoles of P_i/min, per mg dry wt	0.42	0.41	3.23	3.72
Total lipid, % dry wt	24.1	38.9	29.5	75.3
Ganglioside NANA, % dry wt	0.069	0.18	0.074	0.014, 0.039
Lipids^c				
Cholesterol	10.6	14.0	14.1	28.1
Total galactolipid	2.1	1.8	9.9	29.3
Cerebroside	–	–	7.3	24.0
Sulfatide	–	–	1.5	3.6
Total phospholipid	72.3	70.9	62.2	43.0
Phosphatidylcholine	39.9	36.3	29.4	10.9
Ethanolaminephosphatides	18.2	20.1	14.0	17.4
Sphingomyelin	3.2	3.7	7.1	7.1
Phosphatidylserine	3.9	5.2	4.7	6.5
Phosphatidylinositol	4.9	3.5	4.1	0.8

^{a} This value is only a crude approximation.
^{b} Mean values $\pm$ SD of 10 separate preparations.
^{c} All lipid values are expressed as percent of total lipid weight.

the cells to exogenous histolytic enzymes and endogenous lysosomal enzymes, as well as subjecting the cells to hyperosmotic sucrose gradients. Thus it is necessary to determine the effect of the separation procedure on the enzyme under consideration. One can get some idea of this by comparing the freshly minced tissue with the cell suspension just before it is put on the density gradient.

2. In some procedures the technique for obtaining one cell type may be different from that required for another. That is neurons are isolated from rat whole brain and oligodendroglia from calf white matter by a slightly different procedure. Thus, the problems outlined in the previous paragraph are compounded.

3. The separation of oligodendroglia requires significant amounts of white matter as starting material. Therefore present techniques are restricted to larger species. It is known that much enzymatic activity changes during development. In larger species, such as calf, developmental curves are difficult to obtain because of the imprecise age of the animals and the impossibility of performing *in vivo* studies.

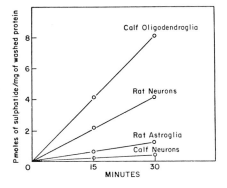

FIG. 2. Time course of sulfatide synthesis by homogenates of isolated cells. Calf oligodendroglia and neurons were isolated from white and grey matter, respectively. Rat neurons were isolated from forebrains of 17-day-old rats. Although absolute activities of cerebroside sulfotransferase varied from one preparation to another, the single experiments shown are representative of the relative activities of one cell type compared to another.

4. The possibility exists that different isoenzymes may be present in specific cell types. This question has not been adequately explored in most cases.

STUDIES OF CELLULAR MEMBRANES

An example of the use of a specific cell type for the study of a particular membrane is the isolation and characterization of the plasma membrane of the calf oligodendrocyte (10).

TABLE 2. *Comparison of calf oligodendroglia membranes*

	Plasma membrane	Myelin
Protein (% dry wt)	60	30
Proteolipid protein	+	+
Basic protein	− (?)	+
Lipid		
cholesterol (%)	19.9	30.8
galactolipid (%)	14.8	22.5
phospholipid (%)	65.2	46.7
Enzymes		
2′,3′-cyclic nucleotide 3′-phosphohydrolase	+	+

This study (Table 2) indicates that the plasma membrane of the oligodendrocyte must change as myelin is formed and compacted. This change is primarily in the introduction of certain lipids (cholesterol and galactolipids) and decrease in phospholipids.

CURRENT STUDIES

Previous studies with isolated cells, particularly those of lipid composition, have not required that the cells be intact and viable at the time of study. Our current efforts are aimed at establishing the conditions required for maintaining cells for short-term culture studies. The goals of this type of study are severalfold:

1. to allow the isolated cells to heal or recover from the damage inherent in the separation procedure
2. to carry out short-term metabolic studies, particularly the synthesis of cell-specific components, such as the synthesis of basic protein or proteolipid protein by isolated oligodendroglia
3. to provide a system for the study of cell-to-cell interaction, and of cell maintenance or growth factors
4. to maintain normal or abnormal cells that could be used as model systems for the study of mechanisms or alterations of neurologic disease

Modification of the original method of Poduslo and Norton has made it possible to maintain cells in culture for short-term (24 to 48 hr) periods of time. With such preparations, incorporation of amino acid into protein or uridine into RNA can be demonstrated (11).

APPLICATION TO HUMAN DISEASE

Abnormal neurons can be isolated from either fresh or frozen human brain (12,13). In addition, recent studies in our laboratory indicate that oligodendroglia can also be obtained from human brain. Applications of these techniques to human disease have been limited. However, indications of an abnormality in Huntington's Chorea have been found by Iqbal (13). In our own laboratory, we were able to obtain oligodendroglia from a human fetus with metachromatic leukodystrophy and found that the cells as well as isolated myelin had increased amounts of the stored lipid, sulfatide (14).

SUMMARY AND INDICATIONS FOR FURTHER RESEARCH

The results to date indicate that enriched fractions of neurons, astrocytes, and oligodendroglia can be obtained from the mammalian nervous system. In addition, neurons and oligodendroglia can be maintained in culture. The stage is now set to ask such questions as (a) Are there constituents that are cell-specific markers? (b) What are the chemical properties of the perikarya of neurons or glial cells? (c) Can chemical abnormalities, which might be masked in studies of whole brain, be detected in enriched fractions? (d) Can specific cell fractions be used for studies of selective vulnerability to exogenous agents such as toxins or viruses? These, and other questions, remain to be explored.

ACKNOWLEDGMENTS

These studies were supported by USPHS Grants NS 08719 and NS 10920 from the National Institute of Neurological and Communicative Disorders and Stroke.

REFERENCES

1. Poduslo, S. E., and Norton, W. T. (1975): Isolation of specific brain cells. In: *Methods of Enzymology,* edited by S. P. Colowick, and N. O. Kaplan, pp. 629. Academic Press, New York.
2. Rose, S. P. R. (1967): Preparation of enriched fractions from cerebral cortex containing isolated, metabolically active neuronal and glial cells. *Biochem. J.,* 102:33–43.
3. Sellinger, O. Z., Azcurra, J. M., Johnson, D. E., Ohlsson, W. G., and Lodin, Z. (1971): Independence of protein synthesis and drug uptake in nerve cell bodies and glial cells isolated by a new technique. *Nature,* 230:253–256.
4. Blomstrand, C., and Hamberger, A. (1969): Protein turnover in cell-enriched fractions from rabbit brain. *J. Neurochem.,* 16:1401–1407.
5. Varon, S., and Raiborn, C. W. (1969): Dissociation, fractionation and culture of embryonic brain cells. *Brain Res.,* 12:180–199.
6. Freysz, L., Bieth, R., Judes, C., Sensenbrenner, M., Jakov, M., and Mandel, P. (1968): Distribution quantitative des divers phospholipides dans les neurones et les cellules gliales isoles du cortex cerebral de rat adulte. *J. Neurochem.,* 15:307–313.
7. Fewster, M. E., Scheibel, A. B., and Mead, J. F. (1967): The preparation of isolated glial cells from rat and bovine white matter. *Brain Res.,* 6:401–408.
8. Poduslo, S. E., and Norton, W. T. (1972): Isolation and some chemical properties of oligodendroglia from calf brain. *J. Neurochem.,* 19:727–736.
9. Benjamins, J. A., Guarnieri, M., Miller, K., Sonneborn, M., McKhann, G. M. (1974): Sulphatide synthesis in isolated oligodendroglia and neuronal cells. *J. Neurochem.,* 23:751–757.
10. Poduslo, S. E. (1975): The isolation and characterization of a plasma membrane and a myelin fraction derived from oligodendroglia of calf brain. *J. Neurochem.,* 24:647–654.
11. Poduslo, S. E., Miller, K., Kroen, C., and McKhann, G. M. (1975): Further studies on isolated brain cells. *Trans. Am. Soc. Neurochem.,* 6:97.
12. McKhann, G. M., Ho, W., Raiborn, C., and Varon, S. (1969): The isolation of neurons from normal and abnormal human cerebral cortex. *Arch. Neurol.,* 20:542–547.
13. Iqbal, D., and Tellez-Nagel, I. (1972): Isolation of neurons and glial cells from normal and pathological human brains. *Brain Res.,* 45:296–301.
14. McKhann, G. M., Poduslo, S. E., Price, D., Tennekoon, G., Miller, K., and Weiner, L. (1974): Fetal metachromatic leukodystrophy: Ultrastructure, cell isolation, chemical pathology, and *in vitro* enzyme replacement. *Trans. Am. Soc. Neurochem.,* 5:134.

The Nervous System, Donald B. Tower, Editor-in-Chief. *Vol. 1: The Basic Neurosciences.* Raven Press, New York, 1975.

Membrane Biochemical Approaches to Altered Muscle Structure and Function

Stanley H. Appel, Allen D. Roses, Richard R. Almon,
Clifford G. Andrew, Peter B. Smith, James O. McNamara, and
David A. Butterfield

Biological membranes are important cellular constituents that modulate a wide range of specialized functions. They are intimately involved in the formation of cell-to-cell contacts and the development of complex and precise cellular networks. They represent a key point for the translation of environmental stimuli into intracellular metabolic events. The membranes of excitable tissue such as nerve and muscle have additional specialization for generation of action potentials and for intercellular communication. One of the significant problems for molecular neurobiology is to develop a coherent picture of how membranes actually perform their physiological tasks. In particular, what are the molecular species responsible for the selective transport of solutes in graded as well as regenerative electrical activity, and what are the molecular properties of the membrane receptors responsible for transducing environmental stimuli?

Our own laboratory has been involved in characterizing the membranes of mammalian skeletal muscle as a model for studying membrane functions in excitable tissue and for characterizing the neural influences on excitable membrane structure. This tissue offers significant advantages since the physiological events resulting in the release of the neurotransmitter acetylcholine, its interaction with a specific receptor in the postsynaptic structure, the development of the end-plate potential, and triggering of the action potential, the coupling between excitation and contraction, and the chemical nature of the contractile elements have been extensively studied. However, the biochemical and molecular properties of the membranes mediating many of these events are incompletely understood.

The entire cycle of muscle function can be divided into four events, three of which intimately involve muscle membranes: (a) excitation (sarcolemma and transverse tubule); (b) coupling (transverse tubule and sarcoplasmic reticulum); (c) contraction; and (d) relaxation (sarcoplasmic reticulum) (Fig. 1). The characteristics of these events are different for at least two types of muscle, namely, fast and slow, and their innervated and denervated states. Thus, muscle tissue offers an opportunity to examine the association of membrane structure in several different functional conditions.

This review describes three phases of our research. Our initial efforts have been to characterize the surface membranes of mammalian muscle and to analyze those macromolecular constituents of potential relevance to the excitable membrane. As a model of an alteration of excitable properties of muscle, we have investigated the human disease, myotonic muscular dystrophy, a condition inherited as an autosomal trait. The widespread expression of this disorder in many organ systems suggested a diffuse membrane involvement and prompted the detailed examination of red cell membranes. We reasoned that, if erythrocyte membranes were involved, we might obviate the difficulties in obtaining sufficient quantities of purified muscle membranes for biochemical analysis. The fruitfulness of this strategy is indicated in the studies reported below. Our final efforts have been directed toward a study of the skeletal muscle acetylcholine receptor. We have characterized definite differences in receptor extracted from normal and denervated muscle. Furthermore, we have found that serum globulins from another human disease, myasthenia gravis, provided a useful tool for

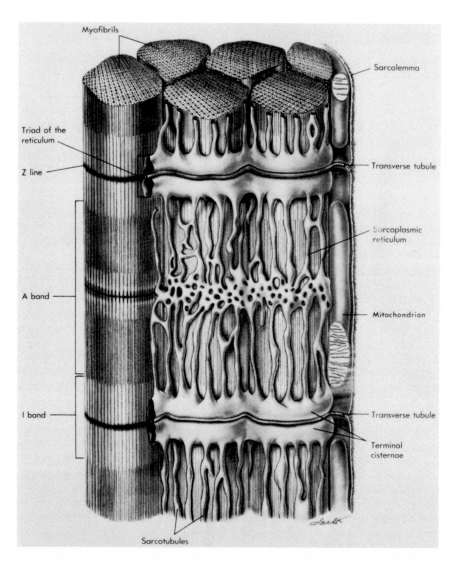

FIG. 1. Schematic representation of muscle morphology, showing the anatomic relationships between sarcolemma, sarcoplasmic reticulum, and transverse tubule (T-system) membranes in a section of a single frog muscle fiber. [Reprinted from S. McNutt and D. Fawcett (1965), *J. Cell Biology,* 25:209 with permission from the Rockefeller University Press.]

investigating the acetylcholine receptor and for approaching the neuromuscular alterations of the disease process.

MUSCLE MEMBRANE FRACTIONATION

In order to approach a biochemical understanding of muscle membranes, a subcellular fractionation scheme was devised to yield enriched fractions for each of the major muscle membrane components. Of the two general schemes available, hypotonic extraction (1) and hypertonic extraction (2), the latter approach was selected because of the relatively greater enrichment in specific surface membrane markers. Our technique was modified from Boegman et al. (3) and consisted of polytron homogenization, sequential extraction with lithium bromide, potassium chloride, and water, and differential and density gradients centrifu-

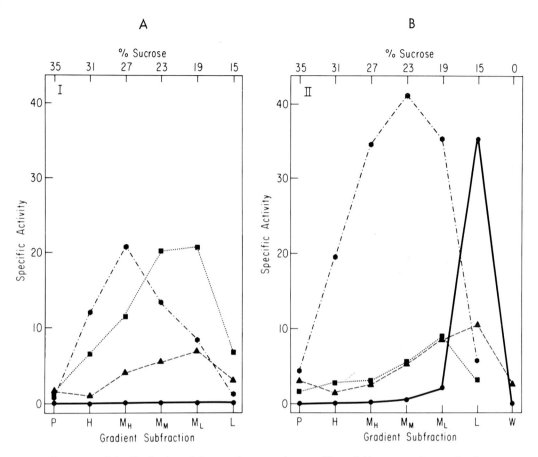

FIG. 2. Summary of the distribution of the membrane marker specific activities on continuous density sucrose gradients. The distribution shown for the three surface membrane markers represent their average from normal and denervated muscle. **A:** Membrane fraction I; **B:** Membrane fraction II. (■··■) Na$^+$K$^+$(Mg^{2+}) ATPase (μmole/hr/mg), sialic acid (nmole/mg), alpha-bungarotoxin binding (pmole/mg); (●··●) Ca^{2+}/Mg^{2+} ATPase (μmole/hr/mg); (▲--▲) lactoperoxidase iodination (cpm $\times$ 10^{-3}/mg); (●—●) protein kinase: endogenous membrane protein phosphorylation (pmole $\times$ 10^{-1}/min/mg).

gation to isolate two major membrane fractions from rat hind limb muscle (4).

Sarcolemmal Membranes

A subfraction highly enriched in fragmented sarcolemma was isolated from the initial nuclear pellet (1,000 $\times$ g, 10 min) and distributed between 19 and 23% sucrose on sucrose density gradients. These membranes were identified as sarcolemma on the basis of their enrichment in a combination of four markers and activities characteristic of surface membrane. These included Na$^+$K$^+$Mg^{2+} ATPase, sialic acid containing macromolecules, acetylcholine receptor, and adenylate cyclase (Fig. 2) (5). As a con-

firmation for the surface nature of the membranes containing these various markers, intact muscle tissue was iodinated by lactoperoxidase after which membrane fractions were prepared. In the sarcolemmal membranes derived from the initial nuclear pellet, the specific activity of the iodination exactly paralleled those of the other surface markers.

Sarcoplasmic Reticulum

A subfraction highly enriched in fragmented sarcoplasmic reticulum was isolated from the "microsomal" fraction (between 9,000 $\times$ g, 10 min and 44,000 $\times$ g, 90 min) and exhibited a broad distribution between 19 and 27% sucrose in the final density gradient. These membranes were identified as sarcoplasmic reticulum on the basis of their enrichment in Ca ATPase and their sodium dodecyl sulfate (SDS) polyacrylamidē electrophoretic polypeptide profile (6,7).

Possible Transverse Tubules — Membrane Protein Phosphorylation

An unexpected finding of this research was the discovery of a third major membrane subfraction distinct from both fragmented sarcolemma and sarcoplasmic reticulum and highly enriched both in lactoperoxidase iodination and in the capacity for membrane protein phosphorylation (Fig. 2). This membrane subfraction was derived from the "microsomal" fraction and layered at the 15% sucrose interface of the density gradient (8). No other membrane fraction contained any significant protein kinase activity. The optimal specific activity of the enzyme in these membranes was 350 pmoles/mg/min. The endogneous muscle membrane protein kinase required Mg, was stimulated by micromolar concentrations of Ca, had a pH optimum between 7.0 and 7.5, and demonstrated a K_m for ATP of 2.6×10^{-5} M. The enzyme was markedly heat labile and demonstrated a linear Arrhenious plot with an apparent energy of activation of 12,100 cal/mole (9). There was no stimulation by cyclic nucleotides, and neither monovalent cations nor various neurotransmitters exerted any effect.

A single polypeptide of approximately 28,000 MW represented the major endogenous substrate of the membrane protein kinase. Following isolation by preparative SDS gel electrophoresis and partial acid hydrolysis, the phosphate group of the phosphorylated 28,000-MW substrate was identified in phosphoserine. The amino acid composition of the substrate was neither strongly acidic nor basic. It had a high content of glycine, glutamic acid, serine, and lysine. Hydrophobic residues constituted only 45% of the total composition (9).

The morphological identity of the membrane subfraction containing protein phosphorylation is unknown. The possibility that it might represent fragmented transverse tubule (T-system) is consistent with its "external surface" localization as defined by lactoperoxidase accessibility,

as well as with what is known about the relative quantity of T-system, representing seven times that of sarcolemma (10). However, it is also possible that the protein kinase-containing vesicles represent surface membranes that have pinched off from the sarcolemma during homogenization, and migrate at a lighter density than other surface markers. Further experiments are in progress to demonstrate the association of the membrane fraction with fragmented transverse tubule membranes.

PHYSIOLOGICAL EFFECTS OF DENERVATION (11)

Membranes were examined from denervated muscle in an attempt to characterize biochemically the altered physiologic parameters noted with the destruction of normal nerve–muscle relationship. Denervated muscles exhibit a proliferation of sarcoplasmic reticulum and T-system. Mitochondria are usually unchanged. Lysosomal proteolytic activity is increased resulting in loss of glycogen, destruction of contractile elements and muscle atrophy. Physiologically denervation results in spontaneous muscle contractions and fibrillations, and there appears to be a relative uncoupling of excitation and contraction as measured by the increase in time necessary for the muscle to reach peak tension. Additional sarcolemmal changes include an increased total membrane resistance and Na permeability, and decreased resting membrane potential, K permeability, rate of action potential rise and fall, and tetrodotoxin sensitivity. In addition, sensitivity to acetylcholine spreads outward from the normal endplate localization over the entire sarcolemmal surface. Finally, the denervated muscle regains its original capacity to receive a nerve fiber and set up another synapse. Many of these effects can be attributed to a loss of the "trophic" factors supplied by nerve although it is also possible that many of these changes are merely related to muscle inactivity (12).

BIOCHEMICAL CHARACTERISTICS OF DENERVATED MEMBRANES

In membrane preparations derived from denervated muscle there were several specific changes. There was a dramatic 10- to 20-fold increase in alpha-bungarotoxin binding to fragmented sarcolemma which confirms the increase and spread of cholinergic receptor demonstrated both pharmacologically and by autoradiography with ^{125}I-alpha-bungarotoxin (13). Although enhanced toxin binding could be demonstrated, no change was detected in the same subfraction either in the levels of the ATPases or in the apparent polypeptide composition. The phospholipid composition of the sarcolemma was only slightly altered with a decrease of phosphatidylethanolamine from 15 to 10% and an increase of phosphatidylcholine from 50 to 57% of total phospholipids. There was a marked increase in the turnover of phosphatidylinositol (PI) in denervated membranes with no changes in the turnover of other membrane phospholipids (14). Such changes in PI turnover were not limited to the sarcolemma but were noted in all membrane subfractions examined. Sialic acid content of the membranes was increased twofold with denervation.

ALTERED PROTEIN PHOSPHORYLATION IN DENERVATED MEMBRANES

Although denervation produced no significant alterations in the electrophoretic polypeptide profile of the sarcolemmal fraction, it had quite distinctive effects on the surface membrane fraction which we hypothetically associate with transverse tubules (9). Three specific polypeptides including the 28,000-MW protein kinase substrate were diminished 60% as quantitated by Coomassie blue staining (Fig. 3). Furthermore, phosphate incorporation into this polypeptide declined 82% after denervation.

The physiological correlate of the muscle membrane protein kinase in normal and denervated membranes is presently unclear. A number of highly purified membrane preparations have been found to contain both membrane protein kinases as well as endogenous protein substrates of phosphate acceptors. Membrane phosphorylation has been described in brain microsomes, synaptosomes, erythrocyte plasma membranes, adenohypophyseal secretory granules and plasma membranes, polymorphonuclear leukocyte and platelet membranes, adrenal cortex endoplasmic reticulum, mammary gland plasma membranes, cardiac sarcoplasmic reticulum, and muscle membranes.

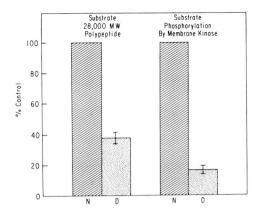

FIG. 3. Denervation alterations of the 28,000-MW polypeptide and its phosphorylation by the endogenous muscle membrane protein kinase. A series of five membrane preparations from both denervated and contralateral limb control muscles were assessed for their content of 28,000-MW polypeptide as quantitated by densitometric scans of Coomassie blue stained gels as well as for their initial rates of phosphate incorporation into this polypeptide. The results are expressed in terms of percent control levels for the five preparations ± SEM (N = normal; D = denervated).

The function of the membrane protein phosphorylation is unknown, although it is thought to be an important physiological modulator of various specialized membrane functions including cation binding, ion and water permeability, secretion, membrane associated enzymatic activities, and membrane excitability. The common denominator in many of these reactions may be the effects of calcium on the membrane.

The unique role of calcium in physiologic concentrations as modulator of the endogenous membrane protein kinase in muscle and the postulated localization in transverse tubule membranes of this reaction may indicate a role for the enzyme in excitation contraction coupling occurring at the transverse tubule sarcoplasmic reticulum junction. The loss of membrane protein phosphorylation following denervation may well relate to the destruction of the normally highly ordered transverse tubule sarcoplasmic reticulum morphology and the possible change in coupling of surface membrane excitation and muscle contraction. Alternatively the decreased protein phosphorylation may relate to altered potassium conductance of denervated transverse tubule membrane and a relative depolarization of the resting membrane potential.

ACETYLCHOLINE RECEPTOR FROM NORMAL AND DENERVATED MUSCLE

Acetylcholine receptor was isolated from rat muscle following Triton X-100 extraction and was monitored by ^{125}I-alpha-bungarotoxin binding and gel permeation chromatography on Sephadex G-200. The radioactive bungarotoxin bound to receptor emerged in the void volume, whereas free radioactive bungarotoxin was considerably retarded. The specificity of this reaction for receptor was confirmed (a) by the specific inhibition of binding by decamethonium, *d*-tubocurarine, and carbamyl choline; and (b) by the 10- to 20-fold increase in binding following denervation (Table 1). Of greatest interest was the dramatic increase in the affinity of binding of alpha-bungarotoxin to the acetylcholine receptor following denervation. The toxin bound to receptor extracted from normal slow and fast muscle demonstrated an affinity constant (K_A) of 10^8 liters/mole (15). The number of receptor sites (N) was approximately 8 pmoles/g of muscle. Both types of denervated muscle possess a single set of binding sites with an affinity constant of 10^9 liters/mole. The number of sites (N) in denervated muscle was 122 to 150 pmoles/g of muscle or approximately 15-fold higher than in normal muscle (Table 1) (15).

At free toxin concentrations between 10^{-10} and 10^{-7} M, the binding of the toxin to the receptor preparations from both normal and denervated muscle clearly approximated the mass law equation for the interaction of one mole of ligand with one mole of identical and independent sites. Because of the differences in binding constant, we suggested that the differences between normal and denervated acetylcholine receptors might reflect differences in conformation. In support of the difference in conformation, we noted that prolonged exposure of extracted normal receptor to Triton X-100 converted all binding from the lower affinity 10^8 liters/mole to the higher affinity 10^9 liters/mole without changing the total number of sites. However, we cannot definitely rule out the possibility that such differences in binding affinity might reflect covalent alterations during the prolonged exposure to Triton X-100.

BINDING OF MYASTHENIC GLOBULIN TO ACETYLCHOLINE RECEPTOR

An additional means of differentiating normal from denervated forms of the receptor came from our studies of serum of patients with myasthenia gravis (16). The serum of many such patients was shown to contain a circulating globulin which bound to the acetylcholine receptor extracted from denervated muscle. There was no reactivity with acetylcholine receptor extracted with detergent from normal innervated rat muscle tissue.

Myasthenia gravis is a neuromuscular disease of man characterized by muscle weakness which increases on exertion and improves with rest. Although numerous electrophysiologic studies have demonstrated the involvement of the neuromuscular junction, it is still not clearly resolved whether the primary site of pathology is the nerve terminal or the muscle end plate. Two recent studies support the physiological and immunological involvement of muscle acetylcholine receptor in myasthenia gravis. Lindstrom and Patrick demonstrated that injection of purified electric tissue acetylcho-

TABLE 1. *Alteration of acetylcholine receptor with denervation*[a]

	A Muscle membrane acetylcholine receptor (pmoles/mg)	B Triton-extracted acetylcholine receptor (pmoles/g of muscle)
Normal	1.04 ± 0.31	8.36 ± 2.09
Denervated	16.87 ± 2.18	128.00 ± 32.00

[a] Column A, membranes from surface enriched rat mixed muscle subfractions were assayed for ^{125}I-alpha-bungarotoxin binding activity (5). Column B, acetylcholine receptor was extracted for ^{125}I-alpha-bungarotoxin binding activity. Results are expressed on the basis of grams of muscle tissue initially extracted (15).

line receptor into rabbits resulted in a flaccid paralysis with electromyographic and pharmacologic similarities to myasthenia (17). Fambrough et al. demonstrated that myasthenic muscle biopsies had only 11 to 30% binding capacity of normal muscle for alpha-bungarotoxin (18).

Our studies showed that myasthenic serum immunoglobulin inhibits the interaction of radioactive alpha-bungarotoxin with the acetylcholine receptor. The serum factor was identified as globulin by its failure to pass through an Amicon 50,000-MW filter, its precipitation by sodium sulfate, its passage through DEAE cellulose without absorption, and its precipitation by rabbit anti-human IgG. Equilibrium experiments demonstrated that myasthenic serum immunoglobulin did not affect the affinity of bungarotoxin binding but did reduce the number of toxin binding sites. The maximal effect observed in saturation levels of myasthenic globulin approached 50%. The titer of this antibody was different in the various patients. A positive result was obtained in 11 out of 15 patients with myasthenia (Table 2). No inhibitory activity was present in control sera which included patients with myopathy, neuropathy, brain tumor, stroke, infection, or drug toxicity (16).

A second assay was developed which involved precipitation of a ^{125}I-toxin–receptor–IgG complex by anti-human IgG (19). The assay was based upon the premise that globulin that binds to the radioactive toxin–receptor complex would be precipitated by antibody against the globulin. Control globulin that had not bound to the complex would also be precipitated by antibody against human IgG but

TABLE 2. *Serum and globulin inhibition of bungarotoxin and binding to acetylcholine receptor*[a]

| | % Control | | |
	50–86%	87–90%	97–105%
Myasthenia gravis	5/15	6/15	4/15
Control	0/15	0/15	15/15

[a] Serum globulin from 15 myasthenic patients or matched controls were incubated with acetylcholine receptor extracted from rat muscle. The inhibition was then monitored by assaying with radioactive bungarotoxin. All samples were normalized to a saline buffer control. With this assay 11/15 myasthenic sera inhibited toxin binding at least 10% (16).

TABLE 3. *Serum globulin interaction with ^{125}I-toxin–acetylcholine receptor complex*[a]

Population	No. patients positive	Pellet/supernatant ratio mean ± SEM
Myasthenic	14/22	0.155 ± 0.015
Control	0/25	0.075 ± 0.004

[a] Detergent extracted acetylcholine receptor was incubated with radioactive toxin and the complex isolated by Sephadex chromatography. The complex was incubated with myasthenic or control sera and the radioactive complex was precipitated with rabbit anti-human IgG globulin. A positive result was any pellet/supernatant ratio greater than 10% (19).

in this instance only a small amount of radioactivity would be nonspecifically pelleted. In four experiments the binding of myasthenic globulin to the denervated acetylcholine receptor could be demonstrated in 14 of 22 myasthenic patients (Table 3). No controls demonstrated any binding. Binding of myasthenic globulin to acetylcholine receptor prepared from human muscle also corresponded exactly to the binding demonstrated with denervated rat acetylcholine receptor.

The binding of myasthenic globulin to denervated rat acetylcholine receptor and to normal human acetylcholine receptor provides evidence for the antigenic similarity of the two receptor populations. Clearly, normal and denervated rat receptors appear to differ with respect to turnover rate, sensitivity to acetylcholine, sensitivity to cholinergic antagonists, and binding myasthenic globulin. Some of these differences reflect variations in the conformation of the receptor protein or the state of receptor aggregation. Other differences are related to antigenic properties of the receptor presently under investigation. It is still unclear what relationship the myasthenic globulin bears to the pathophysiology of the disease process. Nevertheless, these inhibitory globulins should be useful for characterizing the acetylcholine receptor and for investigating the myasthenic disease process.

MEMBRANES AND MYOTONIC DYSTROPHY

As a means of studying membrane structure and function, several diseases of muscle membranes were examined. Myotonic muscular dystrophy was selected as a disorder of humans with widespread independent expression of the metabolic defect involving many organ systems. Cataracts, frontal balding, bony abnormalities, smooth muscle, skeletal muscle, cardiac muscle, endocrine tissue, red blood cells, central nervous system, and gamma globulin metabolism are clearly involved. Physiological investigations have suggested a membrane abnormality as the underlying metabolic defect. No abnormalities in muscle contractile proteins or "relaxing factor" have been demonstrated. Repetitive depolarization of myotonic muscle fibers, even after nerve block or neuromuscular blockade, has led many investigators to localize the defect to muscle sarcolemma.

Although muscle is one of the principal target organs, we initially felt that the presence of atrophy, fibrous tissue, and changes of denervation in muscle might produce multiple secondary biochemical changes. Erythrocytes were used as an easily accessible source of membrane preparations that have no known functional abnormality. The polypeptide profile of red cell membranes were identical in myotonic and control preparations. Furthermore, phospholipid composition, gangliosides, cholesterol, and enzymes such as Mg ATPase, Ca ATPase, and NaKMg ATPase were all normal.

ALTERED PROTEIN PHOSPHORYLATION IN MYOTONIC ERYTHROCYTES

Our initial experiments demonstrated a significant decrease in the phosphorylation of erythrocyte ghost protein using endogenous protein kinase of frozen erythrocyte membrane as the enzyme source (Table 4) (20). The initial failure to demonstrate a difference in the en-

dogenous protein kinase activity of fresh erythrocyte ghosts prompted an examination of the techniques of ghost membrane preparation and isolation. Such an approach appeared warranted since variation of membrane protein phosphorylation with buffer, pH, and method of membrane preparation had been observed with human erythrocytes. The use of ghosts prepared with Mg-free solutions resulted in highly permeable membranes. Endogenous protein kinase activity was more readily demonstrated in this preparation and phosphorylation of band III was significantly decreased in freshly prepared ghosts from patients with myotonic muscular dystrophy (Table 4) (21). This region of the gel is known to consist of several different proteins including the NaK ATPase, and Component A, a minor glycoprotein. The phosphorylation initially appeared to migrate with Component A, but fractionation by Concanavalin A-Sepharose chromatography separated a subfraction which was phosphorylated from one which was not. Such data suggested that Component A may be a diverse group of glycoproteins with possible carbohydrate and apoprotein heterogeneity. Our further investigations are aimed at clarifying the particular glycopeptide being phosphorylated and the differences between the normal and myotonic substrates.

DECREASED MEMBRANE PROTEIN PHOSPHORYLATION IN MUSCLE TISSUE

Following the demonstration of protein phosphorylation in purified fractions of rat muscle membrane, the technical capacity presented itself for evaluation of human muscle biopsy material in myotonic dystrophy. In membrane isolated from human biopsy material,

TABLE 4. *Protein Phosphorylation.* ^{32}P incorporated (pmoles/mg protein)[a]

	Frozen RBC (20)	Fresh RBC Component a (21)	Fresh muscle membrane (22)
Normal	17.5 ± 1.2	2.82 ± 0.17	15.90 ± 1.8
Myotonic	8.7 ± 1.2	2.07 ± 0.22	9.95 ± 1.1

[a] Endogenous membrane protein phosphorylation was assayed in each tissue with ATP^{32} and SDS acrylamide gel electrophoresis according to previously described techniques (20–22). All studies demonstrated a statistically significant difference between myotonic tissue and matched controls.

we were not able to obtain purified membrane fractions because of the limited amount of tissue available. Our biopsies were obtained from six patients with myotonic muscular dystrophy representing six separate families and from "control" patients undergoing operations for femur or hip repair. None of the controls had any known muscle disease. The membranes employed in the assay were known to contain a variable content of sarcolemma, sarcoplasmic reticulum, and other membrane organelles. However, despite the potential heterogeneity of the membrane preparation from different patients, the SDS-polyacrylamide gel electrophoresis pattern of muscle membrane proteins indicated no gross difference between normal and myotonic preparations. Furthermore, activity of adenocyclase and both Mg and NaKMg ATPase were equivalent in normal and myotonic preparations. The membrane protein kinase activity was decreased in all myotonic biopsies (Table 4) (22). Phosphorylation of muscle membrane components was noted in band I of approximately 90,000 MW, band II of approximately 50,000 MW, and band III of approximately 30,000 MW. Phosphorylation of bands II and III was specifically decreased in myotonic membranes compared to controls. Whereas there was considerable variation between the experiments, the protein regions in myotonic membranes were phosphorylated approximately 50% of their control rate. The 90,000 MW was extremely variable and appeared to disappear with extensive washing of the membrane fractions.

Although these data demonstrate a significant alteration in the endogenous membrane associated protein kinase activity of erythrocyte and muscle membranes from myotonic dystrophy, we could not make any definitive statement as to whether the enzyme itself, the specific substrates, or the state of the lipid–lipid or lipid–protein interactions within the membrane were responsible for the altered enzymatic activity. Whether the altered protein phosphorylation of muscle membranes and red blood cells is the primary genetic defect in the disease process is not known. Either a primary or secondary alteration may be associated with an abnormal membrane and either interpretation would support the concept of a diffuse membrane abnormality of myotonic dystrophy.

BIOPHYSICAL STUDIES OF MEMBRANE ABNORMALITY IN MYOTONIC DYSTROPHY

Electron spin resonance spectroscopy was utilized to investigate the possible physical alterations of the membrane. The magnetic measurements of a spin-labeled probe intercalated into the membrane provided a measure of membrane fluidity and polarity. Stearic acid methyl ester with nitroxide groups located at the 5, 12, and 16 positions on the fatty acid alkyl chain were used (23). The results of these studies demonstrated that the physical state of the erythrocyte membrane from patients with myotonic muscular dystrophy was different from that of normal controls. At all levels of the membrane probed by the spin label, myotonic membranes were more fluid and less polar than control membranes. The fluidity difference between normal and myotonic membranes was most apparent near the surface of the membrane while the polarity difference was approximately constant at various depths within the membrane.

SCANNING ELECTRON MICROSCOPY OF ERYTHROCYTES

Morphological characteristics of red blood cells were studied using scanning electron microscopy of unmanipulated cells from patients with myotonic dystrophy and from controls (24). A large increase in the number of stomatocytes over that seen in normal controls was demonstrated. However, similar stomatocytes could be produced in normal cells by adverse conditions such as washing before fixation or extreme pH, although the changes noted in red blood cells from patients with myopathy were more marked. There is no evidence that erythrocytes of myotonic dystrophic patients were misshapen *in vivo*. The stomatocytic shapes were probably the result of intrinsic biochemical membrane differences that respond to fixation in an abnormal manner *in vitro*.

THE SPECIFICITY OF BIOCHEMICAL AND BIOPHYSICAL TESTS IN MYOTONIC DYSTROPHY

To monitor the specificity of these findings, similar studies were undertaken in red blood cells from patients with congenital myotonia

(MC) as a model of myotonia without dystrophy, and from patients with Duchenne muscular dystrophy (DuD) as a model of dystrophy without myotonia. In the assay for protein kinase activity in red blood cell membrane preparations, there was a significant increase in phosphorylation of bands II and III from patients with DuD as well as the DuD carrier state. This pattern of phosphorylation was different from controls and was opposite to that noted in myotonic dystrophy. When red blood cell membranes from two patients with MC were examined, endogenous membrane phosphorylation was found to be identical to control membranes.

With electron spin resonance studies employing stearic acid methyl ester spin labels, patients with DuD were normal. However, patients with MC demonstrated the same significant increase in fluidity noted with myotonic dystrophy (MyD) cells. Morphologic analysis of red blood cells by scanning electron microscopy demonstrated a large increase in the number of stomatocytes in all three conditions, MyD, DuD, and MC.

The decrease in protein phosphorylation was noted only in myotonic dystrophy just as the increase in protein phosphorylation was noted only in DuD. The membrane fluidity changes were the same in both MC and MyD even though the presumed physiological mechanism underlying myotonia is known to be different in the two conditions. Muscle membranes from MC have been reported to demonstrate increased membrane resistance and a decreased conductance to chloride (25), whereas the membrane resistance and chloride conductance was reported as normal in MyD. However, the fluidity changes were noted only in myotonia, since there was no change in membrane fluidity in the nonmyotonic DuD. Finally, abnormal morphology with scanning electron microscopy was found in all three conditions. Thus, the combination of altered protein phosphorylation, electron spin resonance, and scanning electron microscopy permit us to determine which of the three disease states was being examined. However, it is not presently possible to determine whether these results either individually or collectively are specific for these conditions, or whether they might also occur in myopathies or hematological disorders not yet investigated.

FUTURE DIRECTIONS IN MYOTONIA AND DYSTROPHY RESEARCH

The most critical questions remain to be answered: (a) What is the molecular defect responsible for the myotonia? (b) What is the molecular defect responsible for the dystrophy? (c) What is the inborn error of metabolism and to what extent does it either directly or indirectly give rise to the myotonia and the dystrophy? The protein phosphorylation changes, scanning electron microscopy, and electron spin resonance together provide a sensitive and possibly specific assay of the altered membranes. However, further work will be necessary to determine the potential role of the phosphorylation in myotonia or dystrophy. It is encouraging that the altered protein phosphorylation of myotonic dystrophy red blood cells was also noted in muscle tissue. Because protein phosphorylation in rat muscle was confined to a membrane fraction possibly of transverse tubule origin, a similar localization might be postulated for protein phosphorylation of human muscle tissue. The transverse tubule has been implicated as the point where the myotonic discharge may be initiated in goat myotonia when chloride conductance cannot correct the depolarizing influence of potassium in the lumen of the transverse tubule (25). Myotonic dystrophy muscle is not thought to have any alteration in chloride conductance. However, it is possible that a diminution in potassium efflux might give rise to the altered resting membrane potential as well as the myotonic discharges. The decreased protein phosphorylation in human muscle may thus be located in the transverse tubule region and may lead to myotonic activity on the basis of altered potassium flux.

At this juncture our investigations have employed biochemical techniques to explore the pathogenesis of several diffuse membrane disorders of man. It will be of additional value to use the pathological studies to help us understand aspects of normal membrane structure and function. Denervated muscle may provide a model for the biochemical approach to altered action potentials, ionic conductance, tetrodotoxin sensitivity, and altered acetylcholine receptor localization and sensitivity. Myasthenic muscle may help us to understand the possible heterogeneity of receptors, their dynamic interplay, their membrane localization, and their antigenic character. Myotonic dystrophy may shed light on the character of repetitive activity and the role of the transverse tubule in electrical events and excitation–contraction coupling in muscle tissue. All of these approaches provide an opportunity for translating functional alterations of the membrane into biochemical terms and helping to explain normal physiological mechanisms.

ACKNOWLEDGMENTS

We thank Winfred J. Clingenpeel and Michael H. Herbstreith for expert technical assistance and Eleanor H. Chapman and Karen A. Case for expert secretarial assistance. This work was supported by Grant GM01238 from the National Institute of General Medical Sciences; Grants NS12213, NS07872, and NS06233 from the National Institute of Neurological Diseases and Stroke; and Grant 558-D-5 from the National Multiple Sclerosis Society. Richard R. Almon and James O. McNamara were supported by the National Institute of Health Behavioral Medicine Training Grant GM01238. Clifford G. Andrew was supported by the National Institute of Health Biochemistry Training Grant GM00233. Peter B. Smith was supported by the National Institute of Mental Health Biological Sciences Training Grant MH08394.

REFERENCES

1. McCollester, D. L. (1962): A method for isolating skeletal-muscle cell-membrane constituents. *Biochim. Biophys. Acta,* 57:427-437.
2. Kono, T., and Colowick, S. P. (1961): Isolation of skeletal muscle cell membrane and some of its properties. *Arch. Biochem. Biophys.,* 93:520–533.
3. Boegman, R. J., Manery, J. F., and Pinteric, L. (1970): Separation and partial purification of membrane bound Na^+, K^+, Mg^{2+} ATPase and Mg^{2+} ATPase from frog skeletal muscle. *Biochim. Biophys. Acta,* 203:506–530.
4. Andrew, C. G., and Appel, S. H. (1973): Macromolecular characterization of muscle membranes. I. Proteins and sialic acid of normal and denervated muscle. *J. Biol. Chem.,* 248:5156–5163.
5. Andrew, C. G., Almon, R. R., and Appel, S. H. (1974): Macromolecular characterization of muscle membranes II. Acetylcholine receptor of normal and denervated muscle. *J. Biol. Chem.,* 249:6163–6165.
6. Hasselbach, W., and Makinos, M. (1963): Ubor den mechanismus des calciumtransportes durch die membranen des sarkoplasmatischen reticulums. *Biochem. Z.,* 339:94–111.
7. MacLennan, D. H. (1970): Purification and properties of an adenosine triphosphatase from sarcoplasmic reticulum. *J. Biol. Chem.,* 245:4508–4518.
8. Andrew, C. G., Roses, A. D., Almon, R. R., and Appel, S. H. (1973): Phosphorylation of muscle membranes: Identification of a membrane-bound protein kinase. *Science,* 182:927–928.
9. Andrew, C. G., Almon, R. R., and Appel, S. H. (1975): Macromolecular characterization of muscle membranes: Endogenous membrane kinase and phosphorylated protein substrate from normal and denervated muscle. *J. Biol. Chem.,* 250:3972–3980.
10. Peachey, L. D. (1965): The sarcoplasmic reticulum and transverse tubules of the frog's sartorius. *J. Cell Biol.,* 25:209–231.
11. Thesleff, S. (1974): Physiological effects of denervation of muscle. *Ann. NY Acad. Sci.,* 228:89–103.
12. Drachman, D. B., editor (1974): Trophic functions of the neuron. *Ann. NY Acad. Sci.,* 228:3–423.
13. Fambrough, D., Hartzell, H. C., Rash, J. E., and Ritchie, A. K. (1974): Receptor properties of developing muscles. *Ann. NY Acad. Sci.,* 228:47–61.
14. Appel, S. H., Andrew, C. G., and Almon, R. R. (1974): Phosphatidyl inositol turnover in muscle membranes following denervation. *J. Neurochem.,* 23:1077–1080.
15. Almon, R. R., Andrew, C. G., and Appel, S.H. (1974): Acetylcholine receptor in normal and denervated slow and fast muscle. *Biochemistry,* 13:5522–5528.
16. Almon, R. R., Andrew, C. G., and Appel, S. H. (1974): Serum globulin in myasthenia gravis: Inhibition of α-bungarotoxin binding to acetylcholine receptors. *Science,* 186:55–57.
17. Patrick, J., and Lindstrom, J. (1973): Autoimmune response to acetylcholine receptor. *Science,* 180:871.
18. Fambrough, D. M., Drachman, D. B., and Satyamurti, S. (1973): Neuromuscular junction in myasthenia gravis: Decreased acetylcholine receptors. *Science,* 182:294.
19. Almon, R. R., and Appel, S. H. (1975): Interaction of myasthenic serum globulin with the acetylcholine receptor. *Biochim. Biophys. Acta,* 393:66–77.
20. Roses, A. D., and Appel, S. H. (1973): Protein kinase activity in erythrocyte ghosts of patients with myotonic muscular dystrophy. *Proc. Natl. Acad. Sci. USA,* 70:1855–1859.
21. Roses, A. D., and Appel, S. H. (1975): Phosphorylation of Component a of the human erythro-

cyte membrane in myotonic muscular dystrophy. *J. Mem. Biol.* (*In press.*)

22. Roses, A. D., and Appel, S. H. (1974): Muscle membrane protein kinase in myotonic muscular dystrophy. *Nature,* 250:254.

23. Butterfield, D. A., Roses, A. D., Cooper, M. L., Appel, S. H., and Chesnut, D. B. (1974): A comparative electron spin resonance study of the erythrocyte membrane in myotonic muscular dystrophy. *Biochemistry,* 13:5078–5082.

24. Miller, S. E., Roses, A. D., and Appel, S. H. (1975): Scanning electron microscopic studies in muscular dystrophy. *Arch. Neurol.* (*In press.*)

25. Adrian, R. H., and Bryant, S. H. (1974): On the repetitive discharge in myotonic muscle fibers. *J. Physiol.* (*Lond.*), 240:505–515.

The Nervous System, Donald B. Tower, Editor-in-Chief. *Vol. 1: The Basic Neurosciences*. Raven Press, New York, 1975.

Molecular Topography of the Synapse

Henry R. Mahler, James W. Gurd, and Yng-Jiin Wang

The continuing objective of our research (i.e., of the Brain Research Group of the Department of Chemistry, Indiana University) is, and has been for more than 10 years, to understand in biochemical, molecular terms the dynamics of synaptic junctions. We are concentrating on this entity because it is the region that must be the site of communication between nerve cells, both by conduction and by means of trophic interactions.

Our underlying hypothesis is that higher functions of the central nervous system, such as memory and learning, must affect, and in turn be affected by, specific structures fulfilling specific functions and controlling specific events. At the cellular level, it is reasonable to speculate that the structures residing at and defining the synapse, and in particular its membrane system, would constitute prime candidates for any such modification through use. On the molecular level, the hypothesis states that continuing electrical activity in a connected set of neurons can be altered in response to its inputs, and that includes feedback inputs, in such a manner as to produce alterations in the amount, distribution, disposition, structure, rate of formation, or degradation of one or more macromolecules, probably proteins, of the synaptic junction. For this reason, we have concentrated on the isolation and characterization of nerve endings, their membranes, and their constituent proteins, with particular attention to features that lend themselves to, or may reflect, their lasting modification.

ORGANIZATION OF THE SYNAPTIC REGION

Isolation of Synaptosomes and Their Membranes

Techniques for the Isolation of Purified Synaptosomes

Three, not unrelated, objectives underlie contemporary endeavors (including our own) at improving the methodology for the isolation of synaptosomes (nerve ending particles) as free as possible of all contamination by other membranous organelles. First, these particles, retaining as they do most of the structural and morphological elements of the intact nerve ending, including its junctional apparatus, are proving of ever-increasing utility as functional *in vivo* models or analogues in studies on transmitter uptake, release, binding, metabolism, regulation, and so on (1,2). Freedom from contaminants that might interfere with the quantitative aspects of the measured parameters is thus of critical importance. Second, recent studies have indicated that it may be possible to subdivide synaptosomes according to their most important functional attribute, i.e., the nature of the transmitter(s) to which they are geared (2,3). Again, prior removal of possible contaminants may be of critical importance in the actual success of such endeavors. Finally, although it is possible to obtain synaptic plasma membranes (SPM) from relatively crude synaptosomal–mitochondrial preparations by osmotically shocking these particles (4) and subjecting the resultant membrane population to refined isopycnic banding techniques (5–7), it is much easier and more convenient to reduce the contamination level of the resultant SPMs, particularly with respect to microsomal, and mitochondrial, elements to acceptable levels, by appropriate manipulation of the starting material rather than of the eventual product.

The following modifications of the procedures developed in Whittaker's laboratory (1) and still in use by many groups have been found by ourselves and others to produce synaptosomes meeting the criteria just enunciated: (a) Extensive washing of a crude mitochondrial pellet, itself obtained at moderate g forces: we use 10,000 $g \times$ 20 min for its isolation, at least three washes at the same speed, all in 0.32 M sucrose (8); Morgan et al. use 11,500 $g \times$ 25 min (9), also with three washes in the same medium. (b) Substitution of different gradient procedures, combining rate and equilibrium sedimentation, for the separation of synaptosomes from other organelles, especially mitochondria and various bilaminate membranes. We have used zonal sedimentation in continuous sucrose gradients (5,6) as have others (10); relatively pure synaptosomes can be obtained by these methods, but the recovery is poor. For this reason most procedures currently in use have returned to collection of fractions banding at zones of discontinuities in step gradients, but with two additional modifications: (c) The substitution of the nonpermeant polysaccharide Ficoll for sucrose for the construction of isoosmolar gradients, eliminating the shrinkage and shear caused by the use of sucrose (11); and in some procedures, including our own (8), the attainment of density equilibrium by flotation rather than sedimentation. With this modification a single two-step gradient (7.5/15% Ficoll) appears as effective as the multiple-step gradients used in other procedures.

Isolation of Transmitter-Specific Nerve Endings

Ever since the first reported isolation and studies on nerve-ending preparations (synaptosomes) *in vitro,* investigators had anticipated, sometimes explicitly, that it should eventually prove possible to separate different populations of such organelles, each one specific for one, or at least a class of transmitter types. Some success along these lines yielding cholinergic and noncholinergic synaptosomes had already been claimed from de Robertis' laboratory (4) but using somewhat inadequate markers. More recent and critical studies indicate that such separations are indeed feasible. Thus, Snyder and his collaborators (2) have pioneered in the use of rate sedimentation in sucrose gradients to effect the sorting out of synaptosomes apparently specific for various amino acid transmitters from serotonergic and adrenergic ones. Lagercrantz and Pertoft (12) have used isopycnic banding in both sucrose and colloidal silica (Ludox) to isolate highly purified synaptosomes from corpus striatum and hypothalamus enriched in storage vesicles for catecholamines. Bretz et al. (3) have reported on an extensive

investigation of isopycnic banding patterns of synaptosomes in sucrose gradients by means of zonal rotors. Using total postnuclear supernatants of rat forebrain, they obtained three populations banding at modal densities of 1.137 (type α — apparently specific for acetylcholine), 1.149 (type β — specific for GABA and containing glutamate decarboxylase) and 1.165 (type γ — adrenergic, specific for noradrenaline and dopamine, and containing monoamine oxidase in high concentration). Free mitochondria are heavier and are easily resolved at a density of 1.183 g/ml. In our own studies (13), we used cortex from 15-day-old rats to minimize contamination and entrapment by myelin and myelinated axons, isolated and purified synaptosomes by flotation on Ficoll gradients and used a discontinuous gradient of the same material in 0.32 M sucrose for their separation. On centrifugation at 1.2×10^6 g min (2 hr at 10^4 g) two populations were obtained banding at 6/11.5% (P_2B_2) and 11.5/18% (P_2B_3) Ficoll interfaces. The first set was classified as specific for catecholamines on the basis of enrichment in the high-affinity uptake systems (by slices and synaptosomes) for noradrenaline, serotonin, and dopamine (but not choline), and in catechol-O-methyl transferase and dopamine-β-hydroxylase. The second set appeared specific for acetylcholine on the basis of enrichment in its content and uptake (of choline), as well as of choline acetyltransferase. The apparent discrepancy in buoyant densities of the two types of synaptosomes between this study and that of Bretz et al. (3) appears to be due to two effects: the use of Ficoll-sucrose rather than pure sucrose gradients and an alteration in the composition of the synaptosomes in immature animals.

Isolation of Synaptic Plasma Membranes

The isolation of highly purified SPMs has been a continuing concern of research in our (5–8,14), as it has in a number of other laboratories (for citations, see refs. 7,11). All of these methods are based on the findings by Whittaker et al. (1) and de Robertis (4) that synaptosomes could be disrupted by hypoosmolar shock, liberating their synaptoplasm, including its particulate components such as mitochondria and synaptic vesicles, but leaving their limiting

TABLE 1. *Marker activities of representative SPM preparations*

Entity	Ref. (8)[a]	Ref. (9)	Ref. (15)[b]	Ref. (16)[c]
1. Na-K ATPase	~150	103.1	12.0	2.7
2. AChEsterase	4.6[d]	5.34	21	25
3. 5'-Nucleotidase	–	103	2.2	–
4. Succinate dehydrogenase	0.5	0.06	–	–
5. Cytochrome oxidase	0.3[d]	1.60	6	7.4
6. NADPH:cytochrome c reductase	0.6	"0"	–	–
7. acid phosphatase	1.5	0.07	36	–
8. 2',3'-cyclic nucleotidase	–	198	–	130
9. RNA (μg/mg)	2	<1	–	–
10. Protein (mg/g wet weight)	0.2–0.25	0.2–0.25	1.5–2	1

Activities 1, 2, and 3 are considered positive markers for SPM; 4 and 5 are used as negative markers for mitochondrial, 6 and 9 for microsomal, 7 for lysosomal and 8 for myelin contaminants. Units, except for 9, are micromoles substrate consumed $\times$ mg^{-1} protein $\times$ hr^{-1}.

[a] Fraction A-II; contamination by microsomal and mitochondrial elements can be further reduced by varying the buffer composition, particularly during the lysis of synaptosomes (to HEPES, pH 8.4); this treatment, however, reduced the ATPase activity.

[b] Fraction F.

[c] Procedure 1 – without sonication.

[d] From ref. 42.

membrane relatively intact, thus permitting its isolation in a morphologically and functionally competent form. Initially, we developed methods based largely, or solely, on isopycnic banding of these SPMs in continuous sucrose gradients at their characteristic density range of 1.125–1.140 g/ml[1] (29–34% sucrose), using zonal rotors. By selecting narrow cuts, these procedures can yield highly purified SPMs, but are quite wasteful of material – collecting a broader band improves the latter, but at the expense of contamination, particularly by microsomal elements. We have therefore changed our approach and now isolate synaptosomes, purified by extensive washing and flotation on Ficoll gradients (see previous section), and then fractionate the lysed particles on a five-step discontinuous sucrose gradient. The most highly purified SPMs are isolated at the 0.6/0.8 M sucrose interface. This scheme is quite similar to ones developed by other groups (9,15) and has been modified to a very rapid and convenient form (16) with some sacrifice of purity. Success, especially in regard to retention of characteristic marker activities, as well as re-moval of contaminating membranes, is strongly influenced by such details as the choice of buffer in the suspension and fractionation media. Some of the properties characteristic of these preparations are summarized in Table 1. The best preparations probably consist of SPMs contaminated by <10% of extraneous membranes.

Characteristic Components

Integral proteins

The proteins or rather polypeptide subunit composition of plasma membranes is conveniently analyzed by first removing easily detachable (nonintegral, peripheral[2]) proteins by washing, dissociating the remaining integral[2] proteins and phospholipids under strongly denaturing and reducing conditions, and then separating and displaying the resultant subunits by electrophoresis in acrylamide gels in the pres-

[1] It must be remembered that the buoyant density of any particle is not independent of the medium: in the case of SPMs the density equals 1.04 in Ficoll and 1.15 in sucrose–CsCl.

[2] We use the nomenclature proposed by Singer (17). In this scheme integral proteins are further characterized by the extent of their exposure to and penetration into the medium. Highly exposed membrane proteins have been referred to by some workers as peripheral or synonyms thereof. Integral and peripheral are also called intrinsic and extrinsic, respectively.

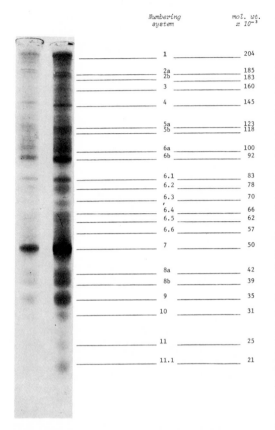

Numbering system	mol. wt. x 10⁻³

(figure labels)

1 — 204
2a — 185
2b — 183
3 — 160
4 — 145
5a — 123
5b — 118
6a — 100
6b — 92
6.1 — 83
6.2 — 78
6.3 — 70
6.4 — 66
6.5 — 62
6.6 — 57
7 — 50
8a — 42
8b — 39
9 — 35
10 — 31
11 — 25
11.1 — 21

FIG. 1. Electrophoretic band pattern of SPM polypeptides under strongly denaturing conditions: 30 μg (*left*) and 60 μg (*right*) were subjected to electrophoresis on SDS-polyacrylamide gels; molecular weights were determined by comparison with standard proteins run under identical conditions.

Glycoproteins

Because of their inherent or perceived capacity for intracell communication, synaptic glycoproteins have received a great deal of recent attention. At least some of the subunits just described either are, or comigrate with, entities stained by the periodic acid-Schiff reaction and thus contain carbohydrate prosthetic groups (8); these are components 4, 5, 6, 6.1, 6.4, and 7, and possibly 2 or 3 and 8. This distribution has also been confirmed by *in vivo* labeling with radioactive fucose (18). In order to learn more about the details of these structures, Gurd developed a method of sequential, lectin affinity chromatography, using the agglutinins from *Lens culinaris* (LcH) and wheat germ (WGA) as the affinity ligands (18). The former interacts most strongly with mannose and glucosamine, the latter with oligomeric *N*-acetyl-glucosamine residues of the prosthetic groups. These, plus fucose, galactose, and galactosamine, in addition to (terminal) sialic acid are known to be the constituents of the carbohydrate moieties of the synaptic glycoproteins and the glycopeptides derived from them (19). Although complete separation was not achieved we observed concentration, especially of component 6 into Fraction D (LcH +, WGA +), 6.1 into Fraction C (LcH +, WGA −) and 7 into Fraction A (LcH −, WGA −).

Transmitters and Receptors

We have concentrated on the identification and characterization of proteins of interest within the context of the transmitter function of acetylcholine. We have isolated various forms (isoenzymes) of acetylcholinesterase, including the one bound to the synaptosomal membrane (20). After purification to homogeneity all these isoenzymes were found to be composed of the same basic subunit, a glycoprotein with a molecular weight of 80,000 (perhaps Component 6.1). The subunit exists in six variants with isoelectric points of 5.51, 5.43, 5.30, 5.21, 5.10, and 5.09, which can be separated by isoelectric focusing. They associate into oligomers, of which the dimer and trimer (molecular weights of 150,000 and 320,000) appear the most important for catalysis.

Salvaterra in our group has been successful

ence of sodium dodecyl sulfate (SDS). When this method is applied to purified SPMs it yields the patterns shown in Fig. 1. Fourteen major bands are obtained [Nos. *1*, 2a,b; *4, 5a,b; 6a,b;* 6.1, *7, 8a,b; 9, 11.1*] with estimated molecular weights (× 10⁻³) of *204*, 185, 183, *145, 120; 100, 92;* 83, *53, 42, 39; 35*, 21; of these, nine, the ones shown in italics, are the principal ones, i.e., those estimated to contribute >5% to the total membrane proteins. In turn, 6 (a and b), 7, and 8 (a and b) together probably account for 30 to 50%. The principal differences between SPMs prepared by our more extensive and the short-cut procedure (16) are reduction in all components between 1 and 5, in 6.2 through 6.6, and in 10, 10.1, and 11, accompanied by an increase in component 6.1 and especially 8a.

in obtaining evidence (21) for the presence of a protein in synaptosomes and SPMs capable of strong and specific interaction with ^{125}I-bunga-rotoxin (at a concentration range of the ligand $\leqslant 10^{-8}$ M). Its subcellular and regional distribution, which coincided with those of other cholinergic markers, its response to cholinergic agonists and antagonists, and its subsynaptic localization in high-resolution autoradiographs all make it appear likely that we are indeed dealing with the muscarinic acetylcholine receptor of the central nervous system (22). Its concentration in beef and rat brain caudate nucleus is 4.9 and 4.0 pmoles/g wet weight of tissue, with cortex about 20% lower in each instance. The enrichment in the SPM fraction is approximately 8- to 10-fold, amounting to a concentration of about 0.3 to 0.5 pmoles/mg protein.

Fibrous Proteins

Based on the earlier studies and speculations of Feit and Barondes (24) and Berl and Puszkin (25), several groups of investigators have recently become interested in the possibility of a close association of fibrous proteins with synaptosomes and their membranes (25–27). These proteins include microtubule protein (tubulin) and actin-like proteins (nerve actin or neurin), as well as homologues or analogues of accessory proteins involved in the mechanochemical transductions associated with actin and tubulin such as myosin (stenin) and dynein, and components of the relaxing complex such as tropomyosin and troponin. By means of a combination of the high-resolution gel system developed by Laemmli (28) and internal standardization with authentic brain tubulin and muscle actin (kindly provided by Professor A. Szent-Gyorgyi), either using staining intensity, or prelabeling with ^{125}I, Crawford has recently been able to demonstrate comigration of a doublet (probably 7 in our standard gels, Fig. 1) with tubulin and of another band (probably 8 a or b) with actin. Using both, gel staining and isotope dilution, we estimate that 21 and 11% of the membrane components in these bands are contributed by tubulin and actin, respectively. We also have considerably more tentative evidence for the presence of dynein in the doublet seen at the top of the gel.

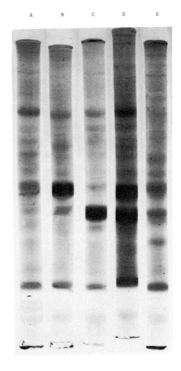

FIG. 2. Identification of microtubule protein and actin among synaptic plasma membrane proteins of rat brain. Samples were electrophorecsed according to Laemmli (28) on 3% stacking, 7.5% running gels. From left to right the gels contain (**A**) synaptic plasma membrane protein (SPM), (**B**) SPM + 27 μg microtubule protein (MTP), (**C**) SPM + 33 μg actin (**D**) SPM + 27 μg MTP + 33 μg actin, (**E**) synaptosomal proteins (similar methodology) of goldfish brain for comparison. (Muscle actin was a gift of Dr. A. Szent-Gyorgyi and MTP was prepared from rat brain according to Shelanski, ref. 53.)

DYNAMICS OF THE SYNAPTIC REGION

Functional Dynamics

Disposition of Major Components

The topographical disposition of proteins on surface membranes can be probed by a variety of means (7,29,30), and we have applied some of these methods to the case of the SPM. The simplest, probably, is based on the assumption (generally verified with these other membranes) that glycoproteins are localized externally, so as to permit their carbohydrate prosthetic groups to penetrate into the surrounding medium, and in fact constitute the antennae for intercell recognition and communication. This means in the present instance that synaptic glycoproteins extend into the synaptic cleft, and this part of the assumption has been shown to be justified by the demonstration that receptors for the lectin Concanavalin A (Con A) are localized in this area (31,32). Thus identification of a membrane subunit as a glycoprotein (see the section on Glycoproteins) suffices to suggest its disposition on the exterior surface of the membrane. Another commonly used method consists of iodination of tyrosine residues in membrane proteins by means of lactoperoxidase; since the enzyme is too large to penetrate through the intact surface membrane into the interior of a cell or organelle, properly controlled application of the technique to intact synaptosomes should label only the exterior proteins of the SPMs derived from them. If, in contrast, the synaptosomes are subjected to hypoosmotic shock prior to iodination this reaction should affect all proteins. The set of experiments therefore serves not only as a means of distinguishing (by difference) interior from exterior proteins but also as an internal control for membrane integrity. In the present instance, we have performed enzymatic iodinations on synaptosomes and derived SPMs obtained from both the complete (8) and abbreviated (16) procedures. The results were qualitatively similar, although, as expected, the introduction of additional steps leads to purer but somewhat less intact membranes and a resulting increase in the amount of iodination of internal proteins. The components definitely identified as being located on the exterior (junctional) side are 4, 5b, 6, 6.1, 6.4, and 7, with the minor protein band 6.4 carrying a disproportionate part of the label.[3] These are the very bands previously identified as glycoproteins. All other bands, but especially components 1, 5a, 8b, 9, 11, and 11.1 are not accessible to iodination and are therefore disposed on the interior surface. Some components, such as 4, 7, and 10, although labeled in intact synaptosomes, take up additional radioactivity after

---

[3] A component with this approximate mobility has been shown by Banker et al. (33) to be very strongly stainable for carbohydrates. Its iodination may therefore involve prosthetic groups as well as proteins.

lysis and thus may span the membrane or else be composed of more than one entity.

Effects of Surface Modification

We have tested the possibility that the glycoproteins of the SPM are involved in high affinity uptake of neurotransmitters by studying the effects of lectin binding and trypsin treatment on this process in synaptosomes (34). Binding of two lectins, Con A and a lectin isolated from the lentil *Lens culinaris,* to synaptosomes does not change the uptake of the putative transmitters: norepinephrine, 5-hydroxytryptamine, dopamine, choline, γ-amino butyrate, and L-glutamate. Although trypsin digestion of surface proteins of synaptosomes has no effect on their uptake of the first five transmitters, it reduces the rate of uptake of L-glutamate. This reduction is not due to synaptosomal lysis or a drastic conformational change of the synaptic plasma membrane since the maximal velocity of high-affinity uptake is reduced drastically from 0.965 ± 0.109 to 0.298 ± 0.045 (nmoles glutamate taken up $\times$ min^{-1} $\times$ mg^{-1} protein), with little attendant change in K_M ($\simeq 1.3 \times 10^{-5}$ M).

Biogenesis

Synthesis of Integral Proteins

The mode of biosynthesis of the SPM has been an object of our studies from the very beginning. The source and mode of insertion of individual membrane subunits constitute most intriguing problems within the context of membrane biogenesis in general. However, in the case of SPM, they become exacerbated, and the question is rendered even more acute, by two considerations: (a) the great distances between the sites of synthesis of most proteins in the cell body and their utilization in the synapse, as well as (b) the possibility, that somehow the secret of synaptic facilitation, or modification through use, must be explicable in terms of structural modifications of the membrane and of its proteins. Even at the most superficial level the problems can be divided into two groups, one dealing with the parameters that govern the synthesis of membrane proteins, the other with its possible mechanisms.

Turnover

One of the more convenient ways of investigating protein synthesis *in vivo* is to look at turnover in the steady state, that is to say in adult animals, where there is no longer any net increase in membrane protein, and the rate of its renewal must keep pace with the rate of its degradation (35). The latter is the parameter actually measured, and this is done by following the decay (anticipated to be first order) of radioactivity in proteins, previously labeled by exposure to an appropriate precursor. By the use of this technique and using uniformly labeled [³H]-leucine as the precursor, studies by von Hungen in our group (36) showed that the total proteins of synaptosomes isolated from rat cortex and the integral proteins of their membranes exhibited turnover with a half life of approximately 20 days. Similar results (half-life ≈ 17 days) were also reported in analogous studies on the membrane proteins of mouse brain by Morris et al. (37). Although encouraging, such results are difficult to interpret for three reasons: (a) They are a measure of only the average rate of turnover and cannot give any information on individual proteins. (b) Even then they are a measure only of that average rate which exhibits first-order decay characteristics; in the present instance only some 20% of the total, with the remainder turning over more rapidly with a more complex pattern. (c) The actual half-lives may be erroneous, largely due to possible reutilization of the precursor or a derivative thereof. In order to gain additional information concerning point (a) and minimize (c) Merel has extended these studies to a determination of the turnover characterization of the major, individual integral proteins of the SPM (38). To this end, she used a SPM fraction isolated by zonal sedimentation on sucrose (6), dissociated and separated its major subunits by electrophoresis on acrylamide in the presence of SDS, and compared their turnover by the modified double isotope techniques of Glass and Doyle (39); arginine labeled in its guanido-group with either ¹⁴C or ³H was used as precursor. At least 10 separate bands were analyzed, all of which were found to turn over with similar kinetics. In the absence of an internal standard, the method does not afford estimates of the absolute half lives, but at the very least we are now able to say that this parameter must be similar for most of the major integral subunits with one important proviso. If any of the bands displayed and separated on acrylamide gels are themselves heterogeneous and composed of entities with half-lives either much more rapid or slower than the main components, these will not be measured. On the basis of recent experiments under conditions that minimize reutilization, the actual half-lives are probably of the order of 5 days (40).

Origin and mechanism

Because of the topological and functional considerations mentioned earlier a great deal of recent attention has been devoted to the possibility that at least some of the proteins of the (presynaptic) SPM may be synthesized in the immediate vicinity of the synapse. Excluding glia as possible sources, three major mechanisms for such synthesis may be considered: (i) Export and transfer from synaptoplasmic mitochondria; (ii) local synthesis by a system sequestered in or on the SPM proper; (iii) synthesis in postsynaptic cell bodies followed by trans-synaptic transfer. Hypothesis (i) can be ruled out out of hand for the majority of polypeptides of the SPM. As already stated they turn over in unison and thus probably share a common site of synthesis. This cannot be the mitochondria for three reasons: (a) synthesis is sensitive to cycloheximide and emetine and insensitive to chloramphenicol, a pattern opposite to that exhibited by mitochondria; (b) the polypeptides synthesized by brain mitochondria upon short exposure to precursors in slices are different from those found in the SPM; (c) the informational capacity of mitochondrial DNA of animals is only sufficient for the specification of < 10 polypeptides; this number of polypeptides is required to satisfy the need of the organelle for its own biogenesis and known proteins implicated in this process. There is thus no significant capacity for export. Import of one or more minor proteins of the SPM from this source is also unlikely for the same reasons and is a complete lack of precedent in other systems; it cannot yet be ruled out entirely, however, particularly if it is supposed that the messenger RNA responsible is of nuclear, rather than mitochondrial, origin. On the basis of evidence currently available, hypothesis (ii) is now also considered unlikely. We have subjected it to an intensive and critical analysis by the following types of experiments (41,42). (a) A qualitative and quantitative analysis of the RNA (an essential component of any protein-synthesizing system) present in highly purified synaptosomes and their membranes showed that in the former the only RNAs were the ribosomal and transfer RNAs characteristic of their mitochondria; using a very sensitive, fluorometric method of analysis, the amount of RNA associated with SPMs was below the limit of detection, i.e., less than 0.5 μg/mg protein. This is considered to be an amount insufficient to support protein synthesis at a significant level. (b) Very little kinetic activity was found of incorporation of label into SPM proteins isolated from cortex slices exposed to radioactive leucine: Finally, the entities responsible for this incorporation were examined by means of high-resolution radioautography. In agreement with the earlier studies by Morgan (43), we found contaminants present in the synaptosomal fraction, consisting of inside-out vesicles studded with ribosomes rather than synaptosomes themselves, to be primarily, or perhaps even exclusively, responsible for the extramitochondrial (emetine-insensitive) protein synthesis of this fraction. None of the studies reported so far rule out hypothesis (iii), but the radioautographic studies would tend to indicate that most of the protein synthesized by this route ends up in the post- rather than the presynaptic portion of the junction.

Glycoproteins

Glycoproteins present a rather special case since one needs to inquire into the origin of both the protein and carbohydrate moieties and needs to entertain the possibility of local processing or modification of the latter. To establish a base line, we asked in a recent study (44), using incorporation of ³H-leucine *in vivo,* if there appeared to be any major difference between proteins and glycoproteins of the SPM with respect to origin, mode of transport, or turnover of their protein components capable of rapid turnover. No major differences were found.

Synthesis of Peripheral and Synaptoplasmic Proteins

Because of the inherent difficulties of using SPMs and their subunits for the determination of protein dynamics, we also decided to investigate isolated, purified proteins, of known function. These studies by Wenthold (45,46) concentrated on the two enzymes involved in the synaptic metabolism of acetylcholine, the membrane-associated acetylcholinesterase and the synaptoplasmic choline acetyltransferase. The turnover of the former was studied by measuring the decay of L-leucine-1-¹⁴C incorporated into these proteins: the observed half-life equaled 2.84 ± 0.13 days. To study the dynamics of the latter, we first had to develop a satisfactory method for its purification and characterization (as a single subunit enzyme with a molecular weight of 62,000) and then used a double-isotope technique (47) for an estimation of its half-life. This parameter equaled 5.2 days, in comparison to a value of 3.8 for tubulin, which was also isolated and studied as an internal standard.

CONCLUSIONS AND OUTLOOK

Comparison of the SPM with Other Membranes

The pattern of polypeptide subunits of the SPM disclosed by this, and parallel investigations elsewhere, is highly complex. However, it is not greatly more so than that of other, *a priori* much more homogeneous, populations of cell surface membranes. This conclusion is borne out quite dramatically by the data of Table 2. Except for erythrocyte plasma membranes (not shown), which because of the highly specialized nature and limited lifetime of their cells of origin clearly represent a special case, the similarities in composition of various plasma membranes, in both their qualitative and quantitative aspects, are much greater than are the differences. Furthermore, at least in mammalian cerebral cortex, as pointed out by our studies (8,42) and those of Wannamaker and Kornguth (53), there is considerable similarity and overlap in patterns between the SPM and membranes concentrated in the microsomal fraction. Some possible explanation for this particular similarity have been discussed by Barondes (11). But even

TABLE 2. Subunits of plasma membranes

Class		Rabbit thymocyte (48)		Rat adipocyte (49,50)			Rat limb muscle (51)			Rat; swine, human SPM (33,52)		
(48)[a]	This work (Fig. 1)	$M_{app}{}^b \times 10^{-3}$	Rel. freq.[c]	$M_{app}{}^b \times 10^{-3}$	Rel. freq.[c]	External[d,e]	$M_{app}{}^b$	Rel. freq.[c]	External[d]	$M_{app}{}^b \times 10^{-3}$	Rel. freq.[c]	External[d]
1.1	1	~250	+	310	++	–	–	–	–	211	–	yes
2	2	~230	++	–	–	–	–	–	–	194	–	–
–	3	–	–	–	–	–	–	–	–	191	+	–
2.1	4	~160	+	178	–	–	150	–	–	156	+	–
2	–	~160	++	143	+	yes	–	–	–	–	–	–
3	–	~160	++	–	–	–	–	–	–	–	–	–
3.0	5	120	++	126	++	–	110	+++ or +[f]	–	124	++	–
1	–	110	++	–	–	–	93	++ or +++[f]	yes	–	–	–
2	6	105	++	100	+++	yes	–	–	–	99	+++	–
4.0	–	80	+++	81	+++	yes	74	++	–	–	–	–
5.0	–	–	–	69	+	–	65	+	–	–	–	–
1	–	–	–	69	+	–	–	–	–	62[d]	+	yes
6.0	7	55	++	55	+	yes	55	+	–	53	+++	yes
1	–	55	+++	–	–	–	–	–	–	–	–	–
7.0	8	44	++	45	++	–	45	+	–	42	++	–
–	9	–	–	40	++	–	–	–	–	36	++	yes
8.0	10	36	++	33	–	–	34	++	–	33	+	–
9.0	11	27	+	25	–	–	–	–	–	26	+	–
10.0	–	21	+	17	–	–	–	–	–	–	–	–
1	–	16.5	+	15	–	–	–	–	–	–	–	–

[a] Modified.
[b] Apparent molecular weight based on mobility of protein standards.
[c] Relative frequency: ++++ ≥20%, +++ 15–20%, ++ 6–10%, + ~5%, no designation 2–5%.
[d] For presence of carbohydrate.
[e] By surface labeling with ^{125}I.
[f] Two separate subfractions.

the homologies between limiting membranes of divergent origin may not really be so surprising, but rather represent the structural correlates of a basic similarity of membrane function. The commonly accepted fluid mosaic model of the structure of a surface membrane (17,29,30) postulates a lipid bilayer forming the substrate for, and facilitating the interaction with and between, proteins of at least three different classes: those exposed to and penetrating the extracellular milieu, those so disposed as to penetrate the interior (cytoplasmic) milieu, and those that span the membrane, with a possible fourth class consisting of proteins entirely within and surrounded by the lipid bilayer. All the functional characteristics of the membrane must be implicit in this structure: its role as an architectonic and functional boundary between the two sides; its vectorial organization permitting selective uptake and release of low molecular weight constituents, sometimes on demand; its ability to couple these processes to ATP generation or hydrolysis; and finally its ability to communicate with and to receive communication from other cells. Even though the detailed nature of the entities involved will differ from cell to cell, the fundamental similarity of the process would argue for an underlying similarity of structure. This homology of structure should then in turn reflect some basic similarity in function. In fact, three of these ubiquitous membrane proteins do appear to represent functionally homologous entities. Thus the bands in the molecular weight range of 200,000 to 250,000 are probably contributed at least in part by myosin-like proteins, those around 45,000 by actin-like components, those at 30,000 and 20,000 by components of the relaxing complex (tropomyosin and troponin), whereas those around 90,000 and 55,000 may contain contributions by the subunits of the $(Na^+ - K^+)$ ATPase and of microtubules.

There is an additional consideration. The studies discussed here have focused on the most prevalent, integral proteins of the membrane. It is entirely conceivable that many proteins concerned with highly specific functions in fact belong to the class of peripheral (detachable, extrinsic) proteins, and it is almost certain that most of them, regardless of their classification, will be present in less than stoichiometric amounts relative to these majority proteins.

Good examples are provided by two proteins that we have been interested in: membrane-bound acetylcholinesterase is a protein that exhibits at least some peripheral attributes (17) and is present in amounts that would almost certainly not show up among the standard pattern; the nicotinic acetylcholine receptor, although perhaps present in high concentrations in the postsynaptic region of cholinergic junctions, will certainly not be detected as a discrete band in the heterogeneous membrane population under study.

In the future we plan to repeat and extend our investigations to SPMs enriched (a) for specific transmitter types and (b) in their pre- or postsynaptic components. Only with such preparations will it be possible to distinguish what is general from what is specific, and in this manner arrive at a model for the topography of the synapse.

ACKNOWLEDGMENTS

This research was supported by U.S. Public Health Service Research Grant NS 08309 from the National Institute of Neurological Diseases and Stroke. H.R.M. is a recipient of a U.S. Public Health Service Research Career Award KO 05060 from the National Institute of General Medical Sciences. We are deeply indebted for their inspiration in thought and deed to all members of the Brain Research Group, past and present, but especially to Prof. Walter J. Moore, who in conjunction with one of us (H.R.M.) initiated this research and was responsible for its joint direction for many years. The results and interpretation represent truly joint and cooperative efforts by a large number of individuals, most prominent among them Drs. C. Cotman, A. Campagnoni, G. Dutton, L. R. Jones, S. Munroe, M. Maguire, W. McBride, S. McGovern, P. Salvaterra, K. von Hungen, F. White, and H. Cohen, A. de Blas, A. Merel, and J. Ondrik.

REFERENCES

1. Whittaker, V. P. (1969) The synaptosome. In: *Handbook of Neurochemistry, Vol. 2*, edited by A. Lajtha, pp. 327–364. Plenum Press, New York; see also Whittaker, V. P. (1973): The biochemistry of synaptic transmission. *Naturwissenschaften*, 60:281–289.

2. Snyder, S. H., Young, A. B., Bennett, J. P., and Mulder, A. H. (1973): Synaptic biochemistry of amino acids. *Fed. Proc.*, 32:2039–2047.
3. Bretz, U., Baggiolini, M., Hauser, R., and Hodel, C. (1974): Resolution of three distinct populations of nerve endings from rat brain homogenates by zonal isopycnic centrifugation. *J. Cell Biol.*, 61:466–480.
4. de Robertis, E., and Rodriguez de Lores Arnaiz, G. (1969): Structural components of the synaptic region. In: *Handbook of Neurochemistry, Vol. 2*, edited by A. Lajtha, pp. 365–392. Plenum Press, New York; see also de Robertis, E. (1967): Ultrastructure and cytochemistry of the synaptic region. *Science*, 156:907–914.
5. Cotman, C., Mahler, H. R., and Anderson, N. G. (1968): Isolation of a membrane fraction enriched in nerve-end membranes from rat brain by zonal centrifugation. *Biochim. Biophys. Acta*, 163: 272–275; also Mahler, H. R., and Cotman, C. W. (1970): Insoluble proteins of the synaptic plasma membrane. In: *Protein Metabolism of the Nervous System*, edited by A. Lajtha, pp. 151–184. Plenum Press, New York.
6. McBride, W. J., Mahler, H. R., Moore, W. J., and White, F. P. (1970): Isolation and characterization of membranes from rat cerebral cortex. *J. Neurobiol.* 2:73–92.
7. Kornguth, S. E., Flangas, A. L., Geison, R. L., and Scott, B. (1972): Morphology, isopycnic density and lipid content of synaptic complexes isolated from developing cerebellums and different brain regions. *Brain Res.*, 37:53–68.
8. Gurd, J. W., Jones, L. R., Mahler, H. R., and Moore, W. J. (1974): Isolation and partial characterization of rat brain synaptic plasma membranes. *J. Neurochem.*, 22:281–290.
9. Morgan, I. G., Wolfe, L. S., Mandel, P., and Gombos, G. (1971): Isolation of plasma membrane from rat brain. *Biochim. Biophys. Acta*, 241:737–751.
10. Day, E. D., McMillan, P. N., Mickey, D. D., and Appel, S. H. (1971): Zonal centrifuge profiles of rat brain homogenates: Instability in sucrose, stability in iso-osmotic Ficoll-sucrose. *Anal. Biochem.*, 39:29–45.
11. Barondes, S. H. (1974): Synaptic macromolecules: Identification and metabolism. *Ann. Rev. Biochem.*, 43:147–168.
12. Lagercrantz, H., and Pertoft, H. (1972): Separation of catecholamines storing synaptosomes in colloidal silica density gradients. *J. Neurochem.*, 19:811–823.
13. McGovern, S., Maguire, M. E., Gurd, R. S., Mahler, H. R., and Moore, W. J. (1973): Separation of adrenergic and cholinergic synaptosomes from immature rat brain. *Febs Lett.*, 31:193–198.
14. Cotman, C. W., Mahler, H. R., and Hugli, T. E. (1968): Isolation and characterization of insoluble proteins of the synaptic plasma membrane. *Arch. Biochem. Biophys.*, 126:821–837.
15. Cotman, C. W., and Matthews, D. A. (1971): Synaptic plasma membranes from rat brain synaptosomes: Isolation and partial characterization. *Biochim. Biophys. Acta*, 249:380–394.
16. Jones, D. H., and Matus, A. I. (1974): Isolation of synaptic plasma membranes from brain by combined flotation-sedimentation density gradient Centrifugation. *Biochim. Biophys. Acta*, 356:276–287.
17. Singer, S. J. (1974): The molecular organization of membranes. *Ann. Rev. Biochem.*, 43:805–833.
18. Gurd, J. W., and Mahler, H. R. (1974): Fractionation of synaptic plasma membrane glycoproteins by lectin affinity chromatography. *Biochemistry*, 13:5193–5198.
19. Gombos, G., Morgan, I. G., Waehneldt, T. V., Vincendon, G., and Breckenridge, W. C. (1971): Glycoproteins of the synaptosomal plasma membrane. *Adv. Exp. Med. Biol.*, 25:101–113.
20. Wenthold, R. J., Mahler, H. R., and Moore, W. J. (1974): Properties of rat brain acetylcholinesterase. *J. Neurochem.*, 22:945–949.
21. Salvaterra, P. M., Moore, W. J., and Mahler, H. R. (1974): ^{125}I-α Bungarotoxin binding to subcellular fractions in brain. *Trans. Am. Soc. Neurochem.* 5:72; also Salvaterra, P. M., Mahler, H. R., and Moore, W. J. (1975): Subcellular and regional distribution of ^{125}I-α bungatotoxin binding in rat brain and its relationship to acetylcholinesterase and choline acetyltransferase. *J. Biol. Chem.*, 250:6469–6475.
22. Eterovic, V. A., and Bennett, E. L. (1974): Nicotinic cholinergic receptors in brain detected by binding of α-[^{3}H]bungarotoxin. *Biochim. Biophys. Acta*, 362:346–355.
23. Feit, H., and Barondes, S. H. (1972): Colchicine-binding activity in particulate fractions of mouse brain. *J. Neurochem.*, 17:1355–1364.
24. Berl, S., Puszkin, S., and Nicklas, W. J. (1973): Actomysin-like protein in brain. *Science*, 179: 441–446.
25. Blitz, A. L., and Fine, R. E. (1974): Muscle-like contractile proteins and tubulin in synaptosomes. *Proc. Natl. Acad. Sci. USA*, 71:4472–4476.
26. Puszkin, S., and Kochwa, S. (1974): Regulation of neurotransmitters release by a complex of actin with relaxing protein isolated from rat brain synaptosomes. *J. Biol. Chem.*, 249:7711–7714.
27. Gaskin, F., Kramer, S. B., Cantor, C. R., Addstein, R., and Shelanski, M. L. (1974): A dynein-like protein associated with neurotubules. *Febs Lett.*, 40:281–286.
28. Laemmli, U. K. (1970): Cleavage of structural proteins during the assembly of the head of bacteriophage T4. *Nature*, 227:680–685.
29. Steck, T. L. (1974): The organization of proteins in the human red blood cell membranes. *J. Cell Biol.*, 62:1–19.
30. Wallach, D. F. H. (1972): The disposition of proteins in the plasma membranes of animal cells: Analytical approaches using controlled peptidolysis and protein labels. *Biochim. Biophys. Acta*, 265:61–83.
31. Matus, A., de Petris, S., and Raff, M. C. (1973):

Mobility of concanavalin A receptors in myelin and synaptic membranes. *Nature [New Biol.]*, 244:278–279.

32. Cotman, C. W., and Taylor, D. (1974): Localization and characterization of concanavalin A receptors in the synaptic cleft. *J. Cell Biol.*, 62: 236–242.

33. Banker, G., Crain, B., and Cotman, C. W. (1972): Molecular weights of the polypeptide chains of synaptic plasma membranes. *Brain Res.*, 42: 508–513.

34. Wang, Y.-J., Gurd, J. W., and Mahler, H. R. (1975): Topography of synaptosomal high affinity uptake systems. *Life Sci.*

35. Schimke, R. T., and Doyle, D. (1970): Control of enzyme levels in animal tissues. *Ann. Rev. Biochem.*, 39:929–976.

36. von Hungen, K., Mahler, H. R., and Moore, W. J. (1968): Protein and RNA turnover in synaptic subcellular fractions from rat brain. *J. Biol. Chem.*, 243:1415–1423.

37. Morris, S. J., Ralston, H. J., and Shooter, E. M. (1971): Studies in the turnover of mouse brain synaptosomal proteins. *J. Neurochem.*, 18:2279–2290.

38. Merel, A. (1973): Protein turnover of synaptic plasma membranes. *Trans. Am. Soc. Neurochem.*, 4:80.

39. Glass, R. D., and Doyle, D. (1972): On the measurement of protein turnover of animal cells. *J. Biol. Chem.*, 247:5234–5242.

40. Sabri, M. T., Bone, A. H., and Davison, A. N. (1974): Turnover of myelin and other structural proteins in the developing rat brain. *Biochem. J.*, 142:499–507.

41. Maguire, M. E. (1973): Isolation and fractionation of synaptosomal populations from rat cerebral cortex. Ph.D. Dissertation, Indiana University.

42. Jones, L. R., Mahler, H. R. and Moore, W. J. (1975): Synthesis of membrane proteins in slices of rat cerebral cortex: Source of proteins of the synaptic plasma membranes. *J. Biol. Chem.*, 250:973.

43. Morgan, I. C. (1970): Protein synthesis in brain mitochondrial and synaptosomal preparations. *Febs Lett.*, 10:273–275.

44. Gurd, J. W., and Mahler, H. R. (1975): Biosynthesis of synaptic plasma membranes: Incorporation of [^{3}H]leucine into proteins and glycoproteins of rat brain synaptic plasma membranes. *J. Neurochem.*

45. Wenthold, R. J., Mahler, H. R., and Moore, W. J. (1974): The half-life of acetylcholinesterase in mature rat brain. *J. Neurochem.*, 22:941–943.

46. Wenthold, W. J. and Mahler, H. R. (1975): Purification of rat brain choline acetyltransferase and an estimation of its half-life. *J. Neurochem.*

47. Bock, K. W., Siekevitz, P., and Palade, G. E. (1971): Localization and turnover studies of membrane nicotinamide adenine dinucleotide glycohydrolase in rat liver. *J. Biol. Chem.*, 246: 188–195.

48. Schmidt-Ulrich, R., Hoelzl Wallach, D. F., and Ferber, E. (1974): Concanavalin A augments the turnover of electrophoretically defined thymocyte plasma membrane proteins. *Biochim. Biophys. Acta*, 356:288–299.

49. Czech, M. P., and Lynn, W. S. (1973): Studies on the topography of the fat cell plasma membrane. *Biochemistry*, 12:3597–3601.

50. Trosper, T., and Levy, D. (1974): Characterization of the surface protein components in adipocyte plasma membranes. *Biochemistry*, 13:4284–4290.

51. Andrew, C. G., and Appel, S. H. (1973): Macromolecular characterization of muscle membranes. I. Proteins and sialic acid of normal and denervated muscle. *J. Biol. Chem.*, 248:5156–5163.

52. Wannamaker, B. B., and Kornguth, S. E. (1972): Electrophoretic patterns of proteins from isolated synapse of human and swine brain. *Biochim. Biophys. Acta*, 303:333–337.

53. Shelanski, M., Gaskin, F., and Cantor, K. (1973): Microtubule assembly in the assembly of added nucleotides. *Proc. Natl. Acad. Sci. USA*, 70: 765–768.

The Nervous System, Donald B. Tower, Editor-in-Chief. *Vol. 1: The Basic Neurosciences*. Raven Press, New York, 1975.

Myelin: Structure and Biochemistry

William T. Norton

The existence of a sheath investing large nerve fibers has been known since the earliest days of light microscopy. Attempts to decipher the nature of this structure have occupied scientists of many disciplines for three centuries. By the end of the 19th century much fundamental knowledge had already been established. Histological studies had shown that myelin was primarily lipoidal in nature, but had a protein component as well, and optical studies had determined the paracrystalline nature of myelin as shown by its birefringence in polarized light. By 1950 the multilayered membrane nature of myelin was established and a fair amount could be inferred about its composition. Our knowledge of the structure, chemistry, and biochemistry of myelin has advanced rapidly in the past 25 years. These advances have been made possible largely through the application of electron microscopy, X-ray diffraction, subcellular fractionation techniques, and newer methods for the study of lipids and proteins. In this chapter I will summarize some of the progress in these areas. It is impossible to treat every subject in the detail one would like, and I apologize for ignoring many important observations and speculations. It has been especially painful for me not to be able to cite all the original references to the exciting biochemical work done in the last few years. Space limitations required a "textbook" format, and I have been forced to refer mainly to comprehensive reviews or to some original articles that include good summaries of a subject. It will be clear that even in this attempt I have not been consistent. For a fuller treatment of some subjects I refer the reader to a number of recent books and reviews (1–10).

The myelin sheath is a greatly extended and modified plasma membrane which is wrapped in a spiral fashion around most large (>0.3–1 μm diam) axons of higher organisms. In mammals, the myelin membranes originate from, and remain part of, the Schwann cell in the peripheral nervous system, and the oligodendroglial cell in the central nervous system. In the mature sheath these membranes have condensed in a compact multilayered structure in which each unit membrane is closely apposed to the adjacent one (see Fig. 1). Each myelin-generating cell furnishes myelin for only a segment of the axon. Between segments short portions of the axon are left uncovered. These periodic interruptions, called nodes of Ranvier, are critical for the function of myelin.

The function of myelin appears well established, its main role being to permit much higher conduction velocities than can occur in a comparably sized unmyelinated fiber (see 11 for review). In a myelinated fiber, conduction occurs by sequential depolarization of the axonal membrane at the nodes resulting in "saltatory" conduction, i.e., the impulse jumps along the fiber from node to node. The only other way nature has provided for increasing conduction velocity is to increase fiber diameter. However, conduction velocity in unmyelinated fibers is proportional to the square root of the diameter, whereas in myelinated fibers it is proportional to the diameter. It can be calculated that if nerves in the spinal cord were not myelinated, and equivalent conduction velocities were maintained, the human spinal cord would need to be as large as a good-sized tree trunk. Besides the space-saving feature, saltatory conduction requires only 1/300th of the sodium flux required for conduction in an unmyelinated nerve of the same diameter and therefore a much greater reduction in energy for equal conduction velocities. Obviously, the evolutionary adaptation of myelin was critical for development of higher nervous systems.

It has always been assumed that the alteration of nervous system function seen in demyelinating diseases is a result of myelin loss. Recently, it has been possible to study the effects of experimental demyelination of nerve conduction (see ref. 12 for review) and it has been con-

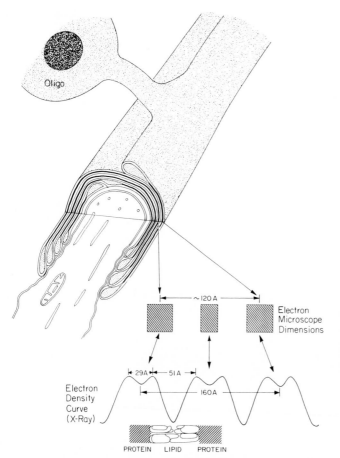

FIG. 1. A composite diagram summarizing some of the structural data on CNS myelin. At the top an oligodendroglial cell is shown connected to its sheath by a process. The cutaway view illustrates the relationship of the myelin to the axon at the nodal and paranodal regions. (Only a few myelin layers have been drawn for the sake of clarity.) The myelin layers can be seen terminating on the axon in structures called lateral loops, which contain glial cytoplasm. At the internodal region, the cross section reveals the inner and outer mesaxons and their relationship to the inner and outer tongues of cytoplasm. The lower part of the figure shows the dimensions of the repeating unit as seen in the electron microscope contrasted with the dimensions and appearance of the electron density curve derived from X-ray diffraction studies of fresh optic nerve. The molecular correlates of the physical data are sketched below. (Reprinted courtesy of Little, Brown.)

firmed that lesions can cause either a complete conduction block or reduce conduction velocity. However, there is still no direct proof that the loss of function in human disorders of myelin is a direct consequence of myelin loss, or that recovery of function in multiple sclerosis, for example, is due to remyelination.

STRUCTURE

Our current view of the structure of myelin is derived mainly from physical techniques. It was known from the polarized light studies of the 19th century that myelin was a highly ordered structure, and as early as 1913 Göthlin showed that there was both a lipid-dependent and a protein-dependent birefringence. Modern studies of myelin structure began with the improved polarized light studies of Schmidt and Schmitt and co-workers (for review see refs.

13 and 14) in the 1930s. These investigations established that myelin was built up of layers, with the lipid components oriented radially, while the proteins were oriented tangentially to the nerve. During the same period, using X-ray diffraction, Schmitt and Bear (13) found that peripheral nervous system (PNS) myelin had a radial repeating unit of 170 to 180 Å, sufficient to accommodate two bimolecular leaflets of lipid together with associated protein. Danielli and Davson had already formulated their concept of the cell membrane as a bimolecular leaflet of lipid coated on both sides with protein, so these early physical studies were interpreted with the awareness of the possible membrane nature of myelin.

The X-ray studies were extended in the 1950s and 1960s by Finean and co-workers (for review see ref. 15). Low-angle diffraction of PNS myelin provided an electron density plot of the repeating unit showing three peaks and two troughs, with a repeat distance of 180 Å. The peaks were attributed to protein plus polar lipid groups and the troughs to lipid hydrocarbon chains. The electron-density plots of this repeating unit were consistent with a protein(a)-lipid-protein(b)-lipid-protein(a) structure in which the lipid is a bimolecular leaflet of about 50 Å thickness and the protein layers (a) and (b) are different from each other in some way.

Similar electron density plots of mammalian optic nerve showed a repeat distance of 80 Å, i.e., adjacent protein layers reacted identically to the X-ray beam. Because 80 Å can accommodate one bimolecular layer of lipid (about 50 Å) and two protein layers (about 15 Å each), this represents the width of one unit membrane, and the main repeating unit of two fused unit membranes is twice this figure, or 160 Å (see Fig. 1).

The conclusions regarding myelin architecture derived from these two techniques are fully supported by electron microscope studies. Myelin is now routinely seen in electron micrographs as a series of alternating dark and less dark lines separated by unstained zones. The stained or osmophilic lines represent the protein layers and the unstained zones the lipid hydrocarbon chains (Fig. 1). The asymmetry in the staining of the protein layers results from the way the myelin sheath is generated from the cell plasma membrane (see the following section). The less dark line (called variously the minor dense line, intermediate period line, or intraperiod line) represents the apposed, outer protein coats of the original cell membrane; the dark, or major period line is the fused, inner protein coats of the cell membrane. Frequently in PNS myelin, but less often in central nervous system (CNS) myelin, the intraperiod line is actually seen to be a double line, indicating that the two outer protein coats of the membrane are probably not fused.

The X-ray diffraction data and the electron microscopic data correlate very well. Studies by both Finean and Robertson showed that PNS myelin, when swollen in hypotonic solutions, separated only at the intraperiod line, and the electron density plots showed that the broadening occurs at the wider of the three peaks in the repeating unit. This combined approach showed the continuity of the apposition of membrane surfaces which comprise the intraperiod

line with the extracellular space and proved that the wide electron density peak in peripheral nerve plots corresponded to the intraperiod lines seen in electron micrographs. It also indicated that the troughs correspond to the light zones between the two dark lines in electron micrographs. From both X-ray and electron microscopic data, it can be seen that the smallest radial subunit that can be called myelin is a five-layered structure of protein–lipid–protein–lipid–protein consisting of two apposed single membranes. This unit, comprising the center-to-center distance between two major period lines, has a spacing in fixed and imbedded preparations of about 120 Å. This repeat distance is lower than the 160 to 180 Å period given by X-ray data because of the considerable shrinkage that takes place during fixation and dehydration.

To the nonexpert the low resolution X-ray diffraction studies of Schmitt and Bear and Finean and co-workers correlated so well with other data on myelin, that the degree of ambiguity in deriving the final electron density plots from the diffraction data was not appreciated. These X-ray studies continue to present challenges and to provoke a surprising amount of controversy. It is now agreed that the phase angles of the first five diffraction orders were correctly assigned by Finean and Burge (see ref. 4). More recent studies by such workers as Blaurock, Worthington, and Caspar are concerned with refining the analysis to higher resolution using more diffraction orders. Two approaches seem to have been made for high-resolution work. One is to assume membrane symmetry and similarities between PNS and CNS myelin. The other is to work with models of the sheath. These two approaches give similar results and indicate that the membrane is asymmetric in the region representing the junction of the lipid bilayer and the protein. Caspar and Kirschner (see ref. 4) interpret this to a difference in the distribution of cholesterol in the two sides of the leaflet. If a direct analysis is carried out, independent of model building, then Worthington (16) obtains an asymmetric plot that is different from any previously obtained but does not have the shoulders attributed to cholesterol. There is as yet no chemical evidence for asymmetry of myelin lipids in the two sides of the leaflet, but such asymmetry has been detected in other membranes. It is clear that the X-ray data are not as straightforward as the earlier studies would indicate and that definitive electron density plots of myelin and their interpretation in terms of molecular structure may be some time in coming. Thus we may expect the low resolution electron density plot shown in Fig. 1 to undergo considerable revision in the future.

MORPHOLOGY OF MYELINATION

The early optical and X-ray diffraction studies gave a good indication that myelin was composed of layers of membranes. The first electron micrographs of tissue fragments published by Sjöstrand and by Fernández-Morán in 1950 clearly indicated the layered nature of myelin. However, not until the use of thin-sectioning techniques could it be discerned how these membranes arose from the cell.

In 1954 Geren (17) showed that before myelination the axon lies in an invagination of the Schwann cell (Fig. 2A). The plasma membrane of the cell then surrounds the axon and joins to form a double membrane structure that communicates with the cell surface (Fig. 2B). This structure, previously noted in unmyelinated fibers and called the "mesaxon," then elongates around the axon in a spiral fashion (Fig. 2B,C). Geren postulated that mature myelin is formed in this jelly-roll fashion; the mesaxon winds about the axon, and the cytoplasmic surfaces condense into a compact myelin sheath (Fig. 2D).

In early electron micrographs, cell membranes appeared as single dense lines, the mesaxon as two lines, and myelin as a series of repeating dense lines 120 Å apart. Robertson (see ref. 18 for review) was later able to show that the Schwann cell membrane is really a three-layered structure composed of two dense lines and a middle light zone (as shown in Fig. 2). When the two portions of this membrane come together to form the mesaxon, the two external surfaces fuse to form a single line (now seen as double) that eventually becomes the myelin intraperiod line. As a mesaxon spirals into the compact myelin layers, the cytoplasmic surfaces of the mesaxon fuse to form the major dense line. It was thus shown beyond doubt that peripheral myelin is morphologically an

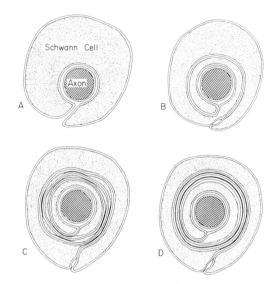

FIG. 2. Myelin formation in the peripheral nervous system. **A:** The Schwann cell has surrounded the axon but the external surfaces of the plasma membrane have not yet fused in the mesaxon. **B:** The mesaxon has fused into a five-layered structure and spiraled once around the axon. **C:** A few layers of myelin have formed but are not completely compacted. Note the cytoplasm trapped in zones where the cytoplasmic membrane surfaces have not yet fused. **D:** Compact myelin showing only a few layers for the sake of clarity. Note that Schwann cell cytoplasm forms a ring both inside and outside of the sheath. (Reprinted courtesy of Little, Brown.)

extension of the Schwann cell membrane. The mesaxon is thus the smallest myelin subunit and has the five-layered structure previously described.

It was reasonable to assume that myelin in the CNS was formed in a similar fashion by the oligodendroglial cell. However, these nerve fibers are not separated by connective tissue nor are they surrounded by cell cytoplasm, and specific glial nuclei are not obviously associated with particular myelinated fibers. In 1960 it was shown independently by Maturana and Peters that central myelin is a spiral structure similar to peripheral myelin; it has an inner mesaxon and an outer mesaxon that ends in a loop or tongue of glial cytoplasm (Fig. 1) (see ref. 2 for a review of this work).

Unlike peripheral nerve, in which the sheath is surrounded by Schwann cell cytoplasm, the cytoplasmic tongue in the CNS is restricted to a small portion of the sheath. It was assumed that this glial tongue was eventually connected in some way to the glial cell, but confirmation was difficult. Finally, Bunge (reviewed in ref. 19) and colleagues showed that the central myelin sheath is continuous with the plasma membrane of the oligodendroglial cell through slender processes. They also showed that one glial cell apparently can myelinate more than one axon. Peters recently calculated that in the rat optic nerve, one oligodendroglial cell myelinates, on the average, 42 separate axons (2).

The actual mechanism of myelin formation is still obscure. In the PNS, a single axon may have up to 100 myelin layers, and it is therefore improbable that myelin is laid down by a simple rotation of the Schwann cell nucleus around the axon. In the CNS, such a postulate is precluded by the fact that one glial cell can myelinate several axons. During myelination, there are increases in the length of the internode, the diameter of the axon, and the number of myelin layers. Myelin is therefore expanding in all planes at once, and any mechanism to account for this growth must assume the membrane system is flexible. It must be able to expand and contract, and layers probably slip over each other.

Isolation

Myelin is present in all parts of the nervous system but is, of course, more concentrated in areas composed mainly of fiber tracts, such as brain white matter and peripheral nerve trunks, such as sciatic nerve, which contain large motor fibers. It comprises a very large part of the tissue in such areas. It can be calculated that mammalian brain white matter is about 50 to 60% myelin on a dry weight basis. Even in the whole brain of an adult rat, myelin is approximately 25% of the dry weight and accounts for more than 40% of the lipid of the brain (20). A human brain, which has a higher ratio of white to gray matter, has an even higher percentage of myelin: an adult brain weighing 1,500 g might contain 120 g of myelin, 35% of the dry weight.

It is obvious that myelin is a very plentiful substance. This fact, combined with its specific physical properties, enables it to be isolated readily in high yield and high purity by conventional subcellular fractionation techniques. These procedures are covered in detail in some recent reviews (21,22). The perfection of these methods more than ten years ago in the laboratories of Davison, Horrocks, Kies, Norton, and others made possible very rapid advances in our knowledge of myelin chemistry and biochemistry and alterations in disease. All of the myelin isolation procedures take advantage of two properties of myelin—large vesicle size and low density. When myelin is homogenized in sucrose solutions of low ionic strengths the myelin peels off the axons and reforms in vesicles of the size range of nuclei and mitochondria, and will therefore sediment with these fractions during differential centrifugation. Because of their high lipid content these vesicles have the lowest intrinsic density of any membrane fraction of the nervous system. Myelin is less dense than 0.85 M sucrose ($d = 1.11$) and will band above this density during isopycnic centrifugation whereas microsomes, nuclei, and mitochondria will migrate through this region. Some subfractions of myelin have densities close to 0.5 M sucrose ($d = 1.065$).

The isolation methods fall into two groups, depending on whether the initial step is differential or density gradient centrifugation. In the former methods myelin is found predominantly in the crude mitochondrial fraction, although a variable amount is also present in the nuclear fraction. The crude mitochondrial fraction is centrifuged on a sucrose step gradient to yield fractions of crude myelin, synaptosomes and mitochondria. In the latter methods the total tissue homogenate is centrifuged on a density gradient to yield a crude myelin layer in the first step. This is accomplished by either overlaying the homogenate in isotonic sucrose (0.32 M) on more dense sucrose and allowing the myelin to migrate down to the interface, or by having the homogenate as the dense layer and allowing the myelin to rise to the interface. Variations have included the use of zonal rotors, mixed Ficoll–sucrose gradients and CsCl gradients.

The crude myelin layer obtained by either of these methods is of varying purity, depending on the tissue from which the myelin is isolated. White matter from adult brain yields reasonably pure myelin; myelin from the whole brain of a very young animal might be quite impure. The major impurities are microsomes and axoplasm trapped in the vesicles during the homogenization procedure. Further purification is generally achieved by subjecting the myelin to hypo-osmotic shock in distilled water. This opens up the myelin vesicles, releasing trapped materials. The larger myelin particles can then be separated from the smaller membranous material by low-speed centrifugation or by repeating the density gradient centrifugation on continuous or discontinuous gradients.

The purity of myelin preparations has generally been determined by the conventional methods used for other cell fractions, i.e., electron microscopy and assay of marker enzymes and other constituents believed to be localized in contaminating structures. There is, however, some ambiguity in the definition of myelin which may confuse attempts to establish purity. We have talked throughout this chapter of myelin as the compact multilayered structure. References to diagrams or electron micrographs show that the morphological definition of the sheath would include, besides this condensed membrane system, varying amounts of the cytoplasm of the generating cell. These pockets of cytoplasm occur adjacent to the axon (the inner tongue), outside the layers (the outer tongue), as well within the layers (Schmidt–Lantermann clefts) and at the nodal region (the lateral loops) (see Fig. 1). The isolation methods are designed to exclude these cytoplasmic constituents and purify only the condensed membrane system. Another source of ambiguity is the fact that these membrane systems appear heterogeneous and can be subfractionated into preparations of similar ultrastructure but of different chemical and biochemical properties (see below for further discussion).

COMPOSITION

It has been known for many years that myelin was a lipid-rich structure, and that it was mainly responsible for the gross chemical differences between gray and white matter; the most striking being the high lipid content and low water content of the latter. Early inferences about myelin composition were made from three types of indirect measurements: comparative analyses of gray and white matter, the measurement of brain constituents during the period of rapid myelination, such as the classic studies of Folch-Pi on mouse brain, and studies of brain and nerve composition during experimental demyelination. From such studies it became generally accepted that proteolipid protein, cerebrosides, and sulfatides were exclusively myelin constituents; that sphingomyelin and the plasmalogens were predominantly myelin constituents; that cholesterol and phosphatidylserine were major, but not exclusively, myelin lipids; and that lecithin was probably not a myelin lipid. These suppositions have now been shown to be only partially correct. Even so, in 1949 Brante was able to calculate that myelin sheath lipids were 25% cholesterol, 29% galactolipids, and 46% phospholipids, figures very close to those obtained by direct analyses of isolated myelin.

Analyses of isolated myelin show it has a much higher lipid: protein ratio than other subcellular fractions. The solids of myelin are 70% to 85% lipid and 15% to 30% protein. The lipids of mammalian CNS myelin are composed of 25% to 28% cholesterol, 27% to 30% galactosphingolipid, and 40% to 45% phospholipid.

No direct determination of water can be made on myelin, although obviously myelin is a relatively dehydrated structure. From X-ray diffraction studies on nerve tissue during drying, Finean determined the water content to be about 40%. This is probably a fairly accurate calculation, and all the data on yields of myelin and the composition of myelin and white matter are consistent with myelin having about 40% water and the nonmyelin portions of white matter having about 80% water, similar to gray matter.

Myelin Lipids

Table 1 lists the composition of bovine, rat, and human myelin compared to bovine and human white matter, human gray matter, and rat whole brain. It can be seen that all the lipids found in whole brain are also present in myelin, i.e., there are no lipids localized exclusively in some nonmyelin compartment except, possibly, cardiolipin. We also know that the reverse is true; that is, there are no myelin lipids that are not also found in other subcellular fractions of the brain. Even though there are no "myelin-specific" lipids, cerebroside is the most typical of myelin. During development, the concentration of cerebroside in brain is directly proportional to the amount of myelin present.

Figures expressed in this way give no in-

TABLE 1. *Composition of CNS myelin and brain*[a]

Substance[b]	Myelin			White matter		Gray matter (human)	Whole brain (rat)
	Human	Bovine	Rat	Human	Bovine		
Protein	30.0	24.7	29.5	39.0	39.5	55.3	56.9
Lipid	70.0	75.3	70.5	54.9	55.0	32.7	37.0
Cholesterol	27.7	28.1	27.3	27.5	23.6	22.0	23.0
Cerebroside	22.7	24.0	23.7	19.8	22.5	5.4	14.6
Sulfatide	3.8	3.6	7.1	5.4	5.0	1.7	4.8
Total galactolipid	27.5	29.3	31.5	26.4	28.6	7.3	21.3
Ethanolamine phosphatides	15.6	17.4	16.7	14.9	13.6	22.7	19.8
Lecithin	11.2	10.9	11.3	12.8	12.9	26.7	22.0
Sphingomyelin	7.9	7.1	3.2	7.7	6.7	6.9	3.8
Phosphatidylserine	4.8	6.5	7.0	7.9	11.4	8.7	7.2
Phosphatidylinositol	0.6	0.8	1.2	0.9	0.9	2.7	2.4
Plasmalogens[c]	12.3	14.1	14.1	11.2	12.2	8.8	11.6
Total phospholipid:	43.1	43.0	44.0	45.9	46.3	69.5	57.6

[a] All average figures obtained on adults in the author's laboratory.
[b] Protein and lipid figures in percent dry weight; all others in percent total lipid weight.
[c] Plasmalogens are primarily ethanolamine phosphatides.

formation about lipid concentrations in either the dry or wet tissue. Thus, while human myelin and white matter lipids have similar galactolipid contents, the total galactolipid is 19.3% of the myelin dry weight but 14.5% of white matter dry weight. These differences are much greater if a wet-weight reference is used. Then galactolipid is 11.6% of myelin but only 4.1% of fresh white matter. As another example, total phospholipids are a larger percent of gray matter lipid than of either myelin or white matter lipids. However, on a total dry-weight basis, phospholipids are 30.2% of myelin, 25.2% of white matter, and 22.7% of gray matter.

Figures in Table 1 show that many of the suppositions of the earlier deductive work are true. The major lipids of myelin are cholesterol, cerebrosides, and ethanolamine phosphatides in the plasmalogen form. However, lecithin is seen to be a major myelin constituent and sphingomyelin a relatively minor constituent. The reason that sphingomyelin was given such prominence as a myelin lipid in the early studies was that it was usually measured as "alkali-stable lipid phosphorus." It was not appreciated that this assay will also measure ethanolamine plasmalogen which is a predominant myelin lipid; therefore, the early figures for sphingomyelin include both lipids. If the data for lipid composition are expressed in mole percent, most of the preparations analyzed so far contain cholesterol, phospholipid, and galactolipid in molar ratios varying from 4:3:2 to 4:4:2. Thus, cholesterol constitutes the largest proportion of lipid molecules in myelin although the galactolipids are usually a greater proportion of the lipid weight.

Central nervous system myelin lipids from a large number of species have been analyzed, including man, ox, rat, and mouse (see refs. 1,2,4–10 for reviews). Much of this work has been carried out in the laboratories of Davison, Eng, Horrocks, Norton, O'Brien, and Smith. The composition of myelin from these species is very much the same. However, there are some obvious species differences. For example, rat myelin has less sphingomyelin than ox or human (Table 1).

Besides the lipids listed in the table, there are several others of importance. If myelin is not extracted with acid organic solvents, the polyphosphoinositides remain tightly bound to the myelin protein, and therefore are not included in the lipid analysis. Eichberg and Hauser have obtained good evidence that the triphosphoinositide of brain which is stable to postmortem hydrolysis is mainly localized in myelin. Triphosphoinositide accounts for between 4% and 6% of the total myelin phosphorus, and diphosphoinositide for 1% to 1.5% of the myelin phosphorus. Although low ganglioside levels have been used as an indicator of myelin purity, work by Suzuki and colleagues has now made it apparent that there is an irreducible amount of ganglioside associated with myelin; which is in the order of 40 to 50 μg of sialic acid per 100 mg of myelin (about 0.15% ganglioside). The myelin gangliosides in the mature animal have a pattern completely unlike the pattern of gangliosides extracted from whole brain; the major monosialoganglioside, G_{M1}, accounts for 80 to 90 mole% of the total myelin ganglioside. Ledeen and colleagues have shown that an unusual ganglioside, sialosylgalactosylceramide, is a major component of human myelin gangliosides, although it is less abundant in other species. This ganglioside is the only one known which is derived from galactocerebroside and which contains appreciable quantities of α-hydroxy fatty acids.

The long-chain fatty residues of myelin are characterized by a very high proportion of fatty aldehydes. These fatty aldehydes, which are derived primarily from phosphatidylethanolamine and, to a lesser extent, from phosphatidylserine, constitute one-sixth of the total glycerylphosphatide fatty residues and 12 mole% of the total hydrolyzable fatty chains of the myelin lipids. The phospholipid fatty acids differ considerably from one phospholipid to another, but are generally characterized by a high oleic acid content and a low level of polyunsaturated fatty acids. The glycosphingolipids, cerebrosides, and sulfatides have two classes of fatty acids — unsubstituted and α-hydroxy — both of which can be saturated or monounsaturated, whereas sphingomyelin has only unsubstituted fatty acids. The sphingolipid acids are primarily long-chain (22 to 26 carbon atoms) with varying amounts of 18:0. For example, human myelin glycosphingolipids have very little α-hydroxy-stearic acid but significant amounts of stearic acid, whereas bovine glycosphingolipids have both. Cerebrosides with unsubstituted acids and hydroxy fatty acids correspond, respectively, to cerasine and phrenosine of the older literature. (See refs. 10 and 11 for discussions of myelin acyl and alkenyl residues.)

The previous discussion on composition refers primarily to myelin isolated from the brain. There is good evidence that myelin isolated from the spinal cord has a considerably higher lipid–protein ratio than that isolated from the brain of the same species. The differences between myelins isolated from different parts of the CNS are not well documented and deserve much further study although Smith has shown that myelins from different brain areas may differ in composition. We do know, however, that myelin from the PNS has a different composition from myelin of the CNS. Peripheral nerve myelin has not received the same extensive documentation primarily because of the technical difficulty of homogenizing peripheral nerve. The few lipid analyses that have been made show that PNS myelin has less cerebroside and sulfatide and considerably more sphingomyelin than CNS myelin (23,24).

Enzymes

It was generally believed that myelin was an inert tissue which contained essentially no enzymatic activity. There are however two enzymes which appear to be relatively myelin specific and can probably be considered myelin markers. The first of these to be found is 2',3'-cyclic nucleotide-3'-phosphohydrolase. All recent work (from the laboratories of Kurihara, Drummond, Mandel, and Braun) confirms that the level of this enzyme in brain correlates very well with the amount of myelin in brain, whether during normal development or in the myelin-deficient mouse mutants, quaking and jimpy. This enzyme, however is low in peripheral nerve where it may be an axolemmal constituent rather than a myelin constituent. Eto and Suzuki have discovered a second enzyme, a cholesterol ester hydrolase, which appears to meet all the criteria for myelin specificity. They have found three distinct hydrolases in brain, but only the one with pH optimum 7.2 is primarily localized in myelin. Nothing is known about the true function of either enzyme in myelin. In fact, even the natural substrate of the 2',3'-cyclic nucleotide-3'-phosphohydrolase is not known. More recently, it has been shown independently in the laboratories of Carnegie, Miyamoto, and Appel that myelin contains a protein kinase capable of phosphorylating basic protein in a cyclic adenosine monophosphate (cyclic AMP)-independent reaction. It is not known whether this is a myelin specific enzyme. The situation with respect to other enzymes is not clear. Myelin has been found to have some nonspecific esterase activity which is retained after extensive purification steps, but the final activity is small relative to the total brain activity. Whether peptidase activity is present is still unsettled. It seems that neutral proteinase activity may not be an intrinsic constituent.

CNS Myelin Proteins

With the availability of purified myelin preparations, the once rather confused picture of myelin proteins began to be clarified somewhat. The studies of myelin proteins were slow in getting started because, with the exception of the "basic protein," the experimental allergic encephalomyelitis (EAE) antigen, the myelin proteins are insoluble in aqueous media and thus are not amenable to study by conventional protein techniques. Rapid advances have been made in this area in recent years. These advances have been due largely to the application of the technique of polyacrylamide gel electrophoresis of proteins dissolved in sodium dodecyl sulfate. This technique permits the separation of proteins according to molecular weight and has made possible the routine analysis of myelin proteins, studies of their synthesis and turnover, and the discovery of new myelin proteins. Myelin proteins can also be partially separated by the solvent fractionation technique of Gonzalez-Sastre and by differential solubility in salt solutions or salt solutions containing detergents using the procedure of Eng et al. As far as the gross composition goes, these various techniques give reasonably consistent results and it is generally agreed that there are three major proteins in myelin: 30% to 50% proteolipid protein; 30% to 35% basic protein and a lower percentage of a higher molecular weight protein doublet soluble in acidified $CHCl_3$–CH_3OH (called Wolfgram protein after its discoverer).

The electrophoresis studies indicate that the protein composition is more complex than this. Besides these three well-known proteins some rodents have an additional smaller basic protein, and all mammals have: a proteolipid-type protein doublet of lower molecular weight than proteolipid protein, at least one glycoprotein, and a family of high molecular weight proteins. These high molecular weight proteins appear to vary in amount depending on the species and

comprise a higher percent of the total in mouse and rat myelin than in bovine and human myelin. For this reason there is some doubt whether all of these high molecular weight proteins are intrinsic myelin components.

The major protein, the classic Folch-Lees proteolipid protein, can be extracted from whole brain with chloroform–methanol (2:1) and can be solubilized in either chloroform or chloroform–methanol even though its lipid content is reduced to less than 10%. It contains about 40% polar amino acids and 60% nonpolar amino acids. This protein has been the subject of much study over the years because of its unusual solubility properties (for an historical review see ref. 25). It, however, remains somewhat of an enigma. Recent work from the laboratories of Lees and of Mandel shows that the proteolipid protein fraction, as isolated from whole brain by solvent extraction, is heterogeneous, although the major component appears to be a single protein of about 24,000 MW. Part of the heterogeneity probably arises from aggregation of subunits. There is a myelin protein, or protein doublet, which runs between basic protein and proteolipid protein on SDS-polyacrylamide gels and which has been called DM-20 by Agrawal et al. This fraction may accompany the proteolipid protein during extraction procedures, but has not yet been well characterized.

Quarles, Brady, and co-workers have discovered that central nervous system myelin contains a small amount of glycoprotein which can be labeled with fucose, glucosamine, or N-acetylmannosamine. This protein runs in the high molecular weight region of SDS-polyacrylamide gels, and undergoes an apparent decrease in molecular weight during development.

The basic protein of myelin has been the most extensively studied because, when it is injected into an animal, it elicits a cellular antibody response that produces an autoimmune disease of the brain called EAE (for reviews, see refs. 5,26,27). This disease involves focal areas of inflammation and demyelination and resembles multiple sclerosis in some respects. The basic protein cannot be extracted from whole brain with organic solvents, but it dissolves when isolated myelin is treated with chloroform–methanol (2:1). It can readily be extracted from myelin or from whole brain by dilute acid or salt solutions, and, when so extracted, it is soluble in water.

The bovine protein is a highly basic protein (isoelectric point greater than pH 12), and it is highly unfolded, with essentially no tertiary structure. It has a molecular weight of around 18,000 and contains approximately 54% polar amino acids and 46% nonpolar amino acids. It has no cysteine and has one mole of tryptophan per mole of protein. This is in contrast to proteolipid protein, which is high in cysteine and methionine as well as being rich in tryptophan. The complete sequences of both human and bovine basic protein have been elucidated by Eylar and co-workers, and the sequence of the human basic protein has been determined independently by Carnegie. These two proteins differ from each other by only 11 residues.

Considerable effort has been devoted to determining which portions of the sequence are necessary for encephalitogenic activity. A small peptide sequence containing the tryptophan is necessary for EAE production in guinea pigs. Another region (residues 45–90) which does not contain tryptophan has been shown by Kibler and colleagues to be encephalitogenic in rabbits but inactive in guinea pigs. Other regions are apparently active in monkeys but not in either guinea pigs or rabbits. It has also been shown that the antibody combining site does not necessarily correspond to any encephalitogenic site. This is a very active area of investigation which is still controversial.

As noted above, mice and rats have a second basic protein, smaller than the encephalitogen. This second protein has been found in some other rodents by Martenson et al., but no clear-cut evolutionary pattern is evident. Martenson and co-workers have shown that the small basic protein has the same N- and C-terminal sequences as the larger, but differs by a deletion of 40 residues.

Since the myelin membrane is asymmetric, i.e., the cytoplasmic (major dense line) and extracellular (intraperiod line) surfaces are different by both X-ray and electron microscopic studies, there has been speculation that one of the major myelin proteins might be preferentially located at one surface. Dickinson et al. found that conditions that remove only basic protein from myelin led to collapse of the structure with disappearance of the intraperiod

line, thus implying a preferential location for this protein. However, the staining procedure of Adams et al. indicated this protein to be largely localized in the major period line (major dense line). Recent work on the peroxidase catalyzed iodination of intact spinal cord myelin by Poduslo and Braun supports the latter conclusion, that basic protein is present at the fusion of the cytoplasmic surfaces of the sheath.

PNS Proteins

These proteins have been extensively studied in the laboratories of Morell, Brostoff, Eylar, Dawson, Brady, and London, and have been shown to have quite different electrophoretic patterns from the proteins of CNS myelin. Three major proteins are present and the two lowest molecular weight proteins are basic proteins. The principal protein has been called variously P_0, J-protein, and X. There are, in addition, one or two proteins of molecular weights intermediate between P_0 and P_1 (the largest basic protein) and several high molecular weight proteins. It is noteworthy that proteolipid protein is absent. The major protein, P_0, has now been characterized as a glycoprotein but is obviously different from the CNS myelin glycoprotein. The larger basic protein, P_1, appears to be identical to the larger basic protein of the CNS. The smaller basic protein, P_2, has a molecular weight of 11,000 to 12,000 and does not have a counterpart in the CNS. It may be the antigen responsible for experimental allergic neuritis (EAN). The proportions of P_1 and P_2 vary considerably between species and in different types of nerves from the same animal. Guinea pig sciatic nerve has, for example, almost no P_2 protein. These results are extremely interesting from the immunologic point of view. It has been supposed that since injections of peripheral nerve could cause EAN but not EAE, that PNS myelin did not have the EAE antigen. However with the finding of the same antigen in both CNS and PNS, it is postulated that the EAE disease-producing site is blocked in the P_1 protein in the intact myelin structure. For a summary of the work on PNS myelin proteins see ref. 28.

Compositional Variations

I have discussed the variation in myelin composition in different species and the substantial differences in protein composition between PNS and CNS myelin of the same species. It has been known since the early work of Autilio et al., that cerebral myelin preparations from a single species which appear reasonably pure by conventional criteria can be subdivided, usually by density gradient centrifugation, into fractions having different chemical composition. The general findings by Adams and Fox, Benjamins et al., and Matthieu et al., among others, is that the heavier subfractions have more high molecular weight proteins and a higher content of enzymes, such as acetylcholinesterase, and other markers believed to be absent in pure myelin. The supposition has been that the heavier fractions are somewhat more contaminated with plasma membranes, axoplasm, axolemma and microsomes than the lighter subfractions. In fact, McIlwain has shown that the acetylcholinesterase present in purified myelin is always localized to exterior portions of multilayered fragments or is in small unit membrane vesicles, suggesting a plasma membrane origin for this enzyme activity. However it is also probable that myelin itself exists in a continuum of different densities, either in the native state or because of disruption during the isolation process.

Another possibility that must be considered is that myelin differs in composition in different areas of the brain. It is well known that spinal cord myelin has less protein and more sphingomyelin than brain myelin, yet both are CNS myelin. It is possible that this difference is related to the phylogenetic age of the two structures. If so then brain structures which myelinate early and are thus phylogenetically older than, for example, cortical structures may produce myelin of a different and more "primitive" composition. Smith has produced some evidence that this is true. Such data may partially explain the results (discussed below) on changes in whole brain myelin during development.

Developing Brain

The developing nervous system is marked by several overlapping periods, each defined by one major event in brain growth and structural maturation. These periods can be determined by following the concentrations of a specific marker. For example, the period of cellular

proliferation can be followed by measuring the amount of DNA per whole brain, and the period of myelination by following a myelin marker such as cerebroside. In the rat, whose CNS undergoes considerable development postnatally, the period of rapid myelination overlaps with this period of cellular proliferation and is one of the most dramatic in nervous system development. The rat brain begins to form myelin at about 10 to 12 days postnatally. At 15 days of age, about 4 mg of myelin can be isolated from one brain. This amount increases sixfold during the next 15 days, and at 6 months of age, 60 mg of myelin can be isolated from one brain (20). This represents an increase of about 1,500% over 15-day-old animals. During the same 5.5 month period, the brain weight increases by 50% to 60%.

It has been proved convincingly in the laboratories of Horrocks, Eng, Davison, Einstein, and Norton that the myelin that is first deposited has a very different composition from that of the adult (see 20 for discussion). As the rat matures, the myelin galactolipids increase by about 50% and lecithin decreases by a similar amount. The very small amount of desmosterol declines, but the other lipids remain relatively constant. In addition, the polysialogangliosides decrease and the monosialoganglioside, G_{MI}, increases to 90% of the total gangliosides. These changes are not complete until the rat is about 2 months old.

All of these studies indicate that there is a continual increase in the amount of myelin in rodent brains throughout the animal's lifetime. For the rat, myelin deposition appeared to be almost solely responsible for the continued increase in brain weight after about 100 days of age. A sensitive indicator of myelin maturation can be obtained by measuring the mole ratio of galactolipid to phosphatidylcholine, the two lipids which undergo the greatest change. In the rat this ratio in cerebral myelin varies from 1.2 at 15 days to 2.8 at maturity.

Morell et al. were the first to show that there is a change in composition of the protein portion as well. At the earliest practical age for study (8 days) mouse brain myelin contains all the known myelin proteins, but the high molecular weight, uncharacterized proteins predominate. The basic protein fraction (sum of both) increases from 18% of the total at this age to 30% at 300 days. Proteolipid protein increases more dramatically from 7% to 27%. Similar results were found by Savolainen et al. for human myelin during development. These studies indicate that basic protein appears in the sheath before proteolipid protein. A study of Adams and Osborne also shows that basic protein appears before proteolipid protein, but the latter increases in amount at a faster rate.

These studies have generally been interpreted as reflecting changes in any one myelin sheath. However it is not known whether the early myelin laid down maintains its singular composition and is diluted by mature myelin of a different composition or whether the inner layers also change. One must also keep in mind the possibility that phylogenetically older areas which myelinate first maintain a different composition throughout.

Little is known about analogous changes in human myelin or about quantitative changes in amount in human brain. It has been stated that myelination is not complete in the neocortex until the end of the second decade, but some neuroanatomists feel myelination is still going on through the 4th and 5th decades of life. Perhaps therefore the picture we get from the rat of continual increase in myelin throughout life is not unique.

Besides these natural variations there are a number of striking compositional changes in myelin seen in a variety of human diseases and in experimental and model conditions. It is beyond the scope of this chapter to discuss these alterations, which have been reviewed in some detail (5,7).

BIOCHEMISTRY

The principal biochemical features of myelin are its high rate of synthesis during the early stages of myelination and its relative metabolic stability in the adult. Although myelin is one of the most stable structures of the body when it is once formed, it is not by any means a completely inert tissue. Recent evidence indicates that some of the earlier conclusions regarding its extreme stability may be incorrect. Before myelination begins, the immature brain has a relatively high concentration of cholesterol and phospholipids, but the amount of cerebroside, the lipid typical of myelin, is extremely low, as is the activity of the enzyme which synthesizes

cerebrosides from UDP-galactose and ceramide. In the mouse the activity of the cerebroside-synthesizing system reaches a peak at 10 to 20 days, coinciding very well with the maximal rate of myelination. Most other lipid synthesizing systems also become most active at this time.

The concept of the metabolic stability of myelin in the adult has been largely developed by the studies of Davison and co-workers (1–3). This concept originated in the classic studies of Waelsch, Sperry, and Stoyanoff in the 1940s (for a review, see ref. 1). They found that heavy water was incorporated slowly into adult brain cholesterol and fatty acids, but was incorporated much more rapidly in young myelinating rats. Davison and colleagues confirmed these observations in much greater detail, using various isotopic labels and several precursors of myelin constituents. Because these constituents were isolated from whole brain, the biochemical behavior of myelin itself had to be determined by inference. Davison and his group then pioneered in the biochemical study of isolated myelin using similar tracer techniques, and the earlier results were found to be valid for the most part. The conclusions from this work were that myelin shows considerably more long-term metabolic stability than do other structures in the nervous system, and that all of the myelin lipids turn over at about the same rate; therefore, the myelin membrane may be metabolized as a unit.

Experiments by Smith and colleagues (10) confirmed the relative metabolic stability of myelin but cast some doubt on the idea that myelin is metabolized as a unit. They showed that lipid precursors are incorporated into myelin and mitochondria at similar rates in young animals but that they are lost much more rapidly from the mitochondrial lipids. This finding is in accord with Davison's earlier work. However, long-term experiments show that the radioactivity is lost from individual myelin lipids at different rates. Three myelin lipids—phosphatidylinositol, lecithin, and phosphatidylserine—have half-lives of 5 weeks, 2 months, and 4 months, respectively, whereas the ethanolamine phospholipids cholesterol, sphingomyelin, cerebrosides, and sulfatides have half-lives of 7 months to more than 1 year. By contrast, the half-lives of the lipids in mitochondria range from 11 days (phosphatidyl-inositol) to 59 days (cerebroside).

The rates of synthesis of these lipids, as determined in short-term experiments, are in agreement with the rates of turnover, phosphatidylinositol and lecithin being labeled more than the others. These observations have been extended by Smith to long-term studies of adult rats, as well as to *in vitro* studies of the myelin of rat spinal cord slices, using ^{14}C-glucose as a precursor in both instances. These experiments also confirm the earlier data—phosphatidyl-inositol and lecithin have the most active metabolism, and sulfatide, cerebroside, sphingomyelin, and cholesterol the least. The incorporation of precursors into myelin *in vitro* is, as might be expected, age dependent—higher activities are present in actively myelinating animals, but considerable uptake can still be measured in slices from 120-day-old animals.

In the past few years some possible explanations for the discrepancies in turnover times obtained by different investigators have been explored. In particular, the nature of the precursor and route of administration seem to be important variables. One of the more interesting recent findings is that there is apparently considerable reutilization of myelin constituents and exchange of constituents between myelin and other brain membranes. For example it has been shown, by Rawlins et al., that in Wallerian degeneration in the PNS cholesterol from the degenerating sheath is retained in the myelin debris and reused for the formation of new myelin. Spohn and Davison, in a study of long term cholesterol metabolism of brain showed that eventually there is a relatively uniform distribution of labeled sterol in all subcellular fractions. They explained these results by suggesting there is a single pool of cholesterol with which all membrane structures, including myelin, readily exchange. A similar conclusion was reached by Jungalwala and Dawson with regard to phospholipid molecules, although a small pool of slowly exchangeable material may also exist. The data by Jungalwala on the long-term persistence of sulfatide in brain membranes indicates that membranes other than myelin have a very slow turnover after long periods, also suggesting exchange, but not complete equilibrium. These

concepts are rather different from the usual way of looking at brain metabolism and may explain the disparate results obtained for myelin protein turnover. If proteins are degraded some precursors may be retained and reutilized, whereas others go into faster turning over pools and on to other metabolic pathways. The implications are, of course, that a slow incorporation or turnover of a particular precursor does not necessarily reflect the true rate of renewal of molecules in the sheath.

Methods for the separation of myelin proteins have now made possible metabolic studies of these individual species. Although the turnover studies make it clear that in general the half-lives of myelin proteins are greater than those of other brain proteins, the half-lives reported vary considerably. For example, the half-life of basic protein in the rat has been reported as 14 to 21 days by D'Monte et al., 21 days by Wood and King, and 42 to 44 days by Smith and, in the mouse, as 95 to > 100 days by Fischer and Morell, depending on the age at injection. Both Fischer and Morell and Smith found that proteolipid protein has generally about the same half-life as basic protein, whereas Wolfgram protein has a shorter half-life; although D-Monte et al. reported a longer half-life. The shorter turnover times for basic and proteolipid proteins are probably less reliable. Smith and Hasinoff have found that the rate of synthesis of these proteins is also roughly in the same order—basic protein and proteolipid protein are labeled more slowly than the high molecular weight proteins of myelin.

Myelin assembly and site of synthesis has been the subject of considerable speculation. It has generally been assumed that synthesis would proceed in an orderly manner, with the parts of the sheath formed early in development segregated from parts formed late. Because it was believed myelin had little metabolic turnover, the inner layers might represent early myelin and outer layers late myelin. Recent autoradiographic studies by Rawlins show that this static picture cannot be true, at least for cholesterol. Young mice were injected with ^{3}H-cholesterol and the sciatic nerves examined after short labeling times. After 20 min, cholesterol was mainly at the outer and inner edges of the sheath, with little at the midzone. After 3 hr, the cholesterol was homogeneously distributed throughout the sheath. These results are consistent with the idea (*vide supra*) that lipids of the sheath continuously exchange with other membranes and with blood, and certainly do not support the concept of a sequential deposition of myelin into unchanging layers. Rawlins suggested that the cholesterol entering the sheath from the inner edge might actually be supplied by the axon. There is now evidence from the work of Giorgi et al. that some myelin proteins in the optic pathway are labeled if precursors are injected into the eye. The current feeling is that any label in the nerve and tract, when corrected for systemic labeling in the noninjected side, represents synthesis in the ganglion cells only. Thus, it is speculated that label in the myelin would come from proteins synthesized in the nerve cell and transported through the axon. The exchange of lipid molecules from axon to myelin seems feasible, but the idea that the neuron synthesizes myelin protein strikes most as an heretical idea. This problem is being actively pursued by several groups including Elam, Autilio-Gambetti et al., and Prensky et al. So far the most likely conclusions are either that the proteins labeled by axoplasmic flow are contaminants rather than intrinsic myelin proteins, or that they are labeled by transported precursors that go from axon to glial cell.

The actual reasons for the greater metabolic stability of myelin compared with other brain constituents are unknown. However we may need to look no farther than the peculiar geometry of the Schwann and oligodendroglial cells. Consider a typical large PNS axon of 5-μm diameter, with a myelin sheath 1.0 μm thick and an internode length of 1,000 μm. Such an axon will have about 50 layers of myelin. A simple calculation shows that the total volume of myelin generated by one Schwann cell is 18,840 μm^3. The total area of a myelin double unit membrane (assuming a thickness of 180 Å or 0.018 μm), if it were unrolled from the axon, is about 1×10^6 μm^2 or 1 mm^2. This enormous amount of membrane is maintained by the remainder of the cell, which may be two orders of magnitude smaller. The situation with respect to the oligodendroglial cell is similar. Although CNS sheaths are thinner and internodes shorter, one cell having a perikaryon volume of about 500 μm^3 myelinates an average

of about 40 such internodes. It can easily be seen that the combination of the physical isolation of most of the sheath from enzymatic systems and the enormous ratio of membrane to cytoplasm may be sufficient to explain the average low metabolic activity.

Investigations of myelin have now reached the stage of maturity where the broad outlines have been defined, most of the easy problems solved, and details are being refined. Myelin is seen to contain more enzymatic activity than suspected, yet the function of these enzymes is obscure. Even the composition of myelin must be reconsidered, as there are obviously myelin fractions of many different compositions. Myelin metabolism is more complex than previously thought, yet this is the simplest membrane in the nervous system. One of the major problems is the relationship of myelin to the generating cell and the mechanisms of its synthesis and assembly. Membrane assembly is a general problem in biochemistry, but the unique character of myelin should give us a better chance to study this process. Myelin is different from other plasma membranes and different from the membrane of its generating cell. There is some evidence for precursor fractions in brain but this is still under investigation. There may be membranes intermediate in composition between the glial cell plasma membrane and myelin, but they may not necessarily be biochemical intermediates. As yet, unfortunately, there are no simple model systems for the study of the myelination process. Organ culture has been a useful tool, but such explants are as complex as the brain itself.

REFERENCES

1. Davison, A. N., and Dobbing, J. (1968): *Applied Neurochemistry*. Davis, Philadelphia.
2. Davison, A. N., and Peters, A. (1970): *Myelination*. Thomas, Springfield, Illinois.
3. Davison, A. N. (1972): Biosynthesis of the myelin sheath. In: *Lipids, Malnutrition and the Developing Brain* (Ciba Foundation Symposium). Elsevier, New York.
4. Mokrasch, L. C., Bear, R. S., and Schmitt, F. O. (1971): Myelin. *Neurosci. Res. Prog. Bull,* 9:439.
5. Morell, P., editor: *Myelin*. Plenum Press, New York. (*In press.*)
6. Norton, W. T. (1975): Myelin. In: *Basic Neurochemistry,* 2nd ed., edited by R. W. Albers,

G. J. Siegel, R. Katzman, and B. W. Agranoff. Little, Brown, Boston.

7. Norton, W. T. (1975): The myelin sheath. In: *The Cellular and Molecular Basis of Neurologic Disease,* edited by G. M. Shy, E. S. Goldensohn, and S. H. Appel. Lea & Febiger, Philadelphia.

8. O'Brien, J. S. (1970): Lipids and myelination. In: *Developing Brain,* edited by H. E. Himwich. Thomas, Springfield, Illinois.

9. O'Brien, J. S. (1970): Chemical composition of myelinated nervous tissue. In: *Handbook of Neurology.* Vol. 7, edited by Vinken, B., and Bruyn, G. North-Holland Publ., Amsterdam.

10. Smith, M. E. (1967): The metabolism of myelin lipids. *Adv. Lipid Res.,* 5:241.

11. Hodgkin, A. L. (1964): *The Conduction of the Nervous Impulse.* Thomas, Springfield, Illinois.

12. McDonald, W. I. (1974): Remyelination in relation to clinical lesions of the central nervous system. *Br. Med. Bull.,* 30:186.

13. Schmitt, F. O., and Bear, R. S. (1939): The ultrastructure of the nerve axon sheath. *Biol. Rev.,* 14:27.

14. Schmitt, F. O. (1959): Ultrastructure of nerve myelin and its bearing on fundamental concepts of the structure and function of nerve fibers. In: *The Biology of Myelin,* edited by S. R. Korey, p. 1. Hoeber-Harper, New York.

15. Finean, J. B. (1969): Biophysical contributions to membrane structure. *Q. Rev. Biophys.,* 2:1.

16. Worthington, C. R. (1973): X-Ray Diffraction Studies on Biological Membranes. In: *Current Topics in Bioenergetics, Vol. 5,* edited by D. R. Sanadi and L. Packer. Academic Press, New York.

17. Geren, B. H. (1954): The formation from the Schwann cell surface of myelin in the peripheral nerves of chick embryos. *Exp. Cell Res.,* 7:558.

18. Robertson, J. D. (1966): Design principles of the unit membrane. In: *Principles of Biomolecular Organization* (Ciba Foundation Symposium), edited by G. E. W. Wolstenholme and M. O'Connor. Churchill, London.

19. Bunge, R. P. (1968): Glial cells and the central myelin sheath. *Physiol. Rev.,* 48:197.

20. Norton, W. T., and Poduslo, S. E. (1973): Myelination in rat brain: Changes in myelin composition during brain maturation. *J. Neurochem.,* 21:759.

21. Spohn, M., and Davison, A. N. (1972): Separation of myelin fragments from the central nervous system. In: *Research Methods in Neurochemistry,* edited by N. Marks and R. Rodnight. Plenum Press, New York.

22. Norton, W. T. (1974): Isolation of myelin from nerve tissue. In: *Methods in Enzymology,* Vol. 31, edited by S. Fleischer and L. Packer, p. 435. Academic Press, New York.

23. Horrocks, L. A. (1967): Composition of myelin from peripheral and central nervous systems of the squirrel monkey. *J. Lipid Res.,* 8:569.

24. O'Brien, J. S., Sampson, E. L., and Stern, M. B. (1967): Lipid composition of myelin from the peripheral nervous system. Intradural spinal roots. *J. Neurochem.,* 14:357.

25. Folch, J., and Stoffyn, P. (1972): Proteolipids from membrane systems. *Ann. NY Acad. Sci.,* 195:86.

26. Eylar, E. H. (1972): The structure and immunologic properties of basic proteins of myelin. *Ann. NY Acad. Sci.,* 195:481.

27. Kies, M. W., Martenson, R. E., and Deibler, G. E. (1972): Myelin basic protein. In: *Functional and Structural Proteins of the Nervous System,* edited by A. N. Davison, P. Mandel, and I. G. Morgan, p. 201. Plenum Press, New York.

28. Brostoff, S. W., Karkhanis, Y. D., Carlo, D. J., Reuter, W., and Eylar, E. H. (1975): Isolation and partial characterization of the major proteins of rabbit sciatic nerve myelin. *Brain Res.,* 86:449.

The Nervous System, Donald B. Tower, Editor-in-Chief. *Vol. 1: The Basic Neurosciences*. Raven Press, New York, 1975.

Sphingolipids of the Nervous System

Kunihiko Suzuki

In the historical perspective, it is probably fair to consider the classical work of Thudichum, almost a century ago, as the beginning of studies of sphingolipids of the nervous system. He laid the foundation for future studies remarkably well with the crude analytical methodologies available at that time. Since then, a great deal of information has been accumulated concerning chemistry, distribution within the nervous system, metabolism, and functional implications of sphingolipids, although large areas of uncertainty still remain for future investigation. During early stages, the major emphasis was on structural identification of various lipid components of the brain, which was then followed by studies of developmental and regional differences, synthetic and degradative pathways, composition of cellular and subcellular fractions, neurological diseases involving abnormal sphingolipid metabolism, immunology, and more recently, possible physiological roles of these complex lipids. Attempts will be made in this chapter to first consider the fundamental aspects of brain sphingolipids and then to select a few highlights of this field in recent years. The field to be covered is vast and therefore the topics and reference citations are inevitably highly selective. Emphasis will be placed on the areas that are actively evolving and that hold potential for future development. A few areas, such as myelin biochemistry or genetic disorders of spingolipid metabolism, are omitted entirely because they are dealt with in other chapters in this volume. Because of the limited space for references, original articles are often not cited. Preference is given to review articles in which original references are found. For the same reason, a series of related studies from a single laboratory may be cited only by the most recent article in the series.

REGIONAL, CELLULAR, AND SUBCELLULAR DISTRIBUTION

Sphingolipids are ubiquitous constituents of the biological membrane, and are present in all regions and cellular and subcellular fractions of the both central and peripheral nervous system. However, the distribution of individual sphingolipids are by no means even. With the advent of modern analytical techniques, sphingolipid compositions of different brain regions, brain cell types and of subcellular fractions have largely been clarified.

The structure of sphingosine, the basic building block of all sphingolipids, was conclusively established largely by Carter and co-workers during the 1950s. Although relatively minor details of the chemical structure of some minor sphingolipids in the nervous system remain to be clarified, all essential aspects have been firmly established, and readers are referred to recent review articles (1,2). The sulfate group of sulfatide had erroneously been thought to be at the 6-position of galactose, but it was corrected relatively recently to the 3-position (3). Identification of minor glycosphingolipids that are related to galactosylceramide were also relatively recent events. They include cerebroside plasmalogen identified by Kochetkov et al., and two types of acylated galactosylceramide, one with the acyl group at C-6 of galactose which was reported by Norton and Brotz, as well as by Kishimoto et al., and the other at C-3 described by Klenk and Löhr. The structures of the important group of sphingolipids, gangliosides, have also been greatly clarified in recent years (4).

The structural characterization of these compounds occurred simultaneously with increasing refinements of cellular and subcellular fractionation procedures and more sophisticated and sensitive analytical methods, including thin-layer and column chromatography, and gas chromatography. A large amount of reliable analytical information is now available concerning distribution of sphingolipids in the nervous system.

Galactolipids

Galactosylceramide and its sulfate ester, sulfatide, constitute most of brain glycosphingolipids containing only galactose as the sugar moiety. It is a reasonable generalization to consider that both of these compounds are localized primarily in the myelin sheath. This is reflected in the analytical findings in that normal adult white matter is much richer in these galactolipids than gray matter. The amount of whole brain galactosylceramide correlated very closely with the yield of myelin in developing rat brain (5). It was known early, however, that their localization in myelin was not exclusive. For example, brain mitochondria contain some sulfatide, although much less than in myelin. More recent developments concerning the extramyelin localization of galactosylceramide suggest some exciting possibilities. Since the myelin sheath is a specialized extension of the oligodendroglial plasma membrane, it was not surprising that the isolated oligodendroglia contained substantial amounts of galactosylceramide and sulfatide (6). The finding of similarly high concentrations of these lipids in isolated axons was surprising (6). The isolated axonal fraction appeared essentially free of myelin, and, although the total lipid content was lower than myelin, the proportions of galactosylceramide and sulfatide within the lipid fraction were similar to those in myelin. Most recently, neurofilaments obtained from isolated axonal fractions were reported to contain similarly large amounts of galactolipids (7). These findings are potentially significant with respect to the question of the neuron–glia interactions, particularly of the events that take place between the axon and the myelin sheath. It is generally postulated that some specific mutual recognition process and metabolic interdependence should exist between them, but the precise nature of such interaction is entirely obscure. Galactosylcera-

mide is the lipid most characteristic of myelin and is present only at very low concentrations in neuronal perikarya (6). Its presence at a high concentration in the axon is therefore quite intriguing. It is also noteworthy in this context that direct evidence that neurons are capable of synthesizing galactosylceramide has been reported by Radin and co-workers.

Gangliosides

Gangliosides, defined as sialic acid-containing glycosphingolipids, have been under intensive studies in recent years. While the nervous system as a whole is rich in gangliosides compared to systemic organs, they show characteristic regional and subcellular distributions. Gangliosides are more highly concentrated in gray matter than in white matter or in the peripheral nerve. The concentration in the white matter is generally 10% to 20% of that in gray matter. This predominant occurrence in gray matter suggests strongly that gangliosides may be primarily localized in neurons. Although as many as 12 different gangliosides have been isolated and characterized from mammalian brains, there are four major gangliosides in the normal brain and others are all minor in quantity (4).

Different cortical regions appear to contain different proportions of the four major gangliosides (8). The frontal tip, precentral, postcentral and superior temporal gyri show similar ganglioside compositions. However, the distribution of gangliosides in the uncal area differ in that G_{M1}- and G_{D1a}-gangliosides are present in much higher concentrations. Other rhinencephalic areas, such as trigonal and cingulate gyri, share the same distribution characteristics of gangliosides. In contrast, the visual cortex is richer in G_{T1}- and G_{D1b}-gangliosides. The cerebellar cortex is uniquely rich in the trisialo-ganglioside, G_{T1}. Within the basal ganglia, the caudate and globus pallidus are relatively richer in G_{M1}- and G_{D1a}-gangliosides, while the thalamus contains much higher proportions of G_{T1}- and G_{D1b}-gangliosides. White matter consistently contains high proportions of G_{M1}-ganglioside, and in human brain, also sialyl-galactosylceramide (9). These analytical data have been in the literature for 10 years, but their potential implications with respect to physiological functions of the brain have not been examined. The peripheral nerve also contains the same four major gangliosides. However, a recent report by Li et al. indicated that a substantial proportion of G_{M1}-ganglioside in the peripheral nerve contains *N*-acetyl-glucosamine in place of the usual *N*-acetylgalactosamine.

The bulk of brain ganglioside can be recovered in the microsomal fraction. Its total amounts in other fractions, such as nuclei, mitochondria, and myelin, are smaller. In terms of the concentration, however, the synaptosome is the richest in ganglioside content (10). Further, it has been established with reasonable certainty that gangliosides are most concentrated within the synaptic membrane but not in the synaptic vesicles (10), despite some earlier suggestions to the contrary. The relative specific concentration of ganglioside in the isolated synaptic membrane is approximately 10, and its distribution is similar to that of acetylcholinesterase, sodium–potassium stimulated ATPase, or adenyl cyclase, and cyclic AMPase. These findings, coupled with the unusual chemical structure of gangliosides with its long hydrophilic and hydrophobic chains, naturally prompted speculations as to the possible role of brain gangliosides in synaptic transmission. Although this idea is interesting, no firm evidence exists as yet for its support.

The ganglioside patterns of brain subcellular fractions are generally similar to that of whole brain, despite the wide variations in the total content. The myelin sheath appears to be an exception. Early on, it was noticed by Norton and Autilio that highly purified myelin fraction contained a small amount of ganglioside. A series of analytical, developmental, and metabolic studies later showed that the mature myelin sheath apparently contains predominantly G_{M1}-ganglioside (11–13). The proportion of G_{M1}-ganglioside in isolated myelin increased during development, reaching 90 mole%. All attempts to localize G_{M1}-ganglioside in nonmyelin contaminants failed, and metabolically G_{M1}-ganglioside in isolated myelin behaved similarly to other myelin lipid rather than to whole brain G_{M1}-ganglioside. Available data indicate that if G_{M1}-ganglioside in the myelin fraction is in nonmyelin contaminants, they must possess the following unusual properties. The impurities are isolated together with myelin

and contain a very high concentration of predominantly G_{M1}-ganglioside, the metabolic activity of which is similar to that of myelin lipids and different from that of other brain gangliosides. Furthermore, the appearance of such impurity must coincide precisely with the process of myelination in time and quantity because the content of ganglioside in the myelin fraction is reasonably constant throughout development. At least in human CNS myelin, another ganglioside, sialylgalactosylceramide appears to be also an important component (9). Its presence was overlooked earlier because this ganglioside was lost during the conventional fractionation procedures involving solvent partitioning. Unlike G_{M1}-ganglioside, which is also present in all other neural fractions, sialylgalactosylceramide appears relatively specific to myelin. Its fatty acid composition is similar to myelin galactosylceramide, containing predominantly normal and α-hydroxylated long chain fatty acids. Most recently, galactosylceramide has been shown to act as the sialyl acceptor from CMP-NeuNAc for biosynthesis of sialylgalactosylceramide (14). Whether gangliosides in the myelin sheath are merely minor structural constituents or whether they might play important roles for maintenance of the unusual structure of the myelin membrane remains to be clarified.

Studies of the ganglioside composition of isolated neural cells—neurons, astrocytes, and oligodendroglial cells—have been largely unrevealing. The ganglioside concentration of isolated neuronal perikarya was no higher than that of glial cells (6). Isolated astrocytes contained approximately twice as much gangliosides as isolated neuronal perikarya. However, the ganglioside concentration in either of these two cell types was far less than that of whole brain. The proportions of individual gangliosides were also similar among the three neural cells. The generally accepted interpretation of these findings is that the uniquely high ganglioside concentration in the neuron is concentrated in the synaptic region away from the perikaryon. Almost all neuronal processes are eliminated during the isolation procedure of neurons. This interpretation is also supported by a microanalytical study on hand-dissected neurons by Derry and Wolfe, who showed the highest concentration of gangliosides in the neuropil adjacent to neuronal perikarya. Another possible interpretation was suggested by Norton and Poduslo. They reasoned that astrocytes contain higher concentrations of gangliosides than neurons because astrocytes as isolated have a much higher ratio of surface area to volume than neuronal perikarya stripped of their processes, resulting in a higher ratio of the plasma membrane.

Glucosylceramide, and Other Minor Sphingolipids

Glucosylceramide is a very minor constituent of adult mammalian brain, although it is an essential precursor and a breakdown product of almost all gangliosides. Careful examinations showed that not only glucosylceramide but other more complex neutral glycosphingolipids that are asialo-derivatives of gangliosides — lactosylceramide (asialo G_{M3}), *N*-acetylgalactosaminyl-galactosyl-glucosylceramide (asialo G_{M2}), and galactosyl-*N*-acetylgalactosaminyl-galactosyl-glucosylceramide (asialo G_{M1}) — are all minor but normal constituents of the brain (15,16). The distribution of glucosylceramide among isolated neural cells has been examined by several investigators (6). It was found by Abe and Norton in all of the three cell types at substantial concentrations. In fact, glucosylceramide was the major monohexosylceramide in both neurons and astrocytes from immature rat brain. The concentration of glucosylceramide in isolated bovine oligodendroglia was in fact higher than that in whole white matter or myelin. Since galactosylceramide is present in isolated neurons and astrocytes also, the general concept of localization of galactosylceramide in myelin — and hence oligodendroglia — and glucosylceramide in neurons is clearly an oversimplification. Abe and Norton also found substantial amounts of lactosylceramide in all three cell types, and much less amounts of trihexosylceramide and tetrahexosylceramide in neurons and astrocytes. In addition, they found that a minor glycosphingolipid, fatty acid ester of galactosylceramide, was a constituent of oligodendroglial cells. The current state of knowledge on lipids of isolated neural cells has recently been reviewed in detail by Norton et al. (6). These authors also make another important observation. Sphingolipid compositions of isolated mammalian neural cells are

entirely dissimilar to those of neurally derived tumor cell lines maintained in tissue culture, such as various lines of neuroblastoma or astrocytoma. The sphingolipids of these cell lines appear to reflect the state of neoplastic transformation rather than their neural origin. Extreme care, therefore, would be required if one wishes to extrapolate findings on cultured neurally derived neoplastic cells to normal neurons or glial cells.

SPHINGOLIPIDS IN DEVELOPING BRAIN

The nervous system is an exceedingly complex organ consisting of at least three major different cell types, which have different functions and which proliferate, migrate, make connections, and otherwise undergo dramatic developmental changes, each with its own biological program and yet interdependent to each other. Concomitantly, highly complex biochemical changes take place, and even considering only sphingolipids, what is now known is undoubtedly crude and oversimplified. Most of the well-controlled data were obtained from developing small mammalian brains. Rats and mice are most appropriate in this regard because the brain of these animals at birth is very immature and is roughly equivalent to that of a midterm human fetus in its developmental stage. Excellent and extensive analytical studies of lipid composition of human brains at different ages are available from Svennerholm, Vanier, and their colleagues (15,16). Regarding developmental changes of cerebral sphingolipids, they can be divided into three general groups — those primarily associated with myelin (galactosylceramide and sulfatide), those associated with neurons (gangliosides), and those which show relatively little developmental changes (glucosylceramide, lactosylceramide).

Galactolipids

A large number of studies are in the literature concerning the changes in cerebroside and sulfatide in developing brain. All data agree that dramatic increases of these two sphingolipids occur concomitant with the period of active myelination. There was a near-perfect linear relationship between the amount of galactosylceramide and the myelin deposition (5). These findings simply affirm the general concept that these galactolipids are primarily localized in myelin. As pointed out above, however, these lipids appear to be present ubiquitously throughout the nervous system, although at much lower concentrations. Reflecting this fact, these galactolipids are detected in the brain well before commencement of myelination when sufficiently sensitive analytical procedures are employed. The two enzymes which catalyze the last steps of synthesis of galactosylceramide and sulfatide, UDP-galactose:ceramide galactosyltransferase and PAPS:galactosylceramide sulfotransferase, both show developmental changes consistent with the analytical findings. Activities of the both enzymes are very low in immature rodent brains. A rapid increase and the peak activity occur corresponding to the initiation and maximum myelination, and the activity declines rapidly thereafter (17,18). Furthermore, most recent study indicated probable presence of a small portion of UDP-galactose:ceramide galactosyltransferase within the myelin sheath (19), although sulfotransferase was reported to be absent in myelin by Jungalwala. Sphingomyelin is present in high concentration in all regions, cellular and subcellular fractions of the brain. Its developmental changes are closest to galactosylceramide, however, because quantitatively myelin deposition represents the period of its most rapid increase.

Gangliosides

In contrast to galactosylceramide and sulfatide, developmental changes of total cerebral gangliosides reflect their primary localization in neurons. Gangliosides are present in neonatal rat brain or human fetal brain at substantial concentrations. The most rapid increase occurs concomitant with the period of rapid proliferation of neuronal networks, approximately at 10 days after birth in rats and probably at or slightly before birth in humans (8,16). Total ganglioside in rat brain reaches a plateau by age 16 days and remains constant thereafter. In addition to the total amounts, the molecular distribution of the four major gangliosides undergoes characteristic changes during development. When the whole rat brain including the cerebellum was examined (8), the molar ratio of G_{T1}- and G_{D1a}-gangliosides was one at birth. Then G_{T1}-ganglioside declined rapidly in pro-

portion while G_{D1a}-ganglioside increased. At 18 to 20 days, the ratio of G_{D1a} to G_{T1} was nearly 3 to 1. After this period, the ratio gradually approached the adult level of 2:1. The other two gangliosides, G_{M1} and G_{D1b}, showed relatively small changes. However, when the cerebellum was not included in the samples (16), a similar inverse relationship appeared to exist between G_{D1a}- and G_{M1}-gangliosides. Discrete anatomical regions may have to be examined to obtain precise changes occurring in the ganglioside patterns in developing brain. Similar changes in ganglioside patterns also occur in human brains with the neonatal period corresponding to the time of the maximum proportion of G_{D1a}-ganglioside. Although these descriptive findings are of considerable interest, their functional significance remains entirely obscure. One recent finding is however intriguing in this regard. Hakomori et al. showed in cultured cell lines that there was a prominent increase in G_{D1a}-ganglioside at the earliest phase of cell to cell contact and that once-increased G_{D1a}-ganglioside decreased when cells were left confluent.

Glucosylceramide and Other Minor Sphingolipids

The third group of sphingolipids is present in the nervous system at relatively small concentrations and does not change as dramatically as galactosylceramide or ganglioside. This group includes glucosylceramide, lactosylceramide and other asialo-derivatives of gangliosides. Presence of these compounds is most conspicuous in immature brains before myelination because of relative lack of galactosylceramide and sulfatide. Careful analyses indicate, however, that these compounds are present even in adult brains at comparable concentrations per unit weight of the brain. Reflecting such finding, the glucosylceramide-synthesizing enzyme, UDP-glucose:ceramide glucosyltransferase, in mouse brain showed no conspicuous developmental changes except for steady gradual decline throughout (17).

GANGLIOSIDE AS RECEPTOR

A substantial proportion of sphingolipid in the nervous system appears to be present as structural components of various membranes, and, as often stated above, their physiological function remains largely obscure. Most of the "theories" go little beyond mere speculations. Gangliosides have been considered to play a role in ion transport across the membrane. The potentially significant speculation regarding the role of ganglioside in transmission of neuronal impulses has been mentioned. Increasing evidence from outside of neuroscience indicates the importance of cell surface glycolipids and glycoproteins in the process of cell to cell recognition, immunological properties, and other functions. Although experimental supports are lacking for most of these hypotheses concerning physiological roles of brain sphingolipids, one area of studies is rapidly developing with promising future. This concerns apparently specific interactions of ganglioside with certain toxins known to affect the nervous system.

Tetanus Toxin

The idea of ganglioside as receptors for certain physiologically active compounds is not necessarily new. van Heyningen and colleagues pointed out early that tetanus toxin binds strongly with brain ganglioside and suggested that ganglioside might be the natural receptor for the toxin (20,21). Upon binding, ganglioside inactivated tetanus toxin. More recent studies indicated that the tetanus toxin binds specifically with those gangliosides with two sialic acid residues located at both the internal and terminal galactose residues (21). Thus, among the major gangliosides, only G_{D1a} and G_{T1} react with the toxin. The binding was potentiated when galactosylceramide was added to the mixture as an auxiliary lipid. Because of the specific requirement for the molecular structure, neuraminidase treatment of G_{T1}- or G_{D1a}-ganglioside abolishes the anti-tetanus toxin capacity of these gangliosides.

Botulinum Toxin

Another bacterial exotoxin, botulinum toxin, produced also by a Clostridium, appears to bind ganglioside (22). The potency of botulinum toxin was not affected by several sphingolipids, including sphingosine, galactosylceramide, glucosylceramide, and other neutral oligohexo-sylceramides, by sterols or fatty acids. It was however rapidly inactivated when incubated with gangliosides. Specificity of this binding was somewhat broad and all gangliosides tested were active. However, there was a positive correlation between the binding potency and the number of sialic acid residues. Thus, the trisialoganglioside, G_{T1}, was the most potent inactivator of botulinum toxin. Unlike for binding of ganglioside and tetanus toxin, galactosylceramide added as an auxiliary lipid was inhibitory to the binding process. While these findings indicate strong interaction between botulinum toxin and ganglioside, additional possible binding of botulinum toxin to sialic acid-containing glycoproteins has not been ruled out.

Cholera Toxin

Although not a neurotoxin, the specific binding of Vibrio cholerae toxin to G_{M1}-ganglioside has recently been studied extensively (23–29). Purified cholera toxin consists of heavy (H) and light (L) subunits. The L subunits appear to be responsible for the initial tight binding of cholera toxin to the surface of the plasma membrane while the H subunit probably mediates its biological activity. Cholera toxin binds with G_{M1}-ganglioside with very high affinity and specificity. Its specificity is such that binding of cholera toxin to G_{M1}-ganglioside is not inhibited by the presence of tetanus toxin which specifically binds to disialo- and trisialogangliosides. G_{M1}-ganglioside is effective at a concentration of 1 ng/ml. When the plasma membrane was treated with neuraminidase, its toxin-binding capacity increased as expected because the enzyme converts polysialogangliosides to G_{M1}-ganglioside. When the membrane glycolipids were extracted, the remainder lost the toxin-binding capacity, which was recovered in the extract. Choleragenoid, which is an inactive derivative of cholera toxin, could competitively block the binding of the active toxin to G_{M1}-ganglioside by its own capacity to bind G_{M1}-ganglioside. Furthermore, when fat cells were incubated with G_{M1}-ganglioside and excess G_{M1}-gangliosides removed, the toxin-binding capacity of the cells increased as the result of incorporation of G_{M1}-ganglioside from the solution into the plasma membrane. These findings indicate strongly that G_{M1}-ganglioside may be the specific receptor for cholera toxin. Cuatrecasas suggested the mechanism of cholera toxin action as "cholera toxin initially forms an inactive toxin–ganglioside receptor complex on the cell membrane, and this complex is transformed into a biologically active complex by a special transition which involves a major, spontaneous relocation of the complex within the two-dimensional structure of the membrane."

Other Receptor Function

At a more physiological level, Woolley and Gommi presented some experimental evidence that G_{D3}-ganglioside (sialyl-sialyl-lactosyl-ceramide) might be the specific serotonin receptor in rat smooth muscle. The specificity appeared high in that other ganglioside species tested were far less active (30). Some of the more recent reports (31) provide some circumstantial evidence that ganglioside might play a role in the synaptic transmission because neuraminidase alters the characteristics of transmission. Such results do not exclude sialic acid-containing glycoproteins as the responsible compounds, however.

IMMUNOLOGY OF BRAIN SPHINGOLIPID

Although there were occasional attempts to study immunological properties of brain lipids during the first half of this century, application of modern immunological techniques was initiated relatively recently in the past 15 years or so. The development of this field up to the late 1960s was reviewed thoroughly by Rapport (32). With the conventional definitions of "antigen" and "hapten," the immunological properties of sphingolipids appear to be limited to those of haptens in that they alone do not induce antibody production, although they react with the specific antibodies once they are produced. The haptenic nature of glycosphingolipids was first clearly defined with lactosylceramide in human cancer tissue by series of studies by Rapport and co-workers. From here it was a relatively short step to the identification of galactosylceramide as the major lipid hapten of the nervous system. As is the case for most lipid haptens, galactosylceramide requires a large excess of auxiliary lipid for formation of the

antigen–antibody complex, and two different antibodies appear to be formed, each requiring different amounts and different ratio (cholesterol:lecithin) of auxiliary lipids. Anti-galactosylceramide antiserum has been reported to demyelinate cultured brain explants (33,34), although this finding is controversial (35). The immunological specificity appears to reside in the carbohydrate residues and anti-galactosylceramide antibody does not react with glucosylceramide, sulfatide, or lactosylceramide.

Since ganglioside is an important neuronal constituent and since it is increasingly implicated in neuronal functions, more attention is being paid to its immunological properties also. Antigenicity of ganglioside is generally low and there are still considerable discrepancies and uncertainties among the data in the literature. Early attempts to obtain anti-ganglioside antibody did not achieve high titers, although Sherwin, Lowden, and Wolfe managed to produce antiserum of a considerable titer by multiple injections. Pascal et al. examined antisera to G_{M1}-, G_{D1a}-, and G_{M2}-gangliosides and showed that the Ouchterlony technique could distinguish G_{M1}- and G_{D1a}-ganglioside, which have terminal galactose, from G_{M2}-ganglioside which has terminal N-acetylgalactosamine. Most recently, Naiki et al. (36) obtained anti-G_{M1} and anti-asialo G_{M1}-ganglioside antibodies by injecting a mixture of both lipids, human red cell glycoprotein and complete Freund's adjuvant to rabbit followed by incomplete Freund's adjuvant 4 weeks later. The IgG fraction contained specific anti-asialo G_{M1}-ganglioside antibody and anti-G_{M1}-ganglioside antibody which however also reacted with asialo G_{M1}- and G_{D1a}-ganglioside. The IgM fraction contained both anti-G_{M1}- and anti-asialo G_{M1}-ganglioside antibodies which cross-reacted with each other and also with G_{D1a}-ganglioside. Specific anti-G_{M1}-ganglioside antibody could be obtained by absorption with asialo G_{M1}-ganglioside. The subject of glycosphingolipid immunology is obviously highly complex, and it will probably take some time before general concensus is reached. Because of the high specificity and high sensitivity that can be achieved by immunological techniques and because of the immunological implication of brain sphingolipid in certain disease states, this area seems sure to attract increasing attention in the future.

SUMMARY

The present status of our knowledge on sphingolipids of the nervous system has been briefly reviewed. The field has moved from structural, chemical, and compositional studies to more functional questions. An integrated approach would be necessary, involving ultrastructural morphology, biochemistry, electrophysiology, immunology, and others. Other than those discussed here, some of the important questions are the exact molecular configurations of sphingolipids within the plasma membrane, particularly in relation to its functional states, genetic control of sphingolipid metabolism, and many others. Recent development of highly sophisticated experimental methodologies in related fields now make it possible to approach some of these questions in a meaningful way.

REFERENCES

1. Rouser, G., and Yamamoto, A. (1969): Lipids. In: *Handbook of Neurochemistry*, Vol. 1, edited by A. Lajtha, pp. 121–169. Plenum Press, New York.
2. Eichberg, J., Hauser, G., and Karnovsky, M. L. (1969): Lipids of nervous tissue. In: *The Structure and Function of Nervous Tissue*, edited by G. H. Bourne, Vol. 3, pp. 185–287. Academic Press, New York.
3. Yamakawa, T., Kiso, N., Handa, S., Makita, A., and Yokoyama, S. (1962): On the structure of brain cerebroside sulfuric ester and ceramide dihexoside of erythrocytes. *J. Biochem.*, 52:226–227.
4. Svennerholm, L. (1970): Gangliosides. In: *Handbook of Neurochemistry*, edited by A. Lajtha, Vol. 3, pp. 425–452. Plenum Press, New York.
5. Norton, W. T., and Poduslo, S. E. (1973): Myelination in rat brain: Changes in myelin composition during brain maturation. *J. Neurochem.*, 21:759–773.
6. Norton, W. T., Abe, T., Poduslo, S. E., and DeVries, G. H. (1975): The lipid composition of isolated brain cells and axons. *J. Neurosci. Res.*, 1:57–75.
7. Schook, W. J., and Norton, W. T. (1975): On the composition of axonal neurofilaments. *Trans. Am. Soc. Neurochem.*, 6:214.
8. Suzuki, K. (1965): The pattern of mammalian brain gangliosides. III. Regional and developmental differences. *J. Neurochem.*, 12:969–979.
9. Ledeen, R. W., Yu, R. K., and Eng, L. F. (1973): Gangliosides of human myelin: Sialosylgalactosylceramide (G₇) as a major component. *J. Neurochem.*, 21:829–839.
10. Breckenridge, W. C., Gombos, G., and Morgan, I. G. (1972): The lipid composition of adult rat brain synaptosomal plasma membranes. *Biochim. Biophys. Acta*, 266:695–707.
11. Suzuki, K., Poduslo, S. E., and Norton, W. T. (1967): Gangliosides in the myelin fraction of developing rats. *Biochim. Biophys. Acta*, 144:375–381.
12. Suzuki, K., Poduslo, J. F., and Poduslo, S. E. (1968): Further evidence for a specific ganglioside fraction closely associated with myelin. *Biochim. Biophys. Acta*, 152:576–586.
13. Suzuki, K. (1970): Formation and turnover of myelin ganglioside. *J. Neurochem.*, 17:209–213.
14. Yu, R., and Lee, S. H. (1975): Biosynthesis of sialylgalactosylceramide (G₇) by mouse brain microsomes. *Trans. Am. Soc. Neurochem.*, 6:145.
15. Svennerholm, L. (1964): The distribution of lipids in the human nervous system. I. Analytical procedure, lipids of foetal and newborn brain. *J. Neurochem.*, 11:839–853.
16. Vanier, M.-T. (1974): Contribution a l'étude des lipides cérébraux au cours du développement chez le foetus et le jeune enfant. Thèse, Université Claude Bernard, Lyon, France.
17. Costantino-Ceccarini, E., and Morell, P. (1973): Synthesis of galactosylceramide and glucosylceramide by mouse kidney preparations. *J. Biol. Chem.*, 248:8240–8246.
18. McKhann, G. M., and Ho, W. (1967): The in vivo and in vitro synthesis of sulfatides during development. *J. Neurochem.*, 14:717–724.
19. Costantino-Ceccarini, E., and Suzuki, K. (1975): Evidence for presence of UDP-galactose: ceramide galactosyltransferase in rat myelin. *Brain Res.*, 93:358–362.
20. van Heyningen, W. E. (1959): Tentative identification of the tetanus toxin receptor in nervous tissue. *J. Gen. Microbiol.*, 20:310–320.
21. van Heyningen, W. E., and Mellanby, J. (1968): The effect of cerebroside and other lipids on the fixation of tetanus toxin by gangliosides. *J. Gen. Microbiol.*, 52:447–454.
22. Simpson, L. L., and Rapport, M. M. (1971): The binding of botulinum toxin to membrane lipids: Sphingolipids, steroids and fatty acids. *J. Neurochem.*, 18:1751–1759.
23. van Heyningen, W. E., Carpenter, W. B., Pierce, N. F., and Greenough, W. B., III (1971): Deactivation of cholera toxin by ganglioside. *J. Infect. Dis.*, 124:415–418.
24. King, C. A., and van Heyningen, W. E. (1973): Deactivation of cholera toxin by a sialidase-resistant monosialoganglioside. *J. Infect. Dis.*, 127:639–647.
25. Holmgren, J., Lönnroth, I., and Svennerholm, L. (1973): Tissue receptor for cholera exotoxin: Postulated structure for studies with G_{M1}-ganglioside and related glycolipids. *Infect. Immunity*, 8:208–214.
26. Cuatrecasas, P. (1973): Vibrio cholerae choleragenoid. Mechanism of inhibition of cholera toxin action. *Biochemistry*, 12:3577–3581.

27. van Heyningen, S. (1974): Cholera toxin: Interaction of subunits with ganglioside G_{M1}. *Science*, 183:656–657.

28. Staerk, J., Ronneberger, H. J., Wiegandt, H., and Ziegler, W. (1974): Interaction of ganglioside $G_{Gtet}1$ and its derivatives with choleragen. *Europ. J. Biochem.*, 48:103–110.

29. Lönnroth, I., and Holmgren, J. (1974): Chemical modification of cholera toxin for characterization of antigenic, receptor-binding and toxic sites. *FEBS Lett.*, 44:282–285.

30. Woolley, D. W., and Gommi, B. W. (1965): Serotonin receptors VII. Activities of various pure gangliosides as the receptors. *Proc. Natl. Acad. Sci. USA*, 53:959–963.

31. Tauc, L., and Hinzen, D. H. (1974): Neuraminidase: Its effect on synaptic transmission. *Brain Res.*, 80:340–344.

32. Rapport, M. M. (1970): Lipid haptens. In: *Handbook of Neurochemistry*, edited by Lajtha, A., Vol. 3, pp. 509–524. Plenum Press, New York.

33. Dubois-Dalq, M., Niedieck, B., and Buyse, M. (1970): Action of anti-cerebroside sera on myelinated nervous tissue cultures. *Pathol. Europ.*, 5:331–347.

34. Fry, J. M., Weissbarth, S., Lehrer, G. M., and Bornstein, M. B. (1973): Cerebroside antibody inhibits sulfatide synthesis and myelination and demyelinates in cord tissue cultures. *Science*, 183:540–542.

35. Seil, F., Smith, M. E., Leiman, A. L., and Kelly, J. M. III (1975): Myelination inhibiting and neuroelectric blocking factors in experimental allergic encephalomyelitis. *Science*, 187:951–953.

36. Naiki, M., Marcus, D. M., and Ledeen, R. (1974): Properties of antisera to ganglioside G_{M1} and asialo G_{M1}. *J. Immunol.*, 113:84–93.

The Nervous System, Donald B. Tower, Editor-in-Chief. *Vol. 1: The Basic Neurosciences*. Raven Press, New York, 1975.

Glycoproteins in the Nervous System

Richard H. Quarles

In the past decade there has been an enormous increase of research on membrane glycoproteins. The development of this field has been prompted in part by technical advances which, for the first time, have enabled workers to study glycoproteins which are tightly bound to insoluble cell membranes. Another factor that has been important in stimulating the growth of this field is the increasing awareness that cell-surface glycoproteins are likely to play critical roles in the interactions of cells with their external environment and with other cells. If the now widespread belief that glycoproteins are involved in intercellular recognition and adhesiveness is correct, these glycosylated macromolecules may be called upon to perform their most demanding roles in the establishment of the complex intercellular relationships of the mammalian nervous system. Many specific cell surface interactions must occur in the developing nervous system as proper neuronal-glial relationships are established and as intricate synaptic connections between neurons or between neurons and target cells are formed. The carbohydrate residues of glycoproteins on the surfaces of neuronal and glial cells are prime candidates to be involved in these processes.

Spiro has provided a readable review of the field of glycoproteins in general (1). In addition, there are reviews (2,3) and even a book (4) emphasizing glycoproteins which are components of cellular membranes. Reviews on glycoproteins of the nervous system have been published by Brunngraber (5,6). The reader is referred to these sources for extensive coverage of the field. In this chapter, I emphasize those aspects of glycoprotein research that are of particular relevance to the development, function, and pathology of neural tissue.

GLYCOPROTEINS AS SURFACE-MEMBRANE COMPONENTS AND THEIR POSSIBLE ROLES IN CELL–CELL INTERACTIONS

Knowledge that glycoproteins are concentrated on cell surfaces has come from a combination of histological studies and biochemical analyses of isolated plasma membranes (2–4). The current ideas of how glycoproteins are integrated into the structure of membranes are derived largely from studies on the red blood cell glycoprotein (7). The portion of the glycoprotein containing the oligosaccharide moieties extends into the external environment of the cell, while the protein is attached to the membrane by a hydrophobic region which penetrates into the lipid rich core of the membrane (Fig. 1). In some cases at least, the glycoproteins are believed to be associated with the intramembranous particles revealed by freeze etching techniques (7).

The concept that glycoproteins play a role in interactions between cells is reasonable in view of their localization on cell surfaces. Part of the experimental evidence for such a role involves the reaggregation of dissociated cells. (See refs. 2,3, and 4, and the chapter in this volume by Barondes for more detailed reviews of this subject.) The earliest experiments of this type were done with different species of marine sponges which can be distinguished by color. When sponges of two different species were dissociated into individuals cells and mixed in suspension, the cells reaggregated to form multicellular groups that were species specific, i.e., of one color. In 1965 Margoliash et al. (9) analyzed a factor released by sponge cells that specifically stimulated the aggrega-

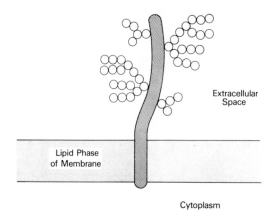

FIG. 1. Schematic representation of the current concept of how glycoproteins are integrated into the structure of cell surface membranes. One part of the polypeptide chain (*hatched structure*) penetrates into the lipid-rich core of the membrane. This portion of the glycoprotein contains a large number of hydrophobic amino acids which interact with the lipids of the membrane. The other end of the protein extends into the external environment of the cell, and it is this portion of the molecule to which the carbohydrate residues (*circles*) are attached. A model of this type was first proposed by Morawiecki (8) for the major glycoprotein of the erythrocyte and later elaborated on by Winzler (2), Marchesi et al. (7), and others. Glycoproteins of other membranes, including those of neural tissue, may be incorporated into membranous structures in a similar manner.

tion of cells of the same species and showed that it contained about 50% amino acids and 50% carbohydrate. There were differences in the carbohydrate compositions of the factors from different species. More recently, an aggregation promoting factor from the marine sponge *Microciona parthena* has been purified and shown to be an acidic proteoglycan complex of several million daltons (10). Reaggregation experiments have now been performed with many different systems including mammalian cells. In some cases, treating cells with agents which would be expected to alter carbohydrate residues, such as periodate or glycosidases, interfered with the specific cellular interactions, a finding in support of the concept of a functional role of oligosaccharides in cell–cell interactions.

Perhaps the most elegant chemical investigation showing the roles of sugar moieties of glycoproteins in recognition phenomena is that of Ashwell and his colleagues (11). In this case

the recognition is not between two cells, but between soluble glycoproteins in the blood and the liver cell plasma membrane. A specific receptor on the liver cell surface interacts with terminal galactose residues on desialylated serum glycoproteins, causing the glycoproteins to be removed from the circulation and taken up by the liver. If the galactose residues are covered with sialic acid, removed, or chemically modified, the binding to the liver cell membrane does not occur, and the serum protein remains in the circulation. Conversely, there are sialic acid groups associated with the membrane receptor which are required for the specific binding of the desialylated serum glycoproteins.

Direct evidence for a role of glycoproteins in recognition or intercellular adhesion in the nervous system is limited. However, reaggregation experiments similar to those described previously have been done with neural cells. β-Galactosidase treatment of embryonic neural retina cells suggested that terminal galactosyl residues were involved in specific intercellular adhesion (12). Recent investigations have been directed toward characterizing the tissue-specific adhesive molecules in the tissue culture supernatants of chicken embryo neural retina and cerebral lobe, respectively (13). Macromolecules in the supernatants which are labeled by ^{3}H-glucosamine and ^{14}C-leucine bind specifically to cells of the same type. Treatment with glycosidases and competition experiments with monosaccharides suggest that the specificity resides at least in part in the oligosaccharide moieties of a complex glycoprotein. Different sugar residues seem to be important for the two different tissues. Reaggregation experiments with cerebral isocortex and cerebellar cortex of developing mouse brain have shown the establishment *in vitro* of structures morphologically resembling the original tissue (14), indicating that highly specific surface recognition occurs in dissociated cells. "Reeler" mouse mutants present a highly disorganized arrangement of cells in the cerebellar cortex, hippocampus, and cerebral isocortex, and this highly ordered *in vitro* alignment of cells does not occur during reaggregation of cells isolated from these animals (14). Such mutants appear to offer a valuable experimental model for elucidating the chemical basis of the intercellular recognition. A number of reviewers have speculated on the possible roles of glycoproteins of the nervous system in cell–cell interactions (15–17), and in some cases specific mechanisms have been proposed.

LOCALIZATION OF GLYCOPROTEINS OF NEURAL TISSUE

Studies on separated cells have shown that glycoproteins are in all of the three major cell types of brain, neurons, astrocytes, and oligodendroglia (18). Most of the glycoproteins of neural tissue are associated with membranes, and subcellular fractionation of brain has shown that they are most concentrated in synaptosomal and microsomal fractions (5). Only small amounts of glycoproteins are found in nuclear, myelin, mitochondrial, and soluble fractions, although the glycoproteins associated with myelin are unique (see below). The microsomal fraction from brain as customarily prepared contains many fragments of axonal, dendritic, and glial surface membranes. Therefore, the results of subcellular fractionation of brain are compatible with a concentration of glycoproteins on cell surfaces. Histochemical techniques also indicate the presence of glycoproteins on neuronal and glial cell surfaces, with a particularly high concentration in the region of the synaptic cleft (19). The high density of glycoproteins at the synapse is consistent with hypotheses that they are instrumental in the formation and maintenance of specific interneuronal connections. Many of the glycoproteins of the synaptic region are synthesized in the neuronal cell body and transported to the nerve ending (20). Also, there is experimental evidence which suggests that some of the glycoproteins synthesized in the neuronal cell body are incomplete, and additional sugars are added at the nerve ending after they are transported down the axon (17). Glucosamine appears to be added to a particular class of glycoproteins at the nerve ending (21). Although the interpretation of these investigations has been questioned (6), modification of glycoproteins in the region of the synapse could play a role in the formation or alteration of synaptic connections during development or learning (17). In order for such a process to occur, biosynthetic glycosyltransferases would have to be present at the nerve endings. Since there are many inherent difficul-

ties in obtaining highly purified subcellular fractions from brain, it is not surprising that there are conflicting results in the literature concerning the possible synaptosomal localization of glycosyltransferases. Much additional work is required before the possible roles of glycoproteins and glycosyltransferases in the formation and maintenance of synaptic junctions can properly be evaluated. Synaptosomal glycoproteins might also be involved in the action of neurotransmitters at synapses, and some studies suggesting this have been summarized in another review (6).

CHEMISTRY AND METABOLISM

Detailed knowledge about the chemistry of glycoproteins of neural tissue has been elaborated slowly for two primary reasons. The first is that attempts to fractionate intact brain glycoproteins have revealed a great deal of heterogeneity (5,15,22,23) making it very difficult to obtain individual components for analysis. Even an individual glycoprotein (i.e., one polypeptide) may not behave uniformly during fractionation procedures due to microheterogeneity in the carbohydrate moieties. The second reason is that most glycoproteins of brain are tightly bound to membranes, and detergents must be used for solubilization, rendering their isolation and characterization difficult. Much of what we know about the chemistry of brain glycoproteins has come from the pioneering efforts of Brunngraber and his colleagues, who overcame the problem of insolubility by treating delipidated tissue with a proteolytic enzyme to produce water soluble glycopeptides. Although this yielded a very heterogeneous mixture of glycopeptides derived from a great number of glycoproteins, much has been learned from fractionating and analyzing the glycopeptides. The results of such experiments have been reviewed in detail (5,6), and indicate that the oligosaccharide moieties of brain glycoproteins resemble those found in other tissues. They contain galactose, mannose, fucose, N-acetylglucosamine, N-acetylgalactosamine, sialic acid, and sulfate. Also, the mechanisms of biosynthesis and degradation of brain glycoproteins are similar to those in other tissues (5,6). Biosynthesis involves activated nucleotide derivatives of sugars, and breakdown is catalyzed by glycosidases which are concentrated in lysosomes. Superimposed upon the biosynthesis of glycoproteins in neurons, however, is the rapid axonal transport of some of the newly synthesized glycoproteins to sites which are often far removed from the place of synthesis in the cell bodies (20).

DEVELOPMENT

If glycoproteins are involved in the establishment of complex intercellular relationships of the nervous system, it might be expected that they would exhibit developmental changes during the period of rapid brain maturation. Such changes have been observed although their precise significance is unclear. Some high molecular weight glycoproteins are synthesized to a greater extent in neonatal mice (22) and rats (23) than in more mature animals. There are differences in the carbohydrate composition of glycopeptides prepared from 15-day-old rat brain in comparison to those from adult brain (24). Recently, it was reported that the amounts of *N*-acetylneuraminic acid and *N*-acetylgalactosamine in the acidic glycopeptides prepared from whole rat brain reach their highest level per mg of lipid-free residue at 5 days of age and then decrease, whereas other sugars continue to increase up to about 30 days of age (25). The dialyzable fucose-labeled glycopeptides of mature rat brain exhibited a slightly higher molecular weight during gel filtration than those from 5-day-old rats (26). The higher molecular weight appeared to be due to a higher sialic acid content since the difference was eliminated by neuraminidase treatment. Although these changes in the carbohydrate composition of glycopeptides are of considerable interest, their functional significance is obscured by the fact that the glycopeptides were derived from a complex mixture of glycoproteins obtained from whole brain.

Another approach to elucidating the involvement of neural glycoproteins in development has been to investigate the glycoproteins of different lines of neuroblastoma in culture. There are several reports (27–29) of differences between the surface glycoproteins of differentiated and undifferentiated neuroblastoma cells. However, relating the results to the development of the intact brain is complicated by the fact that glycoproteins are known to be affected by growth conditions in culture and by oncogenic transformation (3,4).

It would seem that relating the chemical composition of glycoproteins to specific developmental phenomena will require the isolation of individual glycoproteins from well-defined subcellular structures or from particular regions of brain. The chemical composition of these glycoproteins could then be correlated with developmental changes. Also specific antisera to such glycoproteins might be used to obtain information about their function. Precise identification and chemical characterization of the aggregation-promoting factors mentioned previously (13), which are specific for different regions of the brain, will be of considerable interest. Continuation of the work on the purification and characterization of the glycoproteins in synaptosomal plasma membranes (30–32) may provide clues about the mechanism of recognition during synaptogenesis. GP-350, a small molecular weight, soluble, sialoglycoprotein which has been isolated and partially characterized (33), appears to be associated in part with synaptosomal membranes (34). A glycoprotein which our laboratory has shown to be associated with the myelin–oligodendroglial complex is likely to be of importance in neuronal-glial interactions, and it is considered in some detail in the next section.

MYELIN-ASSOCIATED GLYCOPROTEINS

Myelin is formed as an extension of the surface membrane of the oligodendrocyte in the central nervous system (CNS) and of the Schwann cell in the peripheral nervous system (PNS). Although surface membranes are known to be rich in glycoproteins, myelin has generally been assumed to contain little or no glycoprotein. Early indications of the presence of protein bound carbohydrate in myelin (35–37) received little attention. Several years ago in an examination of ^{3}H-fucose-labeled glycoproteins in various subcellular fractions prepared from rat brain, we noted that the myelin fraction contained radioactive glycoproteins with a unique pattern on polyacrylamide gel electrophoresis (38). The pattern of labeled glycoproteins was very different from that in all other subfractions and was dominated by a major peak with an apparent molecular weight of about 100,000 daltons. Subsequently, we were also

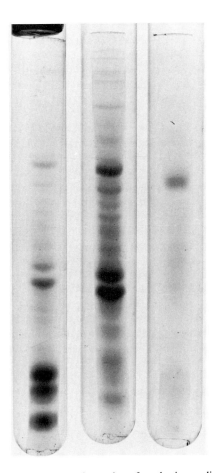

FIG. 2. Separation of proteins of rat brain myelin by polyacrylamide gel electrophoresis. Myelin proteins were solubilized with sodium dodecyl sulfate and electrophoresed on 5% polyacrylamide gels (38). The gel on the left shows total myelin proteins stained with Fast Green. The three bands at the bottom of the gel are the major proteins of CNS myelin; from the bottom to the top they are the small basic protein, the large basic protein, and proteolipid protein, respectively. Also, there are a number of high molecular weight proteins in the upper two-thirds of the gel. These high molecular weight proteins are enriched in the insoluble residue obtained when myelin is extracted with chloroform–methanol (2:1, v/v). The middle gel shows the proteins in this residual fraction after electrophoresis and staining with Fast Green. The gel on the right shows the same fraction stained with periodic acid-Schiff reagent for carbohydrate. The glycoprotein is clearly seen migrating about one-third of the way down the gel.

able to demonstrate this high molecular weight glycoprotein in the myelin fraction by periodic acid-Schiff staining (Fig. 2). The glycoprotein is present in myelin isolated from all species which we have examined, including man. Quantitatively the glycoprotein accounts for only a small percentage of the total protein in the myelin fraction, but numerous experiments have shown that it is genuinely associated with myelin or myelin-related membranes in the brain. Some of the most convincing evidence for the association of the glycoprotein with myelin came from experiments with myelin-deficient mutant mice (39). Jimpy mice have a severe myelin deficit and die between 20 and 30 days of age. Double labeling experiments were done in which 17-day-old Jimpy mice were injected with ^{14}C-fucose, and control mice of the same age were injected with ^{3}H-fucose. The brains from the mutant and normal mice were combined, homogenized together, and myelin was purified from the mixed homogenate. The isolated myelin fraction had the ^{3}H-labeled glycoprotein from the normal mice but little or no ^{14}C-labeled glycoprotein from the mutant mice. In these experiments, there was a substantial amount of normal myelin present during the isolation procedure to potentially trap nonmyelin contaminants from the Jimpy brains. Since the primary difference in the Jimpy brain is an almost complete absence of myelin, these results are strong evidence for the association of the glycoprotein with myelin in normal brain. These and other experiments (38) have convinced us that the glycoprotein is in myelin or myelin related membranes *in situ* and is not in an unrelated contaminant in the isolated myelin fraction.

The low concentration of the glycoprotein in isolated myelin may reflect a selective concentration of the glycoprotein in loose, uncompacted myelin membranes, and possibly in oligodendroglial surface membranes and their region of transition to myelin. Compact myelin, which comprises much of the isolated myelin fraction, may contain little or none of the glycoprotein. Evidence for such a selective localization of the glycoprotein was obtained in experiments in which we separated myelin into light, medium, and heavy subfractions on discontinuous sucrose gradients (40). The light fraction contained primarily large fragments of compact myelin and had the highest concentrations of lipid and myelin basic protein. However, this light fraction had the lowest concentration of the glycoprotein. The glycoprotein was most concentrated in the heavy myelin subfraction which contained a much higher proportion of single membranes without the classical periodicity of myelin. The myelin marker enzyme, 2'3'-cyclic nucleotide 3'-phosphohydrolase, was also most concentrated in the heavy subfraction, and we think that this enzyme and the glycoprotein may have similar localizations in myelin and myelin-related membranes. In addition to the surface membrane of the oligodendrocyte itself, we think it is likely that the glycoprotein is also in the paranodal membranes which are extensions of the oligodendroglial plasma membrane. These paranodal membranes are known to contain particles of about 10 nm diameter which are believed to be involved in the glial-axonal junction (41) and are similar to particles with which glycoproteins are associated in other membranes (7).

This glycoprotein in myelin or oligodendroglial membranes could be of importance in recognition or contact phenomena occurring during the process of myelination. It could be involved in recognition and encirclement of the axon by the oligodendroglial process or in contact relationships between adjacent myelin lamellae as the membranes are layered and compacted. The glycoprotein might be chemically changed or even removed before mature, compact myelin is formed. We have experimental evidence for a chemical alteration of this glycoprotein during the process of myelinogenesis. The glycoprotein in myelin isolated from 14-day-old rats, which are just beginning to myelinate, has a slightly higher apparent molecular weight on sodium dodecyl sulfate-gels than that from mature rats (42) (Fig. 3). This developmental change in the electrophoretic mobility of the glycoprotein might reflect an alteration of its carbohydrate residues which is important for the formation or maturation of myelin. That this change in the glycoprotein is important for myelinogenesis is suggested by studies with Quaking mice. These mutants form only a limited amount of myelin and that which they form is structurally immature. The glycoprotein in the Quaking mice has a higher apparent molecular weight than that in age-matched controls (43). We are currently devising procedures for

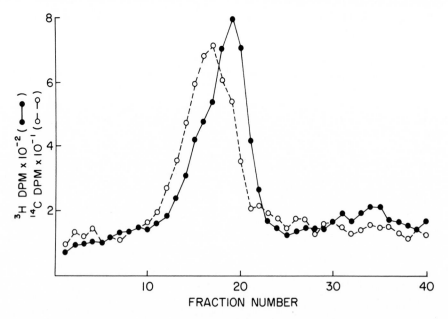

FIG. 3. Developmental change in the myelin-associated glycoprotein of rat brain. Fourteen-day-old rats were injected with ^{14}C-fucose and 22-day-old rats were injected with ^{3}H-fucose. The brains from rats at the two ages were combined, homogenized together, and myelin was prepared from the mixed homogenate. The fraction enriched in glycoproteins was electrophoresed on polyacrylamide gels similar to those shown in Fig. 2. The gel was cut into 1 mm slices and radioactivity determined by double label counting techniques. The figure shows only a 4 cm segment of the gel containing the major glycoprotein. *Open circles,* 14-day myelin labeled with ^{14}C; *closed circles,* 22-day myelin labeled with ^{3}H. (Reproduced from ref. 42 with the permission of Elsevier.)

isolating sufficient amounts of the glycoprotein for chemical characterization and investigation of its antigenic properties. It should soon be possible to relate chemical changes in the glycoprotein to the process of myelin formation. Specific antibodies to' the glycoprotein will be useful for obtaining information about its precise localization and function.

The glycoprotein which is associated with CNS myelin is not present in myelin isolated from the peripheral nervous system. On the other hand, peripheral myelin contains a unique structural protein (not present in CNS myelin) accounting for more than 50% of the protein content. Everly (44), in our laboratory, and Wood and Dawson (45) independently demonstrated that this major structural protein is a glycoprotein. Thus, the glycoproteins of central and peripheral myelin are quite different; CNS myelin has a high molecular weight glycoprotein which is quantitatively a minor component, whereas PNS myelin has a major structural protein which is glycosylated. Nevertheless, the carbohydrate moieties of these different glycoproteins could conceivably perform similar functions in myelin formation and maintenance. In any case, the fact that the glycoproteins associated with myelin are not as heterogeneous as those in other membranes of neural tissue should facilitate their characterization and the elucidation of their function. Also, the interactions between glial and axonal membranes and between adjacent myelin lamellae during myelin formation are probably relatively simple in comparison to the complex interactions which must occur in forming the intricate interneuronal pathways of the developing nervous system. Therefore, we think that the glycoproteins associated with myelin offer a valuable opportunity for investigating the roles of glycoproteins in recognition and contact phenomena within the nervous system.

GLYCOPROTEINS AND PATHOLOGICAL PROCESSES IN THE NERVOUS SYSTEM

In this final section, I discuss the possible importance of glycoproteins for disease processes in the nervous system. It has been shown that glycoprotein material accumulates in some inherited enzyme deficiency diseases. In some cases such as in mannosidosis or fucosidosis,

the missing enzymes catalyze the hydrolytic cleavage of sugars characteristic of glycoproteins. However, in other cases (e.g., Tay-Sachs disease), the pathology has been classified primarily as a lipid-storage process. The nature of the glycoprotein material accumulating in these conditions has been summarized (6).

It is reasonable to expect that glycoproteins will prove important for understanding viral diseases of the nervous tissue. There are a large number of disorders of the nervous system with demonstrated or suspected viral origin. It has long been known that the cell surface receptors for certain viruses are glycoproteins, and in some cases interaction of a virus with its receptor results in chemical alteration of the glycoprotein receptor (2–4). More recent studies have shown that viral transformation of cells results in changes of cell surface glycoproteins (3,4). In the nervous system, altered glycoproteins have been reported in subacute sclerosing leukoencephalitis which is of suspected viral origin (46). A virally altered glycoprotein might initiate pathological events in any number of ways. For example, it could prevent appropriate cell–cell interactions leading eventually to cell death. Alternatively, an altered surface glycoprotein might be seen as a foreign antigen by the host and result in an autoimmune attack against the cell or structure of which it is part. In this connection, we are quite interested in the myelin-associated glycoprotein of the CNS and its possible involvement in the viral or autoimmune aspects of multiple sclerosis and other demyelinating diseases. The involvement of glycoproteins in demyelinating processes is suggested by a large decrease of the myelin-associated glycoprotein of the CNS in a fraction of degenerating myelin isolated from hexachlorophene intoxicated rats (47). Also, the major glycoprotein of peripheral myelin disappears more rapidly than other proteins during Wallerian degeneration of rat sciatic nerve (48).

Finally, glycoproteins may be involved in a type of pathology suggested by the emphasis in this chapter on their probable roles in cell–cell interactions. There are congenital diseases of the brain in which there is abnormal histogenesis. In some cases, these diseases appear to involve abnormal migration of neurons or the failure of neurons to organize properly (41). Some of the latter conditions might be similar in a general way to the "reeler" murine mutants mentioned earlier (14), in which there is an impairment of intercellular recognition. Incorrect oligosaccharide structures on cell surfaces could prevent appropriate recognition and lead to this type of pathology. In any case, it seems clear that as our knowledge about glycoproteins of the nervous system accumulates, increased consideration of their potential roles in pathological processes is merited.

REFERENCES

1. Spiro, R. (1969): Glycoproteins: Their biochemistry, biology, and role in human disease. *N. Engl. J. Med.*, 281:991–1001, 1043–1056.
2. Winzler, R. J. (1970): Carbohydrates in cell surfaces. *Int. Rev. Cytol.*, 29:77–125.
3. Hughes, R. C. (1973): Glycoproteins as components of cellular membranes: *Progr. Biophys. Mol. Biol.*, 26:189–268.
4. Cook, G. M. W., and Stoddart, R. (1973): *Surface Carbohydrates of the Eukaryotic Cell.* Academic Press, London.
5. Brunngraber, E. G. (1969): Glycoproteins. In: *Handbook of Neurochemistry*, edited by A. Lajtha, Vol. 1, pp. 223–244. Plenum Press, New York.
6. Brunngraber, E. G. (1972): Biochemistry, function and neuropathology of glycoproteins in brain tissue; In: *Functional and Structural Proteins of the Nervous System*, edited by A. N. Davison, P. Mandel, and I. G. Morgan, pp. 109–133. Plenum Press, New York.
7. Marchesi, V. T., Jackson, R. L., Segrest, J. P., and Kahane, I. (1973): Molecular features of the major glycoprotein of the human erythrocyte membrane. *Fed. Proc.*, 32:1834–1837.
8. Morawiecki, A. (1964): Dissociation of M- and N-group mucoproteins into subunits in detergent. *Biochim. Biophys. Acta*, 83:339–347.
9. Margoliash, E., Schenck, J. R., Hargie, M. P., Burokas, S., Richter, W. R., Barlow, G. H., and Moscona, A. A. (1965): Characterization of specific cell aggregating materials from sponge cells. *Biochem. Biophys. Res. Commun.*, 20: 383–388.
10. Henkart, P., Humphreys, S., and Humphreys, T. (1973): Characterization of a sponge aggregation factor. A unique proteoglycan complex. *Biochemistry*, 12:3045–3050.
11. Ashwell, G., and Morell, A. G. (1974): The role of surface carbohydrates in recognition and transport of circulating glycoproteins. *Advan. Enzymol.*, 41:99–128.
12. Roth, S., McGuire, E. J., and Roseman, S. (1971): An assay for intercellular adhesiveness. *J. Cell Biol.*, 51:525–531.
13. Balsamo, J., and Lilien, J. (1975): The binding of tissue specific adhesive molecules to the cell surface. A molecular basis for specificity. *Biochemistry*, 14:167–171.
14. Delong, G. R., and Sidman, R. L. (1970): Alignment defect of reaggregating cells in cultures of developing brains of Reeler mutant mice. *Develop. Biol.*, 22:584–600.
15. Bogoch, S. (1968): *The Biochemistry of Memory.* Oxford University Press, New York.
16. Brunngraber, E. G. (1969): The possible roles of glycoproteins in neural tissue. *Persp. Biol. Med.*, 12:467–470.
17. Barondes, S. H. (1970): Brain glycomacromolecules and interneuronal recognition. In: *The Neurosciences, Second Study Program*, edited by F. O. Schmitt, pp. 747–760. Rockefeller Univ. Press, New York.
18. Margolis, R. U., and Margolis, R. K. (1974): Distribution and metabolism of glycoproteins in neuronal perikarya, astrocytes, and oligodendroglia. *Biochemistry*, 13:2849–2852.
19. Rambourg, A., and Leblond, X. X. (1967): Electron microscope observations on the carbohydrate-rich cell coat present at the surface of cells in the rat. *J. Cell Biol.*, 32:27–53.
20. Ochs, S. (1974): Systems of material transport in nerve fibers (axoplasmic transport) related to nerve function and trophic control. In: *Trophic Functions of the Neuron*, edited by D. B. Drachman, *Ann. N.Y. Acad. Sci.*, 228:202–223.
21. Dutton, G. R., Haywood, R., and Barondes, S. (1973): [^{14}C]Glucosamine incorporation into specific products in the nerve ending fraction *in vivo* and *in vitro*. *Brain Res.*, 57:397–408.
22. Dutton, G. R., and Barondes, S. H. (1970): Glycoprotein metabolism in developing mouse brain. *J. Neurochem.*, 17:913–920.
23. Quarles, R. H., and Brady, R. O. (1971): Synthesis of glycoproteins and gangliosides in developing rat brain. *J. Neurochem.*, 18:1809–1820.
24. Holian, O., Dill, D., and Brunngraber, E. G. (1971): Incorporation of radioactivity of D-glucosamine-1-^{14}C into heteropolysaccharide chains of glycoproteins in adult and developing rat brain. *Arch. Biochem. Biophys.*, 142:111–121.
25. Krusius, T., Finne, J., Karkkainen, J., and Jarnefelt, J. (1974): Neutral and acidic glycopeptides in adult and developing rat brain. *Biochim. Biophys. Acta*, 365:80–92.
26. Margolis, R. K., and Gomez, Z. (1974): Structural changes in brain glycoproteins during development. *Brain Res.*, 74:370–372.
27. Brown, J. C. (1971): Surface glycoprotein characteristic of the differentiated state of neuroblastoma C-1300 cells. *Exp. Cell Res.*, 69:440–442.
28. Glick, M. C., Kimih, Y., and Littauer, U. Z. (1973): Glycopeptides from surface membranes of neuroblastoma cells. *Proc. Natl. Acad. Sci. USA*, 70:1682–1687.
29. Truding, R., Shelanski, H. L., Daniels, M. P., and Morell, P. (1974): Comparison of surface membranes isolated from cultured murine neuroblastoma cells in the differentiated or undif-

ferentiated state. *J. Biol. Chem.,* 249:3973–3982.

30. Breckenridge, W. L., Breckenridge, J. E., and Morgan, I. G. (1972): Glycoproteins of the synaptic region: In *Functional and Structural Proteins of the Nervous System,* edited by A. N. Davison, P. Mandel, and I. G. Morgan, pp. 109–133. Plenum Press, New York.

31. Gurd, J. W., and Mahler, H. R. (1974): Fractionation of synaptic plasma membrane glycoproteins by lectin affinity chromatography. *Biochemistry,* 13:5193–5198.

32. Zanetta, J. P., Morgan, I. G., and Gombos, G. (1975): Synaptosomal plasma membrane glycoproteins: Fractionation by affinity chromatography on Concanavalin A. *Brain Res.,* 83:337–348.

33. Van Nieuw Amerongen, A., Van der Eijnden, D. H., Heijlman, J., and Roukema, P. A. (1972): Isolation and characterization of a soluble, glucose containing sialoglycoprotein from cortical grey matter of calf brain. *J. Neurochem.,* 19:2195–2205.

34. Van Nieuw Amerongen, A., and Roukema, P. A. (1974): GP-350, a sialoglycoprotein from calf brain: Its subcellular localization and occurrence in various brain areas. *J. Neurochem.,* 23:85–89.

35. Wolman, M. (1957): Histochemical study of changes occurring during the degeneration of myelin. *J. Neurochem.,* 1:370–376.

36. Margolis, R. U. (1967): Acid mucopolysaccharides and proteins of bovine whole brain, white matter, and myelin. *Biochim. Biophys. Acta,* 141:91–102.

37. Gagnon, J., Finch, P. R., Wood, D. D., and Moscarello, M. A. (1971): Isolation of a highly purified myelin protein. *Biochemistry,* 10:4756–4763.

38. Quarles, R. H., Everly, J. L., and Brady, R. O. (1973): Evidence for the close association of a glycoprotein with myelin in rat brain. *J. Neurochem.,* 21:1177–1191.

39. Matthieu, J.-M., Quarles, R. H., Webster, H. deF., Hogan, E. L., and Brady, R. O. (1974): Characterization of the fraction obtained from the CNS of Jimpy mice by a procedure for myelin isolation. *J. Neurochem.,* 23:517–523.

40. Matthieu, J.-M., Quarles, R. H., Brady, R. O., and Webster, H. deF. (1973): Variation of proteins, enzyme markers and gangliosides in myelin subfractions. *Biochim. Biophys. Acta,* 329:305–317.

41. Livingston, R. B., Pfenninger, K., Moor, H., and Akert, K. (1973): Specialized paranodal and interparanodal glial-axonal junctions in the peripheral and central nervous system: A freeze etching study. *Brain Res.,* 58:1–24.

42. Quarles, R. H., Everly, J. L., and Brady, R. O. (1973): Myelin-associated glycoprotein: a developmental change. *Brain Res.,* 58:506–509.

43. Matthieu, J.-M., Brady, R. O., and Quarles, R. H. (1974): Anomalies of myelin-associated glycoproteins in Quaking mice. *J. Neurochem.,* 22:291–296.

44. Everly, J. L., Brady, R. O., and Quarles, R. H. (1973): Evidence that the major protein in rat sciatic nerve myelin is a glycoprotein. *J. Neurochem.,* 21:329–334.

45. Wood, J. G., and Dawson, R. M. C. (1973): A major myelin glycoprotein of sciatic nerve. *J. Neurochem.,* 21:717–719.

46. Brunngraber, E. G., Brown, B. D., and Chang, I. (1971): Glycoproteins in subacute sclerosing leukoencephalitis: Isolation and carbohydrate composition of glycopeptides from human brain. *J. Neuropathol. Exp. Neurol.,* 30:525–535.

47. Matthieu, J.-M., Zimmerman, A. W., Webster, H. deF., Ulsamer, A. G., Brady, R. O., and Quarles, R. H. (1974): Hexachlorophene intoxication: characterization of myelin and myelin-related fractions in rat during early postnatal development. *Exp. Neurol.,* 45:558–574.

48. Wood, J. G., and Dawson, R. M. C. (1974): Lipid and protein changes in sciatic nerve during Wallerian degeneration. *J. Neurochem.,* 22:631–635.

49. Adams, R. D., and Sidman, R. L. (1968): *Introduction to Neuropathology,* pp. 329–341. McGraw-Hill Book Company, New York.

The Nervous System, Donald B. Tower, Editor-in-Chief. *Vol. 1: The Basic Neurosciences.* Raven Press, New York, 1975.

Membrane Proteins in the Nervous System

Blake W. Moore

It has become apparent that proteins are important in the structural and dynamic functions of cell membranes. Some membrane proteins may have a structural function, that is they may confer a stabilized architecture to a portion of the membrane, for example in controlling or preventing translational motion of particular proteins or other molecules in an area of the membrane in order to maintain its organization for a specific function. Other membrane proteins may have dynamic functions. Some are known to act as receptors on the external surface of the cell, for example, as receptors for insulin and other hormones, receptors for trophic molecules such as nerve growth factor, or receptors which trigger the production of secondary messengers such as cyclic AMP within the cell. Membrane proteins are known to function in regulation of the internal environment of the cell by acting as regulators of permeability or active transport across the cell membrane, such as the Na^+,K^+-ATPase or the proteins involved in galactose transport in bacteria. Membrane proteins have also been implicated in cell–cell recognition processes. It is known, for example, that the carbohydrate groups of membrane glycoproteins are exposed on the external surface of cell membranes and are active as receptors for agglutinins, certain viruses, and blood group antibodies and may be involved in processes of development and differentiation of tissues such as the nervous system. The structure and function of the nervous system must be particularly dependent on membrane properties and, in turn, on membrane proteins. There are, of course, many specific types of membranes with highly specific functions, such as myelin, plasma membranes of glial and neuronal cell bodies, membranes of processes such as axons and dendrites which have specific electrical properties, and synaptic membranes with specific receptors and associated mechanisms, all of which must depend, in their functions, on the presence of specific membrane proteins. Therefore, in working out the function of the nervous system, it would be important to investigate the structural and dynamic properties of the proteins of nervous system membranes.

The architecture of cell membranes, particularly in regard to their proteins, has recently been a very active field of research. The success of recently developed methods for investigating the topography of proteins in red cell membranes, suggests that such methods could be applied to membranes of the nervous system, particularly myelin, synaptic membranes, and membranes of cultured gliomas and neuroblastomas.

Methods for preparation of specific membranes from the nervous system in high purity recently have been improved, particularly the preparation of myelin and synaptic membranes by differential centrifugation methods. A number of cell cultures of cloned glioma and neuroblastoma cells are now available and plasma membranes can be prepared from these in relatively large quantities. Methods for bulk separation of neurons, glia, and axons from the central nervous system, although not entirely satisfactory, have been improved and can be used in the preparation of more or less specific plasma membranes. Methods for solubilization, fractionation, purification and assay of membrane proteins have also been greatly improved.

Therefore, with all of these methods presently available for studying membrane proteins in general, and for purification and isolation of nervous system membranes in particular, it is probable that much will be learned about the structural and dynamic properties of nervous system membranes in the near future.

RED CELL MEMBRANE PROTEINS

Since there are several excellent recent reviews on the properties and arrangement of red cell membrane proteins (1,2), this review attempts only to summarize the major findings in order to provide a background for the discussion of synaptic membrane and myelin proteins which follows. It is generally agreed that, when red cell membranes are solubilized in SDS buffers, and subjected to electrophoresis in SDS-polyacrylamide gels, there are about seven or eight major and several minor protein bands which stain with Coomassie blue (3,4), and there are three or four major glycoprotein bands (3) visualized by PAS staining. The sizes of these major proteins (estimated on SDS gels) range from 15,000 to 250,000 daltons. The largest amount of protein by weight is contained in a protein of about 90,000 daltons which represents about 25 to 30% of the total red cell membrane protein. This protein corresponds to polypeptide III of Steck (3). It reacts, in unlysed red cells, with reagents that do not permeate the membrane (5–12), such as lactoperoxidase-iodide, proteolytic enzymes, and an impermeable imidoester.

The other red cell membrane protein which seems to be exposed at the external surface of the membrane is the major glycoprotein [glycophorin (13) or PAS-1 (3)]. It can be extracted from red cell membranes with lithium diiodosalicylate and contains at least several receptor activities including blood group antigens, those for certain agglutinins, and for influenza viruses. It contains about 55% carbohydrate and 41% protein which is probably a single polypeptide chain (14). The best estimate for the size of this glycoprotein is 29,000 daltons (15). Sequential proteolytic digestion of the membrane in intact red cells indicates that the carbohydrate containing N-terminal end is exposed at the exterior of the cell, the carboxy terminus is exposed to the cytoplasm, and a hydrophobic central region is held within the membrane (16).

The third major protein of red cell membranes is the complex known as "spectrin," which represents about 30% of the membrane protein [polypeptides I and II and probably V of Steck (3)]. It consists of two large polypeptide chains, about 250,000 daltons each, and a smaller component of about 43,000 daltons. The large peptides (I and II) have many of the properties of myosin and peptide V resembles actin (2). It is certain that the two large peptides are not aggregates of a lower molecular weight peptide (17). It has been suggested that spectrin controls lateral mobility of components in the red cell

membrane (2). There are a number of enzymes which seem to be bound loosely to the cytoplasmic side of the membrane such as 3-phosphoglyceraldehyde dehydrogenase.

It is evident that the red cell membrane is a highly asymmetric structure with different proteins, or different parts of the same protein, exposed on the outer and cytoplasmic surfaces. It is reasonable to assume that nervous system membranes possess the same type of asymmetry.

PREPARATION OF NERVOUS SYSTEM MEMBRANES

Myelin

Myelin is produced by oligodendrocytes or Schwann cells, but only in the presence of differentiated neurons, and may be considered to be a specialized type of plasma membrane. Its functions seem to be primarily to maintain the internal environment of the axon and to facilitate axonal conduction. It contains more lipid (about 80% of weight) and less protein (about 18%) than most known plasma membranes.

Myelin is relatively easy to prepare from brain. The most commonly used criterion for purity is electron microscopic appearance with its five-layered structure and periodicity of about 120 Å. The only enzyme marker known to be specific for myelin is 2′,3′-cyclic nucleotide-3′-phosphohydrolase. Another criterion of purity which has been used recently is the pattern obtained on SDS polyacrylamide gel electrophoresis of solubilized myelin proteins. Myelin is generally prepared by differential centrifugation methods (18,19).

Synaptosomes

Generally, synaptic membranes are isolated by first preparing "synaptosomes" or "nerve-ending particles," lysing these by osmotic shock, and then purifying synaptic membranes by centrifugation through a sucrose density gradient. Synaptosomes are usually prepared by a modification of the original methods of Whittaker (20) and DeRobertis (21). Both of these methods involve gentle homogenization of brain in 0.32 M sucrose, a process which results in the pinching off and resealing of nerve endings. The homogenate is spun at $1,000 \times g$ for 10 min which sediments intact cells, nuclei, and debris. The supernatant is then spun at higher speed ($10,000 \times g$ for 30 min) which sediments the so-called "crude mitochondrial" fraction. This fraction is resuspended in 0.32 M sucrose and layered on a discontinuous sucrose gradient consisting of a bottom layer of 1.2 M and a top layer of 0.8 M sucrose. After the gradient is centrifuged, the synaptosomes collect mainly at the 0.8 to 1.2 M interface, the mitochondria pellet at the bottom, and myelin concentrates mainly at the 0.32 to 0.8 M interface. Using this method there is considerable contamination of the synaptosome fraction by mitochondria, myelin fragments and smooth endoplasmic reticulum.

Recently the major improvement in preparation of synaptosomes has been the use of Ficoll rather than sucrose density gradients (22–24). It was shown by Cotman et al. (24) that preparation of synaptosomes by sucrose density gradient centrifugation leads to contamination with glial membrane fragments and that the use of Ficoll gradients overcomes this difficulty. Ficoll, being a high molecular weight polymer, allows for sufficient densities for isopycnic density gradient centrifugation without the disadvantage of high osmolarity of sucrose solutions of sufficient density. One of the contaminants still likely to be present in synaptosomes prepared by Ficoll gradient centrifugation is comprised of membranes derived from the endoplasmic reticulum and recently several improvements have been made in order to get rid of this source of contamination. The method developed by Gurd et al. (26) is essentially the same as the method of Cotman and Matthews (24) except that they add three washes of the crude mitochondrial pellet with 0.32 M sucrose, a modification which reduces the contamination with smooth endoplasmic reticulum. Furthermore they suspend the washed crude mitochondrial pellet in 14% Ficoll, overlay with 7.5% Ficoll and centrifuge; the synaptosomes float up to the interface between the two Ficoll layers and the mitochondria collect as a pellet at the bottom. This modification, they claim, reduces mitochondrial contamination.

Synaptosomes have also been prepared from squid (loligo) (27) and octopus brain (28,29). The main advantage of these preparations, although they do not seem to be as highly purified as the best preparations from mammalian brain, is that they probably consist predominantly of cholinergic nerve endings. Since one of the major disadvantages of the nerve-ending and synaptic membrane preparations made from mammalian brain is that they represent a variety of types of synapses, improvements in preparation of synaptic fractions from cephalopod nervous system would be an important advance.

Synaptic Membranes

In order to prepare subfractions of synaptosomes, they are generally lysed by swelling in hypotonic buffer, releasing the contents (mainly cytoplasm, mitochondria, and synaptic vesicles) and the synaptic membranes are left as "ghosts." This mixture of nerve-ending components has been fractionated by a number of methods, all based on centrifugation in sucrose density gradients. In the original method of Whittaker (30), the gradient is discontinuous. The synaptic membrane fraction prepared by this method is contaminated with other types of membranes, including endoplasmic reticulum and synaptic vesicles.

Two recent improvements, based on the method of Whittaker, that result in much purer preparations of synaptic membranes are the methods of Morgan et al. (22) and of Cotman and Matthews (24). In both adaptations, the synaptosomes are lysed in alkaline hypotonic media, a modification which, according to Cotman and Matthews (24), gives more efficient release of synaptic "ghosts" and results in better separation of synaptic membranes from mitochondria in the sucrose density gradient centrifugation which follows.

The purity of synaptic membranes is difficult to assess since there are no known specific enzyme markers. The enzyme (Na^+,K^+-dependent, ouabain-sensitive) ATPase is present in high activity in synaptic membranes but since it is present in other plasma membranes as well, it is not highly specific. Probably the most reliable criterion is electron microscopic examination with the presence of synaptic complexes as a specific marker for synaptic membranes. In order to fairly estimate contamination by other particles by electron microscopy, sections must be made of the entire depth of the pellet since different particles sediment at different rates.

Cotman (31) has described a method for fixing and preparation of sections for electron microscopic examination of synaptosomes and synaptic membranes. Both Morgan et al. (22) and Gurd et al. (26) have shown that the purity of synaptic membrane fractions depends greatly on the extent of prior purification of the synaptosomes, particularly in the degree of removal of microsomes and mitochondria before the synaptosomes are lysed. This is true, in great part, because the densities of a number of cytoplasmic and other membranes are similar to that of synaptic membranes (26) and they would be difficult to remove after the lysis step.

Recently a method has been described (32) for preparation of synaptic membranes from rat brain by a one-step sucrose density gradient centrifugation procedure. The authors indicate that myelin and mitochondrial contamination are less than 10% and that the synaptic membranes are at least 80% pure. The main advantages of this simpler method are: (1) consistently higher yields of synaptic membrane (about 0.1% of the brain protein); (2) about three times the weight of brain tissue in a single preparation can be handled by this method compared to others.

Synaptic Complexes

Synaptic membranes consist largely of neuronal plasma membranes and what is called the synaptic complex which consists of pieces of pre- and postsynaptic membranes joined by the material in the synaptic cleft; this material stains densely by the usual electron microscopic preparation methods. The material in the synaptic cleft also stains specifically with ethanolic phosphotungstic acid (33). It would obviously be important to be able to strip off most of the neuronal plasma membrane from the synaptic complex and prepare enriched fractions of synapses in order to study composition, properties, and metabolism of proteins specifically bound to the synaptic complex. Kornguth et al. (34,35) have prepared fractions enriched in synaptic complexes by zonal centrifugation of synaptic membrane fractions on cesium chloride gradients.

Cotman et al. (36,37) have prepared an enriched synaptic complex fraction by first purifying synaptic membranes by sucrose density gradient centrifugation. The synaptic membranes are freed from greater than 95% of the mitochondrial contamination by incubating with the tetrazoliun histochemical medium for succinic dehydrogenase which "weights" the mitochondria (38), before the sucrose density gradient centrifugation. Treatment of the membrane with Triton X-100 strips off most of the neuronal plasma membrane, leaving the more resistant synaptic complex intact. The purified synaptic complex fraction can be seen by electron microscopy or by light microscopy after staining with ethanolic phosphotungstic acid (33).

Recently Banker et al. (39) have reported that synaptic complexes, or postsynaptic densities could be prepared by stripping most of the neuronal plasma membrane from synaptic membranes with sodium N-lauroyl sarcosinate. The postsynaptic densities were said to be 85% pure and to consist of 90% protein. Two polypeptides of molecular weights 53,000 and 97,000 daltons predominated.

Bulk Isolation of Neurons, Glia, and Axons from Brain

A number of methods have been developed for the bulk separations of neurons and glia from the central nervous system (40–45). All of these methods end up with fractions which represent cell bodies of neurons, astroglia, or oligodendrocytes with processes sheared off.

The method used by Blomstrand and Hamberger (42) is a modification of the method of Rose (40). A suspension of rabbit cortex is forced through nylon meshes of successively smaller sizes and centrifuged in a discontinuous sucrose-Ficoll gradient.

Poduslo and Norton (45) have improved the method for isolation of oligodendrocytes from calf brain. White matter is minced in a hexose-albumin–phosphate medium (HAP) and subjected to digestion with trypsin. After trypsinization, the cells are spun down, washed, suspended in a 0.9 M sucrose made up in HAP, then pressed through nylon mesh and filtered through a 200 mesh stainless steel screen. Purification of the oligodendroglia was done by centrifugation in a sucrose density gradient. The authors claim that the yield of oligodendroglia was about 11% of the total number of cells in the tissue and that the cell fraction was greater than 90% pure on the basis of electron microscopy. The myelin-specific enzyme 2',3'-cyclic nucleotide-3'-phosphohydrolase was present at a high level of activity, nearly equal to that in purified myelin.

Purified axon preparations have also been prepared from bovine brain (46). A homogenized suspension of white matter in 0.85 M sucrose is centrifuged and the myelinated axons float to the top. When these are allowed to swell in hypotonic buffer, the myelin strips off, leaving axons without myelin or axolemma.

Membranes from Glioma and Neuroblastoma Cell Cultures

A number of clonal lines of gliomas and neuroblastomas from several species are now available (47–49). These are differentiated in the sense that they send out processes (50) under certain conditions, that the neuroblastomas have action potentials (51–53), have some enzymes of neurotransmitter synthesis (50,54,55) and produce certain brain-specific proteins (47–49,56–58). Cell membranes from the C1300 murine neuroblastoma have been purified (59).

PROTEIN COMPOSITION OF NERVOUS SYSTEM MEMBRANES

Methods for Fractionating Proteins of Membranes

The loosely bound, or so-called "peripheral" proteins of membranes can be removed and solubilized preferentially by mild methods such as EDTA treatment (which removes "spectrin" from red cell ghosts), or treatment with chaotropic agents such as lithium diiodosalicylate (LTS). Nonionic detergents such as Triton X-100 also selectively remove certain proteins; for example, the neuronal plasma membrane is stripped preferentially off synaptic membranes by Triton X-100, leaving essentially undissociated the "synaptic complex" as described above.

The most generally used and most successful method for analyzing membrane proteins has been the use of SDS-polyacrylamide gel electrophoresis. The membranes (native or delipidated) are solubilized completely in SDS buffers and the solubilized proteins separated by electrophoresis in SDS gels by any of a number

of systems. It has been shown (60) that most proteins bind identical amounts (on a weight basis) of SDS when the SDS monomer concentration is greater than 0.5 mM. The polypeptide chains generally assume the conformation of a rigid rod whose length is proportional to the molecular weight, and any intrinsic charge on the chain is swamped out by the large number of charges due to bound SDS molecules. If 2-mercaptoethanol or other disulfide-reducing agents are added to the SDS solubilizing buffer, polypeptide chains joined by disulfide linkages can be separated from each other. Therefore, the electrophoretic mobilities of polypeptide chains in SDS-polyacrylamide gels fall in order of molecular weight. The method of Weber and Osborn (61), using phosphate buffers in a continuous electrophoretic system, was one of the original methods used for electrophoresis of polypeptide chains in SDS-polyacrylamide gels and estimation of molecular weights. The method of Fairbanks et al. (3) has been used to fractionate red cell membrane proteins and is a continuous electrophoretic system using Tris and sodium acetate buffers. There are several discontinuous SDS-gel electrophoretic systems which give extremely high resolution in separating polypeptide chains on the basis of molecular weights. The system of Laemmli (62) is one of the best and if this system is used with gradient gels in a slab apparatus, remarkable separations of membrane proteins can be achieved as far as resolution and reproducibility are concerned.

Myelin Proteins

There are probably at least 4 polypeptide chains in myelin as it is usually prepared. The most well characterized protein is "basic" or "encephalitogenic" protein which can be extracted from purified myelin with weak acids. Its molecular weight is about 18,000 daltons and the amino acid sequence from bovine (63) and human (64) sources have been determined.

Folch and Lees (65) first described the proteolipid protein as a component of myelin in 1951. It is a highly nonpolar protein which contains lipid and is soluble in 2:1 chloroform–methanol. The molecular weight of the polypeptide chain of proteolipid is about 25,000 daltons (66). The "Wolfgram protein" is the third class of myelin proteins (67). This protein is soluble in acidified

2:1 chloroform–methanol. A fourth protein characteristic of myelin is the DM-20 protein of Agrawal (68). Finally, there is evidence (69–71) that there is a glycoprotein associated with myelin as a minor component.

Chan and Lees (72) have carefully determined molecular weights of polypeptide chains of myelin by SDS-polyacrylamide gel electrophoresis in the presence and absence of urea. Purified proteolipid protein, prepared by the method of Folch et al. (73) contained four bands with molecular weights of about 40,000, 30,000, 25,000, and 20,000 daltons. The 30,000 dalton band corresponds to the proteolipid protein itself and the 25,000 dalton band to DM-20. They suggest that the other bands may represent various states of aggregation of a monomeric PLP polypeptide chain of molecular weight 5,000.

Synaptic Membrane Proteins

Patterns on Polyacrylamide Gels

Cotman and Mahler (74,75) first subjected synaptic membrane proteins to electrophoresis on polyacrylamide gels by the method of Takayama et al. (76) which utilizes a phenol–acetic acid–urea solvent system in the gels and for solubilizing the membranes. There were five major and a number of minor bands which were seen by this method. Morgan and co-workers (77) extracted synaptic membranes, prepared by their method (22), with first Triton X-100 and then with sequentially increasing concentrations of SDS (0.04%, 0.06%, 0.10%, and 0.2%). Each extract was subjected to SDS-polyacrylamide gel electrophoresis and it was found that the Triton X-100 extracts contained polypeptides of different mobility than those contained in the SDS extracts, with few proteins seemingly in common. Almost all of the glycoproteins, visualized on the gels by PAS stain, were extracted by the Triton X-100. They concluded that the protein patterns of synaptic membranes are much more complex than those of myelin and are of the order of complexity of those of liver plasma membranes.

Gurd et al. (78) prepared synaptic membranes from three strains of mice, using a zonal centrifugation method, and subjected the membrane proteins to polyacrylamide gel electro-phoresis in the phenol–acetic acid–urea system of Takayama et al. (76). They found that there were minor, but reproducible differences between the patterns of DBA and C-57 mice, a finding which suggests that there may be genetically determined variations in synaptic membrane proteins.

McBride and VanTassel (32) prepared synaptosomes by modification of the method of Cotman and Matthews (24). These were osmotically shocked and fractionated on a discontinuous sucrose density gradient to give purified fractions of (1) soluble synaptoplasm proteins, (2) synaptic vesicles, (3) synaptic membranes, and (4) mitochondria. Each fraction was treated with Triton X-100 as described by Cotman et al. (36) to extract the more loosely bound proteins, and then the residue was solubilized completely in SDS–urea–2-mercaptoethanol. The soluble cytoplasmic fraction (S_3, containing mainly cytoplasm from neurons and glia) and the synaptoplasmic fraction from the synaptosome lysate, were first precipitated with TCA and the pellet redissolved in the same SDS–urea–2-mercaptoethanol solvent. Each solubilized fraction was then subjected to SDS-polyacrylamide gel electrophoresis and stained with Coomassie Blue. The gel patterns for the S_3 (cytoplasm) and synaptoplasm fraction were nearly identical, with only quantitative differences, except that there was one minor band in the synaptoplasm fraction not detected in S_3. The patterns of synaptic mitochondria and mitochondria from neuronal and glial cell bodies were similar in having about 22 discernible bands. There were about 20 bands from the synaptic membrane fraction and there were 22 in the synaptic vesicle fraction, 8 of which were not seen in the synaptic membrane fraction, and one of which was present in much greater quantity in vesicles.

Banker et al. (79) prepared synaptic membranes by the method of Cotman and Matthews (24) using the "weighting" method of Davis and Bloom (38) to remove mitochondrial contamination. The membranes were solubilized in SDS and dithiothreitol and subjected to SDS-polyacrylamide gel electrophoresis by the method of Fairbanks et al. (3). At the same time nine polypeptides with molecular weights from 3,000 to 94,000 daltons were used as calibration standards so that molecular weights of synaptic membrane proteins could be estimated. They counted at least 30 bands when gels were overloaded to reveal minor components. They also compared patterns of synaptic membrane proteins prepared by two methods, Cotman and Matthews (24) and Morgan et al. (22) and found that the patterns were similar.

There was very little overlap in patterns from synaptic membranes and those from purified mitochondria. Similarly, major myelin bands were not seen in the patterns of synaptic membranes. The two major polypeptide components of synaptic membranes have molecular weights of 99,000 and 52,400 daltons. Table 1 shows estimates of molecular weights of the predominant polypeptide chains of synaptic membranes. Two major PAS-staining proteins had molecular weights of 62,000 and 52,000 daltons, although these size estimations are only tentative since glycopeptide molecular weights cannot be measured accurately by SDS-gel electrophoresis (17).

Wannamaker and Kornguth (80) prepared synaptic membranes by three different methods, the CsCl gradient zonal centrifugation method (35), the methods of Whittaker and DeRobertis using sucrose density gradients to purify synaptosomes (20,21) and the method of Abdel-Latif (23) which uses a Ficoll gradient to purify synaptosomes. The SDS-polyacrylamide gel patterns [by the method of Weber and Osborn (61)] of human synaptic membrane proteins are similar for the 3 methods of preparation. Human and swine synaptic membranes also give similar patterns with four major polypeptide bands, 92,000, 53,000, 43,000, and 36,000 daltons. These cor-respond closely to bands C6, C7, C8, and C9 seen by Banker et al. (79).

Specific Proteins in Synaptic Membranes

It is known that there are muscle-like proteins in brain; for example, an actomyosin-like protein (neurostenin) (81,82), an actin-like protein (41), and a tropomyosin-like protein (83) have all been isolated from brain. Recently Blitz and Fine (84) have prepared synaptic membranes, synaptic vesicles, and soluble synaptoplasm by the modified method of Cotman and Matthews (24,26). Extracts of the fractions were made in SDS-2-mercaptoethanol and the solubilized proteins separated on SDS-polyacrylamide gels by the method of Weber and Osborn (61). Standards of brain myosin, tropomyosin and myelin, actin, and microtubular protein were run at the same time. The synaptic membrane fraction contained major bands that corresponded to microtubular protein, actin, and tropomyosin. Synaptic vesicles contained no actin or tropomyosin, but contained microtubular protein, many bands in common with synaptic membranes, and an unidentified polypeptide as a major component with a molecular weight of 50,000 daltons, which is close to the size of the subunit of neurofilaments (85). It was suggested that these contractile proteins may be associated with synaptic membranes and take part in the process of neurotransmitter release. Since Ca^{2+} is involved in neurotransmitter release at nerve-endings, and is also involved in contractile processes, and affects the polymerization of microtubular protein (86), this suggestion is plausible.

Glycoproteins in Synaptic Membranes

Recently two papers have appeared showing that glycoproteins are present in synaptic membrane. Gurd and Mahler (87) prepared synaptic membranes by their modification of the method of Cotman and Matthews (26). The membrane fraction was extracted with 1% deoxycholate to solubilize glycoproteins preferentially and the extract chromatographed on affinity columns consisting of *Lens culinaris* (lentil) phytohemagglutinin or wheat germ agglutinin attached to Sepharose. Four fractions containing glycoproteins were obtained (as seen by ^{3}H-fucose

TABLE 1. *Polypeptide composition of synaptic membranes (79)*

Polypeptide	MW (daltons)
C1	211,000
C2	194,000
C3	191,000
C4	156,000
C5	124,000
C6	99,000
C7	52,400
C8	41,500
C9	36,000
C10	33,000
C11	25,800

labeling). The four fractions each had a characteristic lectin specificity. Zanetta et al. (88) prepared synaptic membranes by the method of Morgan (22), lipids were removed by solvent extraction, the delipidated membranes dissolved in SDS-2-mercaptoethanol, and alkylated with iodoacetamide. The extract was subjected to affinity chromatography on concanavalin A-Sepharose columns and the fractions were subjected to SDS-polyacrylamide gel electrophoresis, protein being stained with Coomassie Blue and glycoproteins with PAS. The two largest fractions from the concanavalin A column, one unabsorbed and one loosely absorbed, contained a single major glycoprotein band and several minor ones. The third fraction from the column gave a complex glycoprotein (PAS) pattern and was highly enriched in carbohydrate.

Other Nervous System Membranes

Karlsson et al. (89) separated neurons and glia from rabbit brain and prepared purified plasma membranes from each cell type. They also prepared purified brain mitochondria, microsomes, synaptosomes, and synaptic membranes, and compared the protein composition of all these fractions by SDS polyacrylamide gel electrophoresis. The neuronal, glial and synaptic membrane fractions showed similar polypeptide patterns with major peptides of molecular weights 44,000, 52,000, and 95,000 daltons in agreement with Banker et al. (79). They suggest that the 52,000 dalton peptide may be microtubular protein, in agreement with the work of Blitz and Fine (84), and that the 44,000 may be the glial fibrillary protein of Uyeda et al. (90). Grefrath and Reynolds (91) prepared the axonal membrane from garfish olfactory nerve, which is an unmyelinated nerve with a low population of Schwann cells, by Ficoll sucrose density gradient centrifugation. The membrane was solubilized and the polypeptides, which constitute 28% of the total membrane, were separated by SDS-polyacrylamide gel electrophoresis by the method of Weber and Osborn (61). The gel pattern was relatively simple with peptide chains ranging in molecular weight from 32,000 to 150,000 daltons. One of these (100,000 daltons) was shown to be the Na^+,K^+-ATPase of nerve membrane.

Glick et al. (92) removed surface glycopep-tides from clonal C1300 cell cultures by a two-step trypsinization procedure, the first step at a lower concentration of trypsin than the second. The cells had been grown in the presence of ^3H- or ^{14}C-fucose in order to label the carbohydrate proteins of the glycopeptides. After the trypsinization the released glycopeptides were digested with pronase and the digest examined by Sephadex G-50 chromatography in order to determine if there were differences in glycopeptides released in the two steps of trypsinization. Since there were differences, it was concluded that some of the glycopeptides are more readily removed from the surface of the cells than others and therefore some glycopeptides are probably buried more deeply in the membrane or are less accessible than others. There also seemed to be differences in glycopeptide patterns in clones of axon-forming cells and those of axon-minus cells. Truding et al. (59) compared surface membrane proteins isolated from cultured clonal murine (C1300) neuroblastoma in the differentiated and undifferentiated states. The cells were induced to differentiate, or send out processes, by dibutyryl cyclic 3',5'-AMP, as described above and subjected to SDS-polyacrylamide gel electrophoresis. It was found that, when the cells were grown in radioactive glucosamine, there was preferential incorporation into a glycoprotein with an apparent molecular weight of 105,000 in differentiated cells. Glucosamine was also preferentially incorporated into a soluble protein of the same size in differentiated cells. This preferential incorporation always accompanied differentiation, but could be induced by dibutyryl-cyclic-AMP under conditions where process formation is prevented. When proteins exposed on the cell surface were radioiodinated by the lactoperoxidase method, a protein of molecular weight of 78,000 was shown to be preferentially exposed on the surface of differentiated cells. This effect occurred only when process formation occurred.

Membrane Receptors

Neurotransmitter Receptors

Several excellent reviews on receptors for neurotransmitters, especially acetylcholine receptors, have appeared recently (93–95). The subject will only be briefly mentioned here in relation to the dynamic functions of proteins in nervous system membranes. Most of the work on the nicotinic acetylcholine receptor has been done using the electric organ of the electric eel or torpedo, since there is a high concentration of pure acetylcholine nerve endings in that organ. Changeux et al. and others have studied the acetylcholine receptor in the eel on three levels: (1) at the cellular level in the isolated electroplax (96, 97); (2) at the membrane level, using membrane fragments (98–102); (3) at the molecular level using purified receptors or reconstituted membranes (95,103–107).

At the cellular level (electroplax) a number of electrical parameters (membrane potentials, conductance changes) were measured as a function of acetylcholine and of agonist and antagonist concentrations. Dose response curves were obtained and apparent dissociation constants measured.

Membrane fragments were prepared (108) by homogenizing electroplax in 0.2 M sucrose, a process which breaks the cells, giving membrane fragments which arise from either the innervated (caudal) end of the cell, which is rich in acetylcholinesterase, or the noninnervated (rostral) end, which has the Na^+ pump and is rich in Na^+,K^+-ATPase. These fragments from the innervated end form microsacs which retain the permeability characteristics to Na^+ and K^+ of the original electroplax. The efflux of Na^+ from the microsacs was found to be increased by acetylcholine and acetylcholine agonist (such as carbamylcholine) binding, and inhibited by antagonist (*d*-tubocurarine) binding. Therefore there is an acetylcholine receptor in these isolated membranes, which exhibits the same specificity as the receptor in the electroplax, and there is a mechanism for transduction of the energy of binding of acetylcholine, or an agonist, to permeability or conductance changes in the membrane.

A great amount of work has gone into isolation and characterization of the protein acetylcholine receptor molecule from electric organ. The molecular weight of the polypeptide of the receptor protein seems to be about 40,000 to 45,000 daltons (95,105,107,109). The assay of the nicotinic acetylcholine receptor molecule has been greatly improved by the discovery of specific venom toxins, which bind tightly to the receptor, such as alpha-bungarotoxin (110,111) or cobra toxin.

Attempts have been made to isolate and characterize nicotinic acetylcholine receptors from mammalian brain, using specific toxin binding as an assay (112). Recently it was shown (113) that when a fraction isolated from rat diaphragm muscle, containing the specific endplate nicotinic acetylcholine receptor, was incorporated into artificial phospholipid membranes, the reconstituted membrane became sensitive to acetylcholine in the sense that there was a large increase in ionic conductance.

Snyder et al. (114,115) have studied the glycine receptor of spinal cord. They found that ^{3}H-strychnine, which is an antagonist of the hyperpolarizing action of glycine at spinal synapses, binds to synaptic membrane fragments from spinal cord, and is displaced by glycine and other glycine-like transmitters. They have also shown that Cl^- and other neurophysiologically active anions inhibit the strychnine binding. They suggest that strychnine affects the ionic conductance mechanism for chloride associated with the glycine receptor.

Other Receptors

There is evidence that there are a number of other membrane-bound receptors in the nervous system that are probably proteins. Frazier et al. (116) have shown that there is a receptor for nerve growth factor (NGF) on the surface of the cell membrane of chick sensory or sympathetic ganglia. Bannerjee et al. (117) also found that NGF binds to superior cervical ganglia of rabbit, and that the binding is saturable with an apparent affinity constant of 2 nM.

Finally, there is evidence that there are receptors on nervous system membranes which may be responsible for specific cell–surface recognition phenomena, particularly during development of the nervous system when specific interconnections are formed between classes of neurons. Barbera et al. (118) have prepared ^{32}P-labeled single-cell suspensions of dorsal and ventral halves of retinas from chick embryos. More cells from the dorsal half of the retina bind to the ventral half of the optic tectum and more cells from the ventral half of the retina bind to the dorsal half-tectum. This preferential binding mimics the retinal-tectal projections actually formed during development. Merrel and Glaser (119) isolated plasma membrane fractions from embryonic retina and cerebellum. When ^{3}H-glucosamine-labeled retinal plasma membranes were incubated with retinal or cerebellar cells, about 20 to 21% of the membranes bound to retinal but less than 5% to cerebellar. They conclude that the embryonic cells recognize homotypic membranes. They assume that cell–cell recognition involves a passive recognition site and an active component, both of which reside at the outside surface of the cell membrane, and that this recognition process may be involved in the specific aggregation of like cell types during development. Glycoproteins may be involved since they are known to be present at the outside membrane surface and can act as specific receptors.

A clonal line of rat glioma cells, grown on plates (C6), does not accumulate the nervous system-specific protein, S-100, until the cell cultures enter the stationary phase and become confluent (120). When cell growth was arrested during exponential proliferation, before confluency, by any of several methods, the cells do not accumulate S-100. Stationary phase cultures grown in suspension do not accumulate S-100, and when C6 cells were plated with an equal number of cells from a line that does not produce S-100, the C6 line did not accumulate S-100 either, even at confluency. These results indicate that specific homologous cell–cell contact is required to trigger S-100 accumulation and that therefore the mechanism probably involves cell–cell recognition at the outside membrane surface.

SUMMARY AND CONCLUSIONS

A number of methods have been worked out, applied in large part to red cell membranes, for investigation of the arrangement of proteins in membranes, so that at the present time, much is known about the topography of proteins in this particular membrane. Some proteins are exposed on the external surface, some on the cytoplasmic surface, and some on both. Glycoproteins generally seem to have their carbohydrate portions accessible to the external surface of the membrane so that they can act as receptors with many different functions. These methods, worked out for red cell membranes are and will be applied to nervous system membranes. Also, excellent methods are available, particularly SDS-polyacrylamide gel electrophoresis, for investigating the polypeptide composition of membranes.

The red cell membrane is a relatively simple membrane as far as the number of major polypeptides is concerned. The work that has been done so far suggests that, with the exception of myelin, the polypeptide composition of nervous system membranes is much more complex. However, gel patterns indicate that red cell membranes, myelin, synaptic membranes, and other nervous system membranes have a number of minor components. Red cell membranes and myelin are easier to prepare without contamination from other subcellular fragments than are, for example, synaptic membranes. Also the preparation of nervous system membranes requires a great deal of manipulation, involving homogenization, centrifuging through various concentrations of sucrose or Ficoll, and exposure to a variety of ionic conditions. Finally, it is difficult to assess the purity of a class of membranes, and if they are prepared from mammalian brain, a given class may represent a great variety of cell types. Therefore, the following questions must be asked and, it is hoped, methods must be found to answer them.

(a) How pure and uncontaminated is a membrane preparation?

(b) Does a membrane preparation represent a number of different cell types whose membranes may have differing protein composition or architecture?

(c) Are specific membrane proteins lost during the purification of the membrane?

(d) Are proteins added to the membrane during purification which were not present in the original intact membrane?

(e) Is the topography of a given protein in the membrane changed during the purification of the membrane?

(f) How is the importance of a "minor" polypeptide component of a membrane assessed? That is, is it a contaminant, is it of minor functional importance, or does it represent, although small in quantity, a major function of the membrane?

REFERENCES

1. Guidotti, G. (1972): *Ann. Rev. Biochem.*, 731–752.
2. Singer, S. J. (1974): *Ann. Rev. Biochem.*, 805–833.

3. Fairbanks, G., Steck, T. L., and Wallach, D. F. N. (1971): *Biochemistry*, 10:2606.
4. Rosenberg, S. A., and Guidotti, G. (1969): *J. Biol. Chem.*, 244:5118.
5. Phillips, D. R., and Morrison, M. (1970): *Biochem. Biophys. Res. Commun.*, 40:284.
6. Phillips, D. R., and Morrison, M. (1971): *Biochemistry*, 10:1766.
7. Phillips, D. R., and Morrison, M. (1973): *Nature (New Biol.)*, 242:213.
8. Hubbard, A. L., and Cohn, Z. A. (1972): *J. Cell Biol.*, 55:390.
9. Reichstein, F., and Blostein, R. (1973): *Biochem. Biophys. Res. Commun.*, 54:494.
10. Bretscher, M. S. (1971): *J. Mol. Biol.*, 58:775.
11. Boxer, D. H., Jenkins, R. E., and Tanner, M. S. A. (1974): *Biochem. J.* 137:531.
12. Whiteley, N. M., and Berg, H. C. (1974): *J. Mol. Biol.*, 87:541.
13. Marchesi, V. T., Jackson, R. L., Segrest, J. P., and Kahame, I. (1973): *Fed. Proc.*, 32:1833.
14. Marchesi, V. J., and Andrews, E. P. (1971): *Science*, 174:1247.
15. Grefrath, S. P., and Reynolds, J. A. (1974): *Proc. Natl. Acad. Sci. USA*, 71:3913.
16. Jackson, R. L., Segrest, J. P., Kahane, I., and Marchesi, V. T. (1973): *Biochemistry*, 12:3131.
17. Treyer, H. R., Nozaki, Y., Reynolds, J. A., and Tanford, C. (1971): *J. Biol. Chem.*, 246:4485.
18. Autilio, L. A., Norton, W. T., and Terry, R. D. (1964): *J. Neurochem.*, 11:17.
19. Norton, W. T., and Poduslo, S. E. (1973): *J. Neurochem.*, 21:749.
20. Gray, E. E., and Whittaker, V. P. (1962): *J. Anat. (Lond.)*, 96:79.
21. DeRobertis, E., Pellegrino, DeIraldi, A., Rodriguez DeLores Arnaiz, G., and Salganicoff, L. (1962): *J. Neurochem.*, 9:23.
22. Morgan, I. G., Wolfe, L. S., Mandel, P., and Gombos, G. (1971): *Biochim. Biophys. Acta*, 241:737.
23. Abdel-Latif, A. A. (1966): *Biochim. Biophys. Acta*, 121:403.
24. Cotman, C. W., and Matthews, D. A. (1971): *Biochim. Biophys. Acta*, 249:303.
25. Cotman, C. W., Herschmann, K., and Taylor, D. (1971): *J. Neurobiol.*, 2:169.
26. Gurd, J. W., Jones, L. R., Mahler, H. R., and Moore, W. J. (1974): *J. Neurochem.*, 22:281.
27. Dowdall, M. J., and Whittaker, V. P. (1973): *J. Neurochem.*, 20:921.
28. Jones, D. G. (1967): *J. Cell Sci.*, 2:573.
29. Florey, E., and Winesdorfer, J. (1968): *J. Neurochem.*, 15:169.
30. Whittaker, V. P., Michaelson, I. A., and Kirkland, R. J. A. (1964): *Biochem. J.*, 90:293.
31. Cotman, C. W. (1970): *Brain Res.*, 22:152.
32. McBride, W. J., and VanTassel, J. (1972): *Brain Res.*, 44:177.
33. Bloom, F. E., and Aghajanian, G. (1971): *J. Ultrastruct. Res.*, 34:103.
34. Kornguth, S. E., Anderson, J. W., and Scott, G. (1969): *J. Neurochem.*, 16:1017.
35. Kornguth, S. E., Flangas, A. L., Siegel, F. L.,

Geison, R. L., O'Brien, J. F., Lamar, L., and Scott, G. (1971): *J. Biol. Chem.*, 246:1177.
36. Cotman, C. W., Levy, W., Banker, G., and Taylor, D. (1971): *Biochim. Biophys. Acta*, 249:406.
37. Cotman, C. W., and Taylor, D. (1972): *J. Cell Biol.*, 55:696.
38. Davis, G. A., and Bloom, F. E. (1973): *Anal. Biochem.*, 51:429.
39. Banker, G., Churchill, L., and Cotman, C. (1974): *Trans. Am. Soc. Neurochem.*, 5:109. (Abstract).
40. Rose, S. P. R. (1967): *Biochem. J.*, 102:33.
41. Fine, R. E., and Bray, D. (1971): *Nature (New Biol.)*, 234:115.
42. Bloomstrand, C., and Hamberger, A. (1969): *J. Neurochem.*, 16:1401.
43. Norton, W. T., and Poduslo, S. E. (1970): *Science*, 167:1144.
44. Sellinger, O., Azcurra, J. M., Johnson, D. E., Ohlsson, W. G., and Lodin, Z. (1971): *Nature (New Biol.)*, 230:253.
45. Poduslo, S. E., and Norton, W. T. (1972): *J. Neurochem.*, 19:727.
46. DeVries, G. H., Norton, W. T., and Raine, C. S. (1972): *Science*, 175:1370.
47. Benda, P., Lightbody, J., Sato, G., Levine, L., and Sweet, W. (1968): *Science*, 161:370.
48. Pfeiffer, S. E., Kornblith, P. L., Cares, H. L., Seals, J., and Levine, L. (1972): *Brain Res.*, 41:182.
49. Schubert, D., Heinemann, S., Carlisle, W., Tarikas, H., Kimes, B., Steinback, J. H., Culp, W., and Brandt, B. L. (1974): *Nature*, 249:224.
50. Schubert, D., Humphreys, S., Baroni, C., and Cohn, M. (1969): *Proc. Natl. Acad. Sci. USA*, 64:316.
51. Nelson, P., Ruffner, W., and Nirenberg, M. (1969): *Proc. Natl. Acad. Sci. USA*, 64:1004.
52. Nelson, P. G., Peacock, J. H., Amano, T., and Minna, J. (1971): *J. Cell Physiol.*, 77:337.
53. Harris, A. J., and Dennis, M. J. (1970): *Science*, 167:1253.
54. Blume, A., Gilbert, F., Wilson, S., Farbor, J., Rosenberg, R., and Nirenberg, M. (1970): *Proc. Natl. Acad. Sci. USA*, 67:786.
55. Augusto-Tocco, G., and Sato, G. (1969): *Proc. Natl. Acad. Sci. USA*, 64:311.
56. Herschmann, H. R. (1971): *J. Biol. Chem.*, 246:7569.
57. McMorris, F. A., Kolber, A. R., Moore, B. W., and Perumal, A. S. (1974): *J. Cell Physiol.*, 84:473.
58. Kolber, A. R., Goldstein, M. N., and Moore, B. W. (1974): *Proc. Natl. Acad. Sci. USA*, 71: 4203.
59. Truding, R., Shelanski, M. L., Daniels, M. P., and Morell, P. (1974): *J. Biol. Chem.*, 249:3973.
60. Reynolds, J. A., and Tanford, C. (1970): *Proc. Natl. Acad. Sci. USA*, 66:1002.
61. Weber, K., and Osborn, M. (1969): *J. Biol. Chem.*, 244:4406.
62. Laemmli, U. K. (1970): *Nature*, 227:680.
63. Eylar, E. H., Brostaff, S., Hashim, G., Caccam,

J., and Burnett, P. (1971): *J. Biol. Chem.*, 246: 5770.

64. Carnegie, P. R. (1971): *Nature*, 229:25.
65. Folch, J., and Lees, M. (1951): *J. Biol. Chem.*, 191:807.
66. Green, H. O., and Reynolds, J. A. (1971): *Fed. Proc.*, 30:1065.
67. Wolfgram, F. (1966): *J. Neurochem.*, 13:461.
68. Agrawal, H. C., Burton, R. M., Fishman, M. A., Mitchell, R. F., and Prensky, A. L. (1972): *J. Neurochem.*, 19:2083.
69. Quarles, R. H., Everly, J. L., and Brady, R. O. (1972): *Biochem. Biophys. Res. Commun.*, 47:491.
70. Quarles, R. H., Everly, J. L., and Brady, R. O. (1973):*J. Neurochem.*, 21:1177.
71. Druse, M. J., Brady, R. O., and Quarles, R. H. (1974):*Brain Res.*, 76:423.
72. Chan, D. S., and Lees, M. B. (1974): *Biochemistry*, 13:2704.
73. Folch, J., Webster, G. R., and Lees, M. (1959): *Fed. Proc.*, 18:228.
74. Cotman, C. W., and Mahler, H. R. (1967): *Arch. Biochem. Biophys.*, 120:384.
75. Cotman, C. W., Mahler, H. R., and Hugli, T. E. (1968): *Arch. Biochem. Biophys.*, 126:821.
76. Takayama, K., MacLennan, D. H., Tzagoloff, A., and Stoner, C. D. (1966): *Arch. Biochem. Biophys.*, 114:223.
77. Waehneldt, T. V., Morgan, I. G., and Gombos, G. (1971): *Brain Res.*, 34:403.
78. Gurd, R. S., Mahler, H. R., and Moore, W. J. (1972):*J. Neurochem.*, 19:553.
79. Banker, G., Crain, B., and Cotman, C. W. (1972): *Brain Res.*, 42:508.
80. Wannamaker, B. B., and Kornguth, S. E. (1973): *Biochim. Biophys. Acta*, 303:333.
81. Puszkin, W., Berl, S., Puszkin, S., and Clarke, D. (1968): *Science*, 161:170.
82. Puszkin, S., Nicklas, W. J., and Berl, S. (1972): *J. Neurochem.*, 19:1319.
83. Fine, R. E., Blitz, A. L., Hitchcock, S. L., and Kaminer, B. (1973): *Nature (New Biol.)*, 245: 182.
84. Blitz, A. L., and Fine, R. E. (1974): *Proc. Natl. Acad. Sci. USA*, 71:4472.
85. Davison, P., and Winslow, B. (1974): *J. Neurobiol.*, 5:119.
86. Weisenberg, R. C. (1972): *Science*, 177:1104.
87. Gurd, J. W., and Mahler, H. R. (1974): *Biochemistry*, 13:5193.
88. Zanetta, J. P., Morgan, I. G., and Gombos, G. (1975): *Brain Res.*, 83:337.
89. Karlsson, J. O., Hamberger, A., and Henn, F. A. (1973): *Biochim. Biophys. Acta*, 298:219.
90. Uyeda, C. T., Eng, L. F., and Bignami, A. (1972):*Brain Res.*, 37:81.
91. Grefrath, S. P., and Reynolds, J. A. (1973): *J. Biol. Chem.*, 248:6091.
92. Glick, M. C., Kimhi, Y., and Littauer, U. Z.

(1973): *Proc. Natl. Acad. Sci. USA*, 70:1682.
93. Hubbard, J. I., and Quastel, M. J. (1973): *Ann. Rev. Pharmacol.*, 13:199.
94. O'Brien, R. D., Eldefrawi, M. E., and Eldefrawi, A. T. (1972): *Ann. Rev. Pharmacol.*, 12:19.
95. Karlin, A. (1973):*Fed. Proc.*, 32:1847.
96. Changeux, J.-P., and Podleski, T. R. (1968): *Proc. Natl. Acad. Sci. USA*, 59:944.
97. Blumenthal, R., and Changeux, J.-P. (1970): *Biochim. Biophys. Acta*, 219:398.
98. Kasai, M., and Changeux, J.-P. (1971): *J. Membrane Biol.*, 6:1.
99. Kasai, M., and Changeux, J.-P. (1971): *J. Membrane Biol.*, 6:24.
100. Kasai, M., and Changeux, J.-P. (1971): *J. Membrane Biol.*, 6:58.
101. Cartand, J., Benedetti, E. L., Kasai, M., and Changeux, J.-P. (1971): *J. Membrane Biol.*, 6:81.
102. Duguid, J. R., and Raftery, M. A. (1973): *Biochemistry*, 12:3593.
103. Miledi, R., Molinoff, P., and Potter, L. T. (1971): *Nature*, 229:554.
104. Eldefrawi, M. E., and Eldefrawi, A. T. (1972): *Proc. Natl. Acad. Sci. USA*, 69:1776.
105. Biesecker, G. (1973): *Biochemistry*, 12:4403.
106. Schmidt, J., and Raftery, M. A. (1973): *Biochemistry*, 12:852.
107. Klett, R. P., Fulpius, B. W., Cooper, D., Smith, M., Reich, E., and Loureval, D. P. (1973): *J. Biol. Chem.*, 248:6841.
108. Gautran, M., Israel, M., and Podleski, T. R. (1969): *C.R. Acad. Sci. (D) (Paris)*, 269:1788.
109. Reiter, M. J., Cowburn, D. A., Prives, J. M., and Karlin, A. (1972): *Proc. Natl. Acad. Sci. USA*, 69:1168.
110. Lee, C. Y., and Chang, C. C. (1966): *Mem. Inst. Butantan Simp. Int.*, 33:555.
111. Changeux, J.-P., Rasai, M., and Lee, C. (1970): *Proc. Natl. Acad. Sci. USA*, 67:1241.
112. Bosman, H. P. (1972): *J. Biol. Chem.*, 247:130.
113. Kemp, G., Dolly, J. P., Barnard, E. A., and Wenner, C. E. (1973): *Biochem. Biophys. Res. Commun.*, 54:607.
114. Young, A. B., and Snyder, S. H. (1973): *Proc. Natl. Acad. Sci. USA*, 70:2832.
115. Young, A. B., and Snyder, S. H. (1974): *Proc. Natl. Acad. Sci. USA*, 71:4002.
116. Frazier, W. A., Boyd, L. F., and Bradshaw, R. A. (1973): *Proc. Natl. Acad. Sci. USA*, 70:2931.
117. Banerjee, S. P., Snyder, S. H., Cuatrecasas, P., and Greene, L. A. (1973): *Proc. Natl. Acad. Sci. USA*, 70:2519.
118. Barbera, A. J., Marchesi, R. B., and Roth, S. (1973): *Proc. Natl. Acad. Sci. USA*, 70:2482.
119. Merrel, R., and Glaser, L. (1973): *Proc. Natl. Acad. Sci. USA*, 70:2794.
120. Pfeiffer, S. E., Herschmann, H. R., Lightbody, J., and Sato, G. (1970): *J. Cell Physiol.*, 75:329.

The Nervous System, Donald B. Tower, Editor-in-Chief. *Vol. 1: The Basic Neurosciences.* Raven Press, New York, 1975.

The History of Research on Proteolipids

J. Folch-Pi

The occurrence of *proteolipids*, a group of lipoproteins characterized by solubility in chloroform:methanol mixtures and completely insoluble in water or aqueous solutions, was established by Folch and Lees (1) in 1951, in the McLean Hospital Research Laboratory. Since then, work on proteolipids has been an ongoing project in this laboratory, at times at a slow pace, and at other times with great intensity, according to the rate of probable progress that was anticipated. In recent years, the work on proteolipids has been a major concern of the laboratory. Therefore, it seems proper to select a brief review of proteolipids, as being specially fitting for a book intended to commemorate the 25th anniversary of the establishment of the National Institute of Neurological and Communicative Disorders and Stroke.

The amount of material related to proteolipids is very large and its review, even in concise form, would be several times the length available in this commemorative volume. In addition, there are some recent reviews (2) on the subject, and at least one comprehensive review is in preparation and should appear very shortly. Under these circumstances, it has been decided to devote the bulk of this discussion to the history of the ideas and working hypotheses that we have had at different times on the nature of proteolipids. Besides giving information that hitherto has remained unpublished, this relation will illustrate the continuity of thought in the evolution of a research program of 25 years existence. A secondary aim of this contribution will be to describe some aspects of the problem that have not been properly emphasized heretofore. It is hoped that this article will round up and complete the information available on proteolipids.

THE EVOLUTION OF OUR IDEAS ON THE NATURE OF PROTEOLIPIDS

Discovery and Initial Studies

The discovery of proteolipids was a serendipitic result from work on the development of a satisfactory procedure for the extraction and initial purification of total brain lipids (3).

It had been established that such a procedure required an extracting medium of high solvent power for lipids, and the removal from the extract of the cripplingly large proportion of nonlipids that the solvating power of lipids carried into the extract. Chloroform was clearly the solvent with the widest and most marked ability to dissolve lipids. The addition of methanol provides a solvent mixture which at proper dilution was miscible with the tissue water, thus permitting the direct extraction of the tissue. The presence of methanol in the extract also made possible the removal of nonlipid solutes from the extract by simply layering it under a large volume of water: the methanol at the interface diffused into the water, leaving behind at the interface a chloroform enriched extract which by gravity diffused downwards into the mass of the remaining extract, being replaced at the interface by portions of new extract. This process was continuous and lasted until all the methanol had diffused into the upper water phase. There was an accumulation of a fluff-like material at the interface. The study of the upper water–methanolic phase, the lower chloroformic phase, and the interfacial fluff showed that lipids remained in the lower phase, that nonlipids had diffused quantitatively into the upper phase, and that the fluff was completely soluble in chloroform:methanol. If the upper phase was removed by siphoning, and enough methanol was added to the lower phase, the fluff was dissolved and a reconstituted chloroform:methanol solution was obtained which was free of water soluble substances, i.e., of nonlipids. Only negligible amounts of lipids were lost in the upper phase.

In the next step in the procedure, the solutes in the washed chloroform:methanol extract were recovered by evaporation of the solvents. When the resulting residue was redissolved in chloroform, or chloroform:methanol, part of the residue was insoluble. The study of the portion of the residue that had become insoluble showed that it was constant in yield and composition among parallel evaporations: that it was insoluble in a variety of organic solvents and of aqueous solutions, and that it contained about 12 to 14% N and 0.2 to 0.4% P. By hydrolysis in boiling 6 N HCl, it yielded a mixture of amino acids; i.e., it appeared to be an insoluble protein residue containing small amounts of phospholipids. It was resistant to the action of trypsin, erepsin, pepsin, and papain. By varying conditions of operation, it was found that the insolubilization of this protein material occurred only when the solvent mixture that was being evaporated contained enough water to cause the formation of a biphasic system in the course of the evaporation. It was also found that the extent of the insolubilization depended approximately on the amount of water present in the mixture and that in order to secure quantitative insolubilization of the protein, it was necessary to repeat the operation several times; i.e., the whole residue from the washed extract was redissolved in chloroform:methanol, water added to the limit of miscibility, and the evaporation of the solvents repeated. Three such evaporations usually sufficed for the quantitative insolubilization of the protein material.

At the time it was thought that the protein was part of a protein–lipid complex so structured as to exhibit a hydrophobic surface. (Hence the name proteolipids, to distinguish these substances from plasma lipoproteins which were generally soluble in aqueous media, and insoluble in organic solvents.) The postulated lipoprotein would be a dipole, which would orient itself at the water–chloroform interface: this ordered disposition would render the protein moiety available to the denaturing action of chloroform with the consequent insolubilization of the protein.

The knowledge acquired about some of the properties of proteolipids in operational terms permitted the preparation, by solvent fractionation of the washed total lipid extract from brain, of three different proteolipid-containing fractions (A, B, and C). They varied in yield and proteolipid content with small changes in the procedure followed, and since the pattern of amino acid composition of the different fractions was indistinguishable from one another, it was concluded that the observations did not correspond to the separation of distinct proteolipids, but only to the demonstration that proteolipids were stable through solvent manipulation.

In these initial observations, a screening of different tissues for proteolipid content had shown that proteolipids were specially abundant in central nervous system white matter, followed in order of content by central gray matter, heart muscle, kidney, liver, and skeletal muscle. They were absent from immature central nervous system and they appeared and increased in concentration in the central nervous system in parallel with the onset and increase in myelination. Hence it was postulated that proteolipids in the central nervous system were mainly myelin components.

Similar work from numerous laboratories has eventually established that proteolipids are present in most animal and vegetal tissues, and that they are usually associated with membranous structures (2).

In theory the purification of proteolipids required only their separation from lipids, the establishment of their homogeneity or heterogeneity and, in the latter case, their separation into pure compounds. In practice, the attainment of these goals was severely handicapped by the special properties of proteolipids. On the one hand their peculiar solubility properties made it difficult, if not impossible, to apply to them the rich armamentarium available for the isolation, purification, and identification of proteins; on the other hand, their relative instability limited the application of classical procedures for the isolation of lipids. The difficulties of treating them as lipids were increased by the then as yet not fully appreciated ability of proteolipids to interact with all kinds of lipids.

As a consequence of these severe operational difficulties, little progress was made for several years towards the seemingly simple goal of separating proteolipids from free lipids. Since we were limited to the use of solvent fractionation, countercurrent distribution appeared to be the method of choice. By trial and error, a number of biphasic systems were developed which could be used with proteolipids. It soon became clear that as the proteolipids were separated from lipids by the successive partitions, the overall physical characteristics of the proteolipids changed in the sense that their distribution coefficient did not remain constant, but was affected by the composition of the lipid mixture present in the proteolipid solution. This change robbed any successful countercurrent distribution procedure that we might develop from its main advantage, i.e., from the pattern of distribution as a criterion for homogeneity or heterogeneity of the proteolipids that were migrating along the countercurrent distribution train. The long and arduous work that led to this negative finding resulted far from fallow: It taught us that proteolipids, although unstable in the relatively mild conditions of evaporating the solvents from the original chloroform:methanol extract from the tissue, were remarkably stable under an array of much more drastic circumstances; it permitted the development of a procedure for the easy preparation of sulfatides (4); in the course of the work it had been realized that proteolipids in lipid mixtures could be estimated by absorption at 280 nm in chloroform:methanol; this simple nondestructive procedure replaced the estimation of proteolipids by chemical analysis, which was time-consuming and required sizable amounts of material; finally, the observations made led to the widely used method of Folch et al. (5) for the removal of nonlipid substances from chloroform:methanol tissue extracts. By this procedure the chloroform:methanol tissue extract is washed by addition of one-fifth its volume of water. A biphasic system results, with an upper water–methanolic phase, a mainly chloroformic lower phase, and no fluff at the interphase. The lower phase contains the proteolipids quantitatively. In addition the residue

obtained from this lower phase by evaporation of the solvents is completely soluble in chloroform:methanol, i.e., the process of evaporation has not resulted in insolubilization of the proteolipids.

The Emulsion-centrifugation Procedure for Preparation of Proteolipids

This was the first time that total proteolipids had been obtained in solid form without change in their solubility properties. The residue was tested for solubility in numerous media, in an effort to extract the last opportunity from this novel finding. Among other things it was found that the residue formed emulsions in water readily, by simply standing or shaking at room temperature or at cold room temperature (0 to 6°C). The easy emulsification suggested differential centrifugation as a means of separating proteolipids from lipids, since protein had a higher specific gravity than lipids. This proved to be the case and by repeated centrifugations 98 to 100% of the proteolipid in the starting chloroform:methanol tissue extract was recovered in a sediment consisting of 40% proteolipid and 60% lipids, i.e., a fivefold concentration of proteolipids without loss. The proteolipid protein in the sediment was raised to an average of 60% by solvent fractionation. The eightfold enriched preparation obtained by the emulsion-centrifugation method was a major step in operational terms.

Study of the Nature of the Lipid–protein Linkage in Proteolipids

The variations in the physical properties of proteolipids and their puzzling lability to mild operations in contrast with a high stability in front of other agents, made it imperative to attempt to learn something about the nature of the linkage(s) between the protein and lipid moieties in proteolipids. Our knowledge of this linkage at the time was only in operational terms and negative in nature, in the sense that we could only follow its destruction; i.e., when the linkage was broken, the protein moiety became insoluble and precipitated as an insoluble residue which was resistant to the action of proteolytic enzymes, and insoluble in all the media that had been tried. This was the only means we had to recognize that the linkage had been changed.

In a possible approach to the study of more subtle changes in the nature of the linkage, it was decided to investigate if calcium bridges might play a part in the protein:lipid linkage. The underlying reason for this approach was that brain lipids had been shown to have a high affinity for Ca^{2+} (6). In addition, when $CaCl_2$ was added to an aqueous emulsion of total washed brain lipids, the emulsion was visibly cleared. To approach this question it was decided to test the effect of oxalates and citrates on the properties of proteolipids: portions of washed total brain lipid extract were made into the biphasic system C:M:H_2O 8:4:3 (v/v/v) and varying amounts of citrates or of oxalates were added to the upper phase. It was found (7) that these anions had an effect only when the pH of the upper phase was made slightly alkaline, roughly above pH 8.5. The effect was also obtained with an array of neutral salts that had no special effect of calcium ions. The final conclusion was that the proteolipid linkage was dissociated at slightly alkaline pH and that the extent of this dissociation was roughly proportional to the logarithm of the ionic strength of the medium. It appeared in addition that calcium bridges played no prominent part in the proteolipid linkage.

Chromatography of Proteolipids

The techniques for chromatographic separation of lipids had become feasible during the late 1950s and it appeared indicated to apply this sophisticated technique to the separation of proteolipid. This was successfully accomplished on silicic acid using elution by a discontinuous gradient of C:M:water mixture of increasing polarity, with the final eluant containing HCl at 0.004 N concentration (8). Three or four protein peaks were obtained. Each consisted of 95 to 97% protein and 2 to 5% phospholipids. The amino acid compositions of the different protein peaks were identical or indistinguishable from each other. The phospholipids present in each peak appeared to be inositol-containing phospholipids, mainly diphosphoinositide. On rechromatography, each peak was separated into three peaks, the

most prominent of which corresponded to the position of the mother peak. In brief, the work carried out had shown that chromatography was applicable to the separation of proteolipids, but that the fractions that we had separated were indistinguishable from each other and were otherwise physically not homogeneous, since they separated into several peaks upon rechromatography. The main progress achieved was the preparation of proteolipids with only minimal amounts of lipids, and the observation that the lipid present appeared to be one or more phosphoinositides. Another observation, the importance of which did not become immediately apparent, was made during the routine collection of peaks in the step at which the recovered proteolipid was partitioned in the biphasic system C:M:H_2O, 8:4:3. With the first peaks, the proteolipid remained quantitatively in the lower phase. With the last peak, which had been eluted with an acidified C:M mixture (see above) the proteolipid partitioned between upper and lower phase in a 1:3 ratio. Since HCl had been removed from the medium, the departure from the usual partition indicated a physical change in the material that was collected as the last peak. The fractions from upper and lower phase were not studied at the time because of the scarcity of material.

Concentration of Proteolipids by Dialysis in Organic Solvents

In parallel with the chromatographic work, the total brain white matter proteolipids prepared by the emulsion centrifugation procedure had been submitted to dialysis in chloroform: methanol mixtures using cellophane casings as semipermeable membranes. As expected, the proteolipids were retained by the membrane and the lipids diffused through it (9), along with about $^1/_6$ of the protein material in it. The final undialyzable material proved to contain up to 85% protein, the remaining 15% of material being lipids linked to the protein. Since by chromatography on silicic acid the lipid content was reduced to 2% to 5%, it was obvious that some lipids were bound to the protein moiety by stronger linkages than other lipids.

Independently from us, Murakami et al. had applied successfully dialysis in organic solvents to the preparation of heart proteolipids (10).

Preparation of a Water-Soluble Proteolipid Apoprotein (PLA) by Dialysis in Acidified Solvents

The change in the partition behavior of the proteolipid fraction eluted from silicic acid by the final acidified eluant suggested that the exposure to acid changed the proteolipids rendering them more soluble in polar media than they were prior to exposure to acid. To study this effect further, proteolipids were purified by dialysis in chloroform:methanol containing HCl at a concentration of 0.04 N. It was found that this acidification increased the proportion of diffusable lipids without affecting the undiffusibility of protein. The final undialyzable material consisted of 99 to 100% protein with lipids present below the level of detection, if at all. It was also found that when the dialysis medium was changed from chloroform:methanol to water by gradual passage through mixtures of C:M:water with increasing proportions of water, the undialyzable protein remained in "solution" (11). The proteolipid aqueous solution thus obtained was not very stable, unless it was acidified below pH 5. It could not be lyophilized without losing its solubility. It apparently was highly aggregated, and its ultraviolet spectrum had a high background absorption. The preparation was freely soluble in chloroform:methanol. Unfortunately, the instability of the aqueous solutions of this apoprotein made it impossible to apply to its study the procedures of protein chemistry. On the other hand, it showed that the apoprotein was soluble both in chloroform:methanol and in water and it permitted Zand (12) to show by optical rotatory dispersion measurements that in chloroform:methanol the apoprotein exhibited a high content of α-helix and that in water the α-helix content dropped to a level below detection.

Purification of Proteolipids by Gel Permeation

The use of gel permeation in the purification of proteolipids can be traced to Autilio (13) who, in 1966, used a polysterene gel in the study of central myelin proteins. She was able to isolate, among other fractions, one with the properties of proteolipids. It represented about 55% of total myelin proteins, a value that has been confirmed repeatedly by later workers. With the availability of Sephadex LH20, gel permeation became more practical. In 1967 Mokrasch (14) combined precipitation with ethyl ether with passage through a Sephadex LH20 column. Proteolipid was obtained in the excluded volume as a preparation of composition similar to the preparations obtained by dialysis with neutral solvents. When this preparation was reprecipitated with ethyl ether and then passed through a Dowex 1-X2 column, a product was obtained comparable to the preparations obtained by Matsumoto and coworkers by the use of a silicic acid column.

In 1969 Soto and associates (15) used Sephadex LH20 in the purification of proteolipids from white matter and from gray matter. From the latter they were able to separate a distinct fraction exhibiting many of the properties postulated for an acetylcholine receptor, and for which the function of physiological receptor of acetylcholine was claimed (16). As concerns the general usefulness of Sephadex LH20 columns, Soto and associates reported substantial losses of proteolipid protein on the column and otherwise obtained a distribution of proteolipids among several overlapping peaks. They suggested that Sephadex LH20 acted both through gel permeation and by partition chromatography.

Preparation of a Stable Water-soluble Preparation of Central White Matter PLA

The information gathered by the various lines of work summarized above had brought about a change in our concept of proteolipids. The initial idea had been that proteolipids consisted of a protein core covered by bound lipids, the resulting complex offering a nonpolar surface to the media. When this outer lipid shell was disturbed or removed, the protein core came into contact with chloroform:methanol, which rendered the protein insoluble, as it does with water-soluble proteins in general. The changes in physical behavior of proteolipids were due to loose linking of different lipids to the lipid shell.

With the persistence of the characteristic solubilities of proteolipids upon gradual delipidation, up to and including the fractions obtained by chromatography on silicic acid, the hypothesis of a protein core covered by a lipid shell became increasingly less tenable. The sudden appearance, in the last of the peaks from silicic chromatography, of a proteolipid fraction more polar than the classical proteolipids, and the preparation of the water-soluble apoprotein constituted final proof that our original ideas on the structure of proteolipids required a drastic revision. Indeed we were faced with a protein, the proteolipid apoprotein, which appeared to be natively soluble both in chloroform:methanol mixtures and in water, and which seemed to change conformation with the dielectric constant of the medium. These new ideas had more than a theoretical value. They required a rethinking of the whole approach to the study of proteolipids. It was necessary to define as precisely as possible the procedural limitations in the handling of proteolipids. The first step was to reexamine the procedures of preparation of PLA with a view to the elimination of drastic steps and protracted handling. Since the procedure of choice was dialysis in neutral CM followed by dialysis in acidified CM, a thorough study of dialysis in organic solvents was carried out (2). The final conditions selected involved dialysis in neutral CM, followed by CM:HCl and neutral CM again, to remove the acid. This yielded a stable preparation readily soluble in CM, and with a high α-helix content. On the assumption that the protracted passage of the PLA through media of increasing polarity might be harmful to the preparation, the passage of PLA from CM into water was carried out within one hour by simply placing the CM solution of PLA in a current of nitrogen. As the solvents were removed, they were replaced by water which was added at frequent times to the point of inmiscibility. The end result of this process was an aqueous solution of PLA. This PLA was very stable. It could be dried, without losing its solubility in water, and water solutions up to 3% could be prepared without difficulty. These solutions were water clear, showing little background absorption in the ultraviolet. PLA exhibited a high α-helix content in CM, and about one-half as much in water solution. This change in conformation was readily reversible, and the simple dilution of the aqueous solution of PLA with CM resulted in an increase in α-helix content to the level of the starting PLA in CM (17). The preparation was suitable for physical and chemical studies. It gave essentially single major peaks by ultracentrifugation and moving boundary electrophoresis (2). The molecular weight was high and variable, indicating extensive aggregation. That this was the case was shown by polyacrylamide gel electrophoresis, which showed PLA to contain several different proteins, with a major band first found to correspond to 34,000 to 36,000 daltons (17). Further studies lowered this size to 22,000 to 24,000 daltons (18). Finally, the dialyzable fraction of proteolipids was isolated and found to be identical with the undialyzable proteolipids (19), an observation that suggested a minimal molecular size of PLA of the order of 12,000.

The chemical study of PLA showed it to be devoid of carbohydrates, and to have about 3% of fatty acid radicals combined by ester linkages, presumably to the polypeptide chain itself. These combined fatty acids consist of palmityl, stearyl, and oleyl radicals in the molar ratios 12:5:2 (20).

Current Research on Proteolipids

With this finding, this "microhistory" of our evolving concept of proteolipids may be brought to an end. The substantial progress made in our knowledge of proteolipids since the point summarized above is not as amenable to a meaningful historical perspective. Many laboratories are now involved in work on the chemistry, the metabolism, the biosynthesis, and the possible functions of proteolipids. The results obtained can only be reviewed by detailed consideration of the numerous, and at times, conflicting observations. Such a discussion is clearly outside of the scope of this contribution.

REFERENCES

1. Folch, J., and Lees, M. (1951): Proteolipids, a new type of tissue lipoproteins. Their isolation from brain. *J. Biol. Chem.,* 191:807–817.
2. Folch-Pi, J., and Stoffyn, P. J. (1972): Proteolipids from membrane systems. *Ann. N.Y. Acad. Sci.,* 195:86–107.
3. Folch, J., Ascoli, I., Lees, M., Meath, J. A., and LeBaron, F. N. (1951): Preparation of lipid extracts from brain tissue. *J. Biol. Chem.,* 191:833–841.

4. Lees, M., Folch, J., Sloane-Stanley, G. H., and Carr, S. (1959): A simple procedure for the preparation of brain sulfatides. *J. Neurochem.,* 4:9–18.

5. Folch, J., Lees, M., and Sloane-Stanley, G. H. (1957): A simple method for isolation and purification of total lipides from animal tissues. *J. Biol. Chem.,* 226:497–509.

6. Folch-Pi, J., Lees, M., and Sloane-Stanley, G. H. (1957): The role of acidic lipids in the electrolyte balance of the nervous system of mammals. In: *Metabolism of the Nervous System,* edited by D. Richter, pp. 174–181. Pergamon Press, London.

7. Webster, G. R., and Folch, J. (1961): Some studies of the properties of proteolipids. *Biochim. Biophys. Acta,* 49:399–401.

8. Matsumoto, M., Matsumoto, R., and Folch-Pi, J. (1964): The chromatographic fractionation of brain white matter proteolipids. *J. Neurochem.,* 11:829–838.

9. Lees, M. B., Carr, S., and Folch, J. (1964): Purification of bovine brain white matter proteolipids by dialysis in organic solvents. *Biochim. Biophys. Acta,* 84:464–466.

10. Murakami, M., Sekine, H., and Funahashi, S. (1962): Proteolipid from beef heart muscle. Application of organic dialysis to preparation of proteolipid. *J. Biochem.,* 51:431–435.

11. Tenenbaum, D., and Folch-Pi, J. (1966): The preparation and characterization of water-soluble proteolipid protein from bovine brain white matter. *Biochim. Biophys. Acta,* 115:141–147.

12. Zand, R. (1968): Solution properties and structure of brain proteolipids. *Biopolymers,* 6:939–953.

13. Autilio, L. (1966): Fractionation of myelin proteins. *Fed. Proc.,* 25:764.

14. Mokrasch, L. C. (1967): A rapid purification of proteolipid protein adaptable to large quantities. *Life Sci.,* 6:1905–1909.

15. Soto, E. F., Pasquini, J. M., Placido, R., and La Torre, J. L. (1969): Fractionation of lipids and proteolipids from cat grey and white matter by chromatography on an organophilic dextran gel. *J. Chromatogr.,* 41:400–409.

16. DeRobertis, E., Fiszer, S., and Soto, E. F. (1967): Cholinergic binding capacity of proteolipids from isolated nerve-ending membranes. *Science,* 158:928.

17. Thorun, W., and Mehl, E. (1968): Determination of molecular weights of microgram quantities of protein components from biological membranes and other complex mixtures: Gel electrophoresis across linear gradients of acrylamide. *Biochim. Biophys. Acta,* 160:132–134.

18. Eng, L. F. (1971): Molecular weights of the major myelin proteins. *Fed. Proc.,* 30:1248 (abstr.).

19. Folch-Pi, J. (1971): Nature of the dialyzable brain white matter proteolipid. Third Intern. Meet. Intern. Soc. Neurochem. Abst:239 Publ. Akademiai Kiado. Budapest, Hungary, 1971.

20. Stoffyn, P., and Folch-Pi, J. (1971): On the type of linkage binding fatty acids present in brain white matter proteolipid apoprotein. *Biochem. Biophys. Res. Commun.,* 44:157–161.

The Nervous System, Donald B. Tower, Editor-in-Chief. *Vol. 1: The Basic Neurosciences*. Raven Press, New York, 1975.

Quantitative Histochemistry

Oliver H. Lowry

It has been realized for a long time that there must be profound biochemical heterogeneity underlying the unique structural complexity of brain. This has been a great challenge to the neurochemist. Investigators have responded to this challenge, in a variety of ingenious ways, each with its own virtues and provenance and its own limitations.

There have been three general approaches. The first is to try to localize the tissue constituent by making it visible in some manner in histological sections, e.g., by staining, or making the substance fluorescent, or by radioactive labeling followed by radioautography. Procedures of this sort have become increasingly sophisticated and successful in overcoming formidable problems of diffusion, inactivation of enzymes, and a variety of other artefacts. The results are usually qualitative or semi-quantitative. Nevertheless, this may suffice in many cases.

The second approach is to make bulk fractionations of the tissue into as many component parts as possible (cell bodies, nuclei, mitochondria, synaptosomes, synaptic vesicles, myelin fragments, etc.), followed by appropriate chemical studies. Here also, progressively better procedures have resulted in more nearly homogeneous fractions, less degradation of components, and better assessment of the loss of soluble constituents. There have even been studies of differences in subcellular fractions from different (although relatively large) regions of the nervous system.

The third approach—the oldest—is the subject of this chapter. It consists of the direct quantitative microchemical analysis of identified samples obtained under controlled conditions from specific sites in the nervous system.

Considering the small size of the discrete elements in brain and spinal cord, it seemed at first a hopeless job to push the direct approach far enough to do much good—to achieve by microchemistry much more insight into function than might be learned from chemical studies of whole brain or its major subdivisions. However, it has been possible to develop over the years a general technique which permits analysis of identified samples as small as 10 μm in diameter for a wide variety of enzymes, cofactors, and metabolites. The technique and some of the steps in its development will be described and its place in neurochemistry will be discussed.

The originators of direct quantitative histochemistry were Kai Linderstrøm-Lang and Heinz Holter, who made their beginning in the early 1930s. Their basic style is illustrated by a study of the localization of pepsin in the gastric mucosa (1). Serial frozen sections were cut from a tissue core. Alternate sections (100–200 μg wet weight) were analyzed for pepsin; intervening sections were stained to identify the cells present. Correlation between the distribution of pepsin and the several cell types permitted unequivocal assignment of this enzyme to the chief cells.

David Glick (2) and Alfred Pope were among the first to apply the original Lang–Holter methodology to the nervous system. Pope and associates studied the distribution of dipeptidase, for example, among the layers of the cerebral cortex (3). Although valuable information was obtained, it became evident that the original procedure had to be modified if it were to be applied generally, because adjacent sections in the nervous system may be very dissimilar in cellular composition. This is true for example of the retina; and in 1942 Anfinsen et al. reported a procedure which permitted histological appraisal of each retinal section prior to analysis (4). The sections were dried at −20°C over P_2O_5, usually at atmospheric pressure, and were then lightly stained to permit identification of the layers. The staining was carried out in a bland organic solvent (xylene) which did not inactivate any of three enzymes tested. In some cases, parts of the dry section were trimmed away to leave a more nearly homogeneous sample of the predominant retinal layer present. Because the sections were no longer uniform in volume, each piece was weighed on a microbalance before analysis. With this technique, Anfinsen was able to ascertain the distribution among the retinal layers of an enzyme [cholinesterase (5)] and a coenzyme (NAD) (6).

Since 1942, this general procedure has been progressively refined (7–9). Improvements have been required at all stages of the procedure: isolation of samples, measurement of sample size, chemical analysis.

Isolation of the Sample

In nearly all regions of the nervous system, a microtome section, even a few square millimeters in area, is only slightly less complicated than the brain as a whole. Therefore, the procedure proposed by Anfinsen et al. was modified to permit dissection of small structures out of frozen–dried sections under good visual control. It was found that if ice crystal artefacts were minimized by rapid freezing, and suitable lighting was provided, cell bodies, nuclei and other details were visible in frozen–dried sections without staining (Figs. 1 and 2). This removed the worry that stain or solvent might cause trouble. It was also found that drying was best carried out under vacuum at −35°C to −40°C, because at higher temperatures shrinkage occurred, and at lower temperatures drying time was unnecessarily prolonged. With razor blade splinters mounted on a flexible shaft, it proved to be remarkably easy to isolate, by free hand dissection, samples as small as 10 to 20 μm in diameter. This makes it possible to sample single cell bodies of all but perhaps the smallest sizes.

Pretreatment of the Tissue and Stability of Constituents

The elements of the nervous system are designed to respond rapidly to stimuli and injury. Therefore, in some cases what happens to the sample before analysis may be at least as important as the analysis itself. In the case of most enzymes, the history of the tissue prior to freezing is not critical. Exceptions are enzymes, such as glycogen phosphorylase, which exist in two forms that can be rapidly interconverted. For example, Breckenridge and Norman (10) found that phosphorylase *b* in mouse brain is maximally converted to the *a* form by a few seconds of ischemia.

In contrast to most enzymes, certain metabolites are profoundly influenced by the treatment prior to freezing. P-creatine, ATP, lactate, etc.

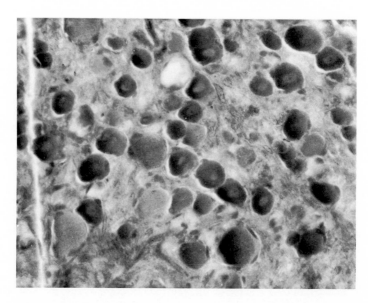

FIG. 1. Frozen–dried, unfixed, unstained 12 μm section of rabbit dorsal root ganglion.

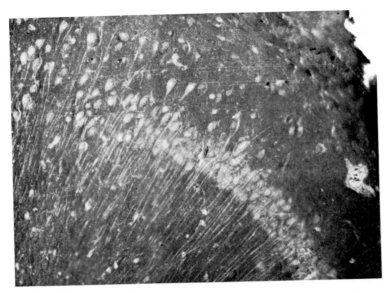

FIG. 2. Frozen-dried, unfixed, unstained 8 μm section of rabbit Ammon's horn.

are dramatically affected by anoxia or anesthesia. The point of the experiment may actually be to determine histochemical differences under different circumstances in the concentrations of constituents that are metabolically labile or affected by stimulation. The fact that heat conductivity is slow in tissues has made it difficult to assess the status of some of these materials in deeper lying structures of unanesthetized large animals. A problem for the future is to find ways around this difficulty.

The usual alternative to dissection from frozen–dried material, is to isolate samples from fresh material. There have been many microchemical studies of single cell bodies (for example) isolated in the fresh state for analysis. This may be satisfactory for stable enzymes, but seems risky for components that are responsive to the state of excitation or metabolic condition.[1]

Even after freezing, enzymatic changes can occur if the temperature is too high. For example, storage for an hour at $-20°C$ has been shown to result in a 20% loss of glucose-6-phosphate in mouse brain (9). Also certain enzymes may deteriorate in a few days at this temperature. In contrast, enzymes and metabolites appear to be indefinitely stable at $-70°C$ or below. Once tissue sections are lyophilized, stability is greatly increased. In dry sections, enzymes and labile metabolites have been shown to be stable for months or years at $-25°C$.

Measurement of Sample Size

The heterogeneity of the brain persists down to its smallest parts. From the histochemical point of view, a 100 μg sample from most parts of the mammalian brain is nearly as complicated as whole brain. Analyses begin to be rewarding with samples of the order of 10 μg (2 μg dry weight) obtained from discrete layers of structures such as the cerebellum. On the other hand, some nerve cell bodies have a dry mass 100,000 times less (0.1–0.2 ng). In each case some measure of sample size is required.

With the original Lang–Holter technique, each sample consisted of an entire microtome section, and its volume was known from its thickness and diameter. This volume provided the analytical basis. Fragments dissected as described above from a dry section vary in

---

[1] This is not meant to imply that there are no situations in which the isolation of cells or parts of cells in the fresh state is desirable. There have been many valuable experiments with surviving isolated nerve cells *in vitro*.

size, and must be measured individually. The volume itself has been used in special cases. This can be estimated from the section thickness and the area of the isolated fragment [measured for example by planimetry of the image projected through a microscope (7)]. Volume is, however, not a convenient or always reliable basis. (Although changes in volume during drying can be prevented, changes in thickness by compression during cutting may occur, particularly with thinner sections.) Initially, the size of the dissected dry samples was estimated from protein content; i.e., protein and some other substance were measured in the same sample (11). This complicated the analyses and was limited by the protein method then available to samples containing at least 1 μg of protein. A far more satisfactory basis has proven to be dry weight. It turned out to be exceedingly easy to measure the dry weight of samples as small as 0.01 μg, and not much harder to measure those as small as 100 pg

(0.0001 μg). The device used is a "fishpole" balance which is merely a fine quartz fiber mounted horizontally (Fig. 3). The sample is placed on the free end, and the resulting displacement is measured with a micrometer ocular in a low power microscope. In spite of its simplicity, this device far outperforms more elaborate balances, because it can be mounted in a very small chamber where air currents are manageable.

Originally, balances of this type were constructed with a small glass pan fastened to the free end on which the sample was placed (7). Later it was found that with samples smaller than 0.05 μg, a pan is unnecessary; surface forces are sufficient to hold the minute tissue fragment to the quartz fiber tip. Weighing is quick (perhaps 30 sec per sample), and accuracy to within 1 or 2% is routine. Because of its porosity, the dry tissue, on removal from vacuum, quickly equilibrates with room air to increase its weight (at 50% humidity) by 5%

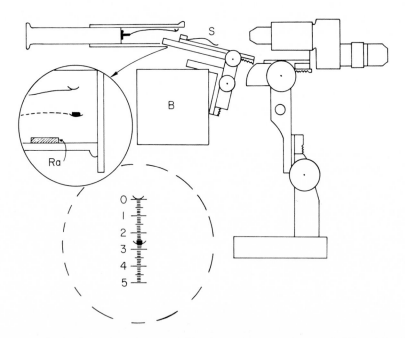

FIG. 3. Arrangement for loading and reading quartz fiber balance. The wooden sample holder is held by spring S to the double rack and pinion loading device shown (a modified stage micrometer). The loader is mounted on a 4 × 4 inch beam (B) which also provides a steady rest for the right hand with which samples are transferred to the balance tip. Transfers are supervised through the wide-angle microscope. The displacement of the balance tip is measured on the micrometer ocular in one eyepiece of the same microscope (see inset). The zero point is adjusted by means of the vertical rack and pinion of the microscope mount. The radium is to dispel static electricity. [Reproduced from Lowry and Passonneau (9).]

from adsorbed moisture and 2% from adsorbed O_2 and N_2.

Chemical Analysis

The major difficulty of quantitative neuro-histochemistry is clearly the analysis itself: to measure the minute amounts of material available, and to provide adequate specificity. The range of sensitivity required varies enormously according to sample size and substance measured. For example, a 5 μg dry sample from the molecular layer of the cerebellum has enough lactic dehydrogenase to produce 10^{-7} moles of pyruvate in an hour, whereas a 0.2 ng cell body may contain only 10^{-16} moles of pre-formed pyruvate—a billion times less.

Initially a variety of titrimetric (3,5) colorimetric, fluorometric, and manometric [Cartesian diver (6)] methods were applied in neurohistochemical studies. These methods did not seem easily adapted to the measurement of amounts of smaller than perhaps 10^{-11} moles (see below, however). Fortunately, an analytical methodology of more general applicability and almost unlimited sensitivity gradually evolved. This has practically displaced other methods in the author's laboratory. Specificity and generality are provided by the common practice of using enzymatic methods linked through one or more steps to a pyridine nucleotide indicator reaction.

Sensitivity is achieved by chemical amplification of the resultant reduced or oxidized NAD or NADP ("enzymatic cycling").

Typical Protocol

An example will illustrate how the system works. This example is taken from a study of the metabolic rate of mouse anterior horn cells, as compared to that of the surrounding neuropil, when stimulated by the shock of decapitation or inhibited by anesthesia (12). One of the components that had to be measured was ATP. The mice, appropriately pretreated, were quick frozen in Freon at $-150°C$. The spinal cords were sectioned (12 μm) at $-20°C$, lyophilized at $-35°C$, and the anterior horn cell bodies (actually their central 12 μm portions) dissected out free-hand and weighed (1–3 ng). (Similar sized samples of surrounding neuropil were also obtained and weighed.)

Each sample was now placed in a 0.01 μl droplet of 0.02 N NaOH, contained under mineral oil in one of 60 holes ("oil-wells") drilled in a Teflon block (about the dimensions of a triple thickness microscope slice, Fig. 4). After heating to destroy enzymes, 0.01 μl was added of a reagent containing all the components (except ATP) necessary to carry out the following sequential enzymatic reactions.

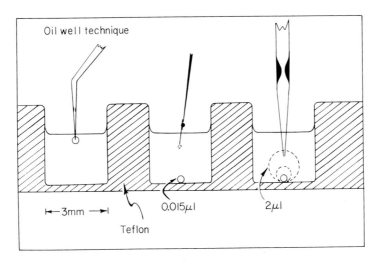

FIG. 4. The oil wells of an oil well rack, and steps in the analysis. A frozen–dried sample is being introduced in the middle well. The volumes indicated are arbitrary. [Reproduced from Lowry and Passonneau (9).]

$$\text{ATP} + \text{glucose} \longrightarrow \text{glucose-6-P} + \text{ADP}$$
$$\text{glucose-6-P} + \text{NADP}^+ \longrightarrow$$
$$\text{6-P-gluconate} + \text{NADPH}$$

After 30 min, when all of the ATP had reacted, the excess NADP^+ was destroyed by adding 0.05 μl of NaOH and heating to 80°C. This left NADPH (which is stable in alkali) equivalent to the original ATP (1 to 3×10^{-14} moles in the case of control cell bodies). This NADPH was then amplified by adding $5\mu l$ of reagent containing all of the components except NADP necessary to carry out the following enzymatic cyclic process:

$$\left.\begin{array}{l}\alpha\text{-ketoglutarate} \\ \text{NH}_4^+ \\ \text{glutamate}\end{array}\right) \left(\begin{array}{l}\text{NADPH} \\ \\ \text{NADP}^+\end{array}\right) \left(\begin{array}{l}\text{6-P-gluconate} \\ \\ \text{glucose-6-P}\end{array}\right.$$

After an hour, because of the high levels of the two enzymes (glutamic and glucose-6-P dehydrogenases) this cycle had gone around about 10,000 times, resulting in the formation of 10,000 molecules of 6-P-gluconate for each molecule of NADPH added.

The cycle was now stopped with heat and alkali and most of the sample (an exact 4 μl aliquot) transferred from the oil well to a fluorometer tube containing 1 ml of reagent with 6-P-gluconate dehydrogenase and an excess of NADP^+.

$$\text{6-P-gluconate} + \text{NADP}^+ \longrightarrow$$
$$\text{ribulose-5-P} + \text{CO}_2 + \text{NADPH}$$

There was now enough NADPH (1 to 3×10^{-10} moles from control cell bodies) to measure by fluorescence. The overall precision was 2 to 4% (standard deviation).

Some of the features of the analytical system may be pointed out.

Sensitivity

In the example given, NADPH was measured at the end by its fluorescence. This is because the fluorometer provides greater sensitivity than the spectrophotometer, by a factor of perhaps 100. (Sensitivity can be increased another 10-fold, if desired, by pretreatment of the NADPH with strong alkali and peroxide.)

More important is the fact that if sufficient amplification had not been achieved above, the cycling step could have been repeated (after destroying with alkali the excess NADP^+ of the last reaction shown). This would give up to 10,000 × 10,000 amplification, and provide sufficient sensitivity to measure 10^{-18} moles of starting material. This is the amount of cyclic AMP in a small cell body, or the amount of product produced by one average enzyme molecule in an hour. (Even a third cycling step would be possible, but it is hard to imagine that so much amplification would be useful at present.)

One might suppose that enzymatic cycling would increase the percentage error. Actually the reverse may be true. By specific amplification of the pyridine nucleotide, extraneous blank fluorescence from tissue or reagents becomes insignificant.

Generality of the Analytical System

There are few natural substances which cannot be linked to an NAD or NADP system. There are literally hundreds of enzymes and metabolites that have already been measured in pyridine-linked systems by biochemists in different fields. In many cases the necessary enzymes are available commercially.

An efficient cycling system is available for NAD (13) as well as for NADP. The cycles obviously do not distinguish between oxidized and reduced nucleotides. This does not matter because NADH and NADPH are unstable in acid but stable in alkali, whereas just the opposite is true for NAD^+ and NADP^+. The differences are remarkable. For example, at pH 2 and 25°C, NADH is 99.99% destroyed in 2 min, without detectable loss of NAD^+; conversely, at pH 13 and 60°C, NAD^+ is 99.99% destroyed in 5 min, without detectable loss of NADH. In consequence, whether the indicator reaction is an oxidation or a reduction, the excess *substrate* nucleotide can be selectively destroyed without detectable loss of the *product* nucleotide.

Volume Reduction

The final fluorometric measurement is made in a large volume, e.g., 1 ml. However, to utilize the high sensitivity of enzymatic cycling, it is necessary to carry out initial steps in much smaller volumes. Otherwise, reagent blank values become excessive. In the example given, the amounts of ATP were in the 10^{-14} mole range. In a volume of 100 μl this would mean concentrations in the order of 10^{-10} M, and meaningful assays would be hopeless. By conducting the first enzyme step in a 0.02 μl volume, concentrations were brought into the 10^{-6} M range, and precise measurements became possible.

Volume reduction presents two problems: precise volume measurement and prevention of evaporation. Fortunately the Lang–Levy constriction pipette [invented by Milton Levy (14) in Linderstrøm-Lang's laboratory] is capable of precise delivery of volumes as small as 0.0001 μl (7). Originally, reactions were carried out in micro test tubes. This is practical with volumes down to about 1 μl, but with smaller volumes, evaporation becomes too troublesome. A simple solution has been to work under mineral oil as described in the example [the "oil-well technique" (15)]. Each oil well serves as a test tube, evaporation is negligible, even with very small volumes, and when heated almost to 100°C. As many successive reagent additions as necessary can be carried out in the same well.

It was seen that the frozen dried sample is passed through the oil into the aqueous droplet (Fig. 4). This maneuver was tried at the suggestion of J.-E. Edström. Although the oil impreg-

nates the sample during passage, on contact with the aqueous droplet the oil is displaced and all of the tissue constituents become accessible to the reagent. This has been repeatedly confirmed with many enzymes (soluble and unsoluble), as well as metabolites and cofactors.

Illustrative Results

Three examples of the use of the system are presented. The first is a record of the levels of two enzymes in nucleus and cytoplasm of dorsal root ganglion cells of the rabbit (Fig. 5). The nucleus and two samples of the cytoplasm were analyzed in each case. Lines join samples from the same cell. In the case of isocitric acid dehydrogenase, the cytoplasm samples were lower in activity than the nucleus in all but one case. The reverse is true for P-fructokinase. Note that, particularly in the case of P-fructokinase, the rather large variation from cell to cell is shared by nucleus and cytoplasm.

The second illustration shows the distribution within dorsal root ganglion cell bodies of the enzyme which synthesizes NAD (Fig. 6). This enzyme which is usually regarded as confined to the nucleus is here shown to be concentrated in the periphery of the cell body. Note that the values represent the sum of preformed plus synthesized NAD, and when correction is made for preformed NAD (see figure legend), essentially zero NAD synthesis is found in the nucleus. Double enzymatic cycling was required to measure the low levels of NAD (see above).

The third illustration shows P-creatine values for anterior horn cell bodies and adjacent neuropil from four mice (Fig. 7). Larger samples from the whole anterior horn were also analyzed. Two mice were nonanesthetized, two were anesthetized with phenobarbital. All were decapitated. One anesthetized and one control were frozen immediately, the other two were frozen after 40 sec. In the zero time anesthetized mouse, P-creatine values were similar in cell bodies, neuropil and whole anterior horn, and in each of these areas P-creatine fell about 65% during the 40 sec of ischemia.

Other analyses showed that when mice are frozen without decapitation, the anterior horn P-creatine level is the same with and without anesthesia, and is equal to that shown here from the zero time anesthetized mouse. It is there-

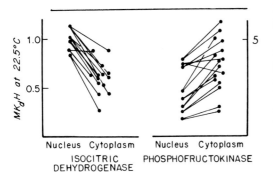

FIG. 5. Distribution of isocitric dehydrogenase and P-fructokinase between nucleus and cytoplasm of individual dorsal root ganglion cell bodies of the rabbit. Points for samples from the same cell body are connected to each other. The nuclear samples ranged from 0.2 to 1.2 ng dry weight, and produced 0.2 to 2 × 10^{-12} moles of product during the 1 hr incubation. Activity is recorded as moles per kg dry weight per hour. [Reproduced from Kato and Lowry (16).]

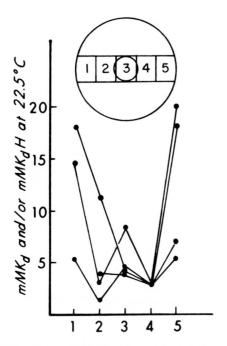

FIG. 6. Intracellular distribution of ATP–NMN adenylyltransferase activity in dorsal root ganglion cell bodies. Each cell body was trimmed to eliminate the cell membrane and a strip was dissected out along the axis through the center as shown in the diagram. The numbers on the abscissa indicate the position of pieces along the strip. (Number 3 is the nucleus.) The sum of DPN formed in 1 hr plus native DPN per kilogram dry weight is shown on the ordinate. Incubation volumes were 0.001 μl. The absolute amounts of DPN in each sample ranged from 2 to 20 $\times$ 10^{-15} moles. Native DPN alone averaged 3.1 mmole/kg in the nucleus and 2.3 mmole/kg in the cytoplasm. Therefore the nucleus itself was practically devoid of enzyme activity. [Reproduced from Kato and Lowry (16).]

fore assumed that the lower values for P-creatine in the zero time nonanesthetized mouse of Fig. 7 (as compared to the corresponding anesthetized animal) are due to the convulsion of the cord resulting from the transection. Freezing is not instantaneous, and appears to have allowed enough time for the intense neuronal activity to be reflected in a fall in P-creatine. It will be seen that the neuropil is most affected, the whole anterior horn less so, and the cell bodies least. By the end of 40 sec, P-creatine was practically zero in cell bodies as well as in the neuropil. Similar differences were observed for ATP, glucose, and glycogen (12), except that ATP and glycogen were little changed by ischemia in the

anesthetized mouse, and some ATP and glycogen were left after 40 sec of ischemia even in the neuropil of the nonanesthetized mouse. Our interpretation is that the intense neuronal activity (and sodium influx) causes much greater sodium pump activity *per unit volume* in the fine fibers of the neuropil (where there is a large relative surface area) than in the cell bodies.

OTHER WAYS OF ACHIEVING SENSITIVITY

In spite of (possibly biased?) personal preference for the analytical methodology described, there are other ways of achieving high sensitivity. There are also important constituents of the nervous system for which enzymatic pyridine nucleotide methods are not yet available. It is not possible to do justice here to all of the various other sensitive methods that have been developed. The following, however, should suffice to illustrate the different kinds of approaches. [Additional methods and details are described by Glick (8) and Osborne (17).]

It has been found possible to increase greatly the sensitivity of colorimetry and fluorometry by working with small volumes under a microscope. The extreme example is probably that of Rotman (18) who measured the activity of single β-galactosidase molecules with a fluorogenic substrate in droplets of about 10^{-6} μl volume dispersed under oil. The limit of measurement with reasonable accuracy was about 10^{-17} moles. Unfortunately, this method does not seem applicable to quantitative histochemistry. However, Galjaard et al. (19) with a less sensitive but more adaptable system have analyzed single frozen dried cells for several hydrolases with fluorogenic substrates. Measurements were made in capillary tubes with a microscope photometer. As little as 5×10^{-14} moles of the liberated fluorescent compound (methyl umbelliferone) could be measured with precision. Ornstein and Lehrer (20) described a spectrophotometric procedure of comparable sensitivity. The original sample in a volume of about 10^{-3} μl was caused to shrink to a volume of 10^{-6} μl with a resulting large increase in optical extinction. Edström and Hyden (21) developed a spectrophotometric method for measuring the base composition of RNA in single nerve cell bodies (10^{-12} mole range). The measurements are made directly on cellulose acetate fibers or strips on which the components had been separated by electrophoresis.

Giacobini (22) succeeded in measuring as little as 10^{-12} moles of CO_2 or O_2 with a micro-modification of the Cartesian diver and applied this to the study of single cell bodies.

Radiometric methods have also been developed and applied to neurohistochemical problems. For example, Buckley et al. (23) measured choline acetylase in single sympathetic ganglion cells by forming acetylcholine with radioactive acetate, and then coprecipitating the acetylcholine with added choline. Sensitivity was sufficient to measure the formation of about 5×10^{-13} moles acetylcholine. McCaman et al. (24) measured acetylcholine itself in single Aplysia neurons by enzymatically substituting radioactive phosphate for acetate. The phosphorylcholine was then separated from the precursor (^{32}P-labeled ATP) and counted; 2×10^{-12} moles of acetylcholine could be measured to about 10%. There are at present no suitable pyridine nucleotide linked enzyme methods for either choline acetylase or acetylcholine.

It is perhaps surprising that pyridine nucleotide linked enzyme methods plus enzymatic cycling are more sensitive than radiometric methods. In the case of ^{14}C there is an absolute limitation, imposed by the long half-life, which makes it difficult to measure much less than 10^{-12} moles of carrier free carbon. With ^{3}H and ^{35}S the limits would be roughly 10^{-14} and 10^{-15} moles, respectively. In the case of ^{32}P, the limit sensitivity would be more impressive: the order of 10^{-18} moles. Even here, serious practical problems may greatly restrict the sensitivity. (Note the relatively low sensitivity of the acetylcholine method above.) Although substantial increases in sensitivity of ^{32}P methods will be possible, it is necessary to separate precursor and product. This may be difficult with the small volumes that would be needed to measure the incorporation, for example, of 10^{-15} moles of ^{32}P.

A recently developed powerful analytical tool is the radioimmunoassay based on the principle of isotope dilution. Using iodinated tyrosyl-succinyl-cyclic GMP as marker, J. A. Ferrendelli (*personal communication*) succeeded in measuring as little as 5×10^{-15} moles of cyclic GMP in individual layers of mouse cerebellum (dissected from frozen–dried sections).

Mass spectrometry, particularly in combination with gas liquid chromatography, is another powerful and sensitive tool that will probably be increasingly applied in neurohistochemical studies. The theoretical sensitivity is exceedingly great, but at present it requires more material, by many orders of magnitude, for a practical quantitative analysis. It should in the future be possible to reduce this discrepancy. Abramson et al. (25) have in fact been able to carry out analyses of nervous tissue for a variety of biogenic amines and amino acids in amounts as small as 10^{-14} moles, and they discuss the possibility of increasing the sensitivity 1,000 fold.

Sensitivity is not the only consideration in choice of methods. In some situations, a colorimetric or fluorometric procedure may be preferable because it is *not* too specific. For example, it may be desirable to measure the distribution of total free amino acids. There are several reagents which produce highly fluorescent derivatives which can be measured *in toto,* or can be separated on a micro scale, to give at least an approximate measure of each of the free amino acids (17).

Comparison Between Quantitative and "Slide" Histochemistry

The maximum "resolution" of direct quantitative histochemistry at present is on the order of 5 μm. The limitation is the initial dissection rather than the analysis, since many substances, enzymes in particular, could be measured in samples as small as 1 μm in diameter. In any event, a resolution of 5 μm is far poorer than that of even the light microscope, let alone the electron microscope. Obviously, when serious artifacts can be avoided, the visualization approach has great advantage. Moreover, a single histochemically stained section may provide as many bits of information as a hundred chemical analyses.

What then does the quantitative approach have to offer? There are at least four things: (1) a high degree of specificity and quantitation, (2) capacity to measure substances present in low concentration, (3) freedom from fixation artifacts, (4) comparative freedom from diffusion problems. An example was given earlier of the measurement of changes in P-creatine and three other components of the energy reserve in cell bodies during ischemia. When the cord was stimulated by decapitation, these metabolites

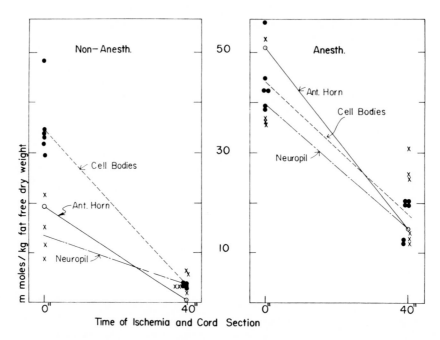

FIG. 7. P-creatine in anterior horn cell bodies, neuropil, and whole anterior horn of four mice. See text for details of pretreatment. Samples averaged 2 ng dry weight and contained 1 to 10×10^{-14} moles of P-creatine except for the lowest points. [Reproduced from Passonneau and Lowry (12).]

fell more slowly in the anterior horn cell bodies than in the surrounding neuropil. This would have been quite difficult to determine with staining histochemistry.

Ideally, visualization and quantitative histochemistry should be used to complement each other. The localization of lactic dehydrogenase might be pinpointed with fluorescent or radioactive antibody. Quantitative methods could give the exact average concentration of the enzyme, the proportion of M and H types, and the concentrations of the substrates and products: lactate, pyruvate, NAD^+, and NADH.

Perhaps the greatest future value of the quantitative histochemical approach to the nervous system may be (a) to validate (or invalidate) visualization histochemistry and (b) to determine local *changes:* rapid transient changes with activity, slower more permanent changes with maturation, adaptation, or learning.

CONCLUSION

Over the past 35 years, the classical quantitative histochemical methodology of Linderstrøm-

Lang and Holter has been adapted to the nervous system. In one current version, the *in vivo* state is preserved as far as possible by quick freezing; samples as small as 5 or 10 μm in diameter are isolated by dissection from frozen dried sections; pyridine nucleotide-linked enzymatic methods combined with enzymatic amplification permit measurement of a wide variety of enzyme activities, metabolites and cofactors in amounts as small as 10^{-16} to 10^{-17} moles. Many other kinds of analytical methods (colorimetric, fluorometric, volumetric, radiometric) have also been developed for neurohistochemical studies. Although somewhat less sensitive, they meet needs not yet met by the pyridine nucleotide methodology.

None of the quantitative histochemical procedures is capable of the high degree of localization possible with direct visualization by staining or radioautography. Nevertheless, in compensation for this deficiency, the quantitative methods supply several kinds of information that are not attainable at present by the visualization methods. Each approach can complement the other to provide a more complete picture of the chemical machinery of the nervous system—how it functions in health and why it may fail to function in disease.

ACKNOWLEDGMENTS

The research in the author's laboratory was supported in part by grants from the U.S. Public Health Service (NS-05221, NS-08862) and the American Cancer Society (P-78).

REFERENCES

1. Holter, H., and Linderstrøm-Lang, K. (1935): The distribution of pepsin the gastric mucosa of pigs. *C. R. Lab. Carlsberg. Ser. Chim.*, 20:1–32.
2. Glick, D. (1938): Cholinesterase and the theory of chemical mediation of nerve impulses. *J. Gen. Physiol.*, 21:431–438.
3. Pope, A. (1952): Quantitative distribution of dipeptidase and acetylcholine esterase in architechtonic layers of rat cerebral cortex. *J. Neurophysiol.*, 15:115–130.
4. Anfinsen, C. B., Lowry, O. H., and Hastings, A. B. (1942): The application of the freezing-drying technique to retinal histochemistry. *J. Cell. Comp. Physiol.*, 20:231–237.
5. Anfinsen, C. B. (1944): The distribution of cholinesterase in the bovine retina. *J. Biol. Chem.*, 152:267–278.
6. Anfinsen, C. B. (1944): The distribution of diphosphopyridine nucleotide in the bovine retina. *J. Biol. Chem.*, 152:279–284.
7. Lowry, O. H. (1953); The quantitative histochemistry of the brain. Histological sampling. *J. Histochem. Cytochem.*, 1:420–428.
8. Glick, D. (1961, 1963): *Quantitative Techniques of Histo- and Cytochemistry.* Vols. I and II. Interscience, New York.
9. Lowry, O. H. and Passonneau, J. V. (1972): *A Flexible System of Enzymatic Analysis.* Academic Press, New York.
10. Breckenridge, B. M., and Norman, J. H. (1962): Glycogen phosphorylase in brain. *J. Neurochem.*, 9:383–392.
11. Lowry, O. H. (1954): Quantitative histochemistry of the brain. I. Chemical Methods. *J. Biol. Chem.*, 207:1–17.
12. Passonneau, J. V., and Lowry, O. H. (1971): Metabolic flux in single neurons during ischemia and anesthesia. In: *Recent Advances in Quantitative Histo- and Cytochemistry,* edited by U. C. Dubach and U. Schmidt, pp. 198–212. Hans Huber, Bern.
13. Kato, T., Berger, S. J., Carter, J. A., and Lowry, O. H. (1973): An enzymatic cycling method for nicotinamide-adenine dinucleotide with malic and alcohol dehydrogenases. *Anal. Biochem.*, 53:86–97.
14. Levy, M. (1936): Studies on enzymatic histochemistry XVII. A micro Kjeldahl assay. *C. R. Lab. Carlsberg. Ser. Chim.*, 21:101–110.
15. Matschinsky, F. M., Passonneau, J. V., and Lowry, O. H. (1968): Quantitative histochemical analysis of glycolytic intermediates and cofactors with an oil well technique. *J. Histochem. Cytochem.*, 16:29–39.
16. Kato, T., and Lowry, O. H. (1973): Distribution of enzymes between nucleus and cytoplasm of single nerve cell bodies. *J. Biol. Chem.*, 248:2044–2048.
17. Osborne, N. N. (1974): *Microchemical Analysis of Nervous Tissue.* Pergamon Press, Oxford.
18. Rotman, B. (1961): Measurement of activity of single molecules of β-D-galactosidase. *Proc. Nat. Acad. Sci. USA*, 47:1981–1991.
19. Galjaard, H., Van Hoogstraten, J. J., De Josselin De Jong, J. E., and Mulder, M. P. (1974): Methodology of the quantitative cytochemical analysis of single or small numbers of cultured cells. *Histochem. J.*, 6:409–429.
20. Ornstein, L., and Lehrer, G. M. (1960): Shrinking droplet cuvette for analysis of microgram quantities of tissue and cellular substances. *J. Histochem. Cytochem.*, 8:311–312.
21. Edström, J.-E., and Hyden, H. (1954): Ribonucleotide analysis of individual nerve cells. *Nature*, 174:128–129.
22. Giacobini, E. (1959): Determination of cholinesterase in the cellular components of neurones. *Acta Physiol. Scand.* 45:311–327.
23. Buckley, G., Consolo, S., Giacobini, E., and McCaman, R. E. (1967): A micromethod for the determination of choline acetylase in individual cells. *Acta Physiol. Scand.*, 71:341–347.
24. McCaman, R. E., Weinreich, D., and Borys, H. (1973): Endogenous levels of acetylcholine and choline in individual neurons of Aplysia. *J. Neurochem.* 21:473–476.
25. Abramson, F. P., McCaman, M. W., and McCaman, R. E. (1974): Femtomole level of analysis of biogenic amines and amino acid using functional group mass spectrometry. *Anal. Biochem.* 57:482–499.

The Nervous System, Donald B. Tower, Editor-in-Chief. *Vol. 1: The Basic Neurosciences*. Raven Press, New York, 1975.

Integrity of Cell Functioning in Cerebral Subsystems

Henry McIlwain

The degree of functional activity that is now readily observable in biopsy samples and surviving tissues from the mammalian brain, would have been most unexpected to many workers 25 years ago.

It includes metabolic responses to electrical stimulation, observations of cell polarization and excitation, recording of electrical responses of individual cells and cell groups, and associated neurotransmitter output and action. In contributing to these developments, our own laboratories have interacted at two or three critical times with those of the NINCDS, and for this reason I am especially pleased to give on this occasion an indication of how these aspects of cerebral functioning have been displayed.

TYPES OF CEREBRAL ISOLATES

Cerebral subsystems adequate for the performance adumbrated form a recent stage in the wider subject of obtaining significant isolates from cerebral systems. Three main stages can be recognized in such endeavours (1). The *first* of these is the isolation of chemical compounds by the criteria of organic chemistry, a theme that began around 1800 and of which Thudichum is the most famous practitioner. The *second* of these broad categories is the isolation of entities which respond to simple organic chemical effectors. A pioneering example here is given by the cerebral dispersions devised by Peters and co-workers (2) on the basis of their response to thiamine. These contained relatively intact subcellular entities and led to early studies of the pyruvate oxidase complex and of mitochondrial oxidative phosphorylation.

Isolates responding to electrical excitation constitute a *third* category in which are represented some of the electrical as well as chemical phenomena of the brain. They were first devised

in the 1950s by the sequence of investigations outlined in Table 1. There was initially sought a cerebral subsystem which responded to convulsive and anticonvulsive agents. No responses were found in cerebral dispersions variously examined; sliced, cell-containing tissues responded to only one convulsant agent, electrical stimulation (3). The electrically stimulated tissues, however, then proved susceptible to anticonvulsants and to many depressant drugs. Responses initially observed were metabolic (4), and it was at this juncture that a fortunate invitation came to visit NINCDB for a period which it was possible, with the help of Donald Tower, to extend and transmute into a time of intensive electrophysiological laboratory work with the collaboration of Dr. Choh-Lu Li.

This gave the opportunity to display important aspects of the functional integrity of isolated tissues of the brain. Initially the neocortex was examined, and resting membrane potentials and spike discharges observed by intracellular micropipette electrodes (5). The potentials attained were investigated in numerous ways, and shown to be susceptible to modification by added cations, substrates, and pharmacological agents. Discovery of the variety of electrical phenomena observable in cerebral isolates, then proceeded by exploring a number of parts of the brain which could be obtained in a condition suitable for *in vitro* maintenance. The criteria for this were at first metabolic, ensuring adequate respiration and substrate utilization. It was found, for example, that conditions giving high respiratory rate did not necessarily maintain energy-rich intermediates, as adenosine triphosphate or phosphocreatine. Glutamic acid, in particular, depleted neocortical tissues of adenosine triphosphate, a depletion associated with entry of sodium ions, and probably the basis for glutamic acid and certain of its analogues acting as excitatory amino acids (6).

TABLE 1. *Selection of cerebral isolates that gave metabolic responses to electrical stimulation*[a]

Selection		
Among:	For:	Selection gave:
Metabolic characteristics maintained in isolation	Those changed *in vitro* by convulsants	Phosphocreatine, ATP, phosphate
Convulsive agents	Those causing change in phosphocreatine	Electrical stimulation (not convulsant drugs)
Metabolic responses	Others changed by electrical stimuli	Respiration with glucose, pyruvate
Tissue preparations	Those with respiration increased by electrical stimulation	Chopped or sliced tissue; not dispersions
Stimulating agents	Those giving responses most susceptible to anticonvulsants	Electrical stimulation (not dinitrophenol, KCl, diguanidines)

[a] Column 1 gives successive characteristics among which selection was made experimentally for the items of column 2; the results of the selections are given in column 3. Thus, the system finally chosen was of cerebral tissues prepared by slicing or chopping, electrically stimulated, and displaying response by changes in respiration, substrate utilization, and tissue phosphates. (1,3,8,17,18).

A SUBSYSTEM GIVING ELECTRICAL RESPONSES TO EXCITATION

The membrane potentials and spike discharges seen in isolated cerebral tissues gave expectation that they would be suitable for more detailed electrical studies, if an investigator could be found who was willing to examine the isolates of biochemical devising, which were then unorthodox material for electrophysiological study. Correspondence with Donald Tower and Choh-Lu Li was again productive — Dr. Chosaburo Yamamoto, a neurophysiological worker from Japan then finishing a visit to Bethesda, was encouraged to return to Japan by way of London and to spend a period here supported by the Medical Research Council.

Initial preparations from the brain of experimental animals showed regrettably little of the promised electrical activity. There ensued much discussion in which we, as biochemists, emphasized the need for rapid preparation of thin, fully oxygenated tissues, and Dr. Yamamoto emphasized the need for ensuring good neural input from a sizable incoming tract in carefully dissected specimens. Fortunately the guinea pig brain carried regions with which both sets of criteria could be fulfilled.

The first success came with the olfactory system (7), which Dr. Yamamoto had already investigated *in situ*. The structural basis for choice of the system had indeed been described in the guinea pig or rat by Cajal, many years earlier. In these species each lateral olfactory tract runs from its olfactory bulb to the piriform cortex while forming part of the surface of the olfactory lobe. It is easily visible as a white strand, about 12 mm long, 0.7 mm wide, and extending to a depth of 0.2 to 0.3 mm in the piriform cortex. It can thus be included, largely intact, in a tissue slice of 20 to 30 mg fresh weight, cut from the piriform cortex at a thickness of 0.35 mm.

This system, prepared from the guinea pig or rat, has proved versatile and dependable for both electrical and chemical studies (8). To prepare it, one or both of the piriform lobes are first obtained as blocks of tissue. From them, a narrow cutting blade and a guide with coverglass insert (8) for supporting the isolate during handling, enables it to be prepared with minimal trauma. A major value of the preparation as it is obtained from a guinea pig or rat is the facility which it offers for stimulation at the formerly anterior portion of the lateral olfactory tract, and observation of electrical responses at points 15 mm away. Conduction in the lateral olfactory tract and postsynaptic events in the surrounding cortex were characterized (7–9) using surface electrodes initially, and subsequently micropipette electrodes which penetrated the isolate to measured distances from its outer surface.

Unit cell firing was readily observed by the micropipette electrodes, and contributed to understanding surface-recorded responses. The isolate was susceptible to a number of neurohumoral agents and drugs. Metabolic responses also were obtained by stimulation of the lateral olfactory tract (l.o.t.), and metabolic responses greater in magnitude were afforded by field stimulation of the whole isolate; this gave a value for the proportion of tissue in the isolate which was activated from the tract. The l.o.t.-piriform cortical isolate has recently formed part of experiments examining potential neurotransmitters, and the variety of responses observable millimeter by millimeter at the surface of the cortex following stimulation of the tract, has

been correlated with anatomical knowledge of underlying structures (10).

OTHER CEREBRAL SUBSYSTEMS AND COMMENTS ON NEURAL ISOLATES

With the encouragement given by exploration of the l.o.t.-piriform cortical isolate, comparable study of several other parts of the brain has commenced. On his return to Japan Dr. Yamamoto, with Dr. Kawai, developed a means of following the input from an optic tract of the guinea pig through the lateral geniculate body to the superior colliculus. Again, a block of tissue was first dissected out, then a slice cut by a glass guide and narrow blade, with connections to an optic tract intact; an isolate of 20 to 25 mg was obtained in 2 to 3 min (11,12). Response at the geniculate and colliculus, to stimulation

TABLE 2. *Responses of isolated cerebral subsystems to electrical stimulation[a]*

Part of the brain	Electrical responses	Other observations
Subcortical white matter; corpus callosum	Conducted impulses	Rodent and human tissues examined; tract section
Lateral olfactory tract-piriform cortex	Pre- and postsynaptic in cortex; negative wave and unit discharges. Frequency-dependent attenuation; posttetanic potentiation	Actions of butobarbital, halothane, ether, scopamine, γ-aminobutyrate, chlorpromazine; output of norepinephrine, serotonin
Optic tract-superior colliculus	Pre- and postsynaptic in brachium and colliculus; negative spike and wave discharges with relatively long and variable latency and refractory period	Some spontaneous and glutamate-induced firing; action of lysergic acid diethylamide; output of serotonin and adenosine
Medulla	—	Metabolic responses
Hypothalamus	—	Actions of Li^+; ouabain, chlorpromazine; output of serotonin
Caudate nucleus	Action potentials modified by previous stimulation; by Ca^{2+}	Dopamine modified action potentials and cell-firing frequency; actions of phenoxybenzamine and methamphetamine
Corpus striatum	—	Actions of Li, tetrodotoxin
Hippocampus: dentate gyrus and associated structures	Negative spike and wave discharges. Rapid response from an electrically coupled synapse	Low-Cl media induces seizure discharges, propagated
Neocortex	Displacement and recovery of membrane potential; spike discharges; transmitted direct cortical response	With human tissues and neoplasms; induced gliosis; numerous drug interactions; release of several neurohumoral agents

[a] For further details and sources of data see the text and references (3,4,8,19–21). Preparations are derived from the rat or guinea pig unless otherwise specified.

at the optic tract was observed *in vitro* by surface electrodes, and also by micropipette electrodes within the superior colliculus. A postsynaptic field potential was suppressed by serotonin, and this action potentiated by lysergic acid diethylamide.

The dentate gyrus and hippocampus of the guinea pig have also afforded a suitable subsystem: taking first, as a block, the hippocampus with dentate gyrus, subiculum and presubiculum (13,14). Transverse sections of this block were made with a fine blade and microscopic observation, following the expected path of the mossy fibers. When maintained *in vitro* and stimulated at the granular cell layer, this subsystem displayed transmission by synapses between mossy fibers and hippocampal neurons.

Responses observed at a pyramidal cell layer were modified by the Mg^{2+} and Ca^{2+} of bathing fluids. Normally, stimulation at the dentate gyrus elicited a spike response and negative wave, but similar stimulation in fluids of diminished chloride content produced a train of afterdischarges of large amplitude, analogous to that of a seizure discharge.

Other isolated cerebral subsystems of which exploration is already yielding data are included in Table 2, which suggests that there is much scope for their further development. The relatively infrequent use made of such subsystems in pharmacological and neurotransmitter studies of the mammalian brain may be judged from a recent appraisal of the neurotransmitters associated with identified neurons there (15).

It is perhaps significant that electrophysiological study of isolated subsystems from the mammalian brain began with biochemical and neurochemical initiative: biochemically satisfactory experimental conditions are prerequisites. Also, biochemists are familiar with an isolate-oriented approach to living systems, which expects an investigator to demonstrate under as wide a range of conditions as possible, including quite simple conditions, any conclusions about chemical processes which he may from indirect evidence deduce are taking place *in vivo*. Thus, when thiamine lack was found to induce deficiencies in cerebral performance, and also the accumulation of lactic acid in the brain, examining isolates led to discovery of a defined coenzyme role for thiamine, increased understanding of carbohydrate metabolism of

the brain, and gave an indication of which parts of the brain were responsible for particular deficiencies in performance (1,2). Present-day neurochemists have perhaps inherited to a greater degree than others in the neurosciences the view transmitted by Sherrington (16) that "matter works itself," including the matter of the adequately supplied mammalian brain and of derived subsystems.

REFERENCES

1. McIlwain, H. (1975): Thudichum lecture: Cerebral isolates and neurochemical discovery. *Trans. Biochem. Soc.*, 3:579–590.
2. Gavrilescu, N., and Peters, R. A. (1931): An *in vitro* effect of antineuritic vitamin concentrates. *Biochem. J.*, 25:2150–61.
3. McIlwain, H. (1951): Metabolic response *in vitro* to electrical stimulation of sections of mammalian brain. *Biochem. J.*, 49:382–393.
4. McIlwain, H. (1956): Electrical influences and the speed of chemical change in the brain. *Physiol. Rev.*, 36:355–375.
5. Li, C-L., and McIlwain, H. (1957): Maintenance of resting membrane potentials in slices of mammalian cerebral cortex and other tissues *in vitro*. *J. Physiol. (Lond.)*, 139:178–190.
6. McIlwain, H., and Bachelard, H. S. (1971): *Biochemistry and the Central Nervous System*. Churchill-Livingstone, London.
7. Yamamoto, C., and McIlwain, H. (1966): Electrical activities within sections from the mammalian brain maintained in chemically-defined media *in vitro*. *J. Neurochem.*, 13:1333–1343.
8. McIlwain, H. (1975): *Practical Neurochemistry*, 2nd ed. Churchill-Livingstone, London.
9. Richards, C. D., and Sercombe, R. (1968): Electrical activity observed in guinea pig olfactory cortex maintained *in vitro*. *J. Physiol. (Lond.)*, 197:667–683.
10. Halliwell, J. V. (1975): Modifications *in vitro* of a synaptic pathway by low temperature. *J. Physiol. (Lond.)*, 245:97–98P.
11. Kawai, N., and Yamamoto, C. (1969): Effects of 5-hydroxytryptamine, LSD and related compound on electrical activities evoked *in vitro* in thin sections from the superior colliculus. *Int. J. Neuropharmacol.*, 8:437–449.
12. Heller, I. H., and McIlwain, H. (1973): Release of ^{14}C-adenine derivatives from isolated subsystems of the guinea pig brain: Actions of electrical stimulation and of papaverine. *Brain Res.*, 53:105–116.
13. Yamamoto, C. (1972): Intracellular study of seizure discharges elicited in thin hippocampal sections *in vitro*. *Exp. Neurol.*, 35:154–164.
14. Yamamoto, C. (1972): Activation of hippocampal neurons by mossy fibre stimulation in thin brain sections *in vitro*. *Exp. Brain Res.*, 14:423–435.

15. Tebecis, A. K. (1974): *Transmitters and Identified Neurous of the Mammalian Central Nervous System*. Bristol, Scientechnica.

16. Sherrington, C. S. (1940): *Man on His Nature*. University Press, Cambridge.

17. Anguiano, G., and McIlwain, H. (1951): Convulsive agents and the phosphates of the brain examined *in vitro*. *Br. J. Pharmacol.*, 6:448–453.

18. Greengard, O., and McIlwain, H. (1955): Anticonvulsants and the metabolism of separated mammalian cerebral tissues. *Biochem. J.*, 61:61–68.

19. Chase, T. N., Katz, R. I., and Kopin, I. J. (1969): Release of ^{3}H-serotonin from brain slices. *J. Neurochem.*, 16:607–615.

20. Katz, R. I., and Kopin, I. J. (1969): Release of norepinephrine and serotonin evoked from brain slices by electrical field stimulation. *Biochem. Pharmacol.*, 18:1935–1939.

21. McIlwain, H., and Snyder, S. H. (1970): Stimulation of piriform and neo-cortical tissues in an *in vitro* flow system: Metabolic properties and release of putative neurotransmitters. *J. Neurochem.*, 17:521–530.

The Nervous System, Donald B. Tower, Editor-in-Chief. *Vol. 1: The Basic Neurosciences.* Raven Press, New York, 1975.

GABA in Nervous System Function — An Overview

Eugene Roberts

Beginning in 1946, for a number of years I was interested in amino acid metabolism in normal and neoplastic tissues in experimental animals. At that time all of the measurements were made by laborious, and not always absolutely specific, microbiological assays. We were the first ones to apply two-dimensional paper chromatographic techniques to extracts of animal tissues for the examination of the distribution of free or easily extractable ninhydrin-reactive constituents. This was a great advance in our ability to study large numbers of samples and to detect tissue constituents for which micromethods previously were not available. Our observations showed that at a particular stage of development each tissue of a particular species, including the different types of blood cells, had a distribution of ninhydrin-reactive constituents that was characteristic for that tissue; whereas quite similar patterns of free amino acids are found in many different types of transplanted tumors in rodents (see ref. 1 for summary).

In the course of the above studies, relatively large amounts of an unidentified ninhydrin-reactive material were found in extracts of fresh mouse, rat, rabbit, guinea pig, human, frog, salamander, turtle, alligator, and chick brains. At most only traces of this material were found in a large number of extracts of many other normal and neoplastic tissues and in urine and blood. The unknown material was isolated from suitably prepared paper chromatograms and a study of the properties of the substance revealed it to be γ-aminobutyric acid (GABA) (2–4). An independent report of the occurrence of GABA in brain tissues was made by Awapara et al. (5). For several years this finding remained a biochemical curiosity and a physiological enigma. My continued efforts to convince neurophysiologists to test GABA on various preparations at the end of their planned experiments met with complete failure. In the first review on the subject (6), I concluded in desperation, "Perhaps the most difficult question to answer would be whether the presence in the gray matter of the central nervous system of uniquely high concentrations of γ-aminobutyric acid and the enzyme that forms it from glutamic acid has a direct or indirect connection to conduction of the nerve impulse in this tissue." However, later in that year, the first suggestion that GABA might have an inhibitory function in the vertebrate nervous system came from studies in which it was found that topically applied solutions of GABA exerted inhibitory effects on electrical activity in the brain (7,8). Then in 1957, the suggestion was made that GABA might have an inhibitory function in the central nervous system from studies with convulsant hydrazides (9,10). Also in 1957, definitive evidence for an inhibitory function for GABA at synapses came from studies that established GABA as the major factor in brain extracts responsible for the inhibitory action of these extracts on the crayfish stretch receptor system (11). Within a brief period, the activity in this field increased greatly so that the research being carried out ranged all the way from the study of the effects of GABA on ionic movements in single neurons to clinical evaluation of the role of the GABA system in epilepsy, schizophrenia, mental retardation, etc. This warranted the convocation of a memorable interdisciplinary conference in 1959 in which we were fortunate in having present most of the individuals who had a role in opening up this exciting field (12). Today there are many lines of evidence that make it seem probable that GABA is a major inhibitory neurotransmitter in the vertebrate central nervous system and in invertebrate central and peripheral nervous systems. On Feb. 17–20, 1975, a small conference was held, the purpose of which was to prepare a book in which the definitive observations made since the time of the previous conference would be given in detail and in which the individuals currently working on various aspects of GABA function or in closely related areas of neurosciences would give their impressions of the leading edges of the work in the field (13). It was hoped that in this way a book would be prepared that would serve a catalytic function in accelerating work in meaningful and possibly new directions.

METABOLISM

GABA is formed in the CNS of vertebrate organisms to a large extent from glutamic acid.[1] The reaction is catalyzed by an L-glutamic acid decarboxylase (GAD). For a number of years, it was assumed that there was only one GAD in the vertebrate organism and that it was located entirely in neurons in the CNS. With more sensitive methods, it was found that GAD activity can be detected in glial cells, kidney, heart, adrenal, and pituitary glands, and in blood vessels. The GAD from beef heart muscle now has been purified to a considerable extent and its properties are being explored in detail. We have purified to homogeneity a neuronal GAD from mouse brain (1). Since the purification was made from a starting material consisting of a crude mitochondrial centrifugal fraction from mouse brain rich in presynaptic endings, we judged this GAD to be largely synaptosomal in origin. It is a B_6-enzyme with a molecular weight of 85,000 and a sharp pH optimum at 7.0. It catalyzes the rapid α-decarboxylation only of L-glutamic acid of the naturally occurring amino acids, and to a very slight extent, that of L-aspartic acid. The physical chemical evidence suggests that GAD may be a hexamer consisting of 15,000 dalton subunits (16). It is highly sensitive to sulfhydryl reagents and study of the effects of a variety of inhibitors on the enzyme suggests minimally the presence of aldehyde, sulfhydryl, and positively charged groups (amino and probably imidazole) at or near the active site of the holoenzyme (17). It is of particular interest that Zn^{2+} was the most potent inhibitor of the 11 divalent cations tested, inhibiting to the extent of 50% at 10 μm. It is hoped that with further work we will be able to characterize

both the active site and to develop specific inhibitors for this enzyme that are not also active on a variety of other B_6 enzymes. Immunochemical studies with antibodies to the purified mouse brain GAD indicated that the rat brain enzyme is most closely related to the mouse enzyme, followed in order by human, rabbit, calf, guinea pig, quail, frog, and trout (18). Henceforth in this paper, when mention is made of GAD, it will be assumed that reference is being made to the neuronal GAD isolated from a synaptosomal preparation. Recent unpublished work in our laboratories indicates that there is a component with GAD activity in whole brain with a much higher molecular weight than the enzyme that already has been purified and that this enzyme possesses very different properties. Work is in progress on the purification of the high molecular weight component, and it remains for the future to determine whether or not it is similar to, or identical with, the GAD being purified from heart muscle (19). The latter enzyme already has been shown to be chemically and immunologically distinct from the synaptosomal GAD.

The reversible transamination of GABA with α-ketoglutarate is catalyzed by an aminotransferase, GABA-T, which in the CNS is found chiefly in the gray matter; but it also is found in other tissues. The products of the transaminase reaction are succinic semialdehyde and glutamic acid. A dehydrogenase is present in excess in brain tissue which catalyzes the oxidation of the succinic semialdehyde to succinic acid, which in turn can be oxidized by the reactions of the tricarboxylic acid cycle. We have succeeded in purifying GABA-T to homogeneity, and its properties are being studied in detail. The enzyme has a molecular weight of 109,-000, a pH optimum of 8.05, and can be split into two unequal subunits with molecular weights of 53,000 and 58,000, respectively (20,21). It is a sensitive sulfhydryl enzyme, being inhibited to the extent of 50% by *p*-chloromercuribenzoate at a concentration of 5×10^{-7} M. Of the keto acids tested, only α-ketoglutarate was an amino group acceptor. However, of a series of amino acids tested, β-alanine showed activity equal to that of GABA as substrate. δ-Aminovaleric and β-aminoisobutyric acids also are effective amino donors. Therefore, GABA-T may be important in several aspects of metabolism of ω-amino

---

[1] Surprisingly recent data indicate that the GABA in the small precursor pool for the formation of homocarnosine in brain probably arises largely from putrescine (14).

acids and not just related to the GABA system. Antibodies to mouse brain GABA-T were found to crossreact with the enzyme from human, calf, mouse, rat, guinea pig, rabbit, and frog (22). Microcomplement fixation tests showed that only the enzyme from rat brain may be very similar to the mouse brain enzyme in terms of protein structure. Accordingly this enzyme seems to be highly species specific.

Steady-state concentrations of GABA in various brain areas normally are governed by the GAD activity and not by the GABA-T. Both GAD and GABA are present in many inhibitory nerves and are distributed throughout the neuron, the GAD being somewhat more highly concentrated in the presynaptic endings than elsewhere. The GABA-T is contained in mitochondria of many neuronal regions, but it seems to be richer in the mitochondria of those neuronal sites onto which GABA might be liberated. Such regions would be expected to exist in perikarya, nerve endings, and dendrites that receive GABA inputs and possibly in the glial and endothelial cells that are in the vicinity of GABA synapses (23).

Recently it has become possible to visualize GAD (24–26) and GABA-T (*unpublished*) on sections of the central nervous system of rat and mouse at the light and electron microscopic levels, employing rabbit antisera to the purified mouse brain enzymes and peroxidase-labeling techniques. This has led to much more definitive data than were hitherto available through cell fractionation studies and, when coupled with similar procedures for enzymes that are rate-limiting in the biosynthesis of other transmitters, eventually could give detailed information of interrelationships of various neuronal systems at the ultrastructural level.

PHYSIOLOGY AND PHARMACOLOGY

There is evidence for presynaptic release of GABA. Stimulation of axons of several nerves inhibiting different lobster muscles was shown to result in the release of GABA in amounts related to the extent of stimulation, whereas stimulation of the excitatory nerve did not produce GABA release (27). Data showing the liberation of GABA on stimulation of specific inhibitory neurons in the vertebrate nervous system are extremely difficult to obtain, but there are many experiments that suggest this does take place (28–31).

An ionic basis of the inhibitory effect of GABA on the postsynaptic regions of vertebrate and invertebrate neurons is known, at least in some instances. Applied GABA alters the membrane conductance to chloride ions with the membrane potential staying near the resting level. GABA also has a presynaptic inhibitory action at the crayfish neuromuscular junction, imitating the action of the natural inhibitory transmitter by increasing permeability to chloride, thus decreasing the probability of release of quanta of excitatory transmitter (32). Recent evidence suggests that GABA also may be a transmitter mediating presynaptic inhibition in a number of regions in the vertebrate CNS (33) and that it acts by producing depolarization of primary afferent terminals. Although it originally was suggested that sodium may be the chief ion involved in the latter mechanism (34), recent data suggest the participation of the chloride ion, instead (35). At this juncture, the reader should be reminded that the key to the action of transmitter substances always lies in the nature of the changes they cause in the conformations of receptive membrane regions and in the consequences of these changes. It is, therefore, conceivable that instances may be found in which GABA may cause changes in permeability to ions other than chloride and that at some membrane sites the effects may be excitatory rather than inhibitory. Indeed, there is evidence suggesting that GABA may be the excitatory transmitter liberated from hair cells onto the first afferent neurons in the inner ear of the bullfrog and skate and in the lateral line canal organ of the toadfish (36). GABA also may be the excitatory sensory transmitter in the olfactory nerve of garfish and pike (37). However, the latter possibilities still must be subjected to rigorous physiological tests.

Detailed quantitative studies of GABA receptors from the physiological point of view have not been undertaken in vertebrate systems because of currently insurmountable technical difficulties. Employing more manageable invertebrate preparations, Hill plots with slopes of approximately two were obtained for GABA concentration-conductance change plots at the crayfish neuromuscular junction (38) and of approximately three for the membrane of locust muscle fibers (39). The latter data appear to be consistent with the interpretation the conductance change consequent to receptor activation is a cooperative phenomenon and occurs only after more than one molecule of GABA is bound to the active site. The above results would make it seem unlikely that simple analogues of GABA would turn out to be the most effective blockers of GABA action at postsynaptic sites. There is as yet no hint about the manner in which chemical or physical interaction of GABA with membranes produces increases in the chloride ion conductance of the membranes. A direct approach to the isolation of the GABA receptor has proven to be difficult because of the unavailability of a high affinity ligand, as α-bungarotoxin is for the nicotinic cholinergic receptors. The cessation of action of a synaptically active substance could be brought about by the removal of the substance from the sensitive sites by destruction, by transport, or by diffusion. In the case of GABA, it is likely that the active transport out of the synaptic gap is the major inactivating mechanism (23). This transport system has membrane binding sites for GABA that are extremely difficult to distinguish unequivocally from those that may be involved in GABA receptor function. Certainly all membrane fractions prepared either from invertebrate or vertebrate preparations contain both types of sites. In addition, there are GABA-metabolizing enzymes (GABA-T, homocarnosine synthetase, GABA transaminidase, etc.) which have affinities for GABA. Therefore numerous problems must be faced when GABA, itself, is used as ligand in studies of the physiological GABA receptor. Nevertheless three intrepid research groups have begun such studies of GABA receptors in cell free systems in crustacean (40) and mammalian nervous systems (41,42).

There is a vast amount of, as yet, poorly correlated data that purport to deal with the roles of GABA in the control of neuronal excitability and behavior in intact animals. Some of the reasons for the difficulties encountered at this level of analysis should be readily apparent to the reader from the preceding discussion. Often measurements of GABA levels of whole brain or of grossly dissected regions are correlated with global phenomena such as occurrence of convulsive seizures, susceptibility to electro-convulsive shock, EEG changes, etc. In line with experience with studies of other putative neurotransmitters such as the catecholamines, serotonin, and acetylcholine, measurements of levels of GABA generally are not functionally meaningful, since decreases or increases in total content may be attributable to many factors not relevant to use of GABA in informational transactions at synapses. Measurements of turnover rates of GABA in specific brain regions would be potentially much more meaningful and functionally significant. However, adequate techniques for performing this kind of measurement have not yet been developed. It is difficult to envision at this time how one could measure specifically the turnover rates of GABA in transmitter pools in specific regions of the brain or spinal cord. A number of the technical tools that are available in comparable studies with the catecholamines and serotonin are not applicable to GABA, which is made from ubiquitously occurring glutamic acid and which is metabolized extremely rapidly, yielding the common and nondescript metabolic products, CO_2 and H_2O.

The use of drugs in the manipulation of the GABA system to date has yielded no substances with the requisite degree of specificity to be able to reach more than very tentative conclusions. The first pharmacologically active compounds to have been studied in relation to the GABA system were the convulsant hydrazides, substances that inhibit GAD, GABA-T, and a host of other B_6 enzymes. These were first related to the GABA system because the hydrazides were shown to inhibit GAD. In some instances it was shown that there were correlations of the extent of lowering of GABA content and decrease of GAD activity in the brains of animals with the occurrence of convulsive states observed either electrographically or by observing overt convulsions. However, other experiments were performed that showed that decreases in GABA levels could be prevented, but that the convulsions attributable to hydrazides would occur nonetheless. It would, indeed, be surprising if there were a perfect correlation of the decrease in GABA content with the occurrence of seizures produced by the hydrazides, since these highly reactive substances can react with carbonyl and other groups present in many simple and complex molecules in tissues, inhibiting enzymes, altering connective tissue structure and permeability of blood vessels, and forming free radicals that can become alkylating agents. They can participate in the formation of a variety of derivatives, which themselves could have enzyme-inhibitory and pharmacological effects. (The degree of complexity of pharmacological action of these substances is illustrated in some detail in ref. 43.) The study of the properties of purified GAD has not yet led to a completely specific chemical inhibitor of the enzyme that could be used for depletion of GABA *in vivo,* but work is continuing in this direction. Antibodies to GAD could be the most specific inactivators of the enzyme, but to date the animals producing antibodies to the injected enzyme have not shown any symptoms at all, suggesting that the antibodies do not pass the blood-brain barrier. Employing various techniques now available for increasing permeability of the barrier to large molecules and/or direct administration of the antibodies into specific brain regions may prove to be of value in the subsequent pharmacological analysis of the GABA system.

Since the convulsants bicuculline and picrotoxin have been shown to have antagonistic effects to GABA on firing rates of neurons in various preparations (see ref. 44), it has become commonplace to infer the demonstration of GABA-mediated synapses in both vertebrate and invertebrate nervous systems on the basis of such effects. However, when conductance measurements were made, it became obvious that neither bicuculline nor picrotoxin is a competitive antagonist of GABA action on postsynaptic membranes at the crustacean neuromuscular junction (45,46). Actually, it appears more likely from current data that picrotoxin, and possibly bicuculline, might react with the anionophore rather than with the GABA receptor, itself. Probably GABA receptors and associated ionophores are closely coupled, but not identical entities. Bicuculline seems not to be antagonistic at all to GABA-induced conductance increases of the postsynaptic membrane of the slowly adapting stretch receptor neuron of the crayfish (47); nor does it block neurally evoked inhibition at the neuromuscular junction in the hermit crab (48), where applied GABA is active. Also,

bicuculline has been found both to antagonize and potentiate effects of GABA on cat cerebral cortical neurons (49).

To illustrate further the complexity of the situation, bicuculline and picrotoxin have been shown to act on the lobster giant axon in such a manner as to cause depolarization and a broadening of the action potential contour, an increase in excitability, and sometimes even repetitive firing (50). In addition bicuculline, but not picrotoxin, has been shown to be a moderately potent competitive inhibitor of brain acetylcholinesterase (51). It was suggested from the latter data and structural considerations that the physiological effect of bicuculline might be found in some instances to be more directly related to a function of the cholinergic system than to the GABA system *in vivo.* In keeping with the latter suggestion, it was found that bicuculline methochloride caused a marked increase in the excitatory effects of acetylcholine applied to neurons in rat brain (52). When seizures were produced in mice either by bicuculline or picrotoxin, brain acetylcholine levels were twice those found in saline-injected controls (53). The above results are obviously complex and seem unlikely to be interpretable on the basis of a single mechanism of action either of picrotoxin or of bicuculline. Obviously, when effects on firing rates of neurons are observed, nonsynaptic actions, as well as synaptic ones, must be considered. To my knowledge there have been no quantitative intracellular studies of GABA-bicuculline and picrotoxin antagonism on conductance changes in vertebrate neurons. Although there often is a close relationship between the generator potential and frequency of firing, it is well known that a variety of chemical and physical changes can produce a dissociation, or uncoupling, between the two. The above results with bicuculline and picrotoxin bring us face to face with the possibility that, at least in some instances, the bicuculline and picrotoxin may be acting at different neuronal membrane sites than those at which GABA exerts its effects. Thus, at this time it appears that a proven potent specific competitive antagonist to GABA at postsynaptic sites has yet to be discovered.

What will be necessary for the development of a rational pharmacology of the GABA system? First of all it is apparent from current work that there may be more than one type of GABA receptor complex (receptor + ionophore). Although GABA plays largely an inhibitory role in the vertebrate central nervous system, it also can play a depolarizing or excitatory one. From experience with other transmitters, it is likely that the nature of the receptor complexes at the sites on which GABA exerts different effects also will differ. Thus included in whatever test systems are used should be examples of sites on which GABA has both inhibitory and excitatory functions. It is quite conceivable that in some instances GABA receptors may be associated with cationophores and in others with anionophores. It is highly desirable to define by electrophysiological methods the nature of the changes in ionic conductance that GABA produces in a particular instance and to study in detail the characteristics of such changes. From a technical point of view, the latter type of information is much more readily obtained in invertebrate preparations than from studies in a vertebrate nervous system.

With a proper choice of the system it is possible to begin to look for antagonists and mimetics of the postsynaptic action of GABA. Sufficient work has already been done with compounds closely related in structure to GABA to indicate that it is unlikely that a simple structural alteration of the linear GABA molecule will yield highly active compounds. As alluded to previously, one should begin to consider molecular structures whose three dimensional configuration possibly will resemble two or three GABA molecules in different arrays, because possibly more than one GABA molecule may be required to trigger the cooperative activation of receptor sites. The butyrophenones, of which haloperidol is the best known example, are interesting in this connection, since most of these substances can be viewed as di-substituted GABA molecules. The possible interaction of cyclic GMP with GABA in the cerebellum and the GABA-enhancing effects of diazepam open new territory for pharmacological investigation of the GABA system (54–56).

From the point of view of therapy, it would be worthwhile to establish conditions by which it would be possible to enhance the inhibitory function of GABA in the nervous system in a variety of clinical conditions such as Huntington's disease (57,58), epilepsy, and schizophrenia (59,60), in which there are some possibilities that there are defects in key inhibitory elements either in the whole brain or in specific regions. However, the administration of GABA-mimetic substances that pass the blood-brain barrier might not prove to be a generally useful strategy, since GABA has been found to be active on membranes of neurons that may not have an input from GABA-releasing nerve endings. The nonspecific flooding of the CNS with such substances might produce chaotic results. An alternative strategy should be sought by which the effect of GABA liberated from nerve endings that normally use GABA as a transmitter could be amplified in pertinent synapses. Because GABA largely is inactivated at synapses by a mechanism that involves the binding of GABA to membranes and the subsequent transport of the GABA out of the synaptic junction, it would seem that substances that can retard the rate of uptake of GABA, while themselves having no GABA-mimetic or GABA-antagonist properties should be sought. This kind of action would be analogous to that proposed for the action of tricyclic antidepressants on catecholamines. Although hundreds of compounds have been tested as inhibitors of GABA uptake in test systems employing brain slices or subcellular particles,

---

→

FIG. 1. Light microscopy of GAD. **A:** Cerebellar cortex. Experimental section treated with rabbit anti-GAD serum: p, Purkinje cell somata; d, Purkinje cell dendrites; g, cerebellar glomerulus; b, basket cell contacting Purkinje cell somata; *long arrows,* GAD-positive terminals contacting Purkinje cell dendrites; *arrow heads,* GAD-positive terminals in molecular layer associated with undetermined structures; *short arrows,* GAD-positive terminals of Golgi type II cells on cerebellar glomerulus. **B:** Cerebellar cortex control section treated with nonimmune rabbit serum. p, Purkinje cell somata; M, molecular layer; G, granule cell layer. **C:** Nucleus interpositus (NI). Experimental section treated with rabbit anti-GAD antiserum; n, neuronal somata; d, dendrite; *short arrows,* GAD-positive terminals on dendrites of NI neurons; *long arrows,* GAD-positive Purkinje cell terminals contacting the somata of NI neurons. × 880.

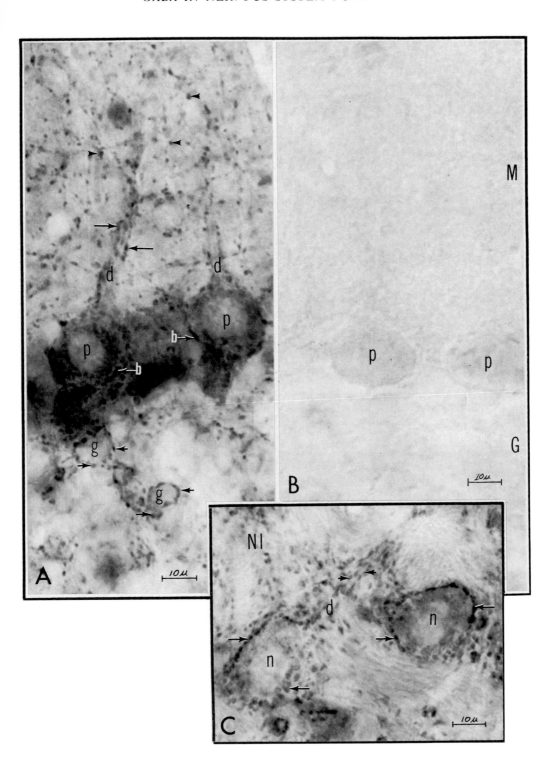

none has yet been found with an affinity approaching that required for such an agent. It is possible that the use of a combination of test systems *in vitro* for the uptake mechanism, employing brain subcellular particles and invertebrate preparations that allow quantitative measurements of responses of nerve membranes to known concentrations of GABA, could be used to approach the development of suitable drugs for use in this field.

TRACKING DOWN THE GABA NEURON

For many years it has been apparent to us that the definitive answers to the localization of GABA neurons only could come by use of immunocytochemical approaches. It was to this end that we purified synaptosomal GAD and obtained antibodies to it. We chose first to attempt to visualize GABA nerve endings in the cerebellum. Although by now the GABA system has been studied with varying degrees of thoroughness in almost every region of the vertebrate CNS, the cerebellum has been by far the most favorable site for investigation of possible substances, which may mediate the activity of neurons with inhibitory functions. More extensive correlative neuroanatomical and neurophysiological analyses have been made of the cerebellum than of any other structure in the vertebrate brain (23,61). The overall function of the cerebellar cortex probably is entirely inhibitory. The only output cells of the cerebellar cortex, the Purkinje cells, inhibit monosynaptically in Deiters' and intracerebellar nuclei. Cells that lie entirely in the cerebellar cortex—the basket, stellate, and Golgi type II cells—are believed to play inhibitory roles within the cerebellum. The basket cells make numerous powerful inhibitory synapses on the lower region of the somata of the Purkinje cells and on their basal processes, or preaxons. The superficial stellate cells form inhibitory synapses on the dendrites of Purkinje cells. The Golgi cells make inhibitory synapses on the dendrites of the granule cells. Afferent excitatory inputs reach the cerebellum by way of the climbing and mossy fibers, which excite the dendrites of the Purkinje and granule cells respectively. The latter are believed to be the only cells that lie entirely within the cerebellum that have an excitatory function. An afferent

inhibitory noradrenergic input is believed to reach the Purkinje cells from cells in the locus coeruleus (62). Even the first comprehensive biochemical laminar analyses of the GABA system suggested the possibility that all of the inhibitory cells of the cerebellum (Purkinje, basket, stellate, and Golgi) might use GABA as transmitter (23), and considerable subsequent experimental work has lent indirect support to this view. Now more direct evidence for the above supposition has come from the immunocytochemical localization of GAD in rat cerebellum, using antibody against the purified mouse brain enzyme. The location of the visualized endings is in complete agreement with the above earlier deductions. At the light level (Fig. 1), the enzyme was visualized in bouton-like punctate structures (24), whereas at the electron microscopic level (Fig. 2) the enzyme was found to be highly localized in certain synaptic terminals in close association with the membranes of synaptic vesicles and mitochondria but not within these organelles (25,26). Similar work is being carried out on spinal cord, hippocampus, retina, basal ganglia, and other regions of the CNS. However, in no instance have the functional relationships been worked out to the same extent as they have been in cerebellum, and, therefore, the immunocytochemical data would tend to have less precise value in terms of elucidating modes of information processing in other neural regions. The visualization of GABA endings in the cerebellum and the other structures cited already has opened new worlds for us. Much more sophisticated questions can be asked and answered by the immunocytochemical approach than by other available techniques. For example, it is interesting to know whether or not nerve terminals which are forming synapses have the transmitter-forming enzymes and, therefore, the potential capacity to synthesize neurotransmitters. If a developing presynaptic terminal has this capacity prior to the early stages of synaptic junction formation (protosynaptic stage), the possibility then exists that the passage of transmitter molecules or of the transmitter-forming enzyme, itself, to receptors on potential postsynaptic membranes might be part of a recognition process that allows for synaptic differentiation of contacts between specified cell types. If, on the other hand,

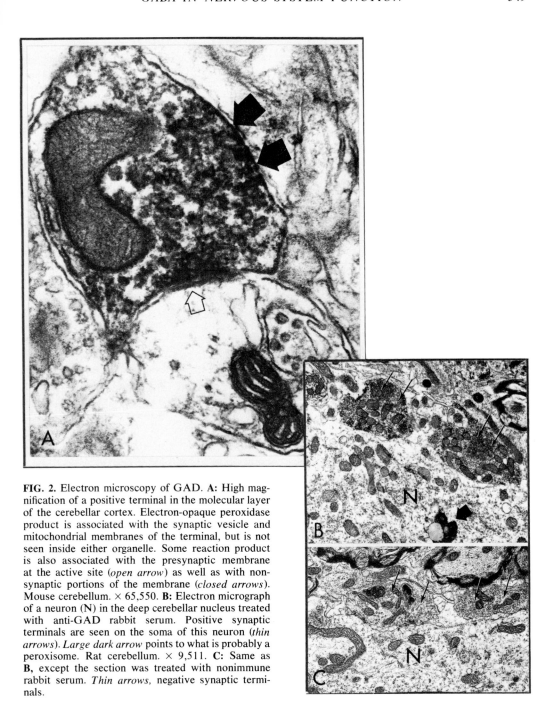

FIG. 2. Electron microscopy of GAD. A: High magnification of a positive terminal in the molecular layer of the cerebellar cortex. Electron-opaque peroxidase product is associated with the synaptic vesicle and mitochondrial membranes of the terminal, but is not seen inside either organelle. Some reaction product is also associated with the presynaptic membrane at the active site (*open arrow*) as well as with non-synaptic portions of the membrane (*closed arrows*). Mouse cerebellum. × 65,550. B: Electron micrograph of a neuron (N) in the deep cerebellar nucleus treated with anti-GAD rabbit serum. Positive synaptic terminals are seen on the soma of this neuron (*thin arrows*). *Large dark arrow* points to what is probably a peroxisome. Rat cerebellum. × 9,511. C: Same as B, except the section was treated with nonimmune rabbit serum. *Thin arrows*, negative synaptic terminals.

transmitter-synthesizing enzyme appears within a presynaptic terminal after a protosynaptic contact is formed, it is possible that the signal for enzyme synthesis may come from the postsynaptic element and that the transmitter enzyme or transmitter molecules may not play a role in synaptic recognition mechanisms. Applying the immunocytochemical method for localization of GAD in a study of developing rat cerebellum (26), we were able to show that

GAD is present in growing neurites in close association with small vesicles prior to the time the neurites make protosynaptic contacts, and that differentiation of these contacts results in a sequestering of GAD into synaptic terminals. The data indicate that the initial signal for GAD synthesis probably predates the establishment of contacts between pre- and postsynaptic elements of a developing synapse. It would be wonderful, indeed, if with antibodies to the GABA receptor in hand, it would be possible to determine when in the developmental sequence the appearance of the receptor takes place!

CONCLUSION

Elsewhere (59,60), I have presented a model of nervous system function that suggests that in behavioral sequences, innate or learned, genetically preprogrammed circuits are released to function at varying rates and in various combinations largely by the disinhibition of the pacesetter neurons whose activity is under the control of tonically active inhibitory command neurons, many of which may use GABA as transmitter. GABA neurons are envisioned to play a key role in nervous system function at all levels, from setting the gain on the sensitivity of sensory receptors to coordinating the function of the systems involved in perceptual integration and in reaching the decisions with regard to which neural circuits should be released for use at a particular time. For example, if in an individual there should be a paucity or defective function of horizontal inhibitory GABA neurons in layer IV of the motor cortex, this individual might be expected to be more susceptible than normal to occurrence of grand mal seizures. If such a problem should exist in the region of the globus pallidus or caudate nucleus, postural control would be expected to be defective. If the GABA system were inadequate in those regions of the hypothalamus dealing with food intake, hyperphagia or anorexia nervosa might result. If GABA neurons in the dorsal horn of the spinal cord were inadequately functional, there might be an inordinately great sensitivity to tactile and thermal stimulation and inadequate spatial and temporal discrimination of the stimuli. If there were a defect in GABA function in the retina, visual

perception and integration might be faulty.

The first known disease in which there appears to be a primary or secondary disturbance in function of the GABA system, Huntington's chorea (57,58), has been reported, and it has been suggested that also in other neurological and mental disorders there may be disturbances in GABA function (59,60). It appears that 25 years after the discovery of GABA as a constituent of rodent brain, in a figurative sense, we finally are "climbing out of the mud." With new tools for visualizing GABA neurons in normal and abnormal material and fine quantitative chemical and physiological test systems now available, it is hoped that the next few years will see greatly accelerated progress in both theoretical and practical aspects of "the GABA problem."

ACKNOWLEDGMENTS

This work was supported in part by USPHS Grants NB-01615 from the National Institute of Neurological Diseases and Blindness and MH-22438 from the National Institute of Mental Health; also in part by support from the Robert Anderson Research Fund.

REFERENCES

1. Roberts, E., and Simonsen, D. G. (1962): Free amino acids in animal tissue. In: *Amino Acid Pools,* edited by J. T. Holden, pp. 284–349. Elsevier, Amsterdam.
2. Roberts, E., and Frankel, S. (1950): γ-Aminobutyric acid in brain. *Fed. Proc.,* 9:219.
3. Roberts, E., and Frankel, S. (1950): γ-Aminobutyric acid in brain: its formation from glutamic acid. *J. Biol. Chem.,* 187:55–63.
4. Udenfriend, S. (1950): Identification of γ-aminobutyric acid in brain by the isotope derivative method. *J. Biol. Chem.,* 187:65–69.
5. Awapara, J., Landua, A. J., Fuerst, R., and Seale, B. (1950): Free γ-aminobutyric acid in brain. *J. Biol. Chem.,* 187:35–39.
6. Roberts, E. (1956): Formation and liberation of γ-aminobutyric acid in brain. In: *Progress in Neurobiology. 1. Neurochemistry,* edited by S. R. Korey and J. I. Nurnberger, pp. 11–25. Hoeber-Harper, New York.
7. Hayashi, T., and Nagai, K. (1956): Action of ω-amino acids on the motor cortex of higher animals, especially γ-amino-β-oxy-butyric acid as a real inhibitory principle in brain. *Internat. Physiol. Congr., 20th, Brussels, 1956. Abstracts of reviews; Abstracts of Communications,* p. 410.
8. Hayashi, T., and Suhara, R. (1956): Substances which produce epileptic seizures when applied

on the motor cortex of dogs, and substances which inhibit the seizure directly. *Internat. Physiol. Congr., 20th, Brussels, 1956. Abstracts of reviews; Abstracts of Communications*, p. 410.

9. Killam, K. F., and Bain, J. A. (1957): Convulsant hydrazides 1: *In vitro* and *in vivo* inhibition of vitamin B_6 enzymes by convulsant hydrazides. *J. Pharmacol. Exp. Ther.*, 119:255–262.

10. Killam, K. F. (1957): Convulsant hydrazides 2: Comparison of electrical changes and enzyme inhibition induced by the administration of thiosemicarbazide. *J. Pharmacol. Exp. Ther.*, 119:263–271.

11. Bazemore, A. W., Elliott, K. A. C., and Florey, E. (1957): Isolation of Factor I. *J. Neurochem.*, 1:334–339.

12. Roberts, E., Baxter, C. F., Van Harreveld, A., Wiersma, C. A. G., Adey, W. R., and Killam, K. F., editors (1960): *Inhibition in the Nervous System and Gamma-Aminobutyric Acid*. Pergamon Press, Oxford.

13. Roberts, E., Chase, T., and Tower, D. B., editors (1975): *GABA and Nervous System Function*. Raven Press, New York.

14. Nakajima, T., Kakimoto, Y., Tsuji, M., Konishi, H., and Sano, Y. (1974): Metabolism of polyamines in mammals-metabolic pathways of putrescine. *Bull. Jap. Neurochem. Soc.*, 13:174–177.

15. Wu, J. Y., Matsuda, T., and Roberts, E. (1973): Purification and characterization of glutamate decarboxylase from mouse brain. *J. Biol. Chem.*, 248:3029–3034.

16. Matsuda, T., Wu, J. Y., and Roberts, E. (1973): Electrophoresis of glutamic acid decarboxylase (EC 4.1.1.15) from mouse brain in sodium dodecyl sulfate polyacrylamide gels. *J. Neurochem.*, 21:167–172.

17. Wu, J. Y., and Roberts, E. (1974): Properties of brain L-glutamate decarboxylase: Inhibition studies. *J. Neurochem.*, 23:759–767.

18. Saito, K., Wu, J. Y., Matsuda, T., and Roberts, E. (1974): Immunochemical comparisons of vertebrate glutamic acid decarboxylase. *Brain Res.*, 65:277–285.

19. Wu, J. Y. (1975): Purification of L-glutamate decarboxylase from beef heart and its differences from the purified brain enzymes. *5th Int. Mtng. of the Int. Soc. Neurochem.*, Barcelona.

20. Schousboe, A., Wu, J. Y., and Roberts, E. (1973): Purification and characterization of the 4-aminobutyrate-2-ketoglutarate transaminase from mouse brain. *Biochemistry*, 12:2868–2873.

21. Schousboe, A., Wu, J. Y., and Roberts, E. (1974): Subunit structure and kinetic properties of 4-aminobutyrate-2-ketoglutarate transaminase purified from mouse brain. *J. Neurochem.*, 23:1189–1195.

22. Saito, K., Schousboe, A., Wu, J. Y., and Roberts, E. (1974): Some immunochemical properties and species specificity of GABA-α-ketoglutarate transaminase from mouse brain. *Brain Res.*, 65:287–296.

23. Roberts, E., and Kuriyama, K. (1968): Biochemical-biophysical correlations in studies of the γ-aminobutyric acid system. *Brain Res.*, 8:1–35.

24. Saito, K., Barber, R., Wu, J. Y., Matsuda, T., Roberts, E., and Vaughn, J. E. (1974): Immunohistochemical localization of glutamic acid decarboxylase in rat cerebellum. *Proc. Natl. Acad. Sci. USA*, 71:269–273.

25. McLaughlin, B. J., Wood, J. G., Saito, K., Barber, R., Vaughn, J. E., Roberts, E., and Wu, J. Y. (1974): The fine structural localization of glutamic decarboxylase in synaptic terminals of rodent cerebellum. *Brain Res.*, 76:377–391.

26. McLaughlin, B. J., Wood, J. G., Saito, K., Roberts, E., and Wu, J. Y. (1975): The fine structural localization of glutamic decarboxylase in developing axonal processes and presynaptic terminals of rodent cerebellum. *Brain Res.*, 85:355–371.

27. Otsuka, M. (1972): γ-Aminobutyric acid in the nervous system. In: *The Structure and Function of Nervous Tissue*, Vol. 4, edited by G. H. Bourne, pp. 249–289. Academic Press, New York.

28. Obata, K., and Takeda, K. (1969): Release of γ-aminobutyric acid into the fourth ventricle induced by stimulation of the cat's cerebellum. *J. Neurochem.*, 16:1043–1047.

29. Jasper, H. H., Khan, R. T., and Elliott, K. A. C. (1965): Amino acids released from the cerebral cortex in relation to its state of activation. *Science*, 147:1448–1449.

30. Mitchell, J. F., Neal, M. J., and Srinivasan, V. (1969): The release of amino-acids from electrically stimulated rat cerebral cortex slices. *Br. J. Pharmacol.*, 36:201–202P.

31. Bradford, H. F. (1970): Metabolic response of synaptosomes to electrical stimulation: release of amino acids. *Brain Res.*, 19:239–247.

32. Takeuchi, A., and Takeuchi, N. (1972): Actions of transmitter substances on the neuromuscular junctions of vertebrates and invertebrates. *Adv. Biophys.*, 3:45–95.

33. Krnjević, K. (1974): Chemical nature of synaptic transmission in vertebrates. *Physiol. Rev.*, 54:418–540.

34. Barker, J. L., and Nicoll, R. A. (1973): The pharmacology and ionic dependency of amino acid responses in the frog spinal cord. *J. Physiol. (Lond.)*, 228:259–277.

35. Nishi, S., Minota, S., and Karczmar, A. G. (1974): Primary afferent neurons: the ionic mechanism of GABA-mediated depolarization. *Neuropharmacol.*, 13:215–219.

36. Flock, Å., and Lam, D. M. K. (1974): Neurotransmitter synthesis in inner ear and lateral line sense organs. *Nature*, 249:142–144.

37. Roskoski, R., Jr., Ryan, L. D., and Diecke, F. J. D. (1974): γ-Aminobutyric acid synthesized in the olfactory nerve. *Nature*, 251:526–529.

38. Takeuchi, A., and Takeuchi, N. (1967): Anion permeability of the inhibitory post-synaptic

membrane of the crayfish neuromuscular junction. *J. Physiol.* (*Lond.*), 191:575–590.

39. Brookes, N., and Werman, R. (1973): The co-operativity of γ-aminobutyric acid action on the membrane of locust muscle fibers. *Mol. Pharmacol.*, 9:571–579.

40. Olsen, R. W., Lee, J., Wanderlich, K., and Reynard, M. (1974): Binding of gamma-aminobutyric acid to crustacean muscle membranes. *Fed. Proc.*, 33:1527.

41. Peck, E. J., Schaeffer, J. M., and Clark, J. H. (1973): γ-Aminobutyric acid, bicuculline, and post-synaptic binding sites. *Biochem. Biophys. Res. Commun.*, 52:394–400.

42. Zukin, S. R., Young, A. B., and Snyder, S. H. (1974): Gamma-aminobutyric acid binding to receptor sites in the rat central nervous system. *Proc. Natl. Acad. Sci. USA*, 71:4802–4807.

43. Roberts, E., Wein, J., and Simonsen, D. G. (1964): γ-Aminobutyric acid (GABA), vitamin B_6, and neuronal function – A speculative synthesis. *Vitamins Hormones*, 22:503–559.

44. Curtis, D. R., and Johnston, G. A. R. (1974): Amino acid transmitters in the mammalian central nervous system. *Ergebn. Physiol.*, 69:97–188.

45. Takeuchi, A., and Onodera, K. (1972): Effect of bicuculline on the GABA receptor of the crayfish neuromuscular junction. *Nature* [*New Biol.*], 236:55–56.

46. Takeuchi, A., and Takeuchi, N. (1969): A study of the action of picrotoxin on the inhibitory neuromuscular junction of the crayfish. *J. Physiol.* (*Lond.*), 205:377–391.

47. Swagel, M. W., Ikeda, K., and Roberts, E. (1973): Effects of GABA and bicuculline on conductance of crayfish abdominal stretch receptor. *Nature* [*New Biol.*], 244:180–181.

48. Earl, J., and Large, W. A. (1972): The effects of bicuculline, picrotoxin and strychnine on neuromuscular inhibition in hermit crabs. *J. Physiol.* (*Lond.*), 224:45–46P.

49. Straughan, D. W., Neal, M. J., Simmonds, M. A., Collins, G. G. S., and Hill, R. G. (1971): Evaluation of bicuculline as a GABA antagonist. *Nature*, 233:352–354.

50. Freeman, A. R. (1973): Electrophysiological analysis of the actions of strychnine, bicuculline and picrotoxin on the axonal membrane. *J. Neurobiol.*, 4:567–582.

51. Svenneby, G., and Roberts, E. (1973): Bicuculline and N-methylbicuculline – Competitive

inhibition of brain acetylcholinesterase. *J. Neurochem.*, 21:1025–1026.

52. Miller, J. J., and McLennan, H. (1974): The action of bicuculline upon acetylcholine-induced excitations of central neurones. *Neuropharmacology*, 13:785–787.

53. Svenneby, G., and Roberts, E. (1974): Elevated acetylcholine contents in mouse brain after treatment with bicuculline and picrotoxin. *J. Neurochem.*, 23:275–277.

54. Ferrendelli, J. A., Chang, M. M., and Kinscherf, D. A. (1974): Elevation of cyclic GMP levels in central nervous system by excitatory and inhibitory amino acids. *J. Neurochem.*, 22:535–540.

55. Mao, C. C., Guidotti, A., and Costa, E. (1974): The regulation of cyclic guanosine monophosphate in rat cerebellum: possible involvement of putative amino acid transmitters. *Brain Res.*, 79:510–514.

56. Mao, C. C., Guidotti, A., and Costa, E. (1975): Inhibition by diazepam of the tremor and the increase of cerebellar cGMP content elicited by harmaline. *Brain Res.*, 83:516–519.

57. Perry, T. L., Hansen, S., and Kloster, M. (1973): Huntington's chorea. Deficiency of γ-aminobutyric acid in brain. *N. Engl. J. Med.*, 288:337–342.

58. Bird, E. D. Mackay, A. V. P., Rayner, C. N., and Iversen, L. L. (1973): Reduced glutamic-acid-decarboxylase activity of post-mortem brain in Huntington's chorea. *Lancet*, 1090–1092.

59. Roberts, E. (1974): Disinhibition as an organizing principle in the nervous system – the role of gamma-aminobutyric acid. *Advances in Neurology, Vol. 5, Second Canadian-American Conference on Parkinson's Disease*, edited by F. H. McDowell and A. Barbeau, pp. 127–143. Raven Press, New York.

60. Roberts, E. (1972): An hypothesis suggesting that there is a defect in the GABA system in schizophrenia. *Neurosci. Res. Prog. Bull.*, 10:468–482.

61. Roberts, E., and Hammerschlag, R. (1972): Amino acid transmitters. In: *Basic Neurochemistry*, edited by R. W. Albers, G. J. Siegel, R. Katzman, and B. W. Agranoff, pp. 131–168. Little, Brown, Boston.

62. Bloom, F. E., and Hoffer, B. J. (1973): Norepinephrine as a central synaptic transmitter. In: *Frontiers in Catecholamine Research*, edited by E. Usdin and S. H. Snyder, pp. 637–642. Pergamon Press, New York.

The Nervous System, Donald B. Tower, Editor-in-Chief. *Vol. 1: The Basic Neurosciences*. Raven Press, New York, 1975.

Some Aspects of Aromatic Amino Acid Metabolism in the Brain, 1975

Gordon Guroff

The past 25 years have seen remarkable increases in the information available about the metabolism of amino acids in the brain and about the effects of amino acids in and out of the brain on brain function. Possibly the most striking progress has been made in the understanding of the role of the aromatic amino acids. This is due to a number of factors including the general fascination of these rather reactive molecules, the drawing together of capable investigators in biochemistry, pharmacology, and clinical medicine to focus on this area, the commercial interest in the biochemistry of these amino acids and their derivatives, and the remarkable properties of the amino acids themselves, especially those such as fluorescence, which lend themselves to sensitive and specific assay measurements.

It will be impossible, within the scope of this short chapter, to deal with the enormous explosion in research in this area. It is possible, however, to outline some of the roles of these amino acids which have been explored profitably and to underline some of the aspects of the biochemistry of these compounds which have been elucidated in the past two or three decades.

ASSAY TECHNIQUES

Initially, perhaps, it would be well to mention the development of assay methods for the amino acids themselves. Clearly, the properties of the amino acids lend themselves to accurate and sensitive measurements. After the development of the specific microbiological assays some methods were presented which took advantage of the unique spectral properties of the aromatics. For phenylalanine, the specific decarboxylation method (1) was followed by the fluorimetric ninhydrin assay (2), which then gave rise to the development of the very useful reagent known as Fluorescamine (3). For tyrosine the colorimetric nitrosonapthol method (4) was then made much more sensitive with a fluorimetric modification (5). And for tryptophan, methods involving the direct reading of fluorescence (6), or the even more sensitive measurements of the fluorescence of the harmine derivative (7), were published. Obviously, the use of the fluorescent properties of these amino acids has led to uniquely useful methodology. Either the posing of biological questions led to the development of methodology or the availability of methodology led to the search for biological questions.

AROMATIC AMINO ACID TRANSPORT

Although covered in detail in another chapter in this volume, it is probably appropriate to say a word or two here about the subject of amino acid transport as it specifically applies to the developments in aromatic amino acid biochemistry. Within the last 20 years it has become apparent that the uptake of amino acids into cells is indeed in the province of biochemistry. The process is known to be catalyzed by some enzyme-like entity on the cell surface, and is clearly specific and energy requiring. This is especially true of amino acid transport into the brain, where the transport systems are more active than in most of the other parts of the body. The work of Lajtha and his colleagues (8) has led to the recognition of some seven separate transport entities for amino acids in the brain and, while the detailed nature of these entities is not known as yet, the specificities of these sites has been delineated. One of them serves the large neutral amino acids, including the aromatics. It has been shown, using tyrosine as the model amino acid, that all the aromatics and some of their analogues are taken into the brain at the same site. Further, these aromatic amino acids compete with each other for entry, and with leucine, isoleucine, and valine as well (9–11). This transport process is known to be structurally and sterically selective and to require energy. Explorations in various laboratories have led to a quantitative picture of the transport system, as well as to an understanding of changes which occur during the development of the animal. Although the transport of amino acids into the brain does not appear to be rate-limiting for either metabolism or protein synthesis, as compared to the transport of glucose which is clearly rate-limiting for metabolism, the uptake of amino acids may very well be crucial to the health of the brain. Certainly, in some pathological states, to be discussed later, the large amounts of specific aromatic amino acids in the blood could restrict the entry of the other amino acids which share that particular site. It has been considered likely by some that this restriction plays a role in the pathological changes occurring in certain diseases of amino acid metabolism.

PHENYLALANINE HYDROXYLASE

Although the enzyme does not occur in brain, phenylalanine hydroxylase has assumed a significant place in the consideration of the chemistry of the brain because its absence, as in phenylketonuria, causes such a great disruption in neurological development and function. The enzyme itself has been studied extensively by Kaufman (12–14) and its mechanism of action, at least in gross outline, is understood. The system for the hydroxylation of phenylalanine in mammalian liver consists of the hydroxylase itself, an unconjugated pteridine cofactor (15), and a pyridine-nucleotide-linked reductase for recycling the pteridine cofactor (16). The hydroxylase from rat liver is a complex, iron-containing protein. It has an as yet uncertain quaternary structure and appears to be stimulated by certain phospholipids and by other specific proteins. The enzyme is a classical mono-oxygenase or hydroxylase requiring molecular oxygen as an oxidant and the tetrahydropteridine as a reductant. The enzyme uses one atom of the molecular oxygen to oxidize the substrate and reduces the second atom to water, using the reduced pteridine as the reductant. The addition of the hydroxyl group induces

the migration of the proton, or, in fact, the migration of some halogen or alkyl substituents, to the adjacent position on the aromatic ring in a reaction sequence which has been called the NIH shift (17). The tetrahydropteridine is truly a cofactor, being present in the liver in small amounts. The second enzyme in the system, dihydropteridine reductase, catalyzes the recycling of the oxidized cofactor using NADH as the ultimate source of electrons.

CONVERSION OF TYROSINE TO NOREPINEPHRINE

As mentioned above, phenylalanine hydroxylase does not occur in brain, although there is evidence that some phenylalanine hydroxylation does take place, catalyzed by other enzymes. Likewise, there is no evidence that the normal degradative pathway for phenylalanine, through tyrosine, hydroxyphenylpyruvic, and homogenistic acids to four-carbon acids, occurs in brain. On the other hand, the pathway of tyrosine metabolism to norepinephrine is present in neural tissue, and the elucidation of this pathway has been one of the most, if not the most, active areas of research in neurochemistry in the past several years. This pathway is of minor quantitative significance in the animal, constituting something on the order of 1% of the total tyrosine metabolism. However, it is the major pathway for tyrosine metabolism in brain and adrenal gland. The pathway, first postulated more than 35 years ago by Blaschko (18), has now been amply verified. This metabolism occurs in the nerve endings of the norepinephrine-containing neurons of the central nervous system, in the peripheral sympathetic nerves, and in the adrenal medulla, as well as in tumors originating in these tissues. Norepinephrine is thus thought to be a transmitter substance for certain neurons of the central nervous system as well as for the sympathetic peripheral system.

TYROSINE HYDROXYLASE

The first enzyme in the pathway, tyrosine hydroxylase, was the last one to be actually observed in the laboratory in cell-free form. For a number of years it was considered possible that the enzyme tyrosinase, which also makes DOPA from tyrosine, was responsible for the first step in the biosynthesis of norepinephrine. However, the distribution of this enzyme in the animal body was quite different than the distribution of norepinephrine. The clean observation of tyrosine hydroxylase by Nagatsu, Levitt, and Udenfriend in 1964 (19) resolved most of the questions. This enzyme is now known to be a mixed-function oxidase, superficially quite similar to phenylalanine hydroxylase in its mechanism of action. It occurs in adrenal gland, in midbrain, and in the

sympathetic nervous system. It uses a reduced pteridine as cofactor, and that cofactor has been identified as the same one that is present in rat liver to serve the phenylalanine hydroxylase, namely, tetrahydrobiopterin. The enzyme also requires molecular oxygen, probably contains ferrous iron, and has been shown to incorporate oxygen into the 3-position of the tyrosine ring (20). It is now clear that the tyrosine hydroxylase reaction is the rate-limiting step for the overall pathway. Further, and as a consequence, it is at this step that the pathway is regulated. The inhibition of the enzyme by catecholamines, including norepinephrine, indicates that the enzyme is under feedback control, and that the catecholamines control the rate of their own synthesis. The mode of inhibition of the enzyme by catecholamines is not clear, but the best data available indicates that the catecholamines compete with the reduced pteridine cofactor and thus cause inhibition (21). In any case, *in vitro* studies on the inhibition of the enzyme by norepinephrine are consistent with any number of studies *in vivo* in which the synthesis of norepinephrine from tyrosine, but not from DOPA, is known to be lowered when the tissue level of norepinephrine is raised. Such a situation can be caused by administration of inhibitors of enzymes involved in the degradation of the catecholamines. Tyrosine hydroxylase is also inhibited by phenylalanine because it uses phenylalanine as a substrate, hydroxylating the tyrosine formed in the meta position to form DOPA. The first observations on this unusual reaction (22) indicated that phenylalanine was a substrate, but a rather poor one compared with tyrosine itself. Further studies have shown that when tetrahydrobiopterin, the natural cofactor, is used instead of the commercially available synthetic 6,7-dimethyltetrahydropteridine, the properties of the enzyme change dramatically, and one of the most interesting of these alterations is the relative activity with phenylalanine as substrate. With the natural cofactor phenylalanine is as good a substrate as is tyrosine (23) for the adrenal enzyme. The enzyme has not been obtained in homogenous form and so a number of questions remain. It has been purified on acrylamide gels in such a way that single bands, presumably pure enzyme, can be used to prepare antibody (24). Such antibody is found not to cross-react with other hydroxylases from the same species, but to inhibit tyrosine hydroxylases from other species.

DOPA-DECARBOXYLASE

DOPA-decarboxylase, the second enzyme in the pathway, seems to be a typical amino acid decarboxylase acting on a large number of related substrates and requiring pyridoxal phosphate for its action. It is not restricted to the nervous system in its distribution, and appears to be in substantial excess of tyrosine hydroxylase in the appropriate sites, and is thus not thought to be a factor in the regulation of the

measurement of pH optima and subcellular distribution suggest that the activities, in brain at least, are on separate molecules (27). A resolution of this debate perhaps must await the complete purification of these activities from the brain.

DOPAMINE-β-HYDROXYLASE

The final step in this pathway is catalyzed by dopamine-β-hydroxylase. This enzyme is, of course, present in brain but has not been thoroughly studied in this tissue because of the difficulties in the assay, and because of the

synthesis of norepinephrine. Correspondingly, inhibitors of the enzyme are not too important pharmacologically since 95% inhibition does not change amine levels. The enzyme has been studied in a number of tissues, most exhaustively by Lovenberg, Weissbach, and Udenfriend (25), who purified the decarboxylase 50- to 100-fold from guinea pig kidney. The kidney enzyme decarboxylates a wide variety of substrates including DOPA, 5-hydroxytryptophan, and histidine. In fact, the enzyme is so non-specific that it has generally been termed "aromatic amino acid decarboxylase" instead of DOPA-decarboxylase. The concept that one enzyme serves in the pathways to both norepinephrine and serotonin, by virtue of its action on both DOPA and 5-hydroxytryptophan, has some substantial implications as far as the regulation and separation of these two important pathways is concerned. Recently, however, some dispute has arisen about the nature of the two activities in the brain, and whether, as in kidney, there is truly only one enzyme. Immunological evidence favors the concept that both activities reside on one protein (26), but some other data involving

presence of potent natural inhibitors. The corresponding enzyme from adrenal medulla has been extensively purified (28). It requires, for its action, molecular oxygen and ascorbic acid. The activity is markedly stimulated by fumaric acid, which is in some way an allosteric activator of the enzyme. Dopamine-β-hydroxylase has a molecular weight of 2.9×10^5 and contains 2 moles of Cu^{2+} per mole of enzyme. Recent work shows that there are four subunits of about 75,000 daltons each (29). The enzyme is a glycoprotein and can be purified by its interaction with the plant lectin, concanavalin A (30). The mechanism of action seems to involve a cyclic oxidation–reduction of the copper component, and the catalysis can apparently be described by a "ping-pong" type of sequential binding to the enzyme (31). The substrate specificity of dopamine-β-hydroxylase is not rigid, since a number of phenylethylamine derivatives will be hydroxylated. In fact, tyramine is a better substrate than dopamine. As a consequence, a number of materials act as competitive inhibitors of the enzyme. The enzyme is also inhibited by a number of copper chelators. One interesting naturally occurring inhibitor is fusaric acid (32). Since the enzyme is not normally rate-limiting for the synthesis of catecholamines, these inhibitors have limited pharmacological significance.

LOCALIZATION OF ENZYMES

Shortly after the early work on tyrosine hydroxylase, it was suggested that all the enzymes in the pathway of norepinephrine synthesis must be contained in a unique particle (33), the function of which would be the coordinated synthesis and movement through the neuron of the transmitter substance. This economical and attractive proposal seems not to represent the actual situation. The evidence against such a concept takes two forms. First, studies on the subcellular distribution of the three enzymes have shown that, although all three can be found in the terminals, only dopamine-β-hydroxylase is truly particle-bound. Tyrosine hydroxylase is found in a bimodal distribution, some being particle bound and some being soluble. The proportion of each depends somewhat on the method of preparation of the tissue. And DOPA-decarboxylase can be found completely in the soluble portion after fairly vigorous homogenization. Thus, dopamine-β-hydroxylase alone of the enzymes seems to be present in the particle which contains the transmitter, and this is consistent with its particle-bound localization in the adrenal gland. A second area of evidence has been the more recent studies on the axonal transport of the three enzymes. Clearly, if all three were in a single particle, they should all move down the axon at the same speed. Just as clearly this is not the case. Work from several laboratories (34–36), although differing a bit in the quantitative aspects of the result, consistently shows that dopamine-β-hydroxylase and the norepinephrine storage particles travel at a rapid rate, tyrosine hydroxylase at a somewhat slower rate, and DOPA-decarboxylase at an even slower rate. Thus, even though the proposal that all the enzymes were contained in the same particle proved not to be the case, the information generated while it was being investigated has added much to our knowledge of these enzymes.

REGULATION OF THE PATHWAY

There are several levels of regulation of the enzymes which synthesize norepinephrine and so any discussion must involve several different physiological conditions. First, in most species there is a developmental increase in the concentration of catecholamines and of the enzymes which synthesize them. This increase parallels the development of the sympathetic nervous system and has its morphological counterpart in the appearance of the catecholamine-containing nerve terminals, which, in most species, are not fully developed at birth. After the pathway is fully developed the regulation of the synthesis is, as mentioned before, at the first and rate-limiting step, tyrosine hydroxylase. The kinetic characteristics of the enzymes in the pathway are such that the K_m of the overall pathway is the K_m of tyrosine hydroxylase since the K_m of the other two are substantially higher. For example, the K_m of tyrosine hydroxylase for its substrate is on the order of 50 μM, the K_m of DOPA-decarboxylase is about 400 μM, and the K_m of dopamine-β-hydroxylase is about 6,000 μM. And since the plasma and tissue concentration of tyrosine is about 100 μM, tyrosine hydroxylase is generally saturated and the others are not. Thus, the rate of tyrosine conversion to norepinephrine is virtually independent of the blood concentration of tyrosine and depends on the activity of tyrosine hydroxylase alone, since as the rate of DOPA production increases the rates of action of the unsaturated DOPA-decarboxylase and dopamine-β-hydroxylase also increase. There are two ways, then, in which the needs of the body can result in an increase in the activity of tyrosine hydroxylase, and, thus, in the synthesis of norepinephrine. First, as mentioned before, the enzyme is subject to feedback inhibition by the end-product, norepinephrine. Stimuli which lower the level of norepinephrine in the nerve terminal instantly produce a rise in the rate of the synthesis of norepinephrine. So it is found that during sympathetic activity, when norepinephrine is liberated at the synapse, more norepinephrine is made from tyrosine. Stimulation of the sympathetic system results very quickly in a markedly increased norepinephrine synthesis from radioactive tyrosine. Conversely, inhibition of monoamine oxidase, which raises norepinephrine levels, decreases norepinephrine synthesis. When the level of tyrosine hydroxylase is measured *in vitro,* however, no increase is found, indicating that what has happened is probably a relief of the end-product inhibition normally present. Since there is no marked change in the overall level of norepinephrine observed, it must be that as sympathetic output increases during stimulation, the concentration of transmitter is maintained by increased synthesis. Thus, a persuasive argument can be made for the concept that the true state of the sympathetic nervous system can not be understood by static measurements of catecholamine levels but only by more complex studies involving the turnover of the sympathetic transmitters.

TRANSSYNAPTIC INDUCTION

More recently it has become clear that prolonged stimulation of sympathetic nerves can lead to an increase in the synthesis of the enzyme proteins in addition to an increase in the level of their activities. Specifically, it has been shown that the synthesis of the enzymes tyrosine hydroxylase and dopamine-β-hydroxylase, but not of DOPA-decarboxylase, is increased by prolonged demand upon the sympathetic nervous system (37). For example, a prolonged cold stress can increase the levels of these enzymes in the superior cervical ganglia. And since this induction can be prevented by decentralizing the ganglia, that is, by cutting the preganglionic cholinergic nerves, this increase in the synthesis of enzyme in the postganglionic neurons clearly depends on the activity of the preganglionic nerves. Since this process goes on in some way across the synapse, it has been termed transsynaptic induction. The exact mechanism of this induction is not known, but it is known that it plays a role in the maintenance of the normal levels of enzyme as well as in the increased levels during sympathetic nerve overactivity, since decentralization produces a fall in the normal levels of these enzymes in adult animals under normal conditions (38).

EFFECT OF NERVE GROWTH FACTOR

An interesting and intriguing development over the past few years has been the observa-

tion that the levels of the enzymes in the pathway to norepinephrine synthesis, at least in the peripheral nervous system, are influenced by the presence of the nerve growth factor. It has been shown that tyrosine hydroxylase and dopamine-β-hydroxylase, but again not DOPA-decarboxylase are specifically induced in the ganglia of young rats by injections of the purified nerve growth factor from mouse submaxillary gland (39). This induction is quite rapid and precedes the generalized growth of the sympathetic nervous system elicited by the nerve growth factor. The induction of tyrosine hydroxylase for instance, occurs within 24 hr and reaches a specific activity 3.5-fold above controls, whereas DOPA-decarboxylase and monoamine oxidase are increased in their total activity, due to the growth of tissue, but not in their specific activity. The induction is quite specific as shown by the failure to observe increases in the specific activity of DOPA-decarboxylase or the even more closely related dihydropteridine reductase (40). The reverse of this regulatory picture also seems to be true; that is, administration of the antibody to nerve growth factor appears to cause a selective decrease in the level of tyrosine hydroxylase before the generalized decrease in protein due to atrophy of the tissue. Whether such effects occur in the norepinephrine-containing neurons in the central nervous system is not known, as are very few of the implications of the nerve growth factor in the central nervous system.

CONVERSION OF TRYPTOPHAN TO SEROTONIN

The conversion of tryptophan to serotonin is a minor pathway in the whole animal, representing perhaps 1% of the total tryptophan metabolism of the body, but it is the major, if not the only, pathway of tryptophan metabolism in the brain. It is catalyzed by two enzymes, tryptophan-5-hydroxylase and 5-hydroxytryptophan decarboxylase. The first of these, tryptophan-5-hydroxylase is present in brain stem, pineal gland, mouse mast cells, and carcinoid tumor (41–43). The enzyme is a mixed-function oxidase, requiring tetrahydropteridine and molecular oxygen as do the tyrosine and phenylalanine hydroxylases. This enzyme is stimulated by high levels of mercaptoethanol

Tryptophan — Tryptophan hydroxylase → 5-Hydroxytryptophan

Tetrahydropteridine → Dihydropteridine

and by ferrous iron. In the case of tryptophan hydroxylase the exact pteridine cofactor present in tissues has not been identified formally. The enzyme is rate limiting for the production of serotonin; but, unlike the tyrosine hydroxylase, which is rate limiting for the synthesis of norepinephrine, tryptophan hydroxylase appears to have a high K_m and is not saturated under normal body conditions. The evidence for this is that elevations in the blood level of tryptophan leads to increases in the tissue content of serotonin. When assayed under optimal conditions the enzyme appears to be primarily in the soluble fraction of the cell. It is known to be localized to some extent in the synaptic portion of the neuron. Phenylalanine and catecholamines inhibit the activity of tryptophan hydroxylase. The latter observation indicates that there is a close relationship between the indole and the catechol pathways of amine formation. Serotonin has been found to repress the synthesis of the hydroxylase, indicating control at the level of synthesis of the enzyme as well as at the level of its activity. Further, prolonged cold stress raises the level of tryptophan hydroxylase in the brain and also raises serotonin concentrations, confirming that enzyme levels can be influenced by environmental alterations. Some initial comparative work aimed at a study of the properties of the brain and the pineal gland tryptophan hydroxylases has shown that the two enzymes are not identical.

The second enzyme, 5-hydroxytryptophan decarboxylase, is the typical, abundant, and ubiquitous aromatic amino acid decarboxylase discussed previously under the section relating to the decarboxylation of DOPA. As mentioned earlier, there has been general agreement for

the last several years that the enzyme in kidney at least was the same for both substrates. Just now, however, there has been some suggestion that, in the brain, which has not been inspected too closely in the past, there are two separate enzymes, one for 5-hydroxytryptophan and one for DOPA.

PTERIDINES

The developments in the hydroxylase field have been paralleled and even prompted by an increasing understanding of the importance and function of reduced, unconjugated pteridines in these hydroxylation reactions. The observations of Kaufman some 15 years ago on the cofactor for phenylalanine hydroxylase were the start of this important series of studies. The early finding that the hydroxylase could use tetrahydrofolic acid as cofactor led to the investigation of the activity of the simple unconjugated pteridines and culminated in the identification of L-erythro-tetrahydrobiopterin, specifically, as the cofactor present in rat liver (15). The further studies in this direction revealed that the quinoid dihydropteridine, among the possible dihydropteridine isomers, was the immediate oxidation product of tetrahydropteridine which was generated in the hydroxylation

L-erythro-Tetrahydrobiopterin

Quinonoid L-erythro-Dihydrobiopterin

reaction (44). These data eliminated folate reductase from consideration as an integral portion of the system since it has no activity against the quinoid form, and, further, detailed the action of the dihydropteridine reductase

5-Hydroxytryptophan — 5-Hydroxytryptophan Decarboxylase → Serotonin + CO_2

in the overall reaction. Thus, the pteridine involvement in the phenylalanine hydroxylase reaction has been quite clear for years. Upon purification of the tyrosine and the tryptophan hydroxylases, a requirement for reduced pteridine was also uncovered. The exact cofactor for the tyrosine hydroxylase in the adrenal is also tetrahydrobiopterin (45). There has been no corresponding study on tryptophan hydroxylase from any source, but it can be anticipated that the cofactor for this reaction in mammals will also be found to be tetrahydrobiopterin. The specificity of the phenylalanine hydroxylase for its cofactor has been studied, and it has been found that tetrahydrobiopterin is by far the most efficient cofactor (46) but that other reduced pteridines can be used as well and quite well. There is no information as yet on the details of the biosynthesis of the pteridine cofactor in mammals. It is an interesting problem for a number of reasons including the pharmacological possibilities for altering the rate of cofactor synthesis. Biochemically speaking, the synthesis of biopterin poses the additional problem of the construction of the methyl side chain, a problem which can not be attacked in the usual bacterial systems used for investigating pteridine biosynthesis, since biopterin has not been shown to occur in the bacteria in which pteridine biosynthesis has been studied. Although recent reports of pteridine biosynthesis in mammalian systems are available, there is none in which the details of the biosynthesis are spelled out.

The relative nonspecificity of the pteridine cofactors, i.e., the high efficiency of the synthetic cofactor 6,7-dimethyltetrahydropteridine, coupled with the difficulty of obtaining pure commercial biopterin, has led to some misconceptions about the actions of the enzymes which use pteridines as cofactors. It is now quite clear that the enzymes which use pteridines exhibit different properties with each of the different pteridines. Initially it was found that the stoichiometry of the hydroxylation reaction was different in the presence of different cofactors (47). Now we also know that the affinity for substrate (48) and for inhibitors (49) is different, in the presence of the natural cofactor from that in the presence of the synthetic. Many other properties of the enzymes change, among the most interesting being the substrate specificity. It has been shown that in the presence of the synthetic cofactor, phenylalanine is a substrate, but a very poor substrate for tyrosine hydroxylase (22). With tetrahydrobiopterin, however, the hydroxylation of phenylalanine to tyrosine proceeds at about the same rate as the hydroxylation of tyrosine to DOPA (23). This means that the direct conversion of phenylalanine to DOPA is an equal, if not preferred, route. In any case, three points should be made about these findings. First, all the data which have accumulated about the hydroxylase enzymes using the synthetic cofactor must be reexamined. Second, the new data probably will turn out to be more understandable in physiological terms. And third, the enzymatic and probably the physical properties of the enzymes change depending upon which of the cofactors is used.

INHIBITION BY *p*-CHLOROPHENYLALANINE

An interesting and useful series of observations have been made regarding an unusual inhibitor of some of the enzymes of aromatic amino acid metabolism. The inhibitor is *p*-chlorophenylalanine, investigated by Koe and Weissman in 1966 (50), and a subject of intense interest ever since. The source of the initial interest was the ability of this inhibitor to deplete brain serotonin almost completely within a few hours. It was quickly shown that the mechanism of this depletion was an inhibition of tryptophan hydroxylase (51). A concomitant inhibition of the liver phenylalanine hydroxylase was also noted (52), but other enzymes, even the closely related tyrosine hydroxylase, are unaffected. The acute behavioral effects of the compound are too complex a subject to be dealt with here, but suffice it to say that the lowering of brain serotonin levels seems to have rather subtle behavioral consequences which are not now fully understood or explored. The mechanism of the inhibition is also an unresolved question. It is known that the *in vivo* inhibition is of two kinds and probably of the same two kinds with both tryptophan and phenylalanine hydroxylases. First, there is a competitive inhibition which is reversible upon dialysis of the preparation (51,52). This lasts for some 6 to 12 hr after administration and can be mimicked by addition of the compound to preparations of the enzyme in the test tube. It is not surprising, in fact, that the compound is a competitive inhibitor since it has been shown that it is a substrate for the phenylalanine hydroxylase (53). After about 12 hr the inhibition, which is generally 80 to 90% effective, becomes irreversible, i.e., dialysis of the preparation made from brain or liver does not restore the activity. By this time little *p*-chlorophenylalanine is left in the tissue anyway, and so the irreversibility by dialysis is not too surprising. It is this irreversible inhibition which (a) cannot be duplicated in the test tube, and (b) cannot currently be explained by any known mechanism. It is known that the return of enzyme activity after several days is due to new enzyme synthesis since the administration of puromycin or of ethionine slows the return of activity (54). But the mechanism of the inhibition itself is unknown. There are published suggestions that the inhibition is due to incorporation of the analogue into the hydroxylase protein (55,56). At the moment, although a slight incorporation of the analogue into cellular protein is not unlikely, it does seem unlikely that such incorporation can explain the inhibition. There are several reasons for this and the reasoning is sometimes a little complex, but it seems clear that the rapidity of the inhibition, even considering the first several hours to be simple competitive inhibition, is incompatible with a mechanism involving incorporation into an enzyme with the turnover time of these hydroxylases. Further, since there is frequently 90% inhibition of activity, there would seem to be a requirement that 90% of the phenylalanines are replaced. And this also appears quite unlikely in view of the very poor incorporation found with this analogue and the general information about amino acid analogues. Nevertheless, until the true mechanism of action is discovered, no suggestion can be completely ruled out.

BEHAVIORAL ASPECTS OF HYDROXYLASE INHIBITION

One final area which has been explored to some extent in the past few years, and which impinges on the inhibitor studies described above, is the question of the effect of large amounts of amino acids on the chemistry of the brain. These questions are obviously motivated by the need to understand the mechanism of damage caused in humans by the high circulating levels of amino acids in certain metabolic disorders. The classic of these is of course phenylketonuria, and, indeed, most of the studies have involved administration of phenylalanine using various routes and various regimens. The earliest work was done by Waisman and his group (57–59) and involved the feeding of 5 or 7% phenylalanine in the diet of rats and monkeys. Although some learning deficits were produced by this means, it was clear from the later work of this group (60) that the animals were suffering from what amounted to intoxication with phenylalanine and that the behavioral problems which they manifested were merely a result of this adverse drug reaction. These behavioral problems disappeared upon removal of the drug and as a consequence had little resemblance to the irreversible damage caused by the clinical condition. Nevertheless, for both theoretical and medical reasons, many people have investigated the biochemical effects in animals of raising the blood levels of various amino acids, especially phenylalanine. For example, the effects of phenylalanine on brain polysome profiles, energy metabolism, cholesterol synthesis, and myelin formation have been studied. Also many experiments have been done on the influence of phenylalanine levels on indole metabolism, especially on serotonin synthesis.

The availability of the inhibitor *p*-chlorophenylalanine allowed the design of studies which were a bit more detailed in scope. Namely, using this inhibitor it was possible to inhibit phenylalanine hydroxylase and to raise phenylalanine levels as well. This manipulation creates a condition somewhat more reminiscent of the clinical state in that phenylalanine levels are raised while tyrosine levels remain normal. Andersen and Guroff (61,62), among others, have studied the effects of inhibiting the hydroxylase in young animals while raising blood phenylalanine levels. Summarizing these studies it seems reasonable to say that the condition in young animals resembles, but is not identical to, that in children with phenylketonuria with regard to their blood amino acid chemistry, their indole metabolism, their seizure threshold (63), and their neuropathology

(64). The chemical picture is not completely accurate since they do not excrete the classical unconjugated phenylalanine metabolites found in the urine of the children (65). In one crucial aspect, though, the model is an interesting one, and that is that the damage is irreversible after a certain point, as is the disease. Many months after the end of the treatment the rats are still hyperactive, still have learning difficulties, and still have neuropathological changes. Further exploration of this model, while perhaps not giving valid or exact information about the disease phenylketonuria, will possibly shed light on the mechanism of the changes caused by altered amino acid levels in young individuals.

REFERENCES

1. Udenfriend, S., and Cooper, J. R. (1953): Assay of L-phenylalanine as L-phenylethylamine after enzymatic decarboxylation: application to isotope studies. J. Biol. Chem., 203:953–960.
2. McCaman, M. W., and Robins, E. (1962): Fluorimetric method for the determination of phenylalanine in serum. J. Lab. Clin. Med., 59:885–890.
3. Udenfriend, S., Stein, S., Bohlen, P., Dairman, W., Leingruber, W., and Weigele, M. (1972): Fluorescamine: A reagent for assay of amino acids, peptides, proteins, and primary amines in the picomole range. Science, 178:871–872.
4. Udenfriend, S., and Cooper, J. R. (1952): The chemical estimation of tyrosine and tyramine. J. Biol. Chem., 196:227–233.
5. Waalkes, T. P., and Udenfriend, S. (1957): A fluorometric method for the estimation of tyrosine in plasma and tissues. J. Lab. Clin. Med., 50:733–736.
6. Duggan, D. E., and Udenfriend, S. (1956): The spectrophotofluorometric determination of tryptophan in plasma and of tryptophan and tyrosine in protein hydrolyzates. J. Biol. Chem., 223:313–319.
7. Hess, S. M., and Udenfriend, S. (1959): A fluorometric procedure for the measurement of tryptamine in tissues. J. Pharm. Exp. Therap., 127:175–177.
8. Cohen, S. R., and Lajtha, A. (1972): Amino acid transport. In: Handbook of Neurochemistry, edited by A. Lajtha, pp. 543–572, Volume 7, Chapter 21. Plenum Press, New York.
9. Chirigos, M. A., Greengard, P., and Udenfriend, S. (1960): Uptake of tyrosine by rat brain in vivo. J. Biol. Chem., 235:2075–2079.
10. Guroff, G., King, W., and Udenfriend, S. (1961): Tyrosine uptake by rat brain in vitro. J. Biol. Chem., 236:1773–1777.
11. Guroff, G., and Udenfriend, S. (1962): Studies on aromatic amino acid and uptake by rat brain in vivo. J. Biol. Chem., 237:803–806.

12. Kaufman, S. (1971): The phenylalanine hydroxylating system from mammalian liver. Advan. Enzymol., 35:245–319.
13. Kaufman, S., and Fisher, D. B. (1970): Purification and some physical properties of phenylalanine hydroxylase from rat liver. J. Biol. Chem., 245:4745–4750.
14. Fisher, D. B., Kirkwood, R., and Kaufman, S. (1972): Liver phenylalanine hydroxylase, an iron enzyme. J. Biol. Chem., 247:5161–5167.
15. Kaufman, S. (1963): The structure of the phenylalanine-hydroxylation cofactor. Proc. Natl. Acad. Sci. USA, 50:1085–1093.
16. Craine, J. E., Hall, E. S., and Kaufman, S. (1972): The isolation and characterization of dihydropteridine reductase from sheep liver J. Biol. Chem., 247:6082–6091.
17. Guroff, G., Daly, J. W., Jerina, D. M., Renson, J., Witkop, B., and Udenfriend, S. (1967): Hydroxylation-induced migration: The NIH shift. Science, 157:1524–1530.
18. Blashko, H. (1939): The specific action of L-dopa decarboxylase J. Physiol. (Lond.), 96:50–51P.
19. Nagatsu, T., Levitt, M., and Udenfriend, S. (1964): Tyrosine hydroxylase. The initial step in norepinephrine biosynthesis. J. Biol. Chem., 239: 2910–2917.
20. Daly, J., Levitt, M., Guroff, G., and Udenfriend, S. (1968): Isotope studies on the mechanism of action of adrenal tyrosine hydroxylase. Arch. Biochem. Biophys., 126:593–598.
21. Udenfriend, S., Zaltzman-Nirenberg, P., and Nagatsu, T. (1965): Inhibitors of purified beef adrenal tyrosine hydroxylase. Biochem. Pharmacol., 14:837–845.
22. Ikeda, M., Levitt, M., and Udenfriend, S. (1965): Hydroxylation of phenylalanine by purified preparations of adrenal or brain tyrosine hydroxylase. Biochem. Biophys. Res. Commun., 18:482–488.
23. Shiman, R., Akino, M., and Kaufman, S. (1971): Solubilization and partial purification of tyrosine hydroxylase from bovine adrenal medulla. J. Biol. Chem., 246:1330–1340.
24. Lloyd, T., and Kaufman, S. (1973): Production of antibodies to bovine adrenal tyrosine hydroxylase: Cross-reactivity studies with other pterindependent hydroxylases. Mol. Pharm., 9:438–444.
25. Lovenberg, W., Weissbach, H., and Udenfriend, S. (1962): Aromatic L-amino acid decarboxylase. J. Biol. Chem., 237:89–93.
26. Christenson, J. G., Dairman, W., and Udenfriend, S. (1972): On the identity of DOPA decarboxylase and 5-hydroxytryptophan decarboxylase. Proc. Natl. Acad. Sci. USA, 69:343–347.
27. Sims, K. L., Davis, G. A., and Bloom, F. E. (1973): Activities of 3,4-dihydroxy-L-phenylalanine and 5-hydroxy-L-tryptophan decarboxylases in rat brain: Assay characteristics and distribution. J. Neurochem., 20:449–464.
28. Friedman, S., and Kaufman, S. (1965): 3,4-Dihydroxyphenylethylamine β-hydroxylase. J. Biol. Chem., 240:4763–4773.

29. Wallace, E. F., Krantz, M. J., and Lovenberg, W. (1973): Dopamine β-hydroxylase: a tetrameric glycoprotein. *Proc. Natl. Acad. Sci. USA*, 70: 2253–2255.

30. Wallace, E. F., and Lovenberg, W. (1974): Studies on the carbohydrate moiety of dopamine β-hydroxylase: Interaction of the enzyme with concanavalin A. *Proc. Natl. Acad. Sci. USA*, 71:3217–3220.

31. Goldstein, M., Joh, T. H., and Garvey, T. Q. (1968): Kinetic studies on the enzymatic dopamine β-hydroxylase reaction. *Biochemistry*, 7: 2724–2730.

32. Nagatsu, T., Hidaka, H., Kuzuya, H., and Takeya, K. (1970): Inhibition of dopamine β-hydroxylase by fusaric acid (5-butylpicolinic acid) *in vitro* and *in vivo*. *Biochem. Pharmacol.*, 19:35–83.

33. Udenfriend, S. (1966): Biosynthesis of the sympathetic neurotransmitter, norepinephrine. *Harvey Lectures*, 60:57–83.

34. Oesch, F., Otten, U., and Thoenen, H. (1973): Relationship between the rate of axoplasmic transport and subcellular distribution of enzymes involved in the synthesis of norepinephrine. *J. Neurochem.*, 20:1691–1706.

35. Wooten, G. F., and Coyle, J. T. (1973): Axonal transport of catecholamine synthesizing and metabolizing enzymes. *J. Neurochem.*, 20:1361–1371.

36. Dairman, W., Geffen, L., and Marchelle, M. (1973): Axoplasmic transport of aromatic L-amino acid decarboxylase (EC 4.1.1.26) and dopamine β-hydroxylase (EC 1.14.2.1) in rat sciatic nerve. *J. Neurochem.*, 20:1617–1623.

37. Thoenen, H. (1972): Comparison between the effect of neuronal activity and nerve growth factor on the enzymes involved in the synthesis of norepinephrine. *Pharmacol. Rev.*, 24:255–267.

38. Hendry, I. A., Iversen, L. L., and Black, I. B. (1973): A comparison of the neural regulation of tyrosine hydroxylase activity in sympathetic ganglia of adult mice and rats. *J. Neurochem.*, 20:1683–1689.

39. Thoenen, H., Angeletti, P. U., Levi-Montalcini, R., and Kettler, R. (1971): Selective induction by nerve growth factor of tyrosne hydroxylase and dopamine β-hydroxylase in the rat superior cervical ganglia. *Proc. Natl. Acad. Sci. USA*, 68:1598–1602.

40. Nikodijevic, B., Yu, M.-Y., and Guroff, G. (1975): *unpublished*.

41. Grahame-Smith, D. G. (1964): Tryptophan hydroxylation in brain. *Biochem. Biophys. Res. Commun.*, 16:586–592.

42. Hosada, S., and Glick, D. (1966): Studies in histochemistry LXXIX Properties of tryptophan hydroxylase from neoplastic murine mast cells. *J. Biochem.*, 241:192–196.

43. Lovenberg, W., Jequier, E., and Sjoerdsma, A. (1967): Tryptophan hydroxylation: Measurement in pineal gland, brainstem, and carcinoid tumor. *Science*, 155:217–219.

44. Kaufman, S. (1964): Studies on the structure of the primary oxidation product formed from tetrahydropteridines during phenylalanine hydroxylation. *J. Biol. Chem.*, 239:332–338.

45. Lloyd, T., and Weiner, N. (1971): Isolation and characterization of a tyrosine hydroxylase cofactor from bovine adrenal medulla. *Mol. Pharmacol.*, 7:569–580.

46. Osanai, M., and Rembold, H. (1971): Cofactor specificity of L-erythrotetrahydrobiopterin for rat liver phenylalanine 4-hydroxylase. *Hoppe-Seyler's Z. Physiol. Chem.*, 352:1359–1362.

47. Storm, C. B., and Kaufman, S. (1968): The effect of variation of cofactor and substrate structure on the action of phenylalanine hydroxylase. *Biochem. Biophys. Res. Commun.*, 32:788–793.

48. Kaufman, S. (1970): A protein that stimulates rat liver phenylalanine hydroxylase. *J. Biol. Chem.*, 245:4751–4759.

49. Ayling, J. E., and Helfand, G. D. (1974): Inhibition of phenylalanine hydroxylase by p-chlorophenylalanine: Dependence on cofactor structure. *Biochem. Biophys. Res. Commun.*, 61:360–366.

50. Koe, B. K., and Weissman, A. (1966): p-Chlorophenylalanine: a specific depletor of brain serotonin. *J. Pharmacol. Exp. Ther.*, 154:499–516.

51. Jequier, E., Lovenberg, W., and Sjoerdsma, A. (1967): Tryptophan hydroxylase inhibition: The mechanism by which p-chlorophenylalanine depletes rat brain serotonin. *Mol. Pharmacol.*, 3:274–278.

52. Lipton, M. A., Gordon, R., Guroff, G., and Udenfriend, S. (1967): p-Chlorophenylalanine-induced chemical manifestations of phenylketonuria in rats. *Science*, 156:248–250.

53. Guroff, G., Kondo, K., and Daly, J. (1966): The production of m-chlorotyrosine from p-chlorophenylalanine by phenylalanine hydroxylase. *Biochem. Biophys. Res. Commun.*, 25:622–628.

54. Guroff, G. (1969): Irreversible *in vivo* inhibition of rat liver phenylalanine hydroxylase by p-chlorophenylalanine. *Arch. Biochem. Biophys.*, 134: 610–611.

55. Gal, E. M., Roggeveen, A. E., and Millard, S. (1970): DL-[2-¹⁴C]p-chlorophenylalanine as an inhibitor of tryptophan 5-hydroxylase. *J. Neurochem.*, 17:1221–1235.

56. Gal, E. M., and Millard, S. A. (1971): The mechanism of inhibition of hydroxylases in vivo by p-chlorophenylalanine: the effect of cycloheximide. *Biochim. Biophys. Acta*, 227:32–41.

57. Auerbach, V. H., Waisman, H. A., and Wyckoff, L. B. (1958): Phenylketonuria in the rat associated with decreased temporal discrimination learning. *Nature*, 182:871–872.

58. Wang, H. L., and Waisman, H. A. (1961): Experimental phenylketonuria in rats. *Proc. Soc. Exp. Biol. Med.*, 108:332–335.

59. Boggs, D. E., and Waisman, H. A. (1962): Effects on the offspring of female rats fed phenylalanine. *Life Sci.*, 8:373–376.

60. Polidora, V. J., Cunningham, R. F., and Waisman, H. A. (1966): Phenylketonuria in rats: Reversi-

bility of the behavioral deficit. *Science*, 151:219–221.

61. Andersen, A., and Guroff, G. (1972): Enduring behavioral changes in rats with experimental phenylketonuria. *Proc. Natl. Acad. Sci. USA*, 69:863–867.

62. Andersen, A., Rowe, V., and Guroff, G. (1974): The enduring behavioral changes in rats with experimental phenylketonuria. *Proc. Natl. Acad. Sci. USA*, 71:21–25.

63. Prichard, J. W., and Guroff, G. (1971): Increased cerebral excitability caused by p-chlorophenyla-lanine in young rats. *J. Neurochem.*, 18:153–160.

64. Avins, L., Guroff, G., and Kuwabara, T. (1975): Ultrastructural changes in rat optic nerve associated with hyperphenylalanemia induced by para-chlorophenylalanine and phenylalanine. *J. Neuropath. Exp. Neurol.*, 34:178–188.

65. Rowe, V. D., Fales, H. M., Pisano, J. J., Andersen, A. E., and Guroff, G. (1975): Urinary metabolites of phenylalanine in the preweanling rat treated with p-chlorophenylalanine and phenylalanine. *Biochem. Med.*, 12:123–136.

The Nervous System, Donald B. Tower, Editor-in-Chief. *Vol. 1: The Basic Neurosciences.* Raven Press, New York, 1975.

The Actomyosin-Like System in Nervous Tissue

S. Berl

Actomyosin, the contractile protein system responsible for muscle contraction, is associated not only with muscle. Its presence in a variety of other cells, some of rather primitive origin, has been established. Its association with the plasmodium of the slime mold *Physarum polycephalum* was first suggested by Loewy (1), and with the ascites sarcoma cell by Hoffman-Berling (2). This protein complex, or its components the actin-like or myosin-like proteins, have now been isolated and characterized from a number of diverse cells such as blood platelets (3) (thrombosthenin), from slime mold (4–6), from acanthamoeba (7,8), from the amoeba of *Dictyostelium discoideum* (9,10), from sea urchin eggs (11), from cultures of fibroblasts (12), and from polymorphonuclear leucocytes (13,14). Actomyosin-like protein in nonmuscle cells in general (15) and in brain in particular (16,17) have been recently reviewed.

Actomyosin-like, actin-like, and myosin-like proteins have been isolated from brains of rat, cat, and cow (18–20) and from cultures of chick sympathetic ganglia and chick brain (21,22). To differentiate between the muscle and brain proteins brain actomyosin was named neurostenin, the brain actin was named neurin and the brain myosin was named stenin (19). In studies of the subcellular distribution of the actomyosin-like protein in brain it was found to be concentrated in the synaptosomal fraction (23–25). Tropomyosin has also been identified in chick brain and sympathetic ganglia cultures (22) and the presence of a Ca^{2+} sensitive component in brain actomyosin has been described (26).

PROPERTIES OF ACTOMYOSIN

The physical and chemical properties of brain actomyosin, actin, myosin, and tropomyosin are very similar to the analagous muscle proteins. Muscle actomyosin enzymatically hydrolyzes ATP to ADP and inorganic phosphate. This catalysis is stimulated by either Mg^{2+} or Ca^{2+}. MgATP is the natural substrate for the enzyme complex. The actomyosin system is composed of a number of proteins; actin and myosin are major constituents. Myosin is a Ca^{2+}-activated ATPase and is inhibited by Mg^{2+}. Actin has no enzyme activity. However, the interaction between actin and myosin results in the formation of the actomyosin complex that now does have Mg^{2+}-stimulated ATPase activity. The active site is associated with the myosin. During contraction of striated muscle the thin actin filaments slide past and interdigitate with the thick myosin filaments resulting in shortening of muscle fibers. The energy for contraction comes from hydrolysis of ATP.

The interaction between actin and myosin is regulated by a calcium sensitive system composed of four proteins, the tropomyosin–troponin complex. In striated muscle the tropomyosin is associated with the actin; three different troponin proteins are associated with the tropomyosin. In the absence of Ca^{2+} (10^{-7} M or less), the troponin–tropomyosin system prevents the interaction of actin and myosin. Upon arrival of a nerve impulse at the neuromuscular junction Ca^{2+} is released (approximately 10^{-5} M). The released Ca^{2+} binds to troponin and inhibits the inhibitory influence of the troponin–tropomyosin system thus permitting the interaction between actin and myosin. The Ca^{2+} in conjunction with troponin–tropomyosin system regulates the interaction between actin and myosin.

The union of actin with myosin results in the development of other chemophysical characteristics in actomyosin which neither protein exhibits alone. One of these characteristics is the phenomenon of superprecipitation which has been described by Szent-Györgyi as contraction without architecture. The occurrence of superprecipitation results in the formation of a dense precipitate in the presence of ATP, Mg^{2+}, and low salt concentrations. This precipitate contracts and shrinks if sufficient protein is present. A second characteristic of actomyosin which neither component exhibits alone is viscometric sensitivity to ATP. The union of actin and myosin in high salt concentration (0.6 M KCl) results in an increase of viscosity. Upon the addition of small amounts of ATP the actomyosin dissociates into actin and myosin with a sharp drop in viscosity. As the ATP is hydrolyzed, the viscosity rapidly rises again.

The properties of the proteins isolated from whole brain that are similar to those of the muscle proteins are listed below.

Brain Actomyosin

(a) Soluble in 0.6 M KCl, insoluble in 0.06 M KCl
(b) ATPase activity stimulated by Mg^{2+} (4+) and by Ca^{2+} (2+)
(c) Superprecipitation
(d) Viscosity sensitive to ATP
(e) Inhibited by sulfhydryl reagents
(f) Not inhibited by ouabain
(g) Dissociates into actin-like and myosin-like components

Brain Actin

(a) Soluble at low ionic strength
(b) No ATPase activity
(c) Stimulates the Mg^{2+}-activated ATPase of muscle and brain myosin
(d) Viscosity increases when mixed with muscle or brain myosin; viscosity sensitive to added ATP
(e) Contains ATP
(f) Exchanges bound ATP with [^{14}C]ATP
(g) Polymerizes with release of phosphate from ATP
(h) Molecular weight of 45,000–47,000
(i) Contains 3-methylhistidine
(j) Forms filaments that can be decorated with arrowhead configurations with heavy meromyosin

Brain Myosin

(a) Soluble in 0.6 M KCl, insoluble in 0.06 M KCl
(b) ATPase activity stimulated by Ca^{2+} but not by Mg^{2+}

(c) Mg^{2+}-ATPase activity stimulated by muscle or brain actin
(d) Viscosity increases when added to muscle or brain actin; viscosity sensitive to added ATP
(e) Molecular weight approximately 220,000 by electrophoresis on SDS polyacrylamide gels
(f) Contains 3-methylhistidine and *N*-ϵ-methyllysine

SYNAPTOSOMAL PROTEINS

Since the subcellular location of the proteins of the complex would provide some indication as to its function in brain, such a study was undertaken (23). The fractionation technique utilized discontinuous ficoll gradients for the purification of the mitochondria and synaptosomal fractions from sucrose homogenates of brain. The synaptosomal fraction was then further separated into synaptic vesicle and synaptosomal membrane fractions by differential centrifugation of osmotically shocked preparations.

Proteins catalyzing Mg^{2+}/Ca^{2+}-activated ATPase activity were extracted, by the method used for the preparation of actomyosin, from the crude nuclear fraction, the microsomal fraction and the synaptosomal fraction. Protein could not be isolated from the purified mitochondrial fraction (although the intact mitochondria did have Mg^{2+}/Ca^{2+}-ATPase activity), or from the myelin fraction. However, the microsomal protein did not have other characteristics exhibited by actomyosin-like proteins. Since the crude nuclear fraction contained cellular debris as well as unbroken cells, it was not surprising that this fraction yielded an ATPase with other characteristics of actomyosin. The protein isolated from the synaptosomal enriched fraction appeared to represent a major portion of the actomyosin-like protein. The Mg^{2+}-ATPase activity of this protein (36 nmoles P_i/mg protein/min) was 4 to 5 times greater than that from either the bovine whole brain (8.0 nmoles P_i/mg protein/min) or the nuclear fraction. The Ca^{2+}-ATPase activity was similarly greater (13.7 versus 4.7 nmoles P_i/mg protein/min). This activity was also greater than that found for the protein prepared from cat or rat whole brain (19). The yield of protein was also increased. Whereas the amount of actomyosin-like protein obtained from rat or bovine whole brain represented approximately 1 to 2% of the total protein, the synaptosomal-enriched fraction yielded 8 to 10% of its total protein as the actomyosin-like protein.

Two characteristics of actomyosin, intrinsic viscosity sensitive to ATP and the phenomenon of superprecipitation were also exhibited by the ATPase extracted from the crude nuclear fraction or the synaptosomal fraction of bovine brain. Dissolved in 0.6 M KCl these proteins did demonstrate a precipitous decrease in relative viscosity upon addition of ATP; it increased again over a period of approximately 20 min. In contrast, the ATPase isolated from the microsomal fraction did not show these changes, although the experiments were carried out at the same time with similar concentrations of protein. The phenomenon of superprecipitation was similarly demonstrated in low ionic strength solution (0.1 M KCl). The protein from the crude nuclear and synaptosomal fractions formed a dense granular precipitate in the presence of Mg^{2+} and ATP. The microsomal protein did not show superprecipitation. Thus by the criteria of Mg^{2+}–Ca^{2+}-stimulated ATPase activity, sensitivity of viscosity to ATP and superprecipitation the actomyosin-like protein appeared to be concentrated in the synaptosomal enriched fraction.

DISSOCIATION OF SYNAPTOSOMAL ACTOMYOSIN

The synaptosomal protein was further characterized by dissociation into actin-like and myosin-like components by zonal centrifugation on a 3 to 30% continuous sucrose gradient containing 0.6 M KI and 1 mM ATP (23). This procedure had been used for the separation of actomyosin from whole brain into these two major components (20). In the presence of 0.6 M KI and ATP the actomyosin dissociates into actin and myosin. The former depolymerizes and the two proteins can be separated by centrifugation since the ratio of molecular weights of the actin to myosin is approximately 47,000 to 500,000. KI had been used by Szent-Györgyi to purify actin from striated muscle as well as from actomyosin.

With this procedure two major bands formed

in the sucrose gradient from synaptosomal actomyosin. The heavier band centered at 0.35 M sucrose and the lighter at 0.15 M sucrose. The heavier band (synaptosomal myosin) was essentially a Ca^{2+}-stimulated ATPase (90 to 330 nmoles P_i/mg protein/min); the lighter band (synaptosomal actin) had little enzyme activity. When the two proteins were added together, the Mg^{2+}-ATPase activity was restored equal to or better than the ATPase activity of the original synaptosomal actomyosin. The Mg^{2+}-ATPase activity was stimulated 8 to 10-fold (from 18–32 to 140–310 nmoles P_i/mg protein/min). In another series of experiments it was found that the synaptosomal actin markedly stimulated the Mg^{2+}-ATPase activity of muscle myosin as well as that of synaptosomal myosin.

The relative viscosity of Band I (synaptosomal myosin) or Band II (synaptosomal actin) from the sucrose gradient was considerably lower than the relative viscosity of the two proteins in the same solution. The addition of ATP then caused a fall in viscosity of the combined solution of the two proteins; this was not exhibited by either protein alone. The viscosity rose over a period of 30 min and responded again with a decline in viscosity upon addition of another small amount of ATP. A similar result occurred when muscle actin was added to synaptosomal myosin. Repetitively, addition of Band II (synaptosomal actin) to muscle myosin increased the relative viscosity of the mixture considerably above that of each in separate solution. The addition of ATP caused a rapid fall in viscosity, which rose again as the ATP was hydrolyzed. Thus by these tests as well, Band I exhibited myosin-like characteristics and Band II exhibited actin-like characteristics. Protein isolated from the microsomal fraction, on the other hand, did not separate into two bands when similarly subjected to zonal centrifugation.

VESICULAR AND MEMBRANE PROTEINS

The distribution of these proteins within the synaptosome was then investigated. Enriched fractions of synaptosomes from rat brain were partially purified on a discontinuous ficoll gradient (23) and presynaptic vesicle and membrane fractions obtained by osmotic shock techniques. These fractions were then extracted as for the isolation of actomyosin-like protein and the proteins thus obtained were centrifuged in sucrose gradients containing 0.6 M KI and 1 mM ATP (24). The protein obtained from the vesicular fraction equilibrated in one major band centered on 0.35 M sucrose. On the other hand, the protein obtained from the membrane fraction equilibrated as one major band at 0.15 M sucrose. These distributions were similar to the bands obtained from actomyosin-like protein from whole brain and from synaptosomal preparations. The vesicle protein, similar to myosin-like protein separated from either whole brain or synaptosomal actomyosin, exhibited Ca^{2+}-ATPase activity (260–550 nmoles P_i/mg protein/min), but little Mg^{2+}-ATPase activity ($\sim$ 30 nmoles P_i/mg protein/min). The membrane protein, similar to actin-like protein separated from either whole brain or synaptosomal actomyosin, demonstrated little enzyme activity. However, the latter enhanced the Mg^{2+}-ATPase activity of the vesicle protein approximately five- to eightfold, but had essentially no affect on the Ca^{2+}-activated ATPase activity. In another series of experiments, it was demonstrated that muscle actin also markedly enhanced as much as 20-fold the Mg^{2+}-ATPase activity of the protein extracted directly from rat brain vesicle fractions by myosin isolation procedures rather than by the sucrose gradient procedure. In corollary experiments, protein isolated directly from membrane preparations by actin isolation methods stimulated markedly the Mg^{2+}-ATPase activity of muscle myosin (17,24).

Because the vesicle fraction yielded mainly myosin-like protein and little actin-like protein and the membrane fraction yielded mainly actin-like protein and little myosin-like protein, the results were interpreted as suggesting that the myosin-like protein is associated with presynaptic vesicles and the actin-like protein with synaptic membrane. These conclusions, however, based on studies of subcellular fractions, are not definitive since these tissue fractions are not pure. The contribution from other subcellular fragments, such as glial or postsynaptic elements that might have been present, requires further evaluation. Other techniques for *in situ* demonstration of the proteins will be required.

Electrophoresis of the membrane protein, purified by column chromatography on Sephadex G-200, and muscle actin in polyacrylamide gels containing sodium dodecyl sulfate (SDS) showed similar rates of migration and one major band (17). Electrophoresis of the protein isolated from the vesicle fraction and purified on Sepharose 4B and muscle myosin also showed similar rates of migration and one major band. The mobility of the proteins in these gels as compared with standard proteins indicated that the molecular weight of the membrane actin was approximately 47,000, similar to that of muscle actin, and the molecular weight of the vesicle myosin was approximately 220,000, similar to the subunit of muscle myosin (17).

The amino acid composition of the brain actin showed it to be an acidic protein similar to that of muscle actin. The brain protein contained 3-methylhistidine (17), an amino acid characteristic of muscle actin. Whether the differences in amino acid composition between the two proteins are significant requires additional analyses. Amino acid analysis of the vesicle protein showed that this protein also contained 3-methylhistidine as well as N-ϵ-methyllysine similar to muscle myosin.

CA^{2+}-SENSITIVE COMPONENT

Another important protein complex associated with muscle actomyosin, the troponin–tropomyosin system was discussed earlier. This complex, in conjunction with Ca^{2+}, controls the interaction of actin with myosin. The removal of Ca^{2+} allows the troponin–tropomyosin system to exert its inhibitory influence on the interaction between actin and myosin while the presence of Ca^{2+} neutralizes this inhibitory influence.

The Ca^{2+}-sensitive component in actomyosin is demonstrated by the addition of the Ca^{2+}-chelator ethylene glycol-bis-(β-aminoethyl ether)-N, N^1-tetracetate (EGTA) to the assay medium. It chelates endogenous Ca^{2+} bound to the troponin system and results in a decrease in the Mg^{2+}-ATPase activity of the actomyosin complex; addition of Ca^{2+} then overcomes the inhibitory effect of the troponin–tropomyosin system and restores the Mg^{2+}-ATPase activity. A similar effect of EGTA and Ca^{2+} on the Mg^{2+}-

ATPase activity of synaptosomal actomyosin from bovine brain has been demonstrated (26). The addition of 1 mM EGTA to the assay system for synaptosomal protein causes a decrease of approximately 50% of the Mg^{2+}-ATPase enzyme activity. The Mg^{2+}-ATPase activity is almost completely restored in the presence of 10^{-6} M free Ca^{2+} generated from a Ca^{2+}-EGTA buffer. Thus the Mg^{2+}-ATPase activity of the synaptosomal actomyosin can be controlled by physiological levels of free Ca^{2+}.

It has been demonstrated that this sensitivity to Ca^{2+} can be removed from muscle actomyosin complex by dialysis of a suspension of the protein complex in a low ionic strength buffer (2 mM Tris–HCl, pH 7.6) against the same buffer. Ca^{2+} sensitivity can then be restored to the desensitized protein complex by reprecipitation of the protein from solution in 0.6 M KCl in the presence of the supernatant from the original protein suspension. The troponin–tropomyosin complex goes into solution during dialysis and can be separated from the actomyosin by centrifugation. It can be recombined with the desensitized actomyosin by precipitation in their mutual presence. This procedure was applied to synaptosomal actomyosin-like protein. It demonstrated the presence of a Ca^{2+}-sensitive component in the brain protein (26). The Mg^{2+}-ATPase activity of the natural synaptosomal actomyosin was inhibited by 1 mM EGTA; this was prevented by the presence of 10^{-5} M free Ca^{2+}. After the dialysis and separation of the protein from its supernatant the protein was no longer affected by EGTA. This response to EGTA and to Ca^{2+} was restored to the desensitized protein by reprecipitation in the presence of the 70,000 $\times g$ supernatant.

The demonstration of Ca^{2+}-sensitivity and its reconstitution requires the presence of dithiothreitol (DTT) during both the desensitization and reconstitution procedure; it is lost if DTT is omitted. This suggests that the integrity of the sulfhydryl groups need to be protected in the brain protein as it is in the muscle protein. The degree of inhibition by EGTA of the Mg^{2+}-ATPase activity of the synaptosomal protein is comparable to that obtained with other actomyosin-like complexes from nonstriated muscle such as uterine smooth muscle, blood platelets and leukocytes; it is less than the almost 100% inhibition obtained with striated muscle actomyosin.

Recently, Fine et al. (22) isolated from chick embryo brain and from cultures of sympathetic ganglia a tropomyosin-like protein very similar to muscle tropomyosin. Substitution of this brain protein for muscle tropomyosin in a calcium regulated actomyosin ATPase system showed that the brain tropomyosin can interact with muscle troponin to confer calcium sensitivity to the Mg^{2+}-activated actomyosin ATPase of muscle. The brain tropomyosin is similar but not identical to the muscle protein; it binds to muscle actin but the binding is weaker; it is of smaller molecular weight (30,000 versus 35,000); paracrystals are formed with $MgCl_2$ but are of shorter periodicity; amino acid composition, although similar, is somewhat different; peptide maps show 8 similar peptides but there are also some differences.

Thus, three contractile proteins, actin, myosin, and tropomyosin are present in brain which are similar to those in muscle actomyosin. However, there is no conclusive evidence that troponin-like elements are also present. Molluscan muscle does not contain troponin; the Ca^{2+}-sensitive sites are not on the tropomyosin but are associated with the myosin molecule and can not be easily separated from it. Since the factor responsible for Ca^{2+}-sensitivity can be easily removed from and restored to the brain actomyosin complex, it is more likely that the Ca^{2+}-sensitive system in brain is similar to that of striated muscle rather than that of molluscan muscle.

In present work, a protein complex conferring Ca^{2+} sensitivity to desensitized brain actomyosin has been isolated directly from bovine brain cortex (27). The method of isolation is essentially similar to that which has been used for direct isolation of troponin–tropomyosin complex from skeletal muscle. The protein complex has neither ATPase activity nor does it generate any MgATPase activity with heavy meromyosin indicating the absence of both an active actomyosin-like and actin-like component. In preliminary studies direct addition of the crude protein preparation to desensitized brain actomyosin (ratio 1:10) in the MgATPase assay medium regenerated 75% of the Ca^{2+} sensitivity observed with the native brain actomyosin. Calcium sensitivity can also be regenerated by coprecipitating the desensitized brain actomyosin with protein complex under conditions of low ionic strength and isoelectric pH. The amount of regeneration is dependent on the amount of protein complex present during the coprecipitation. Purified troponin–tropomyosin complex from skeletal muscle, also, confers Ca^{2+} sensitivity to desensitized brain actomyosin. Electrophoretic analysis on polyacrylamide gels containing SDS of the protein preparations shows the presence of components similar in molecular weights to those present in muscle troponin–tropomyosin complex.

POLYMERIZATION AND INTERACTION WITH HEAVY MEROMYOSIN

Similar to muscle actin as well as nonmuscle actin the brain actin can be polymerized into filaments in the presence of 0.1 M KCl and 1 mM $MgCl_2$. These filaments can be negatively stained with uranyl acetate and visualized by electron microscopy (*unpublished observation*); they are approximately 70 to 80 Å wide. Muscle actin can be decorated with heavy meromyosin (HMM), a fragment of myosin, obtained by tryptic digestion. This protein interacts with actin to form characteristic arrowhead configurations that can be seen in the electron microscope in preparations negatively stained with uranyl acetate. The brain actin was also decorated when interacted with heavy meromyosin (*unpublished observation*). In preliminary studies, synaptosome enriched rat brain fractions were treated with HMM. A tentative interpretation of the results would suggest that the HMM reacted with actin present at both pre and postsynaptic sites.

Chang and Goldman (28), in studies of cultured neuroblastoma cells, were able to demonstrate that HMM could decorate fibers with the characteristic arrowhead formation; they extended down the axon from the cell body to the nerve ending. These preparations do not have synaptic junctions.

CYTOCHALASIN B STUDIES

The fungal metabolite cytochalasin B disrupts many diverse functions that are thought to be of a contractile nature and associated with microfilamentous processes, e.g., cytokinesis, cell locomotion, cytoplasmic streaming, blood clot retraction, and neuronal and glial movements (29). This drug also decreases the intrinsic viscosity of muscle actin, alters the morphology of actin filaments isolated from muscle and blood platelets, inhibits the ATPase activity of acto-meromyosin (30,31), and disrupts the cardiac myofibrils of chick embryo (32). In addition, it inhibits the stimulated release of norepinephrine and dopamine-β-hydroxylase from sympathetic nerve endings (33) and norepinephrine from guinea pig atria (34), as well as hormonal substances.

In our studies we found that cytochalasin B inhibited by approximately 50% the Mg^{2+}-ATPase activity of rat brain synaptosomal actomyosin (35). The inhibition was linear at cytochalasin B concentrations of less than 0.1 mM. The Ca^{2+}-ATPase activity was not inhibited. Cytochalasin B (10^{-4} M) inhibited to a similar degree the Mg^{2+}-ATPase activity of combinations of muscle myosin with muscle actin or brain actin and of brain myosin with muscle actin or brain actin. Since the Mg^{2+}-ATPase activity is dependent upon the interaction of actin with myosin, the data suggest that the drug interferes with this process.

We have also studied the effect of cytochalasin B on the uptake and K^+-stimulated release of radioactively labeled noradrenaline, dopamine, glutamic acid, and GABA by rat brain synaptosomal preparations (35). The drug, at a 10^{-4} M concentration, caused a small, but significant inhibition ($p < 0.01$) on the uptake of norepinephrine (20%) and dopamine (30%), but no effect on the uptake of glutamic acid or GABA. The major effect of the cytochalasin B was on the K^+-stimulated release of the catecholamines. The release of noradrenaline was inhibited 60 to 90% and that of dopamine 22 to 32%. The release of glutamic acid or GABA was unaffected. The mechanisms for uptake or release of the amino acids may be different in some respects from those for the catecholamines.

Based in part on these observations, the suggestion was offered that the effect of cytochalasin B on the stimulated release of catecholamines cited above may be through an affect on the actomyosin-like system in the nerve endings (35) (see section on Function).

COLCHICINE AND VINBLASTINE STUDIES

The alkaloids colchicine and vinblastine were found to inhibit the stimulated release of substances from several different organs, e.g., acetylcholine or nicotine-induced release of catecholamines from the perfused adrenal medulla (36) and the release of norepinephrine and dopamine-β-hydroxylase from sympathetic nerves (33). The action of cytochalasin B was thought to involve the microfilaments at the synapse while the action of colchicine and vinblastine were thought to involve microtubules. We would suggest that the action of the latter two drugs, as well as cytochalasin B, may be mediated through an effect on the actomyosin-like complex at the nerve endings.

Vinblastine can precipitate a number of acidic proteins other than microtubular protein (tubulin). These include muscle actin and actin from neuronal chick embryo cultures (21).

Vinblastine and colchicine also were found to inhibit the Mg^{2+}-ATPase activity of synaptosomal actomyosin (37). Vinblastine (0.1 mM) inhibited the enzyme activity 30% to 50%. The inhibition of enzyme activity was more effective at submaximal concentrations of ATP (0.25 versus 0.50 mM ATP and Mg^{2+}); the ATP appears to offer partial protection to the enzyme. Colchicine was less effective. A 1 mM concentration produced a 35% inhibition in enzyme activity. The Ca^{2+}-ATPase activity was not affected by either drug.

In studies with crude synaptosomal preparations colchicine inhibited the uptake of ^{3}H-dopamine depending upon the dose of alkaloid (37). Colchicine (1 mM) inhibited the uptake of dopamine approximately 50%. In contrast, [^{14}C]glutamate uptake was inhibited only 20% at this concentration of colchicine. Vinblastine was a far more potent inhibitor of uptake of putative transmitters by synaptosomal preparations. At a concentration of 0.1 mM vinblastine, the uptake of GABA, dopamine, and norepinephrine were inhibited approximately 65 to 75%; at 0.05 mM concentration the inhibitory effect was approximately 30 to 50%. Glutamate uptake was unaffected at these drug concentrations.

Vinblastine also decreased the amount of radioactive norepinephrine or dopamine released into the medium upon increasing the external K^+ concentration from 5 to 30 mM when compared with control values. However, this was probably due predominantly to the action of the vinblastine on the nerve ending membranes. It caused leakage of radioactivity into the medium in amounts dependent upon the concentration of the drug. Although the amount of radioactivity released by the elevated K^+ was decreased, the percent of accumulated radioactivity released was unaffected when compared with the amount of radioactivity remaining in the tissue. Again, the release of glutamic acid was not affected until the concentration of vinblastine was raised to 0.25 mM. As in the studies with cytochalasin B, glutamic acid in particular, and GABA to some extent, the uptake and release of the amino acids appear to be different from that of the catecholamines.

The effects of these drugs on the enzyme activity of synaptosomal actomyosin and on uptake and release of the putative catecholamine transmitters are consistent with the concept that they exert their influence via an effect on a membrane component or components, one of which may be the synaptosomal actin.

FUNCTION IN BRAIN

We really do not have any conclusive knowledge as to the function or functions of actomyosin-like protein in any of the nonmuscle systems. In part this is because we do not have an adequate picture of the structural relationships of the actin to the myosin and of their relationships to other cellular structures. These are only well understood in striated muscle systems. In some cells actin-like protein is thought to compose the microfilamentous structures seen close to cell membranes. Even less is known about how and where the myosin-like protein is situated. In comparison with the muscle system and based on a great deal of circumstantial evidence, we assume that these proteins in nonmuscle cells are capable of converting chemical to mechanical energy and provide a motile or contractile force, as in muscle. In blood platelets it is thought to function in clot retraction. In dividing cells (newt, HeLa, echinoderm), the contractile ring formed during cytokinesis is thought to involve actin-like protein. In the slime mold it probably functions in cytoplasmic streaming, and in fibroblasts, polymorphonuclear leukocytes and amoeba it probably functions in motility and as well as in phagocytosis in the latter two cells. It may function in all mobile cells and in the immature nervous system it may very well provide the mechanism for cell migration. The association of the myosin-like protein with the vesicle would place it in the appropriate position for sultatory movement of vesicles down the axon, perhaps associated with the microtubules.

Studies on the subcellular distribution of these proteins in the mature brain, led us to the suggestion that this protein system may function in exocytosis for the quantal release of neurotransmitter substances at nerve endings (24). The hypothesis is that actin is associated with the presynaptic membrane, perhaps as the microfilaments, and myosin with the vesicles. The synaptic vesicles lie in intimate contact with the presynaptic membrane and in response to stimulation, the entrance of Ca^{2+} or its release from membrane would trigger the interaction between actin and myosin, as it does in muscle. Conformational changes in the membranes, perhaps caused by a torsional increase in helical structure, would result in opening of the vesicular and synaptosomal membranes. Transmitter would be released into the synaptic cleft or replace transmitter in the membrane. The action would be terminated by the release or binding of Ca^{2+}. This singular role of Ca^{2+} is in line with the hypothesis of Katz and Miledi (38) that depolarization at the presynaptic terminal causes an increase in the permeability of the terminal to Ca^{2+}, which enters and functions in quantal release of transmitter from vesicles. The similarity between excitation-contraction coupling in muscles and stimulus-secretion coupling in nerve endings and secretory structures was emphasized by Douglas (39). Whether the vesicle is used over again or remains fused with the membrane after a single interaction has received considerable discussion and opinions appear to depend upon the system studied and the experimental condition. Some studies point to the vesicles fusing with the membrane. On the other hand, other studies support the contention that even with extensive stimulation, vesicles may not deplete but may be reused. Whether fusion is a primary or secondary process, is not entirely clear.

Recently, Bray (40) put forth the hypothesis that in the growth cone of the growing neurite contractile proteins are responsible for movement and elongation of the filopodia. In the growth cone there are present numerous tubular vesicles that may come along the microtubules propelled to the neurite tip from their site of synthesis in the cell body. In the filopodia the actomyosin proteins associated with the vesicles and membranes would orient and move the vesicle toward the tip. The vesicle would then fuse with the membrane and result in extension and growth of the neurite.

Other functions, no doubt, can be and will be assigned to the actomyosin-like protein system in nervous tissue. It may also prove to be the case that this protein complex will have more than one function in the nervous system.

REFERENCES

1. Loewy, A. G. (1952): An actomyosin-like substance from the plasmodium of a myxomycete. *J. Cell. Comp. Physiol.,* 40:127–156.
2. Hoffman-Berling, H. (1956): Das kontraktile eiweiss undifferenzierter zellen. *Biochim. Biophys. Acta,* 19:453–463.
3. Bettex-Galland, M., and Luscher, E. F. (1960): Thrombosthenin, the contractile protein from blood platelets and its relation to other contractile proteins. *Advan. Protein Chem.,* 20:1–35.
4. Hatano, S., and Oosawa, F. (1966): Isolation and characterization of plasmodium actin. *Biochim. Biophys. Acta.,* 127:488–498.
5. Hatano, S., and Tazawa, M. (1968): Isolation, purification and characterization of myosin B from myxomycete plasmodium. *Biochim. Biophys. Acta,* 154:507–519.
6. Adelman, M. R., and Taylor, E. W. (1969): Further purification and characterization of slime mold actin. *Biochemistry,* 8:4976–4988.
7. Weihing, R. R., and Korn, E. D. (1971): Acanthamoeba actin: Isolation and properties. *Biochemistry,* 10:590–600.
8. Pollard, T. D., and Korn, E. (1972): The "contractile" proteins of Acanthamoeba castellanii. *Cold Spring Harbor Symp. Quant. Biol.,* 37:573–583.
9. Wooley, D. E. (1970): Extraction of an actomyosin-like protein from amoebae of Dictyostelium discoideum. *J. Cell Physiol.,* 76:185–190.
10. Wooley, D. E. (1972): An actin-like protein from amoebae of Dictyostelium discoideum. *Arch. Biochem. Biophys.,* 150:519–530.
11. Hatano, S., Kondo, H., and Miki-Noumura, T. (1969): Purification of sea urchin egg actin. *Exp. Cell Res.,* 55:275–277.
12. Yang, Y., and Perdue, J. R. (1972): Contractile proteins of cultured cells. *J. Biol. Chem.,* 247:4503–4509.
13. Tatsumi, N., Shibata, N., Okamura, J., Takeu-

chi, K., and Senda, N. (1973): Actin and myosin from leukocytes. *Biochim. Biophys. Acta,* 305: 433–444.

14. Stossel, T. P., and Pollard, T. D. (1973): Myosin in polymorphonuclear leukocytes. *J. Biol. Chem.,* 248:8288–8294.

15. Pollard, T. D., and Weihing, R. R. (1973): Actin and myosin and cell movement. *CRC Crit. Rev. Biochem.,* January:1–65.

16. Berl, S. (1975): Actomyosin-like protein in brain. In: *Advances in Neurochemistry,* edited by B. W. Agranoff and M. H. Aprison. Plenum, New York (*in press*).

17. Berl, S., and Nicklas, W. J. (1975): Contractile proteins in relation to transmitter release. In: *Metabolic Compartmentation and Neurotransmission: Relation to Brain Structure and Function,* edited by S. Berl, D. D. Clarke, and D. Schneider. Plenum, New York (*in press*).

18. Puszkin, S., Berl, S., Puszkin, E., and Clarke, D. D. (1968): Actomyosin-like protein isolated from mammalian brain. *Science,* 161:170–171.

19. Berl, S., and Puszkin, S. (1970): Mg^{2+}-Ca^{2+}-Activated adenosine triphosphatase system isolated from mammalian brain. *Biochemistry,* 9:2058–2067.

20. Puszkin, S., and Berl, S. (1972): Actomyosin-like protein from brain: Separation and characterization of the actin-like component. *Biochim. Biophys. Acta,* 256:695–709.

21. Fine, R. E., and Bray, D. (1971): Actin in growing nerve cells. *Nature New Biol.,* 234:115–118.

22. Fine, R. E., Blitz, A. L., Hitchcock, S. E., and Kaminer, B. (1973): Tropomyosin in brain and growing neurones. *Nature New Biol.,* 245:182–186.

23. Puszkin, S., Nicklas, W. J., and Berl, S. (1972): Actomyosin-like protein in brain: Subcellular distribution. *J. Neurochem.,* 19:1319–1333.

24. Berl, S., Puszkin, S., and Nicklas, W. J. (1973): Actomyosin-like protein in brain. *Science,* 179: 441–446.

25. Blitz, A. L., and Fine, R. E. (1974): Muscle-like contractile proteins and tubulin in synaptosomes. *Proc. Natl. Acad. Sci. USA,* 71:4472–4476.

26. Mahendran, C., Nicklas, W. J., and Berl, S. (1974): Evidence for calcium-sensitive component in brain actomyosin-like protein (neurostenin). *J. Neurochem.,* 23:497–501.

27. Mahendran, C., Nicklas, W. J. and Berl, S. (1975): Partial purification of a protein-complex which confers Ca^{2+}-sensitivity to desensitized neurostenin. *Trans. Am. Soc. Neurochem.,* Vol. 6.

28. Chang, C-M., and Goldman, R. D. (1973): The localization of actin-like fibers in cultured neuroblastoma cells as revealed by heavy meromyosin binding. *J. Cell Biol.,* 57:867–874.

29. Wessels, N. K., Spooner, B. S., Ash, J. F., Bradley, M. O., Ludena, M. A., Taylor, E. L., Wrenn, J. T., and Yamada, K. M. (1971): Microfilaments in cellular and developmental processes. *Science,* 171:135–143.

30. Spudich, J. A. (1973): Effects of cytochalasin B on actin filaments. *Cold Spring Harbor Symp. Quant. Biol.,* 37:585–593.

31. Lin, S., Santi, D. V., and Spudich, J. A. (1974): Biochemical studies on the mode of action of cytochalasin B. *J. Biol. Chem.,* 249:2268–2274.

32. Manasek, F. J., Burnside, B., Stroman, J. (1972): The sensitivity of developing cardiac myofibrils to cytochalasin B. *Proc. Natl. Acad. Sci. USA,* 69:302–312.

33. Thoa, N. B., Wooten, G. F., Axelrod, J., and Kopin, I. J. (1972): Inhibition of release of dopamine-β-hydroxylase and norepinephrine from sympathetic nerves by colchicine, vinblastine, or cytochalasin B. *Proc. Natl. Acad. Sci. USA,* 68:520–522.

34. Sorimachi, M., Oesch, F., and Thoenen, H. (1973): Effects of colchicine and cytochalasin B on the release of ^{3}H-norepinephrine from guinea-pig atria evoked by high potassium, nicotine and tyramine. *Naunyn-Schmiederberg's Arch. Pharmakol.,* 276:1–12.

35. Nicklas, W. J., and Berl, S. (1974): Effects of cytochalasin B on uptake and release of putative transmitters by synaptosomes and on brain actomyosin-like protein. *Nature,* 247:471–473.

36. Poisner, A. M., and Bernstein, J. (1971): A possible role of microtubules in catecholamine release from the adrenal medulla: Effect of colchicine, vinca alkaloids and deuterium oxide. *J. Pharmacol. Exp. Ther.,* 177:102–108.

37. Nicklas, W. J., Puszkin, S., and Berl, S. (1973): Effect of vinblastine and colchicine on uptake and release of putative transmitters by synaptosomes and on brain actomyosin-like protein. *J. Neurochem.,* 20:109–121.

38. Katz, B., and Miledi, R. (1967): The timing of calcium action during neuromuscular transmission. *J. Physiol. (Lond.),* 189:535–544.

39. Douglas, W. W. (1968): The First Gaddum Memorial Lecture. Stimulus-secretion coupling. The concept and clues from chromaffin and other cells. *Br. J. Pharmacol.,* 34:451–474.

40. Bray, D. (1973): Model for membrane movements in the neural growth cone. *Nature,* 244:93–96.

The Nervous System, Donald B. Tower, Editor-in-Chief. *Vol. 1: The Basic Neurosciences*. Raven Press, New York, 1975.

Alterations in the Level and Distribution of Cerebral Amino Acids

Abel Lajtha

In severe nutritional deficiency most organs lose major portions of their constituents, but the brain undergoes only small changes. This and many other examples show the great stability of brain composition in comparison to that of most other organs. Studies, especially those that measure metabolism *in vitro* with labeled isotopes, have established that this stability of the nervous system is dynamic and that the replacement rate of most constituents is surprisingly high. Most recent studies indicate that composition, distribution, and metabolism are not static, thus emphasizing the plasticity of the brain, and that significant changes can occur in a number of physiological and pathological circumstances. The present article briefly discusses some of the alterations that occur in amino acid distribution in the nervous system.

COMPOSITION OF THE CEREBRAL FREE AMINO ACID POOL (1–3)

It has been well established that the composition of the free amino acid pool is specific for the brain, having, for example, a very high content of glutamic acid and related compounds, gamma aminobutyric acid (GABA), aspartate, and glutamine. In a comparison of many species, this composition is found to be very similar. Unlike the level of free amino acids of other tissues, the level in the brain does not change greatly for most compounds even when plasma levels are greatly altered. This maintenance of amino acids may explain why a decrease of brain protein content in the adult does not occur even during prolonged dietary protein deficiency.

Even though we know the composition of the brain's amino acid pools, and a great deal about the mechanisms maintaining their composition, we know very little of what effects may occur when their composition changes. Some aspects may be explainable by preferential metabolic utilization, e.g., the high concentration of the nonessential versus essential amino acids. Because the nonessential amino acids undergo very rapid metabolism, whereas the essential amino acids serve primarily for protein synthesis, with considerable reutilization, the need for a supply of essential amino acids is relatively small.

Obviously, the whole picture is complex, since even a few essential amino acids are rapidly metabolized, and many amino acids are in multiple compartments, with different levels and metabolic fates. If we want to understand changes in level and distribution (for example in relation to neurotransmitter amine formation or myelin metabolism), changes in the composition of various compartments will have to be better understood.

Species and Regional Variations

When the amino acid concentrations of whole brain are arranged in decreasing order, the sequence is surprisingly similar in most species studied. In addition, the absolute concentrations of most compounds seem to be very similar in the species that have been studied (mouse, rat, rabbit, guinea pig, swine, cat, dog, hen, frog, monkey, man). Relatively large species differences have been found for taurine and cystathionine, which suggests that when other compounds are to be so examined (such as acetylaspartate, phosphoethanolamine, peptides) further important differences may be found; but at least the free amino acids that are components of proteins appear to show a great similarity among species.

Although the amino acid content of the whole brain has been studied in detail, the regional amino acid distribution has been measured less often. In general, the distinction mentioned above in considering concentration differences between the nonessential and essential amino acids seems to also occur in their regional distribution. The nonessential amino acid regional distribution is fairly homogeneous. Compounds not present in proteins, such as taurine, cystathionine, carnosine, and homocarnosine, show the greatest regional heterogeneity. The regional heterogeneity is not consistent: Some amino acids are high in cortical areas, others are highest in subcortical structures, or in the cerebellum. Such results may be influenced by the fact that many, especially earlier studies concentrated on the nonessential amino acids because these are at higher levels and are therefore easier to determine. There are very few studies measuring compounds in well-defined specific neuroanatomical areas, but indications from measurements of ganglia are that further hetereogeneity can be expected. In many localized areas the distribution primarily with the putative neurotransmitter amino acids was determined. Large differences were found of glycine, GABA, glutamate, and aspartate levels, especially between dorsal and ventral gray or white matter in the spinal cord. The regional distribution of these putative neurotransmitters indicates that they are highest where they are neurophysiologically functional. This is of interest since the level in the free pool is several orders of magnitude higher than could be deduced from measurements of their high affinity transport constants or from their activity when iontophoretically applied to neurons.

Our knowledge of subcellular distribution of amino acids is scant. Some preparations, such as brain slices, retain many amino acids at levels similar to those in living brain. However, during preparation of subcellular fractions the amino acids of subcellular particles may not be retained well. Just what losses may occur is difficult to determine because techniques are not yet available to measure distribution of amino acids within the cell *in situ* without fixation, and fixation artifacts are not clearly understood. With fixation, autoradiographic studies showed a significant portion of synaptosomes being labeled with GABA and a different set of synaptosomes labeled with glycine. These studies indicate that one third or more of the total synaptosomes may be hypoaminoacidic. Transport studies have indicated some uptake mechanisms present in mitochondria and nuclei, with some

differences between them; and differences in amino acid uptake have also been indicated between neurons and glia. Such differences indicate that many structures in the nervous system can control their internal environment, and the heterogeneity of composition should extend to various cell types and subcellular elements.

THE DYNAMIC STATE OF AMINO ACIDS IN BRAIN (4–6)

Upon the administration of trace amounts of radioactively labeled amino acids, the label rapidly enters the brain from the plasma when physiological levels of the amino acids in the circulation are not increased. This indicates that rapid and simultaneous entry and exit occur, and that the metabolite pools are in dynamic equilibrium rather than in a sequestered, bound state. In addition to exchange, the rapid metabolism of some amino acids and the high rate of incorporation and release from proteins also indicates that a large fraction of metabolites is in a dynamic state. Because of this dynamic state the amino acid pool can be altered, at times rapidly, indicating a plasticity and a vulnerability of brain.

Exchange

The appearance of label from tracer doses administered parenterally was studied in several types of experiments: continuous infusion, lasting for several hours; administration of a bolus, measuring changes during a single passage through the brain; and in experiments in which the pulse was injected intravenously or intraperitoneally. In the short experiments there was a very rapid appearance of label from the essential amino acids and a slow exchange or passage of the nonessential amino acids. The calculated half-life of the essential amino acids via exchange with the circulation was minutes for most compounds. Longer infusion experiments indicated that at least some of the nonessential amino acids are also exchangeable, but because the rate of exchange is lower and the total pool is much larger in the brain, the half-life of these compounds is much longer and can be estimated to be hours or days. Infusion experiments also indicated that the exchange is heterogeneous, that several compartments exist in the various structural elements, and that there may be a significant fraction (varying between 5 and 40%) of the total that exchanges very slowly or not at all. Because of metabolism and incorporation these compartments are not easy to estimate precisely. Indications were found for nonexchangeable compartments, which for most amino acids was less than 15% with brain slices incubated in tracer level of amino acids. Exchange occurs through mediated transport, and it may involve (especially during alterations of amino acid levels in plasma) not only homo-exchange, but also hetero-exchange, the entry of one compound influencing the exit of another compound.

Metabolism

The metabolic rates of turnover of most amino acids in the living brain are not known. The isotopic equilibration between intermediates of the tricarboxylic acids cycle and some nonessential amino acids is very rapid, and therefore ^{14}C from ^{14}C-glucose, for example, appears very rapidly in glutamic acid. The enzyme catalyzing amino transfer between oxoglutarate and glutamate is one of the most active enzymes in the nervous system, and any label in oxoglutarate rapidly equilibrates with glutamate. Because the concentration of glutamate is manyfold higher than that of oxoglutarate, most of the radioactivity appears in glutamate. This reaction in itself does not indicate any net conversion, since for each molecule of glutamate giving rise to oxoglutarate, a molecule of oxoglutarate gives rise to glutamate. The increase of alanine under a number of conditions via amino transfer from glutamate to pyruvate, however, indicates that amino transfer coupled to other metabolic reactions can participate in the net formation or breakdown of amino acids. The rate of appearance of label from leucine and methionine in other compounds in the brain shows metabolism beyond equilibration due to isotope dilution. The rate of catabolism of these two amino acids is such that the content of the pool is metabolized in minutes rather than hours, requiring a constant resupply from the circulation. Perhaps the most reliable estimate of net metabolism arises from measurements of arteriovenous (A-V) differences. These are not easy to perform because of the high rate of blood flow

through the brain: a very small A-V difference (beyond the sensitivity of most measurements) could supply amounts equivalent to the cerebral amino acid pool in minutes. Perfusion experiments also have the drawback of possible changes occurring during the experiments. Only few A-V measurements have been performed and these indicate that there is net amino acid uptake by the brain from the blood.

Metabolism influences both the levels and distribution of amino acids. The high rates of metabolism in the capillary walls may contribute a barrier to entry. It has been proposed that the high activity of GABA aminotransferase and succinic semialdehyde dehydrogenase in the capillaries could be the main barrier to GABA entry to the brain; similarly high monoaminoxidase or high acetylcholinesterase activity in the capillaries may prevent the entry of amines or acetylcholine.

Protein Turnover

Incorporation into, and release from, proteins is a significant part of the exchange of many amino acids. Available evidence indicates that at least 90% of cerebral proteins have half-lives between 4 and 16 days; over 50% are between 4 and 10 days. The fraction of the proteins with half-lives less than 1 day or over 50 days is small, indicating a high rate of turnover for most brain proteins. Since many of the essential amino acids are 200-fold more concentrated in protein-bound form than in the free pool, the turnover rate of the free pool via incorporation into proteins is 200-fold higher than protein turnover, giving a half-life of less than 1 hr for many free amino acids for this exchange. This does not indicate a net utilization of the amino acids in adult brain, which shows no net protein synthesis. However, while the brain is rapidly growing, net deposition of proteins may sequester within an hour an amount of amino acid equivalent to that in the total free pool of the brain. In the young brain the exchange between free and protein bound amino acids is higher than in adults; the higher rate of protein breakdown *in vivo* in young, even during net growth, shows that protein turnover is faster in young brain.

The rate of exchange between the free and the protein-bound forms of amino acids may be close to the rate of exchange between the free pools of brain and plasma. Under such conditions radioactive amino acids entering from the circulation will not reach isotopic equilibrium with the plasma for some time, since protein turnover continuously dilutes the specific activity of brain free pools. This lower specific activity in brain might give us the impression that part of the brain amino acid is nonexchangeable. In experiments measuring the decrease of label in the free pool, if exchange with blood is not very fast the labeled amino acid may be reincorporated into proteins before leaving the brain. This may give the impression of a special pool that is reutilized for protein synthesis and is not freely exchanging with plasma. Although such experiments cannot show whether or not the free pool is compartmentalized, indications are that such heterogeneous compartments with heterogeneous rates of exchange exist. Despite these compartments there is no convincing evidence to indicate that external amino acids are preferentially utilized for brain protein turnover. Indeed, the high rate of protein turnover indicates that alterations in the free pool could easily and rapidly have an effect on protein metabolism.

CHANGES IN DEVELOPMENT (7–11)

The greatest change in the composition of the amino acid pool occurs during development. Although these changes are well established, their connection to developmental functional changes occurring in parallel is not well understood. The control of amino acid levels is not strong in the young brain. Restrictions on the passage of substances into the brain are not absent, and therefore permeability barriers are present. However, for most amino acids, a comparable increase in plasma results in a greater increase in the young brain as compared to that in the adult brain. The major features of cerebral barriers are similar in young and adult; for example, the uptake of essential amino acids is greater than that of the nonessential in both.

Changes in Composition

The changes in the free amino acid pools that have been studied in whole brain as well as in brain regions seem to be similar in all species. Quantitatively, the biggest changes are a de-

crease in taurine and an increase in glutamic acid during development; in newborn, taurine comprises 20% to 40% of the free amino acid pool. Compounds related to glutamic acid in general increase during development (aspartic acid, glutamine, and GABA); glycine and proline mostly decrease. Changes of essential amino acids are smaller and variable, with many showing a small decrease. It cannot be generalized that most essential amino acids decrease with the decreasing rate of protein turnover, nor can it be said that all nonessential amino acids, or the putative neurotransmitters, increase with the increasing functional activity of the brain. This is not too surprising, since each amino acid may have several functions.

The developmental changes are not linear: Amino acids may reach one or two maximal or minimal levels during development. The increase in compounds that exist at higher levels in adult brain (for example, glutamate and related compounds) does not occur in identical periods. When rates of increases are plotted, they show sharp peaks in various developmental stages.

Perinatal Changes

Around birth, very rapid changes occur in a few compounds, for example, taurine, threonine, alanine, and GABA; a 60 to 80% decrease in alanine and a three- to fourfold increase in GABA occur within a few days of birth.

There are perinatal changes in the transport of amino acids. A great increase perinatally is found for uptake of GABA, glycine, taurine, and proline, whereas the uptake of other amino acids does not change greatly. This may indicate not only quantitative but also qualitative changes. In slices, two transport processes could be shown in young for GABA, one of which rapidly disappeared or was "diluted out" in later stages of growth. The developmental changes in transport are not parallel with developmental changes in concentrations. In a comparison of changes of uptake into slice with *in vivo* levels during development, the concentration of GABA and its rate of uptake increase; glycine and taurine levels do not change, although their transport increases; the level of alanine decreases, although its transport does not change. It is easy to see that at the least, the transport capacity, as observed by slice uptake, and the *in vivo* amino acid concentrations are not changing in parallel.

PHYSIOLOGICAL INFLUENCES (12–16)

For the essential amino acids a rapid flux occurs between plasma and brain. The indications are that most of the uptake of these amino acids occurs by active transport. Active transport is even greater for nonessential than for the essential amino acids in brain slices, but these cellular functions that are observed in slices cannot be observed in the living brain. Changes, however, that affect the level of essential amino acids in the blood, or the metabolism of nonessential amino acids in brain, have profound effects on brain metabolite composition.

Nutrition

If a diet is supplied that is greatly enriched in one amino acid, the level of that amino acid will increase greatly in the plasma. If it is one of the amino acids that can penetrate brain, the brain levels also increase. Since amino acids with related structure belong to the same transport class, their altered plasma level will influence the transport of other members of their class. In uptake, primarily competitive inhibition was observed; so the increased plasma level of one amino acid inhibits the uptake by brain of other, related amino acids. In turn, if the level of a number of amino acids of the same transport class are increased in the plasma, they may mutually inhibit each others' uptake so that no increase can occur in brain.

The effect of an increased amino acid concentration within brain, on the movement of related amino acids from the brain, can be either inhibitory or stimulatory. In the former case, the increased concentration causes an increase, and in the latter a decrease, of related amino acids within the tissue. Similar considerations apply to the relationship between extracellular and intracellular amino acids in the brain. Competitive interactions can also occur at cell membranes and membranes of intracellular particles. These localized transport systems may not be saturated at the usual physiological amino acid concentrations, and therefore alterations of extracellular amino acids can influence amino acid influx into cells by several mechanisms. Of particular interest in this respect are recent findings of a daily rhythm, and changes in brain concentrations of tryptophan with nutrition. The consumption of a protein-containing diet raises plasma levels, not only of tryptophan, but of other competing amino acids, resulting in no net increase of brain tryptophan. However, carbohydrate and fat diet increases the plasma tryptophan without changing the levels of other competing amino acids; consequently, such a diet has the effect of increasing brain tryptophan and the brain 5-hydroxytryptamine (5-HT) that is formed from the tryptophan. Although experimentally induced increase or decrease of plasma tyrosine causes changes of brain tyrosine, and therefore causes concomitant changes in L-DOPA, generaly dietary changes do not result in brain tyrosine changes.

It is possible that diet can cause a number of other changes in brain amino acids, but because of the variability and low level of the essential amino acids in brain they have rarely been measured in a statistically significant manner. The changes in tryptophan are of particular interest, not only because they result in similar changes in an important cerebral neurotransmitter, but also because tryptophan may be one amino acid that is rate limiting for protein synthesis. Increased tryptophan may alter protein synthesis at specific sites. Clear evidence for this is yet lacking. The increased rate of conversion of elevated brain tryptophan to 5-HT indicates that changes of amino acid utilization and metabolism could occur when the level of other amino acids are increased in the brain. Enzyme reactions not saturated under physiological conditions would show large changes with increasing or decreasing substrate concentrations. Changes in the free amino acid pool occur in severe protein malnutrition. A number of compounds show some decrease (valine, serine, aspartate; in some regions glutamate and taurine), and there is a striking increase in histidine and homocarnosine.

Endocrine Influences

Changes in amino acids were studied, especially in insulin hypoglycemia, in the hope that changes in amino acids explain the effect of this hormone on brain. Somewhat varying changes were reported, perhaps because of varying experimental circumstances. In general most of the nonessential amino acids (GABA, glutamate, glutamine, alanine, glycine) were decreased. Aspartate was increased, and the major changes occurred in glutamate and alanine. Hyperthyroidism increased most of the nonessential amino acids. These results indicate altered utilization of nonessential amino acids when changes occur in carbohydrate metabolism. When the effects of externally administered hormones on metabolism were studied in the few cases that included brain, comparatively little changes were found in the central nervous system. Despite these negative results, it may be expected that endocrine changes cause an alteration of metabolite levels in brain, particularly with hormones that affect membrane permeability, transport, and metabolism. Effects of those hormones that influence protein metabolism (for example, the administration of growth hormone after hypophysectomy in young animals) is not well established. Such effects of hormones on amino acid transport and protein metabolism that are observed in tissue such as muscle cannot be confirmed in brain. Increases in aminotransferases caused by increased concentrations of amino acids can be observed in liver but not in brain.

PATHOLOGICAL CHANGES (17–24)

The amino acid pool in the brain is altered in many pathological conditions. We have relatively few data available in this area because most of the pathological alterations found in humans cannot be reproduced in animal models. Moreover, it was feared that postmortem changes in human brain would make analysis of pathological samples futile. This, however, need not be the case. It is true that, because a much higher proportion of amino acids are protein bound in brain, any breakdown, perhaps as little as 0.5% of the protein, could double the level of many free amino acids. However, it seems that the postmortem proteolytic breakdown in intact brain tissue is relatively small, and studies of autopsied tissue do yield interesting information.

Aminoacidurias

Among the few pathological changes that have been studied in detail and have also been investigated in animal models, is phenylketonuria. In humans, an approximate fivefold increase of phenylalanine in the brain was reported with a decrease in tyrosine and tryptophan. In spinal fluid several amino acids were increased, including tyrosine and tryptophan. This indicates that high levels of phenylalanine in the plasma competitively decrease the uptake of tyrosine and tryptophan from plasma, while high cerebrospinal fluid (CSF) phenylalanine decreases the transport of related amino acids from the spinal fluid. The inhibition by increased plasma phenylalanine of the uptake of large neutral amino acids by the brain from the plasma, has been confirmed in various systems. In model experiments the feeding of one of a number of amino acids, in excess, decreased the uptake of other members of the same transport class. Other aminoacidurias have been studied less frequently, but the elevated plasma levels of amino acids caused elevated brain levels in most cases (for example, in Maple Syrup Urine disease, the branched chain amino acids were increased in brain; histidine levels were increased in histidinemia). In many cases metabolites of the increased amino acid also increase, but this is not so well-established except in model animal experiments. In one study, galactose also affected free amino acids in brain, decreasing alanine, proline, methionine, and leucine. It can be therefore expected that in pathological alterations of carbohydrate metabolism amino acid distribution may be altered. This does not occur through hexose–amino acid transport interactions; hexoses belong to a separate transport class.

In model systems it was shown in a number of cases that the increased level of an amino acid in brain increases metabolism of related amino acids. Therefore the lowering of cerebral levels of related compounds can be the result not only of restricted uptake from blood, but also of increased cerebral metabolism. Greatly increased levels of amino acids then can have a wide variety of effects; such imbalance can cause inhibition of enzyme activity, and could cause release of lysosomal enzymes, or could have specific effects, such as on myelin lipid or on myelin protein metabolism. It is to be expected that toxic amine formation may also be increased under such conditions.

Brain Damage

One of the principal barriers to substances that are not actively transported is the formation of tight junctions in the capillary endothelium, which prevents large molecular weight compounds from entering the brain. The small amounts of such molecules that do penetrate into the cerebral extracellular space via the spinal fluid or the choroid plexus are prevented intracellular passage primarily by cell membranes. The capillary endothelial barrier, especially, is often altered by diseases of the central nervous system, and the pathological changes in its structural organization most often cause either localized or generalized increased permeability. We know a great deal about increases in permeability that permit the entry of marker substances under a variety of pathological conditions. The changes in the endogenous pools are much less known, and the question is not clear of what role capillary permeability plays in cerebral homeostasis of metabolites. When brain slices are incubated in a medium that has no amino acids, the tissue maintains the composition of the free amino acid pool fairly close to that *in vivo*. Only a few compounds, such as glutamine, leak out, and the amount of others that appear in the medium apparently is produced by autolysis. This indicates that the intracellular pool can be maintained when an extracellular pool is depleted. In turn, the high rate of uptake of most amino acids by slices indicates that any increase in the extracellular levels will cause an increase in the intracellular concentrations.

It is to be expected that damage, even to the capillary endothelium, would be variable, affecting various areas and permeability of various compounds differentially. For instance, osmotic damage to the barrier that causes opening of the tight junctions is reversible, and increased permeation rates, measured by the increased entry of dyes and amino acids, reverts to normal rates in 15 to 30 min. In various edemas (cold-induced, inflammatory, traumatic, associated with anoxia, induced by chemicals such as tryethyltin) ion and fluid changes can often be observed, but the entry of larger molecules can be observed only in those cases of structural damage to the small blood vessels. The discrimination between smaller and larger molecular weight compounds also occurs during recovery from injury, since permeability barriers to large molecules are restored faster than are those that block passage of smaller molecular weight substances.

Permeability changes have been investigated to the greatest extent using brain tumors. There is a great increase in *passive* permeability, since many compounds with different transport characteristics appear equally in the tumor, but not at higher concentrations than in plasma. Initial studies do not indicate any greater capacity of the *active* transport processes, but amino acid uptake rates and changes in pool composition have not yet been established for human tumors. This subject area needs further study because it has been reported that brain tumors do have very low or no GABA, and acetyl aspartate and glutamate may also be lower in comparison to normal tissue. When the neuronal uptake and incorporation of amino acids was compared with that of glia in various experimental systems, the results were somewhat variable, but in general, incorporation was greater in the neurons whereas the uptake of free amino acids was greater in glia. Although some of these results may be due to preparation artifacts, some similar changes can be expected in tumors. Changes in permeability in the pathological conditions, due to glial tumors, for example, and in particular, the increased effect of systemically administered and synaptically active amino acids in induced epilepsy, indicate that changes in brain due to changes in plasma amino acid levels can be observed to a greater extent in the injured than in the normal brain.

ALTERATIONS BY DRUGS (25–27)

A number of drugs affect the cerebral amino acid pool. These changes can be mediated in many ways, among them, by drugs affecting membrane permeability, amino acid metabolism, energy metabolism, or ionic shifts. Thus, it is surprising that amino acid pool changes have been studied only with a few drugs, although effects on amino acid transport have been studied with a large number of pharmaceutical preparations.

Of interest are reports of plasma factors, proteins that influence tryptophan uptake in brain preparations, uptake of which is reported to be altered in schizophrenia. Such studies that await further confirmation could be influenced by alterations in tryptophan binding to albumin in plasma, caused by previous drug treatments or diets.

Chlorpromazine lowers glutamate in particular, as well as some related amino acids (aspartate and GABA); reserpine has somewhat similar effects. Clorpromazine may have multiple effects: it can act as a detergent; it may form mycellar aggregates, with low concentrations stabilizing, and high concentrations lysing, membranes. Drugs that alter catecholamine metabolism (reserpine, lithium, 6-OH dopamine) also lower many of the nonessential amino acids (glutamate, aspartate, alanine, glycine) in specific structures. Ethanol was reported to lower GABA; some changes were reported with other drugs that damage membranes, such as triethyltin.

Damage to capillary permeability caused by noxious chemicals such as mercuric ion caused greater penetration of dyes but reduced the uptake of nonmetabolized amino acid analogues, that is, evidence was obtained for a greater diffusion and a lower degree of active transport.

Alterations During Convulsions

Changes, especially in nonessential amino acids, were studied in detail during experimentally induced seizures and in analysis of human epileptogenic focal tissue. The changes reported depend somewhat on the experimental conditions used to induce seizures. In human epileptogenic cortex, the most specific changes were an increase in glycine and a decrease in taurine and glutamic acid; in surrounding tissue, aspartate and GABA were also lowered. Similar changes were reported in cobalt induced convulsions. When taurine was administered to experimental animals with Co-induced convulsions, the alterations in amino acids were restored, i.e., glutamic acid increased and glycine decreased to normal. These findings led to the trial of taurine in the treatment of epilepsy. Amino acid changes in epilepsy were suggested to reflect an uncoupling between glucose oxidation and amino acid metabolism. Whether the changes that occur in human seizures are normalized by taurine is not clear. With convulsions caused by pentamethylenetetrazole the greatest change observed was an increase in alanine, perhaps by interference with the entry of pyruvate into the tricarboxylic acid cycle. In other experimentally induced seizures, glutamic acid decarboxylase was inhibited, and glutaminase activity increased, resulting in increased glutamate and related compounds. Glutamate also increased during audiogenic seizures.

In addition to changes in metabolism, permeability changes may also occur in convulsions. ^{35}S penetration into electrically activated regions was found during metrazole and strychnine convulsions. However, the degree of metabolic incorporation of ^{35}S was not altered. Similarly, regional entry of albumin indicated altered vascular permeability. These changes, in turn, may be caused indirectly by changes in the supply of oxygen or metabolic energy.

Hypoxia and Hypothermia

The changes in the free amino acid pool after ischemia, hypoxia, or hypothermia are fairly similar: Glutamate and aspartate decrease and GABA increases. These similarities are of interest, since the general effects of hypoxia and hypothermia on metabolism, morphology, and fluid shifts, are very different. Similar effects were found in hibernation, and upon arousal, the amino acid pools returned to normal. Also, in combined anesthesia and hypothermia, glutamate and aspartate were affected, and upon rewarming they changed back, with an overshoot. Hypothermia profoundly affects protein turnover (approximately 6% decrease per degree centigrade), but since protein turnover does not cause net utilization or production of amino acids, turnover rate alterations may not affect the free amino acid pool. Lowering brain temperature also lowers the passage of extracellular markers from the CSF, while under similar conditions the passage of leucine is only slightly altered. These findings indicate a possible change in the extracellular compartment during hypothermia.

MECHANISMS OF CHANGES (28–31)

Perhaps because it is more approachable experimentally, many investigators focused on morphological alterations, especially those that might increase capillary permeability in the brain. Such morphological changes are not likely to result in a major alteration of the cerebral amino acid pool. The nonessential amino acids do not leak out of brain tissue and are highly concentrated and retained in the cells. The concentration difference of the essential amino acids, on the other hand, between brain and plasma, is relatively small. Even if the tissue and plasma would be more "leaky" for these compounds, no great change can be expected.

The two most likely factors involved in pool changes are intracellular metabolism and membrane transport. Both can be influenced in many different ways. The available evidence does not suggest any major change in enzyme concentrations, but indicates that an activation of latent enzyme activity, or an inhibition by the altered substrate levels, or an altered availability of other factors greatly alters the enzyme activity pattern and hence will result in a major shift of amino acid metabolism, with the stimulation of production or inhibition of breakdown greatly increasing particular components, and increased utilization or inhibition of synthesis greatly decreasing others.

That changes in transport can affect amino acid levels was shown measuring competitive interactions of the amino acids in model systems, wherein the increase of one compound interfered with the transport of structurally related compounds belonging to the same transport class. These interactions were observed primarily in uptake experiments measuring amino acid movement from plasma to brain, but similar interactions can occur in other areas and in other directions, e.g., exit from the spinal fluid, or from the brain cells. Heteroexchange or competitive stimulation cannot be excluded among the processes.

In addition to interactions of amino acids within the same transport class, other factors also affect transport rates, e.g., the effect of available energy and ion gradients. Although it is not clearly established what is the primary energy source for active amino acid transport in brain or in other organs, in general a lowered energy supply results in inhibition of transport. Decreased sodium, unidirectional sodium flow, or ion potential gradients affect amino acid flux and distribution.

Changes in available energy levels or in ion distribution may occur locally. However, local and general energy or ion level changes do not affect all amino acids to the same degree. Therefore, alterations are rather specific, and influence a few amino acids or few sites, and may

be even subcellularly localized at membranes of specific particles or cells.

The regional heterogeneity of effects on transport is probably coincident to a similar substrate and regional specificity of metabolic alterations. Most of the enzymes involved in amino acid metabolism (decarboxylases, amino transferases, dehydrogenases) show great heterogeneity in their distribution, latency, inhibition, cofactor requirement, i.e., the decarboxylation of one substrate at specific sites may be altered without concomitant changes of other substrates.

Although we know a great deal about the role of amino acids in protein synthesis, neurotransmission, neurotransmitter production, there are important gaps in our knowledge which prevent us from understanding the mechanism of pathology due to altered amino acid composition. Despite scattered results from some studies, how amino acid levels influence protein turnover or the formation or inhibition of synthesis of specific proteins is not well understood. The function of amino acid catabolism and any effects of the catabolites on brain metabolism and function are not well understood. What, however, has been developed in recent years are the experimental tools to approach and study these problems. A better understanding can be expected, with important contributions, and solutions to the problems of treating of pathological cases well, within the next 25 years of the NINCDS.

REFERENCES

1. Gaull, G. E., Tallan, H. H., Lajtha, A., and Rassin, D. K. (1975): Pathogenesis of brain dysfunction in inborn errors of amino acid metabolism. In: *Biology of Brain Dysfunction,* edited by G. E. Gaull, Vol. 3, pp. 47–143. Plenum Press, New York.
2. Himwich, W. A., and Agrawal, H. C. (1969): Amino acids. In: *Handbook of Neurochemistry,* edited by A. Lajtha, Vol. 1, pp. 33–52. Plenum Press, New York.
3. Osborne, N. N., Wu, P. H., and Neuhoff, V. (1974): Free amino acids and related compounds in the dorsal root ganglia and spinal cord of the rat as determined by the micro dansylation procedure. *Brain Res.,* 74:175–181.
4. Benuck, M., and Lajtha, A. (1975): Aminotransferase activity in brain. In: *International Review of Neurobiology,* edited by C. C. Pfeiffer and J. R. Smythies, Vol. 17, pp. 85–129. Academic Press, New York.

5. Felig, P., Wahren, J., and Ahlborg, G. (1973): Uptake of individual amino acids by the human brain. *Proc. Soc. Exptl. Biol. Med.,* 142:230–236.

6. Lajtha, A., and Marks, N. (1971): Protein turnover. In: *Handbook of Neurochemistry,* edited by A. Lajtha, Vol. 5, pp. 551–629. Plenum Press, New York.

7. Badger, T. M., and Tumbleson, M. E. (1975): Postnatal changes in free amino acid, DNA, RNA and protein concentrations of miniature swine brain. *J. Neurochem.,* 24:361–366.

8. Baxter, C. F. (1968): Intrinsic amino acid levels and the blood-brain barrier. In: *Progress in Brain Research, Vol. 29: Brain Barrier Systems,* edited by A. Lajtha and D. H. Ford, pp. 429–450. Elsevier, Amsterdam.

9. Davis, J. M., and Himwich, W. A. (1973): Amino acids and proteins of developing mammalian brain. In: *Biochemistry of the Developing Brain,* edited by W. Himwich, pp. 55–110. Marcel Dekker, New York.

10. Lajtha, A., and Dunlop, D. (1974): Alterations of protein metabolism during development of the brain. In: *Drugs and the Developing Brain,* edited by A. Vernadakis and N. Weiner, pp. 215–229. Plenum Press, New York.

11. Lajtha, A., and Toth, J. (1973): Perinatal changes in the free amino acid pool of the brain in mice. *Brain Res.,* 55:238–241.

12. Enwonwu, C. O., and Worthington, B. S. (1974): Regional distribution of homocarnosine and other ninhydrin-positive substances in brains of malnourished monkeys. *J. Neurochem.,* 22:1045–1052.

13. Fernstrom, J. D., Madras, B. K., Munro, H. N., and Wurtman, R. J. (1974): Nutritional control of the synthesis of 5-hydroxytryptamine in the brain. In: *Aromatic Amino Acids in the Brain, CIBA Foundation Symposium 22,* pp. 153–173. American Elsevier, New York.

14. Ford, D. H. (1967): Changes in brain accumulation of amino acids and adenine associated with changes in the physiological state. In: *Progress in Brain Research, Vol. 29: Brain Barrier Systems,* edited by A. Lajtha and D. H. Ford, pp. 401–416. Elsevier, Amsterdam.

15. Peng, Y., Gubin, J., Harper, A. E., Vavich, M. G., and Kemmerer, A. R. (1973): Food intake regulation: amino acid toxicity and changes in rat brain and plasma amino acids. *J. Nutr.,* 103:608–617.

16. Roberts, S. (1974): Effects of amino acid imbalance on amino acid utilization, protein synthesis and polyribosome function in cerebral cortex. In: *Aromatic Amino Acids in the Brain, CIBA Foundation Symposium 22,* pp. 299–324. American Elsevier, New York.

17. Agrawal, H., and Davison, A. N. (1973): Myelination and amino acid imbalance in the developing brain. In: *Biochemistry of Developing Brain,* edited by W. A. Himwich, pp. 143–186. Marcel Dekker, New York.

18. Bakay, L. (1972): Alteration of the brain barrier system in pathological states. In: *Handbook of Neurochemistry,* edited by A. Lajtha, Vol. 7, pp. 417–427. Plenum Press, New York.

19. Bulfield, G., and Kacser, H. (1975): Histamine and histidine levels in the brain of the histadinaemic mouse. *J. Neurochem.,* 24:403–405.

20. van Gelder, N. M., Sherwin, A. L., and Rasmussen, T. (1972): Amino acid content of epileptogenic human brain: Focal *versus* surrounding regions. *Brain Res.,* 40:385–393.

21. Warner, K. A., Frohman, C. E., and Gottlieb, J. S. (1972): The effect of the plasma factor on the uptake of amino acids by neural tissue. *Biol. Psychiatr.,* 5:173–180.

22. Wiechert, P., and Göllnitz, G. (1969): Metabolic investigations of epileptic seizures. The concentration of free amino acids in cerebral tissue prior to and during cerebral seizures. *J. Neurochem.,* 16:1007–1016.

23. Winick, M. (1974): Malnutrition and the developing brain. In: *Res. Publ. Assoc. Nerv. Ment. Dis., Vol. 53: Brain Dysfunction in Metabolic Disorders,* edited by F. Plum, pp. 253–261. Raven Press, New York.

24. Wollemann, M. (1974): *Biochemistry of Brain Tumors.* University Park Press, Baltimore.

25. Rapoport, S. I., Hori, M., and Klatzo, I. (1972): Testing of a hypothesis for osmotic opening of the blood-brain barrier. *Am. J. Physiol.,* 223:323–331.

26. Santini, M., and Berl, S. (1972): Effects of reserpine and monoamine oxidase inhibition on the levels of amino acids in sensory ganglia, sympathetic ganglia and spinal cord. *Brain Res.,* 47:167–176.

27. Steinwall, O. (1967): Transport inhibition phenomena in unilateral chemical injury of blood-brain barrier. In: *Progress in Brain Research, Vol. 29: Brain Barrier Systems,* edited by A. Lajtha and D. H. Ford, pp. 357–365. Elsevier, New York.

28. Bennett, J. P., Mulder, A. H., and Snyder, S. H. (1974): Neurochemical correlates of synaptically active amino acids. *Life Sci.,* 15:1045–1056.

29. Franklin, G. M., Dudzinski, D. S., and Cutler, R. W. P. (1975): Amino acid transport into the cerebrospinal fluid of the rat. *J. Neurochem.,* 24:367–372.

30. Lajtha, A. (1968): Transport as control mechanism of cerebral metabolite levels. In: *Progress in Brain Research, Vol. 29: Brain Barrier Systems,* edited by A. Lajtha, and D. H. Ford, pp. 201–218. Elsevier, Amsterdam.

31. Lajtha, A. (1974): Amino acid transport in the brain *in vivo* and *in vitro.* In: *CIBA Foundation Symposium 22,* pp. 25–49. Elsevier, Amsterdam.

The Nervous System, Donald B. Tower. Editor-in-Chief. *Vol. 1: The Basic Neurosciences.* Raven Press, New York, 1975.

Biochemical Strategies in the Study of Memory Formation

Bernard W. Agranoff

That much has been written in the past decade about possible biochemical bases for memory bears witness to the great interest and fascination of scientists and laymen alike for one of the most challenging scientific riddles of our time. Behind this interest lies more than mere curiosity—problems of memory play an increasingly important role in human society. As biomedical advances prolong the viability of our bodies, it becomes more essential that the brain, the organ that the rest of the body subserves, functions sufficiently well to render the added years of lifespan meaningful and useful. That this area of investigation is replete with controversy demonstrates the numerous conceptual and experimental difficulties that still face the investigator. A major problem is that of finding suitable model systems. Human memory, as we ordinarily think of it, is largely verbal and there may not therefore exist a suitable animal counterpart. We, nevertheless, generally assume that understanding the biological basis of the conditioned reflex in lower animals will ultimately lead the way to understanding the biological basis of human behavior. This assumption may or may not prove true, but we are for the present too puzzled and engrossed in the so-called simple animal model to worry, for the time being, about its universality.

Should we not select an even simpler model for study—for example, an isolated neuronal network that will hopefully demonstrate electrophysiological changes that can be formally related to conditioned reflex formation? Although isolated fragments of brain, spinal cord, or ganglia are of great neurobiological interest, they have thus far not served as adequate models of behavior. Electrophysiological changes tend to be of brief duration compared to long-lasting behavioral phenomena. Furthermore, even "simple" systems are extremely complex anatomically. The whole animal, admittedly still more complex, has at least the advantage that its behavioral changes are easily evaluated by a number of generally accepted psychological criteria, including survival of the altered behavioral state over long periods of time.

A BIOCHEMICAL APPROACH—THE USE OF INTERVENTIVE AGENTS

There are possibly only two ways in which one can use biochemical tools to study a complex physiological phenomenon *in vivo.* The first is pharmacological intervention with agents known to have selective biochemical effects. In the case of memory, the independent variable is the observed performance of the experimental subject. The second approach is to search for concomitant biochemical alterations that can be correlated with learning or memory, such as a change in brain composition or metabolism. Although there have been reports of measurable alterations in brain proteins, nucleic acids, and other macromolecular components following various training procedures, claims have more generally been limited to changes in incorporation of an isotopic precursor, such as labeled uridine into brain RNA (1). This latter approach will be discussed below in relation to the blocking agents.

Three species have been predominant in the literature on the use of the various antibiotic blocking agents on memory: the goldfish (2), the mouse (3,4), and the chick (5). In retrospect, this is unexpected, inasmuch as the rat had dominated animal learning studies for many years. I believe that the reasons for this shift include the following:

1. Because "memory bioassays" have great inherent variability, large numbers of subjects

are required. The three experimental subjects are relatively inexpensive (about one-tenth the cost of the rat, in the U.S.).

2. Inbred strains, particularly of the mouse, show less genetic variability than most available rat strains. This might in some instances be reflected in less behavioral variability.

3. In the case of the glutarimide antibiotics, the rat shows an idiosyncratic sensitivity, resulting in high toxicity.

The results of the various studies on memory in the goldfish, mouse, and chick, using a number of different training paradigms, show the following general properties.

1. Inhibition of DNA, RNA, or protein synthesis can be used to block 80 to 100% of the respective synthetic processes for hours without eliciting a significant effect on normal behavior.

2. Under conditions of the block of RNA or protein synthesis, animals show normal acquisition of a novel task but cannot form a permanent memory of what they have learned. In contrast, block of DNA synthesis has no effect on memory.

3. If the blocking agent is administered immediately following training, permanent memory will not be formed, whereas administration of the drug a short time later will have no effect. For example, a goldfish given 20 trials in a shock avoidance task in a single session will demonstrate the learned habit when retested a few days later. If the antibiotic inhibitor of protein synthesis, puromycin, is injected intracranially either before training, or just after training, the animal will perform at about the level of a "naive" subject when retested several days later (6). The same amount of the drug, injected a few hours after training, or at any subsequent time, will have no effect on performance. The period of growing unsusceptibility to the agent just following the training session is referred to as the consolidation period—the time it takes for memory to become fixed. Whether the blocking agents prevent memory from "hardening" or act by blocking the conversion of a temporary, short-term form to a permanent one cannot be distinguished from these experiments.

4. A consolidation gradient can also be obtained by administration of electroconvulsive shock (ECS) at various times after training. For many years, it had been suspected that the early form of memory was "electrical," whereas the long-term form was "chemical." Electroconvulsive shock was believed to destroy the nascent memory by producing electrical storms and silences. At one time it was proposed that the protein inhibitors mediated their effect on memory in a similar way—although no frank convulsions are produced by the antibiotics, such as are seen with ECS, it was possible that puromycin produced "occult seizures" (4). The idea that the various blockers produced amnesia *via* electrical disturbances has in the meantime been generally discredited. Although puromycin does potentiate pentylene tetrazol (PTZ)-induced seizures in the mouse and in the goldfish, the glutarimide antibiotics and actinomycin D do not, yet are amnestic agents (2). Furthermore, PAN (puromycin aminonucleoside) an analogue of puromycin which blocks neither protein synthesis nor memory, shares the property of puromycin of potentiating the PTZ-induced seizures (2).

A curious footnote to this confusion of electrical and antimetabolic actions comes from recent studies in which we have found a proactive effect of ECS on memory in the goldfish (7). Naive subjects are given ECS, allowed to recover, and are trained, all within 2 hr. The subjects, like antibiotic-injected ones, learn normally, but develop a memory loss. In other words, rather than to offer an "electrical" explanation for the action of the antibiotics, we must now ask whether the amnestic effects of ECS have a chemical basis. At least we can say that some lingering process, initiated by the convulsion, and that persists beyond the seizures mediates the amnestic effect.

5. In the fish, one can take advantage of its poikilothermic properties to demonstrate further the chemical nature of memory. Cooling fish following training increases the period of susceptibility to either antibiotic or to ECS-induced amnesia, while warming shortens the consolidation time (2). Cooling, in the absence of an amnestic treatment, for as long as a day, can be administered to mimic the effects of the antibiotic administration on the incorporation of labeled precursor amino acids into brain protein. Following recovery, in this case, there is no observed memory deficit. The block in

macromolecular synthesis must, apparently, take place in the presence of normally ongoing brain metabolism to effect a measurable memory block.

6. Memory fixation is not only time dependent, but can be shown to be sensitive to the animal's environment as well. Goldfish allowed to remain in the training apparatus following training of shock avoidance do not initiate the antibiotic-sensitive step of memory formation: it does not begin until the fish has been returned to its home tank (8). We have interpreted this result to indicate that the lowering of arousal associated with removal from the aversive training setting to a familiar and safe-appearing one is the biological message that triggers fixation. The change in setting is perhaps a physiological way of informing the subject that he has been successful.

ACQUISITION AND THE PREWIRED BRAIN

In the absence of compelling arguments to the contrary, it is only a parsimonious interpretation of the available facts to assume that the information-specific aspects of memory formation are directly related to the complex neuronal network of the brain. It is no more than saying that the most complex information-processing equipment that we know of resides in the most complex known morphological structure. A common, perhaps overworked, reductionist model to illustrate how neurons might mediate behavior depicts two neurons terminating presynaptically on a third. The model requires that one presynaptic neuron represents the conditioned stimulus and the other, the unconditioned stimulus. The postsynaptic neuron mediates the unconditioned response initially. By firing the two neurons in an appropriate temporal sequence, neuron A, initially unable to fire the postsynaptic neuron will, like neuron B now do so permanently. Since, as we have already indicated, the blocking agents do not appear to affect the process whereby the probability of firing is altered, we will not dwell on this aspect of the model, but turn to its use as a conceptual basis for memory based on neuronal connectivity. Although it is doubtful that any single new overt behavior is mediated by alterations in a very small number of neurons, the

model suggests that whatever the number of cells involved, learning may involve relatively minor alterations in the state of preexisting neurons and their synapses. A strict interpretation of this concept suggests that we can evoke only preexisting response routines, in analogy with selective mechanisms of antibody formation. Certainly, we accept the notion of prewired connections in the case of instinctive behavior. An animal raised in isolation still shows species-specific responses following presentation of a natural predator. What we normally regard as brain "plasticity" may be a variant of such prewired behavior in which the animal selects from a diverse number of possible responses. Obviously, a higher degree of selection is required in learning a discrimination task or one which requires a high degree of motor skill for responding, than for the acquisition of a conditioned emotional response, in which the simpler model suffices. For more complex behaviors we must add temporal sequencing of a number of neuronal subunits, a mechanism for reward to inform the animal which response was correct, and also in some instances a message of success that leads to the onset of memory fixation. The "fix signal" may in itself not be task specific. As with the environmental trigger, it may say "whatever just happened, remember it." The possibility is intriguing in that it suggests that the action of the antibiotics may not be on an information specific process.

The question of information specificity is an important one since the antibiotic studies are occasionally quoted to support the idea that memories may be encoded into specific macromolecules, as in the "memory transfer" experiments. For the present, I consider it more likely that the blocking agents do not act on an information-specific process, but on the fixation mechanism itself. By analogy, we might imagine a latent unstable photographic image that has been developed, but not fixed. The fixative must be applied within a short period of time, or else the image will fade. The fixative itself contains no information.

Support for a general fixation mechanism comes from human memory studies. Bilateral hippocampectomy results in a syndrome in which memory may form, but cannot be fixed. Such a lesion has not been demonstrated in subhuman species, although antibiotic-treated animals behave in just this way.

A "fix signal" could be mediated by a neurotransmitter, the diffuse release of which causes fixation in only those synapses which are in a heightened state following acquisition that renders them sensitive to the signal. Alternatively, the agents could be acting at synaptic loci where a "soldering" is converting short-term into long-term memory. As discussed below, resolution of these possibilities may require experiments directed at anatomical localization of the learned response or of the putative fixation signal. Reports from various laboratories of the block of memory formation by drugs that affect catecholamine, indolamine or acetylcholine metabolism may indicate some overlap with the effects of the antibiotics, since the blocking agents could inhibit formation of enzymes of neurotransmitter synthesis. That so many agents have been found effective suggests that there may be many ways to block memory fixation. Since the various reports involve different tasks in different species, it is difficult at present to draw more precise conclusions.

SHORT-TERM MEMORY AND ITS DECAY

The loss of performance that begins following training in antibiotic-treated animals can be viewed as the result of failure to consolidate. What we then see is the decay of the short-term form of memory over the next few hours or days. Short-term memory decay is seen in the goldfish following ECS, giving further support to the proposal that ECS does not destroy memory, but like the antibiotics, causes failure of consolidation.

There are no known agents that selectively block the formation of short-term memory. Such an action might indeed be impossible to demonstrate, as we would not be able to distinguish effects on memory from nonspecific actions such as those produced by drugs that cause a loss of attentiveness, drowsiness, etc. Recently, however, a number of agents have been shown to have an effect on memory distinct from that of ECS or the antibiotics. Lithium, copper, or ouabain, will produce an amnestic response in the chick, if given prior to training, but unlike the antibiotics, has no

effect on memory when given after training. A new phase of memory formation is thus inferred, between acquisition and long-term memory formation, which by further inference is believed to be mediated by synaptic ionic changes (9).

LIMITATIONS AND PROSPECTS FOR MEMORY STUDIES

The number of agents that will block long-term memory formation includes the protein biosynthesis inhibitors puromycin, cycloheximide, acetoxycycloheximide and anisomycin; the RNA biosynthesis blockers, actinomycin D, camptothecin, and alpha-amanitin. Lengthening the list is perhaps not as interesting as finding differential effects, for example, finding agents with selective action on classes of macromolecule synthesis or degradation that will pinpoint further the mechanism of action of the various agents.

A major limitation has been the measurement of memory itself. Performance is the sum of complex interactive behavioral elements. For example, in avoidance conditioning, one can measure associated autonomic response components. In a separate study, we investigated the effect of ECS and puromycin on autonomic conditioning. Fish received a light signal followed by an unavoidable electrical shock. The shock itself, but not the light, caused a temporary cardiac slowing. We were able to condition the animals, i.e., the heart rate eventually decreased on light presentation. They retained this conditioned autonomic response for several days. It turned out not to be blocked by either puromycin or by ECS. It is possible then that the amnestic agents block only the instrumental aspects of learning. We indicated above that such learning might require a higher degree of "selection" of neural circuitry than does the conditioned autonomic response. Instrumental learning might therefore have a greater need for a positive-feedback message of success. If this step is selectively blocked by the antibiotic agents, it could account for the differential sensitivity of instrumental learning relative to the conditioning of the autonomic response.

I am hopeful that the antibiotic interventive approach will be useful in localization studies. We have shown in the monkey (10), that microinjection of cycloheximide can produce regional inhibition of protein synthesis, by means of radioautography. Because these blocks are reversible, chronic experiments are then possible in which selected brain areas can be blocked for varying periods of time, repeatedly. This procedure should be useful for the systematic localization of memory functions in animals in a much more precise fashion than by the surgical lesion approach that has characterized and dominated previous studies attempting to localize higher brain function.

It is in the area of localization, that studies on concomitants of brain function also bear promise for the future. A number of studies have proposed altered labeling of brain macromolecules, usually RNA, as a function of learning. In a typical experiment (1), a mouse is injected intracerebrally with ^{14}C-uridine and is trained, while a yoked-control (exposed to the stimulus, but not trained) is given ^{3}H-uridine. The brains are combined and ^{3}H/^{14}C ratios are surveyed throughout a distribution gradient to seek out a "blip" heralding a novel RNA—the needle in the haystack. This ingenious approach has yielded positive results, of a sort. The needle in the haystack has not appeared—but differences throughout the RNA fractions are seen. If this result can be related to the experiments with blocking agents, it supports a block of an information-*non*specific step, since the observed changes are too massive and global to be related to the learning of a single new task. It is more likely related to the fixation process. It is a great pity that the same behavioral paradigm and strain of animal has not as yet been used with both the antibiotic blocking approach and a labeling experiment. In the goldfish, we have not observed an alteration of RNA or protein labeling specific to learning. Laboratories using the mouse and chick have employed only the interventive approach or the search of concomitants—not both.

In experiments purporting to show changes in RNA synthesis, it remains possible that the investigators are observing alterations in precursor pools rather than *de novo* rates of RNA synthesis. The question of precursor pools in *in vivo* experiments is a thorny one since it is probably not possible to measure the relevant compartments. Whether the changes are due to RNA synthesis or to changes in precursor pool

size, an encouraging aspect of these experiments is the apparent anatomical localization of the effects—the diencephalon in the case of a jump-up task in the mouse, and the roof of the forebrain in an imprinting task in the chick (11). Studies on the anatomical localization of a block of these tasks with antibiotics are in order. Further progress in memory research may well depend on the combined use of several approaches, including the interventive antibiotic studies to indicate *where* and *when* consolidation is taking place in the brain, and concomitant labeling studies to verify *where* and to tell us more about *what* is happening.

In summary, progress in this field leads us to the conclusion that RNA and protein synthesis must be ongoing normally in order for short-term memory of instrumental learning to be converted to a long-term form. Evidence of support of the hypothesis that the antibiotics are blocking the fixation signal rather than an information-containing step is reviewed.

In the introduction, I mentioned the qualitative difference between animal and human memory. At present, a remarkably large part of our knowledge of human memory, particularly those studies where complete neurological documentation is available, tends to be anecdotal. Further progress in understanding human memory may require closer contact between the clinician and the quantitative behavioral scientist. With regard to concomitants of human memory, new trends in noninvasive techniques that couple computer processing with physical tools such as X-ray and gamma emitters give hope that we will eventually be able to evaluate regional cerebral circulation, oxygen consumption, and perhaps even regional protein synthesis in the intact human brain.

REFERENCES

1. Glassman, E. (1969): The biochemistry of learning: an evaluation of the role of RNA and protein. *Annu. Rev. Biochem.,* 38:605.
2. Agranoff, B. W. (1975): Biochemical concomitants of the storage of behavioral information. In: *Biochemistry of Sensory Processes,* edited by L. Jaenicke. Springer-Verlag, Heidelberg.
3. Roberts, R. B., and Flexner, L. B. (1969): The biochemical basis of long-term memory. *Q. Rev. Biophys.,* 2:135.
4. Barondes, S. H. (1970): Cerebral protein synthesis inhibitors block long-term memory. *Int. Rev. Neurobiol.,* 12:177.

5. Mark, R. F., and Watts, M. E. (1971): Drug inhibition of memory formation in chickens I. Long-term memory. *Proc. R. Soc. Lond.* [*Biol.*], 178:439.

6. Agranoff, B. W., and Klinger, P. D. (1964): Puromycin effect on memory formation in the goldfish. *Science,* 146:952.

7. Springer, A. D., Schoel, W. M., Klinger, P. D., and Agranoff, B. W. (1975): Anterograde and retrograde effects of electroconvulsive shock and of puromycin on memory formation in the goldfish. *Behav. Biol.,* 13:467.

8. Davis, R. E., and Agranoff, B. W. (1966): Stages of memory formation in goldfish: evidence for an environmental trigger, *Proc. Natl. Acad. Sci. USA,* 55:555.

9. Watts, M. E., and Mark, R. F. (1971): Drug inhibition of memory formation in chickens II. Short-term memory. *Proc. R. Soc. Lond.* [*Biol.*], 178:455.

10. Eichenbaum, H., Butter, C. M., and Agranoff, B. W. (1973): Radioautographic localization of inhibition of protein synthesis in specific regions of monkey brain. *Brain Res.,* 61:438.

11. Horn, G., Rose, S. P. R., and Bateson, P. P. G. (1973): Monocular imprinting and regional incorporation of tritiated uracil into the brains of intact and split-brain chicks. *Brain Res.,* 56:227.

The Nervous System, Donald B. Tower, Editor-in-Chief. *Vol. 1: The Basic Neurosciences.* Raven Press, New York, 1975.

The "Sign-Post" Function of Brain Glycoproteins: Order and Disorder

Samuel Bogoch

There is an increasing awareness that there is a biochemistry of learning and memory. That awareness has accelerated a direct experimental approach to the brain.

SOME METHODOLOGICAL PROBLEMS

The nervous system is the most complex biological structure known, and the complexity of its function is attested to throughout the ages by all who have attempted to study it. The attempt to understand the biochemistry of learning and memory in an experiment, therefore, presents a formidable challenge. The variables that require control can be divided into biochemical and behavioral. Some of these variables have been discussed by almost all workers in the field, but it is rare that many of them are kept track of in any one experiment. Further, it is likely from the nature of the subject and the unknowns remaining in it at this time, that many of the variables which need attention are as yet unknown.

Some of the behavioral variables will first be discussed. It is only in the last decade that most neurochemists have begun to pay attention to the proposition that the state of activity of the brain must be noted at the time of biochemical measurement. Thus a brain that is asleep is clearly not the same brain as one which is fully awake but at rest, or as one which is awake but active.

The activity composed of running, swimming, flapping of wings, climbing, and other vigorous motor pursuits are different from activities of problem solving intensity accompanied by motor quiescence. Both motor activity and problem solving activity are different from the active state of the brain in states of great motivation and in highly emotional states, especially those in which there is fear.

Further, those states broadly referred to as sleep, rest, motor active, problem-solving-active, motivated-active, emotional-active, (a) have many gradations and (b) usually are each present to different degrees not only in each experiment, but varying throughout the course of longer experiments.

For example what may be called the "swim for your life" type of experiment in which a rat must traverse a stretch of very cold water cannot possibly be thought of in the same light as one in which an apparently happy, well-fed, free-to-move pigeon plays a game with a few buttons, at its own pace. Similarly the "jump or you're going to get it" type of experiment in which the mouse stands on a grid which is periodically electrified to produce a painful and frightening stimulus, and piloerection and defecation are present, is not the same type of experiment as one in which the mouse may leisurely solve a maze problem for a sure reward at the end, with success at solving, or time to solve the key-dependent variable.

It may appear excessive to belabor these points, but even the current literature is full of lofty discussions which compare seemingly disparate biochemical results from two different experiments without noting that they are as different from each other as are those in the above examples.

The influence of strong sensory stimuli in themselves is an important variable.

Another important variable which is still being ignored is that of time. It is foolish to seek for the biochemical equivalent or correlate of a brain process which occurs as quickly as the committing to memory of a telephone number, in the process of axoplasmic flow whose time constant is hours. Figure 1 presented later in this paper emphasizes this point. That is, the incorporation of ^{14}C-glucose into brain glycoproteins in the resting pigeon is different from that in the training, but the pattern of incorporation after 10 min of training is different from each of those at 20, 30, and 60 min of training.

On the structural and biochemical side, in addition to the usual variables of solubility, *in situ* state of components as compared to final isolated products, the effect of changes in blood flow on localized areas of the brain when small brain areas are being compared, measuring concentrations of enough different related and unrelated substances in each experiment, and problems of compartmentation and pool size in radioactive labeling experiments are only a few examples in this area.

Almost all of these methodological problems are soluble by careful attention to detail, careful observation by the experimenter of what is actually happening to the animal, and control of as many variables as possible, or failing that, by comparison of experiments with different groups of variables. Because of the specialized training which most experimenters receive, close collaboration between two people of neurochemical and experimental psychological disciplines is probably best at this time.

PRIMARY AND SECONDARY BIOCHEMICAL PROCESSES IN LEARNING AND MEMORY

An important distinction must be made between energy-generating or membrane-maintaining processes in the nervous system, and the identification of particular molecules and processes which actually mediate the transmission of bioelectrical signal or facilitate storage in a nerve net. The required mechanisms for processing information in the nervous system have been increasingly recognized to involve the following (1): (1) Sensory input reception. (2) Encoding for transmission: transduction from primary sensory modalities to electrochemical equivalents utilized by nervous system cells. (3) Association and abstraction: association with information previously stored, pattern recognition, abstraction, synthesis of new constructs. (4) Storage: (a) Further encoding, or the same as (2)? (b) Same process for short and long duration? (5) Retrieval: remembering–forgetting. (6) Effector consequences of retrieval: further association and abstraction; discharge into thought, lan-

guage; motor and affective accompaniments. (7) Supporting chemical reactions for (1) through (6).

Sites for These Biochemical Processes (1)

The attempt to localize memory, in a biochemical sense, has had certain carryover influences from neuroanatomy and neurohistology. Thus certain efforts concentrate on the notion that memory is mediated by certain distinct brain regions, others on the notion that memory is a totally distributed phenomenon in the brain. Some work focuses on the search for memory traces contained within neurons, or one specific population of neurons; other work concentrates upon axonal change, on the growth of new cell processes, on the formation of new cells, on synaptic events, or on glial cells.

Some Requirements for Prospective Coding Molecules (1)

It is increasingly recognized that information bearing or coding molecules will probably exhibit the following characteristics (4): sufficient heterogeneity, fixed location, development which correlates with learning throughout the life of the organism, impairment in structure or concentration or function in correlation with impairment of memory and learning processes, the ability to demonstrate "recognition" functions, generative and regenerative properties which correlate with memory functions, change with certain forms of behavior, and change with learning.

Some biochemical theories of learning and memory, by molecular type, are listed in Table 1. Although it is not possible to discuss these various theories and the evidence which has accumulated with regard to each, the references in the table indicate some recent thorough reviews.

In addition to the reviews listed in Table 1, the general field of proteins of the nervous system has developed rapidly in the past ten years both in terms of definition of structure and metabolism of individual components. In one volume edited by Lajtha (4), for example, the structure of the nerve growth factor proteins is discussed by Shooter and Varon, axoplasmic

TABLE 1. *Some biochemical theories of memory by molecular type*

Chemical groups	Changes proposed	Theorist	Ref.	Year proposed
Nucleoproteins	Transformation from random to organized configuration	Halstead	(25)	1948
Acetylcholine and acetylcholinesterase	Increase in quantity and activity, respectively	Rosenzweig et al.	(1)	1958
Nucleic acids or proteins	Self-producing macromolecules	Gerard	(25)	1959
Ribonucleic acids	Change in base sequences	Hyden	(25)	1961
	Change in quantity of messenger RNA	Flexner et al.	(25)	1964
Ribonucleic acids or proteins	Change in base sequences or altered amino acid sequences	Gaito	(25)	1961
		Ungar	(3)	1970
Mucoids (glycoproteins and glycolipids) and glycosyl transferases	Change in concentration and activity respectively; carbohydrate plus protein specificity	Bogoch	(1)	1965, 1968
Catecholamines	Modification of protein effects	Roberts et al.	(25)	1970
		Essman	(25)	1973

flow of nerve proteins by Ochs, the effect of drugs on protein synthesis in the nervous system by Clouet, inhibition of brain protein synthesis by Appel, and chemical transfer of learned information by Ungar. In another volume edited by Davison et al. (5) brain-specific proteins are discussed by Moore, by Vincendon et al., by Warecka, and by the present author; neurotubule and neurofilament proteins by Shelanski et al., and by Angeletti; glycoproteins in brain by Brunngraber (see references in Brunngraber to work on their metabolism by Roseman, DiBenedetta, Dische, Barondes, Irwin, Margolis, Quarles and Brady, Forman et al., and Boseman et al.); glycoproteins in synaptic membranes by Breckenridge et al., and myelin lipids discussed by Mehl, by Folch-Pi, by Kies, by Eylar, by Mandel, by Morell et al., and by Marks. Reviews in the present volume will also be relevant to these proteins.

HISTORY OF BRAIN GLYCOPROTEIN AND MUCOID STUDIES

Twenty years ago, the computer analogy to brain function, although limited, was impressive to some, including the author. How-ever, even if this analogy was cogent, there was no notion of how the billions of cells in the brain could form such circuitry. How could all these cells grow together correctly in the first place; and how could these brain circuits be available to new learning?

Since mucoids (carbohydrates attached to proteins and/or lipids to form large molecular weight entities) were beginning to be understood to have a key role in determining the chemistry of "recognition" phenomena (1) in the A, B, O blood group system, and in contact functions of bacteria, the author wondered if they might perform similar functions in the brain (1).

Up to 1963, textbooks of neurochemistry had only a few pages on proteins of the brain. The glycoproteins of the brain were then extracted and found to represent a large and complex fraction of the total brain proteins (6).

The concept that brain glycoproteins are involved in learning processes was developed in studies beginning in 1956 which examined the possibility that the macromolecular carbohydrates in brain have membrane, receptor, and recognition functions. It was demonstrated that a group of substances in the brain with carbohydrate end groups, including the aminoglycolipids and the glycoproteins, have the following properties in common: chemical structural properties that would make them suited to function at membrane surfaces and membrane interfaces (7), properties of viral receptors (8,9), pharmacological specificity (10,11), molecular specificity related to antigen-antibody reactions (12); they occur in high concentration in the brain substance itself (13) and in membranes and synaptosome fractions from brain (14); they show changes in concentration with increasing developmental complexity of the nervous system (1), are disturbed when there is regression of higher brain functions (1,13), and show increases in concentration in particular brain glycoprotein fractions in relationship to operant conditioning training of pigeons (12).

In 1965 when we first demonstrated that the glycoproteins of brain change in concentration during training, I proposed that the glycoproteins and related substances of the brain are involved in information, contact, and communication functions in the nervous system (2). The 10 years of work preceding that study and 3 subsequent years of work on the subject were summarized in the 1968 monograph *The Biochemistry of Memory: With an Inquiry into the Function of the Brain Mucoids* and the "sign-post" theory was proposed (1).

The fine structure of the carbohydrate and amino acid chains of the glycoproteins that appear to be most involved in the brain of the training pigeon was studied in detail (14). The function of glycoproteins in the formation of brain circuitry was discussed (2,14–16), and the role of the brain glycoproteins in cell recognition was detailed in further studies on glycoproteins and brain tumors, where there is a regression of these postulated functions for brain glycoproteins (17).

Further to the study of brain glycoproteins in terms of intercell recognition, studies on the brain glycoproteins in the functionally regressive cerebral states of Tay-Sachs' disease have suggested that here there may be a disturbance of intraneuronal recognition (18).

In the functionally regressive cerebral states observed in the psychoses, our earliest observations on nervous system glycoproteins can be seen from the same perspective. In the case of human cerebrospinal fluid, we found the gly-

coproteins to be present in surprisingly high concentration, to increase with maturation, to show certain deficiencies in psychotic illness, and to return toward normal with recovery (Publications 1957–1967 summarized in Ref. 19). Thus if the brain glycoproteins are indeed involved in establishing functionally correct brain circuitry then disorders of brain glycoproteins may well be responsible for the functional disorders of thought, mood, and behavior.

THE SIGN-POST THEORY OF BRAIN CIRCUITRY

I have proposed (1,2) that the glycoproteins of the nervous system are involved in cell recognition, contact, and position functions and that these properties are responsible for the stable intercell circuitry necessary for information handling and storage by the nervous system. That is, the glycoproteins determine which nerve cells grow together in contact during development to permit transmission, as well as the facility of transmission at a given synaptic junction throughout life.

"A single carbohydrate end group might determine whether or not transmission of an impulse is facilitated between neuron A and B. Consider that in the presynaptic membrane belonging to neuron A there is a glycoprotein, glycoprotein A^1, whose carbohydrate end group can be two types, which determine whether contact is or is not taking place with the postsynaptic membrane belonging to neuron B. Thus, for example, glycoprotein A^1 may exist with its end group a galactosamine residue, but with the postsynaptic membrane B possessing the specific receptor B^1 (possibly, but not necessarily, also a glycoprotein) specific only for a galactose residue. In the resting state A^1 does not combine with B^1 and no synaptic contact results. Thus, although transmission is possible between A and B, it may not occur without facilitation. To state it another way, the threshold for transmission between neurons A and B may be an inverse function of the amount of physical contact between the membranes of A and B; the more contact, the lower the threshold.

A synthetic mechanism, a galactose transferase here taken as only one example, could be present at or in A, which could upon the proper stimulus attach a galactose residue to the galactosamine end group of A^1, thus changing the galactosamine end group to a galactose end group for A^1. This galactose end group of A^1 would combine immediately with receptor B^1, ionically or covalently, the contact between A and B would be increased, the threshold lowered, and transmission between A and B facilitated. It is possible that the 'proper stimulus' for attachment of galactose is the passage of an excitatory impulse of sufficient intensity through A. The question of whether A can fire B will depend upon (1) whether the synthetic reaction necessary to attach the correct end group on A^1 is at hand and immediately available, or if repressed, is able to be derepressed; and (2) whether the receptor B^1 is at hand to react with A^1 galactose. These paired configurations might be laid down with complete or relative specificity by genetic coding mechanisms and realized in the morphogenesis of the nervous system. Thus the chemical specificities of A and B which allow them to grow together in synaptic contact in the first place would be the same specificities determining their contact and the transmission of an impulse between them throughout the life of the organism.

The influence of experience would enter in terms of (1) the frequency of stimuli, or both, passing through A causing it to fire B. That is, the potential to synthesize A^1-galactose may require the activation by strong and/or repeated stimulation. (2) The competitive pathways available. That is, neuron A could transmit to neuron C, A to D, A to E, etc. All might be programmed genetically as possibilities, then a combined selection-instruction mechanism brought to bear by experience to determine which pathway is selected, or which alternative pathways are preferred, and their order of preference. A DNA-specified repression-derepression type of induction requiring experiential input for activation could well be involved for the A^1-galactose transferase reaction. The potential of the system may be quite extensive, as genetically programmed, but each component would require experiential realization in order to perform. That is, the degree of derepression in each instance would be a direct function of experiential input.

For A^1-galactose, it might be necessary to substitute A^1-(glycosaminoglycan)$_n$-galactose, 'n' representing the number of residues actually required to bridge the synaptic cleft so that the molecule A^1 may reach B^1.

Even greater complexity and selectivity could be achieved by having more than one specific glycoprotein and receptor present per synapse, thus A^1, A^2, A^3, A^n, and B^1, B^2, B^3, and B^n.

Chemical coding of information in the brain would thus be visualized as a specific set of instructions determining whether, and under what conditions, each neuron will fire any other accessible neuron. The actual information coded in glycoprotein A^1 could be no more than that required

to define whether or not B^1 would be contacted. The mucoids would thus act as switching mechanisms, 'sign-posts' which route transmission. The mucoids would thus be the chemical basis of the make-break mechanisms of the brain's circuitry, the chemical basis of the establishment of the cluster of specific circuits which constitute a memory trace. They might also underlie specificities of contact between glia and neurons." (2)

The experimental evidence in support of this "sign-post" theory, summarized in the above references, has included the fact that a change in the structure and function of the brain glycoproteins should accompany both the expression of, and the regression of, these higher nervous system functions.

The general field of glycoproteins outside the nervous system grew in the last few years and provided evidence from nonbrain systems relevant to the postulated or demonstrated functions of brain glycoproteins. Thus for example lectins, cell-agglutinating, and sugar-specific proteins are useful in the study of the native glycoproteins of the cell surfaces and of the basic of recognition and contact functions of cells. The properties of glycoproteins on the cell surface are seen to be disturbed in some cancer cells, are thought to be related to transplantation antigens, have been shown to be cell surface receptors for viruses and endotoxins and are involved in the attachment and penetration of the ovum by the spermatozoan (for references see ref. 20).

These various recent confirmations of the role of glycoproteins in cell-surface recognition phenomena outside of the nervous system are clearly relevant to the evidence and hypothesis on glycoproteins of the nervous system.

FURTHER EVIDENCE IN SUPPORT OF THE BRAIN GLYCOPROTEIN "SIGN-POST" THEORY IN LEARNING AND MEMORY

Changes in Glycoprotein 11A in Relation to the "Amount of Learning"

Whereas many experimental protocols have been published for the study of the "all-or-none" acquisition of information in a variety of experimental animals, it is a more difficult task to express a graded response in terms of the amount learned in a given time by an individual subject. In order to approach this problem in the training pigeon, as it might relate to brain glycoproteins, we did the following experiment.

The pigeons were male White Carneaux, maintained at approximately 85% of their free-feeding body weights. The apparatus used was a two-key operant chamber for pigeons according to Ferster and Skinner.

First, all birds were trained to peck equally at the two response keys in order to obtain food reinforcement. After this preliminary training a concurrent VI I VI I schedule was instituted. On this schedule, responding on one key occasionally (on the average of once each minute) resulted in a delay interval of 20 sec that was followed by food. Responding on the other key resulted only in the delay (again, on the average of once each minute). During the 20-sec delay, the experimental chamber was completely dark, and responses were ineffective. Thus, responding on only one of the keys is effective in producing food.

The subjects were run for 21 sessions, each session terminating after 30 reinforcements were received. Following the last session, all subjects were sacrificed by dipping the pigeon into a Dry Ice–acetone bath. Each pigeon brain was coded and extracted individually for brain glycoproteins, and 16 groups separated on column chromatography with Cellex D as previously described (1,2). The chemical analyses, Folin-Lowry quantitative determination of protein, were done "blind" with regard to the performance of each pigeon.

The degree to which the responses deviated from a random 50–50 response to the two keys represented the preference for the correct key. The results of this deviation from random are expressed as deviations from 50, the highest deviation being 50 and the lowest being zero. The pigeons were ranked according to their scores and then divided into three groups: the highest group scoring in the range of 28 to 50, the middle group scoring in the range of 10 to 24, and the lowest group scoring in the range of 0 to 9. Because of the small numbers of subjects in each group, only a trend can be perceived.

The pigeons which demonstrated the highest "amount of learning" had the highest mean amount of brain glycoprotein 11A, 2.63 mg/g

wet weight of brain tissue; those of the middle group had 0.65 mg/g, and those of the lowest group 0.56 mg/g. The concentration of brain glycoprotein 10B did not show any relationship to rank order. Since these were long-term results observed after 21 sessions of training, these results were in confirmation of the earlier results on the changes in brain glycoprotein 10B, which was elevated early, then normal later (1,2).

Carbohydrate Constituents of Pigeon Brain Glycoproteins 10B and 11A

In earlier studies (1,2) it was shown that the carbohydrate constituents of glycoproteins 11A and 10B (10B has two separate fractions, $10B_1$ and $10B_2$, in the pigeon) are quite different from each other, although their amino acid chains appear quite close in composition. Thus, a change from 10B to 11A represents a major structural change in terminal carbohydrate units, which would correlate with the notion that specific kinds of connections are being favored or that entirely new kinds of connections are being formed. Thus, 11A has considerably less hexose and hexosamine than does either $10B_1$ or $10B_2$. These differences are sufficient that specific antibodies have been made to these substances which distinguish between them. This type of specificity is therefore of a sufficiently high order that it might account for specificity of contact between neuronal membranes of two different neurons.

Incorporation of ^{14}C-Glucose into Training and Resting Pigeon Brain Glycoproteins

Glucose labeled in the first carbon was injected intravenously into pigeons at rest, or before they engaged in a training procedure for varying periods of time before sacrifice in a Dry Ice–acetone bath. The brain glycoproteins were extracted and separated as previously described (1,2). (See Fig. 1.)

At rest for 30 min, only slight incorporation was observed in groups 2, 3, and 11B. Much more incorporation was observed at only 10 min of training.

Furthermore, the nature of the most actively labeled groups was a function of time. Thus, at 10-min training, groups 1, 10A, and $10B_1$

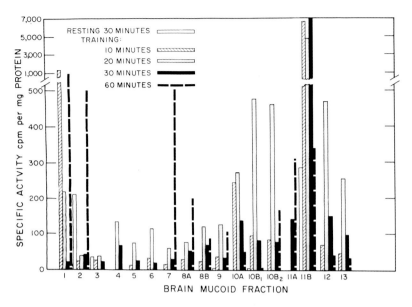

FIG. 1. Incorporation of ^{14}C-glucose into brain mucoids of pigeons.

and at 20 min $10B_2$, 11B, 12, and 13 were most active. At 60 min, groups 1 and 2 associated with the lateral dendritic processes (2) and group 10B proteins associated with astrocytic glia. This indicates that the sequential activity of glycoproteins of different cellular organelles as well as of different cell types (glia and neurons) will require further individual examination.

What is clear is that there is an extremely active turnover of glycosidically bound glucose in the brain glycoproteins of training pigeons, and that much of this activity occurs within minutes. We had previously noted (2) that these changes occurred earlier than those times usually examined in such studies, and the present data confirm the importance of examining discrete and short time periods in relation where possible to specific glycoproteins and specific cell fractions.

While glucosamine was found by one study to be slowly incorporated during training (21), confirmation of our finding of early and rapid incorporation of sugars into brain glycoproteins has been obtained for training mice when tritiated fucose is the subcutaneously injected sugar (22). In further confirmation of both early incorporation (30 min) and the relevance of the functional state, aggregated mice were shown to incorporate both more ^{14}C-glucose and

[14]C-mannose into brain glycoproteins than did isolated mice (23).

Glycoproteins Are in High Concentration at the Synapse

With the development of the new stains for the electron microscope which visualize large molecular weight carbohydrate materials, the periodic acid stains, it has been possible to demonstrate visually the presence in high concentration of glycoproteins at the synaptic cleft. Periodic acid–silver methenamine shows stained material separating nerve and glial processes from each other in the neuropile. Staining of the intercellular space is sharply increased in the region of the synaptic cleft.

With phosphotungstic acid, as with periodic acid–silver methenamine, a stained layer outlines cell and nerve processes. Staining of the intercellular space is enhanced in the synaptic cleft (24).

INVERSE RELATIONSHIP OF MUCOID-CONTACT FUNCTIONS AND DNA REPLICATION: THE REGRESSIVE STATE OF BRAIN TUMORS

Search for the chemical expression of higher information functions of brain cells has led in addition to findings of structural changes in the same molecules upon regression of these higher functions, in brain tumors. The antisera which we have obtained to a brain tumor cell antigen 10B have possible application to both diagnosis and therapy of brain tumors (17). Thus, since only the 10B of reactive astrocytes will combine with injected 10B antisera, it may be possible to outline radioactively a brain tumor for active viewing on screens, or photography for permanent record. Further, if the 10B antibody injected is coupled with chemically or radioactively toxic compounds, or with such compounds which can be activated by chemical or physical means, destruction of cells in the brain tumor area can be much more selective in sparing normal cells than hitherto possible. In addition, if circulating antibody to brain tumor antigen 10B can be detected in human serum, a further diagnostic procedure may become available.

In recent studies of the glycoprotein fraction 10B, an immunologically active component of this fraction now has been purified and named astrocytin (20).

The growth of ependymoma-glioma tumors subcutaneously in the mouse provides the opportunity to study a brain tumor growing outside the nervous system, and at the same time to study the chemistry of the essentially normal brain (and other organs) in the same animal able to be influenced by the subcutaneously growing brain tumor (17). This factor may be responsible for the induction of a precancerous or early cancerous change in normal cells.

The concentration of total protein-bound hexose in brain under the influence of distant tumor is in agreement with the data obtained for human brain tumors. It is also in general agreement with the previous observations that the concentration of protein-bound hexose in brain is greater: (i) the more complex the anatomical structure of the brain, (ii) the more ordered the chemical structure, as in membranes opposed to cytoplasmic cell constituents, and (iii) the more complex or active the functional state of the animal (1,2). Thus, the greater the "experiential" or environmental informational content or activity of a given structure or function, the greater the concentration of protein-bound hexose. The training brain cell, with relatively high experiential informational content, contains more protein-bound hexose (1,2). The tumor cell, with relatively low experiential informational content, but high "genetic" (mitotic) activity, contains less protein-bound hexose.

This relationship has been generalized to the proposition that I have made that when DNA and cell replication functions are stimulated, as in tumors, normal mucoid biosynthesis is inhibited (17). During normal morphogenesis of brain, DNA and cell division would be more active at one stage, and mucoid biosynthesis for specific interneural connections would be more active at another stage.

This postulated inverse relationship of mucoid-contact functions to DNA replication could account for the cessation of DNA synthesis in retinal ganglion cells observed to be correlated with the time of specification of their central connections (see ref. 17). The theory would also be consistent with the reported relationship of malignancy to loss of contact inhibition (see ref. 17) if contact recognition is indeed a function of mucoids. This cell surface difference in malignancy has been related to the presence of an agglutinin with specificity for the N-acetyglucosamine determinant (see ref. 17). If nucleic acid bases, uridine and cytidine, were available either for nucleic acid synthesis or for transferase activity for mucoid synthesis, but not for both simultaneously, then a control mechanism would be at hand for determining which of the two cell functions — replication or contact positioning — occurred.

CONCLUSION

There is a biochemistry of learning and memory. There are methodological problems in its study. There are a number of theories now being explored experimentally. The "sign-post" theory of the function of brain glycoproteins in the establishment of brain circuitry and its relationship to learning and memory are discussed in some detail.

Studies to date provide evidence that the "expression" of brain function in learning and memory is related to the proposed higher recognition functions of the brain glycoproteins. Other studies have demonstrated the "regression" of these higher recognition functions in the loss of carbohydrate moieties of the brain glycoproteins occurring in brain tumors. This, in turn, has led to the extension of the "sign-post" concept to the proposal that mucoid biosynthesis is inversely related to DNA replication. That is, DNA and cell division are inhibited during cell positioning and the formation of intercell contacts (expression of the proposed "sign-post" experiential function), and mucoid biosynthesis is inhibited when DNA and cell division are active (regression of "sign-post" function).

Thus, brain glycoproteins may well be involved in the developmental establishment of normal brain circuitry, and in its daily maintenance and change in relation to experiential input; and disorders in brain glycoproteins may be associated with regressive disorders of higher brain functions as occur in brain tumor and psychoses.

Many other neurochemical systems may participate in both the primary and the secondary biochemical processes in learning and memory.

REFERENCES

1. Bogoch, S. (1968): *The Biochemistry of Memory: With an Inquiry into the Function of the Brain Mucoids.* Oxford University Press, New York.
2. Bogoch, S. (1965): Brain proteins in learning: findings in the experiments in progress discussed at the NRP work session—June 1965. *Neurosci. Res. Progr. Bull.,* 3:38.
3. Ungar, G. (1974): Molecular coding of information in the brain. In: *Biological Diagnosis of Brain Disorders,* edited by S. Bogoch. Plenum Press, New York.
4. Lajtha, A. (ed.) (1970): *Protein Metabolism of the Nervous System.* Plenum Press, New York.
5. Davison, A. N., Mandel, P., and Morgan, J. G. (eds.) (1972): *Functional and Structural Proteins of the Nervous System.* Plenum Press, New York.
6. Bogoch, S., Rajam, P. C., and Belval, P. C. (1964): Separation of cerebroproteins of human brain. *Nature,* 204:73.
7. Bogoch, S. (1958): Studies on the structure of brain ganglioside. *Biochem. J.,* 68:319.
8. Bogoch, S., Lynch, P., and Levine, A. S. (1959): Influence of brain ganglioside upon the neurotoxic effect of influenza virus in mouse brain. *Virology,* 7:161.
9. Bogoch, S. (1960): Interaction of viruses with native brain substrates. *Neurology,* 10:439.
10. Bogoch, S., and Bogoch, E. S. (1959): Effect of brain ganglioside on the heart of the clam. *Nature,* 183:53.
11. Bogoch, S., Paasonen, M. D., and Trendelen-

burg, U. (1962): Some pharmacological properties of brain ganglioside. *Br. J. Pharmacol.,* 18:325.
12. Bogoch, S. (1960): Demonstration of serum precipitin to brain ganglioside. *Nature,* 185 (4710) 392.
13. Bogoch, S. (1962): Aminoglycolipids and glycoproteins of human brain: New methods for their extraction and further study in the sphingolipidoses. In: *Proceedings of the International Conference on the Sphingolipidoses,* edited by S. M. Aronson and B. W. Volk, p. 249. Academic Press, New York.
14. Bogoch, S. (1970): Glycoproteins of the brain of the training pigeon, in *Protein Metabolism of the Nervous System,* edited by A. Lajtha, pp. 535–569. Plenum Press, New York.
15. Bogoch, S. (1969): Brain circuitry and its structural basis. In: *Future of the Brain Sciences,* pp. 104–113. Plenum Press, New York.
16. Bogoch, S. (1969): Nervous system proteins. In: *Handbook of Neurochemistry,* Vol. I., edited by A. Lajtha. Plenum Press, New York.
17. Bogoch, S. (1972): Brain glycoprotein 10B: Further evidence of the "sign-post" role of brain glycoproteins in cell recognition, its change in brain tumor, and the presence of a "distant factor." In: *Functional and Structural Proteins of the Nervous System,* edited by A. N. Davison, I. G. Morgan, and P. Mandel, pp. 39–54. Plenum Press, New York. (Abstr. 3rd Int. Meeting Soc. Neurochem. 1971.)
18. Bogoch, S. (1972): Brain glycoproteins in intercell recognition: Tay-Sachs disease and intraneuronal recognition. In: *Sphingolipids, Sphingolipidoses and Allied Disorders,* edited by B. W. Volk and S. M. Aronson, pp. 127–149. Plenum Press, New York.
19. Campbell, R., Bogoch, S., Scolaro, N. J., and Belval, P. C. (1967): Cerebrospinal fluid glycoproteins in schizophrenia, *Am. J. Psychiatr.,* 123:952.
20. Bogoch, S. (1973): Brain glycoproteins and learning: New studies supporting the "sign-post" theory. In: *Current Biochemical Approaches to Learning and Memory,* edited by W. B. Essman and S. Nakajima. Spectrum Publications, New York.
21. Routtenberg, A., Holian, O., and Brunngraber, E. G. (1971): Memory consolidation and glucosamine-1-C^{14} incorporation into glycoproteins. *Trans. Am. Soc. Neurochem.,* 2:103.
22. Damstra-Entingh, T. D., Entingh, D. J., Wilson, J. E., and Glassman, E. (1974): Environmental stimulation and fucose incorporation into brain and liver glycoproteins. *Pharmacol. Biochem. Behavior,* 2:73–78.
23. Defeudis, F. V. (1973): Effects of *d*-amphetamine on the incorporation of carbon atoms of D-mannose into the brain and sera of differentially housed mice: short-term reversibility of these effects. *Biol. Psychiatr.,* 7:3.

24. Rambourg, A., and Leblond, C. P. (1969): Localisation ultrastructurale et nature du materiel colore au niveau de la surface cellulaire par melange chromique-phosphotungstique. *J. Microsc.* 8:325.

25. Nakajima, S., and Essman, W. B. (1973): Biochemical studies of learning and memory: An historical overview. In: *Current Biochemical Approaches to Learning and Memory,* edited by W. B. Essman and S. Nakajima. Spectrum-Wiley, New York.

The Nervous System, Donald B. Tower, Editor-in-Chief. *Vol. 1: The Basic Neurosciences.* Raven Press, New York, 1975.

Cell Interaction in Mammalian Brain Development

Richard L. Sidman

Two main themes in the general field of modern developmental biology have been control mechanisms governing specific gene products, and cell interactions underlying morphogenesis. Students of the developing central nervous system have focused mainly on cell interactions, since relatively few nervous system-specific products have been identified and even fewer for which analytical methods are sensitive enough to encourage study of control mechanisms. The "cell interactions" theme has yielded rich dividends at an increasing pace during the past 25 years, and I propose to review some of the highlights, ranging from the early interactions that determine the gross shape and regional characteristics of the central nervous system to the more restricted but crucial interactions that specify the detailed branching patterns and synaptic connections among neuronal processes. Several reviews with more complete documentation are available (1–5).

FORMATION OF THE NEURAL PLATE AND NEURAL TUBE

The earliest steps in formation of the central nervous system (CNS), especially in mammals, are shrouded in mystery. The first organ recognized in vertebrate embryos is the chordamesoderm, and almost immediately upon its formation it interacts with the overlying surface epithelium to establish a longitudinal axis and bilateral symmetry in the embryo, and to initiate formation of the nervous system (6). Differences that could specify each site uniquely along that longitudinal axis, perhaps based on the distribution of two inducing agents in gradients of opposite sign, are thought to account for the basically different organization of the forebrain compared with the brainstem and spinal cord and for the further segmental differences within the latter regions (7).

This early interaction may be representative of a whole series of somewhat more restricted interactions that convert flattened sheets of epithelial cells into curved shapes that in turn transform into hollow tubes, cups, and folded layers. To choose one example, at a particular early stage the neuroepithelium of the developing eye cup and the sheet-like lens placode lie in apposition, with the interface occupied by a polysaccharide-containing matrix secreted by one or both of the epithelia. The epithelia at this stage do not increase in area, perhaps because they are "glued" or otherwise interacting, but do continue rapidly to generate new cells, so that the individual cells become taller and thinner, and the sheet as a whole becomes thicker and curved (8). Additional intercellular and intracellular factors seem to contribute to the morphogenetic curvature. The cells are joined laterally near their apices by junctional complexes, and contain both an apical collar of microfilaments capable of purse string-like contractions and a longitudinal array of microfilaments; at interphase each cell has a basally positioned nucleus. As the individual cells assume pyramidal shapes, based on this distribution of organelles and junctional complexes, the whole epithelial sheet would curve (9).

Within the neural plate or its highly curved derivative, the neural tube, all the columnar epithelial cells look alike by light and electron microscopic criteria, and all behave alike in terms of cell generation kinetics as analyzed by autoradiography. The elucidation of basic general principles of cell behavior by which this apparently simple epithelium is transformed into an incredibly complex mature CNS with billions of cells of diverse types interwoven in a variety of patterns reproducible from vertebrate species to species and from individual to individual, is one of the most satisfactory accomplishments of modern neuroscience. The essential features of the problem had been set forth before the turn of the century in the opposing views of His and Schaper (reviewed by Sidman and Rakic, 10) and were finally re-

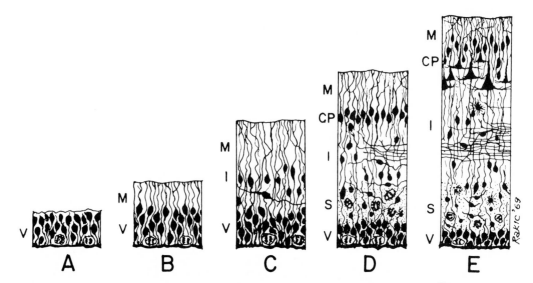

FIG. 1. Semidiagrammatic drawing of the development of the basic embryonic zones and the cortical plate. CP, Cortical plate; I, intermediate zone; M, marginal zone; S, subventricular zone; V, ventricular zone. (From ref. 11.)

solved through the methods and concepts of modern cell and developmental biology in the 1970 report of the Boulder Committee (ref. 11; see also refs. 5 and 10). In virtually all regions of the CNS at one stage of development or another, in all vertebrates examined, one can recognize a series of transient developmental zones, essentially without direct counterpart in the mature CNS (Fig. 1).

The first to form is the *ventricular zone,* composed of elongated epithelial cells, all engaged in the cell generation cycle. The ventricular cells are the sole constituents of the early neuroepithelium. Their nuclei are typically positioned some distance from the dorsal surface of the neural plate or luminal surface of the neural tube when the cells replicate DNA (S phase), and they move toward that surface just before mitosis (G2 phase) and during the early stages of mitosis (M phase). The external cytoplasmic process is withdrawn or broken off as the cell rounds up at the surface for mitosis (12), and the daughter cells then reassume an elongated shape (G1 phase). The outermost segments of their externally directed processes collectively form a cell-sparse *marginal zone,* which is thus receiving and losing processes all the time. For some while the cells divide almost exponentially; then a few, and later progressively more daughter cells become perma-

nently (under normal conditions) postmitotic, leave the ventricular zone, and form an *intermediate zone* at the interface between the sheet-like ventricular and marginal zones. The cells of the early intermediate zone become the neurons that establish the primary circuits of the nervous system as their axons grow outward into the marginal zone. Soon after, additional cells leave the ventricular zone and form a new layer of greater or lesser prominence (depending on the CNS region) between the ventricular and intermediate zones, called the *subventricular zone.* Subventricular cells, like their predecessors, still undergo mitotic divisions, but they are not constrained to a columnar shape and radial orientation, and commonly will undergo considerable further migrations.

A principle repeatedly encountered in study of the developing vertebrate nervous system (in contrast, say, to development in insects) is that shapes and behaviors of individual cells appear to be influenced significantly by neighboring cells that provide the organization of the local milieu. An important property of ventricular cells, recognized in the earliest autoradiographic studies, is that they are randomly distributed with respect to the phases of the cell generation cycle, i.e., they divide asynchronously. Also, the time they spend in the G2 and M phases of the cell generation cycle is relatively short. As a consequence, when a given cell rounds up for mitosis at the ventricular luminal surface, several of its contiguous neighbors will be in the G1 (postmitotic) or S (DNA synthesis) phases of the cycle and will be elongated. As the daughter cells in turn elongate after mitosis, they will be constrained by their neighbors to assume a radial orientation and the uniform polarization of cells in the epithelium will be maintained. The same constraints apply as cells move outward into the intermediate and, probably, into the subventricular zones. Whether the cells influence each other's shape and position by purely mechanical means or by more specialized cell surface interactions is not yet known.

ACQUISITION OF ADDRESSES BY POSTMITOTIC YOUNG NEURONS

The most detailed investigation of the form and behavior of early postmitotic young neurons as they leave the ventricular zone to enter the intermediate zone has been made in the embryonic mouse retina by Hinds and Hinds (12). They reconstructed 69 cells totally and about another 200 cells partially contained within a retinal volume of about $5 \times 10^5 \ \mu m^3$, from serial electron micrograph montages. Among many observations, they noted that both daughter cells of a given mitotic division usually follow the same fate, either to differentiate or to remain in the germinal pool, though sometimes they followed different paths. From statistical analysis of the frequencies of each behavior, they inferred that the decision whether or not to differentiate might be made at any time in the cell generation cycle. Also, they were able to distinguish the differentiating cells cytologically from proliferating cells residing in the ventricular zone, and then followed the permanently postmitotic cells as they withdrew their inward-directed processes, moved outward, and formed a new process which passed externally into the marginal layer and developed axonal properties. Golgi and electron microscopic studies in other regions of the CNS have shown that rounded postmitotic cells come to exhibit a range of variations on the "outward migration" theme, perhaps influenced by whether the decision to differentiate was made before or after mitosis. Thus, some cells form a complete radial process

that reaches the external surface before the nuclear region translocates outward within that relatively fixed cylinder of cytoplasm, while others grow an outward-directed process simultaneously with or even following movement of the nuclear region. The most dramatic radial migrations of whole cells are seen in the primate cerebrum, where bipolar-shaped young neurons a few hundred micrometers in total length may traverse a distance of several thousand micrometers to reach their final addresses in the cerebral cortex (10).

The radial path of the migrating cells is established by a guidance mechanism evolved from the cellular arrangement that earlier constrained ventricular cells and their derivatives to radial columnar positions. At early stages the ventricular cells had appeared to be all of one class, but later, when the CNS tissue becomes thicker (as the neuroepithelium converts from a two-dimensional sheet to a three-dimensional matrix), many of the cells that are now stretched radially across the tissue show cytological properties that denominate them as glial cells. These radial glial cells in their turn serve as guides along which the young neurons invariably migrate as they pass externally toward and into the cerebral cortex. The usefulness, and presumably the necessity, for the guides becomes more apparent when one recognizes that the terrain through which a young neuron moves is not only relatively wide, but is very complex and varied in texture, consisting of a mixture of neuronal and glial processes and blood vessels of various sizes and orientations. The relationship between young neuron and radial guide, then, is not haphazard, but must be based on some kind of recognition between the surface components of the two cell types, or between cell and matrix materials, that allows not only selectivity of contact of these cell types for each other among the many possible choices, but also allows the movement of one cell along the surface of the other. Reconstruction of such migrating cells in the fetal monkey cerebrum indicates that the leading process continuously emits and retracts filopodial "sensors" along one or another radial guide (13), so that the recognition mechanism must operate along most of the length of the radial pathway.

The final position (address) attained by a migrating young neuron must be influenced by further environmental cues. A series of neurons, possibly members of a single clone, usually follows a single radial guide to the cerebral cortex, each neuron soma taking a position distal to its predecessor in a column oriented at a right angle to a surface tangent. In terms of the horizontal laminar organization of the mature cortex, cells of each lamina from inside outward originate at a progressively later time (Fig. 1D compared with 1E). (This is a statistical statement in the case of the normal mouse cortex, where cells destined for several layers arise simultaneously but in proportions that favor deeper layers first; in the monkey neocortex, the cortical lamination reflects the time of origin more exactly.)

Neurological mutant mice provide experimental modifications of development that often are difficult to duplicate by nongenetic means. In the reeler mutant mouse, young neurons fail to acquire their normal cortical addresses, and the data have been interpreted to suggest that another necessary condition is some type of recognition between migrating young neuron and some extrinsic agent, possibly provided by incoming axons of other cells that intercept it along the migration pathway and perhaps influence the final position attained. In reeler, both the migrating neurons and many of the incoming axons lie in abnormal positions at embryonic stages, but it is not yet known which abnormality is the earlier one. It may seem at first surprising that despite the abnormal positions of cells, the basic synaptic circuitry in reeler cortex is curiously close to normal, but on further reflection, this is the outcome one would predict if the cortical addressing mechanism itself, whether in normal or reeler mice, depends on early contact between incoming axon and migrating target neuron.

The radial guidance mechanism reviewed above has another consequence with reference to addressing properties in cortex. In all vertebrates, but especially in mammals, the mature cortical surface is parcellated into territories that are each characterized by distinctive inputs, outputs, intrinsic architecture, and functional correlates. These cortical territories lie in a topographic relation to one another that is consistent across species lines. Since the migrations of neurons from the ventricular and subventricular zones to the cortical plate are

so sharply constrained to the radial vector, it follows that the germinal zones at and near the ventricular surface of the developing CNS must also be parcellated as a two-dimensional mosaic structure. Superimposed on this, and crossing most of the topographic boundaries without interruption, is a smooth spatial gradient system expressed in terms of the relation between time of origin of neurons and their final positions within broad areas of the mature CNS (14). The simplest explanation for these properties, though not the only possible one, is that the gradients reflect the spatial and temporal organization of the essentially two-dimensional germinal zones, whereas the parcellated topographic territories may gain their individuality by a combination of intrinsic genetic properties of the constituent neurons and uniqueness of primary axonal inputs during the migration stages. A relationship yet to be explored is the possible intercellular communication via gap junctions between cells within the germinal area representing a given future cortical territory, but not between cells in different territories.

A very different approach to analysis of the sorting out of diverse cells during development is provided by the reaggregation tissue culture technique worked out by Moscona and others, a potentially powerful experimental method for study of neurogenesis. In a sustained series of studies beginning in 1952, Moscona (15) has examined the properties of cells that allow intercellular recognition, selective adhesion and histogenesis. Embryonic organs are dissociated into suspensions of single cells and allowed passively to make random contacts. Typically they aggregate and then sort out so as to reconstruct their original tissue patterns, after which they may continue to differentiate. Cells of neural tissues, including retina and various parts of cerebral cortex will reassemble in patterns different from each other and with features reminiscent of the region-specific patterns of organization *in vivo*. Further, they form synapses recognized by morphological and electrophysiological criteria, and show some biochemical properties characteristic of differentiating neural tissue. Under appropriate culture conditions, cells of different CNS regions release "aggregation factors" that are specific for the region. These are thought to act at cell surfaces, for lectins and other agents modifying the molecular organization at cell surfaces also affect aggregation behavior. Cells of the reeler mutant cerebrum aggregate in somewhat different patterns than their normal counterparts. These studies, as well as the *in vivo* analyses, have focused attention on the cell surface as a crucial mediator of developmental interactions.

CELL REARRANGEMENTS IN THE DEVELOPING CEREBELLUM

An implication in the studies reviewed in the previous section was that as young neurons migrate toward or reach their final addresses in cortical structures, they make contact with axons destined later to innervate them. The cerebellar cortex, because of the remarkably stereotyped geometry of synaptic relationships among its cells, has proved to be a particularly suitable testing ground for concepts concerning the developmental rearrangement of cells as a requirement for synaptogenesis. Analysis has been most profitable in the fetal monkey, in which the prolonged span of development allows causally related events to be distinguished temporally, and in the mouse, where many of the critical events occur at convenient postnatal ages and several available mutations perturb development selectively.

The most frequent type of synapse in the cerebellar cortex is between a granule cell axon oriented in the longitudinal axis of a cerebellar folium and a series of Purkinje cell dendritic trees oriented transversely in the folium. The granule cell somas lie in the granular layer deep to the Purkinje cell somas, but the granule cell axons pass radially outward and branch at 90° to form fibers that lie parallel to one another in the molecular layer, external to the Purkinje cell somas. The developmental problem is how to insert the very thin (about 0.1 μm in diameter) and very long (1–3 mm) horizontal segments of the granule cell axons into proper position in the molecular layer, how to orient them, and how to coax them to recognize and make synaptic connections with spines on the relevant sectors of Purkinje cell dendrites.

This problem is solved by juxtaposition of the simultaneously growing granule cell axon and Purkinje cell dendrite at the outer border of the marginal zone (incipient molecular layer) even before and while the granule cell soma be-

comes translocated inward past the Purkinje cell dendrites and soma. The evidence based on the findings of several workers during a span of more than 80 years, most notably Ramón y Cajal, Mugnaini, and Förstrønen, and Rakic, is summarized in Fig. 2. Granule cell neurons are generated from a primary fountainhead of subventricular cells that come to form the external granular layer on the outer surface of the cerebellum (10). The early postmitotic granule cell undergoes a remarkable series of changes in shape that transform it from a round form (cell 1, in Fig. 2) through bipolar (cell 2) and tripolar forms (cells 3–5), to the mature granule cell neuron (cells 6,7). A critical event in this sequence is the genesis of the bipolar cytoplasmic processes (cell 2), for these processes always lie in the plane longitudinal to the folium, make direct contact with the distal parts of the growing Purkinje cell dendrites, and differentiate as parallel fiber axons. The position of such an axon relative to the position of the Purkinje cell somas depends on the time when the granule cell differentiates; parallel fibers in the deepest strata of the mature molecular layer belong to the earliest-generated granule cells and those in the most external strata to the last ones formed. With reference to Fig. 1, cell 1 will make a parallel fiber destined to lie external to the fiber of cell 2, and the progeny of cell D, dividing in the left upper corner, will lie still more externally. The Purkinje cell dendrites grow apace through the thickening molecular layer and acquire parallel fiber inputs from each wave of granule cells on progressively more distal parts of the dendritic tree.

Each layer of parallel fibers would seem to gain its orientation by being laid down on the scaffolding provided by the previously generated layer. Yet this would not account for the orientation of the initial layer, and in any case, the idea is contradicted by Altman's experiment in which external granule cells of young rats were partially destroyed by X-irradiation (16). The residual cells regenerated a complete layer, and as some of their progeny differentiated into granule cell neurons, they laid down parallel fibers in abnormal orientations, possibly reflecting the horizontal abnormal migration path of the regenerating cells. The general implication of these studies is that the behavior of a given neuron at any particular stage of development

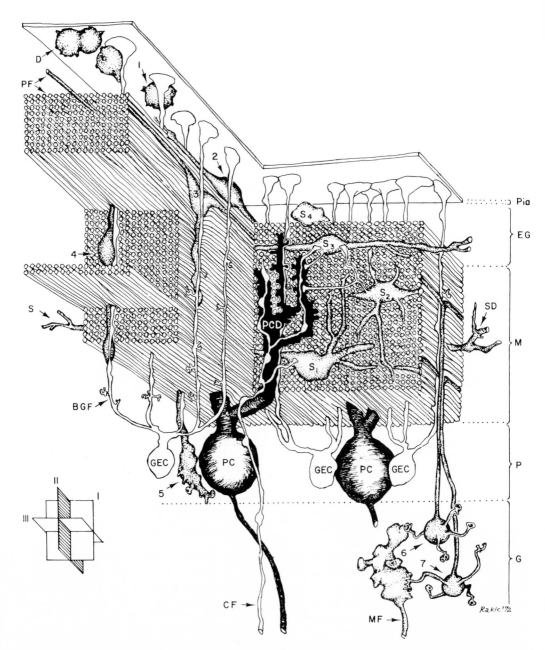

FIG. 2. A "four-dimensional" (time and space) diagrammatic reconstruction of the histogenesis of the cerebellar cortex. The orientation of the drawing is indicated by the figure in the lower left. I, Transverse to the folium; II, longitudinal to the folium; III, parallel to the pial surface. See text for further explanation. BGF, Bergmann glial fiber; D, dividing external granule cell; EG, external granule layer; GEC, Golgi epithelial cell (Bergmann glia); G, granular layer; M, molecular layer; MF, mossy fiber; P, Purkinje layer; PC, Purkinje cell; PCD, Purkinje cell dendrite; PF, parallel fiber; S_{1-4}, stellate cells; SD, stellate cell dendrite. (From ref. 19.)

is strongly influenced by its earlier history and by its local environment.

The further behavior of the normal granule cell, after making its bipolar processes, exemplifies the principle of interaction with other elements in the local milieu. The soma of cell 3 in Fig. 2, and perhaps the somas of even younger cells, are in contact with radially oriented Bergmann glial fibers (the white processes labeled BGF in Fig. 2). Cell 3 is itself making a radially oriented cytoplasmic process that grows along the Bergmann "guide" into the depths of the already complex molecular layer. Next (cell 4) the nuclear part of the neuron transposes within the cytoplasmic cylinder and the cylinder continues to elongate in contact with the Bergmann fiber. The granule cell soma eventually clears the molecular layer (cell 5) and attains a position in the granular layer. The differentiating T-shaped axon spun out behind the soma reflects the migration route, younger cells (e.g., cell 6) having more externally positioned parallel fiber axons than older cells (e.g., cell 7).

The relationship between migrating neuron and radial "guide" may be more than coincidental (17). In the reeler mutant, some Bergmann glial fibers lie obliquely, but young granule cells nonetheless translocate in close contact with them rather than taking the unaccompanied shorter radial route directly across the molecular layer. In the weaver mutant, Rezai and Yoon found that granule cell migration was slowed in heterozygotes and virtually absent in homozygotes, and later Rakic and Sidman found the Bergmann glial fibers to be abnormal at a stage coinciding with and even antedating the expected migration. Although a Bergmann fiber abnormality has been seen by all investigators who have described the young weaver cerebellar cortex, universal agreement has not been reached as to the exact role of the Bergmann fiber or its relevance to the mode of action of the weaver genetic locus (e.g., ref. 18).

Another population of neurons arises in the external granular layer; these are the basket and stellate interneurons of the molecular layer of the cerebellar cortex. They provide a most instructive illustration of the interplay between genetic and environmental factors in development. The somas of the first of these cells to be generated come to lie in the deepest strata of the molecular layer (basket cells), whereas progressively younger cells have somas in progressively more external positions (stellate cells). In considering the determinants of their behavior, it is important to note that some granule cell neurons are generated before the first basket cells, and that granule cells are still being produced for a long time after the last stellate cells are generated.

A probable genetic difference comes to light as one compares the earliest steps in the overt differentiation of granule cells versus interneurons of the molecular layer. The former cells make processes in the longitudinal axis of the folium, as described above, but the latter cells make their processes in the transverse axis of the folium. This reflects either a genetic difference in the ability to recognize and respond to the local milieu or some aspect of earlier history that could have established different behavior for the two classes of neuron. (The difficulty in choosing between these alternatives is but one example of the more general dilemma in defining a means of determining whether a given cell property beyond the transcription–translation level is directly or only indirectly under genetic control.)

It next becomes important to emphasize that several of the differentiated properties of basket and stellate interneurons directly reflect the local cellular environment in which that differentiation took place, and the particular local environment encountered depends in turn on timing relations among several cell types with processes in the molecular layer. The basket and stellate interneurons may actually belong to a common clone. Their volumes and shapes vary systematically according to time of genesis, the earliest cells having the largest volumes and the longest dendrites directed horizontally and externally (e.g., cell S_1 in Fig. 2). Cells generated at intermediate times have smaller volumes and dendrites extending internally and externally (cell S_2), while the youngest cells are the smallest and have horizontal and inward-directed dendrites (cell S_3). The earliest cells to form already lie on a shallow bed of antecedent parallel fibers, and form dendrites at a right angle to the parallel fibers so as, apparently, to maximize the number of parallel fibers contacted. As the parallel fiber bed thickens, the basket cell soma and dendrites become fixed in position, although the dendrites can and do extend outward with the accretion of parallel fibers. Stellate cells, generated later, become fixed in position later, and grow dendritic branches according to the same principle through the available unoccupied parts of the parallel fiber bed. The timing relationships can be marvelously complex, though orderly and explicable in terms of cell kinetics and interactions. Granule cell neurons are generated on a near exponential scale over a lengthy time period, while interneurons of the molecular layer show linear accretion over a shorter period. As a consequence, the interneurons "get ahead" of the granule cells and their parallel fiber axons; later-arising interneurons show progressively longer latent periods between genesis and overt differentiation, the latent period serving to allow the proper local environment to form in order for the stellate cell to respond to it by making its dendritic processes. These concepts, worked out on fetal and neonatal monkey specimens (19), are confirmed in general outline by analysis of mutant mice and other experimentally altered animals in which parallel fibers have failed partially or completely to form, and interneurons of the molecular layer are correspondingly abnormal (17).

DEVELOPMENTAL INTERACTIONS BETWEEN PRE- AND POSTSYNAPTIC ELEMENTS

A few examples of cell relationships have been presented in some detail because they exemplify important general principles of cell interaction in neurogenesis. At a topographically more precise level, we find equally important, though less well defined, interactions that allow functional contacts to develop selectively at sharply limited sites along the extensive surfaces of nerve cells. Genesis of such accurately organized synapses, like previously described aspects of development, also must be controlled by a combination of temporal and geometric factors.

Timing may be critical not only in terms of what components of the potential target cell have developed at the time the putative presynaptic axon reaches it, but also in terms of what other presynaptic elements might be available to compete for occupancy of the target

site. An instructive example is seen in the hippocampus (20), where the relative innervation of pyramidal neurons by ipsilateral versus homologous contralateral inputs varies along the length of the hippocampus. Early-forming neurons are innervated mainly by ipsilateral inputs, which apparently reach them sooner than the corresponding inputs growing the longer distance from the contralateral side; by contrast, later-forming hippocampal neurons are met and innervated by more equal contingents of axons, apparently because these have grown from the two sides to about the same density by the time their target cells have been generated. In other developing cortical areas, it is common for inputs to reach and perhaps to contact their future synaptic partners even before the latter have settled into permanent cortical positions (references sited in 10). The spatial relationships between the growing axon tip of one cell and the growing cytoplasmic processes on dendrites or soma of the target cell appear, despite the inherently static nature of a Golgi or electron microscopic image, to be at one and the same time marvelously intimate and yet unsettled (see illustrations in 21). Some, although probably not all, synapses are initiated at dendritic growth cones or at the tips of transient somatic thorns and may appear later on the dendritic shaft as the dendrite continues to elongate (22) or on the soma or elsewhere as somatic thorns are resorbed (23).

Timing, in itself, would seem an insufficient basis for control of the topographic specificity of synaptogenesis. For example, timing alone does not account for the findings in the cerebellar cortex of heterozygous weaver mutant mice, where newly generated granule cells migrate inward more slowly than normal and many of them remain permanently in the molecular layer. Despite the altered time course of migration and ectopic final position, these neurons become innervated by their usual inputs, the mossy fibers. These axons grow relatively late into the molecular layer, which they normally never reach, and form morphologically "correct" synapses despite the abnormal addresses of their target cells and the delayed timing (17). Presumably some molecular recognition mechanism is involved in synaptogenesis, but there are no firm leads yet as to whether this is based on small molecule gradient systems, intercellular matrices, or specific cell surface components.

Work of recent years has posed the possibility that neurohumoral mechanisms might be used at presynaptic stages, in the genetic conservatism of complex organisms, to allow recognition. The main supporting facts are that monoamines have been demonstrated by fluorescence microscopy in central neurons and their growing axons prior to synaptogenesis (24), and that the gamma aminobutyric acid-synthesizing enzyme, glutamate decarboxylase, is present by immunocytochemical criteria in growing preterminal axon shafts and their growth cones (25). Either the synthetic enzymes or, more likely, their products could be released and recognized selectively by appropriate cells in the milieu. In the case of the cerebellar Purkinje neuron, physiological evidence is available that even before synapse formation target cells are already responsive to exogenous neurohumor (26), and presumably already have the pertinent receptors or other uptake mechanisms.

As synapses are forming and maturing, the pre- and postsynaptic cells may engage in a sequence of interactions that affect not only the synapse itself, but also other cell properties. Cell size, enzyme-specific activities, and other parameters of the postsynaptic cell are reduced in some cases if the synapse is destroyed by section of the presynaptic axon or if the synapse is inhibited pharmacologically (27). There may be striking effects in the opposite direction. Molecules moving up the axon to the cell body in the retrograde direction may mediate the ability of the cell body to know and respond to conditions at the distant axon tip, as has been suggested recently for the protein Nerve Growth Factor in peripheral sympathetic neurons (28). Some classes of presynaptic cells may even die when they are prevented from attaining their major connections (29). Cell death is also a consistent, widespread and surprisingly extensive phenomenon during normal development of many parts of the nervous system (30), although it is not yet clear to what extent this relates to success or failure of synapse formation.

A final principle to emphasize is that mature cells may again express developmental behavior when injured. Focal destruction in the mature mammalian CNS characteristically provokes local regenerative sprouting reactions by injured axons, distant compensatory growth by other axonal branches of the same neurons, and collateral sprouting with local synaptogenesis by intact axons in or near the injury site (31). The initiating signal is almost certainly extrinsic to the injured axons, and the prospect that such reactions might be manipulated so as to encourage an effective regenerative response in the diseased or injured human CNS represents one of the great legacies and challenges from research of the past 25 years to research of the coming decades.

REFERENCES

1. Ramón y Cajal, S. (1960): *Studies on Vertebrate Neurogenesis,* edited by L. Guth (transl.) Charles C Thomas, Springfield.
2. Hochstetter, F. (1929): *Beitrage zur Entwicklungsgeschichte des menschlichen Gehirns. I.* Franz Deuticke, Vienna and Leipzig.
3. Weiss, P. (1955): Nervous system. In: *Analysis of Development,* edited by H. Willier, P. Weiss, and V. Hamburger, pp. 346–401. Saunders, Philadelphia.
4. Jacobson, M. (1970): *Developmental Neurobiology.* Holt, Rinehart and Winston, New York.
5. Sidman, R. L., and Rakic, P. (1975): Development of the human central nervous system. In: *Cytology and Cellular Neuropathology, 2nd edition,* edited by R. D. Adams and W. Haymaker. Charles C Thomas, Springfield *(in press).*
6. Spemann, H. (1938): *Embryonic Development and Induction.* Yale University Press, New Haven.
7. Saxen, L., and Toivonen, S. (1962): *Primary Embryonic Induction.* London.
8. Zwaan, J., and Hendrix, R. W. (1973): Changes in cell and organ shape during early development of the ocular lens. *Am. Zool.,* 13:1039–1049.
9. Schroeder, T. E. (1970): Neurulation in *Xenopus leavis.* An analysis and model based upon light and electron microscopy. *J. Embryol. Exp. Morphol.,* 23:427–462.
10. Sidman, R. L., and Rakic, P. (1973): Neuronal migration, with special reference to developing human brain: A review. *Brain Res.,* 62:1–35.
11. Boulder Committee (1970): Embryonic vertebrate central nervous system: Revised terminology. *Anat. Rec.,* 166:251–262.
12. Hinds, J. W., and Hinds, P. L. (1974): Early ganglion cell differentiation in the mouse retina: An electron microscopic analysis utilizing serial sections. *Dev. Biol.,* 37:381–416.
13. Rakic, P., Stensaas, L. J., Sayre, E. P., and Sidman, R. L. (1974): Computer aided three-dimensional reconstruction and quantitative analysis of cells from serial electron microscopic

montages of fetal monkey brain. *Nature,* 250: 31–34.

14. Angevine, J. B., Jr. (1970): Critical cellular events in the shaping of neural centers. In: *The Neurosciences. Second Study Program,* edited by F. O. Schmitt, pp. 60–72. Rockefeller University Press, New York.

15. Moscona, A. A. (1974): Surface specification of embryonic cells: lectin receptors, cell recognition, and specific cell ligands. In: *The Cell Surface in Development,* edited by A. A. Moscona, pp. 67–99. John Wiley & Sons, New York.

16. Altman, J. (1973): Experimental reorganization of the cerebellar cortex. IV. Parallel fiber reorientation following regeneration of the external granular layer. *J. Comp. Neurol.,* 149:181–192.

17. Sidman, R. L. (1974): Contact interaction among developing mammalian brain cells. In: *The Cell Surface in Development,* edited by A. A. Moscona, pp. 221–253. John Wiley & Sons, New York.

18. Sotelo, C., and Changeux, J-.P. (1974): Bergmann fibers and granular cell migration in the cerebellum of homozygous weaver mutant mouse. *Brain Res.,* 77:484–491.

19. Rakic, P. (1974): Intrinsic and extrinsic factors influencing the shape of neurons and their assembly into neuronal circuits. In: *Frontiers in Neurology and Neuroscience Research,* edited by P. Seeman and G. M. Brown, pp. 112–132. The Neuroscience Institute, Toronto, Canada.

20. Gottlieb, D. F., and Cowan, W. M. (1972): Evidence for a temporal factor in the occupation of available synaptic sites during the development of the dentate gyrus. *Brain Res.,* 41:452–456.

21. Morest, D. K. (1969): The growth of dendrites in the mammalian brain. *Z. Anat. Entwicklungsgesch.,* 128:290–317.

22. Skoff, R. P., and Hamburger, V. (1974): Fine structure of dendritic and axonal growth cones in

embryonic chick spinal cord. *J. Comp. Neurol.,* 153:107–148.

23. Kornguth, S. E., and Scott, G. (1972): The role of climbing fibers in the formation of Purkinje cell dendrites. *J. Comp. Neurol.,* 146:61–82.

24. Olson, L. and Seiger, A. (1972): Early prenatal ontogeny of central monoamine neurons in the rat: fluorescence histochemical observations. *Z. Anat. Entwicklungsgesch.,* 137:301–316.

25. Saito, K., Barber, R., Wu, J.-Y., Matsuda, T., Roberts, E., and Vaughn, J. E. (1974): Immunohistological localization of glutamate decarboxylase in rat cerebellum. *Proc. Natl. Acad. Sci. USA,* 71:269–273.

26. Woodward, D. J., Hoffer, B. J., Siggins, G. R., and Bloom, F. E. (1971): The ontogenetic development of synaptic junctions, synaptic activation and responsiveness to neurotransmitter substances in rat cerebellar Purkinje cells. *Brain Res.,* 34:73–97.

27. Thoenen, H. (1974): Trans-synaptic enzyme induction. *Life Sci.,* 14:223–235.

28. Henry, I. A., Stach, R., and Herrup, K. (1974): Characteristics of the retrograde axonal transport system for nerve growth factor in the sympathetic nervous system. *Brain Res.,* 82:117–128.

29. Cowan, W. M. (1970): Anterograde and retrograde transneuronal degeneration in the central and peripheral nervous system. In: *Contemporary Research Methods in Neuroanatomy,* edited by W. J. H. Nauta and S. O. E. Ebbesson, pp. 217–251. Springer-Verlag, New York.

30. Prestige, M. C. (1970): Differentiation, degeneration, and the role of the periphery: quantitative considerations. In: *The Neurosciences, Second Study Program,* edited by F. O. Schmitt. Rockefeller University Press, New York.

31. Guth, L. (ed.) (1974): Axonal regeneration and functional plasticity in the central nervous system. *Exp. Neurol.,* 45:610–658.

The Nervous System, Donald B. Tower, Editor-in-Chief. *Vol. 1: The Basic Neurosciences*. Raven Press, New York, 1975.

A Comment on the Existence of Motor Unit "Types"

R. E. Burke

Over 50 years ago, Sherrington introduced the concept of the motor unit, recognizing it as a functional entity corresponding to ". . . a so-to-say quantum reaction, which forms the basis, by combinations temporal and numerical, of all grading of the muscle as effector organ . . ." (1). The motor unit is the functional "final common path" upon which converge all the central nervous system processes controlling movement.

The motor unit has two elements, an alpha motoneuron and the group of muscle fibers innervated by it, the latter termed the "muscle unit" portion (see 2). In adult mammals there is little or no double innervation of extrafusal muscle fibers (3), and under normal circumstances all muscle fibers innervated by a given motoneuron are activated by each neuronal action potential, because of the high safety factor for neuromuscular transmission (4). The connection between motoneuron and muscle unit is thus both anatomically exclusive and functionally tight.

SOME QUESTIONS

Restated in a less elegant way than in the first paragraph above, the force output and the rate of force development by a muscle depends on several factors: (a) the number of constituent motor units active; (b) the mechanical characteristics (especially the twitch contraction time and force generated) of the active units; (c) the rates of motoneuron firing; and (d) the preceding history of motoneuron activity which can affect the input-output relations of the muscle unit portion. This description of movement in terms of motor unit action immediately raises a number of questions, such as: What is the range of mechanical properties within a motor unit pool and are there recognizable "types" of motor units? Are motor units in different muscles basically similar or are there specializations depending on the functional role played by the muscle in question? How is motor unit recruitment controlled and what kind of units are active in a given movement? How much plasticity is possible within a motor unit pool in response to altered demands upon it? What properties of motor units are determined genetically and which ones can be modulated by patterns of unit usage?

The list of questions underlying past and future research on motor units could be continued but this chapter mainly discusses recent evidence relating to those above. The available information is quite extensive and, as with many areas of research, can be likened to a partially completed jigsaw puzzle in which the general nature of the sought-after picture is visible despite large and vexing gaps. In a limited space it is possible to touch only on some highlights.

THE UTILITY OF CLASSIFICATION

When faced with populations of elements under study, scientists usually respond by developing systems of classification to organize and communicate observations. The value of a classification system depends on its predictive capacity, that is, its consonance with those properties of the classified elements that are not classification criteria. A system that rapidly becomes fuzzy with added information has little utility. However, it should be recognized that any scheme for grouping elements has an artificial and simplistic nature that may cause loss of information due to a tendency to oversolidify thinking about the system under study. The literature on motor unit and muscle fiber types contains many suggested systems of classification that conflict or can be only partially reconciled (see 5). Having contributed to this situation (e.g., 2,9), I may perhaps be excused for beginning a discussion of motor unit types with the comment that even those systems of classification that are worthwhile should be used skeptically.

It has been known for some time that nominally fast-twitch muscles in mammals contain some muscle units with slow-twitch characteristics. In the early 1960s, Bessou et al. (6) and Henneman and his co-workers (7) provided detailed information about muscle unit properties in cat limb muscles that can be described as heterogeneous, as regards both a broad range of physiological properties exhibited by the units as well as morphological and histochemical diversity of the individual muscle fibers (e.g., 5). The muscle unit population in the cat lumbrical muscle seems best described as a spectrum without clear subgroups, at least with the information presently available (6,8). In contrast the distribution and interrelation of mechanical properties of units in the cat gastrocnemius has led to several suggested classifications based either on twitch contraction times alone (2) or on multiple factor interrelations—a type of cluster analysis (7,9,10).

PHYSIOLOGICAL AND HISTOCHEMICAL PROFILES OF MUSCLE UNITS

There has been a long-standing assumption that the morphological and histochemical profiles of muscle fibers must be meaningfully correlated with their physiological properties, dating from Ranvier's classic work on red and white muscle (see 11,12). This assumption has been reenforced by the broad range of physiological properties of muscle units in histochemically heterogeneous muscle (2,7,12) and the contrastingly narrower range in histochemically homogeneous muscles such as cat soleus (2,13,14). The most direct experimental verification of this hypothesis has been obtained by Lännergren and Smith (15), who studied mechanical responses of single toad muscle fibers in relation to their morphological and histochemical characteristics. Since entire muscle units in the same toad muscle have mechanical properties similar to those of the various types of individual muscle fibers (16), it seems very likely that all of the muscle fibers belonging to a given muscle unit are physiologically identical. The same conclusion has been reached with respect to mammalian muscle units (7), which are at least histochemically homogeneous (9,17), with few exceptions (18,19).

Direct examination of the physiological-histochemical correlations in single mammalian muscle units has recently become possible with development of a technique for marking muscle unit fibers by depletion of intrafiber glycogen upon prolonged stimulation (9,14,17–19). Edström and Kugelberg (18) first demonstrated in the heterogeneous rat tibialis anterior a direct relation between the intensity of unit fiber stain-

TABLE 1. *Comparison of physiological and histochemical profiles in rat and cat motor units*

| Muscle | Type | Physiological profile[a] | | | Histochemical profile | |
		Twitch contraction time (msec)	Twitch tension (g)	Relative fatigue resistance	Myofibrillar ATPase	Oxidative enzyme staining
Rat tibialis anterior (ref. 23,25)	A	12.5	1.8	Sensitive	+++	+
	B	12.5	0.75	Mod. res.	+++	++
	C	12.5	0.4	Res.	(+++?)	(+++?)
Rat soleus (ref. 24)	Fast	18	2.2	Mod. res.	+++	+++
	Intermed.	23	1.8	Res.	++	+++
	Slow	38	1.2	Very res.	+	++
Cat gastrocnemius (ref. 13)	FF	32	43.2	Sensitive	+++	+
	F(int)	30	21.5	Intermed.	+++	++
	FR	43	12.7	Mod. res.	+++	++ − +++
	S	77	2.0	Very res.	+	+++
Cat soleus (ref. 18)	S	97	2.5	Very res.	++	+++

[a] Contraction times and twitch tensions are mean values.

ing for oxidative enzymes and the resistance to fatigue exhibited by the same muscle unit (Table 1; units stimulated in functional isolation by dissection of ventral root filaments). Unfortunately, the most fatigue-resistant units in that study ("C"; see Table 1) were not histochemically identified, but a later study of the heterogeneous rat soleus (19) provided data from all of the muscle unit groups present (Table 1). It is of interest to note that both of these studies used histochemical appearance of unit muscle fibers as the primary criterion for data grouping, and the focus was on how well physiological properties matched with the histochemical groups.

In our laboratory the motor unit populations of the heterogeneous medial gastrocnemius and the homogeneous soleus muscles of the cat have been investigated using the technique of intracellular recording and stimulation of alpha motoneurons, which offers the advantage that intrinsic neuronal properties and the organization of synaptic input can be studied as they relate to the characteristics of the innervated muscle unit (2,9,14,21,22). Our main focus has been on physiological profiles of motor units, and a system of classification based entirely on unit mechanical responses has been developed, which seems to correlate quite closely not only with the histochemical profiles of the muscle unit (9;Table 1) but also with some electrophysiological properties intrinsic to the motoneuron (2,21) and with the organization of synaptic input to the cell (21,22).

MOTOR UNIT TYPES

The classification of motor units into recognizable types seems best accomplished on the basis of muscle unit rather than motoneuron characteristics (2). The motor unit population in the cat medial gastrocnemius muscle can be divided into two major groups, conveniently described as fast twitch and slow twitch, even though twitch contraction time may not be a classification criterion (in fact, we have used a characteristic of unfused tetanic contractions called the sag property as the criterion for making a distinction between fast and slow twitch groups; see ref. 9). The slow-twitch group (making up about 25% of the unit population) appears to contain no detectable subdivisions, and these

units have been referred to as type S. The fast-twitch group, in contrast, contains a spectrum of units that differ from one another primarily in relative resistance to fatigue during a standardized stimulation sequence. In a large series of units from normal cats, the distribution of fatigue resistance has been definitely bimodal, with a large cluster (about 45% of the total population) of units showing considerable sensitivity to fatigue (type FF), another somewhat smaller cluster (about 23%) exhibiting much greater fatigue resistance (type FR), and a few units (about 5%) showing intermediate fatiguability (type F(int)). Table 1 summarizes the interrelations between some aspects of the physiological and histochemical profiles of these unit categories and also includes data for units in the cat soleus muscle, all of which can be classed as type S according to the criteria developed for gastrocnemius units (14).

The diagram shown in Fig. 1 represents an

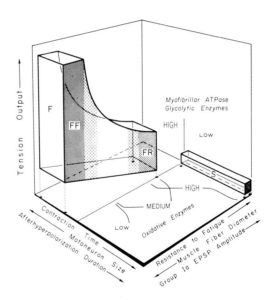

FIG. 1. Three-dimensional diagram showing the interrelation between a variety of physiological and histochemical profiles of muscle units, and of their innervating motoneurons, belonging to motor units of the cat gastrocnemius. The actual data scatter for units classed as fast-twitch (type F) and slow-twitch (type S) are denoted by box-like outlines. Shading on the F group outline indicates the relative numbers of units in different loci, with most units falling into the FF or FR subgroups and fewer [F(int)] into the region intermediate between them. See text for further explanation and references. (Patterned after data display in Fig. 4 of Burke et al., ref. 9.)

attempt to summarize the interrelations between a number of features of the histochemical and physiological profiles exhibited by motor units in the cat gastrocnemius population. It is intended to illustrate the apparent continuum of unit properties within the fast twitch (F) group and brings out the fact that type S units are much more resistant to fatigue than any of the type FR. This method of displaying information provides a useful contrast to tabulation since it emphasizes ranges of data scatter within, as well as between, the clusters recognized as unit types. The fact of such data scatter should be kept in mind when making interpretations as discussed below (see ref. 23).

With respect to the physiological profiles listed in Table 1, there is a tendency for the more slowly contracting muscle units in both rat and cat (see also Fig. 1) to produce less tension on the average and to exhibit greater resistance to fatigue than their fast-twitch counterparts (see also 3,5,7,10,12,15). Tension output is determined by the cross-sectional area of unit fibers and their specific tension output per unit area as well as by the number of fibers belonging to a given unit. The range in tension output among cat gastrocnemius muscle units appears to involve variation in all three factors (24). With respect to physiological-histochemical correlations, there is a trend for faster twitch muscle units to exhibit more intense staining for myofibrillar ATPase activity than is found among slow-twitch unit fibers, as expected from other evidence (see ref. 5) implicating the myosin ATPase reaction as an important determinant of intrinsic speed of muscle contraction. Finally, there is a direct correlation between staining for oxidative enzyme activity and the degree of resistance to fatigue, whereas, conversely, an apparent dependence upon anerobic glycolysis (and presumably on intrafiber glycogen stores) for energy metabolism is associated (e.g., in cat type FF units) with rapid fatigue during repetitive activation (9,15,18,19,20,21).

The above sets of interrelations, complemented by observations on the mechanical, histochemical, and biochemical properties of various whole muscles (e.g., 5,25), lead to the conclusion that at least some of the correlations are causal ones, and that motor unit types based on either physiological or histochemical profiles have utility in that one set of characteristics can

be used to predict the other. However, one may also use the data in Table 1 to point out several disparities between the general trends noted above and specific observations that do not fit them easily. For example, myofibrillar ATPase staining in cat soleus fibers is somewhat more intense than in type S unit fibers of gastrocnemius, even though soleus muscle units contract more slowly on the average (14,23). Oxidative enzyme staining in rat soleus fibers represents another example, in that staining in fibers of the slow units is less intense than in the fast, although the former are in fact much more resistant to fatigue than the latter (19). A given set of criteria for unit typing might be internally consistent for a given muscle unit population but no single set of detailed physiological or histochemical characteristics would suffice for both rat and cat muscle units.

Interspecies differences in the characteristics of motor unit populations are probably closely related to differences in functional roles, such as, for example, the relative prominence of fast contracting, fatigue-resistant units in small rodents with fast movements and sustained patterns of active running (19,20). Gauthier and Padykula (26) have shown that the histochemical mosaic in the diaphragm of small mammals contains a very high proportion of fibers rich in mitochondria (and presumably resistant to fatigue), whereas a large animal like the cow, with much slower rates of breathing and metabolic activity, has uniformaly large diaphragm muscle fibers with few mitochondria, a pattern quite different from that which might be anticipated on a simple fast-slow dichotomy predicted from limb muscle data such as in Table 1 and Fig. 1.

Differences in motor unit populations in various muscles within the same animal presumably also reflect specialization for specific functional roles. The range in tetanic tensions produced by cat gastrocnemius units is over 100-fold from the smallest S unit (less than 1 g) to the largest FF (greater than 100 g). This fits the very wide dynamic range over which this large ankle extensor must operate, from fine postural adjustments during quiet standing to very forceful and rapid contractions during galloping and jumping. Goslow and co-workers (27) have recently discussed the match between muscle unit forces and functional roles in several digit flexor muscles in the cat, showing that muscles probably concerned only with relatively fine movements have a narrower range of tensions (true also of the cat lumbricals; see 6,8) than found in the larger plantaris, which like gastrocnemius can function as an ankle extensor as well as digit flexor.

The above discussion suggests that caution should be exercised in extrapolating detailed results from one motor unit pool to another, particularly across species boundaries. One may then ask how reliable are the motor unit types identified within a given muscle of a given species. Leaving aside consideration of experimental technique, it nevertheless seems likely that some attributes of the motor unit population can vary depending on the activity history of the individual animal tested. For example, Stuart and co-workers (28) have recently found a much less bimodal distribution of fatigue resistance among fast twitch muscle units in cat gastrocnemius than was evident in samples from our laboratory (9; Table 1). This difference in results may be accounted for at least in part by exercise history,

since our animals were caged for at least 6 to 8 weeks prior to experiment, whereas Stuart and colleagues used larger animals that had not been caged for any significant period (Stuart, *personal communication*).

There is rapidly growing evidence that the oxidative enzyme activity and associated resistance to fatigue of skeletal muscle fibers can be increased in parallel by conditioning the animal to endurance exercise (29, see also ref. 31), a modulation that appears to be completely reversible (30). Such changes in oxidative capacity and fatigue resistance are not accompanied by any alteration in fiber myofibrillar ATPase activity, or in the relative proportions of high to low ATPase fibers in the histochemical mosaic, or in whole muscle contraction time (29,31). The evidence suggests that an increased exercise demand can produce a corresponding increase in oxidative enzyme capacity and fatigue resistance among muscle fibers of fast twitch units, with possible intercoversion between units resembling types FF and FR in cat mus-

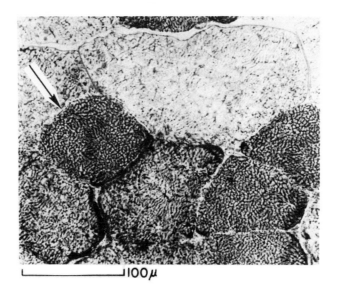

FIG. 2. Oil immersion photomicrograph showing several fibers in cat medial gastrocnemius stained for activity of NADH-diaphorase (see ref. 9). The small fiber indicated by the arrow belonged to a physiologically studied type S muscle unit (identified by glycogen depletion; see text). Note the relatively fine, evenly distributed reticulum of reaction product within the fiber and several similar fibers in the same frame. The indicated S unit fiber lies next to two other fibers, which are also densely stained but in which the reaction product is distributed in larger clumps with subsarcolemmal accumulations and a more broken network. These resemble the staining characteristics of identified type FR unit fibers. The large fiber in the frame, which is lightly stained shows the pattern seen in identified FF muscle units. Note that the irregular distribution of reaction product is also evident in this presumed FF unit fiber. (Unpublished photomicrograph, courtesy of Dr. P. Tsairis, from experiments reported in ref. 9.)

cle but without such interconversion between fast and slow twitch groups (31). The distribution of relative resistance to fatigue among cat fast-twitch muscle units is essentially continuous, as is the distribution of staining intensities for oxidative enzyme activities (Fig. 1; see also 23). In this connection it is of interest that the qualitative pattern of reaction product distribution within fibers of fast-twitch muscle units is different from that observed in fibers of slow units, both in the cat gastrocnemius (Fig. 2; see also refs. 9,23) and in the rat (19). The pattern found after staining for NADH diaphorase (Fig. 2) is relatively fine and evenly distributed in fibers of slow-twitch units (arrow), whereas that in fast-twitch unit fibers is coarser, more irregular, and usually denser at the fiber periphery in both FF and FR unit fibers, despite large differences in overall intensity of stain (Fig. 2; 9).

The evidence available from motor unit populations in cat muscle, summarized in Fig. 1 and discussed above, suggests that the fast- and slow-twitch groups are qualitatively distinct and stable types, between which there is probably no significant interconversion under normal conditions. The fast-twitch subgroups (FF, F(int), and FR) are proposed as useful types, even though the distinctions between them are very likely neither qualitative nor stable under conditions of varying exercise demand. The last statement is made because, as shown in Fig. 1, the FF and FR subgroups which are based on muscle unit physiological profiles are closely correlated with (and therefore predict) other features of muscle unit and synaptic input characteristics. It may be noted, with respect to comments made above about the utility of classification schemes, that relative resistance to fatigue is the only property listed in the diagram in Fig. 1 that is also a parameter of unit classification (see ref. 9).

MOTOR UNIT TYPES AND THE SIZE PRINCIPLE

In an important series of papers in 1965 (12,32), Henneman and co-workers suggested that the anatomical size of alpha motoneurons is a critical parameter of motor unit function, linked on one hand to the relative excitability of the motoneuron and to its place in the order of recruitment and on the other hand to properties of the innervated muscle unit (7,10,12,13). This size principle was a clear formulation of ideas that had been expressed earlier in less detail (e.g., 33,34) and represented a hypothesis eminently suited to experimental test.

The conduction velocities of motoneuron axons and the input resistance presented by the cell to currents passed from a penetrating microelectrode, both physiological indices of anatomical cell size (see ref. 21), are indeed related to muscle unit type, indicating that motoneurons innervating slow-twitch units are generally smaller in size than those innervating fast-twitch units, although there is some size overlap (Fig. 1; 2,21; see also 7,8,10,12,13). There is no difference in the distribution of axonal conduction velocities between the FF and FR groups of cat motor units (9), suggesting no statistical difference in average size of their motoneurons. Figure 1 also shows the general relation found between the duration of post-spike hyperpolarization and both motoneuron size and muscle unit type (2). The after-hyperpolarization is believed to be an important factor controlling motoneuron firing rate and this property can account at least in part for the relatively slow firing of slow-twitch motor units under natural synaptic drive (35). All of these observations are in essential accord with the general size principle formulation.

With regard to the relation between the size of alpha motoneurons and their relative excitability and recruitment order, there is a great deal of evidence that these properties are indeed correlated (36–38), although there is some question about the precision and invariance of the correlation (21,38,39). The anatomical size of a motoneuron, in and of itself, is probably not a causal factor with regard to relative excitability (21,40), but is rather simply one of the many interrelated properties of motor units. Thus the size principle seems to be a useful and convenient shorthand for expressing such information as shown in Table 1 and Fig. 1, rather than a physical explanation for motoneuron usage. The root cause of variations in excitability and of specific orders of motor unit recruitment probably lies in the interaction between a variety of intrinsic motoneuronal properties (size being only one) and the patterns of organization of synaptic input to the same motoneurons (see 21). An illustration of this point

The Nervous System. Donald B. Tower, Editor-in-Chief. *Vol. 1: The Basic Neurosciences.* Raven Press, New York, 1975.

Humoral and Cellular Influences on Neuronal Development

Silvio Varon

In the adult nervous system, nerve cells operate in a generally stable environment and their relatively invariant performances have encouraged a view of fixed and irreversible capabilities of the mature neurons and glia. During development, however, as in pathological or regenerative situations, neural cells have to operate in changing or even abnormal contexts. To understand the dynamic behavior of neurons and glia in any of these situations, one must learn to distinguish between the inherent capabilities of these cells and the extent to which they become expressed under different cellular and humoral environments. In recent years, considerable progress has been made in three main directions.

In Vitro Studies of Neural Tissues

The *in vivo* study of normal neural tissue can rarely distinguish between intrinsic and extrinsic contributions to neural performances. The investigation of neural tissue *in vitro* has provided ways to examine neural cell behavior in simpler contexts, which can be manipulated with regard to both their humoral and their cellular components. Several experimental systems have been used, which progressively diverge from the *in situ* situation and range from organ or tissue cultures to the use of clonal lines from neoplastic neuronal and glial elements. The properties and the validity of these in vitro systems, as well as the substantial contributions they have already provided, have been reviewed recently (1,2), and only two general points need to be restated here.

(a) Neural cells transferred out of their natural habitat do not lose their competence for specialized traits. All neuronal and glial properties described *in vivo* have been observed in one or more *in vitro* systems.

(b) Properties and behaviors observed *in vitro* are instructive with regard to neural properties *in vivo*. Additional cell-specific properties, first identified with an *in vitro* system, have subsequently been confirmed for the tissue *in situ*. Analysis of extrinsic influences regulating neural behaviors *in vitro* have offered pertinent clues to *in vivo* regulatory mechanisms.

Glia–neuron Interrelationships

Neuroscientists have long been intrigued by the concept of a *"neuron–glia unit,"* operating at the morphological, metabolic and functional levels. Such a concept has been encouraged by several *in vivo* studies (see 1). In development, glial cells play roles in neuronal migration, axonal guidance, and, possibly, synaptic selections. In both the developing and the adult neural tissues, the humoral environment of nerve cells is modulated by the glia, and their cellular environment is exclusively supplied by it. Particularly close is the relationship of myelinating glial cells to the neuronal axons, and of satellite glial cells to the neuronal somata. With the advent of neural culture studies, new and better opportunities have been provided to investigate glia-specific properties and glia–neuron relationships (1,2).

One means by which glial cells could affect their partner neurons could be the presentation or delivery to the neurons of specific proteins required for the maintenance and/or regulation of general neuronal performances. "Trophic" or regulatory roles of glial cells, possibly mediated by specific proteins, are at least proposed by several observations in vitro (2). Central and peripheral neurons in monolayer cultures are often seen to fare better in association with other neural cells, though not with cells of non-neural origin. Quality and number of the non-neuronal cells in a mixed neural culture determine specific patterns of intercellular organization, which in turn appear to be critical for the degree to which the neurons will express their properties. Ganglionic or tumoral glial cells, but not fibroblasts, have been reported to solicit massive development of acetylcholine production and cholinergic synapses in sympathetic ganglionic cultures. Cerebral extracts of different embryonic ages promote morphological maturation of different classes of cerebral neurons and glia, and cerebral cell cultures release aggregation-promoting agents that also appear to be both age and tissue specific. Evidence has been provided that glial cultures secrete proteins into their medium, and that neurons may take up protein from their environment. Finally, materials secreted by clonal glial cells have been described to elicit neurite production from clonal neuroblastoma cells.

The Nerve Growth Factor Phenomenon

Some twenty years ago, Levi-Montalcini and her co-workers demonstrated the occurrence of a protein factor that specifically promotes growth and differentiated functions in selected classes of neurons. The term Nerve Growth Factor (NGF) now covers several proteins from different sources which share immunochemical and functional properties, though they may differ in the details of their chemical structures. The discovery and subsequent investigations of the NGF phenomenon have been the object of several reviews (e.g., 3,4), including a very recent one (5) to which this chapter will make frequent reference. The increasing interest of neurobiologists in the NGF phenomenon is amply justified by the presence of NGF in all animal species examined, its identification as a protein agent uniquely directed to neurons, the apparent restriction of its effects to a few selected neuronal classes, and the possibility of viewing it as a model for other, as yet unidentified, neuron-directed protein agents. In addition, NGF provides an unusual opportunity to investigate the role that other tissues may play in neuronal development, maintenance and/or regeneration, and can serve as a tool to probe into the operations of a neuron and the ways by which different parts of its machinery may regulate one another.

It is with several of these more general aspects of the NGF phenomenon that this paper will be concerned. It will discuss the more re-

cent information provided by the study of NGF with regard to its sources, the identification of its target cells and their mode of association with the factor, the role of NGF and its mode of action. In so doing, it will attempt to formulate some models which may encourage a wider perspective on the extrinsic controls to which other developing and mature neurons may be subject.

NGF AND ITS SOURCES

NGF and the Mouse Submaxillary Gland

The richest source of NGF currently known is the submaxillary gland of adult male mice. The mouse submaxillary factor (β NGF) is a highly basic protein, comprising two identical chains (about 13,000 daltons each) whose physicochemical characteristics and amino acid sequence have been determined (5). Substantial structural analogies between NGF and insulin polypeptide chains have raised the possibility of an evolutionary relationship between them (6), a suggestion further encouraged by the similarity of some metabolic responses elicited by the two agents from their target cells (see also section "NGF Effects on RNA and Protein Synthesis").

Another aspect that deserves further investigation is the relationship of NGF to several other proteins present in the adult male mouse submaxillary gland. In the gland extract (7), β NGF occurs in a high molecular weight complex (*7S NGF*) with two other types of subunits, Gamma (8) and Alpha (9). The three subunits have distinctive activities, but all are quantitatively altered by the concurrent presence of the other two proteins. Although several considerations establish the 7S complex as a distinct entity on its own (5), its biological significance remains to be identified and the models suggested thus far are only speculative (9). Moreover, the gland also contains a number of other growth- or differentiation-promoting protein factors, some of which also occur in association with Gamma-like subunits (8). Their storage, like that of NGF, is associated with the development of the intercalate tubuli of the gland, which is strictly dependent on testosterone.

Synthesis, as well as storage, of NGF in the gland has been reported (3), though it need not be within the tubular structure. Even in the adult male mouse, however, the submaxillary gland is not the sole source of NGF (5). Removal of the gland only causes a transient decline of serum levels, and minute amounts of NGF have been demonstrated in most tissue and body fluids of several species. The original discovery of NGF in chick embryo-implanted sarcomata had raised the possibility of a mesenchymal production of the factor (3), and recent observations with cultured fibroblasts of normal as well as tumoral origin have reproposed the candidacy of mesenchymal cells as a generalized source of NGF in the organism (10).

NGF and the Neuroglia

A role of the glial cells in the supply of NGF or NGF-like support to ganglionic neurons has been brought forth by a recent set of investigations (11–13). The two traditional target tissues for NGF are sympathetic ganglia and early embryonic dorsal root ganglia (DRG), and most neurons dissociated from them have been repeatedly shown to require NGF for their survival and neurite production in culture (3). Intact postnatal DRG have exhibited no response to NGF *in vivo* or *in vitro*. However, neurons dissociated from postnatal mouse DRG were found to display the same critical dependence on exogenous NGF as their earlier counterparts, when the dissociation had caused a considerable loss of ganglionic glial cells. Conversely, exogenous NGF was no longer required, and maximal neuronal performance could still be elicited, if the cultures were resupplemented with glial cells from the same DRG source. Under such conditions, the additional presence of exogenous NGF had no further recognizable effects. The neuronal performance could be set at any intermediate level by intermediate supplementations with ganglionic glia, or suboptimal NGF concentrations, or a combination of both. A similar competence of ganglionic nonneuronal cells to substitute for exogenous NGF was verified in the case of the traditional NGF target tissues: sympathetic ganglia from prenatal chick or postnatal mouse and rat, and DRG from embryonic chick. With these cultures, too, the requirement for and the effects of NGF were considerably reduced or entirely abolished by adequate supplementation with nonneurons from the same source.

The NGF-like competence of ganglionic nonneurons was found not only to be restricted to glial cells but to involve some finer specificity with regard to species and/or age of the ganglionic sources. Out of a score of neural and nonneural cell types tested as supplements for purified mouse DRG neurons, in the absence of exogenous NGF, only DRG-derived cells exhibited an NGF-like support capability. Cross-reacting neurons and nonneurons from DRG of chick embryo, neonatal mouse, and neonatal rat indicated that the most effective combination was always the one involving strictly homologous partnerships. A similar selectivity was found in cross tests of neurons and glia from DRG of 10-day fetal, 15-day fetal, and neonatal mice. Sympathetic neurons from chick embryo, neonatal mouse, and neonatal rat also appear to be selectively supported by their own nonneuronal cells (Varon and Raiborn, *unpublished*).

The glial support to ganglionic neurons is not only functionally similar to NGF, it actually involves an NGF-like antigen. In a culture of mouse DRG neurons exclusively supported by homologous glia, neuronal performance is blocked by the presence in the medium of immune globulin specifically directed to the mouse submaxillary β NGF, and so is the performance of chick embryo DRG neurons when exclusively supported by their nonneuronal partners. The immunologically induced block is a graded effect, in that increasing numbers of neurons are affected by increasing concentrations of the agent. The same graded interference with the mouse DRG neuronal performance can be achieved by treating with varying amounts of antibody the glial supplement, before it is presented to the neurons. A fully effective pretreatment requires less than 1 hr exposure to the antibody, it is not affected by an excess presence of normal serum protein, and it survives a mild trypsinization and reseeding of the glial cells. The pretreated glial cells recover their competence only after several hours of incubation in antibody-free medium, apparently with a concomitant release of moderate amounts of antibody, suggesting that the antibody exerted its blocking effect from a location on the glial surface. The NGF-like antigen involved in the glial supportive action has not yet been isolated, and its source and active location remain to be definitely determined. The available data are entirely consistent with an actual production and outward presentation by the glial cells of a glial NGF protein. However, one cannot rule out an alternate possibility that the glia act by capturing an exogenous NGF-precursor, which they activate and effectively deliver to the partner neurons. The species- or age-selective effectiveness of the homologous glia may reflect minor differences in the NGF-antigen produced, or different fits in the mode of delivery of an identical agent, whether produced or modified by the glial cells.

A direct production of NGF (or NGF-like proteins) by glial cells is supported by several other observations (see 2,5). Intracerebral or intraventricular administration of NGF promotes functional recovery after hypothalamic lesion, and accelerates axonal regeneration from catecholamine-containing central neurons. Conversely, antiserum to NGF opposes this axonal regeneration, proposing a physiological role of NGF in the central nervous system (14). Since access to central neurons of blood-borne protein is presumably prevented by the blood-brain barrier, such a central role of NGF would require local, i.e., glial, synthesis of the factor. NGF synthesis by ganglionic glia has also been suggested by observations that rat superior cervical ganglia in explant culture release greater amounts of NGF than those detectable in the initial system, and that the release declines over the first few days in parallel with the degeneration of the ganglionic satellite cells (15). Finally, extracts of a rat glioma grown *in vivo* have been reported to contain both NGF activity and protein constituents closely resembling β NGF in their antigenic and physicochemical properties (16).

Based on the above studies, and several other considerations, the interrelationships among glia, NGF and NGF-related neurons can be formulated within the framework of the following hypothesis. Certain classes of neurons depend on NGF for their survival and the progressive expression of their already built-in differentiated programs (see section "Effects and Role of NGF"). The extent of their performance *in vivo* or *in vitro* reflects the extent to which NGF is available to them. Under optimal availability, neuronal performance will achieve the full potential of the cells, and

additional administration of NGF will fail to elicit any improvement. Under suboptimal NGF availability, neuronal performance is quantitatively restricted and, thus, susceptible of being enhanced by exogenous NGF supplementation. The neurons can derive their NGF from both extraneural and local, i.e., glial, sources. During development the local supply of NGF increases as the local glial cells increase in number, competence and/or effective association with their neurons. With DRG, this may fulfill the entire NGF requirement (DRG neurons have the most conspicuous endowment of satellite cells), and leave no scope for an action by exogenous NGF. With sympathetic ganglia, the indigenous supply may never meet the full neuronal need, and the sympathetic neurons will remain dependent on, and susceptible to, exogenous NGF throughout their lifetime to at least some degree. Whatever the glial contribution in the intact tissue, experimental — or, possibly, pathological — conditions may impose a restriction of it and consequently change or even restore an observable responsiveness to exogenous NGF.

Tentative as this hypothesis may be at present, it raises a number of questions for future investigations. What are the detailed characteristics of the "glial" NGF? How is it delivered to the neurons and what accounts for the observed intercellular selectivity? If NGF production does occur in the glia, is it subject to extrinsic regulation, or even a feedback modulation from the neurons? Is NGF production a property of all glial cells, or one limited to only certain glial categories? If all glial cells cannot produce NGF, do they produce other protein factors with an analogous role with respect to NGF-unrelated neurons? The extent to which the target neurons may depend on the supply of such glial factors could have a critical impact on our understanding of some neuronal pathology in terms of a primary defect of the neuroglia.

NGF AND ITS TARGET CELLS

Target Cell Identification

The study of neural cells *in vitro* has stressed the need to distinguish between intrinsic and extrinsic contributions to a neuronal performance. Thus, observation of a cellular response to NGF may require the concurrence of three elements. One is a programmed susceptibility to NGF action, i.e., a true target nature of the cell. A second element is a restrictive situation where the cell is performing below maximal capacity, so that an increased NGF availability can in fact enhance performance. The third component, particularly applicable *in vitro,* involves permissive experimental conditions that will allow the display by the cell of the response under investigation.

The "programmed" element, and the modulation of its expressibility, will be discussed in the next section. The "restrictive" component is illustrated by the studies of postnatal mouse DRG, where an experimental reduction of ganglionic glia was necessary before exogenous NGF could be shown to be needed and effective. (Another case of restricted conditions is described in section "NGF Effects on RNA and Protein Synthesis".) An example of the third requirement ("permissive" conditions) was also supplied by the studies with mouse DRG cells, and a brief discussion of it may help to dispel any confusion about its implications. In the earlier work (e.g., 11), it had been noted that purified mouse DRG neurons would not perform in glia-free cultures even in the presence of exogenous NGF. Subsequent studies (12) showed that supplementation with any kind of cell, while unable to mimic ganglionic glia as a substitute for NGF itself, would allow the neurons to exhibit their response to exogenous NGF in terms of the culture parameters (attachment, fiber growth, survival). Thus, the presence of other cells was needed to permit the display of the neuronal response rather than the occurrence of an NGF action. It is known, for example, that the attachment abilities of dissociated neurons may differ with different sources, dissociation procedures or culture systems and, indeed, neurons from rat superior cervical ganglia have been cultured with the help of NGF in the near absence of other cells (see 2,5).

Traditionally, NGF has been described to act exclusively on sympathetic ganglionic neurons at all ages, though with progressively declining effects, and on one of the two neuronal populations of DRG but for only a limited period of their embryonic life (3). Because of the reserva-

tions just discussed, it remains possible that other neurons may have failed to display a response to NGF even though they are additional NGF targets. In recent years, the list of cells reported to be responsive to NGF has slowly expanded (see 5) to include postnatal DRG neurons, neurons from trigeminal and gasserian ganglia, catecholamine-containing derivatives of cephalic neural crest, catecholamine-containing central neurons, and—in a few cases—possibly even some nonneural cell types.

NGF Association with the Target Cells

Polypeptide agents are generally assumed to operate from outside the target cells by binding to specific surface receptors and, thus, activating some transduction mechanism. Alternatively, the membrane-bound agent could be internalized by an endocytotic process to reach an intracellular site of action. Considerable evidence acquired over the past 3 years by several independent research groups (see 5) indicates that cells from sympathetic ganglia and embryonic DRG have both surface binding sites specific for NGF and the ability to internalize NGF from humoral or peripheral sources. However, both properties have also been observed for several other neural and nonneural cells (17,18), and a definitive interpretation of their functional roles remains to be reached.

NGF binding displays two ranges of apparent affinity (about 10^9 and 10^6 liters/mole). It remains unresolved whether the two affinity ranges describe two different sets of binding sites, or the occurrence of negative cooperativity between occupied and free sites. The higher affinity matches the range of optimal bioactivity in several ganglionic test systems. Substrate specificity is demonstrated by the lack of competition by other proteins including basic proteins of similar size and the structurally related insulin. In addition, chemical treatment of the NGF protein has resulted in a parallel loss of binding and of biological capabilities, demonstrating their common dependence on certain molecular structures, and at least encouraging the view that NGF binding may be necessary for NGF action. A probable role of the NGF binding sites as true receptors is also indicated by the successful elicitation of ganglionic responses upon presentation of NGF covalently coupled to large particles (sepharose beads, T4-bacteriophage, erythrocytes) and, thus, presumably prevented from entering the cells (see 5).

Intracellular accumulation of radio-NGF has been shown to occur in superior cervical ganglia upon *in vivo* administration of the agent into the blood stream or the anterior chamber of the homolateral eye. The data indicate that such internalization involves uptake at the sympathetic terminals and subsequent retrograde axonal transport to the neuronal somata. A functional significance of the NGF uptake modality is suggested by recent *in vivo* investigations (Hendry, *personal communication*) that correlate enzyme activities in sympathetic ganglia with the availability of NGF in their peripheral innervation fields. *In vitro* DRG studies (18) have also suggested endocytotic intake of exogenous NGF. In addition, they recognized a retention of biological competence by the reextracted NGF, implicated a substrate-specific binding step in the uptake process, and noted that the NGF uptake was accompanied by some release of the accumulated radio material.

Both models—surface and intracellular sites of action—are, therefore, permitted but not definitely proven by the available evidence. It is possible that both "routes" are functionally involved, perhaps to mediate different NGF effects. A more speculative way to merge the two sets of information could be to conceive the action of NGF at the receptor site as the only functional modality, and the intake of peripheral NGF—accompanied by a release at the somal level—as a way to ensure availability of the factor in the immediate local environment of the receptor sites.

The reported occurrence of both modalities of NGF association in all cells tested raises further questions on the nature of their involvement with NGF. Some of these cells may be genuine, though unrecognized, NGF targets (see preceding section) while others may be involved in NGF production and externalization. A third view is suggested by observed correlations between the extent of sympathetic innervation of peripheral tissues and their NGF binding capability (17). In this view, nontarget, NGF-binding cells may act to store the factor either as a general "buffer" system or more specifically to guide or supply NGF-dependent nerve fibers.

Whatever its significance, the presence of NGF binding sites on both responsive and nonresponsive cells indicates that their occurrence is not a sufficient (though, possibly, still a necessary) condition for NGF action. *Responsiveness,* then, must involve other, target-specific, cellular properties. One candidate could be the presence or absence of a follow-up machinery to transduce the association between NGF and binding sites into meaningful cell alterations. Nothing is known at present about the physicochemical characteristics of the surface binding sites or the transduction mechanisms operating in conjunction with them, but a provoking suggestion has been advanced by Levi-Montalcini and co-workers (19) that tubulin-like membrane constituents be involved in both. An alternate requirement for an NGF responsiveness could be the extent to which the cell can bind NGF, i.e., a threshold number of binding sites below which action could not take place. Relevant to this concept may be an observation, recently reported by Revoltella et al. (20), that mouse neuroblastoma cells display a vast increase in functional binding sites for NGF at specified stages of their mitotic cycle. Mouse neuroblastoma cells, despite their sympathetic characteristics, have failed to reveal a response to NGF in several investigations, and it is attractive to speculate that such failure may relate to their having been tested when endowed with subthreshold numbers of binding sites.

NGF AND ITS MODE OF ACTION

Effects and Role of NGF

The *in vitro* effects of NGF on the traditional ganglionic target tissues (3) comprise support or enhancement of general cell functions (biosynthesis of RNA, protein and lipid; energy metabolism), specific neuronal properties (e.g., neurotransmitter enzymes), and production of neurites (hence, the term "nerve" growth factor). It remains to be determined how these several responses are related to one another, and to the initial association of NGF with the target cells.

NGF has been often described (3) as a differentiation agent, promoting selective properties of the responsive neuron, hence presumably altering distinctive transcriptional events to provide the cell with new sets of specific instructions. An alternative view (5) is that NGF promotes the expression of all the properties for which the nerve cell is already programmed. This view is based on several features of the cell responses to NGF, which are firmly established by *in vitro* studies and at the very least compatible with the less readily analyzable *in vivo* observations. First, NGF (or an NGF-like support by other cells) is required for the survival of ganglionic target neurons. Secondly, the requirement is for the continuous presence of NGF. Thirdly, the cellular responses are graded with regard to the NGF levels, up to the maximal responses dictated by the potential of the target cell in a given set of permissive conditions. Fourthly, no responses to NGF have been described other than in terms of earlier or greater expressions of normal traits (5). Finally, NGF appears to play its role over an extended span of the target cell history, from neuroblastic (replicative) to adult stages.

Thus, NGF fits more readily the definition of a modulation agent than that of a differentiation one, with the modulation range stretching between no stimulus (cell death) to optimal stimulus (full cell potential). This view of NGF as a modulating agent is consistent with the interpretation of the roles of extraganglionic and glial NGF already presented in a previous section (see "NGF and the Neuroglia"). It also encourages attempts to identify a central property of the target cell, which could be directly regulated by NGF and in turn responsible for regulating a variety of cell performances.

NGF Effects on RNA and Protein Synthesis

The early view of NGF as a differentiation agent focussed attention to transcriptional events in NGF-treated ganglia. Angeletti et al. (3) reported that DRG incubated with NGF and radioprecursors showed higher accumulation of labeled RNA by 2 hr and of labeled protein by 6 hr than did untreated ganglia, and that the RNA effect was independent of ongoing protein synthesis while the protein effect was blocked by actinomycin D. Based on such observations,

it was proposed that RNA synthesis be the primary site of NGF action with all other responses occurring secondarily, and subordinately, to the RNA response.

Several subsequent studies, however, have called for a reassessment of such a model. Neurite production could still be elicited by NGF, in sympathetic ganglia and in DRG, under actinomycin D-blocked RNA synthesis (21,22). Explanted sympathetic ganglia and unattached DRG (intact or dissociated) both displayed a progressively declining accumulation of labeled RNA and protein when incubated without NGF, and a maintenance of the initial capabilities when provided with the factor (21,22). Radioincorporation into RNA and protein by DRG could also be supported, in the absence of NGF, by treatment with insulin, concanavalin A or serum, although different mechanisms or different cell targets appeared to be involved (23). In particular, NGF and insulin had additive effects, clearly separating the actions of these two polypeptides on DRG cells. These several studies stress the difficulty of interpreting experimental systems where: (a) the "control" material (i.e., the untreated ganglionic tissue or cells) varies within the experimental time span and, through its variation, determines the difference to be measured between treated and untreated samples; and (b) different cell populations are jointly involved, whose behaviors may vary independently with time and be selectively susceptible to different agents.

A partial clarification of the DRG system has been achieved by examining in greater detail the consequences of NGF deprivation *in vitro* (24). DRG cells, supplied with NGF after increasing incubation times without the agent and tested with 1-hr pulses of radioprecursors, revealed two distinct sets of events. An early set of events, developing over the first 6 hr without NGF, is revealed by a decline in the cell capability to label RNA, but not protein. The decline was reversed by a delayed presentation of NGF, however long the delay up to the end of this period. In all cases, the reversal led to full restoration of the incorporation ability displayed by the cells at the start, or retained by them under continuous NGF treatment. The reversal was completely effected by NGF within 10 min of its presentation, providing for the first time an experimental situation where NGF elicits a short-latency biochemical response against a relatively invariant "control" behavior. One should note that over this early period, an NGF effect on ganglionic cells is observable only to the extent to which the NGF-deprived cells have changed, another example—as yet not adequately interpretable—of the "restrictive" situation discussed above (section "Target Cell Identification").

A later set of events occurs if NGF deprivation is prolonged beyond 6 hours. It is revealed by several changes developing concurrently: (a) irreversible decline in RNA labeling, (b) irreversible decline in protein labeling, (c) onset and progression of RNA degradation, and (d) accelerated degradation of protein. The entire set of these later events is prevented by presentation of NGF before 6 hr, only interrupted or delayed when NGF is supplied between 6 and 15 hr, and no longer susceptible to NGF after longer deprivations. The character and timetable of the later events indicate a delayed onset and progression of irreversible damage and/or death of the NGF-dependent ganglionic population, and confirm morphological observations previously reported by several investigators (see 3,5,22). In addition, they suggest that these events are secondary to the persistence or the aggravation of a condition generated within the earlier set of events.

Permeation Effects of NGF

The early and reversible loss of RNA-labeling capability could result from a reversible decline in the rate of RNA synthesis or a reversible decrease in the amounts of radioprecursor available for it. A direct measure of the size and specific activity of RNA precursor pools is, at best, a difficult task in these ganglionic preparations and their interpretation may suffer from the heterogeneity of the cell population. However, considerable evidence has now been accumulated (24,25) that the early set of events and their prevention or reversal by NGF involve primarily changes in the availability of radioprecursor.

Accumulation of acid-soluble radioactivity upon 1 hr pulse of radiouridine was constant in DRG cells under continuous NGF treatment,

declined in the NGF-deprived cells and was rapidly and fully restored upon delayed NGF presentation up to 6 hr, in precise temporal coincidence with the observed behavior of RNA labeling. The ratio of precipitable to soluble radioactivities within each sample was constant across a large number of different experiments and regardless of whether uridine, cytidine, or guanosine were used as radioprecursors. Chromatographic analysis of "soluble radioactivity" from NGF-deprived and NGF-treated cells demonstrated identical qualitative compositions in radiouridine and phosphorylated derivatives (with radio-UTP accounting for over half of the total radioactivity), and each component exhibited the same ratio as the total pool between NGF-treated and control samples. The NGF-induced increase in soluble radioactivity occurred even after pretreatment with actinomycin D or cycloheximide, demonstrating its independence from any NGF consequences on RNA or protein synthesis. Finally, preliminary experiments with labeled 2-deoxyglucose and α-isoaminobutyrate indicate that accumulation of other substrates by the DRG cells is similarly declining in the absence of NGF and promptly restored by its delayed administration. Important ion transfers could also be involved (2,5,25), although they have not yet been investigated.

The NGF-induced rise in intracellular accumulation of exogenous substrates, revealed by the above experiments, must involve changes in transport or retention mechanisms, either of which would reside in the plasma membrane of the target cells. These changes are elicited within minutes of the NGF presentation and can occur in the absence of transcriptional and translational events. Thus, they represent not only a new set of NGF effects occurring independently from those traditionally described for this factor, but the one response among all presently known which is closest in both time and space to the association between NGF and the target cell membrane. This closeness will hopefully provide new opportunities to investigate other changes that NGF may elicit at the membrane level (see 5) within the same time span and, possibly, to sort out the sequential and/or causal relationships among the various membrane events. Perhaps more importantly, the permeation responses to NGF place the NGF phenomenon into a new perspective, closely aligned with the current recognition of plasma membranes as critical mediators of cell regulation. In this perspective, the NGF-induced alterations of the cell membrane can be viewed as the only direct effect of NGF on the target cells, and the other known responses taken to reflect intracellular regulatory mechanisms describing the properties of the cell itself rather than the mode of action of the factor.

The following formulation of a model for the NGF action attempts to bring together several of the concepts described throughout this paper. (a) NGF binds to its receptor sites on the surface of the cells. If an adequate number of receptors are occupied (target cells), changes in the membrane properties are induced, which cause increased intracellular accumulation of several exogenous substrates. (b) Increased availability of certain critical substrates enhances, coordinately or independently, the performance by the target cell of the several tasks for which it is programmed (energy metabolism, biosynthesis of general and cell-specific constituents, neurite production, etc.). (c) NGF deprivation leads to inverse changes in the membrane properties, reducing or cutting off supply of the relevant exogenous substrates. The cell can continue to operate for a time on preexisting intracellular reserves, upon whose depletion deterioration and death occurs.

Such a model, at present, is admittedly only a speculative one, even though it appears to account for all available information. It offers, however, the considerable advantage of stressing a distinction between cellular responses that are instructive on the NGF mode of action, and those that may only describe cell-intrinsic regulation mechanisms. On one hand, therefore, the search for an NGF mechanism becomes focussed on events residing in the membrane. On the other, NGF becomes an invaluable tool to probe into the various machineries operating in a nerve cell and their control systems. Specifically, the model raises the question of which substrates and ions may be critically needed in the various functions of a nerve cell, an area where information is sorely lacking. Lastly, a paradigm is suggested which may help further understanding of the action of other polypeptide agents on neuronal or other responsive cells.

ACKNOWLEDGMENTS

The research work by this author and his collaborators was mainly supported by USPHS grant NB-07606 from the National Institute of Neurological Diseases and Stroke and, in part, by grant E-513 from the American Cancer Society.

REFERENCES

1. Varon, S. (1975): Neurons and glia in neural cultures. *Exp. Neurol. (in press)*.
2. Varon, S., and Saier, M. (1975): Culture techniques and glial-neuronal interrelationships *in vitro. Exp. Neurol. (in press)*.
3. Levi-Montalcini, R., and Angeletti, P. U. (1971): Nerve Growth Factor. *Physiol. Rev.,* 48:534–569.
4. Zaimis, E., and Knight, J. (eds.) (1972): *Nerve Growth Factor and Its Antiserum.* The Athlone Press (Univ. of London), London.
5. Varon, S. (1975): Nerve Growth Factor and its mode of action. *Exp. Neurol. (in press)*.
6. Frazier, W. A., Angeletti, R. H., and Bradshaw, R. A. (1972): Nerve Growth Factor and insulin. *Science,* 176:482–488.
7. Varon, S., Nomura, J., and Shooter, E. M. (1968): Reversible dissociation of the mouse Nerve Growth Factor into different subunits. *Biochemistry,* 7:1296–1303.
8. Greene, L. A., Tomita, J. T., and Varon, S. (1971): Growth-stimulating activities of mouse submaxillary esteropeptidases on chick embryo fibroblasts *in vitro. Exp. Cell Res.,* 64:387–395.
9. Varon, S., and Raiborn, C. (1972): Protective effect of mouse 7S Nerve Growth Factor protein and its Alpha subunit on embryonic sensory ganglionic cells during dissociation. *Neurobiology,* 2:183–196.
10. Oger, J., Arnason, B. G. W., Pantazis, N., Lehrich, J., and Young, M. (1974): Synthesis of Nerve Growth Factor by L and 3T3 cells in culture. *Proc. Natl. Acad. Sci. USA,* 71:1154–1558.
11. Burnham, P. A., Raiborn, C., and Varon, S. (1972): Replacement of Nerve Growth Factor by ganglionic non-neuronal cells for the survival *in vitro* of dissociated ganglionic neurons. *Proc. Natl. Acad. Sci. USA,* 60:3556–3560.
12. Varon, S., Raiborn, C., and Burnham, P. A. (1974): Selective potency of homologous ganglionic non-neuronal cells for the support of dissociated ganglionic neurons in culture. *Neurobiology,* 4:231–252.
13. Varon, S., Raiborn, C., and Norr, S. C. (1974):

Association of antibody to Nerve Growth Factor with ganglionic non-neurons (glia) and consequent interference with their neuron-supportive action. *Exp. Cell Res.,* 88:247–256.

14. Bjerre, B., Björklund, A., and Stenevi, U. (1974): Inhibition of the regenerative growth of central noradrenergic neurons by intracerebrally administered anti-NGF serum. *Brain Res.,* 74:1–18.

15. Johnson, D. G., Silberstein, S. D., Hanbauer, I., and Kopin, I. J. (1972): The role of Nerve Growth Factor in the ramification of sympathetic nerve fibers into the rat iris in organ culture. *J. Neurochem.,* 19:2025–2029.

16. Longo, A. M., and Penhoet, E. E. (1974): Nerve Growth Factor in rat glioma cells. *Proc. Natl. Acad. Sci. USA,* 71:2347–2349.

17. Frazier, W. A., Boyd, L. F., Szutowicz, A., Pullman, M. W., and Bradshaw, R. A. (1974): Specific binding sites for ^{125}I-Nerve Growth Factor in peripheral tissues and brain. *Biochem. Biophys. Res. Commun.,* 57:1096–1103.

18. Norr, S. C., and Varon, S. (1975): Dynamic, temperature-sensitive association of ^{125}I-Nerve Growth Factor *in vitro* with ganglionic and non-ganglionic cells from embryonic chick. *Neurobiology,* 5:110–118.

19. Levi-Montalcini, R., Revoltella, R., and Calissano, P. (1974): Microtubule proteins in the Nerve Growth Factor mediated response. In: *Recent Progress in Hormone Research,* Vol. 30,

edited by R. O. Greep, pp. 635–669. Academic Press, New York.

20. Revoltella, R., Bertolini, L., and Pediconi, M. (1974): Unmasking of Nerve Growth Factor membrane-specific binding sites in synchronized murine C1300 neuroblastoma cells. *Exp. Cell Res.,* 85:89–94.

21. Partlow, L. M., and Larrabee, M. G. (1971): Effects of a Nerve Growth Factor, embryo age and metabolic inhibitors on growth of fibers and on synthesis of ribonucleic acid and protein in embryonic sympathetic ganglia. *J. Neurochem.,* 18:2101–2118.

22. Burnham, P. A., and Varon, S. (1974): Biosynthetic activities of dorsal root ganglia *in vitro* and the influence of Nerve Growth Factor. *Neurobiology,* 3:232–245.

23. Burnham, P. A., Silva, J., and Varon, S. (1974): Anabolic responses of embryonic dorsal root ganglia to Nerve Growth Factor, insulin, concanavalin A or serum *in vitro. J. Neurochem.,* 23:689–697.

24. Horii, Z. I., and Varon, S. (1975): Nerve Growth Factor induced rapid activation of RNA labeling in dorsal root ganglionic dissociates from the chick embryo. *J. Neurosci. Res. (in press).*

25. Horii, Z. I., and Varon, S. (1975): Nerve Growth Factor action on membrane permeation to exogenous substrates in dorsal root ganglionic dissociates from the chick embryo. *(In preparation.)*

The Nervous System, Donald B. Tower, Editor-in-Chief. *Vol. 1: The Basic Neurosciences.* Raven Press, New York, 1975.

Using Immunology to Understand Neurobiology

Michael B. A. Oldstone

An explosion has taken place in immunology. Beginning in the mid 1950s, the accomplishments of its disciples have continually enlarged and diversified leading to the current massive increase in basic research results, many of which are being applied to patients in a variety of medical fields. Unquestionably, future immunologists will use their technology to uncover the secrets of the neural code and to define causes, understand mechanisms and eventually treat and prevent human diseases of the nervous system.

The rapid growth and present practical uses of immunology in biology and in medicine are largely attributable to the formation of the National Institutes of Health. Since the N.I.H. was established, membership in the American Association of Immunologists has tripled. Now more than 40 journals that deal with immunology and allergy mark the achievements in this discipline. Reflected in this rising number of publications is the work of young bioscientists who become trained in its techniques, perfect new ones, and spread their advancements in immunology to other biomedical fields.

In this chapter I shall discuss selected work in which immunologic expertise has been applied to problems of the nervous system, particularly those areas where I believe the greatest progress will be made in the next decade. Specifically, I focus my attention on two major subjects: first, using the groundwork laid by immunology to understand the neural code and organization of the nervous system and, second, reviewing selected aspects of immunologic diseases of the human nervous system.

TOWARD UNDERSTANDING THE NEURAL CODE

One of the mysteries of neurobiology is why one neuron (neuron 1) chooses to come in contact with another neuron (neuron 2) and avoids meeting a third neuron (neuron 3). Although all three neurons may look morphologically similar, they obviously have different purposes and tend to travel with different friends in life. Are all three different, and, if so, what determines their differences? How many dissimilar types are there and what factor(s) accounts for their various orientations? How does a neuron recognize another neuron or an astrocyte, oligodendroglia, or ependymal cell? Simply put, the question is what are the surface antigenic markers for distinguishing neurons from each other and from other cells of the nervous system? Answers to these questions should provide important data for understanding the organization of the nervous system.

The difficulties being experienced by neurobiologists today are similar to those of immunologists who tried to distinguish functional classes and subclasses of lymphocytes. In the early and mid 1960s several investigators demonstrated in birds and then mammals that there were basically two sets of immune responses that were either dependent on or independent from the thymus. Each response involved a different population of lymphocytes (1–4). Soon after, the discovery and utilization of various surface antigenic markers not only allowed one to distinguish between thymus-dependent lymphocytes (T lymphocytes) and thymus-independent or bone-marrow-derived (B) lymphocytes but also to purify these lymphocytes by using specific antisera, rosetting techniques, and density and column procedures (reviewed 5,6). This technology then led to experiments in which the roles of various cells in the immune response were tested by depleting one of the lymphocyte populations and subsequently reconstituting it first to prevent and second to restore the response being tested. Presently with more detailed studies new functional subpopulations were found within each class, i.e., T lymphocytes, T suppressor cells, T helper cells. Unquestionably more digging will uncover more riches which will sharpen our knowledge of the basic immune responses and thus allow us to understand, evaluate, and treat abnormal responses, i.e., increased, decreased, or aberrant immune responses.

These successful methods for studying lymphocytes of the immune system are now being applied in several laboratories to studying cells of the nervous system. At present this field is in its infancy, and the surface antigen markers needed to differentiate various types of neurons or to separate glia from neuronal cells have not yet been found. As expected in this early stage, the work is controversial. However, if the parallel with immunology is complete, exciting and productive days loom in the future in neurobiology.

Several investigators have cloned cells from the central nervous system (CNS) and looked for known "specific" markers for brain cells. Theta (Θ) alloantigen is a marker for T lymphocytes of the mouse, and by absorption studies has been shown to reside on surfaces of mouse thymocytes, and in brain tissues, restricted lymphocyte populations and skin fibroblasts (7,8). Further, antibody to brain (9) can also be used as a marker for T lymphocytes. This has led several investigators to study whether Θ is a marker for unique cells in the nervous system. Utilizing cloned neuroblastoma N18, N115, S20, C1300 cells, ependymoblastoma cells, and astrocytoma cells derived from mouse, rat, and human tissues and employing the techniques of radioimmunoautography, immunofluorescence, and cytotoxic assays, we were unable to demonstrate Θ markers on any of these cells. Nor could we by similar techniques demonstrate S100, 14-3-2 or basic protein on the surfaces of such cells (10). As expected, surface specific histocompatibility antigens were present on all cells studied. Hence, while Θ antigen is present in large amounts in the brain, its precise location remains a mystery to most investigators. With better techniques for separating and harvesting neuronal tissue, increased knowledge of the composition of Θ antigen and more investigators studying the problem, Θ antigen in the brain will be located. Since thymosin, a hormone of the thymus, plays an important role in differentiating B and T lymphocytes, this reagent may play an im-

portant role in controlling Θ expression and activity in CNS tissues.

Surface markers for cells of the nervous system have been reported within the last year. Coakham documented surface antigen(s) common to human astrocytoma cells (11); Schachner reported the occurrence of a glial cell specific surface antigen on three or four mouse methylcholanthrene-induced glioblastomas but not on surfaces of C1300 neuroblastoma cells (12), whereas Akeson and Hersman found large quantities of antigens specific to differentiating neuroblastoma cells in mouse brain (13). Studies in my laboratory in collaboration with Meinke (14) have demonstrated DNA on the cytoplasmic membranes of mouse neuroblastoma cells. The role played by DNA on the surfaces of specific cells is not known, but the possible mechanism of gene amplification is apparent. All these studies, though preliminary and in need of confirmation, nevertheless indicate a surging tide of valuable information forthcoming in neurobiology.

Obtaining specific surface markers for cells of the nervous system has great potential application to the field of medicine and other scientific disciplines. Specific antisera that react with an oligodendroglia but not an astrocyte will allow workers in tissue culturing to identify the cell in question, whereas at present identification of CNS tissue in culture is uncertain and unreliable. In addition, with specific antisera one could select unique cells, i.e., select oligodendroglia in which myelination and demyelination can be studied in depth, and examine them with agents that slow down or accelerate myelination. With surface markers one could ascertain the alignment of nervous tissue cells *in vivo* and shed light on aberrant motor and behavioral mutants seen in animal models and in similar human disorders.

IMMUNOLOGIC DISEASES OF THE NERVOUS SYSTEM

Whereas the use of surface markers in neurobiology is in the embryonic stage, the fact that a host's immune response may cause disorders of the nervous and other body systems is well established. Immunologic injury can occur by two basic mechanisms. First, the components of the immune system (humoral:antibody, complement; cellular:T lymphocytes, macrophages; humoral and cellular:K cells, cytophilic macrophages) react against antigens unique to the tissues where they are located. Second, antibodies can combine with antigens in the blood or other body fluids and form antigen–antibody complexes that cause injury when they become trapped by basement membranes.

CNS Disease Caused by Direct Interaction of Immune Reactants with Nervous System Antigens

The classic example of immunologic injury against CNS tissue caused when the host is sensitized against brain antigens is experimental allergic encephalomyelitis (EAE). Sensitization of animals with whole brain or purified encephalogenic basic protein antigen in adjuvant leads to immunologic attack on CNS tissue resulting in perivascular cell cuffing and tissue injury. Over the years this model has received much attention from neuroimmunologists and neuroimmunopathologists and will not be discussed further here. EAE and its possible relevance to human disease have been reviewed (15,16). Another classic example of immunologic injury mediated by specific tissue antigens is glomerular basement membrane disease. Although studied primarily in experimental animals, basement membrane disease occurs in man, for example in Goodpasture's syndrome. In both experimental animals and humans the injury is directed by antibodies against antigens on basement membranes. Here, in addition to the kidney and lungs, other tissues that are similarly rich in basement membranes are attacked. In fact, recent reports on patients with Goodpasture's syndrome who have mental aberrations suggest that the choroid plexus is injured, resulting in CNS dysfunction. Similarly, injection of experimental animals with choroid plexus elicits basement membrane disease.

CNS Disease Caused by Immune Complexes

We identify immune complex disease by finding antigen–antibody complexes in the circulation or in the injured tissues deposited in a characteristic granular pattern (17). Immune complexes are an important cause of

human disease being recognized as the major cause of glomerulonephritis and vasculitis. Over 80% of all cases of human glomerulonephritis are caused by deposits of immune complexes, although the etiologies of a vast majority of initiating antigens are not yet known.

Since kidneys filter so much blood, the basement membranes of their glomeruli are targets for immune complex deposition. The choroid plexus and the renal glomerulus share many anatomical similarities, and therefore, it seemed logical to investigate whether the choroid plexus in the brain might not also be a privileged site for immune complex deposits and resultant CNS disease. The choroid plexus consists of tufts of capillaries which, like the glomerular basement membrane, contain fenestrated endothelial (on the blood side) basement membranes, interstitial spaces, and epithelial cells (on the cerebral spinal fluid side). Major differences are that the choroid plexus has two basement membranes, wider interstitial space, and cuboidal to columnar epithelial cells, whereas the glomerulus has one basement membrane, a narrower interstitial space, and squamous cell epithelium.

In looking for immune complex deposits Lampert and I first devoted our attention to experimentally induced and naturally occurring immune complex disease in animals and then turned our focus to immune complex disorders of man (18,19). Mice infected *in utero* or at birth with lymphocytic choriomeningitis virus (LCMV) maintain persistent levels of virus in their tissues and blood and mount a continuous host immune response throughout life (20). Such mice show classical manifestations of immune complex disease and have been the best model of its type for study (21). When we observed the choroid plexes of such mice by immunofluorescence, characteristic deposits of host immunoglobulin G (IgG), viral antigen(s), and the third component of complement (C3) in a granular discontinuous pattern were seen. Electron microscopy showed electron-dense deposits similar to those seen in the renal glomeruli. In contrast, a slow infection of the brain associated with Scrapie agent, in which specific immune complexes do not occur, did not produce these deposits in the choroid plexus.

New Zealand mice spontaneously develop circulating complexes such as nuclear antigen–antibody to nuclear antigens, DNA-antibody to DNA and oncornavirus-antibody to oncornavirus. Subsequently nephritis develops after these complexes become trapped in their renal glomeruli. (NZB × NZW)F$_1$ mice are more susceptible than other New Zealand mice to spontaneous immune complex disease and in the former we found immune complex deposits in the choroid plexus with both immunofluorescence and electron microscopy (18). Host IgG and C3 were shown by direct immunofluorescent staining, and the DNA complexed in the choroid plexus was demonstrated by first treating a tissue section with agents that dissociated antigen–antibody bonds, removing the IgG from the complex and finally showing that fluoresceinated antibody specific to DNA stained the complex. In contrast, if the complex was dissociated and then treated with DNAse, the fluoresceinated antibody to DNA did not stain these complexes. Two additional pieces of evidence established that the deposits were immune complexes and were related to the general disease process. First, immune complex deposition in the choroid plexes clearly followed the time sequence of spontaneously occurring circulating complexes in (NZB × NZW)F$_1$ mice (18). Second, when we injected DNA methylated bovine serum albumin into New Zealand white mice, DNA-antibody to DNA and nuclear antigen-antibody to nuclear antigen complexes deposited rapidly and heavily in the choroid plexuses of these mice. Hence, we determined experimentally that immune complexes accumulated in the choroid plexus, as expected, in disorders associated with immune complex disease. Subsequently, immune complex deposits in choroid plexuses have been reported in other models of immune complex disease such as Aleutian disease of mink and acute and chronic serum sickness of rabbits.

Systemic lupus erythematosus (SLE) is the human version of the spontaneous disease of New Zealand mice. Patients with SLE spontaneously develop nuclear antigen-antibody to nuclear antigen and DNA-antibody to DNA complexes in their circulations. These complexes deposit in their glomeruli leading to immune complex glomerulonephritis. Further-

more, 40% to 80% of patients with SLE have aberrant CNS findings ranging from personality difficulties to stupor and coma. In evaluating patients with SLE who died with CNS disease, we (19) and others (22) have found evidence of immune complex deposits in the choroid plexus. Again, Lampert and I could, by immunologic techniques, demonstrate host IgG, C3, and DNA in the immune complex deposits. Still other investigators have found DNA-antibody to DNA complexes in the cerebral spinal fluid of patients with CNS SLE and alterations in a unique complement component (C4) (23) indicating not only the presence of soluble complexes in brain fluids but activation and utilization of complement which is the major effector system fired by antigen–antibody complexes. Thus, it is likely that several manifestations of CNS SLE are due to immune complex disease of the choroid plexus. Techniques are now available to substantiate this diagnosis (measuring hemolytic C4 level and DNA-antibody to DNA complexes in cerebrospinal fluid), and treatment to benefit the patient (steroids) is based on these observations.

Further study in LCMV models suggest that immune complex deposits in the choroid plexus may be a common occurrence during either acute or persistent virus infections in which the host mounts an immune response against the virus and forms virus–antibody immune complexes. This information raises the possibility that transient mental aberrations during many infections or behavioral inconsistencies whose cause is unknown may be due in part to immune complex disease of the choroid plexus with activation of complement or other effector systems. Certainly this possibility can, with the present technology, be confirmed or rejected by careful experimental investigation.

Control of Immune Responses

Since various immune responses can cause disease, understanding the factor(s) controlling such responses is of utmost importance. The history of research in this area clearly demonstrates that basic research results have been adapted to animal models and then to man. Work mainly by Benacerraf and McDevitt (24) showed that immune responses to certain antigens were controlled by genes that were dominant and mapped close to the major histocompatibility loci. Using synthetic antigens as immunogens these investigators showed that although one murine strain made an enhanced immune response, another made a significantly lower response and the offspring from mating the high and low responders made an enhanced immune response. The genetics were then determined by backcrossing hybrids to either parent and showing that the ability to mount a higher immune response and histocompatibility type segregated together. This led Benacerraf and McDevitt to postulate that immune responses to various antigens are controlled by an immune response gene which is dominant and located near the histocompatibility locus.

The next extension of these fundamental observations was the study of animal models in which immune responses led to disease. In all the classical models studied, EAE (25), thyroiditis (26), and acute LCMV infection (27), disease was related to an autosomal dominant gene that segregated with the major histocompatibility marker. These and other experiments were compatible with the idea that diseases associated with immune responses were also associated with certain histocompatibility types.

Currently many investigators are studying histocompatibility systems of man (HL-A markers) related to disease. Those who work with CNS disease are particularly interested in reports of the association of multiple sclerosis with HL-A-3,7 and LD-7a loci and the relationship of paralytic poliomyelitis to an HL-A7 marker. Although these and other conclusions are in some flux and need confirmation, nevertheless, the possibility is exciting that individuals with greater susceptibility to develop disease (or with a greater susceptibility to having more severe disease) can be detected. Others are placing cells bearing these HL-A or LD-7 markers in cultures and studying such cells by various immunologic and virologic parameters.

CONCLUSION

Great productivity in immunology has resulted in techniques and approaches now ripe to be applied to problems in neurobiology. Development of these methods is directly parallel to and associated with the first 25 years of NINCDS existence. The next 25 years of NINDS support should bring a revolution in our understanding of the nervous system and our ability to utilize this information in the treatment of some of the diseases of man.

ACKNOWLEDGMENTS

This is Publication Number 954 from the Department of Immunopathology, Scripps Clinic and Research Foundation, La Jolla, California. This research was supported in part by U.S. Public Health Service Grants AI-09484, AI-07007, Contract No. NO1 CP 53512 within the Virus Cancer Program of the National Cancer Institute, the Violet June Kertell Memorial Grant for Research on Multiple Sclerosis from the National Multiple Sclerosis Society, and National Foundation Grant No. 1–364. I am grateful to Frank J. Dixon under whose sponsorship I first began my studies in immunology.

REFERENCES

1. Warner, N. L., Szenberg, A., and Burnet, F. M. (1962): The immunological role of different lymphoid organs in the chicken. I. Dissociation of immunological responsiveness. *Aust. J. Exp. Biol.*, 40:373–388.
2. Armason, B., Jankovic, B., Waksman, B., and Wennersten, C. (1962): Role of the thymus in immune reactions in rats. II. Suppressive effect of thymectomy at birth on reactions of delayed cellular hypersensitivity and the circulating small lymphocyte. *J. Exp. Med.*, 116:177–186.
3. Parrot, D. M. V., de Sousa, M. A. B., and East, J. (1966): Thymus-dependent areas in lymphoid organs of neonatally thymectomized mice. *J. Exp. Med.*, 123:191–204.
4. Davies, A. J. S., Leuchars, E., Wallis, V., Marchant, R., and Elliott, E. V. (1967): The failure of thymus-derived cells to produce antibody. *Transplantation*, 5:222–231.
5. Raff, M. (1971): Surface markers for distinguishing T and B lymphocytes in mice. *Transplant Rev.*, 6:52–80.
6. Wigzell, H., Hayry, P. (1974): Specific fractionation of immunocompetent cells. Current Topics in Microbiology and Immunology, Vol. 67, pp. 1–42. Springer-Verlag, New York.
7. Reif, A. E., and Allen, J. M. V. (1964): The AKR thymic antigen and its distribution in leukemias and nervous tissues. *J. Exp. Med.*, 120:413–434.
8. Reif, A. E. and Allen, J. M. V. (1966): Mouse

thymic iso-antigens. *Nature (Lond.)*, 209:521–523.

9. Golub, E. (1972): The distribution of brain associated theta antigen cross-reactive with mouse in the brain of other species. *J. Immunol.*, 109:168–170.

10. Joseph, B. S., and Oldstone, M. B. A. (1974): Expression of selected antigens on the surface of cultured neural cells. *Brain Res.*, 80:421–434.

11. Coakham, H. (1974): Surface antigen(s) common to human astrocytoma cells. *Nature*, 250:328–330.

12. Schachner, M. (1974): NS-1 (Nervous System Antigen-1), a glial-cell-specific antigenic component of the surface membrane. *Proc. Natl. Acad. Sci. USA*, 71:1795–1799.

13. Akeson, R., and Herschman, H. (1974): Neural antigens of morphologically differentiated neuroblastoma cells. *Nature*, 249:620–623.

14. Oldstone, M. B. A., and Meinke, W. (*unpublished observations*).

15. Paterson, P. Y. (1966): Experimental allergic encephalomyelitis and autoimmune disease. *Advan. Immunol.*, 5:131–208.

16. Peterson, P. Y. (1969): Immune processes and infectious factors in central nervous system disease. *Annu. Rev. Med.*, 20:75–100.

17. Cochrane, C. G. and Koffler, D. (1973): Immune complex disease in experimental animals and man. *Advan. Immunol.*, 16:195–264.

18. Lampert, P. W., and Oldstone, M. B. A. (1973): Host IgG and C3 deposits in the choroid plexus during spontaneous immune complex disease. *Science*, 180:408–410.

19. Oldstone, M. B. A., and Lampert, P. W. (1974): Immune complex disease in chronic virus infection: Involvement of the choroid plexus. In: *Advances in the Biosciences*, edited by G. Raspe

and S. Bernhard, pp. 381–390. Pergamon Press, Oxford, New York.

20. Oldstone, M. B. A., and Dixon, F. J. (1969): Pathogenesis of chronic disease associated with persistent lymphocytic choriomeningitis viral infection. I. Relationship of antibody production to disease in neonatally infected mice. *J. Exp. Med.*, 129:483–505.

21. Oldstone, M. B. A. (1975): Virus neutralization and virus induced immune complex disease: Virus-antibody union resulting in immunoprotection or immunologic injury—Two different sides of the same coin. In: *Progress in Medical Virology*, edited by J. L. Melnick, vol. 19, pp. 84–119. S. Karger, Basel.

22. Atkins, C., Kondon, J., Zuismorio, F., Friou, G. (1972): The choroid plexus in systemic lupus erythematosus. *Am. Int. Med.*, 76:65–72.

23. Petz, L. D., Sharp, G. C., Cooper, N. R., and Irvin, W. S. (1971): Serum and cerebral spinal fluid complement and serum autoantibodies in systemic lupus erythematosus. *Medicine*, 50:259–275.

24. Benacerraf, B., McDevitt, H. O. (1972): Histocompatibility-linked immune response genes. *Science*, 175:273–279.

25. Williams, R. M., and Moore, M. J. (1973): Linkage of susceptibility to experimental allergic encephalomyelitis to the major histocompatibility locus in the rat. *J. Exp. Med.*, 138:775–783.

26. Vladutiu, A., Rose, N. R. (1971): Autoimmune murine thyroiditis relation to histocompatibility (H-2) type. *Science*, 174:1137–1139.

27. Oldstone, M. B. A., Dixon, F. J., Mitchell, G. F., and McDevitt, H. O. (1973): Histocompatibility-linked genetic control of disease susceptibility: Murine lymphocytic choriomeningitis virus infection. *J. Exp. Med.*, 137:1201–1212.

The Nervous System. Donald B. Tower. Editor-in-Chief. *Vol. 1: The Basic Neurosciences.* Raven Press, New York, 1975.

Immunology of Myelin Basic Proteins

Marian W. Kies

Research on the immunology of myelin basic protein (BP) really began in 1947 with the independent discoveries by Kabat et al. (1) and Morgan (2) that a single injection of whole central nervous system (CNS) tissue combined with complete Freund's adjuvant (CFA)–induced experimental allergic encephalomyelitis (EAE) in monkeys.

What is CFA and why was this observation more significant than the earlier discovery of Rivers et al. (3) that repeated injections of CNS tissue induced an experimental paralysis? CFA is a suspension of heat-killed mycobacteria in mineral oil, usually combined with some emulsifying agent. When a solid antigen or its solution is suspended in or emulsified with CFA the immunologic reactivity of the antigen is greatly enhanced. The encephalitogenic activity of whole CNS tissue, for example, was only evident in experimental animals after months of repeated inoculations (3). However, when the tissue was emulsified with CFA, its encephalitogenic activity became apparent in 2 to 3 weeks after a single inoculation (1,2). The fact that the experimental disease could be induced by a single injection of antigen permitted a systematic investigation of the etiology and pathogenesis of EAE including the purification and characterization of the antigen (BP) (4).

It is noteworthy that the landmark studies of Kabat et al. (1) and Morgan (2) preceded the organization of NINDB (predecessor of NINCDS) by only 3 years and the creation of a new institute dedicated to basic research on neurologic diseases had a significant effect on the research in this field.

Identification of the antigen responsible for EAE afforded the opportunity for studies of immunologic prevention, suppression, and treatment of the experimental disease (5–10). Furthermore, early studies on EAE provided the background and techniques for similar investigations of the basic proteins of peripheral nervous system (PNS) myelin and a second laboratory disease, experimental allergic neuritis (EAN).

EAE and EAN are thought to be manifestations of delayed hypersensitivity to the basic proteins of CNS and PNS myelin, respectively. The pathogenesis of EAN and the identity of the specific antigen that induces it have not been so clearly established as the nature of EAE and CNS-BP. Although EAN is readily induced with whole PNS myelin, its induction with an isolated purified PNS protein is still not completely established (11–14). One of the PNS basic proteins (P-1 or BM) appears to be identical to the CNS-BP (15). The other (P-2 or BF) (16) is less basic than CNS-BP and assumes a rigid β-structure in aqueous solution in marked contrast to the behavior of CNS-BP in solution (17).

Myelin basic protein has been isolated from the CNS of a variety of species, both mammalian and submammalian. In general the amino acid compositions of the various proteins are similar, although there are some substitutions, deletions, and insertions in the proteins derived from different species. Bovine, human, monkey, guinea pig, and rabbit basic proteins have similar amino acid compositions and almost identical electrophoretic behavior. Rat myelin contains two basic proteins that differ in size – the larger having about 40 more amino acid residues than the smaller (18). Chicken, turtle, and frog basic proteins differ significantly from the mammalian proteins in amino acid composition, electrophoretic mobility, and encephalitogenicity in guinea pigs and rats (19). Bovine and human CNS-BP (20,21) and the smaller of the two rat BPs (22) have been completely sequenced and the sequence of large portions of the other BPs (monkey, guinea pig, etc.) is known (23) (Fig. 1).

In spite of our extensive knowledge of BP and the disease that it induces (EAE), we are still unable to define the unique quality that confers on this protein the ability to induce an autoimmune reaction. It is highly charged, presumably occurring in myelin complexed with

His–Gly   Thr
Ac–Ala–Ala–Gln–Lys–Arg–Pro–Ser–Gln–Arg–Ser–Lys–Tyr–Leu–Ala–Ser–Ala–Ser–
                         10

Thr–Met–Asp–His–Ala–Arg–His–Gly–Phe–Leu–Pro–Arg–His–Arg–Asp–Thr–Gly–
        20   30

                    Ile   Ala
Ile–Leu–Asp–Ser–Leu–Gly–Arg–Phe–Phe–Gly–Ser–Asp–Arg–Gly–Ala–Pro–Lys–
                    40   50

                    Ser
Arg–Gly–Ser–Gly–Lys–Asp–Gly–His–His–Ala–Ala–Arg–Thr–Thr–His–Tyr–Gly–
                         60

              Ser   (   )   Ser
Ser–Leu–Pro–Gln–Lys–Ala–Gln–Gly–His–Arg–Pro–Gln–Asp–Glu–Asn–Pro–Val–
        70   80

Val–His–Phe–Phe–Lys–Asn–Ile–Val–Thr–Pro–Arg–Thr–Pro–Pro–Pro–Ser–Gln–
                    90   100

              $(Me)_{0, 1, \text{ or } 2}$
Gly–Lys–Gly–Arg–Gly–Leu–Ser–Leu–Ser–Arg–Phe–Ser–Trp–Gly–Ala–Glu–Gly–
                         110

Gln–Lys–Pro–Gly–Phe–Gly–Tyr–Gly–Gly–Arg–Ala–Ser–Asp–Tyr–Lys–Ser–Ala–
120   130

              Phe
His–Lys–Gly–Leu–Lys–Gly–His–Asp–Ala–Gln–Gly–Thr–Leu–Ser–Lys–Ile–Phe–
              140   150

Lys–Leu–Gly–Gly–Arg–Asp–Ser–Arg–Ser–Gly–Ser–Pro–Met–Ala–Arg–Arg
                    160

FIG. 1. Sequence of bovine BP (40). Arg-106 occurs in three forms: free, mono-, or dimethylated; changes in sequence shown above the line of type are possible substitutions, deletions or insertions in the guinea pig protein.

acidic lipids; its formation in the newborn parallels the development of myelin and formation of the blood–brain barrier; it is immunogenic in the homologous species. Some or all of these characteristics are shared by other proteins of the CNS, notably histones, proteolipids (24), glial fibrillary acid protein (GFAP) (25), and other highly acidic proteins, such as S-100 and 14–3–2 (26). Yet BP, of all the CNS proteins studied, is the only one that has been found to induce CNS tissue damage by appropriate immunization of an animal.

What do we know of its immune reactivity? In guinea pigs, it is nontoxic and induces no histologic damage when injected in saline or incomplete Freund's adjuvant (IFA), an oil-water emulsion containing no mycobacteria. Nevertheless, repeated injections of large amounts in saline (~5 mg daily for 30 days) are immuno-genic, i.e., induce antibody in guinea pigs (27). Minute amounts (≤ 100 μg) combined with 100 μg mycobacteria induce an acute and usually fatal paralytic disease characterized primarily by perivascular inflammatory lesions in CNS white matter (28). Induction of EAE by these small amounts of homologous antigen and CFA is usually not accompanied by detectable amounts of circulating antibody (29). Heterologous antigen appears to be somewhat more immunogenic (30). If the amount of BP and mycobacteria is increased to 0.5 mg and 2.5 mg, respectively, acute and rapidly fatal disease occurs and circulating antibody appears simultaneously with onset of disease (31). Antibody can also be induced in guinea pigs by multiple injections of BP in IFA (10×100 μg) followed by a single injection of BP in CFA (32). In this case antibody is produced without any clinical or histologic evidence of disease. In rats clinical signs of disease are more often accompanied by antibody production than in guinea pigs, but in this species, also, antibody to basic protein can be induced independently of disease and vice versa (30,33–35).

An interesting aspect of EAE in rats is that its clinical and histologic manifestations are much more severe if sensitization with CNS antigen is accompanied by an injection of killed pertussis organisms (36). Because the effect of pertussis is to hasten disease onset and enhance its severity its effect may be to depress rather than enhance antibody production—the rats may die before antibody is produced.

Rabbits, like guinea pigs and rats, are also very susceptible to the encephalitogenic action of purified BP in CFA. However, antibody production following an encephalitogenic injection of BP in CFA is variable, depending perhaps upon whether fatal EAE develops before antibody production gets underway. Kibler and Barnes (37) were unable to correlate antibody production with disease in a series of 49 rabbits. Of the experimental animals sensitized with homologous encephalitogen 60% developed clinical signs of disease; 45% of the latter produced antibody to the encephalitogen. On the other hand, 60% of the clinically negative animals also produced antibody. The authors pointed out that "early appearance of circulating antibody occurred almost exclusively in rabbits that subsequently developed EAE" (37).

If antibodies to BP cannot be correlated with onset or severity of disease in any of these three species, what does their presence signify? Are they protective? Does their production preclude disease induction or vice versa? Or are disease and antibody production independent phenomena? Before one can answer these questions, much more information on antibody production in various species is needed. Therefore we undertook a study of BP-antibody production in guinea pigs. We hoped that an analysis of the mechanisms of antibody induction and the structure of the antigenic determinants might yield information on the significance of antibody in protection and treatment of EAE and the nature of the genetic control of susceptibility to EAE. Although many of the mysteries remain unsolved, it is clear that such an analysis is essential to our understanding of the reactivity of this remarkable protein in any species.

ANTIGENIC SPECIFICITY OF ANTIBODIES TO MYELIN BASIC PROTEIN INDUCED IN GUINEA PIGS

Guinea pigs are known to be extremely sensitive to the induction of delayed hypersensitivity to many antigens. They are also less effective antibody producers than are rats or rabbits. Precipitating antibody is seldom detected in sera of guinea pigs sensitized with homologous (GP)BP and CFA. Therefore, to study production of anti-BP antibody in this species, it was necessary to resort to a technique capable of detecting soluble antigen-antibody complexes. We felt that the primary binding technique developed by Farr et al. (38) was superior to other techniques that depend upon secondary binding phenomena, such as complement fixation (CF), passive cutaneous anaphylaxis (PCA), or passive hemagglutination (HA). All of the latter, which may be more sensitive than radioimmunoassay (RIA), have the disadvantage that detection of antibody depends on some secondary reaction other than binding antigen. For example, a positive PCA reaction depends on the presence of antibody capable of binding to skin; other types of antibody are not detected by a PCA reaction.

The modified Farr technique used in our laboratory for detection of anti-BP antibody involves incubation of ^{125}I-labeled antigen with guinea pig antiserum and subsequent precipitation of the γ-globulin fraction with rabbit or goat anti-guinea pig γ-globulin. Radioactivity retained in the latter precipitate is an indication of specific antigen-antibody binding. By manipulating the proportion of labeled antigen to antiserum and by using the proper controls, one can accurately determine extremely small amounts of antibody. A simplified version of the method can also be used qualitatively for determining the effect of various immunization schedules on antibody production.

With this technique we found (29), as have other investigators (30), that the amounts of BP and mycobacteria usually used for bioassay (1–100 μg BP + 100 μg mycobacteria) induced little antibody. Even with 100 μg of BP, the in-

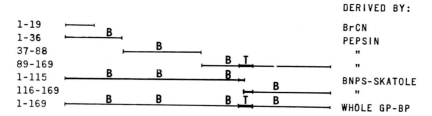

FIG. 2. Specific fragments of BP. Sites of immunological activity in guinea pigs are indicated. B, site that binds specific antibody. T, site that induces EAE; also required for antibody production (?).

cidence of guinea pigs producing detectable antibody is low (9). In order to produce antibody that could be analyzed for specificity, we resorted to a hyperimmunization schedule that involves both priming (repeated injections of BP in IFA) and induction (BP in CFA). The mechanism involved in the conversion of naive lymphocytes to primed lymphocytes, capable of producing antibody is not clear. No antibody is detected after priming alone, yet the primed lymphocytes persist for several months. Antibody is induced in primed guinea pigs by a single injection of BP/CFA even after an interval of 6 months has elapsed between priming and induction.

When antisera induced in primed guinea pigs were analyzed for their ability to bind fragments of BP (Fig. 2) rather than the whole protein, it was found that the specificity of binding varied from serum to serum. Because of this variation in binding specificity, we were able to demonstrate that at least three regions of the molecule contained binding sites that were mutually exclusive (that is, each site was unique and antibodies to a given site did not cross-react with other sites) (39). These sites are located between residues[1] 37 and 88, 89 and 115, and 116 and 169, respectively (Figs. 1 and 2). Such sera were obtained by the use of whole BP for both priming and induction. If GPBP is used for priming but peptides of BP are substituted for induction it is evident that a large part of the molecule (the first 88 residues) is incapable of converting primed lymphocytes to antibody producers (Table 1) even though one of the three binding sites is located in this region. It is noteworthy that the part of the molecule that induces antibody in primed guinea pigs also contains the encephalitogenic site. The fact that antibody induction might have the same structural requirements as induction of EAE is not surprising if one assumes that the effector T-cells and the helper T-cells both are turned on by the same sequence of amino acids, i.e., the nine-residue peptide Phe-Ser-Trp-Gly-Ala-Glu-Gly-Gln-Lys. Experiments are in progress to test this assumption.

The antibodies induced by the combination of priming and induction are present in the absence of EAE or any other evidence of delayed hypersensitivity to BP. In contrast, antibodies induced by a single injection of BP with 2.5 mg mycobacteria are formed in the presence of EAE and delayed hypersensitivity. When the two types of antisera were compared, there was no detectable difference between the binding specificities of the two types (39).

When the comparison between the two methods of producing antibody was extended to the specificity requirements for antibody production it became evident that there was a significant difference. Peptides incapable of inducing antibody in primed guinea pigs (e.g., 1 to 42, 43 to 88, or 1 to 88) were fully immunogenic when injected with 2.5 mg mycobacteria (Ta-

---

[1] Residue numbers are based on the corrected sequence of bovine BP (40).

TABLE 1. *Induction of antibody in guinea pigs preimmunized with BP in IFA and sensitized with either whole GPBP or specific peptides as indicated*

Antigen CFA	% ^{125}I-BP Bound (mean ± SE)
GPBP (1–169)	72.3 ± 6.9
1–88	6.3 ± 0.9
89–169	78.0 ± 4.2
1–115	26.7 ± 4.2
116–169	5.3 ± 0.3

TABLE 2. *Induction of antibody in guinea pigs immunized with either 0.5 mg GPBP or equimolar amount of specific peptide in CFA (2.5 mg mycobacteria)*

Fragment used for immunization	^{125}I-Labeled antigen used for binding % Bound					
	BP	1–36	37–88	89–169	1–115	116–169
Strain 13						
1–36	12	35	1	3	9	1
37–88	11	1	41	3	12	2
1–88	44	44[a]	67	2	45	1
89–169	45	1	1	60	12	28
1–115	55	32[a]	45	21	63	3
116–169	27	5	4	67	6	71
1–169	58	4	43	50	60	8
Strain 2						
1–88	47	18	70	9	46	4
89–169	66	3	5	77	48	57
1–169	63	11	40	57	66	22

[a] 40% Nonresponders

ble 2). We believe the explanation for the difference is the ability of excessive amounts of mycobacteria to bypass some specific T-cell requirement for antibody production. This was suggested by Green et al. (41) in their study of the immunogenicity of poly-l-lysine (PLL) as an explanation for the ability of large amounts of mycobacteria to convert nonresponder to responder guinea pigs.

The results they obtained in their analysis of PLL-susceptible and PLL-resistant guinea pigs are analogous to the results we have obtained

with EAE-susceptible and EAE-resistant guinea pigs: Strain 2 (EAE-resistant) guinea pigs produce very much less antibody than do Strain 13 guinea pigs after priming and induction with whole GPBP (Fig. 3), whereas the two strains produce equivalent amounts of antibody after immunization with GPBP + 2.5 mg mycobacteria (42) (Table 2). We believe this again suggests that induction of antibody in primed guinea pigs requires a specific T-cell, whereas induction of antibody with high levels of mycobacteria does not. Strain 13 T-cells carry this specificity,

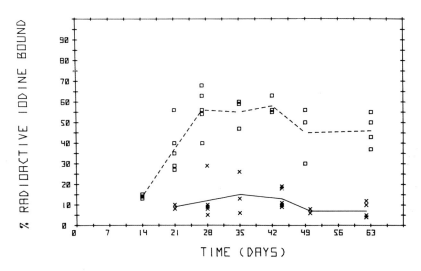

FIG. 3. Induction of antibody in Strain 13 (□----□) and Strain 2 (x——x) guinea pigs preimmunized with BP in IFA and sensitized with BP in CFA.

whereas Strain 2 T-cells do not, or at least are deficient in respect to their activity.

INDUCTION OF ANTIBODY TO BP IN RATS

The specificity of BP antibody in rats has not been analyzed in as much detail as it has been in guinea pigs. Marked differences have been demonstrated, however, between the two species in their response to the encephalitogenic activity of various myelin basic proteins. Thus it would not be surprising to find differences in the immunogenicity of these proteins in the two species as well.

Some interesting examples of biological diversity are readily apparent in these two rodent species: (a) there are two basic proteins in rat CNS myelin in contrast to the single BP in guinea pig CNS myelin; (b) the peptide sequence, which is encephalitogenic in guinea pigs (Phe-Ser-Trp-Gly-Ala-Glu-Gly-Gln-Lys) is inactive in rats — the peptide which is encephalitogenic in rats is located somewhere between residues 43 and 88 (43–45); and (c) all mammalian basic proteins appear to have about the same encephalitogenic activity in guinea pigs, whereas bovine, human, monkey, and rabbit myelin basic proteins, all of which induce EAE in rats, are much less active than GPBP in that species. Martenson et al. (45) have analyzed the weak

activity of the bovine protein in rats and have suggested that there are two encephalitogenic sites in the bovine molecule, which include residues 38 to 42 (Ser-Leu-Gly-Arg-Phe) and residues 109 to 113 (Ser-Leu-Ser-Arg-Phe). The highly active site that is located between residues 43 and 88 in the GPBP molecule is not present in the bovine molecule — minor differences in the sequence of the two proteins have made drastic changes in their encephalitogenicity.

Several papers have been published on BP antibody production in rats (30,33–35,46,47), but very little information is available on the specific sites in the molecule recognized as antigenic in this species. We have found that rats immunized with whole cord, GPBP, or BBP produce antibody which bind to several sites in the molecule (48). Whether these sites are unique (i.e., do not cross-react) is not yet known. It is remarkable that whole cord immunization of rats is as effective as BP immunization for the induction of antibody to BP. This is not the case with guinea pigs (42). There is a difference in the antigenicity of the first 88 residues of the molecule in the two species. Fragment 37 to 88 is more antigenic than Fragment 1 to 42 in guinea pigs, whereas the reverse is true in rats, i.e., Fragment 1 to 42 is bound to a greater extent than Fragment 37 to 88 in the rat sera tested. Some preliminary data showing these

TABLE 3. *Binding specificity of antibody to BP induced in rats*

Strain	Immunizing antigen[a]	\% ^{125}I-Labeled antigen bound					
		1–169 (BP)	1–36 + 1–42	37–88	89–169	1–115	116–169
F 344	10 mg GP cord[b] (day 19)	59 ± 1.7	43 ± 8.9	3 ± 0.8	51 ± 2.5	48 ± 4.2	22 ± 2.6
Lewis	10 mg GP cord[c] (day 16)	61	23	5	39	41	10
Lewis	54 μg BBP[d] (day 14)	35	30	5	12	37	4
Lewis	3.2 μg GPBP[b] (day 21 or 27)	61 ± 1.3	36 ± 6.8	5 ± 1.2	43 ± 3.7	57 ± 3.6	19 ± 3.5
For Comparison GP (NIH)	0.5 mg BBP[b] (day 10 or 11)	55 ± 5.5	9 ± 2.6	26 ± 7.5	53 ± 3.0	62 ± 1.4	13 ± 2.7

[a] Antigen emulsified in CFA; no pertussis used in these experiments. Day of serum collection in parentheses.
[b] Mean ± SE.
[c] Average of 2 sera.
[d] Average of 3 sera.
Normal rat sera bound <8% ^{125}I-labeled antigen.

differences between the two species are shown in Table 3.

IMMUNOGENICITY OF MYELIN BASIC PROTEINS IN RABBITS

Much of the research on BP in rabbits has been on its encephalitogenic activity. The active site for this species is located in the same region of the molecule (between residues 43 and 88) as is the active site for rats (23,43). We know that the two sites are not identical, however, because the bovine Fragment 43 to 88, which is inactive in rats, is fully active in rabbits. Despite the fact that rabbits usually produce antibodies to most antigens without any difficulty, early attempts to produce antibody to BP in rabbits met with variable success. The earliest report was that of Kibler and Barnes (37) cited above. Rauch and Roboz-Einstein obtained precipitating antibody in rabbits with a BP preparation, which they designated FC (49,50), but they were subsequently unable to repeat this with a BP isolated by a different technique (designated G) (51). They did succeed, however, in producing precipitating antibody with preparation G complexed with acidified bovine serum albumen (BSA). These antisera did not cross-react with FC (52).

Hruby et al. (53) induced precipitating antibody in rabbits with large amounts of heterologous BP. These antisera were used very effectively in demonstrating cross-reactivity among preparations of BP from CNS of different species and in the demonstration of species-specific contaminants in purified (but not pure) preparations prepared by several investigators (54,55).

Homologous (rabbit) BP appears to be more encephalitogenic than heterologous BP and therefore less effective as an antigen for induction of antibody. In order to prepare high-titer antiserum with basic protein, it is necessary to prevent the onset of EAE. It is possible to prevent EAE in rabbits by injections of BP in IFA but this procedure is less effective in rabbits than in guinea pigs and the induction of antibody to BP in rabbits is still an unpredictable and uncertain phenomenon. We believe this to be a function of individual variability among rabbits, not an inherent lack of immunogenicity in the BP molecule. We found that schedules that are

very effective in some rabbits [e.g., 1 mg BP + 5 mg mycobacteria injected in multiple sites as suggested by Vaitukaitis et al. (56)] are completely ineffective in others. Several rabbits have also been immunized successfully with a series of 10 injections, the first consisting of 0.5 mg heterologous BP in CFA (2.5 mg mycobacteria) and the nine successive ones consisting of 0.5 mg BP in IFA (three times weekly for 3 weeks). Other rabbits failed to respond at all to this series of injections whereas still others developed EAE without producing antibody. In spite of the variability among individual rabbits, the effort expended in obtaining good antisera has been of considerable value in our research on the pathogenesis of experimental demyelination.

In collaboration with Seil (57,58), we have established the fact that antibody to BP is not the factor responsible for inhibiting myelination *in vitro* which Bornstein et al. (59) found to be present in sera of rabbits immunized with whole CNS tissue.

Rabbit antiserum induced with GPBP in CFA has been used successfully by Eng et al. (60) as a sensitive radioimmunoassay for BP in cerebrospinal fluid of patients with neurologic disease.

Antiserum obtained by immunization of rabbits with partially purified bovine myelin basic protein was found to contain antibody to a protein found in spinal roots, an obvious impurity in the CNS-BP. This enabled us serendipitously to establish the similarity, if not identity, of two nervous tissue antigens isolated independently by two groups of investigators: spinal cord protein antigen (SCP) isolated and purified by Lo and MacPherson (61) and peripheral nerve antigen (BF) described by Uyemura et al. (16,62). BF is the same protein as P-2 isolated by Brostoff et al. (17).

Various rabbit antisera obtained by these and other immunization schedules have been used to investigate the structural specificity of antigenic sites in the molecule in the same way that Driscoll et al. (39) analyzed guinea pig antisera to BP. These studies are still in progress, but it is clear from our data that there are several specific antigenic regions in the molecule.

Other investigators have also studied antigenic specificity of rabbit antisera to BP. Brostoff et al. (40) reported that rabbit antiserum induced with whole BP bound a fragment isolated by liver catheptic digestion (Fragment 1 to 42). The antibody had a low avidity for the fragment relative to its avidity for the whole protein.

Whitaker et al. (63) have reported antigenic sites in the amino terminal (residues 1 to 19) and the carboxy terminal (residues 116 to 169) region of the molecule. These were detected with antisera to BP coupled to albumin. We believe that modification of the BP molecule in order to enhance its antigenicity could also change the nature of the specific antigenic regions in the molecule.

In our experiments, for example, antisera obtained with unaltered BP molecules have contained antibody capable of forming precipitin lines on immunodiffusion with several BP fragments, residues 1 to 88, 43 to 88, 89 to 169, 1 to 115, and 116 to 169. The fact that Whitaker et al. (63) failed to detect binding to a significant portion of the molecule (all of the peptide chain between residues 20 and 116) may simply mean that the binding of albumen to BP blocked this portion of the molecule. It is important to remember that our antisera are selective — not all sera react with all of the fragments. Of special significance is the fact that we detected an antigenic site in Fragment 43 to 88. This region also contains the rabbit encephalitogenic sequence, but the peptide is large enough (45 residues) to contain more than one immunologically active sequence.

SUMMARY

What can one conclude about myelin basic protein and its immunologic reactivity? First, since no pretense is made of having reviewed the literature exhaustively, it would be unfair to draw any definite conclusions. It appears, however, that antibody per se does not induce disease. On the other hand, it appears that antibody and disease induction may be interrelated in the sense that the same portion of the BP molecule that controls proliferation of helper T-cells (which are essential to antibody production) also controls the proliferation of effector T-cells (which damage the target organ) (64). Whether or not the antigenic sites in the molecule are unique to each species (as the encephalitogenic site appears to be) has not been determined.

ACKNOWLEDGMENTS

The author wishes to acknowledge the enormous contribution of many co-workers and collaborators to our research on EAE which began in the Intramural Research Program, NIMH-NINDB. It would be impossible to list all of the investigators whose patience, skill, and hard work have made these last 25 years such a valuable and enjoyable experience. Special thanks are due to Dr. E. C. Alvord, Jr., Dr. R. E. Martenson, Dr. B. F. Driscoll, and Mrs. Gladys Deibler.

REFERENCES

1. Kabat, E. A., Wolf, A., and Bezer, A. E. (1947): The rapid production of acute disseminated encephalomyelitis in rhesus monkeys by injection of heterologous and homologous brain tissue with adjuvants. *J. Exp. Med.,* 85:117–130. Kabat, E. A., Wolf, A., and Bezer, A. E. (1948): Studies on the acute disseminated encephalomyelitis in rhesus monkeys, III. *J. Exp. Med.,* 88:417–426.
2. Morgan, I. M. (1947): Allergic encephalomyelitis in monkeys in response to injection of normal monkey nervous tissue. *J. Exp. Med.,* 85:131–194.
3. Rivers, T. M., Sprunt, D. H., and Berry, G. P. (1933): Observations on attempts to produce acute disseminated encephalomyelitis in monkeys. *J. Exp. Med.,* 58:39–53. Rivers, T. M., and Schwentker, F. F. (1935): Encephalomyelitis accompanied by myelin destruction experimentally produced in monkeys. *J. Exp. Med.,* 61:689–702.
4. Laatsch, R. H., Kies, M. W., Gordon, S., and Alvord, E. C., Jr. (1962): The encephalitogenic activity of myelin isolated by ultracentrifugation. *J. Exp. Med.,* 115:777–788.
5. Alvord, E. C., Jr., Shaw, C. M., Fahlberg, W. J., and Kies, M. W. (1964): An analysis of various types of inhibition of experimental "allergic" encephalomyelitis in the guinea pig. *Z. Immunol. Forsch.,* 126:217–227.
6. Shaw, C. M., Alvord, E. C., Jr., Kaku, J., and Kies, M. W. (1965): Correlation of experimental allergic encephalomyelitis with delayed-type skin sensitivity to specific homologous encephalitogen. *Ann. N.Y. Acad. Sci.,* 122:318–331.
7. Alvord, E. C., Jr., Shaw, C. M., Hruby, S., and Kies, M. W. (1965): Encephalitogen-induced inhibition of experimental allergic encephalomyelitis: prevention, suppression and therapy. *Ann. N.Y. Acad. Sci.,* 122:333–345.
8. Levine, S., Sowinski, R., and Kies, M. W. (1972): Treatment of experimental allergic encephalomyelitis with encephalitogenic basic proteins. *Proc. Soc. Exp. Biol. Med.,* 139:506–510.
9. Driscoll, B. F., Kies, M. W., and Alvord, E. C.,

Jr. (1974): Successful treatment of experimental allergic encephalomyelitis (EAE) in guinea pigs with homologous myelin basic protein. *J. Immunol.,* 112:392–397.

10. Eylar, E. H., Jackson, J., Rothenberg, B., and Brostoff, S. W. (1972): Suppression of the immune response: Reversal of the disease state with antigen in allergic encephalomyelitis. *Nature,* 236:74–76.

11. Bencina, B., Carnegie, P. R., McPherson, T. A., and Robson, G. (1969): Encephalitogenic basic protein from sciatic nerve. *FEBS Lett.,* 4:9–12.

12. Kiyota, K., and Egami, S. (1972): Electrophoretic studies of basic proteins capable of inducing experimental allergic neuritis. *J. Neurochem.,* 19: 857–864.

13. Abramsky, O., Teitelbaum, D., Webb, C., and Arnon, R. (1975): Neuritogenic and encephalitogenic properties of the peripheral nerve basic proteins. *J. Neuropath. Exp. Neurol.,* 34:36–45.

14. Carlo, D. J., Karkhanis, Y. D., Bailey, P. J., Wisniewski, H. M., and Brostoff, S. W. (1975): Allergic neuritis: Evidence for the involvement of the P_2 and P_0 proteins. *Brain Research,* 88:580–584.

15. Brostoff, S. W., and Eylar, E. H. (1972): The proposed sequence of the P_1 protein of rabbit sciatic nerve myelin. *Arch. Biochem. Biophys.,* 153:590–598.

16. Kitamura, K., Yamanaka, T., and Uyemura, K. (1975): On basic proteins in bovine peripheral nerve myelin. *Biochim. Biophys. Acta.,* 379:582–591.

17. Brostoff, S. W., Sacks, H., and DiPaula, C. (1975): The P_2 protein of bovine root myelin: Partial chemical characterization. *J. Neurochem.,* 24: 289–294.

18. Martenson, R. E., Deibler, G. E., Kies, M. W., McKneally, S. S., Shapira, R., and Kibler, R. F. (1972): Differences between the two myelin basic proteins of the rat central nervous system. A deletion in the smaller protein. *Biochim. Biophys. Acta,* 263:193–203.

19. Martenson, R. E., and Deibler, G. E. (1975): Partial characterization of basic proteins of chicken, turtle and frog central nervous system myelin. *J. Neurochem.,* 24:79–88.

20. Eylar, E. H., Brostoff, S., Hashim, G., Caccam, J., and Burnett, P. (1971): Basic Al protein of the myelin membrane. The complete amino acid sequence. *J. Biol. Chem.,* 246:5770–5784.

21. Carnegie, P. R. (1971): Amino acid sequence of the encephalitogenic basic protein from human myelin. *Biochem. J.,* 123:57–67.

22. Dunkley, P. R., and Carnegie, P. R. (1974): Amino acid sequence of the smaller basic protein from rat brain myelin. *Biochem. J.,* 141:243–255.

23. Shapira, R., McKneally, S. S., Chou, F., and Kibler, R. F. (1971): Encephalitogenic fragment of myelin basic protein. Amino acid sequence of bovine, rabbit, guinea pig, monkey, and human fragments. *J. Biol. Chem.,* 246:4630–4640.

24. Folch, J., and Lees, M. B. (1951): Proteolipides, a new type of tissue lipoproteins. *J. Biol. Chem.,* 191:807–817.

25. Eng, L. F., Vanderhaeghen, J. J., Bignami, A., and Gerstl, B. (1971): An acidic protein isolated from fibrous astrocytes. *Brain Res.,* 28:351–354.

26. Cicero, T. J., Cowan, W. M., Moore, B. W., and Suntzeff, V. (1970): The cellular localization of the two brain specific proteins, S-100 and 14–3–2. *Brain Res.,* 18:25–34.

27. Lennon, V. A., *personal communication.*

28. Alvord, E. C., Jr. (1970): Acute disseminated encephalomyelitis and "allergic" neuro-encephalopathies. In: *Handbook of Clinical Neurology, Vol. 9,* edited by P. J. Vinken and G. W. Bruyn, pp. 500–571. North-Holland Publishing Co., Amsterdam.

29. Lisak, R. P., Heinze, R. G., Kies, M. W., and Alvord, E. C., Jr. (1969): Antibodies to encephalitogenic basic protein in experimental allergic encephalomyelitis. *Proc. Soc. Exp. Biol. Med.,* 130: 814–818.

30. Lennon, V. A., Whittingham, S., Carnegie, P. R., McPherson, T. A., and Mackay, I. R. (1971): Detection of antibodies to the basic protein of human myelin by radioimmunoassay and immunofluorescence. *J. Immunol.,* 107:56–62.

31. Kies, M. W., Driscoll, B. F., Seil, F. J., and Alvord, E. C., Jr. (1973): Myelination inhibition factor: Dissociation from induction of experimental allergic encephalomyelitis. *Science,* 179:689–690.

32. Alvord, E. C., Jr., Shaw, C. M., Lisak, R. P., Falk, G. A., and Kies, M. W. (1970): Relationships between antibodies and experimental allergic encephalomyelitis. V. Antibodies and delayed hypersensitivity in production and prevention of experimental allergic encephalomyelitis. *Int. Arch. Allergy,* 38:403–412.

33. Kies, M. W. (1970): Specificity of myelin basic proteins. In: *Protein Metabolism of the Nervous System,* edited by A. Lajtha, pp. 659–670. Plenum Press, New York.

34. Day, E. D., and Pitts, O. M. (1974): The antibody response to myelin basic protein (BP) in Lewis rats: The effect of time, dosage of BP, and dosage of Mycobacterium butyricum. *J. Immunol.,* 113: 1958–1967.

35. Gonatas, N. K., Gonatas, J. O., Steiber, A., Lisak, R., Suzuki, J., and Martenson, R. E. (1974): The significance of circulating and cell-bound antibodies in experimental allergic encephalomyelitis. *Am. J. Pathol.,* 76:529–544.

36. Levine, S., and Wenk, E. J. (1967): Hyperacute allergic encephalomyelitis. Lymphatic system as site of adjuvant effect of pertussis vaccine. *Am. J. Pathol.,* 50:465–483.

37. Kibler, R. F., and Barnes, A. E. (1962): Antibody studies in rabbit encephalomyelitis induced by water-soluble protein fraction of rabbit cord. *J. Exp. Med.,* 116:807–825.

38. Farr, R. S. (1958): A quantitative immunochemical measure of the primary interaction between I*BSA and antibody. *J. Infect. Dis.,* 103:239–262.

39. Driscoll, B. F., Kramer, A. J., and Kies, M. W. (1974): Myelin basic protein: Location of multiple independent antigenic regions. *Science,* 184: 73–75.

40. Brostoff, S. W., Reuter, W., Hichens, M., and Eylar, E. H. (1974): Specific cleavage of the A1 protein from myelin with cathepsin D. *J. Biol. Chem.,* 249:559–567.

41. Green, I., Benacerraf, B., and Stone, S. H. (1969): The effect of the amount of mycobacterial adjuvants on the immune response of Strain 2, Strain 13 and Hartley strain guinea pigs to DNP-PLL and DNP-GL. *J. Immunol.,* 103:403–412.

42. Kies, M. W., Driscoll, B. F., Lisak, R. P., and Alvord, E. C., Jr. (1975): Immunologic activity of myelin basic protein in Strain 2 and Strain 13 guinea pigs. *J. Immunol.,* 115:75–79.

43. McFarlin, D. E., Blank, S. E., Kibler, R. F., McKneally, S., and Shapira, R. (1973): Experimental allergic encephalomyelitis in the rat: Response to encephalitogenic proteins and peptides. *Science,* 179:478–480.

44. Dunkley, P. R., Coates, A. S., and Carnegie, P. R. (1973): Encephalitogenic activity of peptides from the smaller basic protein of rat myelin. *J. Immunol.,* 110:1699–1701.

45. Martenson, R. E., Levine, S., and Sowinski, R. (1975): The location of regions in guinea pig and bovine myelin basic proteins which induce experimental allergic encephalomyelitis in Lewis rats. *J. Immunol.,* 114:592–596.

46. Lennon, V. A., and Dunkley, P. R. (1974): Humoral and cell-mediated immune responses of Lewis rats to syngeneic basic protein of myelin. *Int. Arch. Allergy,* 47:598–608.

47. McFarlin, D. E., Hsu, S. C. L., Slemenda, S. B., Chou, F. C. H., and Kibler, R. F. (1975): The immune response against myelin basic protein in two strains of rat with different genetic capacity to develop experimental allergic encephalomyelitis. *J. Exp. Med.,* 141:72–81.

48. Kies, M. W., Driscoll, B. F., and Levine, S., *unpublished.*

49. Einstein, E. R., Robertson, D. M., DiCaprio, J. M., and Moore, W. S. (1962): The isolation from bovine spinal cord of a homogeneous protein with encephalitogenic activity. *J. Neurochem.,* 9:353–361.

50. Rauch, H. C., and Raffel, S. (1964): Immunofluorescent localization of encephalitogenic protein in myelin. *J. Immunol.,* 92:452–455.

51. Nakao, A., Davis, W. J., and Einstein, E. R. (1966): Basic proteins from the acidic extract of bovine spinal cord. I. Isolation and characterization. II. Encephalitogenic, immunologic and structural interrelationships. *Biochim. Biophys. Acta,* 130:163–170, 171–179.

52. Rauch, H. C., and Einstein, E. R. (1969): Immunogenicity of bovine encephalitogenic protein. In: *Pathogenesis and Etiology of Demyelinating Diseases, Add. ad Int. Arch. Allergy, Vol. 36,* edited by K. Burdzy and P. Kallos, pp. 376–386. S. Karger, Basel.

53. Hruby, S., Alvord, E. C., Jr., and Shaw, C. M. (1969): Relationships between antibodies and experimental allergic encephalomyelitis. I. Production of hemagglutinating and gel-precipitating antibodies in rabbits and guinea pigs. *Int. Arch. Allergy,* 36:599–611.

54. Alvord, E. C., Hruby, S., Hughes, K., Shaw, C. M., and Kies, M. W. (1969): Comparison of organ-specific antigens of the central nervous system. *Int. Arch. Allergy,* 36:276–286.

55. Alvord, E. C., Hruby, S., Shaw, C. M., and Kies, M. W. (1969): Multiplicity of encephalitogenic myelin basic proteins. II. Antigenic determinants related to species of origin and molecular size. *Int. Arch. Allergy,* 36:203–217.

56. Vaitukaitis, J., Robbins, J. B., Nieschlag, E., and Ross, G. T. (1971): A method for producing specific antisera with small doses of immunogen. *J. Clin. Endocrinol. Metab.,* 33:988–991.

57. Kies, M. W., Driscoll, B. F., Seil, F. J., and Alvord, E. C., Jr. (1973): Myelination inhibition factor: Dissociation from induction of experimental allergic encephalomyelitis. *Science,* 179: 689–690.

58. Seil, F. J., Kies, M. W., and Bacon, M. (1975): Neural antigens and induction of myelination inhibition factor. *J. Immunol.,* 114:630–634.

59. Bornstein, M. D., and Raine, C. S. (1970): Experimental allergic encephalomyelitis. Antiserum inhibition of myelination *in vitro. Lab. Invest.* 23:536–542.

60. Eng, L. F., Lee, Y. L., Kies, M. W., and Miller, L. E. M., *unpublished.*

61. Yo, S.-L., and MacPherson, C. F. C. (1972): Studies on Brain antigens. V. Purification and partial characterization of an antiencephalitogenic spinal cord protein (SCP). *J. Immunol.,* 109: 1009–1016.

62. Uyemura, K., Tobari, C., Hirano, S., and Tsukada, Y. (1972): Comparative studies on the myelin proteins of bovine peripheral nerve and spinal cord. *J. Neurochem.,* 19:2607–2614.

63. Whitaker, J. N., Jen Chou, C. H., Chou, F. C. H., and Kibler, R. F. (1975): Antigenic determinants for rabbit antibody to myelin encephalitogenic protein. *Fed. Proc.,* 34:1035.

64. Driscoll, B. F., and Kies, M. W. (1975): Induction of antibodies to homologous myelin basic protein in guinea pigs. *Fed. Proc.,* 34:967.

The Nervous System, Donald B. Tower, Editor-in-Chief. *Vol. 1: The Basic Neurosciences*. Raven Press, New York, 1975.

Correlation of Delayed Skin Hypersensitivity and Experimental Allergic Encephalomyelitis Induced by Synthetic Peptides

Ellsworth C. Alvord, Jr., Cheng-Mei Shaw, Sarka Hruby, Rosemarie Petersen, and Frederick H. Harvey

Experimental allergic encephalomyelitis (EAE) has been studied intensively for the past 30 years, ever since the introduction of Freund's adjuvants made the experimental analyses feasible by decreasing the incubation period from many months to 1 to 3 weeks. The major fields of interest that have been exploited include immunology (especially mechanisms of delayed-type hypersensitivity), biochemistry (especially proteins of myelin), pathology (especially mechanisms of demyelination), and clinical medicine (especially the hope that the experimental model will throw some light on the etiology, pathogenesis, treatment, and prevention of multiple sclerosis and other demyelinating diseases). Our own studies, first with Dr. Lewis D. Stevenson at Cornell University Medical College and then with Dr. Marian W. Kies at the National Institutes of Health, have touched on all of these major fields of interest, and even casual review of the periodic summaries of the state of the art (2–11) provides fascinating documentation of the advances in biomedical research during the past several decades.

One of the most controversial areas at the moment concerns the precise immunochemical mechanisms underlying the production of the disease itself. Why should only one protein in central nervous system (CNS) myelin be capable of producing EAE when there are many more proteins that are also uniquely segregated from the rest of the body and theoretically capable of being autoantigens? Even more than that, why should only one or a few particular sequences of amino acids within this one protein be capable of producing the disease when there are several other sequences that are known to be at least equally antigenic but nonencephalitogenic? And why should sequences that are encephalitogenic in one species be nonencephalitogenic in another?

To summarize briefly, one can say that EAE is generally regarded as due to delayed-type hypersensitivity to one or more encephalitogenic determinants within the specific myelin membrane encephalitogenic protein (MMEP), a linear polypeptide of about 170 residues containing several encephalitogenic determinants and several antigenic determinants (12). In spite of a remarkably accurate correlation between the onset of EAE and the size of delayed-type skin reactions to whole homologous MMEP (6,13), it is not yet known whether the encephalitogenic determinants are themselves also antigenic.

The recent availability of synthetic encephalitogenic peptides (14,15) has made possible the following tests, from which we conclude that at least one but not all of the antigenic determinants responsible for the homologous skin reaction is in the tryptophan-containing nonapeptide, which is encephalitogenic in the guinea pig. Encephalitogenicity requires more than antigenicity, but much more work will be required to define exactly how much more and why.

MATERIALS AND METHODS

Induction of EAE

EAE was induced by the single intracutaneous injection over the sternum of 0.1 ml of a water-in-oil emulsion containing 0.1 mg heat-killed *M. tuberculosis* and varying amounts (0.01–10 nM) of synthetic peptides. Groups of five guinea pigs were injected simultaneously

TABLE 1. *Synthetic peptides used in this study (numbering according to alignment 66, ref. 1)*

114	115	116	117	118	119	120	121	122	123	124	Code no.	Source
Ser	Arg	Phe	Ser	Trp	Gly	Ala	Glu	Gly	Gln	Arg	14b, I	Westall-Eylar, Bury-Beckman (human sequence)
Ser	Arg	Phe	Ser	Trp	Gly	Ala	ILEU	Gly	Gln	LYS	11a	Westall-Eylar (Ileu-substituted bovine sequence)
Ser	Arg	Phe	ALA	Trp	Gly	Ala	Glu	Gly	Gln	LYS	13a	Westall-Eylar (Ala-substituted bovine sequence)
—	—	Phe	Ser	Trp	Gly	Ala	Glu	Gly	Gln	Arg	A,B,C,	Young (human sequence)

with the same emulsion, skin-tested at 10 or 12 days (see below), and observed for a maximum of 30 days or until paralyzed, when they were killed, perfused with buffered 10% formalin, and the brain and spinal cord examined histologically after staining with hematoxylin and eosin and with gallocyanin and darrow red (16), a new myelin sheath stain which does not require differentiation and which gives very precise stains of myelin and early breakdown droplets of myelin. A combined score of the *in vivo* and postmortem observations yielded a disease index for each animal, maximum of 10, and an average for each group (17).

Synthetic Peptides

The synthetic peptides varied in their amino acid sequences and length and were identified only by code numbers (Table 1) at the time of testing. The original numbering of the human sequence (18), of the bovine sequence (14,15), and of the corresponding sequences with single amino acid substitutions has been altered to permit direct comparisons across species lines according to alignment 66 in the *Atlas of Protein Sequences and Structure 1972* (1).

Skin Tests

Ten or 12 days after injection of the emulsion, skin tests were performed as follows: 0.1 ml of a saline solution containing 0.015 mg of a standard guinea pig MMEP (preparation #260, ref. 13) was injected intracutaneously in the previously shaved skin of one side of the back (flank). A positive control (0.001 mg PPD obtained from Merck, Sharp & Dohme) was similarly injected on the other side. The reactions were examined 20 hr later and the maximum and minimum diameters (mm) of erythema and the degree of induration noted.

TABLE 2. *Association of 10-day skin reactions[a] with onset of EAE*

Day of onset of EAE	No. of guinea pigs showing skin reaction with average diameters			Total
	0–5.5 mm	6–9.5 mm	10–15 mm	
10–13	0	0	1	1
14–17	4	4	0	8
18–30	6	1	0	7
Asympt., hist. pos.	11	1	1	13
Asympt., hist. neg.	21	3	0	24
Total	42	9	2	53

[a] Average diameter of the delayed skin reactions to guinea pig encephalitogenic protein (MMEP #260, ref. 13) injected 10 days after sensitization with synthetic peptides.

TABLE 3. *Association of 12-day skin reactions[a] with onset of EAE*

Day of onset of EAE	No. of guinea pigs showing skin reaction with average diameters			Total
	0–5.5 mm	6–9.5 mm	10–15 mm	
12–15	14	15	3	32
16–19	9	21	1	31
20–30	2	0	0	2
Asympt., hist. pos.	7	8	0	15
Asympt., hist. neg.	33	5	0	38
Total	65	49	4	118

[a] Average diameter of delayed skin reactions to guinea pig encephalitogenic protein (MMEP #260, ref. 13) injected 12 days after sensitization with synthetic peptides.

RESULTS

In the first test (Table 2), the association between the sizes of the delayed skin reactions 10 days after sensitization and the onset of EAE 1 week later was poor, largely because of the late onset of EAE and the large number of negative skin reactions. On the hypothesis that the synthetic peptides were less effective stimuli than the whole MMEP, the tests were repeated,

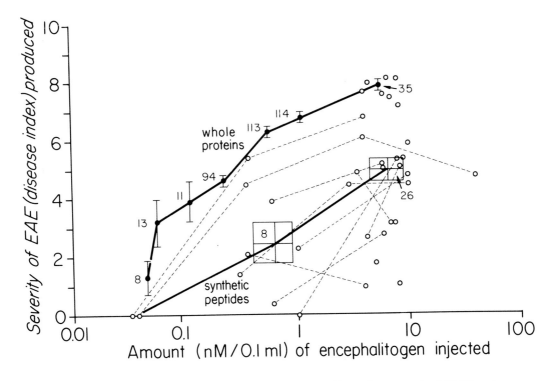

FIG. 1. Severity of EAE, expressed as disease index (18), induced by various amounts of 17 different preparations of four active synthetic peptides (cf., Table 1) with multiple assays of particular preparations being connected by dashed lines. The mean of these assays (heavy line) ± SEM (thin lines for both severity of EAE and amounts of peptides injected) and the number of assays in groups of five guinea pigs are compared with the mean (± SEM) results obtained with 25 consecutive bovine and 75 guinea pig preparations of whole MMEP (original individual results reported in Fig. 41 of ref. 6).

TABLE 4. *Demyelination[a] induced by synthetic peptides as compared with whole MMEP*

		Degree of demyelination							
		0		mild		marked		Total	
		pep.	MMEP	pep.	MMEP	pep.	MMEP	pep.	MMEP
A. Degree of inflam.	mild	2	1	1	0	3	1	6	2
	marked	5	0	1	0	3	3	9	3
B. Day of onset	12–17	6	1	2	0	4	4	12	5
	18–24	1	0	0	0	2	0	3	0
C. Day of death	12–17	6	1	2	0	4	4	12	5
	18–24	1	0	0	0	2	0	3	0
	Total	7	1	2	0	6	4	15	5

[a] Numbers of guinea pigs matched by severity of inflammation and days of onset of EAE and days of death.

allowing an additional 2 days for sensitization to occur. In these tests (Table 3), there was a remarkably close association between the size of the delayed skin reaction and the onset of EAE during the following week ($\chi^2 = 44.75$ for the data combined into a 2×4 table; with 6 degrees of freedom; $p < 0.01$). There was no apparent difference between the skin-reaction-inducing and the EAE-inducing activities of the 17 different preparations of the four sequences of synthetic peptides tested, but these data are too voluminous to report in detail.

The degree of EAE induced by various amounts of the 17 different preparations of these four peptides in a total of 36 bioassays is indicated in Fig. 1. For comparison are included the results obtained with 75 consecutive preparations of guinea pig and 25 consecutive preparations of bovine MMEP in a total of 388 bioassays as individually previously reported (see Fig. 41 in ref. 6). Although most of the synthetic peptides were only 1 to 10% as active as the whole MMEP, at least two of the three assays of the most active synthetic preparation were quite comparable to the average MMEP preparation.

The degrees of demyelination induced by these synthetic peptides and by whole MMEP were estimated blindly and independently by two of us on gallocyanin-stained sections of samples of guinea pigs matched as closely as possible for degree of inflammation (as seen in H & E stained sections) and in days of onset of and death from EAE. These double matchings obviously and markedly decreased the numbers of guinea pigs that could be compared for degrees of demyelination after being matched by these other criteria for severity of EAE. Table 4 indicates that there was generally much less demyelination in otherwise comparable lesions induced by these peptides; however, at least some of the peptide-sensitized guinea pigs had as marked demyelination as did most of the MMEP-sensitized animals.

DISCUSSION

The present results clearly demonstrate a good correlation between the degree of delayed skin reactivity and the onset of EAE within the following week if sufficient time is allowed for sensitization to occur (compare Tables 2 and 3) and if the skin reactions are induced by the homologous (guinea pig) whole MMEP in order to avoid detecting other antigenic determinants in heterologous MMEP. Additional tests with other synthetic peptides, of varying lengths and with varying single amino acid substitutions, will be necessary to refine the association between the two immunological reactions (EAE and cutaneous delayed-type hypersensitivity) induced by these peptides before one can be certain that the hypothesis of Hashim and Schilling (19) is correct, i.e., that the antigenic determinant is the C-terminal 5/9 of the encephalitogenic determinant. More specifically, on the basis of peptides derived from MMEP, Hashim and Schilling (19) suggest that the sequence of amino acid residues responsible for induction of delayed-type hypersensitivity is x-x-x-Gln-Lys (or Arg). This sequence is a part of the longer encephalitogenic sequences, x-x-Trp-x-x-x-x-Gln-Lys(or Arg) in guinea pigs (15,16,20–22) and x-x-Tyr-x-x-x-x-Gln-Lys (or Arg) in rabbits (23). Thus, of special interest will be the testing of a peptide without tryptophan, or with the tryptophan blocked, since this amino acid is necessary for induction of EAE in the guinea pig (15).

One should note that the presently reported skin reactions are generally smaller than those obtained with the same skin test antigen, MMEP #260 (13), applied to guinea pigs sensitized to various whole MMEPs, as previously reported (Table 8 of ref 6). Strong reactions (10 to 15 mm in diameter) occurred in 208 of 466 (45%) of those animals sensitized with MMEP and becoming sick within the next week (6), as compared to only 4 of 63 (6%) of the presently reported animals sensitized with synthetic peptides (Table 3). These differences suggest that the whole homologous MMEP has more antigenic determinants than the one contained in the synthetic peptides used in the present experiments. On the other hand, the percentages of false negatives and false positives (i.e., all those exceptions to the general rule that a positive skin test predicts the onset of EAE within the next week) are about the same, 40 of 208 (19%) and 165 of 591 (28%) in Table 8 of ref. 6 as compared to 23 of 63 (37%) and 13 of 53 (25%) in Table 3, respectively.

When one considers all the possible complications of synthesis of peptides, such as deletions, side chain formation, incomplete removal of blocking agents, inactivation of side groups, etc. (F. C. Westall, J. Young, and A. E. Bury, *personal communications*), the degree of encephalitogenic activity of these synthetic peptides may become more acceptable than Fig. 1 implies at first glance. Although some investigators (14,22) have reported activities of synthetic peptides (at least some of which were aliquots of some used in the present experiments) to be identical to the whole MMEP on an equimolar basis, most of our assays (Fig. 1) and most of those of other investigators (15,20) have indicated much less activity. Since the precise chemical proof of just what was wrong with each preparation is extremely difficult to establish and since bioassays are inherently quite variable, especially near the 50% effective dose (*cf.* Fig. 41 in ref. 6), one could take the optimistic attitude that it is remarkable that any synthetic peptide has any activity, rather than the opposite, that the synthetic ones do not account for anywhere near the total activity of the whole molecule. We can confirm the observations of Hoffman et al. (22) that these synthetic peptides generally do not evoke as much demyelination, even when one compares lesions of similar duration and degree of inflammation (Table 4). However, since at least some peptide-sensitized animals do show severe demyelination, it seems likely that some accessory factor for the induction of maximal sensitization and disease in most of the animals has not yet been recognized or established for these peptides, as compared to the whole MMEP.

The direct experiment of skin-testing with 0.0001 to 0.05 mg of various peptides was not attempted in the present experiments, because others (20) have obtained only negative reactions. Furthermore, rather extensive experiments would be necessary to determine the optimal concentration of each peptide to be used in the skin test. Equimolar concentrations would not be expected to be effective by analogy with some of our MMEP preparations, which required 0.5 mg rather than the 0.015 mg required with our reference standard (13). Such failures may result from many factors, especially too rapid diffusion of the peptides from the injection site. In addition, if large amounts of peptide were injected, inhibition of EAE (24) might occur, thus abrogating the expected correlation. That the size of a molecule (as well as its antigenic specificity) is also important in detecting certain immunologic reactions is well known from studies of haptens, and Nagai (21) has recently demonstrated blast cell transformation by a synthetic decapeptide (with the human sequence from residues 115 to 124) when coupled to Sepharose 4B beads and not when used in a simple solution.

The converse, the demonstration of reactions of delayed hypersensitivity to nonencephalitogenic tryptophan-blocked heterologous (bovine) MMEP (14,15,25), is just exactly what one would expect: the species-specific antigenic determinant(s) and the hapten introduced by blocking the tryptophan are different from and stronger than the species-nonspecific encephalitogenic determinant. This was also shown in our original demonstration of the species-specific reactions being much larger and correlating poorly with the induction of EAE (13). Indeed Bergstrand (26–28) has recently reported antigenic determinants on several peptide fragments of the heterologous (bovine) encephalitogenic protein injected into rabbits and guinea pigs. Lennon et al. (20) also used heterologous (human) peptides and proteins injected into guinea pigs. One cannot tell if these investigators were also detecting species-specific antigenic determinants which may be located near the encephalitogenic determinant. If they had simultaneously tested with homologous (guinea pig) preparations, as in the presently reported experiments, and if they had noted smaller or equal reactions, they would have been able to resolve this important relationship between immunogenicity and encephalitogenicity.

SUMMARY AND CONCLUSION

In summary, then, as the result of testing 17 preparations of four different synthetic peptides in guinea pigs for ability to induce delayed skin reactions to whole homologous MMEP and to induce EAE with accompanying demyelination, one can conclude that the synthetic peptides generally do not induce all of the features of EAE induced by whole MMEP. That is, the molar dose-response curve for severity of EAE, the degree of delayed-type hypersensitivity (size of skin reactions) and the degree of demyelination (even when matched for degree of inflammation and onset of EAE) are generally less than seen following sensitization to whole MMEP. In spite of these deficiences, a correlation persists between the size of the skin reaction and the onset of EAE during the following week, if one allows sufficient time for sensitization to the synthetic peptide to occur and if one skin-tests with whole homologous MMEP. Future work will be directed at further definition of the quantitative and qualitative differences which exist between the effects of small peptide components of MMEP and of the whole MMEP itself, looking not only for specific encephalitogenic and antigenic regions but also for "helper" or adjuvant regions of the molecule. Just how EAE and MMEP will fit into the overall scheme of neurological diseases remains to be seen.

ACKNOWLEDGMENT

Supported in part by U.S. Public Health Research Grants Nos. 5 RO1 NS 03147–15 from the National Institute of Neurological Diseases and Stroke, and National Multiple Sclerosis Society Grant 427-E-12. We wish to thank Dr. Fred C. Westall (The Salk Institute of Biological Studies, San Diego, California 92112), Dr. Edwin H. Eylar (Lincroft, New Jersey), Dr. Janis Young (The Space Sciences Laboratory, University of California, Berkeley, California 94702), and Ms. Anna E. Bury (Spinco Division, Beckman Instruments, Inc., Palo Alto, California 94304), for supplying the synthetic peptides which made this study possible.

REFERENCES

1. Dayhoff, M. O. (1972): *Atlas of Protein Sequence and Structure 1972, Vol. 5.* Natl. Biomed. Res Found., Wash., D.C.
2. Stevenson, L. D., and Alvord, E. C., Jr. (1947): Allergy in the nervous system, a review of the literature. *Am. J. Med.,* 3:614–620.
3. Alvord, E. C., Jr. (1959): Summary and concluding remarks. In: *"Allergic" Encephalomyelitis,* edited by M. W. Kies and E. C. Alvord, Jr., pp. 518–557. Charles C Thomas, Springfield.
4. Alvord, E. C., Jr. (1965): Pathogenesis of experimental allergic encephalomyelitis: Introductory remarks. *Ann. N.Y. Acad. Sci.,* 122:245–255.
5. Alvord, E. C., Jr. (1966): Presidential Address: The relationship of hypersensitivity to infection, inflammation and immunity. *J. Neuropath. Exp. Neurol.,* 25:1–17.
6. Alvord, E. C., Jr. (1968): The etiology and pathogenesis of experimental allergic encephalomyelitis. In: *The Central Nervous System, Some Experimental Models of Neurological Diseases,* edited by O. T. Bailey and D. E. Smith, pp. 52–70. Williams and Wilkins, Baltimore.
7. Alvord, E. C., Jr. (1968): Hypersensitivity states affecting the nervous system. *The Biologic Basis of Pediatric Practice,* edited by R. E. Cooke and S. Levine, pp. 1251–1266 (vol. 2). Also in: *Pathology of the Nervous System,* edited by J. Minckler, pp. 2244–2259, Vol. 3, 1972. The Blakiston Div., McGraw-Hill Book Co., Inc., New York.
8. Alvord, E. C., Jr., Shaw, C. M., Lisak, R. P., Falk, G. A., and Kies, M. W. (1970): Relationships between antibodies and experimental allergic encephalomyelitis, V. Antibodies and delayed hypersensitivity in production and prevention of experimental allergic encephalomyelitis. *Int. Arch. Allergy,* 38:403–412.

9. Alvord, E. C., Jr. (1970): Acute disseminated encephalomyelitis and 'allergic' neuro-encephalopathies. In: *Multiple Sclerosis and Other Demyelinating Diseases, Vol. 9: Handbook of Clinical Neurology,* edited by P. J. Vinken and G. W. Bruyn, pp. 500–571. North-Holland Publishing, Amsterdam.

10. Alvord, E. C., Jr. (1972): Impression of the conference. In: *Multiple Sclerosis, Immunology, Virology and Ultrastructure,* edited by F. Wolfgram, G. W. Ellison, J. G. Stevens, and J. M. Andrews, pp. 569–592. Academic Press, New York.

11. Alvord, E. C., Jr., Shaw, C. M., Hruby, S., and Petersen, R. (1975): Neuro-allergic reactions in primates. In: *The Aetiology and Pathogenesis of the Demyelinating Diseases,* edited by T. Yonezawa, *Acta Neuropath. Suppl. (in press).*

12. Alvord, E. C., Jr., Hruby, S., Petersen, R., and Kies, M. W. (1975): An analysis of antigenic determinants within myelin membrane encephalitogenic protein. In: *The Aetiology and Pathogenesis of the Demyelinating Diseases,* edited by T. Yonezawa. Acta Neuropath. Suppl.

13. Shaw, C. M., Alvord, E. C., Jr., Kaku, J., and Kies, M. W. (1965): Correlation of experimental allergic encephalomyelitis with delayed-type skin sensitivity to specific homologous encephalitogen. *Ann. N.Y. Acad. Sci.,* 122:318–331.

14. Eylar, E. H., Caccam, J., Jackson, J. J., Westall, F. C., and Robinson, A. B. (1970): Experimental allergic encephalomyelitis: Synthesis of disease-inducing site of the brain protein. *Science,* 168:1220–1223.

15. Westall, F. C., Robinson, A. B., Caccam, J., Jackson, J., and Eylar, E. H. (1971): Essential chemical requirements for induction of allergic encephalomyelitis. *Nature,* 229:22–24.

16. Augulis, V., and Sepinwall, J. (1971): Use of gallocyanin as a myelin stain for brain and spinal cord. *Stain Tech.,* 46:137–143.

17. Alvord, E. C., Jr., and Kies, M. W. (1959): Clinicopathologic observations in experimental "allergic" encephalomyelitis, II. Development of an index for quantitative analysis of encephalitogenic activity of "antigens." *J. Neuropath. Exp. Neurol.,* 18:447–457.

18. Carnegie, P. R. (1971): Amino acid sequence of the encephalitogenic basic protein from human myelin. *Biochem. J.,* 123:57–67.

19. Hashim, G. A., and Schilling, F. J. (1973): Allergic encephalomyelitis: Characterization of the determinants for delayed type hypersensitivity. *Biochem. Biophys. Res. Commun.,* 50:589–596.

20. Lennon, V. A., Wilks, A. V., and Carnegie, P. R. (1970): Immunologic properties of the main encephalitogenic peptide from the basic protein of human myelin. *J. Immunol.,* 105:1221–1230.

21. Nagai, Y. (1974): Chemical and immunological studies on experimental allergic encephalomyelitis antigen, 2. The significance of cellular immunity in the pathogenesis of EAE. In: *Studies on the Etiology, Treatment and Prevention of Multiple Sclerosis (National MS Study Team, Ministry of Welfare, Japan, 1973),* edited by Y. Kuroiwa, pp. 195–199. Ministry of Welfare, Japan.

22. Hoffman, P. M., Gaston, D. D., and Spitler, L. E. (1973): Comparison of experimental allergic encephalomyelitis induced with spinal cord, basic protein and synthetic encephalitogenic peptide. *Clin. Immunol. Immunopath.,* 1:364–374.

23. Shapira, R., Chou, F. C.-H., McKneally, S., Urban, E., and Kibler, R. F. (1971): Biological activity and synthesis of an encephalitogenic determinant. *Science,* 173:736–738.

24. Shaw, C. M., Fahlberg, W. J., Kies, M. W., and Alvord, E. C., Jr. (1960): Suppression of experimental "allergic" encephalomyelitis in guinea pigs by encephalitogenic proteins extracted from homologous brain. *J. Exp. Med.,* 111:171–180.

25. Spitler, L. E., von Muller, C. M., Fudenberg, H. H., and Eylar, E. H. (1972): Experimental allergic encephalitis: Dissociation of cellular immunity to brain protein and disease production. *J. Exp. Med.,* 136:156–174.

26. Bergstrand, H. (1972): Localization of antigenic determinants on bovine encephalitogenic protein. Studies in rabbits with the blood leukocyte transformation test. *Eur. J. Immunol.,* 2:266–269.

27. Bergstrand, H., and Kallen, B. (1972): Localization of antigenic determinants on bovine encephalitogenic protein. Studies in guinea pigs with macrophage migration inhibition. *Cell. Immunol.,* 3:660–671.

28. Bergstrand, H. (1972): Localization of antigenic determinants on bovine encephalitogenic protein. Studies with a second set of protein fragments and the macrophage-migration-inhibition technique in guinea pigs. *Eur. J. Biochem.,* 27:126–135.

The Nervous System, Donald B. Tower, Editor-in-Chief. *Vol. 1: The Basic Neurosciences.* Raven Press, New York, 1975.

The Development of Immunology and Its Application to Neuroscience

Dale E. McFarlin

In the 25 years since NINCDS was founded, there has been extensive growth in the field of immunology. The understanding of basic concepts in immunology such as the characterization of surface components on the lymphocyte membrane may have direct application to the understanding of the nervous system. The field of immunology has also provided insight into many diseases of the peripheral and central nervous system which may have an immunopathological basis or are associated with an immunological abnormality. Furthermore, immunological methods provide sensitive and specific mechanisms for the analysis of the nervous system. The purposes of this chapter are to review (a) highlights in the development of the field of immunology that have occurred in the last 25 years, (b) immunological studies that have contributed to the understanding of nervous system structure, function, and pathology, and (c) areas in which immunopathology may directly contribute to the presence of nervous system disease.

DEVELOPMENT OF IMMUNOLOGY

Historical Aspects (1)

The science of immunology grew out of the observation that individuals who survive certain infectious diseases seldom have a second attack of the disease during their lifetime. There are many such records in the ancient Greek, Chinese, and Arabic writings. Subsequently in the 18th century, the practice of inoculation with cowpox infectious material resulted in prevention of smallpox. Over the next 100 to 150 years, the germ theory of disease was developed. In parallel the host mechanisms for combating diseases were studied, and a number

of immunoprophylactic measures were developed. Vaccines that prevented animal diseases were developed in Pasteur's laboratory, and finally in 1885 the dramatic prevention of rabies in a boy who had been bitten by a rabid dog was carried out by immunization with attenuated rabies virus. In the decades that followed, the mechanisms responsible for protection against infectious organisms were extensively studied and a number of mechanisms were elucidated including the following.

Humoral Immunity

The presence of specific serum factors that occurred after the onset of infection with a given agent and that would suppress infection by some microorganisms when passively administered to another host. These substances, called antibodies, were found to be highly specific.

Cell-Mediated Immunity

In a systematic study of immunity to tuberculosis, Koch in the 1890s described delayed skin test reactions in immune animals. Investigations of this type of immunity recognized that it was different from that mediated by antibody and used biological tests, such as skin testing, for its characterization. The studies of Landsteiner and Chase demonstrated that delayed skin test sensitivity could be possibly transferred with immunologically competent cells. This resulted in the term "cell-mediated immunity" (CMI) which is used to indicate reactions of this type. Many antigens evoke a CMI; in addition, this type of immunity leads to the rejection of foreign histocompatibility antigens on tissue grafts and the rejection of tumor antigens on the surface of neoplastic cells in some systems.

Phagocytosis

Since the classic description of Metchnikoff, the phagocyte has been recognized as an important defense against certain microorganisms. These ameboid cells are present in the blood and known as monocytes. They are also present in various tissues where they have specialized names. In the nervous system they are commonly referred to as microglia.

Advances over the Past 25 Years in the Field of Immunology

Rapid growth of basic immunology has occurred (2); it is obviously impossible to summarize this field. Nine areas which have direct bearing on the nervous system are briefly outlined.

Establishment of the Dual Arms of the Immune Response

The above classical approaches to immunity have been extended and it is now common knowledge that immune function is mediated by two subpopulations of immunologically competent cells or lymphocytes. Early in embryonic life, stem cells pass through the thymus and differentiate into thymus-derived lymphocytes (T-cells) that are responsible for cell-mediated immunity. Alternatively, in fowls, primitive cells pass through the bursa of Fabricius and differentiate into bone marrow-derived lymphocytes (B-cells) which produce antibody. It is felt that there is an equivalent in man to the bursa that provides the milieu for the differentiation of B-cells. Support for the dual arms of the immune response comes from animal experiments. In rodents or aves, neonatal thymectomy is followed by reduced cell-mediated immunity and other functions mediated by T-cells. Alternatively, bursectomy in birds results in reduced numbers of B-cells and accordingly decreased immunoglobulins. Support for the dual system of immunity comes from analysis of human immunodeficiency diseases. In Bruton's agammaglobulinemia there is impaired immunoglobulin production while CMI is intact. This can best be explained by postulating a defect of the bursa equivalent in man. In contrast, in the di George syndrome in which there is a failure of thymus development, there is impaired CMI. In Swiss agammaglobulinemia both arms are impaired which is therefore consistent with a defect in stem cells.

Elucidation of the Structure and Function of the Immunoglobulin Molecules

Human immunoglobulins occur in five different classes, each of which has characteristic physicochemical, immunochemical, and biological properties. Immunoglobulin G (IgG) is present in the highest concentration in the serum and cerebrospinal fluid (CSF). Its structure is the prototype for the immunoglobulins and consists of four peptide chains (two heavy chains and two light chains). Each IgG molecule contains two sites (Fab) that specifically react with antigen; these consist of the variable regions of the light and heavy chains. Presumably, changes in the primary sequence of the variable regions of the Fab portions are responsible for antibody specificity. The Fc portion of the heavy chains is responsible for certain biological activities, such as complement fixation and tissue binding.

Development of Radioimmunoassay

Routine methods for detection of antigen–antibody reactions include precipitation, neutralization, agglutination, and complement fixation. Farr demonstrated that antibody could be used to detect minute amounts of radiolabeled antigen. This original description was based on using an antigen (bovine albumin) that was soluble at 50% saturated ammonium sulfate. Following incubation of radiolabeled antigen and antibody the immune complexes were precipitated with 50% saturated ammonium sulfate. The percent binding proved to be a sensitive index of the amount of antigen and antibody present. Subsequently, a double antibody technique was developed to precipitate antigen–antibody complexes. Furthermore, it was demonstrated that unlabeled antigen competed with labeled antigen for binding with the labeled antibody, in a quantitative and predictable manner. This permitted the use of radioimmunoassay (RIA) for the detection of minute amounts of antigens. As a consequence RIA has extensive use in the identification and quantitation of hormones, enzymes and a number of proteins to be discussed below.

Development of Techniques to Detect Antigen in Tissues

Antigen–antibody reactions are highly specific and sensitive. Techniques have been developed in which specific antibody is coupled to markers such as fluorescein and used to identify antigens in tissue. Similar techniques for electron microscopy have been developed to identify antigens at the ultrastructural level. These make use of specific antibody coupled to electron-dense markers or enzymes, such as peroxidase, that generate electron-dense material.

Definition of the Complement System and Its Function

The complement system is now known to consist of more than a dozen proteins that are activated in sequence. Furthermore, the activation of some of these proteins causes significant biological activities, such as increasing vascular permeability, stimulating the contraction of smooth muscle, and promoting the chemotaxis which leads to an infiltration of leukocytes into tissues (3).

Development of in vitro Methods for the Detection and Analysis of CMI

As pointed out above, it is established that T-cells produce CMI. This is believed to occur in a sequence of events. First, there is a reaction between thymus-derived lymphocytes and the antigen against which the lymphocytes are sensitized. Second, T-cells release a number of factors, collectively known as lymphokines, which produce CMI. Some of the biological activities of the lymphokines, such as inhibiting the migration of macrophages, can be easily measured and used to assess CMI *in vitro*. T-cells also react with surface antigens and produce toxicity. *In vitro* techniques for measuring this phenomenon have been developed.

Role of T-cells in Regulation of Immune Response

It has recently been recognized that in addition to producing CMI, T-cells have other important functions; they cooperate with B-cells in the production of antibody (4). Certain subpopulations of T-cells also cooperate or help other subpopulations of T-cells produce CMI. Thymus-derived lymphocytes that suppress the immune response and presumably are operative in the control of immune response have been demonstrated. It is now believed by many immunologists that there are a number of subpopulations of T-cells with different biological functions. Some immunologists are of the opinion that subpopulations of T-cells are at different stages of differentiation and that regulatory effects on the immune response are mediated through soluble factors.

Elucidation of Mechanisms Responsible for Immunopathology

It has long been recognized that damage to the host can result from the immune response. The mechanisms for host damage are currently divided into four categories: (a) anaphylaxis produced by IgE; (b) cytotoxicity produced by binding of antibody to antigen on the surface of cells and subsequent activation of complement; (c) the deposition of immune complexes and complement with subsequent activation of the complement system; and (d) CMI due to reaction between T-lymphocytes and surface antigens.

Immunogenetics

In certain animal systems it is now well established that the immune response to some antigens is under control of genes known as immune-response (Ir) genes; these are linked to genes which control the expression of histocompatibility antigens (5). The mechanisms by which Ir genes influence the immune response is unknown. It is known that closely linked histocompatibility antigen genes are expressed on the lymphocyte membrane surface. Hence it has been postulated that immune response gene products may influence the recognition of antigen by lymphocyte receptors.

IMMUNOLOGY AND THE NERVOUS SYSTEM

Use of Immunological Methods to Study the Nervous System

(a) The techniques used for localization of antigen in tissues described above had been applied extensively to study the nervous system. Using immunofluorescent and electron microscopic techniques, the components of myofibrils have been studied under different physiological conditions (6). Specific antibody has been used to characterize the distribution of enzymes which decarboxylate alpha-amino acids to amines which have neurotransmitter function (7). Immunoelectron microscopy using peroxidase coupled to the Fab portion of antibody has revealed that the autoantibody in myasthenia gravis localizes to the sarcoplasmic reticulum (8). This technique has also been valuable in the characterization of infection by different strains of measles virus one of which is related to subacute sclerosing panencephalitis (9). The use of antibody for identification of antigens on the surface of nervous system cells is still in its infancy. Recently, antigens unique to mouse neuroblastoma cells (10) and to mouse methylcholanthrene-induced glioblastoma (11) have been described. Similarly Coakham has reported antigenic determinants common to human astrocytoma cells (12). The application of such methods to the study of central nervous system differentiation and function is an exciting new field and is more fully discussed elsewhere in this volume. (see chapter by Oldstone.)

(b) Immunological techniques are used to quantitate tissue and serum components. A number of enzymes and hormones (13) are now routinely measured by these methods. The low levels of ceruloplasm in Wilson's disease, of betalipoprotein in abetalipoproteinemia, of alphalipoprotein in analphalipoproteinemia, and of IgA in ataxia-telangiectasia (A-T) are now routinely assessed by immunological methods. In diseases in which there is an enzyme deficiency, it is of major importance to establish whether the defect is due to an absence of the enzyme, an inactive form of the enzyme, or even the absence of the cofactor. In myophosphorylase deficiency and in myophosphofructokinase deficiency these enzymes were demonstrated to be absent by immunological methods revealing that these diseases are the consequence of primary enzyme deficiency. RIA can be used to measure immunoglobulins in small volumes of neat cerebrospinal fluid.

(c) Neurological diseases associated with abnormalities of the immune system not necessarily linked to the pathogenesis. Abnormalities

of the immune system may be sensitive indicators of multisystem diseases involving the nervous system. Such immunological abnormalities may be important for both diagnosis and investigation. For example, in myotonic dystrophy serum immunoglobulin-G (IgG) is low in the majority of patients. This is due to a hypermetabolism of IgG as opposed to decreased synthesis (14). Additional study of the mechanisms responsible for IgG hypermetabolism may provide information as to the underlying defect in myotonic dystrophy. In A-T serum immunoglobulin-A (IgA) is frequently low or absent because of a failure in differentiation of IgA producing cells, which parallels a developmental defect in many organs including the central nervous system. Not only is the IgA deficiency important in the recognition and diagnosis of an A-T, but further study of the defect in differentiation of the B cells which produce IgA may provide information about the defect in differentiation of the nervous system (15).

(d) Diseases with an immunopathological basis (discussed in this and the following four paragraphs) include conditions in which the immune response contributes to pathology. There are animal diseases in which one of the immunopathological mechanisms outlined in section on advances in the past 25 years may primarily be involved. An example in which antibody may produce disease is experimental myasthenia gravis produced by immunizing rabbits with acetylcholine receptor from *Electrophorus electricus* (16). Secondly, experimentally induced immune complexes can produce tissue damage in the kidneys and lungs. There is recent evidence that immune complexes can be trapped in the choroid plexus and possibly result in pathology (17). Thirdly, in mice, infected with lymphocytic choromeningitis virus, the CMI response against virus presumably produced immunopathology and death. In a similar fashion CMI response against this virus in 4-day-old rats leads to cerebellar hypoplasia (18). Experimental allergic encephalitis (discussed elsewhere — see chapter by Kies) is believed, but has not been proven to be T-cell mediated.

Also, there are human diseases possibly having immunopathological counterparts. There are data (discussed in the chapter by Arnason) supporting an immunopathological basis in polyneuritis, myasthenia gravis, and dermatomyositis. The underlying mechanisms operative in these diseases have not been established, however, it is sufficient to point out that these diseases respond to immunosuppressive therapy. In multiple sclerosis an immunopathological reaction either to a host or a viral antigen has long been postulated. Despite extensive investigation, this disease remains one of the major unsolved mysteries in neurology. In systemic lupus involving the central nervous system, evidence has been presented that immune complexes can be trapped in choroid plexus (19) and result in infiltration of inflammatory cells in a manner similar to that seen in the kidneys and lungs. There is evidence that circulating immune complexes occur in other diseases, including polyneuritis, multiple sclerosis, and juvenile dermatomyositis. It has not been established whether there is a human counterpart to the animal models of lymphocytic choromeningitis virus infection cited above. However, it has been postulated that CMI response against many viruses may lead to damage of the host. In all diseases in which there is immunological overactivity contemporary knowledge about regulation of the immune response (section on advances in the past 25 years) raises questions as to whether the immunological overactivity is the consequence of decreased suppressor T-cell activity.

Immunodeficiency. An impaired immune response predisposes to infection. Hypogammaglobulinemia, due to B-cell deficiency predisposes to encephalitis (20). In diseases in which there is chronic T-cell deficiency, progressive multifocal leukoencephalopathy, a demyelinating disease due to atypical infection by human papova viruses results. It is of interest that this group of viruses also has oncogenic properties. Patients who are chronically immunosuppressed to prevent graft rejection following transplantation have a higher incidence of brain tumors (21). This fact is frequently quoted as evidence that immunological surveillance plays a role in the regulation of cancer. It is possible that additional study of such patients will provide important information about the normal host mechanisms for control of neoplastic cells.

Human immunogenetics. Because of animal studies linking the immune response to histocompatibility genes, extensive investigation of the human histocompatibility antigens in various diseases in man has been undertaken. The human histocompatibility system consists of HLA antigens that are serologically defined (SD) and others determined by mixed lymphocyte cultures (LD). The SD antigens 3 and 7 are higher in multiple sclerosis (22), 27 in subacute sclerosing panencephalitis, 1 and 8 in myasthenia gravis (23), and 3 and 7 in patients who developed paralysis after polio virus infection (24). In addition the study of the LD antigens in human disease has just begun. In one report LD-7A (22) was detected in 60% of patients with multiple sclerosis. The significance of these findings in human diseases at this time is unclear, however, in view of the basic findings in animal studies such observations cannot be ignored in planning of future studies of diseases of unknown etiology. It is conceivable that the occurrence of certain human diseases is closely related to the genes linked to histocompatibility antigens. It is also possible that the presence of such a gene may determine the course of the disease. For example, Arnason and co-workers have reported that patients presenting with optic neuritis who lack SD 7 and 3 may have a different clinical course from those who have these antigens.

Prevention of neurological diseases by immunotherapy. As emphasized in the introduction, immunology has always been concerned with preventing diseases, particularly those of an infectious etiology. Many examples could be cited; two which have occurred over the past 25 years come immediately to mind and deserve emphasis: (a) *Prevention of poliomyelitis.* In the 7 years following introduction of the vaccine against polio, it has been estimated that 154,000 clinically apparent cases were prevented. This includes 12,500 deaths, 36,400 cases with severe paralysis, and 58,100 cases with moderate paralysis. This obviously constitutes a tremendous saving to society in human terms. In addition an attempt has been made to calculate the net economic gain for the seven year period outlined above; this has been estimated to be 6 billion dollars (2). Unquestionably, the cumulative savings now after approximately two decades are considerably greater. (b) *Prevention of kernicterus.* In the past a significant cause of infant brain damage was kernicterus resulting from Rh incompatibility. Brain damage in infants having kernicterus can be prevented by exchange transfusion. However, in recent years it has been established that the administration of anti-Rh antibody to Rh-negative mothers shortly after giving birth to Rh-positive infants will prevent sensitization to Rh antigens (26). Although unestablished, it is felt that the anti-Rh antibody results in rapid clearance of the Rh-positive red blood cells and blocks immunization. Through these measures it is possible to prevent the development of Rh sensitization, kernicterus, and the resulting brain damage.

FUTURE RELATIONSHIP BETWEEN IMMUNOLOGY AND THE NERVOUS SYSTEM

The full potential for using immunological techniques to study the nervous system structure has only begun. Undoubtedly, more extensive use of such techniques will provide important information about surface interaction between cells and differentiation discussed in Oldstone's chapter. A second important area is characterization of the immune response against agents which cause persistent infection in the nervous system. For example, subacute sclerosing panencephalitis is undoubtedly related to the measles virus, which is composed of six polypeptide chains (27). However, both the immune response to the various components and subcomponents of this agent and the effect of this virus upon the host immune response are not known. Recent experimental evidence indicates measles infection can suppress T-cell helper function (28). Extensive study of this agent is indicated as each year large masses of individuals are immunized with attenuated living measles virus. There is no question that this practice results in the prevention of acute encephalitis which follows natural measles infection; however, the long-term sequelae are not known; it is conceivable that such practice could predispose to subacute sclerosing panencephalitis or even possibly to multiple sclerosis as there are preliminary data linking multiple sclerosis to measles virus. Hence, extensive study of the immunology and the molecular biology of this agent is essential. It is conceivable that a vaccine capable of inducing immunity could be developed by using peptide from measles as has been shown with adenovirus capsid antigens (29). This would abrogate the necessity for living virus vaccines. Information from studies of this type should be extremely relevant to all chronic diseases of unknown etiology involving the nervous system, which may have an infectious or immunological component.

It is now established that the spongioform encephalopathies can be transmitted to experimental animals and are probably caused by infectious agents. Evidence of any host response against such agents is totally lacking. This seems somewhat paradoxical, but may indeed result in an ideal host parasite relationship from the point of view of the causitive agent. More extensive study of the immunology of these diseases is indicated. It is conceivable that an immune response against the constituent agents could be induced and provide protection.

There are many areas in which immunology can be applied to the study of the nervous system and the disease processes that affect it. All of the progress which has been made to date and is beginning to emerge at an increasing rate was preceded by advancement in the basic areas of research. This fact should not be lost sight of in planning future research. Although there are without question many challenges for applied immunological research, these can only be met and undertaken with the support of strong and continuing basic research.

REFERENCES

1. Humphrey, J. H., and White, R. G. (eds.) (1971): *Immunology for Students of Medicine*. Blackwell, Oxford.
2. Waksman, B. H. (1971): Immunology as a basic and applied science. *J. Immunol.,* 107:617–642.
3. Ruddy, S., Gibli, I., and Austen, K. F. (1972): The complement system of man. *N. Engl. J. Med.,* 287:489–494.
4. Gershon, R. F. (1974): T-cell control of antibody production. In: *Contemporary Topics in Immunobiology*, edited by M. D. Cooper and N. Warner, pp. 1–40. Plenum, New York.
5. Benacerraf, B., and McDevitt, H. O. (1972): Histocompatibility-linked immune response genes. *Science,* 175:273–278.
6. Pepe, F. (1968): Analysis of antibody staining patterns obtained with striated myofibrils in fluorescence microscopy and electron microscopy. *Int. Rev. Cytol.,* 24:193–231.
7. Cooper, J. R., Bloom, F. E., and Roth, R. H.

(1974): *The Biochemical Basis of Neuropharmacology.* Oxford University Press, New York.

8. Mendell, J. R., Whitaker, J. N., and Engel, W. K. (1973): The skeletal muscle binding site of antistriated muscle antibody in myasthenia gravis: An electron microscopic immunohistochemical study using peroxidase conjugated antibody fragments. *J. Immunol.,* 111:847–856.

9. Dubois-Dalcq, M., Barbosa, L. H., Hamilton, R., and Sever, J. L. (1974): Comparison between productive and latent subacute sclerosing panencephalitis viral infection in vitro. An electron microscopic and immunoperoxidase study. *Lab. Invest.,* 30:241–250.

10. Akeson, R., and Herschman, H. (1974): Neural antigens of morphologically differentiated neuroblastoma cells. *Nature,* 249:620–623.

11. Schachner, M. (1974): NS-1 (Nervous System Antigen-1), a glial-cell-specific antigenic component of the surface membrane. *Proc. Natl. Acad. Sci. USA,* 71:1795–1799.

12. Coakham, H. (1974): Surface antigen(s) common to human astrocytoma cells. *Nature,* 250:328–330.

13. Yalow, R. S. (1973): Radioimmune assay methodology application to problems of heterogeneity of peptide hormones. *Pharmacol. Rev.,* 25:161–178.

14. Wochner, R. D., Drews, G., Strober, W., and Waldmann, T. (1966): Accelerated breakdown of IgG in myotonic dystrophy: A hereditary error of immunoglobulin metabolism. *J. Clin. Invest.,* 45:321–329.

15. McFarlin, D. E., Strober, W., and Waldmann, T. (1972): Ataxia-telangiectasia. *Medicine,* 51:281–314.

16. Patrick, J., and Lindstrom, J. (1973): Autoimmune response to acetylcholine receptor. *Science,* 180:871–872.

17. Cochrane, C. G., and Koffler, D. (1973): Immune complex disease in experimental animals and man. *Advan. Immunol.* 16:195–264.

18. Cole, G. A., and Nathanson, N. (1974): Lymphocytic choriomeningitis: Pathogenesis. In: *Progress in Medical Virology,* edited by J. Hotchin, pp. 94–110. S. Karger, Basel.

19. Atkins, C., Kondon, J., Zuismorio, F., and Friou, G. (1972): The choroid plexus in systemic lupus erythematosus. *Ann. Int. Med.,* 76:65–72.

20. Preud'Homme, J. L., Griscelli, C., and Seligmann, M. (1973): Immunoglobulins on the surface of lymphocytes in fifty patients with primary immunodeficiency diseases. *Clin. Immunol. Immunopathol.,* 1:241–256.

21. Schneck, S. A., and Penn, I. (1970): Cerebral neoplasms associated with renal transplantation. *Arch. Neurol.,* 22:226–233.

22. Jersild, C., Dupont, B., Fog, T., Hansen, S., Nielsen, L. S., Thomsen, M., and Svejgaard, A. (1973): Histocompatibility linked immune response determinants in multiple sclerosis. *Trans. Proc.,* 5:1791–1796.

23. Feltkamp, T. E. W., Van Den Berg-Loonen, P. M., Nijenhuis, L. E., Oosterhuis, H. J. G. H., Engelfriet, C. P., Van Rossum, A. L., and Van Loghem, J. J. (1975): Relations between HL-A antigens, myasthenia gravis and autoantibodies. In: *Studies on Neuromuscular Diseases,* edited by K. Kunze and J. E. Desmedt, pp. 180–185. S. Karger, Basel.

24. Morris, P. J., and Pietsch, M. C. (1973): A possible association between paralytic poliomyelitis and multiple sclerosis. *Lancet,* II:847–848.

25. Arnason, B. G. W., Fuller, T. C., Lehrich, J. R., and Wray, S. H. (1974): Histocompatibility types and measles antibodies in multiple sclerosis and optic neuritis. *J. Neurol. Sci.,* 22:419–428.

26. Clarke, C. A. (1968): Prevention of rhesus isoimmunization. *Lancet,* II:1–4.

27. Hall, W. W., and Martin, S. J. (1974): The biochemical and biological characteristics of the surface components of measles virus. *J. Gen. Virol.,* 22:363–374.

28. McFarland, H. F. (1974): The effect of measles virus infection on T and B lymphocytes in the mouse. *J. Immunol.,* 213:1978–1983.

29. Couch, R. B., Kasel, J. A., Pereira, H. G., Haase, A. T., and Knight, V. (1973): Induction of immunity in man by crystalline adenovirus type 5 capsid antigens. *Proc. Soc. Exp. Biol. Med.,* 143:905–910.

The Nervous System, Donald B. Tower. Editor-in-Chief. *Vol. 1: The Basic Neurosciences*. Raven Press, New York. 1975.

Invertebrate Nervous Systems and the Mechanisms of Behavior

Eric R. Kandel

The usefulness of invertebrate neurons for analyzing cellular problems, such as the mechanisms of the resting potential, the action potential, and synaptic excitation and inhibition, has encouraged neural scientists to use the invertebrate nervous system to examine more complex problems including the patterns of interconnections between systems of neurons and how various patterns of interconnections generate different classes of behavior. Such descriptions are also essential for understanding how learning occurs and may some day be useful for understanding behavioral abnormalities. In addition, research on the organization of invertebrate nervous systems is relevant to genetic studies of the nervous system. By specifying the precision involved in the interconnections among neurons and the rules determining their functional expression, these studies may provide a blueprint of what genetic and developmental processes must accomplish.

The invertebrate nervous systems offer several clear advantages for behavioral and developmental studies. First, the number of neurons that make up the nervous systems of most invertebrates is relatively small, about 10^5 compared to the 10^{12} neurons of the mammalian brain. This reduction in number greatly reduces the task of describing the functional architecture of a behavior and of relating an individual neuron to a given behavior. Second, many invertebrate neurons are invariant and can be repeatedly identified from animal to animal. As a result, the developmental history of individual neurons can be followed. In addition, the same neuron can be studied in a variety of functional states.

In this brief summary I review the major features of research on the invertebrate nervous system by focusing first on the morphological features of invertebrate central ganglion, and the morphological and functional approaches to the analysis of cellular interconnections. I will then consider the organization of afferent systems and motor systems and the use of invertebrates for studying behavioral modifiability.

MORPHOLOGY OF INVERTEBRATE GANGLIA

The central neurons of higher invertebrates, such as insects, crustaceans, molluscs, and worms, are characteristically clustered together in ganglia. These connect to symmetrical ganglia, by means of commissures, to other ganglia by means of connectives, and to the periphery by means of mixed (afferent and efferent) nerves. Often the two symmetrical ganglia fuse, forming a single unit, and, in addition, several of the head ganglia usually fuse to form the brain.

As in all nervous systems, the substance of the invertebrate ganglion is divided into two zones, cellular and fibrous. In vertebrates the two zones are intermingled, and axons enter into the cellular zone. In invertebrates the zones are separated. The cell bodies of invertebrate neurons are gathered in a rind around the outside of the ganglion. This cellular region is devoid of axons and synapses. Each neuron sends its axon into a central region, the neuropile, where interconnections between neurons are made.

This characteristic segregation of higher invertebrate ganglia into a peripheral cell-body region and a central neuropile provides certain experimental advantages. For example, the location of the cell bodies on the outer surface often makes it possible to see individual cells in the intact ganglion under the dissecting microscope, and as a result, cells may be identified by a number of visual, as well as functional, criteria.

Invertebrate neurons are often large, ranging from 100 to 1000 μm in diameter and can therefore be readily penetrated with microelectrodes for neurophysiological studies. In addition, they can also be dissected out by hand for biochemical studies. In certain invertebrates, the cell bodies contain chemosensitive receptors which appear to be similar to those found in the neuropile. Thus the cell body, although free of synapses, provides an experimental synaptic membrane for detailed studies of the pharmacology of functional properties. As a result of these several advantages, the transmitter biochemistry and pharmacology of certain invertebrate preparations, such as the lobster and the mollusc *Aplysia,* are quite advanced. (The structure of the invertebrate nervous system is reviewed in Bullock and Horridge (3).)

ANALYSIS OF THE INTERCONNECTIONS BETWEEN CELLS

Morphological Analysis of the Neuropile

The purpose of a morphological analysis of the neuropile is to understand the structural basis of organized neural action by describing the three-dimensional architecture of the neuropile—the course taken by the interconnecting fibers and their various subgroupings as well as the fine structure of the synaptic contacts.

Neuropile architecture is complex but seems to be organized into patterns that recur not only within the same central nervous system (CNS) but in the CNS of differing organisms. For example, there is considerable similarity in the structure of the neuropile in the retinas of arthropods, cephalopod molluscs, and vertebrates, and in the olfactory systems of arthropods and vertebrates. Unknown are the patterns of functional interconnections resulting from different patterns of neuropile organization and how functional and neuropile patterns relate to behavior. To answer these questions several behavioral systems will have to be analyzed in morphological and physiological detail.

A number of promising new techniques for the morphological study of the invertebrate neuropile based on intracellular injection of a marker substance have recently been introduced. One class of useful marker substances are the fluorescent procion dyes that bind covalently to macromolecules within the cell. Another technique is based on the intracellular injection of cobalt chloride which can then be

precipitated in the cell as cobalt sulfate, an electron-opaque marker, following treatment of the ganglion with ammonium sulfate. The advantage of these techniques is that one or more cells can be selectively injected and their processes traced without the confusion normally introduced by conventional stains that are taken up arbitrarily by many cells. This technique has been used to study the geometry of certain identified cells in lobster, crayfish, and insect ganglia, by reconstructing a cell shape through serial sections. By injecting a given cell in different ganglia, it was found that, despite some microheterogeneity in their finer branches, the general pattern of branching of the individual cells studied was quite characteristic. Moreover, by studying different cells and tracing their process it was possible to begin an analysis of the organization of the neuropile. The technique has also been used to identify the location of the cell body of an identified axonal process.

Whereas these techniques are useful for light microscopic studies, a major need exists for techniques that permit electron microscopic identification of the synapses of identified cells. Attempts along these lines involve injection of either labeled material (amino acids, fucose) or electron-dense markers (horseradish peroxidase). Intracellular marking techniques are reviewed in Kater and Nicholson (6).

Functional Analysis of the Neuropile

The purpose of this analysis is to describe the function of the anatomical interconnections between cells in a ganglion. This analysis is facilitated in certain invertebrate ganglia because the synaptic connections between neurons and their follower cells are often detectable electrophysiologically by stimulating the neuron with an intracellular electrode and by recording the elementary postsynaptic potential it produces in the follower cell with another intracellular electrode. This technique is essentially an extension of the electroanatomical mapping used successfully in the vertebrate nervous system for examining connections between populations of neurons. With this technique a number of direct connections of several identified interneurons and their follower cells have been mapped in *Aplysia;* the interconnections between sensory neurons and their followers have been mapped in the leech ganglion and the intra- and interganglionic connections between the Retzius cells have been specified. Also specified have been the interconnections between receptor cells in the eye of the nudibranch *Hermissenda* and the horseshoe crab *Limulus,* the connections of the giant cell in the gastroesophageal ganglia of the nudibranch *Ansiodoris,* and the interconnections of cells in the crustacean cardiac ganglion.

These studies can suggest what factors determine the functional expression of interconnections between cells in a neuronal population. For example, in the abdominal ganglion of *Aplysia,* the connections of one identified neuron have been traced to 14 identified and 20 to 30 unidentified follower cells. The connections between were examined both electrophysiologically and pharmacologically to determine the following four questions: Must a neuron be specialized for inhibition or excitation or can it be multivalent? Does the neuron conform to Dale's principle and release the same transmitter from all of its terminals? Is the sign of the synaptic action determined by the chemical structure of the transmitter substance released by the presynaptic neuron, or by the nature of the receptor located on the postsynaptic? And must the postsynaptic cell have only one receptor to the same chemical transmitter substance, or can it have more than one receptor?

Examination of the various synaptic actions produced by the different branches of the neuron showed it to be multiactioned and to mediate inhibition to the follower cells in one region, excitation to cells of another region, and conjoint excitation–inhibition to a cell in a third region. All of these synaptic actions could be accounted for by a single transmitter substance, acetylcholine, that was released by the different branches of the interneuron interacting with different receptors. The different receptors to acetylcholine determined the sign of the synaptic action by controlling different ionic conductance mechanisms: Na^+ for excitation, Cl^- for one type of inhibition, K^+ for another type, and Na^+ and Cl^- for conjoint excitation–inhibition. Some postsynaptic cells had two receptors to the same transmitter. Similar findings have been made in the buccal and pleural ganglia of *Aplysia*. In each case, the functional expression of cholinergic transmission in this neural population was shown to be determined by the type of receptor and the combination of receptors in the postsynaptic cell. For review, see Kandel and Gardner (5).

Specificity of Neuron Cell Number and of Interconnections

Studies of development and regeneration in vertebrates suggest that individual neurons may be invariant and their connections specific. However, in vertebrates the number of neurons is large, and it is difficult to determine the precise resolution of this specificity. The availability of identifiable cells in invertebrates has permitted a partial resolution of this problem. Maps have now been provided of identified cell bodies in annelids, crustaceans, insects, and gastropod molluscs, and of identified fibers in nerves and connectives of a number of arthropods, in particular, the crayfish. From these maps it appears that the large identified neurons are constant not only in size, relative position, morphological, electrophysiological, and biochemical properties but also in their central interconnections. Thus in these cells these properties are genetically specified. However, the evidence on the invariant properties of smaller invertebrate neurons is less clear.

AFFERENT AND MOTOR SYSTEMS

The availability of identifiable cells has also permitted a detailed exploration of the functional organization of afferent and motor systems. As a result, a number of principles have emerged. Two features, common to the organization of both afferent and motor systems, are particularly important. (a) In both systems neurons code for position. In the motor system they code for position of movement, and in the sensory system they code for the position of the sensory input on the body surface. (b) In both systems many units abstract only certain critical aspects of the stimulus.

Afferent Systems

Sensory information coming either from independent receptors or from receptor aggregates undergoes a series of transformations within the central nervous system. C. A. G. Wiersma (8) and colleagues have done the most detailed studies of sensory interneurons (in the somatosensory and the visual system of the crayfish), and their findings are probably representative of most arthropods.

Afferent interneurons in both sensory systems respond to a large variety of spatial combinations of sensory input. For example, in the somatosensory system a given stimulus activates a large number of parallel units. Some interneurons respond to tactile stimulation of a single abdominal segment; others respond to stimulation of that segment and one or more adjacent segments; and still others may respond to tactile stimulation of any segment of the entire abdomen, and so forth. Thus, the tactile-receptive surface is represented by a series of unique, individual elements, some with very localized receptive fields and others with broad and overlapping receptive fields. Similarly the optic nerve contains a number of identifiable interneurons, each with a uniquely specifiable receptive field. Some units have a moderately restricted field, such as a small segment of a retinal quadrant, whereas other units have a broad and overlapping field and respond to stimulation over a hemiretina or even over a whole retina. In addition, a number of interneurons only respond to complex stimuli and appear to abstract certain features of the sensory input. For example, one type of fiber responds only to moving stimuli. When the animal moves its eye, these fibers are inhibited and do not fire, despite the fact that there is movement of the visual field across the eye. These units thus discriminate between real movement in the visual world and apparent movement resulting from motion of the eye. Another class of visual fibers, space-constant fibers, alters their receptive field as a function of the position of the animal in space. The space-constant fiber responds to stimuli in relation to their vertical coordinate in real space, independent of the locus of stimulation of the eye. This is apparently accomplished by means of proprioceptive input that inhibits the output of the appropriate portion of the potential receptive field. Units having similarly complex receptive fields have also been described in the vertebrate CNS. [For review, see Wiersma (8).]

Motor Systems

The control of movement in higher invertebrates has also been most extensively investigated in arthropods. Because of the arthropod exoskeleton, one can fix leads on the body surface and implant electrodes in muscle or around peripheral nerves without significantly interfering with the movement of the animal. The motor system also consists of relatively few units. For example, in the crayfish the motor supply to a single muscle typically consists of one inhibitor and one to five excitors, each with a different distribution and action. The extracellularly recorded action potential of each of the motor fibers to a given muscle is often distinctive and can be distinguished from its neighboring axons, so that in some experimental conditions the whole population can be studied simultaneously.

There is general agreement that postural adjustments involve proprioceptive reflexes, but a major question in the study of motor systems is to what degree are motor sequences reflexly controlled or centrally controlled. Does cyclical locomotor behavior require proprioceptive feedback from peripheral structures for its maintenance and timing, or is the central nervous system capable of producing these patterns without information from the periphery?

The earlier work of F. W. Mott and C. Sherrington had suggested that locomotion results from information conveyed centrally from the periphery by the immediately preceding sensory input. Each phase of movement was thought to be triggered by a particular pattern of input from peripheral receptors. This view has now been shown to be incorrect for several locomotor patterns in invertebrates. The most detailed of these studies has been that of Donald Wilson on the flight of locusts. Wilson (9) showed that elimination of all phasic sensory feedback from the wings did not disrupt the normal phase pattern of flight; it only produced a decrease in wingbeat frequency. Similarly, with the wing receptors intact, the tonic head-hair receptors could be removed and normal flight still be retained. In the absence of both wing receptors and head-hair receptors, normal flight was not maintained, but a normal wing phase pattern could be restored, at reduced wingbeat frequency, by electrical stimulation anywhere in the CNS from brain to abdominal cord. To be successful for maintaining flight, the central stimulation did not have to be patterned in any way. Random stimuli containing no information for the timing of units worked perfectly well. Direct stimulation of sensory nerves similarly indicated that phasing of the input was not necessary for a phased motor output. These data indicate that peripheral control and patterned feedback cannot explain wing movements in the locust. Instead, the patterned action of locust wing movements is produced by a pattern generator located in the central nervous system.

Given an inherent central program for locust flight, why does the animal need stretch reflexes at all? Wilson's studies suggest that, in the locust flight system, proprioceptive reflexes and exteroceptive sensory information supplement the preprogrammed information built into the CNS so that the motor output can be modified. The need for modification may range from a fundamental mistake in the central program, such as provided by an inherent asymmetry in the output pattern, to a more transient change in the environmental condition for flight, as might be produced by an alteration in wind direction. Thus the nervous system has genetically programmed into it nearly everything that can be anticipated prior to actual flight. The sensory inputs supplement this built-in information about the body and the environment that either cannot be anticipated genetically or which is needed to compensate for minor genetic or developmental errors. As a result of the interaction of genetic and sensory mechanisms, the insect flight-control system is quite stable and overcompensated. No single motor or sensory structure appears uniquely necessary for stable flight. Only as more and more of the entire flight system is damaged is flying ability progressively reduced.

Evidence now also exists for a central control of motor sequence in a number of other invertebrate locomotor systems, including control of the thoracic and abdominal appendages of the crayfish, the cicada song, the cricket song, the control of heartbeat in crustacea, the copulatory movements in the praying mantis, the respiration of insects, and eye movement in crabs.

Perhaps the most dramatic finding to emerge from recent studies of the invertebrate motor system is the discovery that single command elements can trigger complete preprogrammed motor sequences. Release of a central preprogrammed motor sequence requires the existence of elements within the central nervous system capable of triggering behavioral sequences. Command elements appear to be present in insects, crustaceans, molluscs, and annelids.

The discovery of command elements began with the analysis of the giant fiber system in the crayfish. In 1938, Wiersma first showed that a single electrical stimulus applied to any one of the four giant fibers could produce a complete escape response, consisting of turning in of the eyestalk, forward movement of the antennae and legs, pulling upward of the swimmerets (leglike structures), and a strong tail flip. In addition, inhibition of leg movement occurs. Each of the four giant fibers apparently synapses in every ganglion of the nerve cord and brings a similar, although not identical, peripheral output into play.

Later, Wiersma discovered a single fiber in the circumesophageal commissure which on repetitive stimulation triggered the defensive reflex. This reflex consists of the animal becoming opisthotonic and raising its claws and head while supporting its body on its tail and fourth and fifth thoracic legs.

More recently Wiersma and colleagues, and Kennedy and Davis (7) have described command elements that produce leg and abdominal movements, abdominal postural adjustments, and rhythmic beating of the swimmerets.

From analyses of a number of command fibers in crayfish, several generalizations have emerged. (a) Command fibers generally exert a widespread effect, controlling a total block or sequence of behavior. (b) More than one fiber can initiate a particular behavioral sequence, and there is often overlap in the effector actions mediated by a number of different command fibers. (c) Despite the overlap in effector actions among several command elements, it is often possible to distinguish differences in their detailed field of action, suggesting that the movement produced by each element may be unique. [For review, see Kennedy and Davis (7).]

FUNCTIONAL MODIFIABILITY OF GANGLIA

As a result of the advantages that invertebrates offer for studying the mechanisms of simple behaviors, they have recently also been used to examine the cellular mechanisms of modifications of behavior. In particular, a number of studies have been directed toward analyzing habituation, which is the waning of a response that is repeatedly evoked, and dishabituation, which is the recovery of an habituated response following an extraneous stimulus. The most detailed of these has been the analysis of the defensive withdrawal of the gill in the sea hare (*Aplysia*), and of the escape response in crayfish. In *Aplysia* the reflex is controlled by one ganglion (the abdominal), and its neural circuit has been largely specified. Tactile receptors in the mantle and siphon skin activate sensory fibers that make monosynaptic, as well as polysynaptic, excitatory connections with motor neurons that innervate the gill. In both *Aplysia* and crayfish, cellular studies indicate that habituation involves a plastic change leading to a depression in excitatory synaptic transmission between the afferent fibers and the motoneuron due to a decrease in transmitter quantal output. In *Aplysia* dishabituation involves a restoration of the effectiveness of excitatory transmission at this set of synapses due to an increase in quantal output. In each case the sensitivity of the receptor is unaffected. Both of these short-term modifications in behavior involve changes in the functional expression of previously existing connections. The capability for these modifications seems built into the functional neuronal architecture of the behavior.

On the basis of these recent studies on the invertebrate nervous system, it appears that many neurons and their connections are genetically determined and so the functional architecture for basic perception and motor coordination is specified. What appears not to be specified are some quantitative aspects of the functional expression of previously established connections.

The study of the neuronal control of behavior and the mechanisms of its modification is merely beginning. A number of studies are now under way using the habituation paradigm that illustrate that habituation can readily be prolonged to last several weeks. In *Aplysia* the results suggest that the mechanisms for long-term memory of this modification represent an extension of those involved in the short-term process.

Moreover, a number of laboratories are beginning to use invertebrates to examine more complex behaviors such as feeding which are not only interesting in their own right but are highly contingent on the motivational state of the animal. Thus, studies such as these may provide insight into the neuronal mechanisms of arousal, motivation, and other "state" variables. [For review, see Kandel (4).]

DIRECTIONS FOR FUTURE RESEARCH

I have here considered only studies that combine cellular neurophysiological and behavioral approaches. However, much will be learned in the future from combining behavioral and genetic techniques. Molecular biologists have been highly successful in dissecting the cellular functions in bacteria by using gene changes (mutations) in which one element is altered at a time. It thus seemed only natural to some molecular biologists that the nervous system might also be successfully analyzed by the appropriate use of mutants. In an important series of studies, Seymour Benzer (2) has begun to dissect the neural network underlying behavior in the fly *Drosophila* using behavioral mutants. Benzer now has mutants with a variety of behavioral abnormalities, including visual disturbances, abnormalities in circadian rhythm and sexual behavior, muscular dystrophies, and sudden cessation of development. He has found that mutations can alter behavior in a variety of ways using a variety of mechanisms. These can affect the development and function of sensory systems, motor systems and central integrative systems. Mutations thus provide a powerful means for examining the component parts of a normal behavioral system. This approach promises to revolutionize behavioral genetics and in so doing will shed much light on the neural mechanisms of behavior and of *genetically determined abnormalities of behavior*. [For review, see Benzer (2); Bentley and Hoy (1).]

In addition, studies of behavior and their modifications in invertebrates may make it possible to develop model systems for the study of *socially determined behavioral abnormalities of behavior*. For example, invertebrates such as *Aplysia* show normal withdrawal reflexes in a normal environment. But if exposed to an environment where they receive noxious stimuli, twice a day for 10 days, they become highly overresponsive to previously neutral stimuli and remain so for several weeks after their return to the normal environment. Insofar as an animal's response is less appropriate for the current demands of its environment and more determined by earlier events in its history— these inappropriate responses can be considered abnormal and provide potential models for behavioral abnormalities. This approach is only beginning but it should be possible to develop a family of different behavioral abnormalities in invertebrates that could provide insight into clinical problems. Moreover, by combining genetic, behavioral and cellular neurophysiological approaches one might be able to determine how genetic and social (behavioral) factors interact in determining given behavioral abnormalities.

To move in these directions and analyze the results meaningfully however, much work will have to be expanded. In particular there is a surprising lack of rigorous and imaginative studies of invertebrate behavior. If invertebrates are to provide useful systems for studying learning and behavioral abnormalities a major effort will have to be made in this area. We know much more about almost all aspects of the behavior of the white rat (whose neural mechanisms are difficult to analyze) than we do about the leech, lobster, and *Aplysia,* animals whose nervous system makes them suitable for cellular studies of behavior.

REFERENCES

1. Bentley, D., and Hoy, R. R. (1974): The neurobiology of cricket song. *Sci. Am.,* 231:34–44.
2. Benzer, S. (1973): The genetic dissection of behavior. *Sci. Am.,* 229(6):24–37.
3. Bullock, T. H., and Horridge, G. A. (1965): *Structure and Function in the Nervous System in Invertebrates,* Vol. 2. W. H. Freeman Co., San Francisco.
4. Kandel, E. R. (1974): An invertebrate system for the cellular analysis of simple behaviors and their modifications. In: *The Neurosciences Third Study Program,* edited by F. O. Schmitt and F. G. Worden, pp. 347–370. The MIT Press, Cambridge.
5. Kandel, E. R., and Gardner, D. (1972): The synaptic actions mediated by different branches of a single neuron. *Neurotrans. Res. Publ. A.R.N.M.D.,* 50:91–144.
6. Kater, S. B., and Nicholson, C. (1973): *Intracellular Staining in Neurobiology.* Springer-Verlag, New York.
7. Kennedy, D., and 'Davis, W. J. (1976): The organization of invertebrate motor systems. In: *The Cellular Biology of Neurons,* edited by E. R. Kandel, Section 8, Vol. 1 of *Handbook of Physiology.* American Physiological Society, Bethesda.
8. Wiersma, C. A. G. (1966): Integration in the visual pathway of Crustacea. *Symp. Soc. Exp. Biol.,* 20:151–177.
9. Wilson, D. M. (1968): The flight-control system of the locust. *Sci. Am.,* 218(5):83–90.

Subject Index

Subject Index

A

Acetylcholine
  axoplasmic transport of, 141-142
  cyclic AMP and, 388-390
  cyclic GMP and, 388
  in denervation, 446
  as neurotransmitter, 363-364, 409-411
Acetylcholine receptor (AChR)
  ACh binding by, 323-324, 328
  affinity labeling of, 324-325
  antibodies to, 328-329, 658
  in denervation, 448-449
  disulfide bond in, 324-325
  in excitable membranes, 161
  molecular weight of, 327-328
  in myasthenia gravis, 448-449
  neurotoxin binding, 324
  purification of, 325-327, 511
  in reconstituted membranes, 329
  subunits of, 327-328
Acetylcholinesterase (AChE)
  axoplasmic transport of, 137
  isoenzymes of, 458
  localization of, 365
  of synaptosomes, 458-459
N-acetyltransferase
  of pineal gland, 396-399
  β-adrenergic receptor and, 396
Actin, of brain, polymerization of, 570-571
Actomyosin
  Ca^{++} component, 565, 568-570
  properties of, 565-566
  cytochalasin B and, 570

Actomyosin (*contd.*)
  of synaptosomes, 566-567
  of vesicles, 567-568
Actomyosin-like proteins
  function of, 571-572
  properties of, 565-570
  subcellular distribution of, 572
Adenosine
  as neurotransmitter, 385
Adenylate cyclase
  adrenergic receptors and, 385
  of CNS, 382-383
  catecholamine sensitivity of, 382-383
  neural function of, 381-382
  regulation of, 383
Adrenergic receptor, 374-379
α-Adrenergic receptors
  cyclic AMP and, 384
β-Adrenergic receptors
  N-acetyltransferase and, 396
  cyclic AMP and, 384, 396-397
  of pineal gland, 395-399
  supersensitivity of, 397
Amacrine cells
  of retina, 93-94, 97-99
Amino acid transport
  blood-brain barrier and, 283-287, 553-554
  brain development and, 287
Amino acids
  aromatic, metabolism of, 553-562
  behavior and, 561-562
  in brain injury, 580-581
  in development, 578-579
  drug alterations in, 581-582
  dynamic state of, 576-577
  effect on cyclic AMP, 385